Davidson's

Radiology of the Kidney and Genitourinary Tract

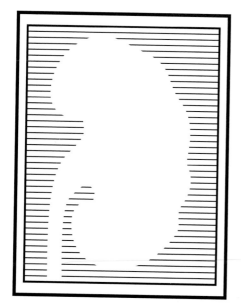

Davidson's

Radiology

of the

Kidney

and

Genitourinary

Tract

Alan J. Davidson, M.D.

Visiting Distinguished Scientist
Department of Radiologic Pathology
American Registry of Pathology
Armed Forces Institute of Pathology
Washington, District of Columbia

David S. Hartman, M.D.

Professor of Radiology
Department of Radiology
Penn State College of Medicine
The Milton S. Hershey Medical Center
Hershey, Pennsylvania

Peter L. Choyke, M.D.

Chief, Magnetic Resonance Imaging
Department of Radiology
National Institutes of Health
Bethesda, Maryland

Brent J. Wagner, M.D.

Visiting Scientist
Department of Radiologic Pathology
American Registry of Pathology
Armed Forces Institute of Pathology
Washington, District of Columbia

W.B. SAUNDERS COMPANY
A Division of Harcourt Brace & Company

Philadelphia
London   Toronto   Montreal   Sydney   Tokyo

THIRD EDITION

W.B. SAUNDERS COMPANY
A Division of Harcourt Brace & Company

The Curtis Center
Independence Square West
Philadelphia, Pennsylvania 19106

Library of Congress Cataloging-in-Publication Data

Davidson's radiology of the kidney and genitourinary tract / Alan J. Davidson . . .
[et al.].—3rd ed.

p.   cm.

Rev. ed. of: Radiology of the kidney and urinary tract / Alan J. Davidson,
David S. Hartman. 2nd ed. c1994.

Includes bibliographical references and index.

ISBN 0–7216–7144–6

1. Kidneys—Radionuclide imaging.   2. Kidneys—Radiography.
I. Davidson, Alan J. Radiology of the kidney and urinary tract.
[DNLM: 1. Kidney Diseases—radiography.   2. Kidney Diseases—
radionuclide imaging.   3. Urogenital Diseases—radiography.
4. Urogenital Diseases—radionuclide imaging.   WJ 302 R1292 1999]

RC904.5.R32D38 1999   616.6′10757—dc21

DNLM/DLC   98–9758

DAVIDSON'S RADIOLOGY OF THE KIDNEY AND GENITOURINARY TRACT

ISBN 0–7216–7144–6

Printed in the United States of America.

Last digit is the print number: 9   8   7   6   5   4   3   2   1

Preface

This book has been written to provide the reader with an informed, organized, and efficient approach to the radiologic diagnosis of diseases of the kidney and genitourinary tract, the retroperitoneum, and the adrenal glands in adulthood as well as in infancy and childhood.

As in previous editions, two concepts have been fundamental. First, the organizational approach taken is that of the radiologist's point of view—how the greatest amount of information can be derived from a given set of careful observations and applied to the resolution of a well-formed clinical question. Second, based on our shared years of analyzing the genitourinary archives of the Department of Radiologic Pathology at the Armed Forces Institute of Pathology, we adhere to the concept that an informed interpretation of any radiologic modality requires a thorough understanding of the underlying pathologic process—acknowledging pathology as the "mother church" of radiology.

We have attempted to be comprehensive in scope yet not exhaustive in detail. The text follows closely the "Recommendation for Resident Curriculum in Genitourinary Tract Radiology" as adopted by the Society of Uroradiology. Interventional procedures, extracorporeal shock wave lithotripsy, and renal transplantation, however, are not included.

Section I, Techniques and Anatomy, discusses the excretion of the iodinated contrast material used in uroradiology, the hazards that attend its use, and the precautions needed to minimize adverse reactions. The first part also covers the proper performance and application of excretory urography, ultrasonography, computed tomography, magnetic resonance imaging, angiography, and radionuclide imaging. The final chapter in Section I presents the normal radiologic anatomy of the kidney and ureter. Here, the embryogenesis and anatomy of a single prototypic renal lobe are used as a model for understanding the radiologic appearance of the entire kidney and its ureter and their anomalous development. A thorough familiarity with the material in Section I is fundamental to the radiologic evaluation of the upper urinary tract and retroperitoneum.

Section II, Renal Parenchymal Disease, is based on analysis of the manner in which pathologic processes alter renal size and contour and the *inherent* distribution of a given disease or abnormality. This approach results in a group of categories called "diagnostic sets," each of which contains a limited number of abnormal states that have common features of renal size, contour, and lesion distribution. Other radiologic observations, such as the appearance of the pelvocalyceal system, the papillae, and the nephrogram, are used to differentiate entities within each diagnostic set. Major radiologic findings for specific diseases are summarized in charts throughout each chapter. Each chapter concludes with a summary section on differential diagnosis.

Although a list of abnormal conditions constitutes each diagnostic set, the reader is urged not to treat these as "gamuts" to be memorized. While gamuts may have rhyme, they do not necessarily have reason. Assignment of entities to each diagnostic set has been rationally derived by consideration of specific pathologic and clinical features; these must be understood thoroughly for the system to work. It is difficult, nevertheless, to fit all diseases neatly into any system of classification. The approach used in Section II is no exception. Some assignments to diagnostic sets are based on arbitrary considerations, such as the most common form of presentation of each entity, the stage at which the radiologist is most likely to encounter the abnormality in the usual clinical setting, and the *typical* distribution of a specific lesion. For example, angiomyolipoma is discussed as a cause of unifocal, unilateral enlargement of the kidney rather than as multifocal and/or bilateral lesions because the former is the common presentation and the latter is uncommon. Acute cortical necrosis is placed in the diagnostic set of bilaterally enlarged, smooth kidneys because the radiologist is more likely to see this condition early on in its evolution rather than at a time when chronic renal failure and small kidneys develop. Similarly, listing reflux nephropathy in the diagnostic set of small kidney with unifocal scar recognizes the fact that a single scar is the elemental lesion; multifocal and/or bilateral lesions may occur as chance events that are randomly distributed.

The five chapters of Section III, The Pelvocalyceal System and Ureter, describe abnormalities of these structures as they appear to the radiologist, using the same approach as that for Section II, Renal

Parenchymal Disease. The first three chapters discuss abnormalities by their site of origin in the upper urinary tract; intraluminal, mural, and renal sinus–periureteral space. The concluding two chapters analyze the meaning of the pelvocalyceal system and ureter that are abnormally dilated or effaced.

Section IV, The Lower Urinary Tract, presents in two chapters the normal anatomy, anomalies, and diseases of the bladder and urethra, except for trauma. Here, the emphasis is on the limited number of radiologic abnormalities that develop in response to a wide variety of pathologic processes. This gives rise to broad differential diagnoses rather than the more precisely defined diagnostic groupings found in other chapters of the book.

Section V, The Retroperitoneum and Adrenal, discusses the relevant normal anatomy and diseases in these two areas that have been so strikingly elucidated by modern imaging methods. Each of these subjects lends itself well to pattern analysis and the concept of diagnostic sets.

Section VI, The Genital Tract, is new to this edition and reflects the remarkable advances that have occurred in recent years in imaging the ovary, adnexa, and the uterus in the female and the prostate, seminal vesicles, testis, and scrotum in the male. Four chapters are devoted to these topics.

Section VII contains three essays on topics that are either not included in other parts or that require integration of material from diverse chapters. These subjects include nephrographic analysis, diagnostic strategies in evaluating renal masses, and the radiologic assessment of the kidneys and genitourinary tract in the traumatized patient.

For readers so inclined, the Appendix contains an historical review of the development of contrast material and data on the chemistry of compounds previously and currently used to opacify the urinary tract, including low-osmolality agents.

The bibliographies for each chapter have been structured to provide the reader with both detailed references that support the text and a starting point for independent search of the literature. In most chapters, references that provide an historical perspective are included as well.

Each of the four authors has critically assessed all of the material in this book for accuracy, timeliness, and validity. It is our hope that these chapters, taken together, will help the reader develop a solid understanding and enjoyment of the contemporary radiologic evaluation of the kidney and genitourinary tract—and that, in turn, patients will be served efficiently and well.

ALAN J. DAVIDSON
DAVID S. HARTMAN
PETER L. CHOYKE
BRENT J. WAGNER

Acknowledgments

A task that began nearly three decades ago—which produced *Radiologic Diagnosis of Renal Parenchymal Disease* in 1977, *Radiology of the Kidney* in 1985, and *Radiology of the Kidney and Urinary Tract* 2/e in 1994—is now complete with the publication of this book, which has been expanded to include the female and male genital tract. A large number of people are owed a debt of gratitude for their support of this effort.

Each of us has had the good fortune and honor to serve as faculty in the Department of Radiologic Pathology at the Armed Forces Institute of Pathology in Washington, D.C. Our professional lives have been singularly enriched in this unique environment. Fathollah K. Mostofi, Charles J. Davis, Jr., and Isabelle A. Sesterhann, three of the world's most eminent uropathologists, and Clara S. Heffess, Chief of Endocrine Pathology, have been patient, accessible teachers as well as research collaborators. Our students, residents in radiology from nearly all educational institutions in the United States and Canada as well as many in Europe, the Middle East, and Latin America, have been at the core of our intellectual growth and pleasure. And, by no means least, we hold an enduring gratitude and affection for our colleagues in the Department of Radiologic Pathology who have shared with us their collegiality, integrity, and selfless support as well as their academic excellence.

Hundreds of educational institutions have enrolled their residents as students in the Armed Forces Institute of Pathology Course in Radiologic-Pathologic Correlation since its inception over 50 years ago. As a result of the support of the chairpeople and the program directors of these departments of radiology and the earnestness of our resident-students, nearly 400 new cases are now accessioned each year in the uroradiologic archives of the Department of Radiologic Pathology. This is the material—with complete radiologic, clinical, and pathologic documentation—on which our research and teaching are based. We have borrowed freely from this valuable and unique collection in illustrating this book. We are grateful to all who have directly or indirectly made these contributions. In addition, many colleagues have generously allowed the use of fine illustrations from their personal experience to supplement the text. Each is acknowledged individually in the legend to the illustration.

The research and publications of our fellow members of the Society of Uroradiology also underlie much of the information contained in this book. We are indebted to these colleagues for their extensive contribution to the literature and for the rich professional relationship that we share with so many. We also express our appreciation to Philip J. Kenney, who contributed so much to our professional lives during the 1996–1997 sabbatical year that he spent as Distinguished Scientist at the Armed Forces Institute of Pathology.

Finally, Lisette Bralow, Vice President and Editor in Chief; Jeff Gunning, Production Manager; Scott Filderman, Copy Editor; Walt Verbitski, Illustration Coordinator; Ellen Zanolle, Designer; Linda Van Pelt, Indexer; and Sally Grande, Marketing Manager, are W.B. Saunders Company staff who have lent welcome support and expert guidance at each stage of the writing and production of this book. We are most pleased by the long association that *Davidson's Radiology of the Kidney and Genitourinary Tract* and its predecessors have enjoyed with this leading medical publishing house.

Contents

Davidson's

Radiology of the Kidney and Genitourinary Tract

TECHNIQUES AND ANATOMY

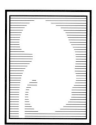

CHAPTER 1

Diagnostic Uroradiologic Techniques

CONTRAST MATERIAL
    Physiology of Excretion
    Practical Considerations
    Adverse Reactions

EXCRETORY UROGRAPHY
ULTRASONOGRAPHY
COMPUTED TOMOGRAPHY
MAGNETIC RESONANCE IMAGING
ANGIOGRAPHY

This chapter describes the principal diagnostic methods for studying the kidneys and surrounding structures. Presented first are the events that follow the intravenous administration of iodinated contrast material and their influence on the quality of the excretory urogram and computed tomogram of the kidney. Following that is a discussion of the hazards associated with the use of contrast material and the means by which these may be minimized or treated. The remaining sections review the technique, applications, and limitations of excretory urography, ultrasonography, computed tomography, magnetic resonance imaging, and angiography. Nuclear medicine techniques are discussed in Chapter 2.

The discussion on contrast material covers both the ionic, monomeric high osmolality compounds and the various nonionic and ionic forms of low osmolality agents. The chemical characteristics of these compounds are described in the Appendix.

CONTRAST MATERIAL

Physiology of Excretion

Following the rapid intravenous injection of a bolus of contrast material, a peak plasma level is reached almost immediately. This is followed by a rapid decline (Fig. 1–1). Plasma level decline is multifactorial. An immediate drop is due to initial rapid mixing in the vascular compartment. Concomitantly, there is loss of plasma contrast material by diffusion into the extravascular, extracellular fluid space. Finally, decrease in plasma contrast material levels occurs from renal excretion, the third factor contributing to the plasma decay curve illustrated in Figure 1–1.

One of the most important determinants of the diagnostic quality of an excretory urogram is the level of contrast material present in the plasma and available to the kidney for excretion. The concept of "high dose" urography is based on the phenomenon demonstrated in Figure 1–2. In that illustration, the 10-minute plasma concentration of sodium diatrizoate is shown to have a positive linear correlation (r = .85) with the amount of contrast material (adjusted for body surface area) injected in patients with normal renal function. These data clearly indicate that a dose can be calculated precisely to achieve any given plasma level.

All contrast material, regardless of osmolality, is excreted by glomerular filtration alone. Rear-

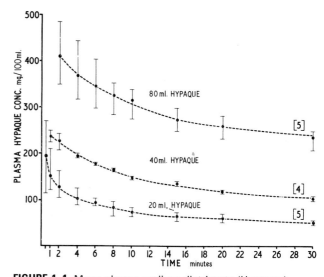

FIGURE 1–1. Mean plasma sodium diatrizoate (Hypaque) concentrations and range of values following intravenous injection of varying volumes. Figures in brackets represent the number of subjects studied. The decline in plasma level represents vascular mixing, extravascular diffusion, and renal excretion. (From Cattell, W. R., Fry, I. K., Spencer, A. G., and Purkiss, P.: Br. J. Radiol. *40*:561, 1967. Reproduced with kind permission of the authors and the *British Journal of Radiology*.)

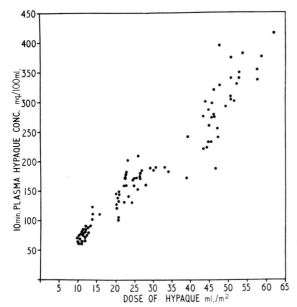

FIGURE 1–2. Plasma sodium diatrizoate (Hypaque) concentration related to dose expressed as mL/m² body surface. A positive correlation between dose and 10-minute plasma levels is shown. (From Cattell, W. R., Fry, I. K., Spencer, A. G., and Purkiss, P.: Br. J. Radiol. *40*:561, 1967. Reproduced with kind permission of the authors and the *British Journal of Radiology*.)

rangement of the mathematical equation expressing the glomerular filtration rate brings out the importance of the relationship between the plasma level of contrast material and the glomerular filtrate:

$$GFR = UV/P$$

where GFR = glomerular filtration rate (mL/min)
U = concentration of contrast material in urine (mg/mL)
V = flow rate of urine (mL/min)
P = plasma concentration of contrast material (mg/mL)
rearranges into:

$$UV = GFR \times P$$

Clearly, the diagnostic quality of an excretory urogram is a function of UV, the amount of iodine-containing contrast material excreted by the kidney in a volume of urine that distends the pelvocalyceal system and ureters. It is important to note that of the determinants of UV, contrast material plasma concentration (P) is the only variable that the radiologist can manipulate by adjustment of dose. Glomerular filtration rate is a given value in any individual, although it varies with each patient.

Another important determinant of the diagnostic quality of an excretory urogram is the volume of urine formed to distend the pelvocalyceal system and ureters. A collapsed collecting system does not reflect surrounding anatomic structures and may obscure abnormalities within its lumen. Adequate distention is basic to optimal urographic technique

and can be achieved by a mechanical device such as a ureteral compression balloon, by taking advantage of the diuretic effect of the urographic contrast material, or by both. High osmolality contrast material is a potent osmotic diuretic because it freely dissociates into two particles when in solution. The iodine-bearing anion is an osmotically active, nonreabsorbable solute that produces a diuresis of salt and water. The degree of diuresis produced varies directly with the dose administered. However, considerably less diuretic effect occurs following the use of sodium salts than after the use of meglumine salts. The cation meglumine is not reabsorbed by the renal tubules to any significant degree and thus provides added osmotic force within the tubule lumen to potentiate the diuretic effect of the nonreabsorbable anion. The cation sodium, on the other hand, is freely reabsorbable by the renal tubules. The additional available sodium in the proximal tubule following the use of a sodium salt enhances water reabsorption. For this reason, a smaller urine volume and higher urine concentration of contrast material follow the use of the sodium salt when compared with a meglumine salt of contrast material. One important difference between low and high osmolality agents is the markedly reduced osmotic diuretic effect of the former compared with the latter. This is true for nonionic monomers and dimers as well as for the ionic dimers. Decreased urine volume translates into enhanced radiodensity of the pelvocalyceal system and ureter because there is less dilution of the iodine-bearing molecule by urine. Decreased urine volume also means less distention of the pelvocalyceal system with low osmolality agents compared with ionic, high osmolality compounds. As a result, when using low osmolality contrast material, ureteral compression to distend the pelvocalyceal system is particularly important to compensate for the relatively small volume of urine being formed by the kidneys.

The foregoing considerations represent events that occur in the proximal renal tubule where the volume of glomerular filtrate is reduced by approximately 85 per cent. The final concentration of contrast material is influenced further by additional water reabsorption, which takes place in the distal tubules and collecting ducts. Here, the major influence on water reabsorption is the level of activity of antidiuretic hormone. This, in turn, reflects the state of hydration. The well-dehydrated, volume-depleted individual will experience less of a diuresis following contrast material injection and will excrete a higher concentration of this material than the volume-expanded individual. Dehydration, on the other hand, potentiates the risk for contrast material–induced nephrotoxicity.

Practical Considerations

With this knowledge of the physiology of contrast material excretion, what can the radiologist do to maximize the diagnostic information derived from the excretory urogram or contrast material–enhanced computed tomogram of the kidneys?

Regarding the choice of high osmolality ionic contrast material, it is clear that sodium salts, rather than meglumine salts, provide a higher concentration of radiopaque material in the urine. Additionally, there is some evidence that fewer adverse reactions occur with sodium salts than with meglumine salts.

Two differences of practical importance are apparent when the physiology of excretion of low osmolality contrast material is compared with that of high osmolality compounds. First, radiopacity of urine is greater with low osmolality agents because a smaller urine volume yields higher iodine concentration. Although this is generally considered advantageous, a high level of radiodensity carries the undesirable potential of obscuring small filling defects in the pelvocalyceal system. Second, reduced osmotic diuresis results in less distention of the pelvocalyceal system than occurs with high osmolality contrast material. Effective ureteral compression and, in some cases, a slight delay in filming sequences to allow time for more urine to form can compensate for this effect. For the same reason—high iodine concentration related to low urine flow rates—maximum density of the nephrogram produced by low osmolality contrast material may be greater and its appearance slower when compared with that of high osmolality agents.

Historically, dehydration was advocated as a means of maximizing the radiodensity of urine during excretory urography. This was an important adjunct at a time when convention restricted the dose of contrast material. In fact, dehydration is now considered a risk-potentiating factor for contrast material–induced nephrotoxicity, particularly in patients with pre-existing renal disease, hyperuricemia, or dysproteinemia. In contemporary practice, patients given contrast material should normally be hydrated. This is discussed further in a following section.

How does one determine an appropriate dose of contrast material? First, it is best to think of dose in terms of grams of iodine administered rather than volume of injectate, because iodine content is the basic determinant of radiopacity, and the various products available vary considerably in their iodine concentration. Second, as emphasized previously, it is useful to relate the dosage to body size.

In adults, it is generally agreed that in the presence of normal renal function, a total dose of 15 to 25 gm of iodine will provide satisfactory opacification. This represents approximately 300 mg of iodine per kilogram of body weight. In the most commonly used forms of contrast material of both high and low osmolality, a dose of 1.0 mL/kg of body weight will result in this dosage range, as noted in Table 1–1. In patients who are obese or who have a great deal of gas and feces, the dose can be increased, either initially or by reinjection of an additional amount of contrast material after the examination has been started and the initial films found inadequate. Historically, it has been demonstrated in adults that a single dose of 4 mL/kg of 50% or 60% diatrizoate resulted in distinct discomfort, including tremors, irritability, and tachycardia. Thus, the convention evolved of limiting total dose for excretory urography to 2 mL/kg; in addition, many workers in this field arbitrarily limit the total volume of injectate to 170 to 200 mL. Some evidence exists, in fact, that at very large doses of high osmolality contrast material, urinary concentration of iodine levels off and may even diminish as a result of the osmotic force of the radiopaque solute interfering with osmotic gradients in the cortex and medulla. This phenomenon is, presumably, of less importance with low osmolality contrast material. Renal failure presents a special problem in dosage determination and is discussed subsequently.

In the pediatric patient, the intravenous dosage of contrast material should be based on weight, as represented in the following schedule for ioversol

TABLE 1–1. Commonly Used Contrast Material for Excretory Urography and Computed Tomography

Generic Name	Trade Name	SODIUM CONTENT (mEq/mL)	IODINE CONTENT (mg/mL)	OSMOLALITY (mOsm/kg H$_2$O)
Ionic Monomers (Ratio 1.5):				
Sodium diatrizoate	Hypaque 50	0.8	300	1515
Meglumine and sodium diatrizoate	Renografin 60	0.16	292	1420
Sodium iothalamate	Conray 400	1.05	400	2300
Meglumine iothalamate	Conray		282	1400
Nonionic Monomers (Ratio 3):				
Iopamidol	Isovue 300		300	616
Iohexol	Omnipaque		300	709
Ioversol	Optiray		320	702
Iopromide	Ultravist		300	620
Ionic Dimer (Ratio 3):				
Meglumine and sodium ioxaglate	Hexabrix	0.15	320	600
Nonionic Dimer (Ratio 6):				
Iodixanol	Visipaque	0.48	320	290

68% (R. Lebowitz, Children's Hospital, Boston, personal communication, 1998):

Weight	Dose
Up to 11.0 kg	3.0 mL/kg
11.0 to 23.0 kg	2.0 mL/kg
23.0 to 45 kg	50 mL
>45 kg	1 mL/kg

A maximum of 3 mL/kg is used. This applies to the smallest patients and represents an upward adjustment in dose in the premature or normal newborn, in whom there is normally a reduction in glomerular filtration rate. Solid food is withheld for 4 hours prior to the administration of contrast material, but liquids are not restricted. Low osmolality agents in infants minimize cardiovascular complications from excessive volume expansion, as discussed subsequently.

The plasma concentration of contrast material is affected materially by the speed of injection. Figure 1–3 illustrates the significant difference in peak and sustained plasma concentration following a rapid single injection when compared with a 15-minute infusion of contrast material. For equivalent total doses, it is apparent that the slow, 15-minute administration never produces as high a plasma level as a rapid, 30- to 90-second injection. In addition, the slow infusion technique has no impact on either urine flow rate or urine sodium diatrizoate concentration when compared with the rapid bolus injection technique. The use of drip infusion technique is therefore unjustified except, perhaps, for its convenience. Patients at risk for contrast material–induced cardiotoxicity are an exception to this generalization. Here, risk is related directly to the speed of injection. It is important to avoid having contrast material reach the myocardium as a bolus. In this group, then, the total dose of contrast material should be delivered over a 2- to 3-minute period. This subject is discussed in greater detail in the following section on contrast material hazards.

Adverse Reactions

Untoward reactions to contrast material can be separated into two major categories: adverse systemic reactions and organ toxicity. The first group can be further subdivided into nonidiosyncratic and idiosyncratic. In the organ toxic reactions, the kidney, heart, and lungs are the organs susceptible to clinically manifested damage by urographic contrast material.

Adverse Systemic Reactions. Systemic reactions to contrast material vary from mild and inconsequential (heat and nausea) to life-threatening and fatal (bronchospasm, hypovolemic hypotension, laryngeal edema, or cardiac arrest). Collection of comprehensive epidemiologic data on serious reactions is hindered by their infrequency, methodologic weaknesses inherent in collaborative multi-institutional studies, nonuniform systems of classification, risk factors that vary with different study populations, and availability and effectiveness of therapeutic measures that may prevent a life-threatening reaction from becoming a fatal one. Despite these limitations, it is generally held that the overall prevalence of adverse systemic reactions of *all* types may be as high as 13 per cent of patients exposed to high osmolality intravenous contrast material and approximately 3 per cent of those exposed to low osmolality intravenous contrast material. This reflects the common occurrence of minor reactions, which account for approximately 98 per cent of all reactions. Intermediate and severe reactions are much less common.

From an epidemiologic perspective, the convention is to classify reactions according to their clinical severity: minor, intermediate, severe, and fatal. These are outlined in Table 1–2. Minor reactions are of limited duration and consequence and usually require no treatment. Nausea, vomiting, a sensation of warmth, and very mild rash are examples. These occur in up to 10 per cent of individuals exposed to high osmolality contrast material, with the highest prevalence in young adults. The use of low osmolality contrast material reduces the overall prevalence of adverse systemic reactions substantially. Most of this is accomplished by up to a 7-fold decrease in minor reactions. The magnitude of reduction varies considerably among specific minor symptoms. Intermediate reactions are those that cause concern for the well-being of the patient and require some form of therapy, which is rapidly effective. Extensive urticaria, angioneurotic edema, bronchospasm, laryngospasm, and hypotension are included in the category. No precise data are avail-

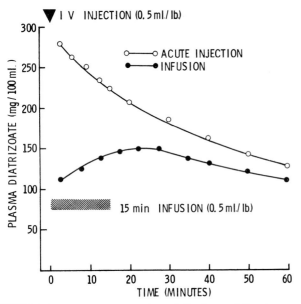

FIGURE 1–3. Plasma concentration of diatrizoate following rapid bolus injection and slow drip infusion. Drip infusion does not produce the same maximal level of contrast material as is achieved by direct injection. (From Cattell, W. R.: Invest. Radiol. 5:473, 1970. Reproduced with kind permission of the author and *Investigative Radiology.*)

TABLE 1–2. Clinical Classification of Adverse Reactions to Urographic Contrast Material

ADVERSE REACTION	MINOR	INTERMEDIATE	SEVERE
Systemic			
Idiosyncratic	Mild urticaria	Extensive urticaria Angioneurotic edema Bronchospasm Laryngospasm Hypovolemic hypotension	Cardiopulmonary collapse Pulmonary edema Bronchospasm Laryngospasm Hypovolemic hypotension
Nonidiosyncratic	Nausea Vomiting Heat Injection site pain Tachy/bradycardia	(?) Hypotension secondary to vasodilation	
Organ Toxic	Tachy/bradycardia	Oliguria/anuria Azotemia Myocardial ischemia Cardiac arrhythmia Bronchospasm	Ventricular tachycardia/ fibrillation Myocardial infarction

able for the frequency of intermediate reactions, but their pattern of age distribution appears to be similar to that of minor reactions. Severe reactions are defined as those that threaten life and require intensive treatment. Cardiopulmonary collapse, pulmonary edema, severe forms of bronchospasm, laryngeal edema, and severe hypotension fall into this category. Earlier reports of the prevalence of severe reactions to high osmolality contrast material varied from 1:3000 to 1:4500 (Ansell et al., 1980; Hartman et al., 1982). Later studies indicate that severe reactions with high osmolality agents are as frequent as from 1:200 to 1:1000 (Lasser and Berry, 1987; Palmer, 1988; Katayama et al., 1990; Caro et al., 1991). The use of either low osmolality contrast material or a corticosteroid pretreatment regimen, discussed subsequently, has been variably reported to reduce the prevalence of severe adverse reactions to a range of from 1:640 to 1:2500 (Lasser and Berry, 1987; Katayama et al., 1990; Caro et al., 1991). Evidence also suggests a reduction in the prevalence of severe adverse reactions when a corticosteroid pretreatment regimen is combined with low osmolality contrast material (Lasser et al., 1994). Unlike minor and intermediate reactions, severe reactions appear to occur uniformly in all age groups, with perhaps a slightly greater frequency among young adults. The literature, however, is not without conflict on this issue. The reported frequency of fatal reactions to high osmolality contrast material has varied between 1:14,000 and 1:110,000. The former figure is most likely inaccurate. The most generally accepted range has been between 1:40,000 and 1:110,000. However, the large study of Katayama and colleagues (1990) failed to document any fatalities unequivocally due to contrast material in nearly 170,000 patents exposed to high osmolality contrast material and an approximately equal number of patients exposed to low osmolality contrast material. The changing data on mortality rates likely reflect the inherent safety of both high and low osmolality agents as well as improved availability and effectiveness of therapy for severe adverse reactions to both categories of contrast material.

The preceding discussion addresses only the frequency and clinical manifestations of adverse systemic reactions to intravenous contrast material, not the pathogenesis of reactions. To this end, systemic reactions are divided into two groups: nonidiosyncratic and idiosyncratic, or anaphylactoid.

Nonidiosyncratic Reactions. Nonidiosyncratic reactions are the consequence of physical and chemical characteristics of the contrast material, such as hyperosmolality, single-valence cations, and the intrinsic chemotoxicity of an iodinated benzoic acid derivative. Low osmolality contrast material is particularly effective in reducing the prevalence of nonidiosyncratic reactions, reflecting the paramount role of osmolality as a cause of this type of reaction. Examples of physicochemical systemic reactions include vasodilation, tachycardia, bradycardia, hypotension, and flushing. Specific organs or tissues may be the site of nonidiosyncratic reactions to contrast material. Examples include venous endothelium damage at the site of injection, nausea and vomiting, transient alterations in heart rate or rhythm, change in renal blood flow and glomerular filtration rate, and deformity of circulating red blood cells. In general, nonidiosyncratic reactions to contrast material are limited in nature and are of minor clinical importance.

Idiosyncratic Reactions. The clinically important adverse systemic reactions to contrast material are idiosyncratic, or anaphylactoid. These comprise those intermediate, severe, and fatal reactions with clinical features usually seen with allergic reactions. They include urticaria, angioneurotic edema, bronchospasm, laryngospasm, cardiopulmonary collapse, pulmonary edema, and hypotension. Although these reactions resemble allergies in their clinical manifestations, they are neither antigen-antibody–mediated nor the result of initial exposure and subsequent sensitization. Thus, it is proper to characterize this phenomenon as idiosyncratic or anaphylactoid rather than allergic or anaphylactic. Reactions in this category are the same whether provoked by either high or low osmolality contrast material, but they are less frequent for the latter. Idiosyncratic reactions are more often associated with intravenous rather than intra-arterial injection of contrast material.

The mechanisms that cause idiosyncratic response to contrast material have not been completely elucidated. The overwhelming body of investigational evidence points to complement activation, release of vascular mediators, and a coagulation disturbance as the biochemical basis for these reactions. The reader is referred to sources listed in the bibliography at the end of the chapter for a more detailed explanation of this subject.

Prophylaxis. What can be done to minimize the risk and consequences of adverse systemic reactions to contrast material? The nonidiosyncratic effects are of little clinical consequence. Paradoxically, the greatest impact of low osmolality contrast material is to reduce the frequency of adverse reactions in this category. When using high osmolality contrast material, some measures can be taken to mitigate nonidiosyncratic reactions. For example, venous endothelial irritation leading to arm pain can be avoided by selecting a large vein for injection, by flushing the vessel with saline after injection, or, if important, by using a meglumine salt rather than the more irritating sodium salt. Similarly, the likelihood of nausea and vomiting can be lessened by a prolonged injection time.

Idiosyncratic adverse systemic effects, on the other hand, are a major concern. Every effort must be undertaken by the radiologist to minimize the likelihood of their occurrence or, once they develop, their consequence. Because a precise understanding of the mechanism involved does not exist, only limited means are available to accomplish this. These include screening patients for epidemiologically determined risk factors, using empirically derived prophylactic measures, and having available and being familiar with all necessary measures for treating a reaction.

Data derived from patients exposed to high osmolality contrast material have identified certain risk factors that indicate an increased likelihood of an idiosyncratic adverse systemic reaction occurring with greater frequency than in the general population (Ansell et al., 1980; Katayama et al., 1990). A patient with a history of allergy is four to five times more likely to develop a severe, adverse idiosyncratic systemic reaction to contrast material than one without such a history. Included in this risk group are patients with a history of hay fever, hives, eczema, and various other allergies to substances such as seafood and penicillin. Current or remote asthma increases the risk of a severe reaction by as much as 8-fold, and a history of prior reaction to urographic contrast material is associated with an 11-fold increase in the risk of a severe

reaction, when compared with that of a population without this history. Increased risk for severe reactions has also been associated with female gender (Lang et al., 1995). These risk factors remain valid for patients exposed to low osmolality contrast material, although the frequency of reactions is less than that provoked by high osmolality contrast material. These data strongly militate for taking a careful history of all patients before administration of either high or low osmolality contrast material and instituting prophylactic measures when appropriate, as discussed below. However, because most adverse reactions to contrast material occur in individuals without any history of allergy or a prior reaction to contrast material, it is important to remember that a negative screen is no assurance that a reaction will not occur. Further, intravenous injection of a test dose of contrast material has not been validated as an effective screen for potential reactors.

In patients who are judged to be at increased risk because of a significant history of allergy or a prior contrast material reaction, the need for a diagnostic test that requires contrast material should be reassessed. Alternative measures, such as ultrasonography or magnetic resonance imaging, may provide the necessary diagnostic information. If the need for an iodinated contrast material–enhanced test remains justified, a low osmolality agent should be used.

Adrenal corticosteroids have been shown to reduce the frequency of severe idiosyncratic adverse systemic reactions in a general population without identified risk factors to a level similar to that achieved by low osmolality contrast material (Lasser and Berry, 1987; Lasser, 1988; Lasser et al., 1994). These observations apply to the high-risk population only by implication. A typical protocol is hydrocortisone, 100 mg (or its equivalent dose in other forms of corticosteroids, such as methylprednisolone, 32 mg) administered orally or parenterally at least 12 hours before injection of contrast material. Some radiologists advocate two doses, one at 24 hours and another at 12 hours before contrast material administration. An initial dose of corticosteroid given less than 12 hours before contrast material administration is thought to be ineffective. This is the same protocol that could be used in the general low-risk population in lieu of low osmolality contrast material.

In any high-risk patient, it is advisable to maintain an open intravenous line during the contrast material examination as an access route for further medication if an adverse reaction develops. Although low osmolality contrast material and, presumably, a pretreatment protocol of adrenal corticosteroids provide a measure of protection, a major reaction may still develop, and vigilance should not be relaxed. If there is extreme concern for a life-threatening reaction, the presence of a resuscitation team at the time of injection should be considered.

Antihistamines have not been generally accepted

as an effective preventative measure in high-risk patients, although theoretically both H₁ and H₂ receptor antagonists may have a role in the prevention of contrast material reactions. Likewise, the possibility exists that epsilon-aminocaproic acid may reduce the risk of reaction. Rapid injection of contrast material is no more likely to precipitate an idiosyncratic reaction than is a slow injection.

Treatment. The treatment of idiosyncratic adverse systemic reactions is determined by their nature and their severity. Minor reactions, by definition, are not treated. Antihistamines (H₁ receptor antagonists such as diphenhydramine) are often advocated for intermediate cutaneous reactions. However, this category of drugs has its own inherent risks, such as drowsiness developing in the ambulatory patient responsible for driving an automobile. These considerations lead some authorities not to recommend antihistamines as a treatment for minor or intermediate adverse contrast material reactions. Clearly, antihistamines have no role in the active treatment of major reactions.

Adrenal corticosteroids, as discussed previously, are used principally for prophylaxis in high-risk individuals, if at all. This category of drugs is not a first line of therapy in the treatment of adverse systemic reactions of any severity that have already developed.

The treatment of intermediate and severe adverse systemic reactions is determined by the nature of the reaction. These fall into four categories: (1) severe urticaria, (2) isolated hypovolemic hypotension, (3) isolated airway compromise due to bronchospasm, and (4) anaphylactoid reactions characterized by severe and progressive combinations of both hypotension and airway compromise (Bush and Swanson, 1991; Cohan and Ellis, 1997).

Severe urticaria is best treated with an H₁ antihistamine such as diphenhydramine in an intravenous or intramuscular injection of 25 to 50 mg. H₂ antihistamines (cimetidine or ranitidine) have also been advocated, although their efficacy is less well established.

Hypovolemic hypotension is associated with tachycardia and is the result of fluid loss through increased capillary permeability, which is part of the pathophysiology of adverse idiosyncratic reactions. The same mechanism accounts for the occasional appearance of pulmonary edema. Treatment of this reaction requires placing the patient in Trendelenburg's position and administering nasal oxygen and normal saline or Ringer's lactate for large volume fluid replacement. Central venous pressure should be monitored as an index of the volume of fluid required to restore blood pressure to normal and to avoid the complications of fluid overload, especially in patients with pre-existing compromised cardiac function. In most cases, fluid replacement is the only measure required to correct hypotension. If pharmacologic intervention is required because of the ineffectiveness of fluid replacement, a beta-adrenergic vasopressor in the form of dopa-

mine is ideal. However, the complicated nature of this therapy requires expertise that is usually beyond that of a radiologist. Instead, subcutaneous epinephrine (0.2 to 0.3 mL of 1:1000 solution) may be used.

Hypotension associated with bradycardia is usually vasovagal in origin and not an idiosyncratic adverse systemic reaction to contrast material per se *except in a patient treated with a beta blocker that prevents a normal tachycardic response to hypovolemia*. Vasovagal-mediated bradycardic hypotension is a common form of hypotension seen in a radiology department under a variety of circumstances unrelated to contrast material exposure. Atropine (0.5 to 2.0 mg intravenously), not epinephrine, is the appropriate pharmacologic intervention for this phenomenon if simple measures of Trendelenburg's positioning, oxygen, and volume expansion are not effective.

Mild to intermediate forms of isolated airway compromise due to bronchospasm can be treated either by epinephrine administered subcutaneously in incremental doses of 0.2 to 0.3 mL of 1:1000 solution or by one or two inhalations of a beta-agonist bronchodilator such as albuterol, metaproterenol, or terbutaline. Signs and symptoms must be carefully assessed to determine the need for additional increments. Severe and/or accelerating airway compromise due to bronchospasm or angioneurotic edema often requires a slow intravenous injection of 1 to 2 mL of 1:10,000 epinephrine.

For anaphylactoid reactions, intravenous epinephrine should be administered slowly to maximize its beta-adrenergic effect and to reduce the alpha-adrenergic effect. An initial dose of 1.0 mL of 1:10,000 epinephrine may be followed by additional doses as needed. Oxygen should be administered and blood volume restored with the rapid intravenous infusion of normal saline or Ringer's lactate.

In any of the above treatment regimens in which epinephrine is administered, particular caution should be exercised with patients who are elderly or hypoxic, which are two risk factors in which epinephrine may induce severe cardiac arrhythmia. Epinephrine should be avoided in patients who are medicated with noncardioselective beta-blocking agents such as propranolol (Inderal). The desired beta-adrenergic effect of epinephrine may be blocked in such patients with deleterious complications resulting from unopposed alpha-agonist effects.

Idiosyncratic reactions manifested as cardiopulmonary collapse require that the radiologist be expert in basic cardiopulmonary resuscitation. Diagnostic tests requiring exposure to contrast material should take place only in an environment that provides both the expertise and the facilities for the effective treatment of this most serious complication. The radiologist's role in this setting can then be limited to first-line measures, such as administering epinephrine, instituting fluid replacement, and performing basic cardiopulmonary resuscitation.

Organ Toxicity. The kidney, heart, and lung are susceptible to damage by contrast material. In the absence of a basic understanding of the mechanisms involved, these organ toxic responses are best defined by the clinical disorders that result.

Nephrotoxicity. Oliguria or anuria with or without azotemia is the clinical manifestation of contrast material damage to the kidneys. Two very different pathogenetic mechanisms lead to this disorder: one is acute tubular necrosis; the other is acute obstruction of tubule lumina by precipitated solutes or proteins.

Nephrotoxicity in the form of acute tubular necrosis occurs mainly in patients with low flow states (congestive heart failure, hypotension), generalized vascular disease (arteriosclerosis, nephrosclerosis), or pre-existing renal failure (such as chronic glomerulonephritis, diabetic nephropathy). Dehydration potentiates the risk for nephrotoxicity and should always be avoided in patients receiving contrast material, particularly those with risk factors for nephrotoxicity. On the contrary, hydration reduces, but does not eliminate, the risk of contrast material–induced nephrotoxicity. Theory and some clinical evidence support the concept that nephrotoxicity is also influenced by time and dosage factors, with a large amount of contrast material (50 gm or greater) given as a single dose imparting the highest risk.

Speculation about the pathogenesis of contrast material–induced acute tubular necrosis has centered on two possibilities. Evidence for a direct toxic effect on proximal tubule cells by contrast material includes induction of enzymuria, reduction in sodium transport by the toad bladder, decreased extraction of para-aminohippuric acid, and vacuolization of tubule cells by these agents. A second body of data suggests that the renal damage that follows exposure to contrast material is a result of ischemia from either vasoconstriction or sludging of red blood cells in the microcirculation.

Diabetic nephropathy is a particularly important risk factor for contrast material–induced acute tubular necrosis. Studies have demonstrated a prevalence of 9 per cent for contrast material–induced nephrotoxicity in patients with diabetic nephropathy with baseline serum creatinine levels of greater than 1.7 mg/dL (Parfrey et al., 1989; Schwab et al., 1989). It is necessary to emphasize, however, that the unique risk of nephrotoxicity in the diabetic patient is limited to those with pre-existing diabetic nephropathy. The nonazotemic diabetic patient and, possibly, the nondiabetic patient with pre-existing renal insufficiency are not at increased risk for contrast material–induced nephrotoxicity when the examination is performed using standard precautions regarding dose and hydration (Shieh et al., 1982; Parfrey et al., 1989).

The other form of contrast material–induced nephrotoxicity is due to an acute obstruction of tubule lumina by precipitation of abnormal urinary proteins in patients with multiple myeloma, by Tamm-Horsfall proteins in dehydrated newborns or infants, or by uric acid precipitation in individuals with very high serum uric acid levels. Contrast material has a uricosuric effect, presumably as a result of inhibition of uric acid reabsorption by the renal tubules. Consequently, its use in patients with marked hyperuricemia potentiates the risk for acute urate nephropathy. A large fluid intake, alkaline diuresis, and reduction of serum uric acid by allopurinol are specific measures that reduce the risk of this complication. The risk of acute myeloma nephropathy and Tamm-Horsfall nephropathy can be minimized by ensuring that dehydration does not occur when at-risk patients are exposed to contrast material.

Precautions. How should a patient be approached when any of the above risk factors are identified? First, the need for a radiologic study requiring contrast material must be reassessed. Often other studies can provide the necessary information. This is particularly true in the diagnostic evaluation of the azotemic patient in whom ultrasonography, unenhanced computed tomography, or, less commonly, magnetic resonance imaging, usually provide all of the information needed to make important management decisions.

If, however, the indication for a diagnostic study using iodinated contrast material remains, hydration appropriate to the patient's general physical condition should be maintained. Bowel purges should be avoided, and only the meal immediately preceding the examination should be withheld. The dose of contrast material should be held to the minimum necessary to obtain the desired information. The specific amount will vary with conditions unique to each patient and cannot be strictly prescribed. Claims that low osmolality compounds reduce the prevalence of contrast material–induced nephropathy have not been unequivocally established (Schwab et al., 1989; Barrett and Carlisle, 1993; Rudnick et al., 1995).

Although nephrotoxicity has been reported in patients exposed to a total dose of only 30 gm of iodine, most reported cases have been associated with at least twice that amount. Furthermore, diagnostic studies should be conducted and scheduled to avoid repeated exposure to contrast material without adequate intervals for observation and recovery.

Protocols for protection against contrast material–induced nephrotoxicity have been proposed and merit attention. One consists of a prescribed amount of intravenous hydration for 12 hours before and during the examination, a moderate dose of contrast material, and mannitol infusion 60 minutes after exposure to the contrast material (Anto et al., 1981). Other protocols use an infusion of normal saline at a rate of 550 mL/h during angiographic procedures (Eisenberg et al., 1981) or an infusion of mannitol and furosemide in the period surrounding contrast material exposure and careful maintenance of hydration (Berkseth and Kjellstrand, 1984). Obviously, patients with medical conditions requiring a controlled fluid intake (congestive heart failure or cerebral edema) should not be subjected to these approaches without special consideration.

Removal of contrast material by natural excretory routes is slow in the patient with renal failure. Pathways for extrarenal, or *vicarious*, excretion include small bowel mucosa, the hepatobiliary system, and salivary glands. Contrast material excreted by these routes becomes concentrated and detectable in the colon (Fig. 1–4). Rapid removal may be desirable for patients with a serious adverse systemic reaction or nephrotoxicity. This can be done by either hemodialysis or peritoneal dialysis.

Clinical or laboratory evidence of contrast material nephrotoxicity may not become apparent in the first 24 hours after exposure. The serum creatinine level in some patients who develop this complication does not peak until 6 days after exposure. Detection requires careful surveillance of serum creatinine

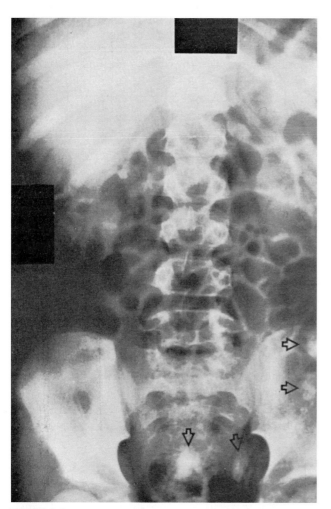

FIGURE 1–4. Extrarenal excretion of contrast material in a youth with acute glomerulonephritis and blood urea nitrogen of 160 mg/dL. Opacification of distal descending and sigmoid colon is present on a film taken 32 hours after intravenous injection of contrast material *(arrows)*. A faint nephrogram persists.

and urinary output during this period. Most patients with contrast material–induced acute tubular necrosis eventually return to baseline levels of renal function.

Contrast material–induced nephrotoxicity may be complicated by lactic acidosis in patients with non–insulin-dependent diabetes mellitus receiving the oral antihyperglycemic drug metformin hydrochloride (Glucophage). Concern over this possible untoward effect has led to the practice of withholding metformin before or at the time of intravascular injection of contrast material and not resuming this drug until baseline renal function has been documented 48 hours or more after the contrast material examination is completed (Dachman, 1995; Rotter, 1995; Bush and Bettmann, 1998). However, a point of view has been expressed that this precaution should be applied only to diabetic patients with pre-existing impairment of renal function (Pond et al., 1996)

Cardiotoxicity. Contrast material can induce cardiac arrhythmias, conduction abnormalities, and myocardial ischemia. Patients at risk include those with pre-existing myocardial, atherosclerotic, or valvular disease and those with existing conduction disturbances. Major cardiac arrhythmias and ischemia have been noted in 18 per cent of patients with cardiac disease and in 5 per cent of healthy individuals with no history of heart disease who were exposed to contrast material during excretory urography (Pfister and Hutter, 1980). Arrhythmias occur more frequently than ischemia. Premature ventricular contraction is the most common cardiac arrhythmia induced by contrast material; ventricular tachycardia and fibrillation are the most severe. Atrioventricular block has also been observed. An increase in cardiac rate leading to an increased oxygen requirement is the likely basis for ST segment depression and symptoms of ischemia.

Many symptoms, such as chest pain, loss of consciousness, and cardiac arrest, traditionally have been classified as adverse systemic reactions to contrast material. In fact, these symptoms are likely manifestations of cardiotoxicity. Similarly, the mortality rate for contrast material usage, historically thought of as the result of idiosyncratic systemic reactions, is undoubtedly composed of a significant cardiotoxic element.

The pathogenesis of contrast material–induced cardiotoxicity has not been established. The sudden introduction of a hypertonic volume load, direct toxicity to the myocardium, and stimulation of neural reflex pathways have been suggested as causative factors.

Precautions. When contrast material is administered to a patient at risk for cardiotoxicity, a low osmolality compound should be used and a bolus injection avoided. This precaution reflects the likelihood that cardiac toxicity is related to hyperosmolality, time, and dosage factors. Injection rates of 1 mL/s can reduce the incidence of cardiotoxicity, as will even slower infusions over a 10- to 15-minute period. Electrocardiographic monitoring during the examination may also be considered an adjunctive precaution in high-risk patients.

Excessive volume expansion in the newborn or infant is a risk when high osmolality contrast material is used. This cardiovascular complication can be essentially avoided by the use of low osmolality agents in an appropriate weight-adjusted dose, as previously discussed.

Pulmonary Toxicity. Subclinical bronchospasm, manifested by decreased forced expiratory flow rates, occurs frequently with exposure to contrast material in both normal and allergic patients. As yet it is unclear whether this reaction is caused by direct pulmonary toxicity or by the mechanisms that mediate idiosyncratic adverse systemic reactions. This phenomenon occurs more often with slow infusion of the meglumine salt than with bolus injection of the sodium salt. Neither an important clinical implication for this pulmonary reaction nor the effect of low osmolality contrast material has been established.

EXCRETORY UROGRAPHY

The goal of excretory urography—to obtain clinically useful information about the urinary tract and its related structures—requires that each examination be designed to meet unique needs. The elements that contribute to a successful study include an adequate dose of contrast material; a film to record the nephrogram; a sequence of films for assessing the dynamics of urine formation and propulsion; adequate distention of the opacified pelvocalyceal system; use of oblique, prone, and upright positions; use of tomography; reinjection of contrast material, if needed; and minimization of risks to the patient. Some of these have already been discussed in the earlier sections on use of contrast material.

Film Sequence

A preliminary film is a fundamental part of an examination using contrast material. This film should be exposed after the patient voids. It is then evaluated by the radiologist for proper radiographic technique and patient positioning; the presence of radiodense structures in areas of the urinary tract that may subsequently be obscured by the excreted contrast material; and assessment of organ systems other than the urinary tract.

The exact number and type of preliminary films are determined by the patient's individual circumstances. A single film of the abdomen that includes the pubis bone (the KUB film) may suffice in some patients, whereas in others an additional film coned to the kidney is needed. A full set of tomograms may be of value in a patient suspected of having small kidney stones. When tomograms are anticipated, a single preliminary cut one-third of the anteroposterior diameter from the table top is use-

ful to determine technique. Finally, an oblique preliminary film is essential for localization of radiodense structures that overlie the kidney (see discussion in Chapter 14). All exposures should be made after the patient fully exhales to minimize the geometric distortion of the renal image that occurs when deep inspiration causes descent and ventral rotation of the lower poles of the kidneys.

It is of great practical advantage during excretory urography to obtain a film of the kidneys as soon as possible after the administration of contrast material, preferably at 1 minute when using a high osmolality compound and somewhat later when low osmolality contrast material has been injected. It is at this time that a relatively large amount of contrast material in the proximal tubules renders radiodense the entire renal parenchyma, causing the urographic nephrogram. This is the most opportune time for the evaluation of renal size, position, contour, and parenchymal integrity (Fig. 1–5). A tomogram at this time is often useful, too.

The number and sequence of films used in excretory urography, following injection of contrast material, must be individualized to each patient. A 5-minute film without compression provides useful information about the rate of urine formation. Oblique films, including those obtained with tomographic technique, may provide important evidence of contour abnormalities, deformities of the papillae or calyces, or abnormalities of the collecting system. Prone or upright films are of value in assessing obstruction. As described in Chapter 27, a sequence of films is needed for time-density analysis of the nephrogram and the dynamics of collecting system opacification. This is a useful exercise in elucidating certain renal abnormalities and a fundamental process in diagnosing obstructive uropathy. In some circumstances, such as preoperative screening of patients undergoing prostatic or gynecologic surgery, a single film exposed 8 to 10 minutes after injection of contrast material will suffice; the most useful information is derived from films obtained within the first 15 minutes after injection of contrast material. After this point, reinjection may be of value if a particular suspicion must be tested.

A complete routine for an excretory urographic examination includes the following:

- 1–3 minute anteroposterior (11 × 14-inch [28 × 35-cm] film)
- 5-minute anteroposterior (11 × 14-inch film)
- Apply ureteral compression
- 10-minute anteroposterior, right and left posterior oblique (11 × 14-inch film)
- Release compression
- Postcompression anteroposterior, right and left posterior oblique (14 × 17-inch [35 × 43-cm] film)
- Upright postvoid anteroposterior (14 × 17-inch film)

Tomograms should be obtained as required at any stage of the examination.

Adequate distention of the pelvocalyceal system

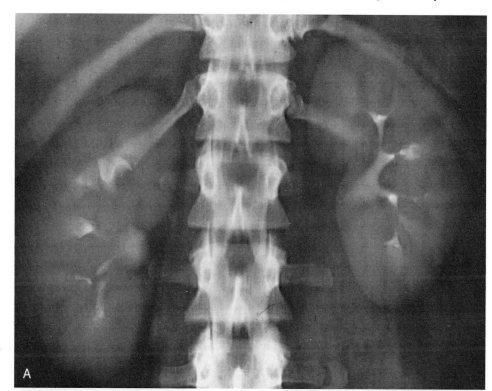

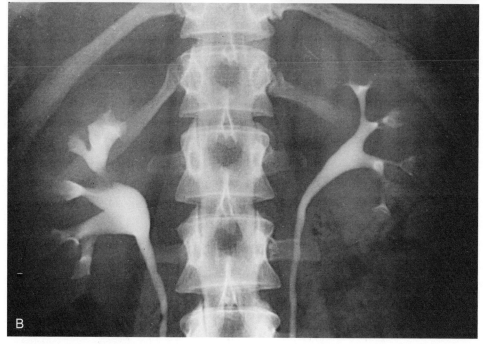

FIGURE 1–5. Normal excretory urogram performed with low osmolality, nonionic contrast material.

A, Tomogram obtained at approximately 90 seconds after injection of contrast material. The nephrographic phase is fully developed, permitting assessment of renal size, contour, and parenchyma.

B, Radiograph obtained approximately 10 minutes later. The pelvocalyceal systems and proximal ureters are opacified and distended by effective ureteral compression. The nephrogram has diminished in density.

is an essential component of the well-performed excretory urogram (see Fig. 1–5). This is effected, in part, by the diuresis that is induced by contrast material, especially high osmolality compounds. Additionally, external compression of the ureter by two small inflatable rubber balloons is a simple and effective way of producing distention. The balloons are held in place by a plastic foam block and a band that passes around the patient. The ureters are compressed at the point at which they pass over the sacral prominence. The most effective commercial devices are those that have two separate balloons that permit mobility, allowing the patient to be placed in an oblique position. External compression should be avoided in patients with possible urinary tract obstruction, recent abdominal or urinary tract surgery, ostomies, abdominal tumor, ureteral stone, or abdominal aortic aneurysm. Ureteral compression is of particular importance in patients given low osmolality contrast material to compensate for the low diuretic effect of these agents.

Value of Tomography. Tomography has been

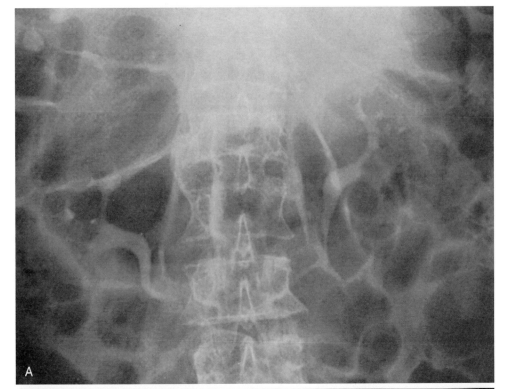

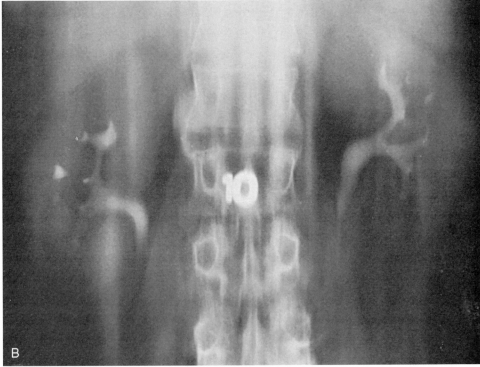

FIGURE 1–6. Value of tomography during excretory urography in a patient with poor bowel preparation. Sodium diatrizoate 50%, 1.0 mL/kg body weight.
A, Details of the kidneys on a 5-minute film are obscured by bowel gas.
B, Tomogram eliminates impediments seen in *A*.

widely recognized as a valuable adjunct to excretory urographic diagnosis. Historically, a great body of literature has tended to categorize nephrotomography as something distinct from excretory urography. However, there is no need to view nephrotomography as a mysterious procedure, separate from routine excretory urography. Tomography during excretory urography should be applied whenever anatomic information is obscured because of overlying bowel content or faint visualization in impaired renal function or simply to acquire better anatomic definition (Figs. 1–6, 1–7). Tomography should be used the moment the need is determined.

To perform this study, exposure factors that allow discrimination of small differences in density must be chosen. Kilovoltage in the 60- to 75-kV range with a variable mAs is considered ideal. Arc may be varied from 10 to 50 degrees, depending on the

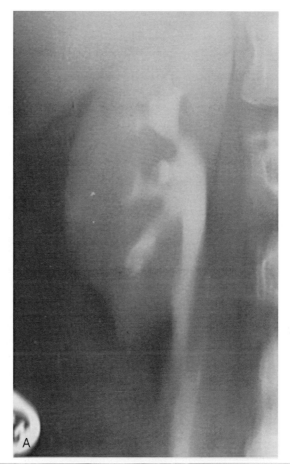

FIGURE 1–7. The use of tomography for improved detail is illustrated in a patient with a depression in renal contour of the right lower pole due to an old infarct.
  A, Tomogram.
  B, Standard film in which the deformity is not well defined.

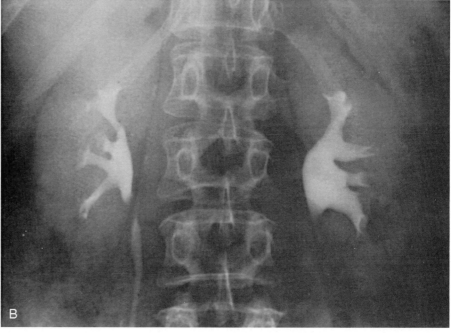

desired thickness of the cut. Often it is valuable to inject additional contrast material immediately before the tomogram. Oblique projections are frequently helpful, and thick-section tomography (zonography) is often sufficient. Computed tomography–derived guidelines based on abdominal thick-

ness are available for accurate determination of tomographic levels (Rhodes et al., 1987).

ULTRASONOGRAPHY

Real-time ultrasonographic imaging systems are used for examination of the kidneys and surrounding structures. Mechanical-sector or phased-array scanners have the particular advantage of being able to image through small acoustic windows such as the intercostal spaces.

The highest frequency transducer that allows adequate visualization of the kidneys should be used. Usually, a 3.5–4–MHz transducer is effective in adults, whereas a 5-MHz transducer works well in most children.

One fundamental aspect in the assessment of the kidneys by ultrasonography is comparing the echogenicity of renal parenchyma with that of the liver and spleen. To make this analysis valid requires compensation for the exponential attenuation of sound as it penetrates the tissue. This is the function of the time-gain-compensation curve, which must be set to produce a uniform intensity of echoes throughout the entire thickness of the homogeneous reference tissue. For renal ultrasonography, the reference tissue is the liver. When the time-gain-compensation curve is properly set, the echogenicity of normal renal parenchyma should be equal to or less than that of the liver at equal depths from the transducer. This criterion maximizes the specificity of ultrasonography in the evaluation of patients for renal parenchymal disease although the sensitivity remains low. As a generality, then, renal parenchymal echogenicity greater than that of the liver reliably indicates renal disease, whereas that which is equal to or less than that of the liver does not. Comparison of relative renal-hepatic echo intensities may be distorted by the interposition of fluid (ascites or a cystic lesion) between the liver and kidney or by intrinsic alterations of hepatic echogenicity by diffuse liver disease.

Ultrasound examination of the kidney should be performed on hydrated patients with empty bladders. Some ultrasonographers claim that hydration enhances differentiation of the cortex from the medulla and increases the likelihood of visualizing the pelvocalyceal system through diuresis. Additionally, a low-grade obstruction is more likely to be detected in a diuretic rather than an antidiuretic state induced by dehydration. On the contrary, a full bladder may impede the flow of urine across the vesicoureteral junction and produce a false impression of obstruction. Therefore, when a full bladder is visualized in the clinical setting of hydronephrosis, the bladder should be emptied and the upper tract re-examined.

The right kidney is best examined using the liver as an acoustic window. The patient is usually placed in a left posterior oblique or supine position. Longitudinal images are obtained along the anterior axillary line, and transverse images are obtained along intercostal and subcostal spaces. Deep inspiration, to position the kidney below the ribs, is often a useful technique in examining the right kidney. Both longitudinal and transverse images are sequentially recorded. Generally, three longitudinal and transverse (upper, middle, and lower) images are obtained.

The left kidney is more difficult to examine than the right because the overlying contents of the gastrointestinal tract often block sound transmission. The most feasible acoustic approach to the left kidney is through the spleen. This requires putting the patient in a right-side-down decubitus position or a right anterior oblique prone position so the transducer can be placed over an intercostal space along the posterior axillary line. Deep inspiration is particularly valuable during imaging of the lower pole of the left kidney. The posterolateral approach to the left kidney results in coronal images.

Accurate measurement of renal length depends on obtaining an image that includes the extreme limits of both the upper and lower poles of the kidney on a single image. The complete examination of the kidney also includes examination in two projections at right angles to each other, evaluation of the vascular pedicle and inferior vena cava, and assessment of the contralateral kidney and the retroperitoneum.

Some ultrasonographic evaluations require assessment of renal vessels with Doppler ultrasound. Duplex ultrasonography is especially useful in confirming flow within the renal veins or inferior vena cava. The Doppler cursor is placed within the vessel image, and venous tracings are sought. Renal artery tracings are generally quite difficult to obtain. The cursor can be placed within the image of the renal parenchyma or renal masses for the purpose of determining vascularity. Color flow imaging greatly speeds evaluation by aiding in the detection of vessels.

COMPUTED TOMOGRAPHY

Computed tomography displays renal anatomy and disease in the transverse plane, thereby overcoming a major limitation of excretory urography by eliminating the effect of overlying tissues. This technique is also ideal for the study of the renal sinus and the retroperitoneum.

In addition, the superior density discrimination of computed tomography over standard radiography is particularly advantageous in assessing urolithiasis and nephrocalcinosis, in determining the nature of renal masses, and in diagnosing renal, subcapsular, and retroperitoneal hemorrhage. The enhanced density discrimination also makes computed tomography desirable for studying patients who should not be exposed to contrast material because of a high risk of adverse systemic reaction or those who can tolerate only a minimal dose of contrast material because of risk of nephrotoxicity.

The ability to derive information about renal perfusion and function from dynamic computed tomographic scanning is another distinct advantage of computed tomography over other diagnostic uroradiologic techniques. This technique can also be applied to study the vascular nature of a renal tumor.

The specific technique for performing computed tomography of the kidneys is determined in part by the characteristics of the available equipment. A standard examination should consist of contiguous sections of approximately 5-mm thickness that extend through the entire length of the kidney. Thinner sections—for example, 3-mm thickness—are used for specific circumstances, such as the search for very small calcifications or fat within a tumor. Oral contrast material is not required for evaluation of the kidneys but is used in many institutions for simultaneous evaluation of the gastrointestinal tract.

Spiral computed tomography techniques offer some advantages over standard computed tomography techniques, especially by eliminating misregistration artifacts due to respiration when scanning the entire kidney in a single breath-hold. This may be of use in the detection of small lesions, including small calcific deposits. The faster examination time is also of particular advantage in the setting of acute trauma and in documenting the transit of contrast material as discussed below. Technical parameters for spiral computed tomography vary. In general, 5-mm collimation with a 1:1 pitch is used routinely but adjusted to individual circumstances. Some degradation in image quality may be associated with the helical mode in comparison to images acquired by standard computed tomography.

Computed tomography of the kidneys is ideally performed both before and after administration of contrast material, assuming no contraindication to the latter. A rapid intravenous injection of a bolus of contrast material is preferable to a slow drip infusion for several reasons. These include optimal detection of difference in the pattern of nephrographic enhancement between the two kidneys (as might be sought in suspected renal artery stenosis), visualization of major renal arteries and veins (as, for example, might be of value in the detection of renal vein invasion by carcinoma), and simply for reproducibility of technique. The volume of contrast material for computed tomography is in the range of 100 to 150 mL of a solution containing an iodine concentration of 300 mg/mL. A mechanical injector allows rapid, consistent administration of contrast material without exposing the operator to radiation.

The very fast rate of image acquisition in spiral computed tomography may yield images of the kidney that fail to fully document the progression of contrast material as it passes from the renal microvasculature through the nephrons and collecting ducts and into the collecting system, ureters, and bladder (Fig. 1–8) (see Chapter 27 for discussion of the nephrogram). Scan times after contrast material injection must be selected in the context of the clinical problem that is being investigated. Repeat or delayed scans are often required. For example, "early" scanning is required for vascular evaluation, whereas a delay of approximately 90 seconds may be needed to detect a richly vascularized mass within homogeneously enhanced renal parenchyma. Obviously, only scans that are even more delayed permit evaluation of the collecting system, ureters,

and bladder. Delayed scans may be of particular value in specific diseases as, for example, in urinary tract obstruction or acute pyelonephritis (see Chapter 9).

Specialized applications of computed tomography can be performed in specific clinical circumstances. Spiral scanning with multiplanar reconstruction of images and without contrast material enhancement can be used to evaluate the patient with acute flank pain for hydronephrosis, urolithiasis, or extrarenal abnormalities. Additionally, computed tomographic angiography incorporates thin-section spiral scanning techniques during and immediately following the injection of a bolus of contrast material to provide three-dimensional reconstruction of images that may demonstrate abnormalities of the renal arteries or veins or vascular malformations or create "road maps" for preoperative planning (Fig. 1–9).

MAGNETIC RESONANCE IMAGING

Magnetic resonance imaging of the kidney and retroperitoneum is a useful alternative to computed tomography in patients in whom the use of iodinated contrast material is contraindicated because of an increased risk of adverse reaction or nephrotoxicity, in characterizing renal masses, in staging carcinoma of the kidney, and in defining the precise anatomy of a tumor in the perirenal space. Although each examination should be tailored to the patient's unique clinical problem, a renal magnetic resonance imaging study should include a T1- and T2-weighted image in at least one plane and a T1-weighted image in at least one plane after contrast material enhancement (Fig. 1–10). Fast gradient echo pulse sequences now allow the acquisition of such images in a time-efficient manner and can replace older spin-echo methods.

Field strength is not a significant factor in obtaining good renal images, although higher field strength does enable more flexibility in scan techniques. Image quality is very dependent on the motion compensation or suppression program of a particular magnetic resonance unit. T1-weighted (TR 300–500 msec; TE 5–20 msec) spin-echo spoiled gradient echo images generally provide the highest quality images. Before contrast material enhancement, the cortex is usually higher in signal intensity than the medulla (corticomedullary ratio = 1.2 to 1.5), depending on the patient's age and hydration status. Fat suppression after contrast material administration should be employed because this improves the ability to detect and characterize renal lesions. Breath-held T1 gradient echo images significantly improve image quality by reducing motion. A T2-weighted (TR 1500–3000 msec; TE 60–120 msec) spin-echo image or fast spin echo (TR 2000–5000 msec; TE 100–150 msec; echo train 8–16) is usually obtained in the axial plane. The medulla is slightly higher in signal intensity than the cortex, owing to its higher water content. This se-

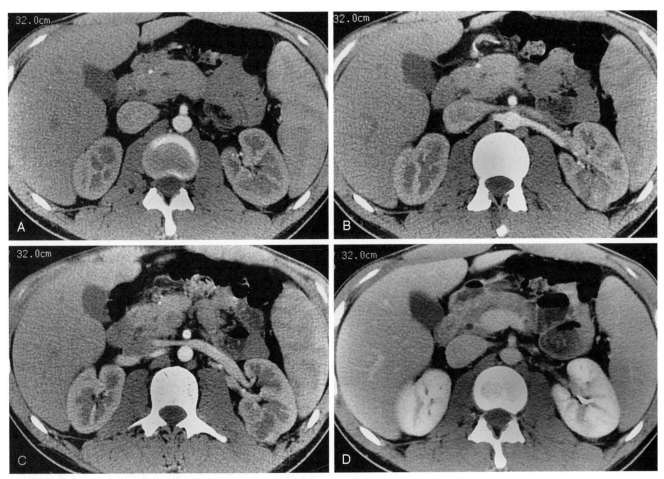

FIGURE 1–8. Helical computed tomogram, contrast material–enhanced.

A, Upper pole image obtained at 15 seconds demonstrates parenchymal enhancement limited to the renal cortex ("cortical nephrogram").

B, C, Early images obtained in the midportion of the left kidney also demonstrate enhancement of the left renal artery and vein as well as the aorta and superior mesenteric artery.

D, Upper pole image obtained at approximately 120 seconds after contrast material injection demonstrates enhancement of both renal cortex and medulla ("urographic nephrogram") as well as opacification of the pelvocalyceal system ("pyelographic phase").

(Same case illustrated in Fig. 27–3.)

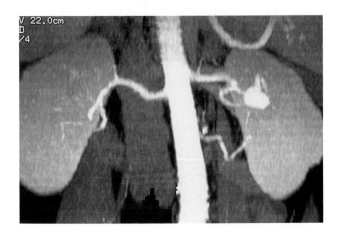

FIGURE 1–9. Computed tomographic arteriogram. Maximum intensity projection (MIP) reconstruction of helical acquisition during rapid bolus administration of intravenous contrast material demonstrates an aneurysm of the left renal artery. (Same patient illustrated in Figs. 6–8 and 16–21.)

quence permits evaluation of cystic and solid masses, although it alone cannot discriminate between these two. Magnetic resonance imaging is limited in the urinary tract by an inability to detect calcifications and the nonspecificity of signal intensity.

Gadolinium chelates are used as contrast material to evaluate masses considered indeterminate by other modalities or in place of iodinated contrast material when it is contraindicated. Gadopentate dimeglumine, gadoteridol, or gadodiamide (0.1 mmol/kg) can be either infused slowly and followed by conventional T1-weighted spin-echo images (with fat suppression, if available) or delivered as a bolus with dynamic image acquisition. The latter approach permits evaluation of the enhancement properties of a focal renal lesion or estimation of the degree of functional impairment associated with hydronephrosis or parenchymal abnormalities. As

with all enhancement techniques, pre– and post–contrast material studies must use exactly the same imaging parameters to detect meaningful differences in signal intensity. There are two types of dynamic images: the rapid spin echo and the rapid gradient echo. In the former, imaging time is decreased by shortening repetition times and halving Fourier's transformation. Even shorter repetition times are possible with dynamic gradient-echo images, allowing for breath-holding. In either case the images obtained after a bolus of contrast material are similar to those obtained with dynamic computed tomography. Dynamic images are obtained during breath-holding. With T2*-weighted sequences, such as gradient-echo images with narrow flip angles (less than 30 degrees) and a long TE in relation to TR, renal parenchyma decreases in signal intensity with progressive renal concentration of contrast material. This enhancement pattern is

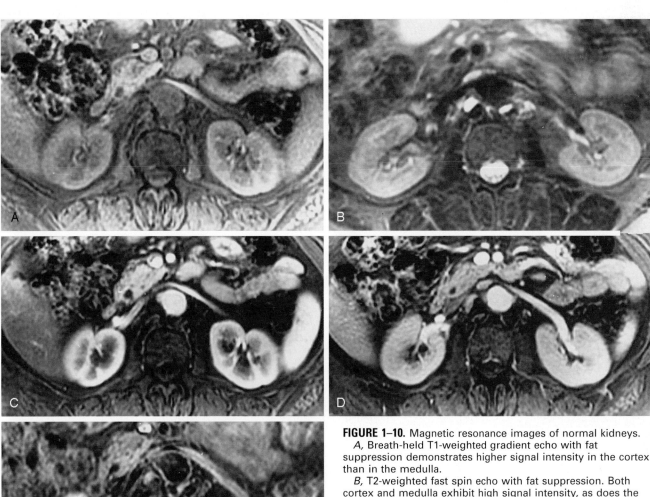

FIGURE 1–10. Magnetic resonance images of normal kidneys.

A, Breath-held T1-weighted gradient echo with fat suppression demonstrates higher signal intensity in the cortex than in the medulla.

B, T2-weighted fast spin echo with fat suppression. Both cortex and medulla exhibit high signal intensity, as does the cerebrospinal fluid within the spinal canal.

C, Early phase dynamic enhanced spoiled gradient echo image with fat suppression. There is intense enhancement of the cortex representing the cortical nephrogram.

D, Late phase enhanced gradient echo image with fat suppression demonstrates the nephrographic phase of contrast material excretion.

E, Delayed T1-weighted spin echo image with fat suppression demonstrates the pyelographic phase of enhancement of the pelvocalyceal system.

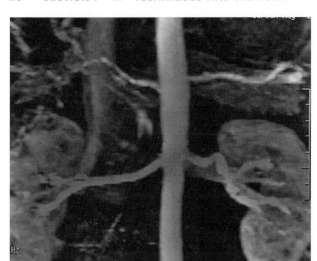

FIGURE 1–11. Magnetic resonance angiogram used for surgical planning prior to nephrectomy. This image was obtained with a 3D spoiled gradient echo technique during the injection of 0.2 mmol/kg of a gadolinium chelate. Single renal arteries are present bilaterally.

more complex than seen with iodinated contrast material–enhanced computed tomography and is susceptible to changes in relation to the patient's hydration status.

To evaluate the inferior vena cava for thrombus, thin, gradient-echo images are obtained. These "bright blood" techniques demonstrate high signal within a normal caval lumen. Using maximal intensity projection (MIP), a magnetic resonance venogram can be created. If gradient-echo images are unavailable, T1-weighted images with presatura-

tion pulses inferior to the plane of section should be employed. However, this "dark blood" technique is susceptible to slow flow artifacts that can mimic thrombus. The two techniques can complement each other.

Magnetic resonance imaging techniques continue to evolve. Faster imaging techniques such as echo planar imaging may be of particular importance in the abdomen, where motion artifact can be "frozen" by images of 50 to 100 msec in duration. Magnetic resonance angiography has potential application for the noninvasive assessment of renal artery stenosis, for presurgical "road mapping," and for assessment of vascular malformations (Fig. 1–11). In addition to anatomic information, magnetic resonance angiography also may provide quantitative renal artery flow measurements.

ANGIOGRAPHY

Angiography of the kidney is performed by Seldinger's technique. The discussion in this section is limited to aspects unique to renal arteriography and venography and applies to either film radiography or digital image recording.

Arteriography

A complete examination of the arterial supply to the kidney includes an aortogram and selective renal arteriograms of all renal arteries.

Aortography. For aortography, the distal curve and side hole placement of the catheter should be designed to promote mixture of contrast material with blood and to minimize the amount of contrast material flowing into the celiac and superior mesenteric arteries (Fig. 1–12). Contrast material is in-

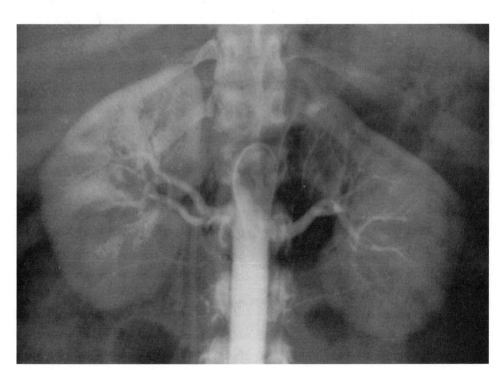

FIGURE 1–12. Aortogram for renal blood vessels. The catheter has been placed to direct the contrast material into the renal arteries and the distal aorta, thus avoiding opacification of the celiac and mesenteric arteries.

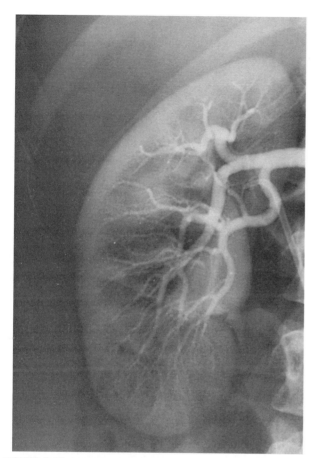

FIGURE 1–13. Selective right renal arteriogram magnified 1.5 times.

jected at 20 mL/s for 2 seconds. A typical image sequence is three images per second over a 3-second period and one image per second over a 4-second period. The initial study is usually done using the anteroposterior projection, but 20- to 30-degree posterior oblique sequences are often used, particularly when searching for stenotic lesions of the proximal renal arteries. It is often best to determine optimal oblique positioning by turning the patient under direct fluoroscopic observation. Careful coning of the recorded image to the margins of the kidneys greatly enhances diagnostic quality.

Selective Renal Arteriography. Selective renal arteriography is performed with a catheter shaped to conform to the renal artery. The orifice of the desired renal artery is sought at the level of origin identified in an initial aortogram. If an aortogram is not done, most arteries can be located by moving the catheter up and down a segment of the aorta from the upper margin of L-1 to the lower margin of L-2. Often, continuous clockwise or counterclockwise torque must be applied to the catheter to keep the catheter tip pointing in a lateral direction. Insertion of the catheter into the renal artery is signaled by a sudden lateral movement of the catheter tip. Injection of 2 to 3 mL of contrast material under fluoroscopic control verifies accurate positioning and ensures that the tip is not pointed into the arterial wall. This procedure may have to be repeated in kidneys with more than one renal artery.

The amount of contrast material used in selective renal arteriography depends on the size of the kidney and the renal blood flow. An average total dose is 10 mL administered over 1.5 seconds. This should be increased in patients with high-flow states, as in vascular renal carcinoma or conditions with arteriovenous shunting. The rate of image recording varies with the state of renal blood flow. A sequence for average flow is four images per second over a 2-second period, two images per second over a 2-second period, and one image per second over a 6-second period. Usually, an anteroposterior and posterior oblique projection are obtained for each kidney, but the actual approach is determined by individual circumstances. Again, the value of careful collimation for achieving superior-quality images cannot be overemphasized. Magnification and subtraction techniques may be employed to search for very small or obscured lesions (Fig. 1–13).

Venography

Inferior vena cavography should be performed before selective catheterization of the renal veins when venous thrombosis is suspected. Selective catheterization of the renal veins is best done with a catheter having good torque control, that is, one that is both larger and stiffer than those used for arterial studies. A single shape usually suffices for both veins. However, the left renal vein is much longer than the right, and a long-limbed catheter may be required in special circumstances. Two side holes may be placed just proximal to the tip of the catheter. A selective renal venogram is performed with contrast material injected at a rate of 10 mL/s over a 3-second period. An image recording sequence of two images per second over a 5-second period is suitable for most circumstances. The examination is usually performed in the anteroposterior projection.

One impediment to satisfactory visualization of the renal veins is that blood flow from the kidney washes out the injected contrast material. Techniques to reduce this effect include reduction of renal blood flow by performing Valsalva's maneuver, by injecting epinephrine into the renal artery immediately before injecting contrast material into the renal vein, or by using balloon-occluding selective catheters. Epinephrine is given in a dose of 5 to 10 mg,* injected into the ipsilateral renal artery and followed in 10 to 20 seconds by a selective renal venogram.

---

*Add 1.0 mg epinephrine to 500 mL normal saline. Each milliliter contains 2 mg epinephrine.

BIBLIOGRAPHY
Contrast Material

Alexander, R. D., Berkes, S. L., and Abuelo, J. G.: Contrast media–induced oliguric renal failure. Arch. Intern. Med. *138*:381, 1978.

Almén, T.: Development of nonionic contrast media. Invest. Radiol. 20(Suppl.):S2, 1985.

Andrews, E. J., Jr.: The vagus reaction as a possible cause of severe complications of radiological procedures. Radiology 121:1, 1976.

Ansari, Z., and Baldwin, D. S.: Acute renal failure due to radiocontrast agents. Nephron 17:28, 1976.

Ansell, G., Tweedie, M. C. K., West, C. R., Evans, P., and Couch, L.: The current status of reactions to intravenous contrast media. Invest. Radiol. 15(Suppl.):S32, 1980.

Anto, H. R., Shyan-Yih, C., Porush, J. G., and Shapiro, W. B.: Infusion intravenous pyelography and renal function: Effects of hypertonic mannitol in patients with chronic renal insufficiency. Arch. Intern. Med. 141:1652, 1981.

Bahlmann, J., and Krüskemper, H. L.: The excretion of iodine-containing x-ray contrast material in patients on intermittent haemodialyses. In Proceedings, IV International Congress of Nephrology, Stockholm, 1969. Basel, Switzerland, Karger, 1970.

Barrett, B.J.: Contrast nephrotoxicity. J. Am. Soc. Nephrol. 5:125, 1994.

Barrett, B. J., and Carlisle, E. J.: Metaanalysis of the relative nephrotoxicity of high- and low-osmolality iodinated contrast media. Radiology 188:171, 1993.

Barrett, B. J., Parfrey, P. S., McDonald, J. R., Hefferton, D. M., Reddy, E. R., and McManamon, P. J.: Nonionic low-osmolality versus ionic high-osmolality contrast material for intravenous use in patients perceived to be at high risk: Randomized trial. Radiology 183:105, 1992.

Berg, G. R., Hutter, A. M., and Pfister, R. C.: Electrocardiographic abnormalities associated with intravenous urography. N. Engl. J. Med. 289:87, 1973.

Berkseth, R.O., Kjellstrand, C.M.: Radiologic contrast-induced nephropathy. Med. Clin. North Am. 68:351, 1984.

Bettmann, M. A.: Clinical summary with conclusions: Ionic versus nonionic contrast agents and their effects on blood components. Invest. Radiol. 23(Suppl. 2):S378, 1988.

Bettmann, M. A.: Guidelines for use of low-osmolality contrast agents. Radiology 172:901, 1989.

Bettmann, M. A.: Ionic versus nonionic contrast agents for intravenous use: Are all the answers in? Radiology 175:616, 1990.

Bettmann M. A.: Intravascular contrast agents: Current problems and future solutions—a review. Acta Radiol. 37:3, 1996.

Bettmann, M. A., Heeren, T., Greenfield, A., and Goudey, C.: Adverse events with radiographic contrast agents: Results of the SCVIR Contrast Agent Registry. Radiology 203:611, 1997.

Brezis, M., and Epstein, F. H.: A closer look at radiocontrast-induced nephropathy. N. Engl. J. Med. 320:179, 1989.

Brismar, J., Jacobsson, B. F., and Jorulf, H.: Miscellaneous adverse effects of low- versus high-osmolality contrast media: A study revised. Radiology 179:19, 1991.

Bush, W. H., and Bettmann, M. A.: Update on metformin (Glucophage) therapy and the risk of lactic acidosis: Change in FDA-approved package insert. Bull. Am. Coll. Radiol. 54:15, 1998.

Bush, W. H., and Swanson, D. P.: Acute reactions to intravascular contrast media: Types, risk factors, recognition, and specific treatment. AJR 157:1153, 1991.

Byrd, L., and Sherman, R. L.: Radiocontrast-induced acute renal failure: A clinical and pathophysiologic review. Medicine 58:270, 1979.

Caro, J. J., Trinade, E., and McGregor, M.: The risks of death and of severe nonfatal reactions with high- vs low-osmolality contrast media: A meta-analysis. AJR 156:825, 1991.

Cattell, W. R.: Excretory pathways for contrast media. Invest. Radiol. 5:473, 1970.

Cattell, W. R., Fry, I. K., Spencer, A. G., and Purkiss, P.: Excretion urography: I. Factors determining the excretion of Hypaque. Br. J. Radiol. 40:561, 1967.

Cohan, R. H., and Ellis, J. H.: Iodinated contrast material in uroradiology: Choice of agent and management of complications. Urol. Clin. North Am. 24:471, 1997.

Cohan R. H., Ellis J. H., and Garner W. L.: Extravasation of radiographic contrast material: Recognition, prevention, and treatment. Radiology 200:593, 1996.

Cohan, R. H., Leder R. A., and Ellis, J. H.: Treatment of adverse

reactions to radiographic contrast media in adults. Radiol. Clin. North Am. 34:1055, 1996.

Cohan R. H., Sherman L. S., Korobkin M., Bass J. C., and Francis I. R.: Renal masses: Assessment of corticomedullary-phase and nephrographic-phase CT scans. Radiology 196:445, 1995.

Curry, N. S., Schabel, S. I., Reinheld, C. T., Henry, W. D., and Savoca, W. J.: Fatal reaction to intravenous nonionic contrast material. Radiology 178:361, 1991.

Dachman A. H.: New contraindication to intravascular iodinated contrast material. Radiology 197:545, 1995.

Dahl, S. G., Linaker, O., Mellbye, AA, and Sveen, K.: Influence of the cation on the side effects of urographic contrast media. Acta Radiol. (Diagn.) 17:461, 1976.

Davies, P., Roberts, M. B., and Roylance, J.: Acute reactions to urographic contrast media. Br. Med. J. 2:434, 1975.

Dawson, P.: Chemotoxicity of contrast media and clinical adverse effects: A review. Invest. Radiol. 20(Suppl.):S84, 1985.

Dawson P.: The non-ionic dimers—some theoretical and clinical considerations. Eur. J. Radiol. 5:S103, 1995.

Dean, P. B., and Kormano, M.: Intravenous bolus of ^{125}I labelled meglumine diatrizoate: Early extravascular distribution. Acta Radiol. (Diagn.) 18:293, 1977.

Diaz-Buxo, J., Wagoner, R. D., Hattery, R. R., and Palumbo, P. J.: Acute renal failure after excretory urography in diabetic patients. Ann. Intern. Med. 83:155, 1975.

Dunnick N. R., Cohan R. H.: Cost, corticosteroids, and contrast media. AJR 162:527, 1994.

Eisenberg, R. I., Bank, W. O., and Hedgcock, M. W.: Renal failure after major angiography can be avoided with hydration. AJR 136:859, 1981.

Ellis J. H., Cohan, R. H., Sonnad S. S., and Cohan N. S.: Selective use of radiographic low-osmolality contrast media in the 1990s. Radiology 200:297, 1996.

Federle, M. P., Willis, L. L., and Swanson, D. P.: Ionic versus nonionic contrast media: A prospective study of the effect of rapid bolus injection on nausea and anaphylactoid reactions. J. Comput. Assist. Tomogr. 22:341, 1998.

Feldman, H. A., and McCurdy, D. K.: Recurrent radiographic dye induced acute renal failure. JAMA 229:72, 1974.

Fountaine, H., Harnish, P., Andrew, E. and Grynne, B.: Safety, tolerance and pharmacokinetics of iodixanol injection, a nonionic, isosmolar hexa-iodinated contrast agent. Acad. Radiol. 3:S475, 1996.

Fry, I. K., Cattell, W. R., Spencer, A. G., and Purkiss, P.: The relation between Hypaque excretion and the intravenous urogram. Br. J. Radiol. 40:572, 1967.

Furukawa, T., Ueda, J., Takahashi, S., and Sakaguchi, K.: Elimination of low-osmolality contrast media by hemodialysis. Acta Radiol. 37:966, 1996.

Gafter, V., Creter, D., Zevin, D., Catz, R., and Djaldetti, M.: Inhibition of platelet aggregation by contrast media. Radiology 132:341, 1979.

Gerstman, B. B.: Epidemiologic critique of the report on adverse reaction to ionic and nonionic media by the Japanese committee on the safety of contrast media. Radiology 178:787, 1991.

Goldsmith, S. R., and Steinberg, P.: Noncardiogenic pulmonary edema induced by nonionic low-osmolality radiographic contrast media. J. Allergy Clin. Immunol. 96:698, 1995.

Golman, K., and Almén, T.: Contrast media–induced nephrotoxicity: Survey and present state. Invest. Radiol. 20:592, 1985.

Gomes, A. S., Lois, J. F., Baker, J. D., McGlade, C. T., Bunnell, D. H., and Hartzman, S.: Acute renal dysfunction in high-risk patients after angiography: Comparison of ionic and nonionic contrast media. Radiology 170:65, 1985.

Greganti, M. A., and Flowers, W. M., Jr.: Acute pulmonary edema after the intravenous administration of contrast media. Radiology 132:583, 1979.

Halpern, J. D., Hopper, K. D., Arredondo, M. G., and Trautlein, J. J.: Patient allergies: Role in selective use of nonionic contrast material. Radiology 199:359, 1996.

Harkonen, S., and Kjellstrand, C. M.: Intravenous pyelography in nonuremic diabetic patients. Nephron 24:268, 1979.

Harkonen, S., and Kjellstrand, C. M.: Contrast nephropathy. Am. J. Nephrol. 1:69, 1981.

Hartman, G. W., Hattery, R. R., Witten, D. M., and Williamson, B., Jr.: Mortality during excretory urography: Mayo Clinic experience. AJR 139:919, 1982.

Jensen, N., and Dorph, S.: Adverse reactions to urographic contrast medium: Rapid versus slow injection rate. Br. J. Radiol. 53:659, 1980.

Katayama, H., Yamaguchi, K., Kozuka, T., Takashima, T., Seez, P., and Matsuura, K.: Adverse reactions to ionic and nonionic contrast media: A report from the Japanese committee on the safety of contrast media. Radiology 175:621, 1990.

Kaye, B., Howard, J., Foord, K. D., and Cumberland, D. C.: Comparison of the image quality of intravenous urograms using low-osmolar contrast media. Br. J. Radiol. 61:589, 1988.

Kelley, W. M.: Uricosuria and x-ray contrast agents. N. Engl. J. Med. 284:975, 1971.

Kennison, M. C., Powe, N. R., and Steinberg, E. P.: Results of randomized controlled trials of low- versus high-osmolality contrast media. Radiology 170:381, 1989.

Khoury, G. A., Hopper, J. C., Varghese, Z., Farrington, K., Dick, R., Irving, J. P., Sweny, P., Fernando, O. N., and Moorhead, J. F.: Nephrotoxicity of ionic and non-ionic contrast material in digital vascular imaging and selective renal arteriography. Br. J. Radiol. 56:631, 1983.

Knapp, M. S.: Renal failure after contrast radiography. Br. Med. J. 287:3, 1983.

Kormano, M.: Volume of distribution of contrast media in blood. Acta Radiol. (Diagn.) 20:33, 1979.

Lamki, L. M. and Barron, B. J.: Low-osmolar contrast agents in patients with renal insufficiency. Am. J. Roentgenol. 168:1615, 1997.

Lang, D. M., Alpern, M. B., Visintainer, P. F. and Smith, S. T.: Gender risk for anaphylactoid reaction to radiographic contrast media. J. Allergy Clin. Immunol. 95:813, 1995.

Lasser, E. C.: Pretreatment with corticosteroids to prevent reactions to IV contrast material: Overview and implications. AJR 150:257, 1988.

Lasser, E. C., and Berry, C. C.: Pretreatment with corticosteroids to alleviate reactions to intravenous contrast material. N. Engl. J. Med. 317:845, 1987.

Lasser, E. C., and Berry, C. C.: Nonionic versus ionic contrast media: What do the data tell us? AJR 152:945, 1989.

Lasser, E. C., Berry, C. C., Mishkin, M. M., Williamson, B., Zheutlin, N. and Silverman, J.M.: Pretreatment with corticosteroids to prevent adverse reactions to nonionic contrast media. AJR 162:523, 1994.

Lasser, E. C., Lang, J., Sovak, M., Kolb, W., Lyon, S., and Hamblin, A. E.: Steroids: Theoretical and experimental basis for utilization in prevention of contrast media reactions. Radiology 125:1, 1977.

Lasser, E. C., Lyon, S. G., and Berry, C. C.: Reports on contrast media reactions: Analysis of data from reports to the U.S. Food and Drug Administration. Radiology 203:605, 1997.

Lawrence, V., Matthai, W., and Hartmaier, S.: Comparative safety of high-osmolality and low-osmolality radiographic contrast agents. Invest. Radiol. 27:1, 1992.

Lawton, G., Phillips, T., and Davies, R.: Alterations in heart rate and rhythm at urography with sodium diatrizoate. Acta Radiol. (Diagn.) 23:107, 1982.

Littner, M. R., Rosenfield, A. T., Ulreich, S., and Putman, C. E.: Evaluation of bronchospasm during excretory urography. Radiology 124:17, 1977.

Littner, M. R., Ulreich, S., Putman, C. E., Rosenfield, A. T., and Meadows, G.: Bronchospasm during excretory urography: Lack of specificity for the methylglucamine cation. AJR 137:477, 1981.

Madowitz, J. S., and Schweiger, M. J.: Severe anaphylactoid reaction to radiographic contrast media: Recurrence despite premedication with diphenhydramine and prednisone. JAMA 241:2813, 1979.

Magill, H. L., Clarke, E. A., Fitch, S. J., Boulden, J. F., Ramirez, R., Siegle, R. L., and Somes, G. W.: Excretory urography with iohexal: Evaluation in children. Radiology 161:625, 1986.

McClennan, B. L.: Ionic versus nonionic contrast media: Safety, tolerance and rationale for use. Urol. Radiol. 11:200, 1989.

McClennan, B. L.: Low-osmolality contrast media: Premises and promises. Radiology 162:1, 1989.

Mikkonen, R., Kontkanen, T. and Kivisaari, L.: Acute and late adverse reactions to low-osmolal contrast media. Acta Radiol 36:72, 1995.

Miller, D. L., Chang, R., Wells, W. T., Dowjat, B. A., Malinovsky, R. M., and Doppman, J. L.: Intravascular contrast media: Effect of dose on renal function. Radiology 167:607, 1988.

Mindell, H. J., and Gibson, T. C.: ECG abnormalities during excretory urography: The effect of stress. AJR 150:1327, 1988.

Moore, R. D., Steinberg, E. P., Powe, N. R., Brinker, J. A., Fishman, E. K., Graziano, S., and Goplan, R.: Nephrotoxicity of high-osmolality versus low-osmolality contrast media: Randomized clinical trial. Radiology 182:649, 1992.

Morcos, S. K., and Einahas, A. M.: Advances in the understanding of the nephrotoxicity of radiocontrast media. Nephron 78:249, 1998.

Murphy, K. J., Brunberg, J. A., and Cohan, R. H.: Adverse reactions to gadolinium contrast media: A review of 36 cases. Am. J. Roentgenol. 167:847, 1996.

O'Reilly, P. H., Jones, D. A., and Farah, N. B.: Measurement of the plasma clearance of urographic contrast media for the determination of glomerular filtration rate. J. Urol. 139:9, 1988.

Owens, A., and Ennis, M.: Arrhythmias occurring during intravenous urography. Clin. Radiol. 31:291, 1980.

Palmer, F. J.: The RACR survey of intravenous contrast media reactions final report. Australas. Radiol. 32:426, 1988.

Parfrey, P. S., Griffiths, S. M., Barrett, B. J., Paul, M. D., Genge, M., Withers, J., Farid, N., and McManamon, P. J.: Contrast material–induced renal failure in patients with diabetes mellitus, renal insufficiency or both: A prospective controlled study. N. Engl. J. Med. 320:143, 1989.

Pfister, R. C., and Hutter, A. M.: Cardiac alterations during intravenous urography. Invest. Radiol. 15(Suppl.):S239, 1980.

Pond, G. D., Smyth, S. H., Roach, D. J., and Hunter, G.: Metformin and contrast media: Genuine risk or witch hunt? Radiology 201:879, 1996.

Postlethwaite, A. E., and Kelley, W. N.: Uricosuric effect of radiocontrast agents: A study in man of four commonly used preparations. Ann. Intern. Med. 74:845, 1971.

Powe, N. R.: Low- versus high-osmolality contrast media for intravenous use: A health care luxury or necessity? Radiology 183:21, 1992.

Purkiss, P., Lane, R. O., Cattell, W. R., Fry, I. K., and Spencer, A. G.: Estimation of sodium diatrizoate by absorption spectrophotometry. Invest. Radiol. 3:271, 1968.

Rahimi, A., Edmondson, R. P. S., and Jones, N. F.: Effect of radiocontrast media on kidneys of patients with renal disease. Br. Med. J. 282:1194, 1981.

Rosovsky, M. A., Rusinek, H., Berenstein, A., Basak, S., Setton, A. and Nelson, P. K.: High-dose administration of nonionic contrast media: A retrospective review. Radiology 200:119, 1996.

Rotter, A., New contraindication to intravascular iodinated contrast material. Radiology 197:545, 1995.

Rudnick, M. R., Berns, J. S., Cohen, R. M. and Goldfarb, S.: Nephrotoxic risks of renal angiography: Contrast media-associated nephrotoxicity and atheroembolism—a critical review. Am. J. Kidney Dis. 24:713, 1994.

Rudnick, M. R., Berns, J. S., Cohen, R. M., and Goldfarb, S.: Contrast media–associated nephrotoxicity. Semin. Nephrol. 17:15, 1997.

Rudnick, M. R., Goldfarb, S., Wexler, L., Ludbrook, P. A., Murphy, M. J., Halpern, E. F., Hill, J. A., Winniford, M., Cohen, M. B., and Vanfossen, D. B.: Nephrotoxicity of ionic and nonionic contrast media in 1196 patients: A randomized trial. Kidney Int. 47:254, 1995.

Schwab, S. J., Hlatky, M. A., Pieper, K. S., Davidson, C. J., Morris, K. G., Skelton, T. N., and Bashore, T. M.: Contrast nephrotoxicity: A radiological controlled trial of a nonionic and an ionic radiographic contrast agent. N. Engl. J. Med. 320:149, 1989.

Shehadi, W. H.: Contrast media adverse reactions: Occurrence, recurrence and distribution patterns. Radiology 143:11, 1982.

Shehadi, W. H., and Toniolo, G.: Adverse reactions to contrast media. Radiology 137:299, 1980.

Shieh, S. D., Hirsch, S. R., Boghell, B. R., Pino, J. A., Alexander, L. J., Witten, D. M., and Friedman, E. A.: Low risk of contrast media–induced acute renal failure in nonazotemic type 2 diabetes mellitus. Kidney Int. 21:739, 1982.

Siegle, R. L., and Gavant, M. L.: Comparison of iodixanol with iohexol in excretory urography. Acad. Radiol. 3:S524, 1996.

Spring, D. B., Bettmann, M. A., and Barkan, H. E.: Deaths related to iodinated contrast media reported spontaneously to the U.S. Food and Drug Administration, 1978–1994: Effect of the availability of low-osmolality contrast medial. Radiology 204:333, 1997.

Spring, D. B., Bettmann, M. A., and Barkan, H. E.: Nonfatal adverse reactions to iodinated contrast media: Spontaneous reporting to the U.S. Food and Drug Administration, 1978–1994. Radiology 204:325, 1997.

Stacul, F., and Thomsen, S.: Nonionic monomers and dimers. European Radiol. 6:756, 1996.

Talner, L. B.: Does hydration prevent contrast material renal injury? AJR 136:1021, 1981.

van der Molen, A. F.: Low-osmolar contrast agents in patients with renal insufficiency. Am. J. Roentgenol. 168:1615, 1997.

Wolf, G. L., Arenson, R. L., and Cross, A. P.: A prospective trial of ionic vs nonionic contrast agents in routine clinical practice: Comparison of adverse effects. AJR 152:939, 1989.

Yamaguchi, K., Katayama, H., Takashima, T., Kozuka, T., Seez, P., and Matsuura, K.: Prediction of severe adverse reactions to ionic and nonionic contrast media in Japan: Evaluation of pretesting. Radiology 178:363, 1991.

Techniques

Aronberg, D. J.: Techniques. In Lee, J. K., Sagel, S. S., and Stanley, R. J. (eds.): Computed Body Tomography. New York, Raven Press, 1983, pp. 9–36.

Berdon, W. E.: Contemporary imaging approach to pediatric urologic problems. Radiol. Clin. North Am. 29:605, 1991.

Cochran, S. T.: Applications of spiral CT in genitourinary imaging. Acad. Radiol. 5:380, 1998.

Ekelund, L., Sjoqvist, L., Thuomas, K. A., and Asberg B.: MR angiography of abdominal and peripheral arteries—Techniques and clinical applications. Acta Radiol. 37:3, 1996.

Elseviers, M. M., Deschepper, A., Corthouts, R., Bosmans, J. L., Cosyn, L., Lins, R.L., Lornoy, W., Matthys, E., Roose, R., Vancaesbroeck, D., et al.: High diagnostic performance of CT scan for analgesic nephropathy in patients with incipient to severe renal failure. Kidney Int 48:1316, 1995.

Engelstad, B. L., McClennan, B. L., Levitt, R. G., Stanley, R. J., and Sagel, S. S.: The role of pre-contrast images in computed tomography of the kidney. Radiology 136:153, 1980.

Farrés, M. T., Lammer, J., Schima, W., Wagner, B., Wildling, R., Winkelbauer, F., and Thurnher, S.: Spiral computed tomographic angiography of the renal arteries: A prospective comparison with intravenous and intraarterial digital subtraction angiography. Cardiovasc. Intervent. Radiol. 19:101, 1996.

Gedroyc, W. M. W.: Magnetic resonance angiography of renal arteries. Urol. Clin. North Am. 21:201, 1994.

George, C. D., Vinnicombe, S. J., Balkissoon, A. R. A., and Heron, C. W.: Bowel preparation before intravenous urography: Is it necessary? Br. J. Radiol. 66:17, 1993.

Hattery, R. R., Williamson, B., Jr., Hartman, G. W., LeRoy, A. J., and Witten, D. M.: Intravenous urographic technique. Radiology 167:593, 1988.

Katzberg, R. W.: Urography into the 21st century: New contrast media, renal handling, imaging characteristics and nephrotoxicity. Radiology 204:297, 1997.

Kauczor, H., Schwickert, H.C., Schweden, F., Schild, H. H., and Thelen, M.: Bolus-enhanced renal spiral CT: Technique, diagnostic value and drawbacks. Eur. J. Radiol. 18:153, 1994.

Keogan, M. T., Kliewer, M. A., Hertzberg, B. S., Delong, D. M., Tupler, R. H., and Carroll, B. A.: Renal resistive indexes: variability in Doppler US measurement in a healthy population. Radiology 199:165, 1996.

King, B. F.: MR angiography of the renal arteries. Semin. Ultrasound CT MR 17:398, 1996.

Lewis-Jones, H. G., Lamb, G. H. R., and Hughes, P. L.: Can ultrasound replace the intravenous urogram in preliminary investigation of renal tract disease: A prospective study. Br. J. Radiol. 62:977, 1989.

Page, J. E., Morgan, S. H., Eastwood, J. B., Smith, S. A., Webb, D. J., Dilly, S. A., Chow, J., Pottier, A., and Joseph, A. E. A.: Ultrasound findings in renal parenchymal disease: Comparison with histological appearances. Clin. Radiol. 49:867, 1994.

Platt, J. F., Rubin, J. M., Bowerman, R. A., and Marn, C. S.: The inability to detect kidney disease on the basis of echogenicity. AJR 151:317, 1988.

Resnick, M. I., and Rifkin, M. D. (eds.): Ultrasonography of the Urinary Tract, 3rd ed. Baltimore, Williams & Wilkins, 1991.

Rhodes, R. A., Fried, A. M., Lorman, J. G., and Kryscio, R. J.: Tomographic levels for intravenous urography: CT-determined guidelines. Radiology 163:673, 1987.

Roberg-Wade, A. P., Hosking, D. H., MacEwan, D. W., and Ramsey, E. W.: The excretory urogram bowel preparation—Is it necessary? J. Urol. 140:1473, 1988.

Rosenfield, A. T., Rigsby, C. M., Burns, P. N., and Romero, R.: Ultrasonography of the urinary tract. In Pollack, H. M. (ed.): Clinical Urography. Philadelphia, W. B. Saunders Co., 1990, pp. 319–386.

Rubin, G. D.: Spiral (helical) CT of the renal vasculature. Semin. Ultrasound CT MR 17:374, 1996.

Saunders, H. S., Dyer, R. B., Shifrin, R. Y., Scharling, E. S., Bechtold, R. E., and Zagoria, R. J.: The CT nephrogram: Implications for evaluation of urinary tract disease. Radiographics 15:1069, 1995.

Schuster, G. A., Nazos, D., and Lewis, G. A.: Preparation of outpatients for exploratory urography: Is bowel preparation with laxatives and dietary restriction necessary? AJR 164:1425, 1995.

Semelka, R. C., Kettritz, U., and Brown, E. D.: Kidneys, adrenal glands and retroperitoneum. In Edelman, R. R., and Hesselink, J. R., (eds.): Clinical Magnetic Resonance Imaging, vol. 2. Philadelphia, W. B. Saunders, 1996, pp. 1513–1563.

Semelka, R. C., Shoenut, J. P., Kroeker, M. A., MacMahon, R., and Greenberg, H. M.: Renal lesions: Controlled comparison between CT and 1.5-T MR imaging with nonenhanced and gadolinium-enhanced fat suppressed spin-echo and breath-hold FLASH techniques. Radiology 182:425, 1992.

Siegelman, E. S., Gilfeather, M., Holland, G. A., Carpenter, J. P., Golden, M. A., Townsend, R. R., and Schnall, M. D.: Breath-hold ultrafast three-dimensional gadolinium-enhanced MR angiography of the renovascular system. AJR 168:1035, 1997.

Wells, P. N. T.: Doppler ultrasound in medical diagnosis. Br. J. Radiol. 62:399, 1989.

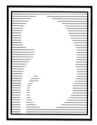
Radionuclide Imaging of the Kidney, Urinary Tract, and Adrenal Gland

Radionuclide imaging plays a major role in the assessment of renal and adrenal function and anatomy. For the kidney, it is the only imaging technique currently available that reliably provides information on blood flow, nephron function, and urine drainage. Although techniques such as dynamic computed tomography and magnetic resonance imaging are beginning to adopt methods originally intended for nuclear medicine, renal scintigraphy remains a robust and useful clinical tool.

A variety of terms are used for radionuclide imaging of the kidneys. These include renal scan, renogram, renography, scintigraphy, differential function study, clearance study, or more simply, "nukes." Special adaptations of radionuclide renography include diuretic renography, also known as the furosemide washout test (which evaluates the obstructed versus nonobstructed nature of a dilated collecting system), and renovascular hypertension studies, or angiotensin-converting enzyme inhibitor (ACEI) renography, for renovascular hypertension.

Flow studies refer to the early images obtained immediately after the bolus administration of a radiopharmaceutical agent and are often included as part of the formal renogram.

In the adrenal gland, unique properties of specific radiopharmaceuticals provide valuable information in the diagnosis of adenoma/hyperplasia and in pheochromocytoma/paraganglioma.

This chapter reviews the radiopharmaceuticals and equipment used in imaging the kidneys and adrenals and the clinical conditions in which these techniques are applied.

EQUIPMENT

Large field-of-view gamma cameras with low energy all-purpose (LEAP) collimators are most commonly employed for radionuclide renal imaging. Single photon emission computed tomography (SPECT) should be available to allow the rapid acquisition of 3-dimensional and 2-dimensional multiplanar images. The latter are especially useful in parenchymal imaging and in localizing focal abnormalities within the kidney using labeled white blood cell studies.

A variety of renogram software is widely available. These programs require the technologist to identify the kidney and appropriate background activity for calibration. The software then automatically generates flow and clearance curves. Analysis includes the ability to display clearance curves and to calculate time to maximum area under the curve and half-time (clearance time) of renal activity.

RENAL IMAGING

Radiopharmaceuticals

The isotope in most common use for renal nuclear studies is technetium 99m (^{99m}Tc). This isotope has the desirable properties of producing a relatively high gamma photon energy (140 keV), high image quality and resolution, and a short (6 hour) half-life that results in almost complete decay by 24 hours. The biologic half life of ^{99m}Tc compounds is even shorter due to renal excretion.

Agents that are primarily filtered through the glomeruli and are neither secreted nor reabsorbed by the tubules are considered *glomerular* agents. A typical example is technetium 99m–labeled diethylenetriaminepentacetic acid, or ^{99m}Tc-DTPA. The small size of this molecule combined with its low protein-binding characteristics enables it to be freely filtered by the glomerulus. In addition to providing information on glomerular filtration rate, ^{99m}Tc-DTPA is also used to assess renal blood flow and urinary excretion. Thus, it provides a global assessment of renal function including prerenal, renal, and postrenal causes of renal dysfunction.

Agents that are excreted principally by the renal tubules constitute another class of renal radiopharmaceuticals. An example is orthoiodohippurate (OIH) or iodohippuran, which is rapidly excreted by tubular secretion. OIH can be labeled with iodine-125 (^{125}I), iodine-123 (^{123}I), or iodine-131 (^{131}I). ^{123}I has the advantages of better image quality and lower radiation dose (shorter half-life) but the disadvantages of higher cost and a short shelf life. OIH is thus most commonly labeled with ^{131}I. OIH is a general-purpose agent that allows the calculation of differential renal function predominantly reflecting tubule function. OIH is also uniquely suited to measure effective renal plasma flow because of its high extraction efficiency. By measuring radioactivity in the blood and urine, OIH can be used to calculate effective renal plasma flow. As with any radiopharmaceutical agent labeled with an iodine isotope, patients should receive a saturated solution of potassium iodide or Lugol's solution before the examination in order to block uptake of ^{131}I to the thyroid. Technetium 99m–labeled mercaptylacetyltriglycine, or ^{99m}Tc-MAG$_3$, is an agent that, like iodohippuran, is almost exclusively excreted via tubule secretion. The imaging characteristics of this agent are very favorable, and images of good quality can be obtained even with rather poor renal function. ^{99m}Tc-MAG$_3$ is somewhat more expensive than ^{99m}Tc-DTPA but generally provides better image quality. The use of ^{99m}Tc-MAG$_3$ in some physiologic assessments of renal function remains controversial because of its complex excretory mechanisms.

Radiopharmaceuticals that either bind to or are retained by the renal parenchyma constitute another class of renal agents. Technetium 99m–labeled dimercaptosuccinic acid, or ^{99m}Tc-DMSA, is one such example that binds to proximal tubules. Maximal renal uptake occurs within 3 to 6 hours after injection. Because this agent does not accumulate in damaged tissue, it is particularly effective in depicting lesions caused by infection or infarction. Moreover, ^{99m}Tc-DMSA can be used to distinguish between neoplasms and renal "pseudotumors," such as lobar dysmorphism or a prominent septum of Bertin, as discussed in Chapter 3. Its role in this regard, however, has been largely supplanted by computed tomography. Technetium 99m–labeled glucoheptanate, or gluceptate (^{99m}Tc-GHA), is another agent that binds to the proximal portion of the nephron. Approximately 80 per cent of ^{99m}Tc-GHA is filtered through the glomerulus, and the remaining 20 per cent binds to the proximal tubule cells.

For imaging renal infections and lymphoproliferative disease, indium 111 (^{111}In)–labeled white blood cells and gallium 67 citrate (^{67}Ga-citrate) are most commonly employed. ^{111}In is labeled to a patient's white blood cells *in vitro,* following which the blood cells are injected back into the patient. The white blood cells migrate to areas of inflammation, thereby localizing the site of infection. The labeling process is somewhat expensive and time-consuming, but the test has the advantage of relatively rapid results in comparison with that of gallium scans. ^{67}Ga-citrate accumulates in inflammatory cells over a period of days. Imaging can usually be performed within 24 to 48 hours of injection, but high background activity in the bowel, liver, and/or spleen often makes difficult the detection of abdominal disease.

Often the clinical situation of the patient requires the assessment of several aspects of renal function at one time: perfusion, filtration, tubule function, and excretion. No single agent is ideal for all these functions, so compromises are necessary. ^{99m}Tc-DTPA and ^{99m}Tc-MAG$_3$ are the two most common general-purpose agents. ^{99m}Tc-DMSA is reserved for parenchymal studies. Because of the complex excretory pathways of ^{99m}Tc-GHA, its usage is controversial; some experts advocate its widespread use, whereas others suggest a more limited role. Orthoiodohippurate is generally considered highly accurate for estimating effective renal plasma flow, but it is generally reserved for the research setting.

CLINICAL APPLICATIONS

Blood Flow

Blood flow to the kidney can be assessed by administering a bolus injection of a radiopharmaceutical agent and measuring its uptake in the kidneys on dynamically acquired images (Fig. 2–1). A variety of radiopharmaceuticals can be used for this purpose including ^{99m}Tc-DTPA, ^{99m}Tc-MAG$_3$, and ^{99m}Tc-GHA. The long half-life of ^{131}I-OIH limits its usefulness in blood-flow measurement.

Images are acquired at 1 frame/s for the first minute after injection and then at 1 frame/30 s for about 30 minutes. By the first minute, the "first pass" has reached the kidney, and subsequent activity reflects recirculation. Region-of-interest measurements are obtained from the kidneys, aorta, and the surrounding background in order to generate time-activity curves. The vascular phase of the study (beginning within 60 seconds of injection) reflects renal perfusion. Decreased perfusion results in a lower rate and amplitude of enhancement. Normally, the kidneys rapidly accumulate the radiopharmaceutical agent because the vascular resistance of the renal bed is very low. With decreased perfusion the normal, nearly vertical enhancement slope is replaced by a slower, less intense rise in radioactivity. Good hydration and an empty bladder are important adjuncts to a successful examination, as are a supine patient position and posterior images to improve signal to noise.

Renal infarction due to embolism or trauma can be detected with all of the perfusion agents (Fig.

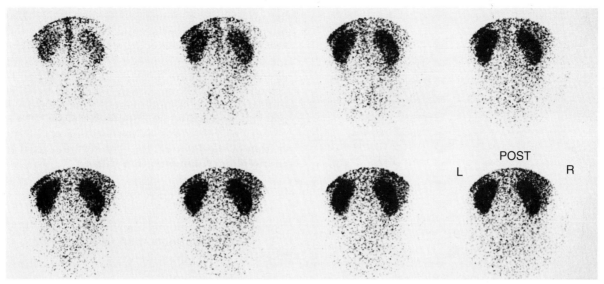

FIGURE 2–1. Normal blood flow to the kidneys is demonstrated on a ^{99m}Tc-MAG$_3$ renogram with images obtained every 2 seconds.

2–2). Radionuclide imaging is usually reserved for cases in which there is severe renal dysfunction and iodinated contrast media is contraindicated. Renal transplants are commonly imaged with these studies to evaluate the integrity of the arterial anastomosis and to detect flow changes due to rejection.

Renal Function

A common question posed by clinicians is, "How much residual renal function is present?" Obviously, this question is overly simplistic to the extent that renal function depends on a variety of parameters including the status of blood flow and perfusion pressure, glomerular filtration, tubule function, fluid resorption in the collecting ducts, and drainage of the collecting system and ureter. Nonetheless, the estimation of global function remains an important

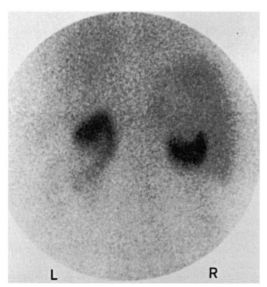

FIGURE 2–2. Multiple emboli. Three-hour ^{99m}Tc-GHA image showing focal areas of no uptake.

measure of renal reserve and is of practical clinical consequence.

To measure renal function in this context, a variety of agents are appropriate: ^{99m}Tc-DTPA, ^{99m}Tc-MAG$_3$, ^{99m}Tc-GHA, and ^{123}I- or ^{131}I-OIH, which, again, has the limitation of a long half-life. After injecting one of these agents and acquiring the dynamic-phase perfusion scans, additional images are obtained every 30 seconds for approximately 20 to 30 minutes. Region-of-interest measurements are used to generate time-activity curves (Fig. 2–3). The following curve parameters are considered important: time to peak, slope of uptake, clearance half-time, and percent clearance at 20 minutes.

One of the most useful measures of renal function is the so-called *differential renal scan*, which calculates the per cent uptake of radionuclide for each kidney over the first several minutes after injection. To avoid overestimating renal function due to a dilated collecting system, this assessment must be performed with a whole kidney region-of-interest measurement 1 to 3 minutes after injection, that is, after the vascular phase but before excretion into the collecting system. Differential function is calculated by dividing the activity for each kidney (corrected for background) by the total counts of both kidneys (corrected for background). It should be noted that there is a normal 5 per cent variation between kidneys, so only changes greater than about 10 per cent (i.e., 60 per cent vs. 40 per cent) are usually considered significant. Unfortunately, if this test is performed while a kidney is obstructed, the degree of damage may be overestimated. Only after obstruction is relieved can an accurate assessment of renal function be made.

The accuracy of global renal function determinations decreases as renal function deteriorates, in part because of an increased dominance of background activity. ^{99m}Tc-GHA, for instance, has an alternate route of excretion through the biliary sys-

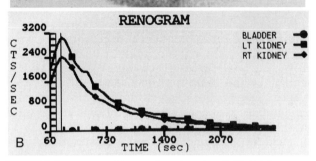

FIGURE 2–3. Radionuclide renal study using ^{99m}Tc-MAG$_3$.
A, Scan demonstrates normal collecting systems.
B, Renogram. There is prompt bilateral clearance of the radionuclide.

tem when renal function is abnormal. This can obscure the kidneys. ^{99m}Tc-DMSA is ideal for global renal function determinations because of its minimal excretion by glomerular filtration and the consequent lack of interference from collecting system activity.

Acute tubular necrosis causes progressive parenchymal accumulation of ^{99M}Tc-MAG$_3$ and ^{131}I-Hippuran, whereas ^{99m}Tc-DTPA shows normal arterial flow with decreased excretion (Fig. 2–4). In severe acute tubular necrosis, arterial flow can be adversely affected, leading to a pattern that overlaps many other medical causes of renal failure.

Renal function studies are of value in neonates with a suspicion of a mass or hydronephrosis. Complete absence of function supports a diagnosis of multicystic dysplastic kidney, as discussed in Chapter 11 (Fig. 2–5). In hydronephrosis, on the other hand, some function is usually demonstrable if scans are acquired over a long period of time.

Radiopharmaceuticals can be used to determine global glomerular filtration rate and effective renal plasma flow by acquiring blood and urine samples without imaging. ^{99m}Tc-DTPA is the agent of choice

for measuring glomerular filtration rate. For this purpose, the patient should be well hydrated and have an empty bladder prior to the study. Separate intravenous lines are used to inject the radionuclide agent and to draw blood samples. After a 1-hour period of equilibrium, timed blood and urine collections are obtained, and urine flow is measured over several consecutive 20-minute intervals. The radioactivity of the sample is used in lieu of the concentration of the ^{99m}Tc-DTPA. The formula used to calculate glomerular filtration rate is:

$$GFR = UV/P$$

where GFR = glomerular filtration rate (mL/min)
U = urine concentration or radioactivity of the filtration agent (mg/mL)
V = urine flow rate (mL/min)
P = plasma concentration or radioactivity of the filtration agent (mg/mL)

^{99m}Tc-DTPA determination of glomerular filtration rate is highly correlated with inulin clearance.

Glomerular filtration rate can also be estimated by analysis of images obtained with a gamma camera in lieu of sampling blood and urine for radioactivity. It should be kept in mind that gamma camera–based determinations are estimates of glomerular filtration rate rather than direct measurements. Nevertheless, these values can be the basis for obtaining comparative glomerular filtration rates between two kidneys.

Urinary Tract Obstruction

It is well known that collecting systems can be dilated without being obstructed, as discussed in Chapter 17. Moreover, some collecting systems are dilated because of minor narrowing of the ureter, whereas others are equally dilated because of complete or near-complete urinary tract obstruction. Diuresis renography is a useful test for investigating the dilated urinary tract to distinguish between obstructed and nonobstructed forms of dilatations and, further, to assess the degree of obstruction when present.

Diuresis renography is performed in a manner similar to that of conventional renography. A large field-of-view gamma camera is used with a LEAP collimator. The patient usually lies supine for the study but can be in a semierect or sitting position, if needed. The patient must be well hydrated and the bladder emptied before the examination if false-positive results due to dehydration or a distended bladder are to be avoided. An indwelling catheter may be necessary in some cases. ^{99m}Tc-MAG$_3$ is the agent of choice, but ^{99m}Tc-DTPA can be used if cost is a consideration. Approximately 20 minutes after injection of the radiopharmaceutical agent, furosemide is injected at a dose between 20 and 80 mg in adults or 1 mg/kg in children. Serum creatinine

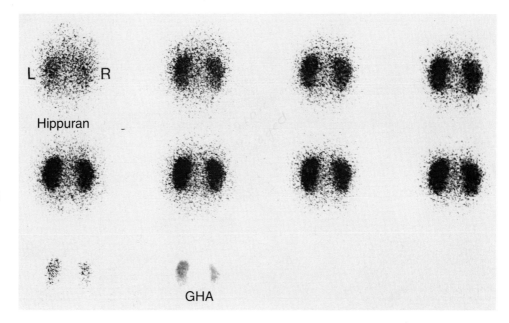

FIGURE 2–4. Acute tubular necrosis. The ¹³¹I-Hippuran scan, represented by images in the upper two rows, demonstrates rapid parenchymal accumulation and no excretion of the radionuclide. The lower row depicts images from a study done with ⁹⁹ᵐTc-GHA in the same patient. There is minimal uptake and no excretion. (Courtesy of Mailine Chew, M.D., Ralph K. Davies Medical Center, San Francisco, California.)

level is a determinant of the dose required. The furosemide-induced diuresis in the normal kidney results in a rapid decline in radioactivity as the radiopharmaceutical agent is washed out of the collecting system by increased urine flow. A dilated but unobstructed collecting system exhibits a washout pattern that is similar to normal. In contrast, an obstructed kidney continues to accumulate radioactivity as a reflection of the inability of the collecting system to empty (Fig. 2–6). Visual inspection of the curve is accurate in most cases. However, the degree of obstruction can be quantified by calculating the time needed for radioactivity to decline to half of its peak activity, called the *T½ of clearance*. A generally accepted normal value for T½ is less than 10 minutes. A T½ of greater than 20 minutes is abnor-

mal and indicates obstruction. When the T½ is between 10 and 20 minutes the result is considered indeterminate for obstruction and must be interpreted within a particular clinical context. Indeterminate results may indicate the need for other studies, such as the pressure/flow urodynamic test of Whitaker, which is discussed in Chapters 15 and 17. It should be kept in mind that these threshold values are not absolute and may be modified somewhat to accommodate specific clinical situations.

False-positive results in diuresis renography can be caused by inadequate hydration or impaired renal function (glomerular filtration rates below 15 mL/min), either of which mute the diuretic response to furosemide. A false-positive result may also occur when an unobstructed system is so mas-

FIGURE 2–5. Multicystic dysplastic kidney. ⁹⁹ᵐTc-DMSA renal scans. The image in the left panel was obtained immediately after injection of the radionuclide and demonstrates multiple photopenic areas that correspond to cysts *(arrow)*. The right panel demonstrates images obtained after a delay of several hours, in which there is no renal function on the left side and normal renal function on the right side.

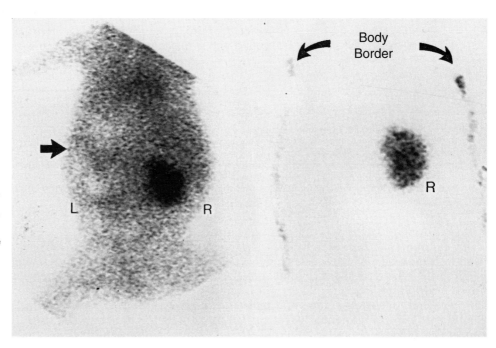

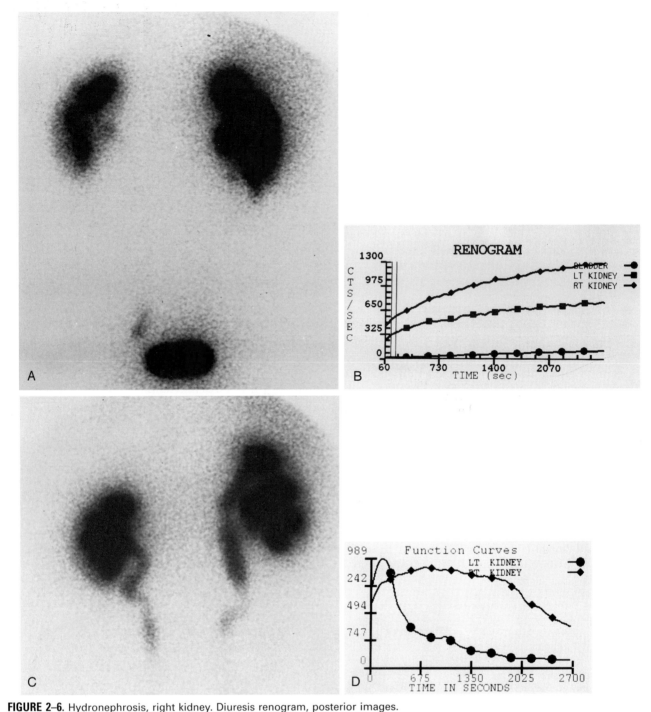

FIGURE 2–6. Hydronephrosis, right kidney. Diuresis renogram, posterior images.

A, 20 minutes after injection of ^{99m}Tc-MAG$_3$ there appears to be bilateral partial obstruction with marked accumulation of radiotracer in the collecting systems.

B, The renogram demonstrates steadily accumulating activity in both kidneys, a finding consistent with partial obstruction.

C, Following furosemide there is more activity in the ureters bilaterally, although both collecting systems remain dilated.

D, Renogram after furosemide demonstrates that the right kidney has delayed emptying (T1/2 = 28 min), whereas the left kidney empties normally (T1/2 = 4 min).

sively dilated that radioactivity clears very slowly despite a diuresis. A distended bladder, especially in children who are sedated, may interfere with upper tract emptying and distort the accuracy of the washout measurements. Catheter drainage should be used in a patient who cannot voluntarily empty the bladder. Finally, refluxing ureters may increase radioactivity in the renal pelvis and give rise to a false-positive interpretation. This problem can be avoided, however, by careful examination of the images for the sequence of changes within the bladder and ureter.

In some patients, an initial rapid elimination phase after furosemide is followed by a sudden flat-

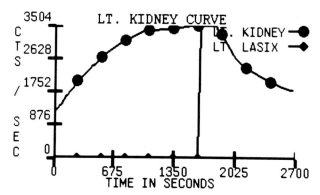

FIGURE 2–7. Diuresis renogram. Normal response to furosemide washout in a patient with a dilated renal pelvis. Note gradual accumulation of radionuclide in the left kidney prior to furosemide. After furosemide is administered (vertical black line), activity rapidly diminishes (T1/2 = 7 min).

tening or even a rise in the excretion curve. This response is known as *Homsy's sign* or the *delayed double peak* sign and is an indicator of intermittent hydronephrosis.

Applications of furosemide renography include the evaluation of those dilated upper urinary tracts in which the presence or absence of obstruction cannot be resolved by standard excretory urography (with or without diuresis) or computed tomography, the evaluation of the persistently dilated urinary tract following surgical correction of an obstruction, investigation of reflux versus obstruction as an explanation for a dilated system in children, assessment of the degree of obstruction in patients with masses or tumors, or assessment of ureteral stent patency (Fig. 2–7).

Parenchymal Imaging

Acute and chronic renal infection can lead to both perfusion defects and scars, depending on a variety of circumstances that are discussed in Chapters 5 and 9. Radionuclide renography is particularly well suited to the detection of these abnormalities when agents that bind to normal tubule epithelium are used. Two such agents are ^{99m}Tc-DMSA, which binds to normal proximal tubules over a period of 2 to 3 hours, and ^{99m}Tc-GHA. In acute pyelonephritis, blood flow to involved lobar or sublobar portions of the kidney is diminished as the acute inflammatory infiltrate increases the interstitial pressure. Focal, wedge-shaped defects are seen (Fig. 2–8). In reflux nephropathy, or chronic pyelonephritis, a dense scar replaces normal nephrons and collecting tubules, which also leads to a focal failure of uptake of radionuclide agents (see Fig. 2–8B). SPECT imaging is helpful in visualizing these lesions.

Radionuclide imaging is particularly well suited to the follow-up of children with acute infection and to assess the totality and progression of renal disease in children with chronic reflux. Defects may be large or small, single or multiple, unilateral or bilateral.

Parenchymal imaging is also useful in confirming that a mass suspected on other imaging modalities of being a pseudotumor functions as normal tissue and, therefore, does not represent a true mass (Fig. 2–9). A renogram using ^{99m}Tc-DMSA demonstrates normal parenchymal uptake in a pseudotumor. On the other hand, there is little or no uptake in a true mass. Pseudotumors are discussed in Chapters 3 and 5.

FIGURE 2–8. Acute pyelonephritis evolving into reflux nephropathy in the left kidney of a 5-year old girl. ^{99m}Tc-DMSA radionuclide scan, left posterior oblique projections. Same patient illustrated in Figure 5–6.

A, Initial scan during acute phase. There is diminished radionuclide uptake in the upper pole in a sharply defined, full-thickness distribution.

B, Follow-up scan 14 months after acute infection. A deep surface scar has developed in the upper pole. (Courtesy of Massoud Majd, M.D., Children's National Medical Center, Washington, D.C.)

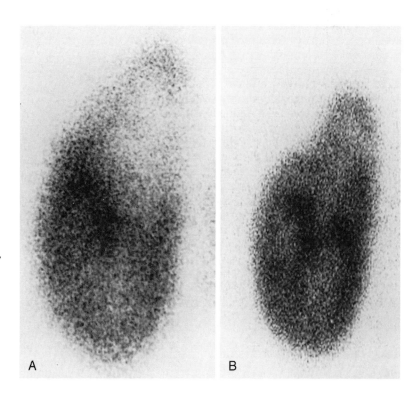

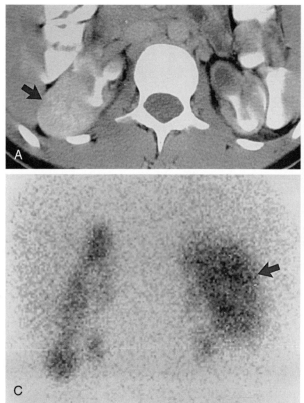

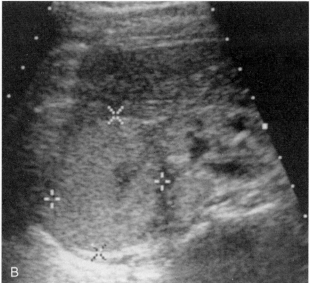

FIGURE 2–9. Reflux nephropathy, bilateral, with a pseudotumor due to focal nodular compensatory hypertrophy in the right kidney.

A, Computed tomogram, contrast material–enhanced. Both kidneys demonstrate focal contour scars overlying dilated, retracted calyces. There is normal, homogeneous enhancement of the pseudotumor in the upper pole of the right kidney *(arrow).*

B, Ultrasonogram, right kidney, longitudinal projection. The dilated calyces and decreased renal parenchyma are noted in the lower portion of the kidney. The focal hypertrophied normal tissue constituting the pseudotumor is outlined by cursors.

C, Radionuclide scan, posterior projection. Radionuclide uptake by the pseudotumor is normal *(arrow)*. Note small size and contour scars of the kidneys.

Same patient illustrated in Figure 5–15.

Infection

In addition to the application of radionuclide imaging to patients with acute pyelonephritis and reflux nephropathy (chronic pyelonephritis), ^{67}Ga-citrate or ^{111}In-labeled white blood cells may be of value in identifying the site of an obscure infection. With ^{111}In-labeled white blood cells, imaging at 6 to 24 hours is required to obtain sufficient activity at the site of infection. Even longer delays of 24 to 72 hours are required for ^{67}Ga-citrate studies to allow for reduction of blood-pool activity and the differentiation of the kidney from bowel contents. Further, ^{67}Ga-citrate has relatively poor imaging characteristics due to its several high energy peaks (93, 184, 296 keV). These disadvantages are offset, in part, by the low cost of the agent and extensive experience with its use in this setting. Both ^{111}In and ^{67}Ga have a higher radiation dose than the parenchymal imaging agents discussed previously and are, thus, considered less suitable for children. Parenthetically, gallium scans may also demonstrate diffuse or multifocal increase in renal activity in patients with lymphoma.

Renovascular Hypertension

When sustained high diastolic blood pressure associated with a main or major branch renal artery stenosis reverses following correction of the stenotic lesion, the hypertension is classified as *renovascular*. In older patients, renovascular hypertension usually is caused by atherosclerosis, whereas in younger patients renal arterial dysplasia is a more common cause. Although renal artery stenosis accounts for less than 3 per cent of all patients with hypertension, it may be the etiologic factor in as many as 45 per cent of patients in specialty clinics for refractory hypertension. Therefore, a substantial number of patients with essential hypertension will undergo diagnostic testing for renovascular hypertension during the course of their illness. Other aspects of renal ischemia are discussed in Chapter 6.

It is important to make a distinction between an arterial stenosis leading to renovascular hypertension and an incidental stenosis of the renal artery. Stenosis of the renal artery is common and may not result in hypertension. Therefore, the purpose of the angiotensin-converting enzyme inhibitor (ACEI) renogram is to identify patients with physiologically significant lesions.

Signs and symptoms that help differentiate renovascular hypertension from essential hypertension are recent onset of hypertension with a diastolic blood pressure greater than 105 mm Hg, sudden worsening of long-standing hypertension, well-controlled hypertension that becomes refractory to treatment, peripheral vascular disease, an abdominal bruit, moderate to severe hypertension under the age of 25 years, refractory hypertension on adequate drug therapy, hypertension associated with progressive renal failure when treated with an angiotensin-converting enzyme inhibitor, hypokalemia, hyperreninemia, and hyperaldosteronemia.

The renin-angiotensin system plays a major role in the pathophysiology of renovascular hypertension. Diminished renal blood flow leads to a decrease in glomerular filtration. In response, renin is released from the juxtaglomerular apparatus and converts circulating angiotensinogen to angotensin I. Angiotensin-converting enzyme is produced by the lung and catalyzes the conversion of angiotensin I to angiotensin II, which is a constrictor of efferent glomerular arterioles. This has the effect of maintaining glomerular filtration. This same mechanism that helps to compensate for the diminished glomerular function also causes increased peripheral arterial resistance that, in turn, leads to systemic arterial hypertension. Angiotensin II also causes the adrenal gland to release aldosterone, which exacerbates hypertension by promoting sodium and water retention. Prolonged hypertension eventually leads to progressive nephrosclerosis and, ultimately, end-stage renal disease.

The administration of an ACEI to a patient with renal vascular hypertension reduces the conversion of angiotensin I to angiotensin II and thereby blocks vasoconstriction of the efferent arterioles of the glomeruli. As efferent arterioles dilate, the pressure differential across the glomerular membrane decreases, and there is a reduction in glomerular filtration rate. An analogy can be made to soaker hoses used in gardens. If the open end of the soaker hose is manually compressed, the water is forced through the small soaker holes, thus providing water for the garden. This is the same as the kidney's compensatory maintenance of glomerular filtration rate through efferent arteriolar constriction in the presence of renal ischemia. If, however, the end of the soaker hose is unoccluded, the water preferentially flows out the end, and only minimal amounts of water emerge from the small holes along the hose. This corresponds to the reduction in glomerular filtration pressure when a patient with renovascular hypertension responds to an ACEI by efferent arteriolar dilatation.

This background provides the rationale for the ACEI renogram. A radionuclide agent, such as ^{99m}Tc-MAG$_3$, ^{99m}Tc-DTPA, or ^{131}I-OIH, is used to perform a standard renogram. A subtle asymmetry in the clearance curve of the abnormal kidney compared with that of the contralateral kidney may be noted even before an ACEI is administered. These findings might include a reduction in the initial uptake of the agent, a blunted peak, and prolonged clearance. Often, however, this pattern is not accentuated enough to differentiate normal from abnormal function. If, however, the renogram is repeated following administration of an ACEI, renal uptake

and clearance of the radiopharmaceutical agent is greatly reduced on the side with significant ischemia. Thus, the sensitivity of the modified renogram in detecting renovascular hypertension is greatly increased.

There are some practical considerations to the performance of ACEI renography. One commonly used inhibitor, captopril, is administered orally in a fasting patient and reaches a peak effect between 60 and 90 minutes. Enalapril, also commonly used, is injected intravenously and achieves a peak level within 15 minutes. Blood pressure must be monitored during these studies. Because the test relies on evoking differences between a baseline renogram and an ACEI-challenged renogram, two separate studies are required. This can be accomplished with either a 2- or a 1-day protocol. In the 2-day protocol the patient receives the ACEI renogram on the first day. If the renogram curve is abnormal, the examination is repeated the following day without an inhibitor to determine if the difference is attributable to the drug. If, however, the ACEI renogram is normal—that is, there is little difference between the clearance curves of the two kidneys—the test is considered negative on the first day, and the patient need not return for the second study. In a 1-day study, 1 to 5 mCi of ^{99m}Tc-DTPA or ^{99m}Tc-MAG$_3$ is administered as a baseline study. Several hours later, an ACEI is administered and a second renogram is performed using 5 to 10 mCi of ^{99m}Tc-DTPA or ^{99m}Tc-MAG$_3$. The addition of an inhibitor for the second study should accentuate the differences in function between a normal kidney and an ischemic kidney. This method is generally preferred because it is more convenient for the patient.

Pitfalls of ACEI renography include dehydration (the patient should be orally hydrated before study), poor renal function, and chronic use of an ACEI. If the patient is being treated with an inhibitor on a daily basis, the drug should be withheld for 3 to 5 days prior to the study. Chronic administration of a diuretic may also make a patient refractory to the effect of an ACEI and thereby reduce the sensitivity of ACEI renography.

Interpretation of the ACEI renogram varies with the radionuclide agent used. With a glomerular agent, such as ^{99m}Tc-DTPA, uptake is decreased compared with that of the normal kidney, and the two curves do not overlap. In contrast, a tubule agent, such as ^{99m}Tc-MAG$_3$ or ^{131}I-OIH, demonstrates prolonged retention of activity in the parenchyma due to poor washout. Whereas the normal kidney continues to excrete the radionuclide, the affected kidney accumulates activity, and the curves may actually cross each other. Thus, unilateral parenchymal retention after ACEI is the most important criterion for positivity when a tubule agent is used (Fig. 2–10).

ACEI renography is very specific for the diagnosis of renovascular hypertension, with only a 5 per cent false-positive rate in the general population of hypertensive patients. Sensitivity has been re-

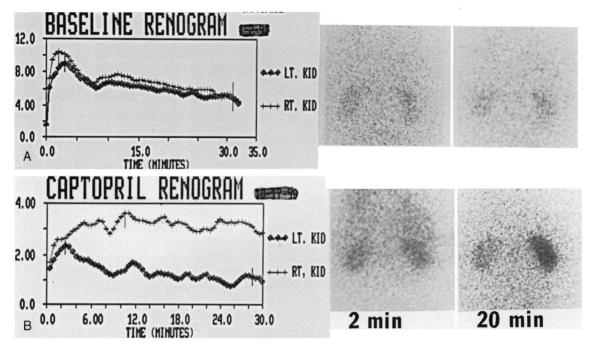

FIGURE 2–10. Renovascular hypertension due to right renal artery stenosis. Captopril-enhanced ^{131}I-Hippuran scans and renograms. *A,* A baseline study demonstrates normal 2- and 20-minute scans and normal time-activity curves for both kidneys. *B,* Repeat scans and renogram after administration of captopril demonstrate marked parenchymal retention of radionuclide by the right kidney and persistently normal findings in the left kidney.

ported at up to 96 per cent. To be cost-effective the test should primarily be employed in patients who are a moderate-to-high risk for renovascular hypertension and who are candidates for correction of a detected lesion. Note that a stenosis that is not functionally significant may be missed with this test. The reliability of ACEI renography in patients with bilateral disease or renal failure is decreased.

Vesicoureteral Reflux

In conventional cystography used to investigate vesicoureteral reflux, a catheter is placed in the bladder and filled with radiopaque contrast material; following removal of the catheter, the patient voids under fluoroscopic observation for urine reflux from the bladder into the upper urinary tract. This technique, although effective, exposes the patient to relatively high radiation doses because it is performed under fluoroscopy.

An alternative to radiographic voiding cystography is the radionuclide cystogram, in which an agent, such as ^{99m}Tc–sulfur colloid diluted in normal saline, is instilled in the bladder. Using sequential gamma camera images, the kidneys and ureters are constantly monitored for refluxing urine. Because ^{99m}Tc-pertechnetate and ^{99m}Tc-DTPA may be absorbed through the bladder wall if the wall is inflamed, ^{99m}Tc–sulfur colloid is the radiopharmaceutical agent of choice for this procedure. Images are obtained continuously every 10 to 15 seconds during filling of the radiopharmaceutical agent and every 1 to 2 seconds during voiding. This results in better surveillance for vesicoureteral reflux while decreas-

ing radiation exposure by up to 200 times, as compared with conventional cystography. Moreover, the sensitivity of the radionuclide method is superior to that of conventional methods because it allows constant monitoring (Figs. 2–11, 2–12). Conventional cystograms are still needed to evaluate the male urethra for posterior urethral valves, but the majority of studies of reflux can be replaced with radionuclide cystography. Grading of vesicoureteral reflux observed by radionuclide cystography is identical to that used for conventional voiding cystography, as discussed in Chapter 5 (see Table 5–1).

A postvoid image is usually obtained. The volume of the bladder and the residual volume after voiding can be calculated by measuring the change in count rate before and after voiding and relating to the voided urine volume. Thus, the residual bladder volume (RBV) can be calculated:

$$RBV = U \times \text{Residual cpm}/(\text{Initial cpm} - \text{residual cpm})$$

where U = voided urine volume

Incidental Information from Other Radionuclide Studies

Information about the kidneys can often be obtained from radionuclide studies that are not directly intended for evaluating renal function. The best example of this is the radionuclide bone scan. ^{99m}Tc-methyldiphosphonate and other bone-scanning chelates are predominately incorporated into the bone matrix. However, during the blood-pool

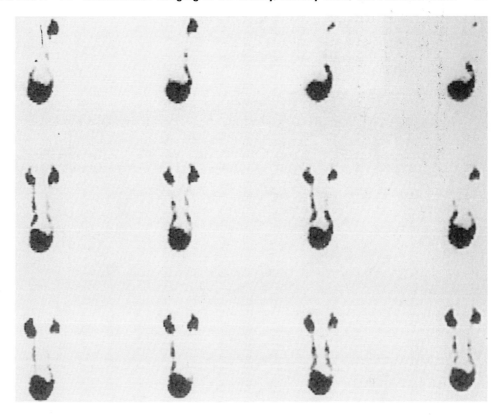

FIGURE 2–11. Vesicoureteral reflux. Cystogram performed with ^{99m}Tc–sulfur colloid. Images obtained sequentially from top left to bottom right demonstrate, first, right-sided (posterior view), then bilateral Grade IV–V reflux.

phase a considerable fraction of the bone-scanning agent is excreted by the kidneys. This provides incidental information about the function of the kidneys, which should always be evaluated when interpreting a bone scan. Among the most common

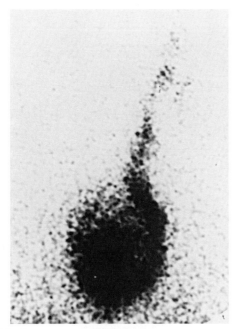

FIGURE 2–12. Vesicoureteral reflux. Cystogram performed with ^{99m}Tc–sulfur colloid in a 9-year-old girl with urinary tract infection. Grade III vesicoureteral reflux is indicated by faint activity in the collecting system. (Kindly provided by Massoud Majd, M.D., Children's National Medical Center, Washington, D.C.)

incidental findings are absence or ectopia of one kidney, hydronephrosis, and masses representing cysts or tumors. Although the bone scan provides no renal functional information, it nevertheless alerts clinicians to the presence of occult disease. One example is the patient with prostate cancer who, on routine bone scan, will show obstruction of a ureter due to extracapsular extension of the cancer (Fig. 2–13).

Practically all other agents have some element of renal excretion; by carefully examining the entire scan useful information can be gleaned (Fig. 2–14).

ADRENAL IMAGING

Two radionuclide agents are employed in imaging of the adrenal gland: iodine 131-labeled 6-beta-iodomethylnorcholesterol (NP-59) and ^{131}I-labeled metaiodobenzylguanidine (MIBG). Additional aspects of adrenal gland imaging are discussed in Chapter 22.

Adenoma/Hyperplasia

NP-59 is a cholesterol analog that is taken up in the adrenal cortex (Fig. 2–15). It, therefore, has an affinity for functional cortical adrenal adenomas and adrenal hyperplasia. Dexamethasone suppression is necessary to decrease native adrenal function and allow abnormal function to be detected. The test takes up to a week to complete and is still considered experimental.

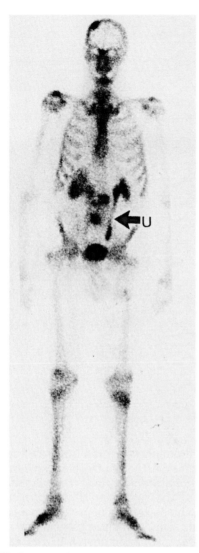

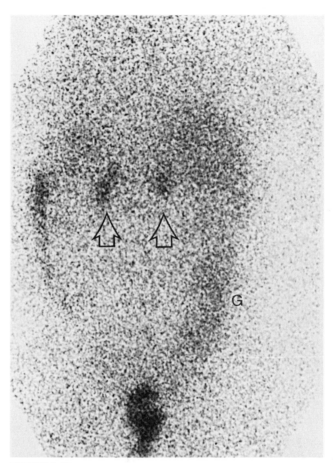

FIGURE 2–15. Normal NP-59 study (^{131}I). There is uptake by both adrenal glands *(arrows)* and residual activity from unbound ^{131}I in gut (G).

FIGURE 2–13. Obstructed ureters *(U, arrow)* demonstrated during a bone scan in a patient with carcinoma of the prostate metastatic to bone and retroperitoneum.

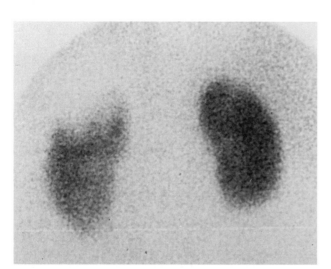

FIGURE 2–14. Incidental diagnosis of a renal cell carcinoma in the early phase of a ^{99m}Tc-MDP bone scan. Soon after injection most radioactivity is still in the kidneys, and excellent renal scans are obtained. The absence of activity in the upper pole of the left kidney corresponds to the tumor.

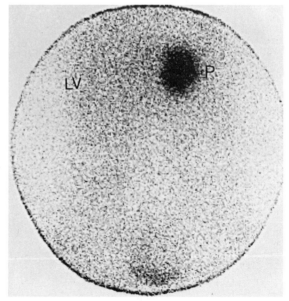

FIGURE 2–16. Pheochromocytoma. ^{123}I-MIBG scan. There is marked uptake of radionuclide by the tumor (P) in the left adrenal gland. Note diminished liver activity (LV). (Courtesy of Dayan Sandler, M.D., and Robert Hattner, M.D., University of California, San Francisco.)

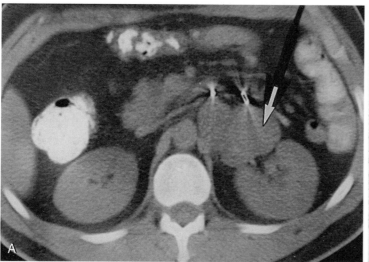 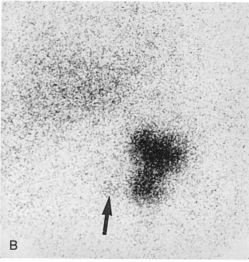

FIGURE 2–17. Metastatic pheochromocytoma detected by MIBG in a patient with prior adrenalectomy.
A, Computed tomogram, unenhanced. Multiple enlarged lymph nodes are present in the retroperitoneum *(arrow)*.
B, MIBG scan, coronal anterior view. There are multiple confluent nodules of tumor within the lymph nodes, confirming that they represent metastatic nodes. Note the faint activity across the midline in small nodes not identified by the computed tomogram *(arrow)*.

Pheochromocytoma/Paraganglioma and Neuroblastoma

MIBG is used widely in the evaluation for a pheochromocytoma or paraganglioma, and it is efficacious in the staging of a neuroblastoma. Benzylguanidine is a guanethidine analog that is incorporated into the neurosecretory vesicles of adrenal medullary cells. A pheochromocytoma, paraganglioma, and neuroblastoma incorporate MIBG, making this agent a very specific indicator for these tumors (Fig. 2–16).

MIBG is usually labeled with ^{131}I and requires 24 to 72 hours to incorporate into the neurosecretory granules. A number of drugs can compete with the uptake of MIBG. Among the most notable are tricyclic antidepressants, phenothiazines, calcium channel blockers, sympathomimetics, and some chemotherapeutic agents. In addition to localizing a pheochromocytoma within the adrenal gland, MIBG studies are also helpful in identifying extra-adrenal sites, such as Zuckerkandl's organ or metastatic foci in lymph nodes or other organs (Figs. 2–17, 2–18). Normal activity is seen in the heart, salivary glands, spleen, and liver.

A positive MIBG study may occur in familial syndromes that are associated with bilateral pheochromocytomas or paragangliomas. These include neurofibromatosis, von Hippel-Lindau disease, and multiple endocrine neoplasia syndrome, MEN II. MIBG uptake by one or more of these lesions may militate for surgical removal.

Organs that overlie the adrenal gland, such as the liver, spleen, and bowel, may give rise to interpretive problems. A pheochromocytoma or paraganglioma less than 2 cm in diameter may be difficult to visualize because of the poor lesion-to-background ratio. A poorly differentiated malignant pheochromocytoma may also fail to take up the agent.

For tumors larger than 2 cm, MIBG is more than 90 per cent sensitive and more than 95 per cent specific. False-positives are unusual and include neoplasms such as neuroblastomas, carcinoid, and medullary carcinoma of the thyroid.

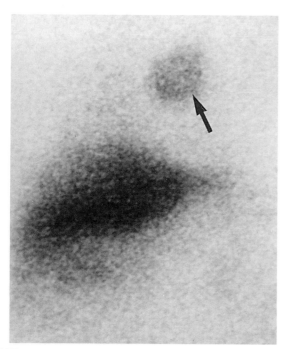

FIGURE 2–18. Paraganglioma within the mediastinum in a patient with episodic hypertension and cardiac arrhythmia. A computed tomogram of the adrenals was normal. MIBG scan, coronal view. The site of the paraganglioma within the mediastinum near the aortic root is apparent *(arrow)*. Activity within abdomen is the liver.

BIBLIOGRAPHY

Blaufox, M. D.: Procedures of choice in renal nuclear medicine. J. Nucl. Med. *32*:1301, 1991.

Blaufox, M. D., Hollenberg, N. K., and Raynaud, C. (eds.): Radionuclides in Nephrourology. Basel, Karger, 1990.

Bratt, C. G., Larsson, I., and White, T.: Scintillation camera renography with ^{99m}Tc DTPA and ^{131}I Hippuran. Scand. J. Clin. Lab. Invest. 41:189, 1981.

Fine, E. J.: Interventions in renal scintigraphy. Semin. Nucl. Med. 21:116, 1991.

Freeman, L. M., and Lutzker, L. G.: The kidneys. In Freeman, L. M. (ed.): Freeman and Johnson's Clinical Radionuclide Imaging, vol. 1. Orlando, Florida, Grune & Stratton, 1984, pp. 725–924.

Sfakianakis, G. N., Vonorta, K., Zilleruelo, G., Jaffe, D., and Georgiou, M.: Scintigraphy in acquired renal disorders. In Freeman, L. M. (ed.): Nuclear Medicine Annual. New York, Raven Press, 1992, pp. 157–224.

Taylor, A., Jr., Eshima, D., Fritzberg, A. R., et al.: Comparison of iodine-131 OIH and technetium-99m MAG3 renal imaging in volunteers. J. Nucl. Med. 27:795, 1986.

Taylor, A., Jr., and Nally, J. V.: Clinical applications of renal scintigraphy. Am. J. Roentgenol. 164:31, 1995.

Thrall, J. H., and Ziessman, H. A.: Nuclear Medicine: The Requisites. Genitourinary System. Mosby-Year Book, St. Louis, 1995, pp. 283–320.

Radiopharmaceuticals

Anghileri, L. J., Crone-Escanye, M. C., Thouvenot, P., Brunotte, F., and Robert, J.: Mechanisms of gallium-67 accumulation by tumors: Role of cell membrane permeability. J. Nucl. Med. 29:663, 1988.

Chervu, L. R., Freeman, L. M., and Blaufox, M. D.: Radiopharmaceuticals for renal studies. Semin. Nucl. Med. 4:3–22, 1974.

de Lange, M. J., Piers, D. A., Kosterink, J. G. W., van Luijk, W. H. J., Meijer, S., de Zeeuw, D., and van der Hem, G. K.: Renal handling of technetium-DMSA: Evidence for glomerular filtration and peritubular uptake. J. Nucl. Med. 30:1219, 1989.

Dubovsky, E. V., and Russell, C. D.: ^{99m}Tc MAG$_3$: Multipurpose renal radiopharmaceutical. In Freeman, L. M. (ed.): Nuclear Medicine Annual. New York, Raven Press, 1991.

Eshima, D., and Taylor, A., Jr.: Technetium-99 (^{99m}Tc) mercaptoacetyltriglycine: Update on the new ^{99m}Tc renal tubular function agent. Semin. Nucl. Med. 22:61, 1992.

Lee, H. B., and Blaufox, M.D.: Mechanism of renal concentration of technetium-99m glucoheptanate. J. Nucl. Med. 26:1308, 1985.

Tsan, M. F., and Scheffel, U.: Mechanism of gallium-67 accumulation in tumors. J. Nucl. Med. 27:1215, 1986.

Blood Flow

Fine, E. J.: Interventions in renal scintirenography. Semin. Nucl. Med. 21:116, 1991.

Renal Function

Blanchi, C.: Measurement of the glomerular filtration rate. Prog. Nucl. Med. 2:21, 1972.

Blaufox, M. D., Aurell, M., Bubeck, B., Fommei, E., Piepsz, A., Russell., C., Taylor, A., Thomsen, H. S., and Volterrani, D.: Report of the radionuclides in nephrourology committee on renal clearance. J. Nucl. Med. 37:1883, 1996.

Blaufox, M.D., Potchen, E. J., and Merrill, J. P.: Measurement of effective renal plasma flow in man by external counting methods. J. Nucl. Med. 8:77, 1967.

Brochner-Mortensen, J.: Current status on assessment and measurement of glomerular filtration rate. Clin. Physiol. 5:1, 1985.

Bubeck, B.: Radionuclide techniques for the evaluation of renal function: Advantages over conventional methodology. Curr. Opin. Nephrol. Hypertens. 4:514, 1995.

Bubeck, B., Brandau, W., Steinbaecher, M., et al.: Technetium-99m-labeled renal function and imaging agents. II. Clinical evaluation of Tc-99m MAG3 (Tc-99m mercaptoacetylglycine). Nucl. Med. Biol. 15:109, 1988.

Burbank, M. K., Tauxe, W. N., Maher, F. T, et al.: Evaluation of radioiodinated Hippuran for the estimation of renal plasma flow. Proc. Staff Meet. Mayo Clin. 36:372, 1961.

Fine, E. J.: Assessment of acute and chronic renal failure, evaluation of renal function and disease with radionuclides. In Blaufox, M. D. (ed.): The Upper Urinary Tract, 2nd ed. Basel, Karger, 1989, p. 316.

Hall, J. E., Guyton, C., and Farr, B. M.: A single-injection method for measuring glomerular filtration rate. Am. J. Physiol. 232:F72, 1977.

Klopper, J. F., Hauser, W., Atkins, H. L., et al.: Evaluation of 99m Tc-DTPA for the measurement of glomerular filtration rate. J. Nucl. Med. 13:107, 1972.

Piepsz, A., Ham, H. R., and DuPont, A. G.: Renal blood flow in renal disease and hypertension: Evaluation of renal function and disease with radionuclides. In Blaufox, M. D. (ed.): The Upper Urinary Tract, 2nd ed. Basel, Karger, 1989, p. 163.

Schlegel, J. U., and Hamway, S. A.: Individual renal plasma flow determination in two minutes. J. Urol. 116:282, 1976.

Tauxe, W. N.: Determination of glomerular filtration rate of single-plasma sampling technique following injection of radioiodinated diatrizoate. J. Nucl. Med. 27:45, 1982.

Tauxe, W. N., Dubovsky, E. V., Kidd, T., Jr., et al.: New formulas for the calculation of effective renal plasma flow. Eur. J. Nucl. Med. 7:51, 1982.

Tauxe, W. N., Maher, F. T., and Taylor, W. F.: Effective renal plasma flow: Estimation from theoretical volumes of distribution of intravenously injected 131-I orthoiodohippurate. Mayo Clin. Proc. 46:524, 1971.

Urinary Tract Obstruction

Brown, R. K., Bahn, D. K., Walters, B. L., Karazim, J. J., Reidinger, A. A., Shei, K. Y., Morgan, A. W., Hurd, D. B., Gontina, H., and Kling, G. A.: Nuclear scintigraphy in the evaluation of renal colic. Clin. Nucl. Med. 15:11, 1990.

Conway, J. J.: "Well-tempered" diuresis renography: Its historical development, physiologic and technical pitfalls and standardized technique protocol. Semin. Nucl. Med. 22:74, 1992.

Fine, E. J.: Interventions in renal scintirenography. Semin. Nucl. Med. 21:116, 1991.

Homsy, Y. L., Saad, F., Laberge, I., Williot, P., and Pison, C.: Transitional hydronephrosis of the newborn and infant. J. Urol. 144:579, 1990.

Kass, E. J., Majd, M., and Belman, B.: Comparison of the diuretic renogram and the pressure perfusion study in children. J. Urol. 134:92, 1985.

Kullendorff, C. M., and Evander, E.: Renal parenchymal damage on DMSA scintigraphy in pelviureteric obstruction. Scand. J. Urol. Nephrol. 23:127, 1989.

O'Reilly, P. H.: Diuresis renography: Recent advances and recommended protocols. Br. J. Urol. 69:113, 1992.

O'Reilly, P., Aurell, M., Britton, K., Kletter, K., Rosenthal, L., and Testa, T.: Consensus of diuresis renography for investigating the dilated upper urinary tract. J. Nucl. Med. 37:1872, 1996.

Parkhouse, H. F., and Barratt, T. M.: Practical pediatric nephrology: Investigation of the dilated urinary tract. Pediatr. Nephrol. 2:43, 1988.

Roarke, M. C., and Sandler, C. M.: Provocative imaging: Diuretic renography. Urol. Clin. North Am. 25:227, 1998.

Upsdell, S. M., Testa, H. J., and Lawson, R. S.: The F-15 diuresis renogram in suspected obstruction of the upper urinary tract. Br. J. Urol. 69:126, 1992.

Parenchymal Imaging

Felson, B., and Moskowitz, M.: Renal pseudotumors: The regenerated nodule and other lumps, bumps, and dromedary humps. AJR 107:720, 1969.

Jackson, J., Blue, P., and Ghaed, N.: Glomerular filtration rate determined in conjunction with routine renal scanning. Radiology 154:203, 1985.

LaFrance, N., Drew, H., and Walker, M.: Radioisotopic measurement of glomerular filtration rate in severe chronic renal failure. J. Nucl. Med. 176:1927, 1988.

Lee, V. W., Allard, J., Foster, J., Sheahan, K., and Franklin, P.: Functional oncocytoma of the kidney: Evaluation by dual tracer scintigraphy. J. Nucl. Med. 28:1911, 1987.

Leonard, J. C., Allen, E. C., Goin, J., and Smith, C. W.: Renal cortical imaging and the detection of renal mass lesions. J. Nucl. Med. 20:1018, 1979.

Mulligan, J. S., Blue, P. W., and Hasbargen, J. A.: Methods for measuring GFR with technetium 99m DTPA: An analysis of several common methods. J. Nucl. Med. 31:1211, 1990.

Perrone, R., Steinman, T., and Beck, G.: Utility of radioisotopic filtration markers in chronic renal insufficiency: Simultaneous comparison of ^{125}I-iothalamate, [169]Yb-DTPA, [99m]DTPA, and inulin. Am. J. Kidney Dis. 16:224, 1990.

Pollack, H. M., Ewdell, S., and Morales, J. O.: Radionuclide imaging in renal pseudotumors. Radiology 111:639, 1974.

Russell, C. D., Taylor, A., and Eshima, D.: Estimation of technetium-99m MAG₃ plasma clearance in adults from one or two blood samples. J. Nucl. Med. 30:1955, 1989.

Infection

Conway, J. J.: The role of scintigraphy in urinary tract infection. Semin. Nucl. Med. 18:308, 1988.

Jakobsson, B., and Svensson, L.: Transient pyelonephritic changes on (99m)technetium-dimercaptosuccinic acid scan for at leasst five months after infection. Acta Paediatr. 86:803, 1997.

Lantto, E. H., Lantto, T. J., and Vorne, M.: Fast diagnosis of abdominal infections and inflammation with technetium-99-m-HMPAO labeled leukocytes. J. Nucl. Med. 32:2029, 1991.

Linton, A. L., Richmond, J. M., Clark, W. F., Lindsay, R. M., Driedger, A. A., and Lamki, L. M.: Gallium 67 scintigraphy in the diagnosis of acute renal disease. Clin. Nephrol. 24:84, 1985.

MacKenzie, J. R.: A review of renal scarring in children. Nucl. Med. Commun. 17:176, 1996.

Majd, M., and Rushton, H. G.: Renal cortical scintigraphy in the diagnosis of acute pyelonephritis. Semin. Nucl. Med. 22:98, 1992.

Majd, M., Rushton, H. G., Jantausch, B., and Wiedermann, B. L.: Relationship among vesicoureteral reflux, P-fimbriated Escherichia coli, and acute pyelonephritis in children with febrile urinary tract infection. J. Pediatr. 119:578, 1991.

Pike, M. C.: Imaging of inflammatory sites in the 1990s: New horizons. J. Nucl. Med. 32:2034, 1991.

Rubin, R. H., Fischman, A. J., Callahan, R. J., Khaw, B. A., Keech, F., Ahmad, M., Wilkinson, R., and Strauss, H. W.: ^{111}In-labeled nonspecific immunoglobulin scanning in the detection of focal infection. N. Engl. J. Med. 321:935, 1989.

Rushton, H. G.: The evaluation of acute pyelonephritis and renal scarring with technetium 99m-dimercaptosuccinic acid renal scintigraphy: Evolving concepts and future directions. Pediatr. Nephrol. 11:108, 1997.

Smellie, J. M., Shaw, P. J., Prescod, N. P., and Bantock, H. M.: [99m]Tc dimercaptosuccinic acid (DMSA) scan in patients with established radiological renal scarring. Arch. Dis. Child. 63:1315, 1988.

Strife, C. F., and Gelfand, M. J.: Renal cortical scintigraphy: Effect on medical decision making in childhood urinary tract infection. J. Pediatr. 129:785, 1996.

Verber, I. G., and Meller, S. T.: Serial ^{99m}Tc dimercaptosuccinic acid (DMSA) scans after urinary infections presenting before the age of 5 years. Arch. Dis. Child. 64:1533, 1989.

Verboven, M., Ingels, M., Delree, M., and Piepsz, A.: [99m]Tc DMSA scintigraphy in acute urinary tract infection in children. Pediatr. Radiol. 20:540, 1990.

Wallin, L., and Bajc, M.: Typical technetium dimercaptosuccinic acid distribution patterns in acute pyelonephritis. Acta Paediatr. 82:1061, 1993.

Wallin, L., Helin, I., and Bajc, M.: Kidney swelling: Findings on DMSA scintigraphy. Clin. Nucl. Med. 22:292, 1997.

Renovascular Hypertension

Blaufox, M. D.: The role and rationale of nuclear medicine procedures in the differential diagnosis of renovascular hypertension. Nucl. Med. Biol. 18:583, 1991.

Blaufox, M. D., Middleton, M. L., Bongiovanni, J. A., et al.: Cost efficiency of the diagnosis and therapy of renovascular hypertension. J. Nucl. Med. 37:171, 1996.

Bourgoignie, J. J., Rubbert, K., and Sfakianakis, G. N.: Angiotensin-converting enzyme-inhibited renography for the diagnosis of ischemic kidneys. Am. J. Kidney Dis. 24:665, 1994.

Chen, C. C., Hoffer, P. B., Vahjen, G., Gottschalk, A., Koster, K., Zubal, I. G., Setaro, J. F., Roer, D. A., and Black, H. R.: Patients at high risk for renal artery stenosis: A simple method of renal scintigraphic analysis with Tc-99m DTPA and captopril. Radiology 176:365, 1990.

Davidson, R. A., Barri, Y. M., and Wilcox, C. S.: The simplified captopril test: An effective tool to diagnose renovascular hypertension. Am. J. Kidney Dis. 24:660, 1994.

Dondi, M., Fanti, S., De Fabritis, A., Zuccalá, A., Gaggi, R., Mirelli, M., Stella, A., Marengo, M., Losinno, F., and Monetti, N.: Prognostic value of captopril renal scintigraphy in renovascular hypertension. J. Nucl. Med. 33:11, 1992.

Dondi, M., Monetti, N., Fanti, S., Marchetta, F., Corbelli, C., Zagni, P., De Fabritis, A., Losinno, F., Levorato, M., and Zuccalá, A.: Use of technetium-99m-MAG₃ for renal scintigraphy after angiotensin-converting enzyme inhibition. J. Nucl. Med. 32:424, 1991.

Erbsloh-Moller, B., Dumas, A., and Roth, D.: Furosemide [131]I Hippuran renography after angiotensin converting enzyme inhibition for the diagnosis of renovascular hypertension. Am. J. Med. 90:23, 1991.

Gates, G. F.: Glomerular filtration rate: Estimation from fractional renal accumulation of 99m Tc-DTPA (stannous). Am. J. Roetgenol. 138:565, 1982.

Grenier, N., Trillaud, H., Combe, C., Degrèze, P., Jeandot, R., Gosse, P., Douws, C., and Palussière, J.: Diagnosis of renovascular hypertension: Feasibility of captopril-sensitized dynamic MR imaging and comparison with captopril scintigraphy. Am. J. Roentgenol. 166:835, 1996.

King, B. F., Jr.: Diagnostic imaging evaluation of renovascular hypertension. Abdom. Imaging. 20:395, 1995.

Mann, S. J., Pickering, T. G., Sos, T. A., et al.: Captopril renography in the diagnosis of renal artery stenosis: Accuracy and limitations. Am. J. Med. 90:30, 1991.

Middleton, M. L., Bongiovanni, J. A., and Blaufox, M. D.: Evaluation of renovascular hypertension. Curr. Opin. Nephrol. Hypertens. 2:940, 1993.

Pedersen, E. B.: Angiotensin-coverting enzyme inhibitor renography: Pathophysiological, diagnostic and therapeutic aspects in renal artery stenosis. Nephrol. Dial. Transplant. 9:482, 1994.

Pickering, T. G.: Diagnosis and evaluation of renovascular hypertension: Indications for therapy. Circulation 83(2 Suppl.):1147, 1991.

Prigent, A.: The diagnosis of renovascular hypertension: The role of captopril renal scintigraphy and related issues. Eur. J. Nucl. Med. 20:625, 1993.

Setaro, J. F., Saddler, M. C., Chen, C. C., et al.: Simplified captopril renography in diagnosis and treatment of renal artery stenosis. Hypertension 18:289, 1991.

Taylor, A., Nally, J., Aurell, M., Blaufox, D., Dondi, M., Dubovsky, E., Fine, E., Fommei, E., Geyskes, G., Granerus, G., et al.: Consensus report on ACE inhibitor renography for detecting renovascular hypertension. J. Nucl. Med. 37:1876, 1996.

Vesicoureteral Reflux

Goldraich, N. P., Ramos, O. L., and Goldraich, I. H.: Urography versus DMSA scan in children with vesicoureteric reflux. Pediatr. Nephrol. 3:1, 1989.

Monsour, M., Azmy, A. F., and MacKenzie, J. R.: Renal scarring secondary to vesicoureteric reflux: Critical assessment and new grading. Br. J. Urol. 60:320, 1987.

Strife, J. L., Bisset, G. S., III, Kirks, D. R., Schlueter, F. J., Gelfand, M. J., Babcock, D. S., and Han, B. K.: Nuclear cystography and renal sonography: Findings in girls with urinary tract infection. AJR 153:115, 1989.

Van den Abbeele, A. D., Treves, S. T., Lebowitz, R. E., Bauer, S., Davis, R. T., Retik, A., and Colodny, A.: Vesicoureteral reflux in asymptomatic siblings of patients with known reflux: Radionuclide cystography. Pediatrics 79:147, 1987.

Incidental Findings

Bihl, H., Sautter-Bihl, M. L., and Riedasch, G.: Extrarenal abnormalities in ^{99m}Tc DTPA renal perfusion studies due to hypervascularized tumors. Clin. Nucl. Med. *13*:590, 1988.

Bocchini, T., Williams, W., and Patton, D.: Radioscintigraphic demonstration of unsuspected urine extravasation. Clin. Nucl. Med. *14*:421, 1989.

Datz, F. L. (ed.): Gamuts in Nuclear Medicine. East Norwalk, Connecticut, Appleton & Lange, 1987, p. 26.

Hurwitz, G. A., Mattar, A. G., Bhargava, R., Driedger, A. A., Hogendoorn, P., and Wesolowski, C. A.: Renal uptake of ^{201}Tl in hypertensive patients undergoing myocardial perfusion imaging. Clin. Nucl. Med. *15*:88, 1990.

Lin, D. S.: "Missing" one kidney. Semin. Nucl. Med. *21*:167, 1991.

Macpherson, R. J., and Leithiser, R. E.: Serendipitous diagnosis of childhood xanthogranulomatous pyelonephritis in a child with osteomyelitis. Pediatr. Radiol. *17*:159, 1987.

Shih, W. J., DeLand, F. H., and Biersack, H. J.: Serial bone scintigrams demonstrating obstructive uropathy and nephropathy due to transitional cell carcinoma of the urinary bladder. Radiol. Med. 7:203, 1989.

Williamson, S. L., Seibert, J. J., Tryka, A. F., Glasier, C. M., and Williamson, M. R.: Renal imaging on liver-spleen scans. Clin. Nucl. Med. *12*:831, 1987.

Adrenal Imaging

Edeling, C. J., Frederiksen, P. B., Kamper, J., and Jeppesen, P.: Diagnosis and treatment of neuroblastoma using metaiodobenzylguanidine. Clin. Nucl. Med. *12*:632, 1987.

Geatti, O., Fig, L., and Shapiro, B.: Adrenal cortical adenoma causing Cushing's syndrome: Correct localization by functional scintigraphy despite nonlocalizing morphological imaging studies. Clin. Nucl. Med. *15*:168, 1990.

Gross, M. D., and Shapiro, B.: Scintigraphic studies in adrenal hypertension. Semin. Nucl. Med. *19*:122, 1989.

Gross, M. D., Shapiro, B., Bouffard, J. A., Glazer, G. M., Francis, I. R., Wilton, G. P., Khafagi, F., and Sonda, L. P.: Distinguishing benign from malignant adrenal masses. Ann. Intern. Med. *109*:613, 1988.

Ikeda, D. M., Francis, I. R., Glazer, G. M., Amendola, M. A., Gross, M. D., and Aisen, A. M.: The detection of adrenal tumors and hyperplasia in patients with primary aldosteronism: Comparison of scintigraphy, CT, and MR imaging. AJR *153*:301, 1989.

Jonckheer, M. H., Mertens, J., Ham, H. R., and Piepsz, A.: Consolidating the role of I-MIBG-scintigraphy in childhood neuroblastoma: Five years of clinical experience. Pediatr. Radiol. *20*:157, 1990.

Kazerooni, E. A., Sisson, J. C., Shapiro, B., Gross, M. D., Driedger, A., Hurwitz, G. A., Mattar, A. G., and Petry, N. A.: Diagnostic accuracy and pitfalls of [iodine-131]6-beta-iodomethyl-19-norcholesterol (NP-59) imaging. J. Nucl. Med. *31*:526, 1990.

Shapiro, B., Fig, L. M., Gross, M. D., and Khafagi, F.: Radiochemical diagnosis of adrenal disease. CRC Lab. Sci. *27*:265, 1989.

Velchik, M. G., Alavi, A., Kressel, H. Y., and Engelman, K.: Localization of pheochromocytoma: MIBG, CT and MRI correlation. J. Nucl. Med. *30*:328, 1989.

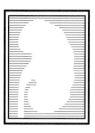

CHAPTER **3**

Radiologic Anatomy and Anomalies of the Kidney and Ureter

The adult kidney and ureter, perhaps more than any other mammalian organ, retain evidence of the series of temporal and structural events that occur during their fetal development. A review of the embryogenesis of the kidney and ureter in this book, therefore, is no routine attempt at completeness. The reader is urged to acquire a knowledge of the process, described in the first section of this chapter, to achieve a better understanding of the architecture of the renal lobe as the basic unit for studying the gross morphology of the kidney. The section on the anatomy of the single lobe is followed by a discussion of the kidney as a union and partial fusion of many lobes. Next, variations in the anatomy of the papillae, which are of fundamental importance in the genesis of acute renal infection and scarring, are presented in detail. This material is then related to uroradiologic landmarks and measurements. The final section describes anomalous development of the kidney and ureter. The anatomy of the lower urinary tract is discussed in Chapters 19 and 20, and that of the retroperitoneum, including the renal sinus, and that of the adrenal gland are presented, respectively, in Chapters 21 and 22. Chapters 23 through 26 include details of genital tract anatomy and anomalies.

EARLY EMBRYOGENESIS OF THE KIDNEY AND URETER
Pronephros

The human excretory system has its origin in the plate of embryonic mesenchyme known as the *inter-*

mediate mesoderm. The first evidence of urinary tract development is a cellular condensation visible between the second and sixth somites of the 10-somite embryo. This occurs at the end of the 3rd week of gestation. Because of the cervicodorsal position of these early excretory structures, they have been termed the *pronephroi*, meaning forward, or head, kidney (Fig. 3–1A). No excretory function occurs at this stage, and the pronephros involutes after a very short time. The only potential importance of the pronephroi is the occasional mediastinal cyst, which may develop as a vestige of this developmental phase of the excretory system.

Mesonephros

The second of the three phases of excretory system development begins with the differentiation of tissue, the *mesonephros*, immediately caudal to the involuting pronephros. In this stage, the intermediate mesoderm on each side of the midline is asymmetrically divided by a longitudinal cleft into a narrow medial structure, the *mesonephric (wolffian) duct*, and a broad lateral portion, the *nephrogenic cord*. This process occurs at slightly more than 3 weeks of gestation, between the 9th and 13th somites of the 20-somite embryo, and progresses caudally. Communication with the cloaca is established within the next few days (29 somites).

The *mesonephroi* are supplied by a series of paired vessels, the rete arteriosum urogenitale, which originate from the aorta and iliac arteries.

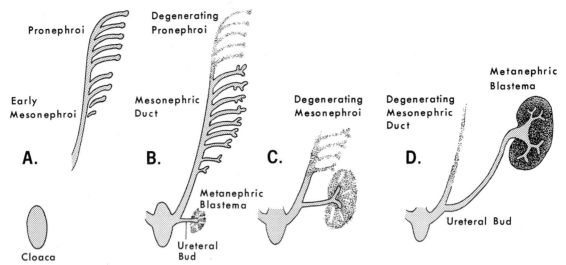

FIGURE 3–1. Schema of successive stages of the embryogenesis of the kidney and ureter from pronephros *(A)* and mesonephros and appearance of the ureteral bud *(B)* to division of the ureteral bud and development of the metanephric blastema into the mature kidney *(C and D).*

In the laterally situated nephrogenic cord, vesicles form and differentiate into functioning glomeruli and tubules, which drain directly into the mesonephric (wolffian) duct. All in all, some 40 to 42 pairs of glomeruli form in the mesonephros. However, only 30 to 32 are present at any one time because those formed earliest, in the cranial aspect, degenerate at the same time as new glomeruli are formed caudally. These events are illustrated in Figure 3–1*B* and *C*.

With time, all the mesonephric glomeruli degenerate. Remnants of the tubules and mesonephric duct, on the other hand, persist in both sexes as genital structures listed in Table 3–1. These are discussed in detail in Section VI, The Genital Tract, of this book.

Ureteral Bud and Metanephros

All the events described to this point occur at a site somewhat remote from where the kidney will eventually develop. Even though the pronephric and mesonephric stages do not directly influence the anatomic form of the definitive excretory organ, they are essential to the development of a small diverticulum at the caudal end of the mesonephric duct, first noted in the 5-week-old embryo. This structure is the *ureteral bud*, and its appearance signals the start of the development of the definitive ureter and kidney, the latter also known as the *metanephros*.

The ureteral bud has two components of growth: elongation and division. As the ureteral bud elongates, the interaction between the specialized cells at its distal tip, known as the ampulla, and the surrounding *metanephric blastema*, moves progressively anterior and cephalad from its initial sacral location, eventually placing the developing kidney in the upper lumbar region (see Fig. 3–1*C* and *D*). The elongated portion of the ureteral bud eventually becomes the ureter, the thin-walled muscular tube that propels urine from the developing metanephros to the bladder as it evolves from the cloaca.

The metanephros is derived from two cell types. The first is the ureteral bud itself; the second is the metanephric blastema. The metanephric blastema differentiates into nephrons and renal connective tissue under the inductive influence of the advancing point, the ampulla, of the ureteral bud. The ureteral bud is the "prime mover" in this process, inasmuch as the metanephric blastema alone will not develop nephrons unless contacted by the ampulla. Potter (1972) ascribed the following four activities to the ampulla of the ureteral bud: anterior

TABLE 3–1. Fate of Mesonephric Structures in the Adult

MALE		FEMALE	
Mesonephric Tubules	**Mesonephric Ducts**	**Mesonephric Tubules**	**Mesonephric Ducts**
Efferent ductules of testes (connecting seminiferous tubules to epididymis)	Vas deferens Seminal vesicle Ejaculatory duct	Epoöphoron* Paroöphoron*	Complete involution
Epididymis Paradidymis			

*Inconstant, functionless structures in the mesosalpinx.

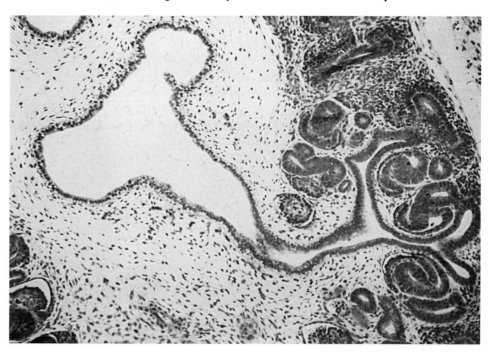

FIGURE 3–2. Photomicrograph of the early development of a human kidney. The ureteral bud is the bifurcating tubular structure that is dilated centrally. The ureteral bud divides peripherally and induces the formation of nephrons from metanephric blastema, seen as dark-staining tissue on the right.

extension, division, induction of nephrons from the metanephric blastema, and establishment of communications between the nephrons from the metanephric blastema and the collecting tubules derived from the ureteral bud.

The process of ureteral bud division is the focus of the remainder of this section. Division is always dichotomous and occurs from the first appearance of the ureteral bud, at approximately 5 weeks of gestation, to the last division in the periphery of the renal medulla, at 5 months of gestation. The first three to five generations of tubes produced by this process dilate to form the renal pelvis; the next three to five generations expand to form the calyces, papillae, and cribriform plates; and the last six to nine generations become the collecting tubules. Understanding this process provides an important foundation for understanding the radiologic anatomy of the kidney.

Development of the Renal Pelvis and Infundibula

Renal function begins when the metanephric blastema, under the inductive influence of the ureteral bud ampullae, starts differentiating into nephrons. This occurs at approximately 7 weeks of gestation. The existing ureteral bud branches at this time begin to dilate, presumably as a result of the accumulation of urine. These dilating branches become the renal pelvis (Fig. 3–2).

The pattern of early ureteral bud branching has an important bearing on the features of the adult kidney. As illustrated in Figure 3–3, more divisions of the ureteral bud occur in the polar than in the interpolar regions of the kidney. Quantitatively, four to five generations of ureteral bud branches contrib-

ute to the formation of each polar region of the renal pelvis, whereas only two to three generations are present in the interpolar region when the pelvis starts forming. The tip of each branch, it should be remembered, is the active portion of the dividing ureteral bud. With substantially more ureteral bud branches inducing nephron formation in the polar regions, it is easy to see why the renal parenchyma normally is thicker in the poles than in the central (interpolar) region of the kidney.

The infundibula that connect the pelvic elements to the calyces are derived from the next generation of ureteral bud branches after those that form the pelvis. These tubular structures do not dilate. It should be pointed out that infundibula have traditionally been called "major calyces," although in fact they are not calyces at all. *Calyx* is the Latin term for cup or chalice. Sherwood and Williams (1973) noted that, properly, this word should be reserved for the structure surrounding the papilla, commonly called the "minor calyx." The "major calyx" is, in

DEVELOPMENT OF RENAL PELVIS

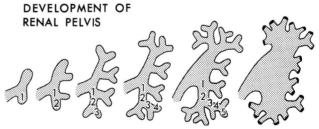

FIGURE 3–3. Schema of early divisions of the ureteral bud. Four to five divisions form the polar regions, and two to three generations form the interpolar area. Dilatation and subsequent assimilation of individual branches occur as urine formation begins. (Modified from Potter, E. L.: Normal and Abnormal Development of the Kidney, 1972, with kind permission of the author and Year Book Medical Publishers.)

fact, a simple tubular conduit, embryologically a part of the renal pelvis, that links the calyx to the common chamber of the renal pelvis.

Development of the Calyces and Papillae

Following the generations of ureteral bud branches that dilate to form the renal pelvis and the infundibula, another series of three to five generations appears. According to Potter (1972), these branches differ from their predecessors in that they are formed one from the other in rapid succession. The rapidity of the dichotomous branching in this series results in little time for growth and elongation of the individual tubes. As a result, three to five generations of very short tubules are produced; these expand to form the cavity of the calyx.

The early calyx has the configuration of multiple, dilated, short fingers. With progressive distention, the calyx undergoes transformation into a saclike cavity. Dilatation is believed to progress as a result of urine filling many short tubules that open into a space having the infundibulum as a single outlet to the pelvis. As nephrons grow, there is both an increase in the bulk of tissue adjacent to the calyx and in the volume of urine formed. The dilating calyx thus becomes interposed between developing nephrons on one side and the enlarging renal pelvis on the other. The net effect is to flatten the calyceal sac and to force the margins of the space to pouch outward and partially encompass the lower ends of the collecting ducts. Thus, a cuplike structure, or calyx, is formed.

Subsequent branching is slower, allowing time for the ducts to elongate considerably. These tubules become the *papillary ducts of Bellini*, which enter the calyx through the *cribriform plate* covering the surface of the papilla. (The cribriform plate is discussed further in the section below, Anatomy of the Papillae.)

The progression of events in the formation of a calyx and papilla is illustrated in Figure 3–4.

Development of the Collecting Tubules and Nephrons

The papillary duct is formed from the ureteral bud branch that is immediately distal to those that have formed the calyx and cribriform plate. A single papilla bears 10 to 20 of these ducts opening into the calyx. Potter estimated that the papillary ducts belong to the 11th generation of divisions from the original ureteral bud. Each of these 10 to 20 ducts at the papillary tip gives rise to another seven to eight generations of structures known as *collecting tubules*. One can easily visualize, then, the beginning formation of the conical renal lobe extending outward from the papillary tip. All that is lacking at this point is the investiture of this bundle of collecting tubules with a cloak of nephrons.

As the ampullae of the collecting tubules elongate and divide, they do so in close contact with the solid

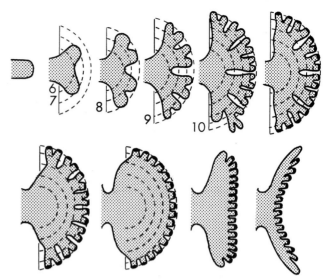

FIGURE 3–4. Schema of the sixth to tenth generations of ureteral bud branches, which form by rapid division. These develop into the calyx. With time, the ducts dilate, and the resultant cavity becomes invaginated by the expanding lobe. (Modified from Potter, E. L.: Normal and Abnormal Development of the Kidney, 1972, with kind permission of the author and Year Book Medical Publishers.)

mass of the metanephric blastema, the anlage of the glomerulus, the proximal convoluted tubule, the loop of Henle, and the distal convoluted tubule. Collectively, these structures constitute the *nephron*. The distal convoluted tubule communicates with the last generation of collecting tubules to establish the final union of the two tissue groups, which combine to form the definitive kidney. Each of the collecting tubule branches eventually has eight to nine nephrons attached to it. There is controversy over the details of how the nephron differentiates into its several components and the various patterns of attachment to the collecting tubule. These differences of opinion, however, are beyond the scope of this book.

Development of the Renal Lobe

There are two consequences of the continued elongation and division of the collecting tubules. First, the mass of formed renal tissue expands centrifugally, in the shape of a cone, from each papilla. Second, the major portion of the nephrons induced by the advancing collecting tubules is arranged peripherally to the collecting tubules rather than intermingled with them. As a result, a central zone of collecting tubules, the *medulla*, is formed. It becomes completely surrounded by a dense zone of nephrons, the *cortex*, which invests the medulla completely, except at the papillary tip.

The sharp demarcation between the ureteral bud derivatives (papillary ducts and collecting tubules) in the medulla and metanephric blastema derivatives (nephrons and connective tissue) in the cortex is striking. Some intermixing does occur, however; loops of Henle and connective tissue extend into the

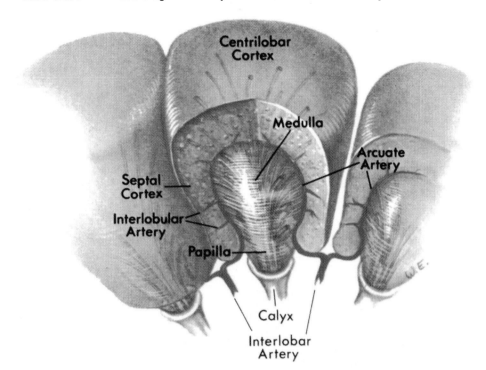

FIGURE 3–5. Diagram of the archetypical renal lobe.

medulla. Actually, the loops of Henle associated with the earliest collecting tubule branches extend deep into the papillae. The vascular supply of the nephrons is also found in the medulla. Intermixing occurs in the cortex when the terminal branches of the collecting tubules extend outward in a radial pattern known as *cortical rays*.

It is of fundamental importance for the reader to recognize that this process of lobe formation occurs simultaneously at each site where a calyx has been formed. Basically, the number of lobes that form is determined by the number of calyces; the size of each lobe is determined by the number of papillary ducts draining into each calyx. In the adult, however, there is not a one-to-one relationship between calyces and papillae. It is common to have an arrangement in which a calyx drains two, three, or occasionally more papillae. In the fetus, on the other hand, the definitive number of primary lobes, averaging 14 per kidney, is established by the end of the 4th month of gestation. At this point, before continuing with the final events that transform these independent units into the adult kidney, it is useful to consider the architecture of the individual renal lobe.

ARCHITECTURE OF THE RENAL LOBE

The archetypical renal lobe consists of medulla, cortex, draining calyx, and vascular system, as illustrated in Figures 3–5 and 3–6.

As has already been described, the conical medulla is composed of collecting tubules (derived from ureteral bud divisions) and proximal and distal convoluted tubules, loops of Henle, and connective tissue (arising from the metanephric blastema). The

arterial blood supply to the medulla comes chiefly from the vasa recta, a system of postglomerular vessels derived from the efferent arterioles of the juxtamedullary cortex (see Fig. 3–6; Fig. 3–7). These vessels follow the descending limb of the

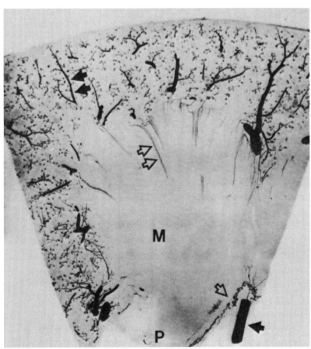

FIGURE 3–6. Microradiograph of a renal lobe from a human kidney injected post mortem with barium. The vasa recta of the medulla are sparsely opacified, whereas the cortical vasculature is well defined. M, medulla; P, papilla; single solid arrow, arcuate artery; double solid arrows, interlobular artery; single open arrow, spiral artery to papilla; double open arrows, vasa recta.

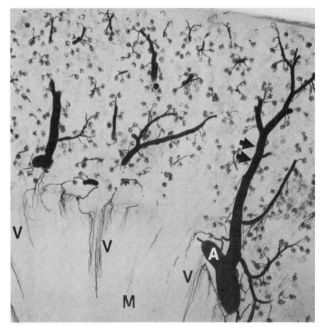

FIGURE 3–7. Enlargement of Figure 3–6 demonstrates details of cortical vascular anatomy. Afferent arterioles branch from the large interlobular arteries and supply glomerular tufts. Vasa recta can be seen in the corticomedullary region. V, vasa recta; A, arcuate artery; arrows, interlobular artery; M, medulla.

loops of Henle through the medulla and into the papillae and return with the ascending loop, where drainage into an interlobular or arcuate vein occurs. Under normal circumstances, the medulla receives less than 20 per cent of the total renal blood flow through this system. The remaining blood flow perfuses the cortex. This difference in regional perfusion is the basis for the radiologic appearance of the medulla as a relatively radiolucent structure surrounded by the opacified lobar cortex during the early nephrographic phase of a dynamic contrast material–enhanced computed tomogram, magnetic resonance image, or renal arteriogram (Fig. 3–8). The papilla also receives blood directly from the arterial branches of the interlobar artery, the *spiral arteries*, in addition to the vasa recta (see Fig. 3–6).

The cortex of the renal lobe is the cloak of dense tissue that in the pristine lobe completely surrounds the medulla except at its papillary tip. Composed largely of nephrons derived from the metanephric blastema, the cortex is interrupted at regular intervals by linear bands, called *cortical rays*, representing straight terminal branches of collecting tubules extending into cortical tissue from the medulla. The portion of the cortex that forms the base of the lobe has been called the *centrilobar cortex* by Hodson (1972); that which surrounds the sides of the medulla is called the *septal cortex*. The distinction between these two is of considerable importance. The centrilobar cortex is invariably present in the adult and is an important border-forming urographic landmark, whereas the septal cortex in the adult kidney is variably present and not always

discernible during radiologic studies enhanced by contrast material. The reader will undoubtedly recognize that the septal cortex is, in fact, what is popularly called the *column of Bertin* or *Bertini*. It is both useful and correct to speak of this structure as either the "septal cortex" or the "septum of Bertin."* In its most internal extension, the septal cortex reaches the level of the papilla. Here, it may have a slight bulbous enlargement, as shown in Figure 3–5, which, if accentuated to some degree, is one explanation for the so-called renal pseudotumor, discussed later in this chapter. As mentioned earlier, the cortex receives approximately 80 per cent of the total renal blood flow through the interlobular arteries, which give rise to the afferent arterioles (see Fig. 3–7).

In the archetypical renal lobe there is a single calyx into which a single papilla is invaginated. These two structures form the innermost landmarks of the renal lobe. In addition, they serve as a reference point for the central axis of the renal lobe, an imaginary line that extends from the tip of the papilla to the midpoint of the centrilobar cortex. The concept of a central axis will be of importance in subsequent chapters in which the impact of various pathologic processes on the renal lobe is discussed.

Each lobe receives its blood supply from *interlobar*, or *segmental*, *arteries* that branch into *arcuate arteries* while still passing through the fat of the renal sinus. The arcuate artery enters the renal substance adjacent to the papilla of the lobe and runs along the corticomedullary junction, periodi-

---

*Hodson (1972) has provided an engaging, brief reconstruction of how Bertin's original description of this structure, using the French word for "internal partition" (*cloison*), has been transformed into the current imprecise term *column*.

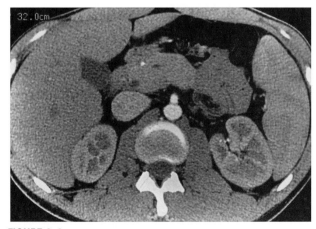

FIGURE 3–8. Angiographic or cortical nephrogram demonstrated in a contrast material–enhanced helical computed tomogram. The centrilobar and septal cortices are opacified, whereas the medulla of each lobe remains unenhanced. This reflects predominant blood flow to the cortex. The angiographic or cortical nephrogram is seen in the first few seconds following arrival of a bolus of contrast material into the renal artery and is essentially a vascular phenomenon.

cally giving off branches, the *interlobular arteries*, which extend into the cortex at right angles to the arcuate artery. Several arcuate arteries serve each lobe in a pattern that allows perfusion of the lobe's full circumference. The interlobular arteries, in turn, give rise to the *afferent arterioles*, which supply the glomeruli and, in the juxtamedullary cortex, the vasa recta as well. Although the preceding description applies to a single lobe, in reality each interlobar artery supplies arcuate vessels to two adjacent lobes, and these have a roughly mirror image distribution, as shown in Figure 3–5.

LATE DEVELOPMENT OF THE KIDNEY: THE KIDNEY AS A WHOLE

The development of the renal lobes continues beyond the cessation of ureteral bud branching at approximately 20 weeks. By the 28th week of gestation the individuality of each lobe is most pronounced. At this time most fetal kidneys have 14 lobes, also known as *renunculi*. Some have as few as 8 lobes; very few have more than 14. Inspection of the kidney at this stage reveals deep surface clefts that delineate the margins of the lobes (Fig. 3–9). In fact, the lobes can be manually separated with ease. At this stage, characteristically, there are seven anterior and seven posterior lobes. A longitudinal groove composed of fibrous tissue, which is well developed by the 28th week of gestation, separates the anterior from the posterior groups.

Calyceal development at this stage corresponds to the pattern of lobar clefts. In most fetal kidneys that have been studied at this stage of development, there were seven anterior and seven posterior calyces, each with a single draining papilla. That is to say, each calyx corresponded exactly with the papilla of each lobe.

Events following the 28th week of gestation result in varying degrees of assimilation of the independent lobes. A reduction in the number of calyces, papillae, and surface lobar clefts follows. Fusion of calyces occurs to a greater degree than does fusion of papillae, resulting in a lower number of individual calyces than papillae by the time of birth. Sykes (1964) reported a mean of 9.0 calyces and 11.4 papillae in a series of kidneys studied at full term. He also noted that the average number of calyces and papillae (respectively, 8.7 and 10.7) was slightly lower in the adult, indicating that fusion continues following birth. It is this process of fusion that results in the so-called compound calyx into which two, three, and occasionally more papillae drain. Thus, the calyx loses its one-to-one relationship with an individual lobe and may drain multiple adjacent lobes. The impact of assimilation on the anatomy of the cribriform plate is discussed in the following section, Anatomy of the Papillae.

Another result of lobar fusion is the disappearance of the septal cortex in many areas (Fig. 3–10). Where fusion is most complete, the septal cortex is lost entirely, and the medullary portions of adjacent lobes abut each other directly, with no landmarks left to note the site of the previous septal cortex. Where lobar fusion is absent, the septal cortex remains extended into the renal sinus and fuses with the septal cortex of the adjacent lobe, and the relationship of single calyx to single papilla remains. Intermediate degrees of fusion also occur, in which the septal cortex persists to varying depths between lobes.

Fusion varies in different parts of the kidney according to a predictable pattern. A greater degree of lobar fusion occurs in the polar regions than in the interpolar region of the kidney. Lobes frequently fuse completely in both the upper and lower poles, and anterior lobes characteristically fuse with posterior lobes. As a result, large compound calyces with absent septal cortex are the rule rather than the exception in the polar regions. This is true to an even greater degree in the superior pole than in the inferior pole. Fusion in the interpolar region of the kidney rarely occurs between anterior and posterior lobes and, as noted previously, is generally less frequent than in the polar regions. Thus, in the middle part of the kidney, single calyces are seen frequently during excretory urography, and the septal cortex is visualized regularly on contrast material–enhanced renal images with both computed tomography and magnetic resonance imaging. On the kidney surface, lobar fusion is manifested as a loss

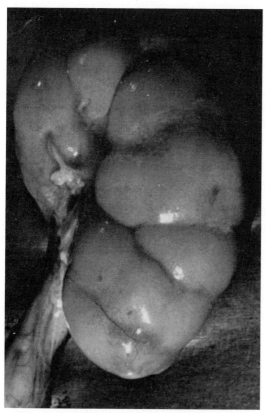

FIGURE 3–9. Fetal kidney. Note deep clefts delineating margins of each lobe. (Courtesy of H. Z. Klein, M.D., University of California, San Francisco.)

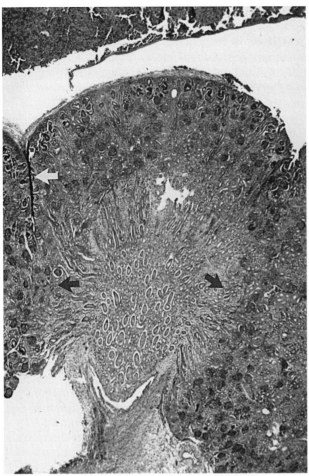

FIGURE 3–10. Photomicrograph of a lobe from a fetal kidney that has developed beyond the 28th week of gestation. The process of lobar assimilation is manifested by the fusion of the septal cortex of adjacent lobes *(black arrows)* and the obliteration of the deep cleft of connective tissue that previously separated adjacent lobes, a residual portion of which remains *(white arrow)*. The papilla and calyx of the lobe remain unfused.

of clefts, which for uncertain reasons is most noticeable on the posterior surface.

The renal artery, derived from the mesonephric artery, originates from the upper lumbar level of the aorta and bifurcates into anterior and posterior branches at a variable point between the aorta and hilum of the kidney. The anterior branch generally perfuses the ventral and upper polar regions, whereas the posterior vessel usually perfuses the dorsal and lower polar regions. The branches of the ventral and dorsal arteries, the interlobar arteries, traverse the fat of the renal sinus and at the level of the calyx give rise to the arcuate arteries that penetrate the renal lobe between the cortex and the medulla (Fig. 3–11). The arcuate arteries continue along the corticomedullary junction, periodically giving off perpendicular branches (the interlobular arteries) that run to the cortex (see Figs. 3–6 and 3–7). Most arcuate arteries are end-arteries, although a few may communicate with capsular arteries by way of an interlobular artery. Arcuate

arteries are visualized in all normal angiograms, whereas interlobular arteries are only occasionally identifiable as discrete structures. A normal renal artery has a smooth wall and gentle curves and overlaps other vessels, tapers gradually, and has a multiplicity of branches. Blood vessels extend to the periphery of the normal kidney (Fig. 3–12).

The middle-sized and large veins of the kidney parallel arteries and are similarly named. Interlobular veins drain the cortex, become arcuate veins, and then become interlobar and segmental veins. Unlike the renal arteries, the veins of the kidney freely anastomose. The arcuate veins form complete arches along the corticomedullary junction. Their opacification vividly depicts lobar architecture (Fig. 3–13).

Features of the fused kidney are shown schematically in Figure 3–14.

ANATOMY OF THE PAPILLAE

In the fully developed kidney, papillae have either a simple or a compound form. The shape of the simple papilla is that of a cone whose convex surface projects into the calyceal lumen. This form is unchanged from that of the embryonic kidney in which each papilla drains urine from a single lobe into a single calyx. The compound papilla has a complex shape composed of flat, concave, or cleftlike profiles projecting into the calyceal lumen (Figs. 3–15 and 3–16). The compound papilla is the result of the partial fusion of lobes, papillae, and calyces that begins after the 28th week of gestation. Urine entering a compound papilla is formed in two or more adjacent, partially assimilated lobes and flows into a compound, or partially assimilated, calyx.

The cribriform plate is the surface of the papilla perforated by the openings of the papillary ducts of Bellini, through which urine passes, normally from collecting ducts into the calyx. There are two basic shapes of papillary duct openings: narrow and slitlike, and round and open (see Figs. 3–15 and 3–16). The narrow, slitlike opening is seen mainly on simple papillae and on those portions of compound papillae that are least distorted by fusion. The slitlike shape is thought to favor closure of the orifices of the papillary ducts in the presence of elevated intrapelvic pressure, thus preventing the reflux of urine into the collecting ducts of the medulla.

The round, open type of orifice, on the other hand, is the result of distortion by fusion. In some kidney specimens, these orifices may be open enough to permit direct visualization of the early branches of the collecting duct system. It is generally held that when pelvic pressure is elevated, the round, open-duct orifice is incapable of preventing reflux of urine from the pelvocalyceal system into the collecting ducts and tubules. This is so-called *intrarenal reflux*. It is likely, also, that these orifices provide access for bacteria in pelvocalyceal urine to enter collecting ducts and tubules in the absence of reflux.

It is clear that variations in the shape of papillary

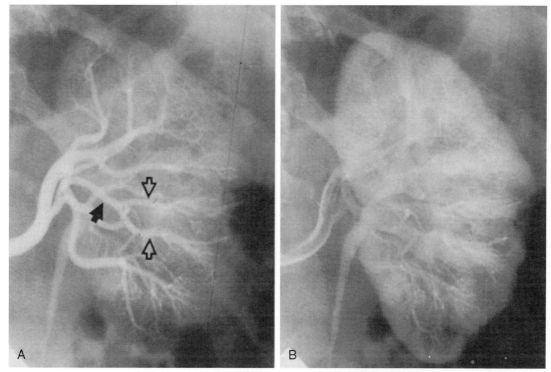

FIGURE 3–11. Normal renal arteries and angiographic or cortical nephrogram. Division of the main renal artery into anterior and posterior branches is followed by branching into interlobar arteries *(closed arrow).* The arcuate arteries *(open arrows)* form at the level of the calyx and run along the corticomedullary junction. The cortex is opacified during the angiographic or cortical nephrographic phase and surrounds the relatively radiolucent medulla.
   A, Selective renal arteriogram. Arterial phase.
   B, Selective renal arteriogram. Late arterial and early nephrographic phase.

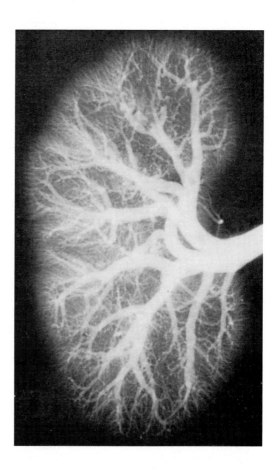

FIGURE 3–12. Radiograph of a barium-injected normal human kidney. Normal arteries are characterized by smooth walls, gentle curves, overlapping of vessels, gradual tapering, and a multiplicity of fine branches. Vessels extend to the periphery of the kidney.

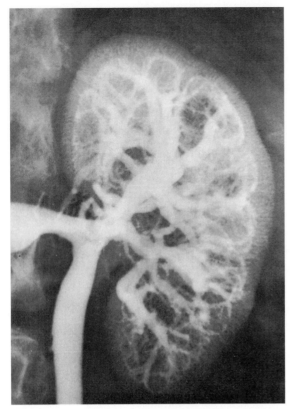

FIGURE 3–13. Normal renal venogram performed with a balloon-occluding technique. Veins parallel arteries but freely anastomose and form complete arches along the corticomedullary junction. Interlobular veins are opacified. (Courtesy of J. Rösch, M.D., University of Oregon, Portland.)

duct orifices are related to the embryogenetic process of fusion and that mixtures of shapes are found on both simple and compound papillae. In addition, both papillary profile and orifice shape can be altered by acquired abnormalities, such as recurrent episodes of increased intrapelvic pressure or the development of scars in portions of the lobe. This subject is discussed further in Chapter 5 in relation to the pathogenesis of reflux nephropathy.

Papillae vary in size as well as shape. Large papillae are of no clinical significance (Fig. 3–17).

URORADIOLOGIC LANDMARKS

Ureter

The length and course of the ureter represents ureteral bud growth by elongation during embryogenesis. The proximal two-thirds of the normal ureter is situated in the perirenal space, where it extends from the ureteropelvic junction to the point of its passage through the cone of fused anterior and posterior renal fascia at the caudal margin of the perirenal space (see Chapter 21). Thereafter, the distal one-third of the ureter traverses the extraperitoneal space of the pelvis to its termination at the lateral margin of the interureteric ridge of the bladder.

As the ureter extends distally from the ureteropelvic junction, it lies anteromedial to the medial margin of the lower pole of the kidney and lateral to the superior portion of the psoas muscle. Near the lower pole of the kidney, the ureter moves medially to a position anterior to the psoas muscle. Within the extraperitoneal space of the pelvis, the ureter passes anterior to the common iliac artery in the region of the first sacral ala. From this point, the ureter usually curves in a broad arc that extends laterally to a point near the ischial spine and then medially to its entry into the bladder.

Most proximal ureters are situated within a vertical zone delineated by the lateral margin of the lumbar vertebral pedicles and the tips of lumbar transverse processes. However, there are marked individual and racial variations in the course of normal ureters, and neither the vertebral pedicle medially nor the transverse process laterally serves as an absolute standard for normalcy. The position of the ureter is likely to be more medial in individuals of African origin than in those of other races (Adams et al., 1985). The detection of ureteral deviation and its various causes are discussed in Chapters 16, 19, and 21.

Kidney

Many of the anatomic features of the renal lobe are best seen during excretory urography. The opacified calyx and the radiolucent indentation of the papilla mark the apex of the lobe. The cuplike configuration of the calyx, with its acute forniceal angle, is the result of the papillary parenchyma's impression on what was a saclike space in the early embryo. The angle remains sharp as long as the volume of papillary tissue and hydrostatic calyceal pressure are

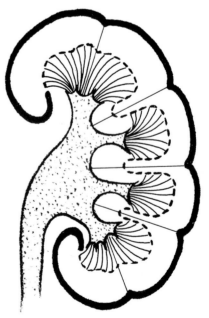

FIGURE 3–14. Schema of kidney after lobar fusion. Note greater degree of assimilation in both poles, represented by compound calyces and loss of septal cortex. The interpolar region tends to retain individual lobes, septal cortex, and fetal surface lobulation.

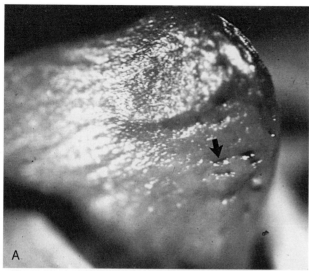

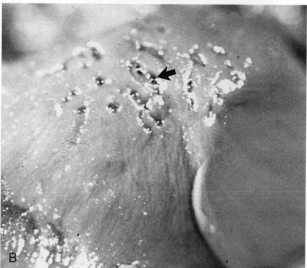

FIGURE 3–15. Simple and compound normal papillae from human kidney.

A, Simple papilla. The papillary duct orifices *(arrow on one representative example)* are narrow and slitlike.

B, Compound papilla has orifices *(arrow on one representative example)* that are round and open as a result of fusion of adjacent papillae.

normal. When disease processes reduce the amount of papillary tissue or when urine pressure in the calyx increases, the angle of the fornix widens. The centrilobar cortex of the base of the lobe forms a portion of the border of the kidney. The distance between the papillary tip and the outer margin represents the medulla *and* cortex of the lobe and is a useful representation of the *amount* of renal parenchyma in the lobe.

The radiologist can see this best during the nephrographic phase of the excretory urogram, which depicts the lobar parenchyma (both cortex and medulla) as a homogeneous density, representing contrast material in the lumina of the nephrons and collecting tubules of the lobe. Replacement of lobar parenchyma by abnormal tissue disturbs the homogeneity of the nephrogram. The lateral mar-

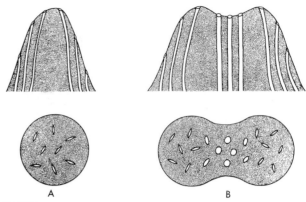

FIGURE 3–16. Schema of papillary duct opening in profile and *en face.* The single cone-shaped pyramid *(A)* has narrow slitlike openings that prevent intrarenal reflux. Compound papillae *(B),* formed as a result of lobar assimilation, have open, round orifices that permit reflux of calyceal urine into the collecting ducts.

gins of the lobe are occasionally detectable during excretory urography by a slight notching of the renal contour, termed *fetal lobation.* This represents the point at which the centrilobar cortex of one lobe abuts that of an adjacent lobe. A line drawn from this notch in the renal contour toward the renal

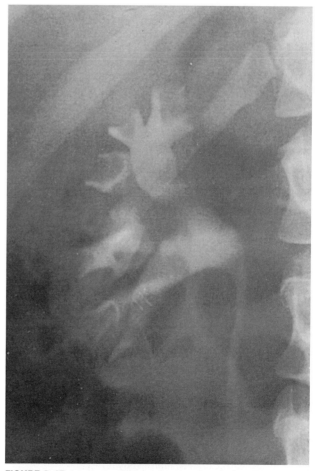

FIGURE 3–17. Large papillae as a normal variation. The papillae are uniformly large; the calyces are normal. Excretory urogram.

sinus will approximate the septal cortex of the two adjacent lobes. In practice, the determination that a renal contour defect is due to fetal lobation, rather than disease-induced scarring, often can be made when the surface indentation is both sharply notched in shape and located between calyces rather than opposite a calyx (Fig. 3–18). A cortical defect opposite a calyx, particularly one that is broad-based, represents pathologic loss of lobar tissue. The most direct visualization of the septal cortex occurs during renal angiography, when both the interlobar and arcuate arteries and the cortex itself are selectively opacified (see Fig. 3–11) or during the early phase of dynamic, contrast material–enhanced computed tomograms.

In the fused adult kidney there is a more or less constant grouping of calyces in each of the three regions of the kidney. Therefore, a group of calyces, often compound, serves each of the two polar regions, and a third group drains the interpolar region of the kidney (Fig. 3–19). This is understandable because the calyces, being ureteral bud derivatives, are essential to the formation of their adjacent renal tissue. One should also recognize that not only are there three regional groups of calyces but also that the amount of renal tissue drained by each group is proportionate to that in the remainder of the kidney. This is the expected pattern because all the calyces are derived from the same generation of ureteral bud branches and begin their structural formation at the same time. As a result, calyces and papillae maintain a remarkably constant spatial relationship to each other within the sinus of the kidney. Thus, a line connecting the

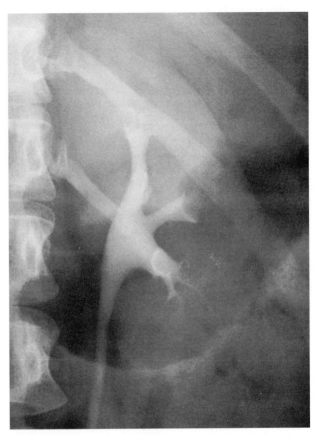

FIGURE 3–19. Normal pelvocalyceal anatomy illustrating the distribution of calyces into three groups subserving, respectively, the upper polar, interpolar, and lower polar regions. Excretory urogram.

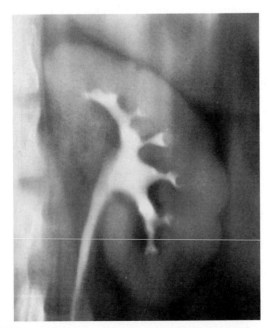

FIGURE 3–18. Characteristic fetal lobation along lateral margin of kidney. Notches in contour are sharply angulated and occur between two calyces rather than overlying a calyx. These notches represent the lateral margins of adjacent lobes. (Courtesy of Robert R. Hattery, M.D., Mayo Clinic, Rochester, Minnesota.)

most peripheral papillae, one to the other, will depict an arc, the *interpapillary line*, which is smooth, conforming in shape to the external contour of the kidney. These features are schematized in Figure 3–20.

The interpapillary line was described by Pendergrass in 1943. This measurement is of fundamental importance in the urographic diagnosis of renal disease. In the normal kidney, the thickness of parenchyma lying between the interpapillary line and the outer margin of the kidney is uniform in the interpolar region and expands symmetrically in both poles (Fig. 3–21). Even in the presence of variations in normal contour, such as hepatic or splenic impressions on the renal contour, the arc of the interpapillary line maintains a close parallel relationship with the renal contour, as illustrated in Figures 3–22 and 3–23. Disturbance of this relationship is a sensitive indicator of change in the parenchymal bulk (either gain or loss) and also permits assessment of whether an abnormal process causing such change in bulk is diffuse or focal.

Opacification of the papillae occurs as an integral part of the nephrogram. Because the countercurrent mechanism concentrating urine is maximal in the papillary region, the papillae are sometimes denser than the remainder of the renal parenchyma. This normal phenomenon is termed *papillary blush*. Oc-

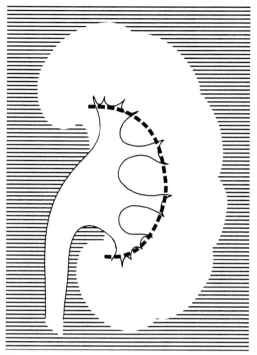

FIGURE 3–20. Schema of the fused kidney as seen during urography. Note the grouping of calyces for each of three regions (upper and lower polar and interpolar), the symmetry between the interpapillary line and the outer margin of the kidney, and the constancy of renal parenchymal thickness, with widening at both poles.

casionally during contrast material–enhanced studies, individual or groups of collecting ducts appear as discrete linear structures radiating from the papillary tips into the medulla for a short distance. This appearance may simulate papillary striations seen in medullary sponge kidney (see Chapter 13). However, in the absence of other evidence for medullary sponge kidney, such as nephrocalcinosis or cysts communicating with collecting ducts, these linear striations are considered normal. Visualiza-

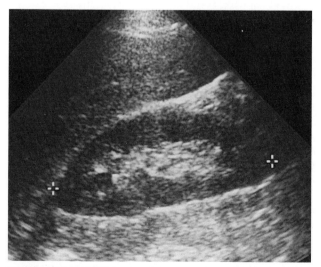

FIGURE 3–21. The thickness of the renal parenchyma is uniform, with slight increases in thickness in the polar regions. Ultrasonogram, longitudinal section.

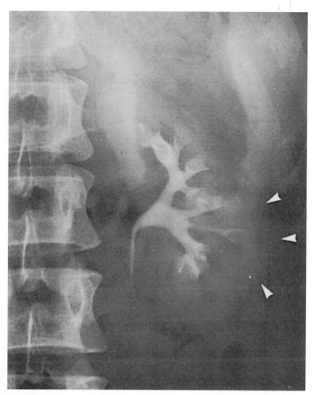

FIGURE 3–22. The constancy of the relationship of the interpapillary line to the renal contour is illustrated in a case of prominent "dromedary hump" (arrows) in which the subservient draining calyx extends outward so that the thickness of renal parenchyma remains constant in the interpolar region. This finding indicates a normal state rather than a growing mass, which would displace the calyx away from the periphery of the kidney.

tion of collecting ducts in papillary tips is seen more frequently with low osmolality contrast material than with high osmolality agents.

The anterior and posterior lobes in the interpolar region do not in fact directly overlie each other. Rather, these two groups are offset, which results in the anterior papillae being situated laterally relative to the posterior papillae. Because of this arrangement, the calyces of the anterior lobes project laterally and are seen in profile on anteroposterior radiographs of the kidney. Those calyces that lie medially in this projection belong to the posterior lobes and usually are seen en face. This pattern is shown schematically in Figure 3–24 and illustrated in Figures 3–25 and 3–26. Thus, the reader should keep in mind that urographic landmarks and measurements such as the interpapillary line, parenchymal thickness, and renal contour are usually determined from images of the anterior part of the kidney and are a sampling of a portion of the kidney, not a representation of the whole organ. This limitation, of course, does not apply to cross-sectional images produced by ultrasonography, computed tomography, or magnetic resonance imaging.

Fetal kidneys can be visualized on ultrasound examination as early as 14 menstrual weeks as paired hypoechoic structures on either side of the

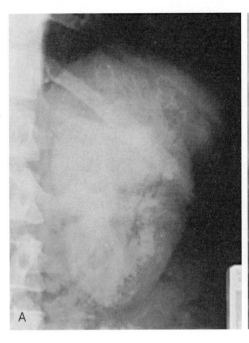
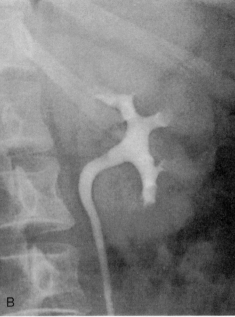

FIGURE 3–23. Splenic impression on upper pole causing apparent distortion of renal contour on 1-minute nephrographic film in frontal projection *(A)*. A later film in the left posterior oblique projection *(B)* established normal interpapillary line and renal parenchymal thickness. (Courtesy of Department of Diagnostic Radiology, Hammersmith Hospital, London, England.)

fetal spine on a cross-sectional image of the abdomen. As the fetus ages, the renal sinus appears as a linear area of echogenicity slightly greater than that of the renal parenchyma. By 30 weeks of gestation, the hyperechoicity of the septal and centrilobar cortex relative to medullary tissue frequently permits differentiation of these two components of the renal parenchyma. Fetal lobation and the pelvocalyceal system are routinely seen at this stage of development as well.

The cortex of the neonatal and infant kidney is often more hyperechoic than the medulla (Fig. 3–27). This reflects the increased size and cellularity of glomeruli during the first few months of life.

X-RAY BEAM

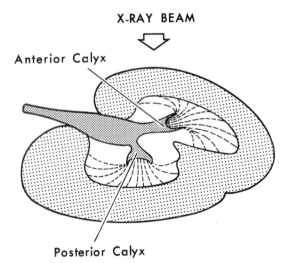

FIGURE 3–24. Schema of transverse section of the interpolar region of the kidney. In the frontal projection, the anterior calyces are lateral to the posterior calyces and are seen in profile. The posterior calyces are seen *en face.* (Modified from Hodson, C. J.: Br. J. Urol. *44:*246, 1972, with kind permission of the author and the *British Journal of Urology.*)

After 6 months of age, the difference in echogenicity between the cortex and the medulla is reduced.

On renal ultrasound examinations, especially of the right kidney in children, a straight echogenic line between the renal sinus and the ventral surface of the upper portion of the kidney may sometimes be identified. This structure, which often expands at the surface of the kidney into a triangular echogenic focus, has been variably called the *renal parenchymal junctional line*, the *hyperechogenic triangle* and *line*, or the *parenchymal interjunctional line* (Fig. 3–28). Occasionally, the hyperechogenic line runs in a posterior and inferior direction. It is uncommon to identify this structure in the left kidney, in the newborn in whom there is usually a paucity of renal sinus fat, and in adults. It is clear that the hyperechogenic triangle and line represent an extension of fat from the renal sinus to the surface of the kidney. Presumably, this fat is deposited along the interface of adjacent lobes that did not undergo fusion during embryogenesis, perhaps along a plane between the anterior and posterior groups of lobes. The fact that these are infrequently seen in adults may be taken as evidence for continued fusion of lobes after birth.

The position of the kidneys in the retroperitoneum follows a general pattern. The upper pole of the kidney is more medially and posteriorly situated than the lower pole. Because the lower pole calyces are less dependent than the upper pole calyces when the patient is in the supine position, they may not fill well with contrast material, which has a higher specific gravity than urine. This sometimes causes nonopacification of the lower pole calyces and a false assumption of disease. In this case, ureteral compression or prone or upright films are useful means to opacify the lower pole collecting system. Most kidneys are positioned somewhere be-

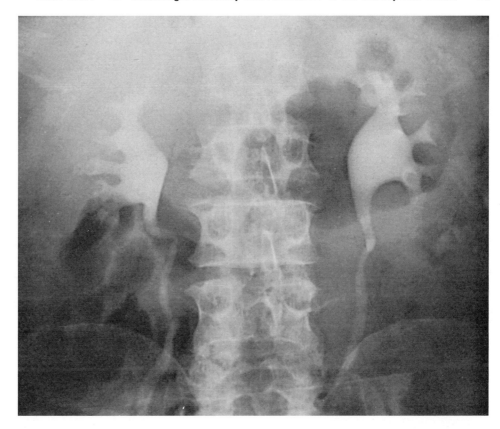

FIGURE 3–25. Difference in position and projection of anterior and posterior calyces is well illustrated in the left kidney. The lateral calyces seen in profile are anterior; the medial ones seen *en face* are posterior. Because of this relationship, measures of parenchymal thickness and renal contour represent a sampling of anterior lobes.

tween the first and third lumbar vertebrae. The pattern for renal position is so variable, however, that meaningful quantification is not possible. Fortunately, the position of the kidney in the retroperitoneum is not of major importance as an aid in the diagnosis of renal disease, although displacement may signal a retroperitoneal mass (see discussion in Chapter 21).

RENAL SIZE

Renal size as a clue to the nature of the pathologic process affecting the kidney is one of the major themes of this book. Unfortunately, a basic frustration encountered in adult uroradiology is the absence of valid standards for assessing the significance of a set of measurements in a given individual. The problem is not inherent in the kidneys; in

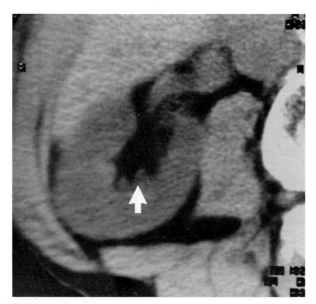

FIGURE 3–26. Transverse cross section of the right kidney demonstrates the lateral position of the anterior portion of the kidney relative to the posterior lobes. Note also the anterior projection of a papilla from the posterior portion of the kidney *(arrow)* and the anteromedial position of the renal sinus. Computed tomogram, unenhanced.

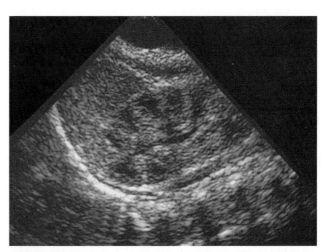

FIGURE 3–27. Normal neonatal kidney. Ultrasonogram. The cortex is usually more echogenic than the medulla during the first 6 months of life.

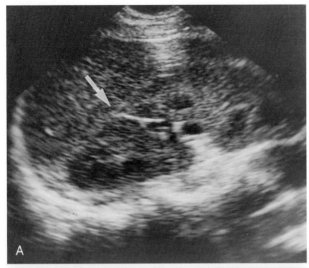

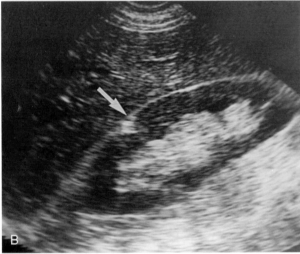

FIGURE 3–28. Hyperechogenic line and triangle in two normal adult kidneys.

A, A well-defined hyperechogenic line extends from the renal sinus to the anterior surface of the upper pole of the kidney.

B, A hyperechogenic triangle of tissue is present on the anterior surface of the upper portion of the kidney. (From Dalla Palma, L., et al.: Br. J. Radiol. *63*:680, 1990. Reproduced with kind permission of the author and the *British Journal of Radiology.*)

fact, there is close correlation between renal mass and such factors as body build and age. Rather, the problem reflects weaknesses in traditional radiographic methods, such as enlargement of the renal silhouette due to object-film distance and foreshortening of renal length and width caused by rotation of the kidney on both longitudinal and transverse axes as it moves with respiration. Another major problem is that standard radiographic methods permit only two-dimensional measurement of a variably shaped organ. The third dimension, thickness, eludes imaging of the kidney by means of radiographs. Further, true renal size varies with the state of hydration and in response to contrast material. One can readily appreciate the difficult task of

determining renal volume from a radiograph of the abdomen or an excretory urogram.

Another weakness that applies to radiography as well as to ultrasonography, computed tomography, and magnetic resonance imaging is that measurements based on overall length, width, and thickness assume a constant normal ratio between the parenchyma and other internal structures of the kidney such as the pelvocalyceal system and renal sinus fat. Clearly, standards based on measurements of normal kidneys cannot be applied to conditions such as hydronephrosis, cyst, tumor, or proliferation of sinus fat, in which overall bulk is preserved at the expense of renal parenchyma.

The advent of cross-sectional reconstructive techniques such as ultrasonography, computed tomography, and magnetic resonance imaging has obviated many, although not all, of the aforementioned problems. The following paragraphs discuss the approaches that have been proposed as useful guidelines for the determination of normal renal size in adults. Studies on normal kidney size in infants and children have been more thorough than those in the adult. These latter studies are discussed at the end of this section.

Methods proposed for evaluating kidney size using traditional radiography or excretory urography have been either too cumbersome for clinical use or have been statistically invalid because of a wide range of normal values (Vuorinen et al., 1960; Karn, 1962; Möel, 1956, 1961; Ludin, 1967; Griffiths et al., 1975). However, some practical observations can be derived from these studies, which have established the greater size of the male kidney compared with the female kidney and the usually larger size of the left kidney compared with the right one. Also well established is a remarkable tendency toward symmetry in the size, shape, and thickness of parenchyma between the two kidneys of an individual (once the normal tendency of the left kidney to be slightly larger than the right is taken into account) and the decrease in renal size that occurs as part of the normal aging process. Marked alterations in the symmetry of an individual's kidneys, particularly of the thickness of renal parenchyma, should be regarded with suspicion (Hodson, 1960).

Ultrasonography, of all imaging techniques, is particularly applicable to the measurement of renal size, although some measurement-to-measurement variation does occur. The ultrasound image is undistorted by magnification and is a true measurement of renal dimension. In addition, views of the kidney can be generated in planes that allow easy measurement of length, width, and thickness. Renal volume can then be determined from these values, using the equation for an ellipsoid (Jones et al., 1983) or a modification of it (Hricak and Lieto, 1983). These same theoretical advantages apply to magnetic resonance imaging, although systematic studies have not been reported using this modality.

Computed tomographic data on adults relating renal parenchymal thickness, the transverse diame-

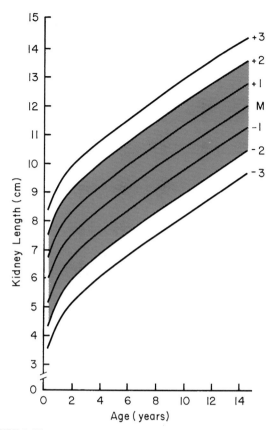

FIGURE 3–29. Graph of kidney length versus age based on excretory urograms in children. The plots include three standard deviations above and below the mean. One standard deviation = 0.785 cm. (From Currarino, G., et al.: Radiology *150*:703, 1984. Reproduced with kind permission of the author and *Radiology*.)

ANOMALOUS DEVELOPMENT OF THE KIDNEY AND URETER

Development of a normal kidney and ureter requires formation, elongation, and division of a ureteral bud; simultaneous induction of metanephric blastema into nephrons; dilatation and assimilation of early generations of ureteral bud divisions; and formation of independent renal lobes, most of which eventually fuse. This process begins in the caudal portion of the embryo when each ureteral bud encounters two parasagittal ridges of metanephric tissue situated medial to the umbilical arteries. As nephrogenesis progresses, the two kidneys separate laterally, and the pelvis and proximal ureter of each rotate medially toward the midline from an initial ventral position. However, a disturbance in any of these complex, concurrent developmental steps can produce anomalies in the shape, number, or position of the kidney and/or ureter. This section describes these anomalies. Other developmental abnormalities, such as multicystic dysplastic kidney, calyceal diverticula, megacalyces, ureteropelvic junction obstruction, megaureter, and ureterocele, are discussed in other chapters, in which their presentation is more consistent with the organization of this book.

Anomalies in Renal Form or Position

A disturbance in the separation of the two ridges of the metanephric blastema, in ureteral bud induction of metanephric tissue, or in the ascent and rotation of the kidney results in anomalous renal form or position. This type of anomaly is sometimes associated with anomalies of the ipsilateral genital organ or other organ systems or with genetic disorders such as Turner's syndrome, trisomy in identical twins, Fanconi's anemia, and Laurence-Moon-Biedl syndrome.

Agenesis. In agenesis, absence of a kidney is due to failure of a ureteral bud to form at all, failure of a growing ureteral bud to encounter and induce metanephric tissue, or absence of metanephric blastema. In the first situation, the ipsilateral trigone and ureteral orifice are also absent, a cystoscopic finding also described as hemitrigone. In the latter two situations, which are induction failures, a ureter of varying length ends blindly, usually in association with renal dysgenesis, as discussed below and in Chapter 11. Renal arteries and veins are absent in renal agenesis. With agenesis of the left kidney, the splenic flexure of the colon occupies the renal fossa on the same side, whereas the hepatic flexure migrates into the ipsilateral renal fossa when right-sided renal agenesis occurs. Renal agenesis often coexists with other anomalies. In particular, unilateral agenesis may be associated with absence of the ipsilateral adrenal gland and with abnormalities of ipsilateral genital structures. In males, these include cyst of the seminal vesicle, absent vas deferens, hypoplastic or absent testes, and hypospadias

---

ter of the vertebral body, and age have been formulated into a reference table of normal values (Gourtsoyiannis et al., 1990). A decrease in renal parenchymal thickness of about 10 per cent per decade has been found in both men and women throughout adulthood.

It is quite obvious that there are a number of approaches to determining normal renal size in the adult. Quantitative data are available and are useful to a certain point. More often than not, however, the qualitative evaluation of renal symmetry and uniformity of parenchymal thickness will be of greatest usefulness in any given individual.

The measurement of normal kidney size in infancy and childhood is subject to fewer vagaries than in the adult. Mean length related to age has been determined for excretory urography by Currarino and colleagues (1984). These data are reproduced in Figure 3–29. Nomograms relating sonographic kidney length to age, height, and weight have been determined by Han and Babcock (1985) and are reproduced in Figure 3–30. Ultrasonographic standards have also been established to relate kidney length to body weight in premature infants (Schlesinger et al., 1987; Fig. 3–31) and for fetal kidneys (Patten et al., 1990).

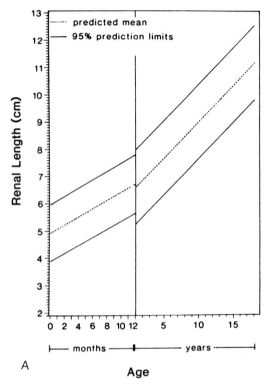

A

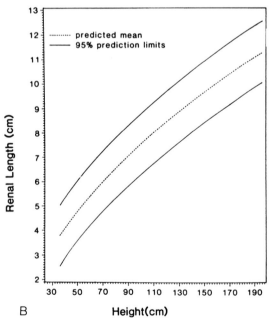

B

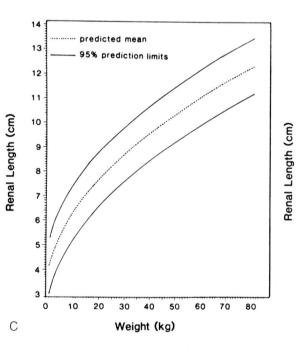

C

FIGURE 3–30. Graphs of maximum renal length versus age *(A)*, height *(B)*, and weight *(C)* based on ultrasonograms in children. (From Han, B. K., and Babcock, D. S.: AJR *145*:611, 1985. Reproduced with kind permission of the authors and the *American Journal of Roentgenology*.)

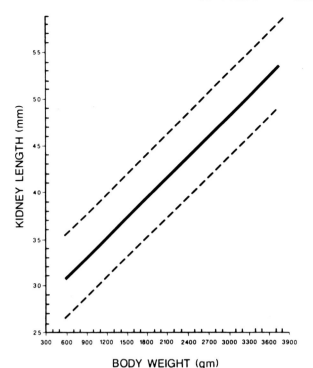

FIGURE 3–31. Nomogram for kidney length versus body weight derived from ultrasonograms in premature infants. The solid line represents the mean and the dotted line the 95 per cent confidence limits. (From Schlesinger, A. E., et al.: Radiology *164*:127, 1987. Reproduced with kind permission of the author and *Radiology*.)

(Fig. 3–32). In females, renal agenesis may be associated with uterine anomalies (agenesis, hypoplasia, unicornuate, bicornuate) or aplasia of the vagina (see Chapter 24).

Dysgenesis. Renal dysgenesis or dysplasia is a designation for undifferentiated renal tissue that has no resemblance to either normal kidney or kidney with acquired disease. When dysgenesis exists as an isolated event, the diagnosis is pathologic and does not have a radiologic counterpart. However, dysgenesis is often associated with multiple cysts in the affected kidney and atresia of the ureter, a condition known as *multicystic dysplastic kidney*. Additionally, dysgenesis is sometimes associated with anomalies in contralateral urinary tract structures. This subject is discussed in detail in Chapter 11.

Hypoplasia. The hypoplastic kidney results from a quantitative deficiency in the ureteral bud and metanephric primordia. This anomaly is discussed in Chapter 6 as one of the causes of the unilateral small, smooth kidney.

Ectopia. The position of the kidney and the associated length of the ureter are determined by the extent of ureteral bud elongation. Normally, the kidney is located in the abdomen, adjacent to the upper three lumbar vertebrae. When elongation of the ureteral bud ceases at a stage earlier than normal, the kidney is positioned in the pelvis or at the sacral or lower lumbar levels, and the ureter is of appropriate length (Figs. 3–33, 3–34, and 3–35). On

rare occasions, the kidney is intrathoracic. A true intrathoracic kidney occurs on the left side more often than on the right side and must be distinguished from displacement of the kidney into the thorax by means of a congenital or acquired diaphragmatic hernia. Ectopic kidneys are perfused by aberrant arteries from the aorta or from iliac arteries.

During elongation a ureteral bud may cross the midline either accompanied by the ipsilateral metanephric blastema or encountering the contralateral metanephric ridge. Here, the total renal mass becomes situated on one side of the abdomen. In this condition, known as crossed ectopia, the distal ureter inserts into the trigone on the side of origin (Fig. 3–36). Renal tissue in crossed ectopia is usually fused. Rarely are the two kidneys separate from each other. Invariably, ectopia is associated with aberrant renal arteries. Ectopia by itself is of no clinical significance.

Fusion. Fusion anomalies reflect disturbances in the early stage of renal organogenesis when both metanephric ridges lie adjacent to the midline. Presumably, fusion is a failure of separation of the ridges. *Lumps, cakes,* and *discs* are a few of the many terms used to describe the forms of fused kidneys (see Fig. 3–36), with *horseshoe kidney* the most frequently encountered form (Fig. 3–37). Here, the lower poles of both kidneys are joined by either renal or fibrous tissue. Rarely are they joined at the upper poles. Features of a horseshoe kidney include medial deviation of the lower poles, incomplete ascent (ectopia), and aberrant renal arteries. The fused lower pole is usually situated just caudal to the origin of the inferior mesenteric artery. The collecting systems and proximal ureters of a horseshoe kidney are located more ventral than normal. Occasionally, aberrant arteries cross and obstruct the proximal ureter or ureteropelvic junction on one or both sides. As a result, hydronephrosis, infection, and stone formation may complicate a horseshoe kidney (Fig. 3–38). An increased prevalence of Wilms' tumor has also been noted as another potential complication of horseshoe kidney. The perirenal spaces on both sides of the abdomen communicate with each other in a horseshoe kidney.

Rotation. Failure of medial rotation of the kidney during ascent is the cause of rotational anomalies. Most frequently, the collecting structures remain ventral to the renal parenchyma (Fig. 3–39). Very uncommonly, rotation occurs laterally on the long axis of the kidneys. This results in the renal artery and vein crossing the ventral surface of the kidney. Even more rare is longitudinal axis rotation beyond the medial position. In this circumstance, the pelvocalyceal system is directed toward a dorsal or dorsolateral position, and the renal artery and vein run over the dorsal surface of the kidney. Rotation on the anteroposterior axis of the kidney, although very rare, leads to a transverse position. Anomalies of ectopia, fusion, and rotation frequently coexist.

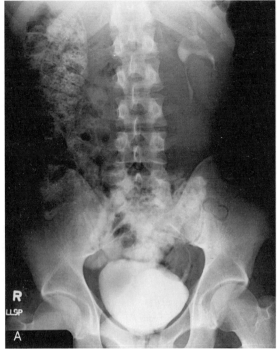

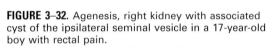

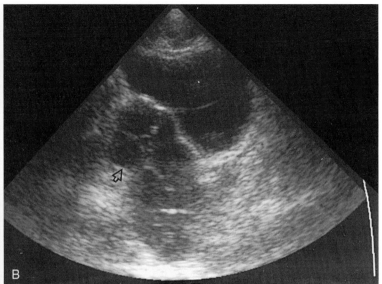

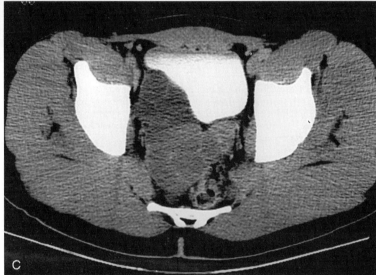

FIGURE 3–32. Agenesis, right kidney with associated cyst of the ipsilateral seminal vesicle in a 17-year-old boy with rectal pain.

A, Excretory urogram. The right kidney is absent, and there is compensatory hypertrophy of the left kidney. A mass effect is present on the right superolateral aspect of the bladder.

B, Ultrasonogram. Transverse projection. There is a multiloculated cyst *(arrow)* in the region of the seminal vesicle.

C, Computed tomogram, contrast material–enhanced. The seminal vesicle cyst impresses on the bladder.

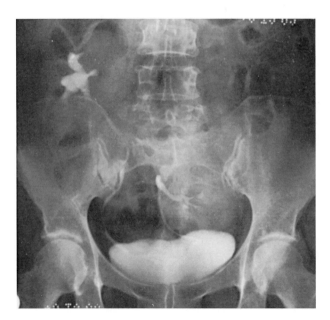

FIGURE 3–33. Bilateral renal ectopia. The left kidney is situated in the pelvis, whereas the right kidney is at the level of the lower lumbar vertebral segments. Excretory urogram.

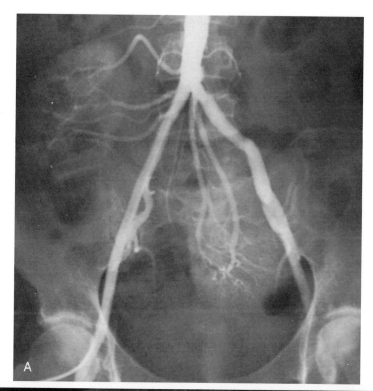

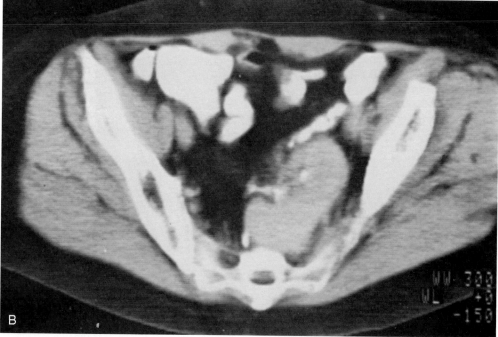

FIGURE 3–34. Renal ectopia. The left kidney is at the level of the sacrum and derives its arterial supply from a renal artery arising from the distal aorta.

   A, Aortogram. Note multiple aberrant renal arteries to a low-lying left kidney.

   B, Computed tomogram, contrast material–enhanced.

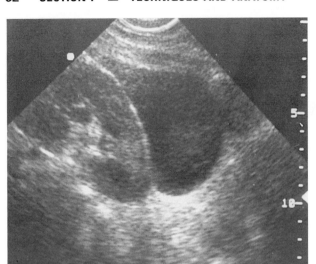

FIGURE 3–35. Renal ectopia. The kidney is situated in the pelvis cranial and posterior to the bladder. Ultrasonogram, sagittal section.

Anomalies in Number

Abnormality in the number or pattern of division of ureteral buds is the basis of this category of upper urinary tract anomalies.

Supernumerary Kidney. More than two kidneys and ureters form in the presence of an extra number of independent ureteral buds or from multiple early branches of a single ureteral bud. Any of these variations are extremely rare. Supernumerary kidneys are usually, though not invariably, caudal to the normal kidneys and hypoplastic.

Multiplications. Multiple ureteral buds arising

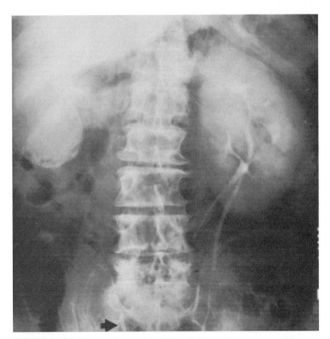

FIGURE 3–36. Crossed ectopia. The right ureter crosses the midline at the lower lumbar vertebral level and drains renal tissue fused with the left kidney. Note the orthotopic position of the right distal ureter *(arrow)*. Excretory urogram.

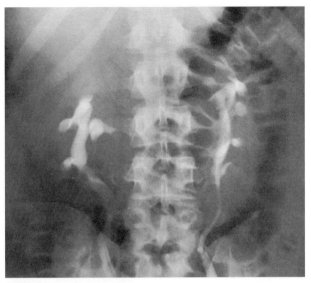

FIGURE 3–37. Renal fusion. Horseshoe kidney. The lower poles of each kidney are oriented medially, and the pelvis is placed laterally. Excretory urogram.

independently from the mesonephric duct or as early branches of a single ureteral bud are frequently encountered anomalies of the urinary tract. Complete duplication of the ureters draining a single kidney results from two ipsilateral, independent ureteral buds forming simultaneously from the mesonephric duct or very early branching of the ureteral bud with incorporation of each branch into the cloaca as separate structures. The moiety draining the upper pole has an ectopic distal insertion at a point caudal and medial to that of the moiety draining the lower pole. The sites of insertion of ectopic ureters in males and females are listed in descending order of frequency in Table 3–2. The lower pole moiety inserts either at the normal, or orthotopic, site in the trigone of the bladder or more cranial and lateral than the normal site, where it is susceptible to vesicoureteral reflux. These relationships are expressed in the Weigert-Meyer law and illustrated schematically in Figure 3–40. The upper pole moiety is susceptible to obstruction either as a complication of the ectopic insertion or by an aberrant artery crossing its ureteropelvic junction. The ectopic ureteral orifice may prolapse into the blad-

TABLE 3–2. Sites of Insertion of Ectopic Ureters in Descending Order of Frequency

MALES	FEMALES
Trigone	Trigone
Bladder neck	Bladder neck
Prostatic utricle	*Urethra
Seminal vesicle	*Vestibule
Ejaculatory duct	*Vagina
Vas deferens	*Cervix/uterus
	*Gartner's duct
	*Distal to urogenital diaphragm and associated with incontinence

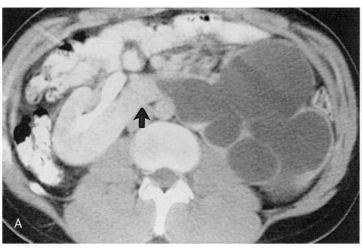

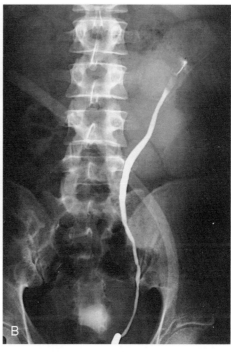

FIGURE 3–38. Horseshoe kidney with left-sided ureteropelvic junction obstruction.

A, Computed tomogram, contrast material–enhanced. There is marked hydronephrosis of the left kidney. Note medial position of the lower pole of the right kidney and fused tissue *(arrow).*

B, Retrograde pyelogram demonstrates an obstruction at the left ureteropelvic junction.

FIGURE 3–39. Failure of rotation and incomplete ascent of left kidney. The left renal pelvis remains ventral to the parenchyma, reflecting failure of medial rotation. Excretory urogram.

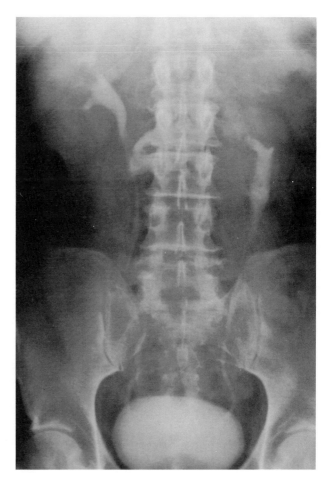

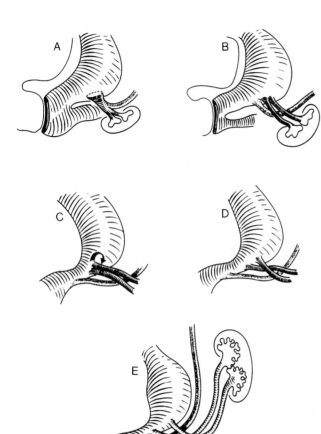

FIGURE 3–40. Embryologic development of complete duplication of the ureter and pelvocalyceal system.

A, There is early bifurcation of the ureteral bud.

B, The common portion of the distal mesonephric duct and ureteral bud are absorbed into the urogenital sinus such that the orifice of the mesonephric duct is caudal and medial to those of the two ureteral orifices.

C through *E,* There is continued absorption of the ureters into the trigone associated with medial rotation of the ureter draining the upper pole around the ureter draining the lower pole. (From Maizels, M.: Normal and anomalous development of the urinary tract. In Walsh, P. C., Retik, A. B., Vaughan, E. D., Jr., and Wein, A. J.: Campbell's Urology, 7th ed. Philadelphia, W. B. Saunders, 1998, p. 1576.)

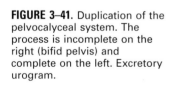

FIGURE 3–41. Duplication of the pelvocalyceal system. The process is incomplete on the right (bifid pelvis) and complete on the left. Excretory urogram.

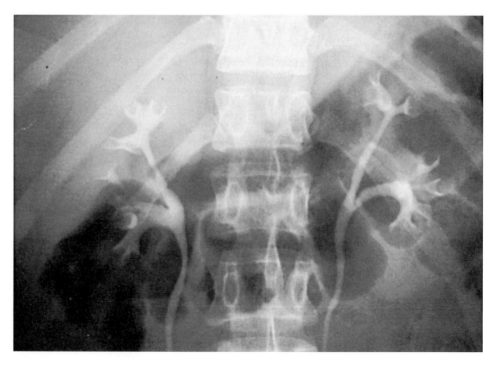

der, a condition known as ectopic ureterocele. The lower pelvocalyceal system moiety drains both the lower pole and the interpolar portion of the kidney and is subject to an increased incidence of vesicoureteral reflux when the intramural segment of its distal ureter is shortened by virtue of a slightly ectopic insertion. A kidney with a duplicated system is larger than normal, reflecting the influence of two ureteral buds inducing metanephric blastema. Kidneys with more than two independent ureters have rarely been reported. Duplication anomalies are discussed further in Chapters 9 and 15.

Duplication limited to the proximal portion of an otherwise unduplicated distal ureter with normal insertion into the bladder is the most common of the anomalies associated with ureteral bud division (Fig. 3–41). Here, the first division of the elongating ureteral bud occurs earlier than normal, and the two branches continue to elongate before beginning the series of branches that ultimately lead to formation of the pelvocalyceal system. Early first branching causes duplication of the distal ureter. Late duplication is seen as a bifid pelvis. The most cephalic branch of a duplicated ureter usually drains only the upper pole, whereas the remainder of the kidney is drained by the larger, inferior collecting system. Sometimes, the superior moiety of a duplicated ureter ends abruptly. This represents failure of the ureteral bud to encounter or induce metanephric blastema, a condition known as *blind-ending ureter* or *ureteral diverticulum* (Fig. 3–42). Rarely, one encounters more than two branches of a single ureter.

Duplication of a ureter, either complete or incomplete, is a precursor of abnormal placement of renal lobes or lobar dysmorphism. This is discussed in detail at the end of this section.

Abortive Calyx. A blind-ending, short outpouching of the renal pelvis is sometimes seen, usually in kidneys with a duplex collecting system. This diverticulum-like structure, believed to represent an abortive calyx, occasionally arises from the infundibulum draining the upper pole rather than directly from the pelvis itself. The direct relationship between this structure and the pelvis, or infundibulum, distinguishes it from a calyceal diverticulum, which arises from a calyceal fornix. The termination of an abortive calyx is blunt or spiked and is never invaginated by a papilla, as would be seen in a microcalyx or a calyx draining a dysmorphic lobe.

It is likely that an abortive calyx represents a ureteral bud branch that failed to continue to divide. This unusual structure must be distinguished from acquired diseases of an infundibulum or calyx, such as tuberculosis or tumor, that might mimic the appearance of this anomaly.

Unicalyceal (Unipapillary) Kidney. A small number of kidneys have been described as unicalyceal or unipapillary. The hallmark of this anomaly is a single collecting structure centrally located in the renal sinus and draining the entire kidney. This

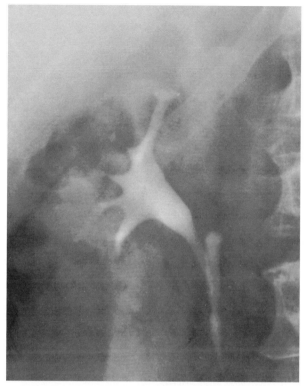

FIGURE 3–42. Blind-ending ureter. The superior moiety of a duplicated ureter ends abruptly. This represents failure of the ureteral bud to encounter or induce metanephric blastema. This is also known as ureteral diverticulum. Excretory urogram.

malformation is sometimes associated with absence of the contralateral kidney, hypertension, proteinuria, azotemia, or anomalies of other organ systems. Histologic study of a limited amount of material has demonstrated reduced numbers of nephrons with enlargement of individual glomeruli and tubules, a condition referred to as *oligomeganephronia*.

It is likely that the single collecting structure represents the renal pelvis and that calyces and papillae are absent owing to the failure of a complete set of ureteral bud branches in the 6th to 10th generations. In essence, the kidney is a single lobe whose ducts of Bellini drain directly into the pelvis.

Anomalies of Lobar Anatomy (Pseudotumor)

In a previous section of this chapter, the early, orderly arrangement of independent lobes into dorsal and ventral groupings and their subsequent fusion into an adult kidney form was described. During this process, a number of events may occur that distort the prototypical pattern of the kidney. One external cause is pressure from the adjacent spleen that changes the shape of the left kidney. Other distortions are due to the persistence of fetal features, the dominance of a part of a lobe, or the aberrant location of an entire lobe—normal variations that may simulate a tumor by causing either a focal bulge in the renal contour or a focal displacement of the pelvocalyceal system. For this reason, these distortions have been designated as renal pseudotumors. It is important to recognize the features that distinguish these normal variants from neoplasia if a costly and complex investigation or needless surgery is to be avoided. Usually, differentiation can be achieved by recognizing the characteristic radiologic features that are described below. Doubtful cases can virtually always be resolved by radionuclide imaging, using agents excreted by the renal tubules to demonstrate that the suspected mass is composed of normal tissue.

Splenic Impression. Flattening of the left kidney along its lateral or upper polar margin is frequently present (Fig. 3–43; see Fig. 3–22). Presumably, this impression on the renal contour is made by the spleen during the development of the left kidney. A bulge in the lateral margin of the kidney, just inferior to the flattened splenic impression, is a frequently associated finding that has been referred to as "dromedary hump." The normal nature of this variant shape is affirmed by the uniform thickness of the renal parenchyma between the surface of the kidney and the interpapillary line, particularly in the area of the bulge. Oblique films are often necessary to confirm this.

Fetal Lobation. The adult kidney sometimes retains sharp ridges on its surface, representing the sites where the septal cortices from two adjacent lobes abut (see Fig. 3–18). The centrilobar cortex between these ridges may be prominent and may be confused with neoplasm. This can be avoided by recognition of the characteristic features of fetal lobation, described earlier in this chapter.

Hilar Bulge. The parenchyma that composes the medial part of the kidney just above and below the sinus is often prominent, sometimes to the extent of causing focal displacement of the polar collecting system. This distortion is most frequently encountered in the suprahilar region of the left kidney.

Large Septum or Cloison of Bertin and Lobar Dysmorphism. There is a group of renal pseudotumors that is characterized by focal displacement of the collecting system within a kidney of normal contour. These pseudotumors usually occur in the presence of partial or complete duplication of the pelvocalyceal system, with the mass effect seen most frequently, although not invariably, in the area between the upper and interpolar portions of the kidney. In many instances, what causes the mass effect is normal septal cortex tissue that has persisted during lobar fusion and in the process has become relatively prominent (Figs. 3–44 and 3–45). This situation has been termed *large column of Bertin, large cloison, focal cortical hyperplasia, benign cortical rest, cortical island,* and *focal renal hypertrophy. Large septum* or *cloison of Bertin* is the most accurate term. In addition to their usual location in a partial or complete duplicated collecting system, these "masses" have a pattern of contrast material enhancement that is characteristic of cortex rather than medulla. Large cloisons are drained by calyces that are connected to the midportion of the pelvis by short infundibula (see Fig. 3–44). Sometimes, a papilla arises from the enlarged cortical tissue directly into the pelvis or an infundibulum. This form of aberrant papilla may be confused with a nonopaque filling defect in the collecting system.

Lobar dysmorphism is another form of pseudotumor that is very similar to large cloison (Fig. 3–46). Here, a complete, although diminutive, lobe is situated atypically, deep within the renal substance. As with a large cloison, this occurs in the region of a partial or complete duplication of the collecting system and will focally displace the pelvis or calyces. The presence of a complete lobe, rather than septal tissue alone, is suggested by a well-formed, although diminutive, calyx in the central portion of the mass. The normal lobar structure is well illustrated by angiography, which demonstrates early

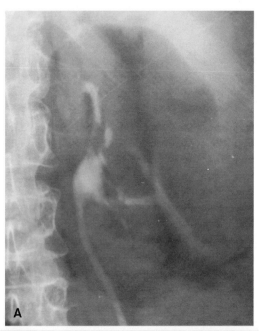

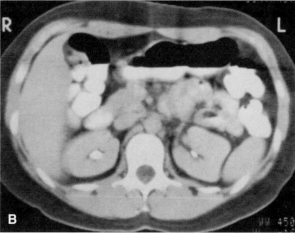

FIGURE 3–43. Splenic impression. Two different cases in which an enlarged spleen has effaced the lateral margin of the left kidney, producing a pseudotumor.

A, Excretory urogram.

B, Computed tomogram, contrast material–enhanced.

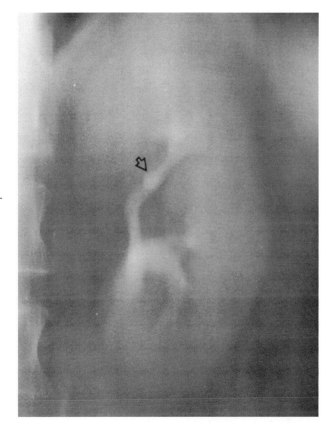

FIGURE 3–44. Pseudotumor due to large septum (cloison) of Bertin. The renal tissue projects between the moieties of a duplicated system and slightly displaces the upper pole collecting system. Note the characteristic calyx draining into the upper pole infundibulum *(arrow)*. Excretory urogram.

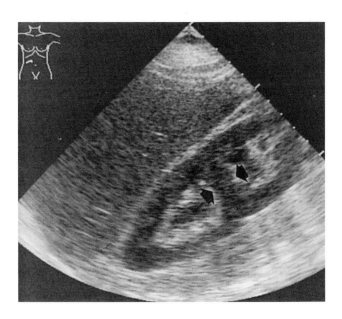

FIGURE 3–45. Pseudotumor due to large septum (cloison) of Bertin. The cortical tissue *(arrows)* projects between the two hyperechogenic regions of the renal sinus that contain the duplicated pelvocalyceal system. (From Dalla Palma, L., et al.: Br. J. Radiol. *63*:680, 1990. Reproduced with kind permission of the author and the *British Journal of Radiology.*)

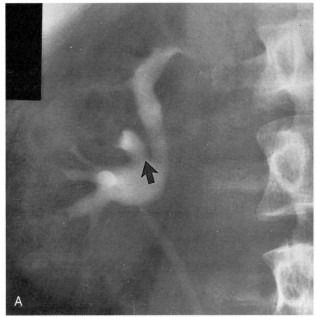

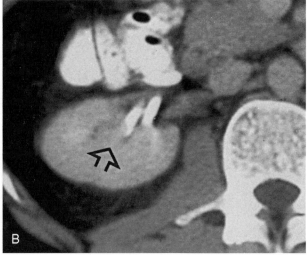

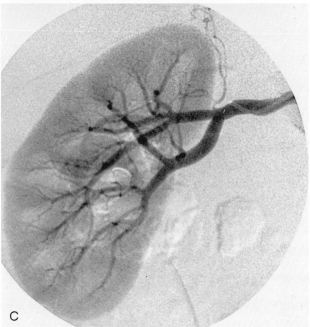

FIGURE 3–46. Pseudotumor due to lobar dysmorphism.
A, Excretory urogram. There is a medially situated calyx and infundibulum associated with the superior portion of a bifid pelvis *(arrow)*.
B, Computed tomogram, contrast material–enhanced. The dysmorphic lobe is dorsal and medial and comprises normally enhancing parenchyma *(arrow)*.
C, Selective renal arteriogram, arterial phase. Normal vascularity is present.

opacification of the septal cortex surrounding a relatively radiolucent medulla, the central location of the microcalyx and papilla, and a set of arcuate arteries serving the diminutive lobe. In clinical practice, the normal nature of the tissue causing this form of pseudotumor can be confirmed by radionuclide techniques when necessary.

Nodular Compensatory Hypertrophy. In the presence of focal renal scarring from infection or ischemia, areas of unaffected normal tissue will undergo compensatory hypertrophy, giving rise to a pseudotumor. This nodular pattern of renal enlargement is seen in severe cases of multifocal reflux nephropathy (see Fig. 5–15). Focal enlargement of deeply situated septal cortex has also been described in analgesic nephropathy (see Chapter 13).

Recognition of these pseudotumors as a component of a pathologic process should not be difficult.

Anomalies of Renal Arteries

Aberrant renal arteries arise from the aorta between T-11 and L-4 and occur in approximately 25 per cent of all individuals. They are persistent mesonephric vessels and usually perfuse one of the poles. Uncommonly, the aberrant artery may enter the kidney directly in the region perfused through an accessory renal hilum (Fig. 3–47).

Anomalies of Renal Veins

In approximately 85 per cent of individuals, a single vein forms in the right renal hilum and follows a

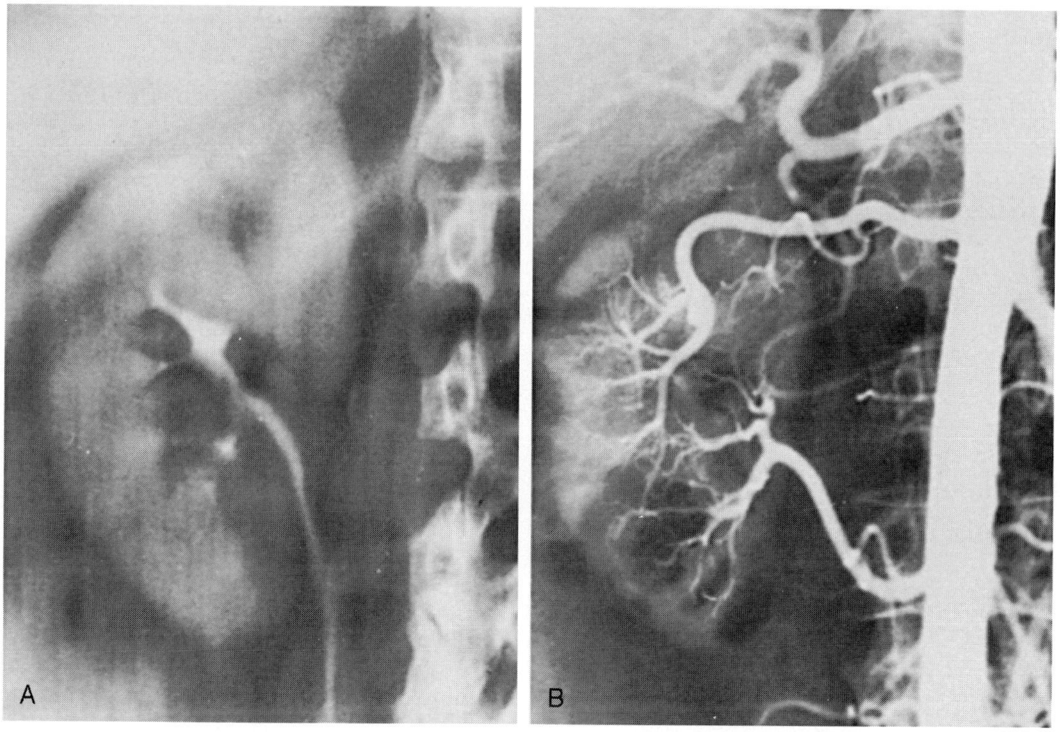

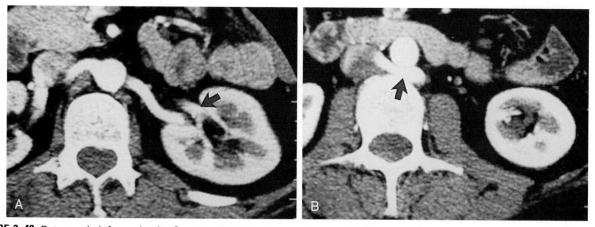

FIGURE 3–47. Aberrant renal arteries with accessory renal hilum. The kidney is perfused by two renal arteries arising directly from the aorta. The superior vessel enters the upper pole through an accessory hilum.
  A, Excretory urogram. Tomogram.
  B, Aortogram. (Courtesy of T. F. Stephenson, M.D., St. Mary's Hospital, Rochester, New York, and AJR *132*:765, 1979.)

slightly oblique cephalad course to its junction with the inferior vena cava. Multiple right renal veins occur in approximately 15 per cent of the population. Capsular, ureteric, and retroperitoneal veins usually drain into the right renal venous system, whereas the right adrenal and gonadal veins usually drain directly into the inferior vena cava.

The left renal vein arises in the left renal hilum, follows a horizontal course between the aorta and the superior mesenteric artery, and drains into the inferior vena cava. A single, preaortic left renal vein, which is encountered in approximately 80 per cent of patients, receives tributaries from the ipsi-

lateral adrenal and gonadal veins as well as the inferior phrenic, capsular, and ureteric veins. Anastomoses also exist between the left renal vein and the hemiazygos and ascending lumbar veins. The most common anomaly of the left renal venous system is a *circumaortic renal vein,* which has been reported in up to 16 per cent of individuals. Here, the common renal vein that arises in the renal hilum bifurcates into a ventral and dorsal limb. The ventral limb, which is often dominant, follows the preaortic course of a normal renal vein and receives adrenal and gonadal venous blood. The dorsal limb passes in an inferomedial direction, crosses behind

FIGURE 3–48. Retroaortic left renal vein. Computed tomogram, contrast material–enhanced.
  A, Image obtained at the level of the left renal hilus demonstrates origin of the left renal vein *(arrow).*
  B, Image obtained at the level of the lower pole of the kidney demonstrates the retroaortic course of the renal vein *(arrow).*

the aorta, and enters the inferior vena cava in the lower lumbar region. A second anomaly, *retroaortic left renal vein*, has been reported in up to 3 per cent of the population. In this variant, a single left renal vein follows an inferomedial course behind the aorta and drains into the lower lumbar portion of the inferior vena cava (Fig. 3–48; see Fig. 21–44). In the retroaortic renal vein, the left adrenal and gonadal veins join as a single structure that follows the usual preaortic course of the normal left renal vein. In either the circumaortic or retroaortic anomaly of the left renal vein, cross-sectional images of the retroaortic component may simulate lymphadenopathy.

Retrocaval Ureter

A retrocaval ureter is due to anomalous persistence of the posterior cardinal vein during the develop-

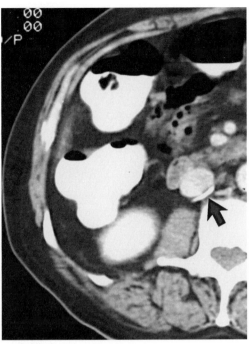

FIGURE 3–50. Retrocaval ureter. Transverse cross section at the level of the lower pole of the right kidney demonstrates the proximal ureter as it passes posterior to the inferior vena cava *(arrow).* Computed tomogram, contrast material–enhanced.

ment of the inferior vena cava. As a result, the right ureter deviates sharply from its normal position lateral to the inferior vena cava and passes posterior and medial to the inferior vena cava at the level of the third or fourth lumbar vertebral bodies. From this point distally, the ureter partially encircles the vena cava as it moves anterior and then lateral to the vena cava to resume its normal position (Figs. 3–49 and 3–50).

In many instances, the retrocaval ureter is asymptomatic. However, obstruction at the site of proximal deviation can cause flank pain or be complicated by urinary tract infection.

BIBLIOGRAPHY

Anatomy

Ablett, M. J., Coulthard, A., Lee, R. E. J., Richardson, D. L., Bellas, T., Owen, J. P., Keir, M. J., and Butler, T. J.: How reliable are ultrasound measurements of renal length in adults? Br. J. Radiol. *468*:1087, 1995.

Adams, E. J., Desai, S. C., and Lawton, G.: Racial variations in normal ureteric course. Clin. Radiol. *36*:373, 1985.

Bischel, M. D., Blustein, W. C., Kinnas, N. C., Valaitis, J., and Rubenstein, M.: Solitary renal calix. JAMA *240*:2467, 1978.

Brandt, T. D., Neiman, H. L., Dragowski, M. J., Bulawa, W., and Claykamp, G.: Ultrasound assessment of normal renal dimensions. J. Ultrasound Med. Biol. *1*:49, 1982.

Carter, A. R., Horgam, J. G., Jennings, T. A., and Rosenfield, A. T.: The junctional parenchymal defect: A sonographic variant of renal anatomy. Radiology *154*:499, 1985.

Cohen, H. L., Cooper, J., Eisenberg, P., Mandel, F. S., Gross, B. R., Goldman, M. A., Barzel, E., and Rawlinson, K. F.: Normal length of fetal kidneys: Sonographic study in 397 obstetric patients. AJR *157*:545, 1991.

Currarino, G., Williams, B., and Dana, K.: Kidney length corre-

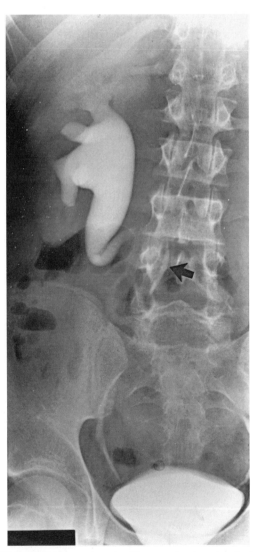

FIGURE 3–49. Retrocaval ureter. The proximal ureter deviates sharply in a cranial direction and then courses medial to the right pedicle of the fifth lumbar vertebral body *(arrow)* before resuming a normal position at the pelvic brim. Excretory urogram.

lated with age: Normal values in children. Radiology 150:703, 1984.

Dalla Palma, L., Bazzocchi, M., Cressa, C., and Tommasini, G.: Radiological anatomy of the kidney revisited. Br. J. Radiol. 63:680, 1990.

DeSanctis, J. T., Connolly, S. A., and Bramson, R. T.: Effect of patient position on sonographically measured renal length in neonates, infants and children. AJR 170:1381, 1998

Dinkel, E., Ertel, M., and Dittrick, M.: Kidney size in childhood: Sonographical growth charts for kidney length and volume. Pediatr. Radiol. 15:38, 1985.

Dorph, S., Sovak, M., Talner, L. B., and Rosen, L.: Why does kidney size change during I.V. urography? Invest. Radiol. 12:246, 1977.

Effman, R. L., Ablow, R. C., and Siegel, N. J.: Renal growth. Radiol. Clin. North Am. 15:3, 1977.

Elkin, M.: Radiology of the urinary tract: Some physiological considerations. Radiology 116:259, 1975.

Emamian, S. A., Nielsen, M. B., Pedersen, J. F., and Ytte, L.: Kidney dimensions at sonography: Correlation with age, sex, and habitus in 665 adult volunteers. AJR 160:83, 1993.

Emamian, S. A., Nielsen, M. B., Pedersen, J. F., and Ytte, L.: Sonographic evaluation of renal appearance in 655 adult volunteers—correlation with age and obesity. Acta Radiol. 29:482, 1993.

Ferrer, F. A., McKenna, P. H., Bauer, M. B., and Miller, S. F.: Accuracy of renal ultrasound measurements for predicting actual kidney size. J. Urol. 157:2278, 1997.

Fine, H., and Keen, E. N.: Some observations on the medulla of the kidney. Br. J. Urol. 48:161, 1976.

Frimann-Dahl, J.: Normal variations of left kidney. Acta Radiol. 55:207, 1961.

Gourtsoyiannis, N., Prassopoulos, P., Cavouras, D., and Pantelidis, N.: The thickness of the renal parenchymal decreases with age: A CT study of 360 patients. AJR 155:541, 1990.

Griffiths, G. J., Cartwright, G., and McLachlan, M. S. F.: Estimation of renal size from radiographs: Is the effort worthwhile? Clin. Radiol. 26:249, 1975.

Han, B. K., and Babcock, D. S.: Sonographic measurements and appearance of normal kidney in children. AJR 145:611, 1985.

Hinman, F., Jr.: Atlas of UroSurgical Anatomy. Philadelphia, W.B. Saunders Co., 1993.

Hodson, C. J.: Hypertension of renal origin. In McLaren, J. W. (ed.): Modern Trends in Diagnostic Radiology. New York, Paul B. Hoeber, 1960, pp. 124–134.

Hodson, C. J.: The lobar structure of the kidney. Br. J. Urol. 44:246, 1972.

Hodson, C. J., and Mariani, S.: Large cloisons. AJR 139:327, 1982.

Hoeltl, W., Hruby, W., Aharinejad, S.: Renal vein anatomy and its implications for retroperitoneal surgery. J. Urol. 143:1108, 1990.

Hoffer, F. A., Hanabongh, A. M., and Teele, R. L.: The interrenicular junction—a mimic of renal scarring on normal paediatric sonograms. AJR 145:1075, 1985.

Howlett, D. C., Greenwood, K. L., Jarosz, J. M., MacDonald, L. M., and Saunders, A. J. S.: The incidence of transient renal medullary hyperechogenicity in neonatal ultrasound examination. Br. J. Radiol. 70:140, 1997.

Hricak, H., and Lieto, R. P.: Sonographic determination of renal volume. Radiology 148:311, 1983.

Jones, T. B., Riddick, L. R., Harpen, M. D., Dubuisson, R. L., and Samuels, D.: Ultrasonic determination of renal mass and renal volume. J. Ultrasound Med. Biol. 2:151, 1983.

Karn, M. N.: Radiographic measurements of kidney section area. Ann. Hum. Genet. 25:379, 1962.

Kasike, B. L., and Umen, A. J.: The influence of age, sex, race and body habitus on kidney weight in humans. Arch. Pathol. Lab. Med. 110:55, 1986.

Kenney, I. J., Wild, S. R.: The renal parenchymal junctional line in children: Ultrasonic frequency and appearances. Br. J. Radiol. 60:865, 1987.

Korenchevsky, V.: Natural relative hypoplasia of organs and process of aging. J. Pathol. 54:13, 1942.

Lewis, E., and Ritchie, W. G. M.: A simple ultrasonic method for assessing renal size. J. Clin. Ultrasound 8:417, 1980.

Ludin, H.: Radiologic estimation of kidney weight. Acta Radiol. (Diagn.) 6:561, 1967.

McCrory, W. W.: Developmental Nephrology. Cambridge, Massachusetts, Harvard University Press, 1972.

Miletic, D., Fuckar, Z., Sustic, A., Mozetic, V., Stimac, D., and Zauhar, G.: Sonographic measurement of absolute and relative renal length in adults. J. Clin. Ultrasound 26:185, 1998.

Möel, H.: Size of normal kidneys. Acta Radiol. (Diagn.) 46:640, 1956.

Möel, H.: Kidney size and its deviation from normal in acute renal failure: A roentgen diagnostic study. Acta Radiol. (Diagn.) 56(Suppl. 206):5, 1961.

Ohlson, L.: Normal collecting ducts and visualization of urography. Radiology 170:33, 1989.

Oliver, J.: Nephrons and Kidneys: A Quantitative Study of Developmental and Evolutionary Mammalian Renal Architectonics. New York, Harper & Row, 1968.

Patriquin, H., Lefaivre, J. F., Lafortune, M., Russo, P., and Boisvert, J.: Fetal lobation: An anatomo-ultrasonographic correlation. J. Ultrasound Med. 9:191, 1990.

Patten, R. M., Mack, L. A., Wang, K. Y., and Cyr, D. R.: The fetal genitourinary tract. Radiol. Clin. North Am. 28:115, 1990.

Pendergrass, E. P.: Excretory urography as a test of urinary tract function. Radiology 40:223, 1943.

Potter, E. L.: Normal and Abnormal Development of the Kidney. Chicago, Year Book Medical Publishers, 1972.

Ransley, P. G.: Intrarenal reflux: Anatomical, dynamic and radiological studies. Part I. Urol. Res. 5:61, 1977.

Ransley, P. G., and Risdon, R. A.: Renal papillary morphology in infants and young children. Urol. Res. 3:111, 1975.

Ransley, P. G., and Risdon, R. A.: Reflux and renal scarring. Br. J. Radiol Suppl. 14, 1978.

Ransley, P. G., and Risdon, R. A.: The renal papilla, intrarenal reflux and chronic pyelonephritis. In Hodson, J., and Kincaid-Smith, P. (eds.): Reflux Nephropathy. New York, Masson Publishing, 1979, pp. 126–133.

Saxton, H. M.: Opacification of collecting ducts at urography. Radiology 170:16, 1989.

Schlesinger, A. E., Hedlund, G. L., Pierson, W. P., and Null, D. M.: Normal standards for kidney length in premature infants: Determination with US. Radiology 164:127, 1987.

Scott, J. E., Hunter, E. W., Lee, R. E., and Matthews, J. N.: Ultrasound measurement of renal size in newborn infants. Arch. Dis. Child. 65:361, 1990.

Sherwood, T. and Williams, D. I.: Post-obstructive renal atrophy, megacalices, hydrocalices. Conversations Radiol. 1:5, 1973.

Sykes, D.: The correlation between renal vascularization and lobulation of the kidney. Br. J. Urol. 36:549, 1964.

Sykes, D.: The morphology of renal lobulations and calices and their relationship to partial nephrectomy. Br. J. Surg. 51:294, 1964.

Thakur, V., and Watkins, T.: Is kidney length a good predictor of kidney volume? Am. J. Med. Sci. 313:85, 1997.

Thomsen, H. S., Larsen, S., and Talner, L. B.: Papillary morphology in adult human kidneys and in body and adult pig kidneys. Eur. Urol. 9:170, 1983.

Thornburn, G. D., Kopald, H. H., Herd, J. A., Hollenberg, M., O'Morchoe, C. C., and Barger, A. C.: Intrarenal distribution of nutrient blood flow determined with krypton[85] in the unanesthetized dog. Circ. Res. 13:290, 1963.

Troell, S., Berg, V., and Johansson, B.: Renal parenchymal volume in children: Normal value assessed by ultrasonography. Acta Radiol. 29:127, 1988.

Tublin, M. E., Tessler, F. N., McCauley, T. R., and Kesack, C. D.: Effect of hydration status on renal medulla attenuation on unenhanced CT scans. AJR 168:257, 1997.

Verschuyl, E. J., Kaatee, R., Beek, F. J. A., Pasterkamp, G., Bush, W. H., Beutler, J. J., vanderVen, P. J. G., and Mali, W. P. T. M.: Renal artery origins: Location and distribution in the transverse plane at CT. Radiology 203:71, 1997.

Verschuyl, E. J., Kaatee, R., Beek, F. J. A., Patel, N. H., Fontaine, A. B., Daly, C. P., Coldwell, D. M., Bush, W. H., and Mali, W. P. T. M.: Renal artery origins: Best angiographic projection angles. Radiology 205:115, 1997.

Vuorinen, P., Pyykönen, L., and Antilla, P.: A renal cortical index obtained from urography films. Br. J. Radiol. 33:622, 1960.

Wald, H.: The weight of normal adult human kidneys and its variability. Arch. Pathol. Lab. Med. *23*:493, 1937.

Ward, J. P., Franklin, D. A., and Wickham, J. E. A.: A computer-based technique for measurement of renal parenchymal area on intravenous urograms. Br. J. Radiol. *49*:836, 1976.

Whitehouse, R. W.: High- and low-osmolar contrast agents in urography: A comparison of the appearances with respect to pyelotubular opacification and renal length. Clin. Radiol. *37*:395, 1986.

Yeh, H. C., Halton, K. P., Shapiro, R. S., Rabinowitz, J. G., and Mitty, H. A.: Junctional parenchyma: Revised definition of hypertrophic column of Bertin. Radiology *185*:725, 1992.

Anomalies

Beckmann, C. F., and Abrams, H. L.: Circumaortic venous ring: incidence and significance. AJR *132*:561, 1979.

Cook, W. A., and Stephens, F. D.: Fused kidneys: Morphologic study and theory of embryogenesis. Birth Defects *13*:329, 1977.

Cope, J. R., and Trickey, S. E.: Congenital absence of the kidney: Problems in diagnosis and management. J. Urol. *127*:10, 1982.

Dacie, J. E.: The "central lucency" sign of lobar dysmorphism (pseudotumour of the kidney). Br. J. Radiol. *49*:39, 1976.

Decter, R. M.: Renal duplication and fusion anomalies. Pediatr. Clin. North Am. *44*:1323, 1997.

Feldman, A. E., Pollack, H. M., Perri, A. J., Jr., Karafin, L., and Kendall, A. R.: Renal pseudotumors: An anatomic-radiologic classification. J. Urol. *120*:133, 1978.

Feldman, A. E., Rosenthal, R. S., and Shaw, J. L.: Aberrant renal papilla: A diagnostic dilemma. J. Urol. *114*:144, 1975.

Fernbach, S. K., Feinstein, K. A., Spencer, K., and Lindstrom, C. A.: Ureteral duplication and its complications. Radiographics *17*:109, 1997.

Friedland, G. W.: Congenital anomalies of the urinary tract. In Friedland, G. W., et al. (eds.): Uroradiology: An Integrated Approach. New York, Churchill Livingstone, 1983, pp. 1349–1519.

Friedland, G. W., and DeVries, P.: Renal ectopia and fusion: Embryologic basis. Urology *5*:698, 1975.

Gluer, S., Kluth, D., Reich, P., and Lambrecht, W.: The development of common nephric duct and its significance in upper urinary tract abnormalities. Pediatr. Surg. Int. *8*:34, 1993.

Hohenfeller, M., Schultz-Lampel, D., Lampel, A., Steinbach, F., Cramer, B. M., and Thuroff, J. W.: Tumor in the horseshoe kidney: Clinical implications and review of embryogenesis. J. Urol. *147*:1098, 1992.

Kellman, G. M., Alpern, M. B., Sandler, M. A., and Craig, B. M.: Computed tomography of vena caval anomalies with embryologic correlation. RadioGraphics 8:533, 1988.

Kunin, M.: The abortive calix: Variations in appearance and differential diagnosis. AJR *139*:931, 1982.

Lafortune, M., Constantin, A., Breton, G., and Vallee, C.: Sonography of the hypertrophied column of Bertin. AJR *146*:53, 1986.

Leekam, R. N., Matzinger, M. A., Brunelle, M., Gray, R. R., and Grossman, H.: The sonography of renal columnar hypertrophy. J. Clin. Ultrasound *11*:491, 1983.

Mesrobian, H.-G. J., Kelalis, P. P., Hrabovsky, E., Othersen, H. B., Jr., deLorimer, A., and Nesbeth, B.: Wilms tumor in horsehoe kidneys: A report from the national Wilms tumor study. J. Urol. *133*:1002, 1985.

Murphy, B. J., Casillas, J., and Becerra, J. L.: Retrocaval ureter: Computed tomography and ultrasound appearance. J. Comput. Tomogr. *11*:89, 1987.

N'Guessan, G., and Stephens, F. D.: Supernumerary kidney. J. Urol. *130*:649, 1983.

Peterson, J. E., Pinckney, L. E., Rutledge, J. C., and Currarino, G.: The solitary renal calyx and papilla in human kidneys. Radiology *144*:525, 1982.

Pollack, H. M., Edell, S., and Morales, J. D.: Radionuclide imaging in renal pseudotumors. Radiology *111*:639, 1974.

Sarajlic, M., Durst-Zivkovic, B., Svoren, E., Vitkovic, M., Batinic, D., Bradic, I., and Vuckovic, I.: Congenital ureteric diverticula in children and adults: Classification, radiological and clinical features. Br. J. Radiol. *62*:551, 1989.

Stephenson, T. F., and Paul, G. J.: Accessory renal hilus. AJR *132*:765, 1979.

Webb, J. A. W., Fry, I. K., and Charlton, C. A. C.: An anomalous calyx in the mid-kidney: An anatomical variant. Br. J. Radiol. *48*:674, 1975.

RENAL PARENCHYMAL DISEASE

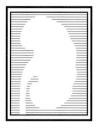

4

A Systematic Approach to the Radiologic Diagnosis of Parenchymal Disease of the Kidney

The anatomic information presented in the preceding chapter is but one of two necessary elements in organizing an orderly approach to the radiologic study of renal disease. The other is understanding how the many different pathologic processes that affect the kidney may manifest themselves radiologically. Obviously, some diseases of the kidney produce lesions detectable only by electron or light microscopy; others are best diagnosed by characteristic abnormalities of renal function or urine content. In these circumstances, the radiologist's role, if any, is limited to defining broad categories, such as acute or chronic, or to excluding other disease processes. On the other hand, radiology is unique among the clinical disciplines in its ability to reveal the kidney as a whole *in vivo*. Analysis of kidney size, contour, nephrogram, calyceal and papillary morphology, and many other features detectable by a variety of imaging modalities may at times provide a more precise clinical diagnosis than can be achieved by microscopic study of needle biopsy tissue or by measurement of various renal function tests.

What is necessary, then, is for the radiologist to organize his or her knowledge of how the kidney responds to various diseases within a framework of what might be detectable by radiologic techniques. This can be accomplished in three ways. First, the impact of a given disease on renal size can be evaluated because many diseases cause either an increase or a decrease in renal bulk. Second, the appearance of the nephrogram and/or the renal contour can be used as an index of the distribution of lesions within the kidney. For example, diseases that cause a loss of renal tissue characteristically limited to a part or all of a lobe produce focal scars in the contour of the kidney. On the other hand, a smooth renal contour and a homogeneous nephrogram will be preserved by processes that are uniformly distributed throughout the entire kidney regardless of the impact on renal size. Other diseases, particularly those that increase renal bulk, inherently affect only portions of the kidney, either in one region or as a multifocal process. These patterns are reflected radiologically as either unifocal or multifocal nephrographic abnormalities with or without unifocal or multifocal bulges in the renal contour. Third, a determination can be made as to whether a given disease characteristically affects the kidney unilaterally or bilaterally. Thus, renal *size, nephrogram/contour,* and *laterality of involvement* provide points of departure for developing an orderly routine for analysis of radiologic images and for establishing an organized categorical framework for the radiologic diagnosis of renal parenchymal disease.

In the sections that follow, pathologic processes are studied in terms of how they alter tissue bulk and their distribution within the renal parenchyma. These considerations provide the basis for classifying a large number of diseases according to their effect on renal size, nephrogram, and contour. These "pathologic-radiologic" categories are refined further by distinguishing diseases that are inherently unilateral from those that are inherently bilateral in their effects. These smaller groups are designated *diagnostic sets.* Finally, radiologic features (called "secondary uroradiologic observations") other than size, nephrogram/contour, and laterality of involvement are used to identify individual diseases within each diagnostic set.

Before proceeding, however, it should be pointed out that in the course of disease, the kidney often will progress from a large to a small size, inevitably passing through an intermediate period in which its size is within the radiologic limits of normal. Likewise, the development of contour abnormalities, such as scars, is not an overnight phenomenon. The reader should therefore keep in mind that assigning each disease to a radiologic classification based on size, nephrogram/contour, and laterality is perforce somewhat arbitrary and likely to be controversial—but also convenient, efficient, and quite accurate. Assignment of each disease to its diagnostic set has been based either on its most commonly presenting form or on the state of activity during which the radiologist is most likely to encounter it in a clinical setting.

PATHOLOGIC-RADIOLOGIC CONSIDERATIONS

Processes Leading to Loss of Renal Tissue

Reflux Nephropathy (Chronic Atrophic Pyelonephritis). Reflux nephropathy involves extensive tubule atrophy and loss, leukocytic infiltration, and marked fibrosis. The lesion tends to be distributed through the full thickness of all or part of a renal lobe, from centrilobar cortex to papilla. Other areas of the lobe adjacent to the lesion may be normal. The combination of dense fibrosis and full-thickness involvement causes a focal reduction and complete disorganization of the affected renal tissue. Retraction occurs at the external margin of the lobe, at the centrilobar cortex, and at the papillary tip. This is seen radiologically as a focal contour depression overlying a calyx that has become dilated because of papillary retraction and scarring.

The lesion of reflux nephropathy is occasionally limited to a part or the whole of a single lobe, usually in one of the poles of an otherwise normal kidney. Often, however, multiple foci are found in one or both kidneys. In this situation, the disease occurs and progresses independently at each site. Therefore, although reflux nephropathy is inherently a focal disease of a single renal lobe, it may be found at random in many areas of the kidney, producing a radiologic image of multiple contour depressions overlying dilated subservient calyces. Normal tissue occupies intervening areas. This process is illustrated diagrammatically in Figure 4–1.

Lobar Infarction. Lobar infarction also causes tissue loss but in a significantly different manner from that seen in reflux nephropathy. When one or more interlobar or arcuate arteries are occluded, infarction develops in the peripheral portion of the lobe, because this part is perfused by fewer vessels than the inner lobe, and these vessels are end-arteries. The infarcted area is seen on a cut section of the lobe as a triangular area, with its base on the centrilobar cortex and its apex extending to a variable depth into the medulla. If more than one of the interlobar or arcuate arteries subserving the involved lobe is occluded, the cortical base of the infarct is likely to be situated in the middle of the centrilobar cortex, whereas if only a single vessel is involved, the infarcted area will be eccentrically located on one margin of the centrilobar cortex. Attention to the limited area subserved by each arcuate artery in Figure 3–5 provides an explanation for this pattern.

FOCAL LOSS OF RENAL TISSUE

Reflux Nephropathy

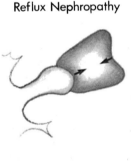

Lobar Infarction

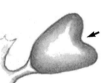

Papillary Necrosis

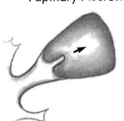

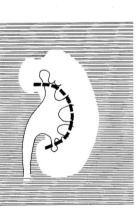

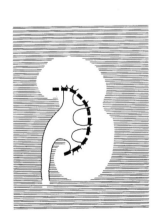

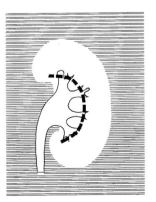

FIGURE 4–1. Patterns of lobar response to diseases producing focal loss of renal substance.

In addition to the peripheral distribution of the infarct lesion, it is characteristic of infarction to cause tissue loss by a "dropping out" of nephrons without a significant fibrotic response. This is in sharp contrast to the important role of fibroblasts in the production of the reflux nephropathy scar. The scar that forms in lobar infarction, therefore, is a reflection of tissue loss due to the disappearance of the dead tubules, not active retraction secondary to fibrosis. This scarring process, plus the peripheral location of the lesion in the lobe, leaves the papilla undisturbed. Thus, the radiologic hallmark of lobar infarction is a contour defect overlying a normal papilla and calyx. This may occur either singly or at multiple foci, depending on the number of vessels randomly involved. Figure 4–1 schematizes this pattern.

Papillary Necrosis. Papillary necrosis is a pathologic process that occurs in the papillary portion of the medulla. The remainder of the lobe is involved only in a very advanced state of certain forms of the disease. Commonly, multiple papillae in one or both kidneys are abnormal, although the process occasionally may be limited to a single lobe.

Papillary necrosis begins with a stage of necrobiosis of the loops of Henle and the vasa recta at the tip of the papilla. This progresses to frank necrosis with a patchy distribution that eventually involves all elements of the papilla. These stages can be detected radiologically, beginning with simple enlargement of an otherwise normal papilla in the earliest period and progressing to include the appearance of fine projections of contrast material extending along the side of the involved papilla, irregularity of the papillary surface, medullary cavitation, and ultimately a complete slough of the papilla. The latter stage is illustrated in Figure 4–1. A late process, related only to the more fulminant forms of papillary necrosis associated with analgesic nephropathy, may involve the entire lobe with fine fibrosis of the interstitial tissue with chronic inflammatory cell infiltrates and tubule loss or atrophy. This stage of chronic interstitial nephritis produces uniform wasting of the entire kidney, which is seen radiologically as a global decrease in kidney size in addition to the usual abnormalities of papillary necrosis.

Global Tissue Loss. The global tissue loss category represents a large group of diseases that, apart from their characteristic smallness, lack distinguishing radiologic features. This category is a catchall for a number of specific diseases that vary widely in their histologic appearance, etiologic factors, and clinical significance. One common feature that binds these entities together in a pathologic-radiologic classification is the global distribution of their lesions. Tubule atrophy and a fine interstitial fibrosis account for much of the generalized tissue wasting, regardless of whether the pathologic process primarily involves arterioles, glomeruli, tubules, or the interstitium. Radiologically detectable

TABLE 4–1. Pathologic-Radiologic Classification of Entities Associated with Both Focal and Global Loss of Renal Tissue: Normal to Small Kidney

Lobar Tissue Loss
Reflux nephropathy (chronic atrophic pyelonephritis)
Lobar infarction
Papillary necrosis

Global Tissue Loss
Ischemia due to major arterial stenosis/aneurysm
Generalized arteriosclerosis
Benign and malignant nephrosclerosis
Atheroembolic renal disease
Chronic infarction
Chronic glomerulonephritis
Acquired cystic kidney disease
Radiation nephritis
Hereditary nephropathies
Congenital hypoplasia
Postobstructive atrophy
Postinflammatory atrophy
Reflux atrophy
Amyloidosis (late)
Arterial hypotension

focal scars and calyceal-papillary distortion are not features of disease in this category.

Table 4–1 includes a list of abnormalities that produce the indeterminate radiologic findings of small kidneys with smooth contours. Each of these in its usual form will present a radiologic picture of a normal-to-small–sized kidney with a smooth contour, although variations in this basic pattern do occur in certain diseases. These are discussed specifically in later chapters of this book.

Decreased excretion of contrast material is frequent and reflects the impairment of renal function commonly seen in many of these diseases. Renal parenchyma, as depicted by the interpapillary line, is, of course, thin. An occasional response to parenchymal tissue loss is proliferation of fat around the pelvis, infundibula, and calyces in the renal hilus, causing lack of distensibility and attenuation of the collecting system. One exception to these generalizations regarding tissue loss in the indeterminate small kidney is the kidney that shrinks as a result of arterial hypotension and depletion of renal blood volume, rather than loss of parenchyma per se. Radiologic changes seen in the global tissue loss category are schematized in Figure 4–2.

Processes Leading to Increase in Renal Bulk

Processes that increase renal bulk are either diffuse throughout the kidney, causing *global enlargement*, or confined to one or more regions and appear as *focal* or *multifocal* nephrographic and contour abnormalities.

Global Tissue Gain. This category, like the global tissue loss group, is an indeterminate pathologic-radiologic category in which the tissue response to disease tends to produce global enlargement of the organ, with preservation of a smooth

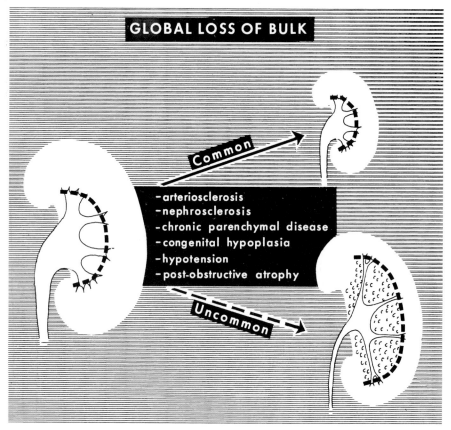

FIGURE 4–2. Patterns of response to diseases causing global loss of renal bulk. In addition to the decrease in renal size, the smoothness of the renal contour and the normal pelvocalyceal relationships are preserved. Uncommonly, wasted tissue is replaced by central fat deposition, with less decrease in overall renal size.

contour and, with the single exception of obstructive uropathy, a normal pelvocalyceal-papillary relationship, as shown in Figure 4–3. Many widely varying mechanisms produce this form of diffuse, smooth renal enlargement. They include parenchymal deposition of abnormal proteins, abnormal accumulation of either edema or blood in the interstitium, neoplastic or inflammatory cell infiltrates, and proliferative and necrotizing disorders of the glomerulus and microvasculature. Numerous miscellaneous conditions also cause global enlargement of the kidney. Table 4–2 is a list of the specific entities that comprise this category.

In addition to an enlarged renal silhouette and smooth borders, other radiologic abnormalities found in the global tissue gain category include increased thickness of the renal parenchyma and attenuation or effacement of the calyces, infundibula, and renal pelvis. These conditions occur when the relatively nondistensible renal capsule no longer accommodates the increased bulk of cells, fluid, or protein deposits. These changes are presented schematically in Figure 4–3.

Regional Tissue Gain. When a pathologic process arises in a specific component of the lobe but by nature is expansive and perhaps destructive, renal enlargement also occurs. In this situation, the enlargement is regional (polar or interpolar) and sometimes multiple. These diseases are grouped un-

der the category *regional tissue gain* in a pathologic-radiologic classification because they produce single or multiple (focal/multifocal) nephrographic abnormalities and concordant lobulations in the renal contour. Table 4–3 lists the entities included in the focal/multifocal normal-to-large–sized kidney category.

A number of radiologic observations serve to distinguish many of these diseases from each other. Figure 4–4 illustrates the radiologic features that distinguish a cyst, a tumor, and an obstructed upper pole infundibulum. These diagnostic features and others are in Chapter 12.

Renal Parenchymal Disease with Normal Size and Contour

Finally, attention must be paid to renal disorders that simply do not fit into a schema for the pathologic-radiologic classification of kidney disease based on abnormal size and nephrogram/contour. The only radiologic abnormality of one major group is deposition of calcium in the renal parenchyma—nephrocalcinosis. This occurs in association with hypercalcemia, in certain metabolic disorders, as a result of cystic dilatation and urine stasis in collecting ducts or dystrophic calcification in necrotic papillae, or as a response to nephrotoxic drugs.

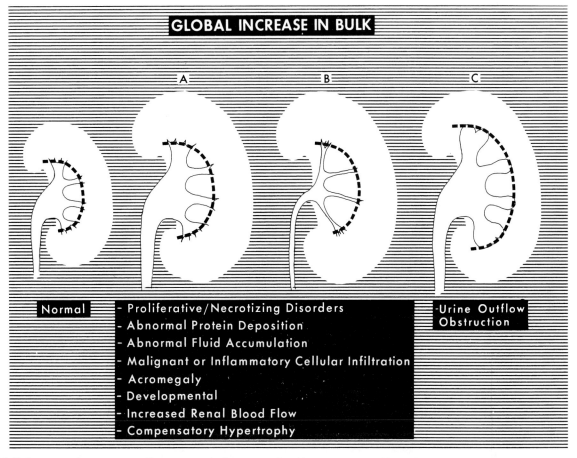

FIGURE 4–3. Patterns of response to diseases producing generalized increase in renal bulk. Pattern A is most common and illustrates the smooth contour, thickened renal parenchyma, and preservation of normal pelvocalyceal relationships. Pattern B occurs when the pelvocalyceal system is effaced by surrounding abnormal cells, fluid, or protein deposits. Only in urine outflow obstruction is the pelvocalyceal system dilated, as shown in pattern C.

FIGURE 4–4. Illustrations of radiologic patterns seen with some of the diseases causing focal increases in renal bulk. Also illustrated are the different nephrographic patterns, which allow distinction among these entities. Rarely, a tumor has a homogeneous nephrogram.

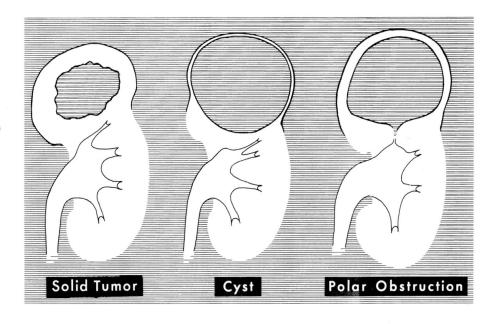

TABLE 4–2. Pathologic-Radiologic Classification of Entities Associated with Global Increase in Renal Bulk: Normal to Large Kidney

Protein deposition	Thrombotic
Amyloidosis	thrombocytopenic
Multiple myeloma	purpura and hemolytic-
Interstitial fluid accumulation	uremic syndrome
Acute tubular necrosis	Wegener's granulomatosis
Obstructive uropathy	Focal glomerulonephritis
Acute arterial infarction	associated with subacute
Renal vein thrombosis/	bacterial endocarditis
stenosis	HIV-associated nephropathy
Acute cortical necrosis	Miscellaneous
Neoplastic cell infiltration	Autosomal recessive
Leukemia	(infantile) polycystic
Inflammatory cell infiltration	kidney disease
Acute interstitial nephritis	Acromegaly
Acute pyelonephritis	Duplicated pelvocalyceal
Xanthogranulomatous	system
pyelonephritis	Compensatory hypertrophy
Proliferative/necrotizing	Nephromegaly associated
disorders	with cirrhosis,
Acute	hyperalimentation,
glomerulonephritides	diabetes mellitus, and
Polyarteritis nodosa	Beckwith-Wiedemann
(microscopic form)	syndrome
Allergic angiitis	Nephroblastomatosis
Anaphylactoid purpura	Acute urate nephropathy
(Henoch-Schönlein	Hemophilia
syndrome)	Homozygous S disease
Lung hemorrhage and	Fabry's disease
glomerulonephritis	Glycogen storage disease
(Goodpasture's	(Type I)
syndrome)	Paroxysmal nocturnal
Systemic lupus	hemoglobinuria
erythematosus	Bartter's syndrome
Diabetic	Physiologic response to
glomerulosclerosis	contrast material and
	diuretics

There are still other entities that do not fit naturally into a schema based on size and contour change. Such is the situation with *renal tuberculosis* and *brucellosis*, in which calyceal and papillary ulceration occurs as the earliest manifestation. Only late in the course of these diseases does the radiologist detect the multiplicity of parenchymal abnormalities that may alter size and contour. Thus, it seems appropriate to place renal tuberculosis and brucellosis in the category of diseases that do not affect renal size or contour while recognizing fully that this classification does not apply to advanced cases.

Similarly, the focal tissue loss associated with *papillary necrosis*, described previously and illustrated in Figure 4–1, is usually limited to the papillae and alters kidney size or contour in only one of the several causes of renal papillary necrosis, namely very advanced analgesic nephropathy.

Diabetes insipidus is yet another disorder included in this category because the abnormally large urine output associated with this abnormality produces marked dilatation of the pelvocalyceal system, often without other radiologic abnormalities.

Table 4–4 lists those entities that, according to

this approach, are in the category of parenchymal diseases having no effect on renal size or contour.

The overview presented in this section is admittedly unorthodox, for it views pathologic processes through the radiologist's looking glass. Thus, diseases of manifestly dissimilar pathogenesis, and at times distinctive histopathologic appearance, are lumped together in categories based on radiologic expressions held in common. Despite its unorthodoxy, this approach clearly is useful in distinguishing some entities that by other criteria might prove indistinguishable from each other. The next section refines this classification one step further.

URORADIOLOGIC ELEMENTS AND DIAGNOSTIC SETS

In the final analysis, the goal of the radiologist is to establish the correct diagnosis as efficiently as possible and in the best interest of the patient. There are many different morphologic and functional aspects of the kidney that can be imaged and evaluated. Of these, kidney size and nephrogram/contour have been the criteria used up to this point in the development of a pathologic-radiologic classification of renal disease. Each of the entities listed in Tables 4–1 through 4–4 inherently is either a bilateral or a unilateral process, although on occasion an inherently unilateral process may affect two kidneys more or less by chance. By incorporating the criterion of laterality into the pathologic-radio-

TABLE 4–3. Pathologic-Radiologic Classification of Entities Associated with Regional Increase in Renal Bulk: Normal to Large Kidney

Tumors
  Malignant
    Adenocarcinoma
    Invasive transitional cell carcinoma
    Wilms' tumor
    Metastases
    Medullary carcinoma
    Sarcomas (liposarcoma, fibrosarcoma, myosarcoma, hemangiosarcoma)
  Benign
    Oncocytoma
    Angiomyolipoma
    Multilocular cystic nephroma
    Mesoblastic nephroma
    Mesenchymal (lipoma, fibroma, myoma, hemangioma)
    Juxtaglomerular cell tumor
Simple cyst/localized cystic disease
Focal hydronephrosis
Focal pyelonephritis/Abscess
Malakoplakia
Congenital cystic disease
  Autosomal dominant (adult) polycystic kidney disease
  Tuberous sclerosis complex
  von Hippel-Lindau disease
  Multicystic dysplastic kidney
Arteriovenous malformation

TABLE 4–4. Pathologic-Radiologic Classification of Entities that Present with Uroradiologic Abnormalities Other than Abnormal Renal Size or Abnormal Nephrogram/Contour

Nephrocalcinosis
Hypercalcemic states
   Hyperparathyroidism
   Milk-alkali syndrome
   Hypervitaminosis D
   Sarcoidosis
   Prolonged immobilization
   Metastatic carcinoma to bone
   Humoral hypercalcemia of malignancy
Metabolic disorders
   Renal tubular acidosis
   Hyperoxaluria
   Bartter's syndrome
Structural abnormalities
   Medullary sponge kidney
   Papillary necrosis
Miscellaneous
   Nephrotoxic drugs (triamterene, amphotericin B)
   Furosemide (in premature infants)

Parenchymal diseases seen initially or primarily as papillary and/or calyceal abnormalities
Papillary necrosis
Tuberculosis
Brucellosis
Diabetes insipidus

TABLE 4–5. Diagnostic Set: Small, Scarred, Unilateral

Reflux nephropathy (chronic atrophic pyelonephritis)
Lobar infarction

TABLE 4–6. Diagnostic Set: Small, Smooth, Unilateral

Ischemia due to major arterial stenosis/aneurysm
Chronic infarction
Radiation nephritis
Congenital hypoplasia
Postobstructive atrophy
Postinflammatory atrophy
Reflux atrophy

TABLE 4–7. Diagnostic Set: Small, Smooth, Bilateral

Generalized arteriosclerosis
Benign and malignant nephrosclerosis
Atheroembolic renal disease
Chronic glomerulonephritis
Acquired cystic kidney disease
Hereditary nephropathies
   Hereditary chronic nephritis (Alport's syndrome)
   Medullary cystic disease
Amyloidosis (late)
Arterial hypotension

logic classifications, useful working tools called diagnostic sets can be defined.

Primary Uroradiologic Elements

Renal size, nephrogram/contour, and laterality of involvement become the three *primary uroradiologic elements* on which the following diagnostic sets are based:

NORMAL TO SMALL KIDNEY
   Small, scarred, unilateral
   Small, smooth, unilateral
   Small, smooth, bilateral
NORMAL TO LARGE KIDNEY
   Large, smooth, bilateral
   Large, smooth, unilateral
   Large, multifocal, bilateral
   Large, multifocal, unilateral
   Large, unifocal, unilateral

Diagnostic Sets

Tables 4–5 through 4–12 rearrange diseases listed in the pathologic-radiologic classifications (see Tables 4–1 through 4–4) according to these diagnostic sets. Assignment of each condition is made on the basis of usual rather than invariable forms of presentation. Exceptions do exist and are noted in the classification. In the absence of absolute upper and lower limits of "normal" for renal size, one must always think in terms of "normal to large" or "normal to small." The latter caveat also applies to

TABLE 4–8. Diagnostic Set: Large, Smooth, Bilateral

Proliferative/necrotizing disorders
   Acute glomerulonephritides
   Polyarteritis nodosa (microscopic form)
   Systemic lupus erythematosus
   Wegener's granulomatosis
   Allergic angiitis
   Diabetic glomerulosclerosis
   Lung hemorrhage and glomerulonephritis (Goodpasture's syndrome)
   Anaphylactoid purpura (Henoch-Schönlein syndrome)
   Thrombotic thrombocytopenic purpura and hemolytic-uremic syndrome
   Focal glomerulonephritis associated with subacute bacterial endocarditis
   HIV-associated nephropathy
Amyloidosis
Multiple myeloma
Acute tubular necrosis
Acute cortical necrosis
Leukemia
Acute interstitial nephritis
Autosomal recessive (infantile) polycystic kidney disease
Acute urate nephropathy
Glycogen storage disease Type I (von Gierke's disease)
Physiologic response to contrast material and diuretics
Homozygous S disease
Paroxysmal nocturnal hemoglobinuria
Hemophilia
Nephromegaly associated with cirrhosis, hyperalimentation, and diabetes
Acromegaly
Fabry's disease
Bartter's syndrome
Beckwith-Wiedemann syndrome
Nephroblastomatosis

TABLE 4–9. Diagnostic Set: Large, Smooth, Unilateral

Renal vein thrombosis/stenosis
Acute arterial infarction
Obstructive uropathy
Acute pyelonephritis
Xanthogranulomatous pyelonephritis
Compensatory hypertrophy
Duplicated pelvocalyceal system

TABLE 4–10. Diagnostic Set: Large, Multifocal, Bilateral

Autosomal dominant (adult) polycystic kidney disease
Tuberous sclerosis complex
von Hippel-Lindau disease
Lymphoma

TABLE 4–11. Diagnostic Set: Large, Multifocal, Unilateral

Malakoplakia
Multicystic dysplastic kidney

TABLE 4–12. Diagnostic Set: Large, Unifocal, Unilateral

Malignant neoplasms
Adenocarcinoma
Invasive transitional cell carcinoma
Wilms' tumor
Metastasis
Medullary carcinoma
Sarcoma
Benign neoplasms
Oncocytoma
Angiomyolipoma
Multilocular cystic nephroma
Mesoblastic nephroma
Mesenchymal/Juxtaglomerular cell tumor
Non-neoplastic masses
Simple cyst/localized cystic disease
Focal hydronephrosis
Focal pyelonephritis/Abscess
Arteriovenous malformation

situations in which diseases are evolving from "large" to "small" as part of their natural history. The reader should also keep in mind that the term *smooth*, when used to describe renal contour, implies a global or generalized distribution of a pathologic process within the renal parenchyma, giving rise to a homogeneous nephrogram. Also, in a few special situations, such as arteriosclerosis, the hypertensive nephroscleroses, and analgesic nephropathy–associated papillary necrosis with chronic interstitial nephritis, focal contour deformities may be superimposed on the basic pattern of a smooth contour. These are discussed in detail in later chapters.

Secondary Uroradiologic Elements

Once having determined which diagnostic set most appropriately matches the primary uroradiologic observations, further distinction among the diseases listed in that set can be made by evaluating additional features, referred to in this text as *secondary uroradiologic elements*. These include the following:

PAPILLAE
   Enlarged (global or focal)
   Effaced (global or focal)
   Retracted (global or focal)
   Irregular
   Disrupted (cavity, tract, or slough)
   Cystic dilatations
   Striations
   Decreased number
   Normal
COLLECTING SYSTEM
   Dilated (global or focal)
   Attenuated (global or focal)
   Irregular
   Displaced
   Absent
   Replaced
   Disrupted
   Strictured
   Notched (including proximal ureter)
   Duplicated
   Decreased number (calyces)
   Opacification time (equal, disparate, or delayed)
   Increased density of contrast material
   Prolonged retention of contrast material
   Normal
PARENCHYMAL THICKNESS (DISTANCE BETWEEN INTERPAPILLARY LINE AND RENAL MARGIN)
   Wasted (global or focal)
   Expanded (global or focal)
   Normal
NEPHROGRAM
   Absent
   "Rim"
   Wedge-shaped defect
   Local replacement
      Margin (smooth or irregular)
      Wall (thin or thick)
      "Beak" deformity
   Striated lucencies
   Time-density relationship (persistently faint, immediately and persistently dense, or increasingly dense)
   Contrast material density (absent, diminished, increased)
   Normal
CALCIFICATION
   Diffuse
   Focal
   Cortical
   Medullary

Papillary
Curvilinear
Peripheral
Nonperipheral
"Tramline"
Pelvocalyceal stone
COMPUTED TOMOGRAPHIC ATTENUATION
  VALUE/MAGNETIC RESONANCE SIGNAL
  INTENSITY
  Related to renal parenchyma, urine, fat,
    blood, calcium, urate, iron
  Change with time
  Unenhanced
  Contrast material–enhanced (including
    dynamic sequences)
ECHOGENICITY
  Hyperechoic relative to liver (focal, dif-
    fuse)
  Hypoechoic (focal, diffuse)
  Anechoic
  Sound transmission (increased, de-
    creased, absent)
  Specular interfaces
MISCELLANEOUS
  Retroperitoneal space
  Kidney mobility
  Scoliosis
  Baseline focal renal fat lucency
  Doppler flow characteristics

As an example of how this approach is applied, the diagnostic set "large, smooth, unilateral" can be analyzed. Obstructive uropathy is the only one of the six entities included in this set (see Table 4–9)

that has the combination of a nephrogram that becomes increasingly dense over time and delayed opacification of a globally dilated collecting system. When the contralateral kidney is small or absent, compensatory hypertrophy is the likely explanation for a kidney that appears entirely normal except for its size. A duplicated pelvocalyceal system is an obvious explanation for smooth renal enlargement. If smooth enlargement is accompanied by global effacement of the collecting system and diminished density of contrast material, abnormal interstitial fluid or cells (as occurs in acute renal venous thrombosis, acute infarction, or severe acute pyelonephritis) are suggested. The first of these diagnoses becomes the likely one if the nephrogram becomes increasingly dense over time and contains striae. In this manner, secondary uroradiologic observations lead either to a specific diagnosis or to a narrowing of possible choices within a given set.

The chapters that follow in this Section II are organized around each of the diagnostic sets. Entities are defined pathologically, and their clinical setting is briefly presented. Radiologic abnormalities are discussed in detail, and typical findings are summarized in chart form. Each chapter concludes with a differential diagnosis of the conditions discussed. Parenchymal diseases in which renal size and contour remain normal are included in a separate chapter. The emphasis throughout this presentation is on urography, computed tomography, and ultrasonography. Angiographic, radionuclide, and magnetic resonance imaging data are summarized when applicable.

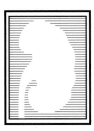

5

Diagnostic Set: Small, Scarred, Unilateral

REFLUX NEPHROPATHY
LOBAR INFARCTION
DIFFERENTIAL DIAGNOSIS

Two major diseases of the renal parenchyma—reflux nephropathy (chronic atrophic pyelonephritis) and lobar or segmental infarction—are characterized by a focal loss of renal substance that produces surface scars and may eventually reduce kidney size. In both diseases, the abnormality is localized to all or part of a renal lobe. It is for this reason that both diseases are placed in a "unilateral" diagnostic set. It should be realized, however, that these processes occur as random events. In practice, therefore, the classic abnormality described for each of these entities may be detected in multiple sites of one or both kidneys; in the latter instance, it can cause renal failure.

REFLUX NEPHROPATHY

Definition

Hodson (1959) first suggested that the diagnosis of what was then called chronic pyelonephritis be based on findings seen in the kidney as a whole rather than on microscopic features alone. The gross anatomic features of this disease, he believed, best reflect the marked coarse fibrosis so characteristic of this process, its focal or multifocal distribution with intervening areas of normal tissue, and the fact that the process involves the full thickness of the renal lobe, leading to a deep surface scar overlying a deformed calyx.

To emphasize this feature of tissue destruction with involvement of the full thickness of renal parenchyma, Hodson suggested the use of the term *chronic atrophic pyelonephritis*, and it is this nomenclature that prevailed until new concepts on pathogenesis led to the designation *reflux nephropathy*.

The specific criteria for the diagnosis of reflux nephropathy (chronic atrophic pyelonephritis) are as follows:

1. The disease process is centered in the medulla, with scar formation eventually affecting the whole thickness of the renal substance.
2. There is irregular surface depression over the involved area.
3. Retraction of the subservient papilla with secondary widening of the surrounding calyx occurs.
4. The widened calyx has a smooth margin, although its shape may be variable.
5. The renal tissue adjacent to the involved area is normal or hypertrophied, with a sharp margin between normal and abnormal portions.
6. The distribution of lesions is unifocal or multifocal and involves one or both kidneys.
7. There is reduction in overall size of the involved kidney.

Some of these features are illustrated in Figure 5–1. It should be readily apparent that this definition of reflux nephropathy assigns an important role to the radiologist in the diagnosis of this disease; the morphologic criteria are only detectable during life by radiologic means.

It is now understood that the full-thickness lobar or sublobar scar of reflux nephropathy evolves from one or more episodes of acute pyelonephritis and that this sequence of events occurs both in the absence as well as the presence of vesicoureteral reflux. Acute infection leading to fibrosis occurs in all age groups. However, the characteristic pronounced surface depression overlying a deformed papilla and calyx is more apt to develop during infancy and childhood, presumably because growth of normal portions of the kidney continues. Adults, on the other hand, usually do not develop this deformity of renal contour and calyx despite full-thickness lobar or sublobar fibrosis precisely because the kidney already has reached its full growth potential at the time of the initial acute infection.

The pathologic findings of reflux nephropathy also may be caused by renal infection secondary to urinary tract obstruction or in acquired forms of

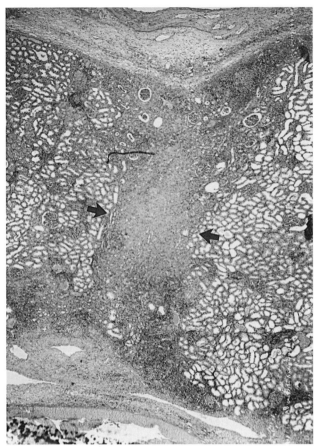

FIGURE 5–1. Reflux nephropathy (chronic atrophic pyelonephritis). Photomicrograph. A tangential section through a renal lobe demonstrates dense scar *(arrows)* extending from the surface of the kidney above to the pelvocalyceal lining below. The entire thickness of the renal lobe is involved and retracted. Note the sharp margin between normal and abnormal tissue. The scar represents the end stage of a process that began as acute pyelonephritis in the collecting ducts comprising one or more medullary rays.

vesicoureteral reflux in the adult, as well as in focal obstruction of papillae in patients with renal papillary necrosis or urolithiasis.

Acute pyelonephritis, the antecedent to reflux nephropathy, is discussed in detail in Chapter 9.

Clinical Setting

Advanced cases of bilateral reflux nephropathy classically present in young adulthood, most often among women, frequently with symptoms of hypertension and chronic renal failure. Although the majority of these patients are not able to provide a history of urinary tract symptoms before the final illness, the disease seen in the adult is usually the end stage of a process that began as episodes of acute pyelonephritis in infancy and early childhood. Any discussion on the pathogenesis of reflux nephropathy, therefore, must begin in the early years of life.

Gram-negative bacteria, particularly *Escherichia coli*, are most frequently implicated in acute kidney

infection, which in some patients will ultimately lead to reflux nephropathy. Vesicoureteral reflux, until recently, has been considered the dominant mechanism by which bacteria ascend from the lower to the upper urinary tract. It is now recognized that vesicoureteral reflux accounts for infection of the upper urinary tract in only a portion of patients with acute pyelonephritis. Nevertheless, severe reflux is still considered an important, although by no means the only, risk factor for the development of reflux nephropathy. Bacteria, once in the pelvocalyceal system, gain access to the renal parenchyma through the papillary orifices of the collecting ducts, a process known as *intrarenal reflux*. Bacteria in the urine, their ascent to the upper urinary tract, and their introduction into the renal parenchyma, therefore, are the three elements essential to the development of reflux nephropathy.

Vesicoureteral reflux occurs principally as a function of the length and the angle of insertion of the portion of the distal ureter that passes through the wall of the bladder and tunnels beneath the mucosa before terminating at the trigone. Reflux is more likely to occur when this intramural segment is short and the angle of insertion is wide. Conversely, the longer the submucosal segment and the more acute its angle of insertion, the less likely is reflux to occur. Elongation of this segment as a characteristic of normal growth and development in the infant and young child explains the well-established observation that the frequency of vesicoureteral reflux is inversely related to age. This means that vesicoureteral reflux spontaneously ceases as the intramural portion of the distal ureter lengthens and its angle of insertion becomes more acute during normal growth and development.

Vesicoureteral reflux is a potential source of damage to the renal parenchyma only when it is severe enough to cause the return of a large volume of bladder urine to the renal pelvis under conditions of elevated pressure. This applies to Grade IV or higher reflux, using the system of grading outlined in Table 5–1 (also refer to Fig. 5–2). Two forms of renal damage may follow. In the first form, high-pressure, large-volume reflux *alone* causes varying

TABLE 5–1. Grading of Vesicoureteral Reflux

GRADE	DESCRIPTION
I	Ureter only
II	Ureter, pelvis, calyces
	No dilatation
	Normal fornices
III	Ureter, pelvis, calyces
	Mild dilatation
	Normal fornices
IV	Ureter, pelvis, calyces
	Moderate dilatation/tortuosity
	Unsharp fornices
	Normal papilla
V	Gross distention
	Effaced papilla

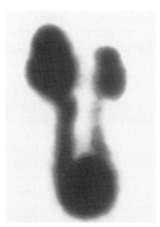

FIGURE 5–2. Vesicoureteral reflux, Grade V, bilateral. ^{99m}Tc-pertechnetate voiding cystogram. Refluxed urine fills the markedly dilated ureters and pelvocalyceal systems (same patient illustrated in Figure 17–13). (Courtesy of Massoud Majd, M.D., Children's National Medical Center, Washington, D.C.)

are delivered to the upper urinary tract where, in combination with intrarenal reflux, the process is initiated that will ultimately result in focal parenchymal scars and other pathologic features that characterize reflux nephropathy (Fig. 5–3).

Reflux of urine from the collecting system into the renal lobe—intrarenal reflux—occurs at sites at which the shape of the orifices of Bellini's ducts on the papillae have been deformed by the process of lobar fusion (Fig. 5–4) (see discussion in Chapter 3). Oval and wide openings allow urine to pass into the collecting ducts that extend through the entire thickness of the renal lobe. Papillary orifices that are narrow and slitlike prevent this passage of urine when elevated pelvocalyceal pressure due to high-volume vesicoureteral reflux is present. Because the duct orifices on any given papilla vary in shape as a function of fusion (compounding), intrarenal reflux may occur in a part, or parts, of a lobe but not necessarily in an entire lobe. The following features explain the pathologic characteristics of reflux nephropathy: full-thickness involvement (reflux into collecting ducts that extend from papillary tip to cortex); partial lobar involvement with adjacent normal tissue (a refluxing orifice next to a nonrefluxing one, each draining an adjacent set of collecting ducts); and a higher frequency of reflux nephropathy scars in the poles of the kidney than

degrees of pelvocalyceal system dilatation and global renal wasting, a condition termed *reflux atrophy* or *diffuse reflux nephropathy*. (This is discussed in Chapters 6 and 17.) In the second form, major vesicoureteral reflux coexists with infected urine. Here, reflux is the means by which the bacteria

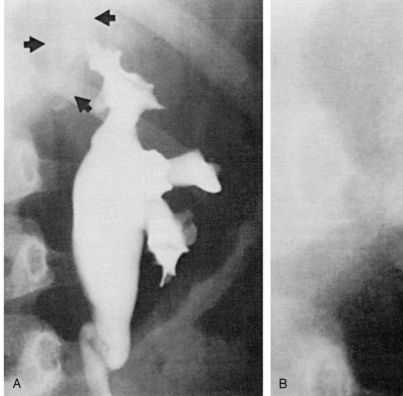
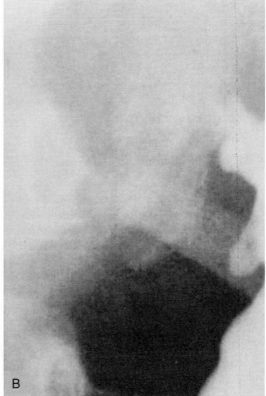

FIGURE 5–3. Reflux nephropathy. Early stage in a young girl with recurrent urinary tract infection.
 A, Voiding cystourethrogram. Vesicoureteral reflux, Grade IV. There is widening of the collecting system and intrarenal reflux into the medial portion of the upper pole *(arrows).*
 B, Photographic enlargement of medial portion of upper pole seen in *A.* Fine linear dense striations through the full thickness of the parenchyma represent intrarenal reflux of opacified urine into collecting ducts. Combined with infected urine, this causes acute pyelonephritis.
 (Courtesy of Gerald Friedland, M.D., Stanford University School of Medicine, Stanford, California.)

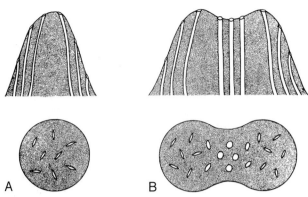

FIGURE 5–4. Schema of papillary duct opening in profile and *en face.* The single cone-shaped pyramid *(A)* has narrow slitlike openings that prevent intrarenal reflux. Compound papillae *(B),* formed as a result of lobar assimilation, have open, round orifices that permit intrarenal reflux of calyceal urine into the collecting ducts.

in the interpolar region (more compound papillae in the poles).

Nonrefluxing papillary orifices can convert to refluxing orifices as a result of elevated pressure of calycine urine, as occurs with vesicoureteral reflux, ureteral obstruction, or disordered peristalsis. Thus, intrarenal reflux may be acquired as well as developmental due to lobar papillary fusion.

Reflux nephropathy is the end stage of acute pyelonephritis induced by bacteria in the collecting system gaining access to the collecting ducts of the renal lobe (see Fig. 5–3). The earliest tissue response is an acute tubulointerstitial nephritis in the affected portion of the renal lobe. This is identical clinically and pathologically to uncomplicated acute pyelonephritis seen in adulthood, as discussed in Chapter 9. The early acute inflammatory stage of reflux nephropathy, occurring in infancy and childhood, does not alter the radiologic appearance of the renal contour or the papillae. Capillary perfusion and glomerular filtration in the affected portion of the lobe are impaired, however, by the interstitial infiltrate of white blood cells and the accumulation of pus in the collecting ducts that are part of the acute inflammatory response. Imaging abnormalities at this stage are detected using radionuclide or radiologic modalities that reflect perfusion. With persistent or recurrent infection with or without reflux, the early inflammatory infiltrate is eventually replaced by fibroblasts and scar formation throughout the full thickness of the lobe, as illustrated in Figure 5–1. Retraction of the renal surface and the subjacent papillae follows (see discussion in Chapter 4). This process may progress through childhood or arrest at any time in its evolution if either the infection of the urine is eliminated or the vesicoureteral reflux ceases as a result of normal maturation or surgical intervention. By the midchildhood years or earlier, the lesions are fully developed and no longer progressive. If enough renal mass is involved, proteinuria and renal failure develop.

The question of whether reflux nephropathy develops from the combination of vesicoureteral and intrarenal reflux without infection of urine remains unanswered. Most of the clinical and laboratory evidence indicates that infection is essential in producing the fully developed picture of reflux nephropathy. The Ask-Upmark kidney, also known as segmental renal hypoplasia, is possibly a reflection of this uncertainty. The Ask-Upmark kidney has the gross morphologic appearance of reflux nephropathy and similar clinical characteristics. A focal, full-thickness scar overlies a retracted papilla and widened calyx. Its microscopic appearance, however, differs from that of reflux nephropathy. Coarse fibrosis is absent. Glomeruli are few, if present at all. Dilated, colloid-filled tubular structures that resemble thyroid tissue predominate, and there is marked sclerosis of medium-sized arteries. One explanation for this lesion is that it develops from intrarenal reflux of sterile urine, perhaps even during intrauterine development of the kidney. (Aspects of the Ask-Upmark kidney as a form of focal hypoplasia are discussed in the section Congenital Hypoplasia in Chapter 6. The possible relationship between vesicoureteral reflux in the fetus and renal dysplasia is addressed in Chapter 11.)

Clinically, urinary tract infection occurs most frequently in girls and women and, in the first year of life, in uncircumcised male newborns. The combination of urinary tract infection and severe reflux may express itself by repeated episodes of fever, flank pain, frequency, and dysuria. Often, however, patients have nonlocalizing symptoms such as lethargy and abdominal pain in addition to fever. Of particular importance is the well-documented fact that many young children have bacteriuria and urographic evidence of renal scars, *even though they are asymptomatic.* Presumably, these represent occult cases of urinary tract infection with or without vesicoureteral reflux.

Radiologic Findings

The earliest radiologic findings of reflux nephropathy are identical to those of acute pyelonephritis, as described in Chapter 9. Contrast material–enhanced computed tomography or ^{99m}Tc-DMSA radionuclide renography demonstrates a normal-sized to enlarged, smooth kidney with a sharply defined, nonenhancing or radionuclide-deficient zone extending through the full thickness of the renal parenchyma in one or more portions of the kidney (Figs. 5–5, 5–6). This corresponds to the infected lobar or sublobar segments where perfusion is impaired by the increased interstitial pressure associated with the acute inflammatory infiltrate. When multiple sublobar segments are involved, the nephrogram is striated (see Fig. 5–5). If delayed computed tomographic scans are obtained, the sites of nephrographic deficiency may become abnormally dense and persistent as contrast material slowly accumulates in tubules and collecting ducts that

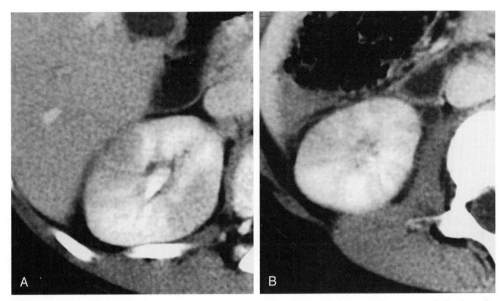

FIGURE 5–5. Acute pyelonephritis in the right kidney of a 7-year-old girl with acute upper urinary tract infection. Computed tomogram, contrast material–enhanced.

A, In the upper pole, there are two sharply defined, full-thickness nephrographic defects, one ventrolateral and the other dorsomedial.

B, In the lower pole, the defects are striated in appearance, representing multiple sublobar areas of involvement. Areas that fail to enhance represent diminished perfusion due to acute inflammatory infiltrate (same patient illustrated in Figure 9–35).

(Courtesy of Massoud Majd, M.D., Children's National Medical Center, Washington, D.C.)

FIGURE 5–6. Acute pyelonephritis evolving into reflux nephropathy in the left kidney of a 5-year old girl. ^{99m}Tc-DMSA radionuclide scan, left posterior oblique projections.

A, Initial scan during acute phase. There is diminished radionuclide uptake in the upper pole in a sharply defined, full-thickness distribution.

B, Follow-up scan 14 months after acute infection. A deep surface scar has developed in the upper pole (same patient illustrated in Fig. 2–8).

(Courtesy of Massoud Majd, M.D., Children's National Medical Center, Washington, D.C.)

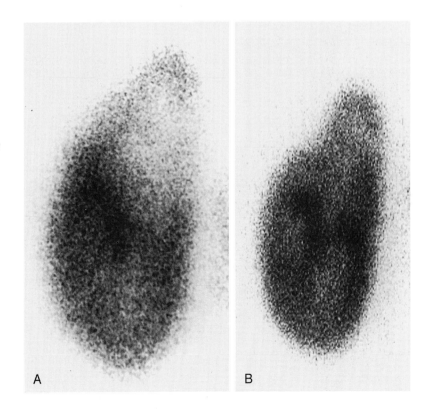

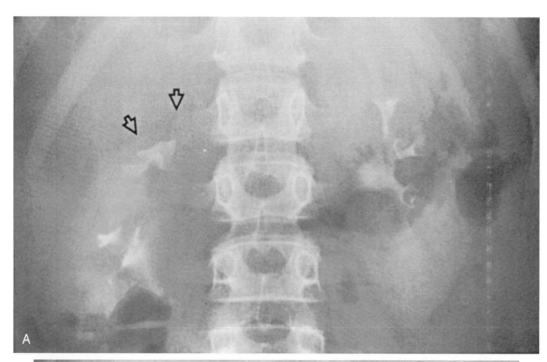

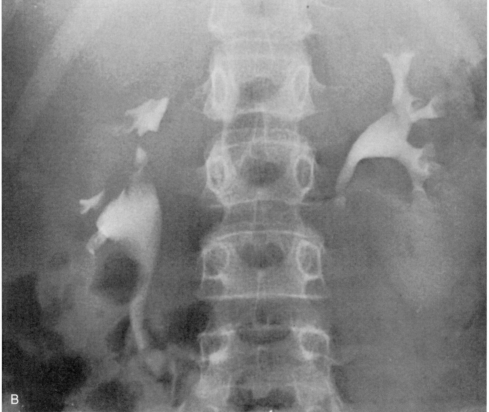

FIGURE 5–7. Excretory urogram performed on an 11-year-old girl with recurrent urinary tract infections and vesicoureteral reflux into the right pelvocalyceal system (same patient illustrated in Fig. 17–14).
  A, There is decreased growth of the right kidney, particularly in the upper pole *(arrows).*
  B, Focal contour scars and calyceal dilatation have not yet developed.

are plugged with inflammatory cells (see Fig. 9–36). Gray-scale ultrasonography may demonstrate enlargement of the kidney but otherwise lacks diagnostic sensitivity in the early stage of renal infection unless Doppler techniques demonstrate diminished perfusion to the involved portions of the kidney (see Fig. 9–39).

In children with persistent or recurrent infections, imaging studies may depict inhibition of growth in affected regions of the kidney. This is seen as a reduction in parenchymal thickness (Fig. 5–7) and is most frequently present in the upper renal pole. This stage, which is intermediate between early acute pyelonephritis and late scar formation, can be detected by careful comparison of parenchymal thickness of the suspected abnormality with other poles. Normally, poles are symmetrical in thickness.

After repeated episodes of acute infection, retraction of the papilla with dilatation of its adjacent calyx and a surface depression appear. This deformity develops predominantly during infancy and childhood, possibly reflecting continued normal or, in some cases, hypertrophied growth of the uninvolved parts of the kidney and absence of growth in the fibrotic, scarred portions of the kidney. This age-related pattern of contour and calyceal deformity may also reflect the spontaneous disappearance of reflux known to occur as children mature. Scar formation can also be arrested by eradication of infection following antibiotic therapy without an antireflux surgical procedure also being performed. Scarring, nonetheless, may progress after the successful treatment of infection.

The radiologic picture of reflux nephropathy discovered in the adult usually reflects the severity of the disease during childhood. When the disease process has been naturally self-limited, or when successful medical or surgical therapy has minimized damage, the radiologic abnormality is limited to a slight thinning of parenchyma in one area, without contour scarring or calyceal deformity due to retraction of the papilla. A conclusive radiologic diagnosis of reflux nephropathy based on these minimal findings cannot be made because this picture is similar to that seen in ischemic or postinfarction states (Fig. 5–8). On the other hand, the fully developed pattern of reflux nephropathy may go undetected until adulthood, especially in patients who remain asymptomatic because of limited disease. The development of the deformities of reflux nephropathy *de novo* in the adult points to urinary tract infection complicated by such factors as stone formation, renal papillary necrosis, obstruction, or neuropathic bladder with vesicoureteral reflux (Fig. 5–9).

Reflux nephropathy can be diagnosed with confidence only when the radiologic pattern reflects "full-thickness" destruction and scarring of all or part of a lobe (i.e., a cortical depression overlying a retracted papilla whose calyx is secondarily dilated). In some individuals, this abnormality will be present at one site (Figs. 5–10, 5–11, 5–12); in others, a number of foci in one or both kidneys will be present (Figs. 5–13, 5–14). In the most severe circumstance (a young patient with hypertension, progressive renal failure, and renal osteodystrophy), severe bilateral contour defects with corresponding papillary retraction and calyceal widening will be present (Fig. 5–15). Even though this pattern is present in both kidneys, involvement is characteristically asymmetric. The margin of the calyx remains

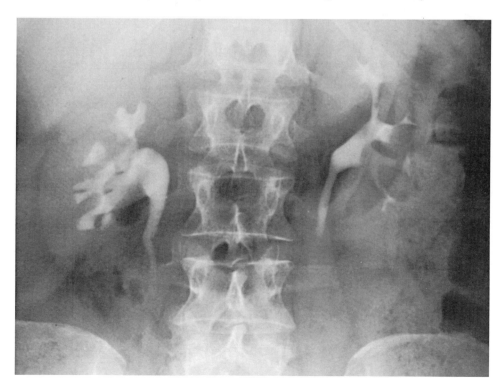

FIGURE 5–8. Excretory urogram in an infection-free, asymptomatic young adult woman who had a right ureteral reimplantation during childhood for reflux and infection. The right upper pole is reduced in thickness, particularly laterally, but does not have a focal scar. Slight calyceal deformity in the region probably represents atrophy from previous reflux. These findings represent minimal damage from reflux nephropathy in childhood.

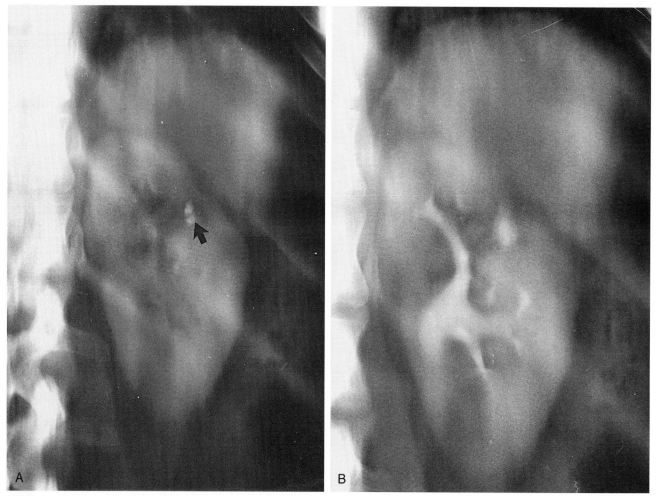

FIGURE 5–9. Chronic atrophic pyelonephritis developing in a single focus in a 49-year-old woman as a result of localized calculi.
  A, Early nephrogram. Tomogram. Two calculi *(arrow)* are clustered in a single calyceal/papillary unit in the upper pole with an overlying parenchymal scar.
  B, Excretory urogram. Tomogram. Calyceal dilatation is present.
  (Courtesy of E. Stephen Amis, M.D., Albert Einstein School of Medicine, New York, New York.)

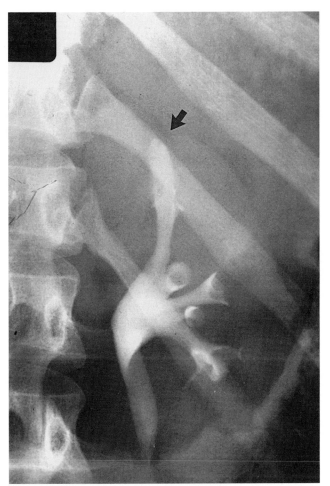

FIGURE 5–10. Reflux nephropathy in a 26-year-old woman who had a urinary tract infection in childhood. The abnormality is limited to a focal contour scar overlying a smoothly dilated calyx in the upper pole *(arrow)*. (Courtesy of Professor Thomas Sherwood, M.B., University of Cambridge, Cambridge, England.)

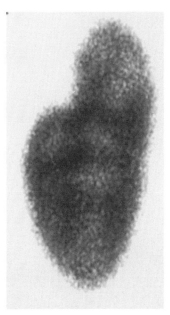

FIGURE 5–11. Reflux nephropathy. ^{99m}Tc-DMSA radionuclide scan, left posterior oblique projection. There is a single focal scar in the dorsolateral aspect of the left kidney. (Courtesy of Massoud Majd, M.D., Children's National Medical Center, Washington, D.C.)

smooth, even when dilatation is advanced, a feature that differentiates reflux nephropathy from calyceal dilatation due to tuberculosis or renal papillary necrosis, in which the margin of the cavity is apt to be irregular.

A few additional miscellaneous observations about advanced reflux nephropathy should be noted. Occasionally, marked peripelvic sinus fat accumulates as destruction of renal tissue advances. This is detectable, as central renal lucency on a preliminary film, by characteristic fat attenuation values or signal intensity on computed tomography or magnetic resonance images, respectively, or as increased echogenicity of the central sinus complex on an ultrasonogram. In this circumstance, a thin mantle of renal parenchyma surrounds the expanded deposit of fat in the renal sinus. When advanced reflux nephropathy affects only one kidney, contralateral compensatory hypertrophy is present. Focal areas of compensatory hypertrophy of unaffected parenchyma may develop as pseudotumors adjacent to scars (see Fig. 5–15). Although microscopic nephrocalcinosis is commonly seen in reflux

---

REFLUX NEPHROPATHY TYPICAL FINDINGS

Primary Uroradiologic Elements

Size: small
Contour: focal or multifocal scar
Lesion distribution: usually unilateral

Secondary Uroradiologic Elements

Papillae: retracted
Calyces: dilated
Parenchymal thickness: wasted (intermediate, late); focal compensatory hypertrophy
Nephrogram: deficient enhancement (lobar, sublobar; full-thickness; may be striated)
Echogenicity: increased central sinus complex
Vascularity/perfusion: absent (early)

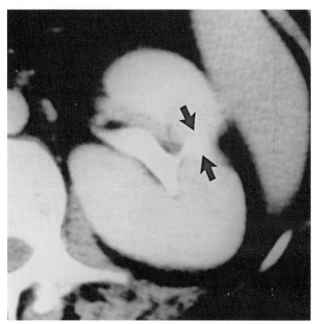

FIGURE 5–12. Reflux nephropathy. Computed tomogram, contrast material–enhanced. There is a single focal scar closely overlying a dilated, retracted calyx *(arrows)*. (Courtesy of Philip Kenney, M.D., University of Alabama at Birmingham, Birmingham, Alabama.)

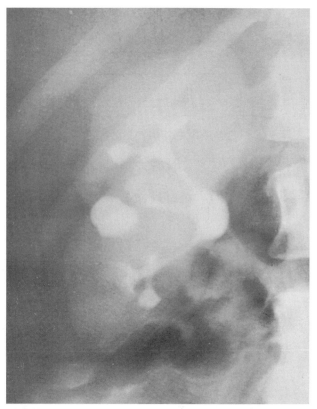

FIGURE 5–13. Reflux nephropathy. Excretory urogram demonstrates advanced changes in multiple areas of the right kidney. Varying degrees of severity and nonuniform distribution are characteristic of this abnormality.

nephropathy, its radiologic detection is unusual. Finally, it is unusual to detect abnormalities in either contrast material density or urine volume, even in patients with severe functional impairment due to advanced disease.

Ultrasonography demonstrates the focal retraction of the renal surface and underlying dilated calyx, as does excretory urography, computed tomography, and magnetic resonance imaging (see Figs. 5–14 and 5–15*B*). Increased echogenicity may be noted where perirenal fat fills the depressions on the surface of the kidney.

The radiologic evaluation of a child for reflux

nephropathy beyond the stage of acute pyelonephritis has the double objective of detecting significant vesicoureteral reflux and assessing the renal parenchyma for retarded growth or scar formation. The additional obligation of follow-up is imposed if either is present. Vesicoureteral reflux can be investigated by either voiding cystourethrography or radionuclide cystography. Kidney structure can be

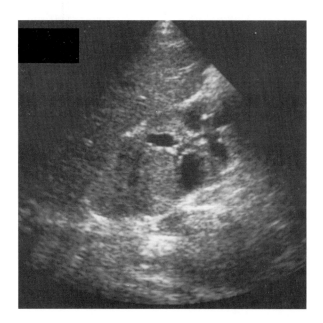

FIGURE 5–14. Reflux nephropathy, right kidney. Ultrasonogram, sagittal projection. There are multiple foci of scars overlying dilated calyces. (Kindly provided by Ulrike Hamper, M.D., and Sheila Sheth, M.D., The Johns Hopkins University, Baltimore, Maryland.)

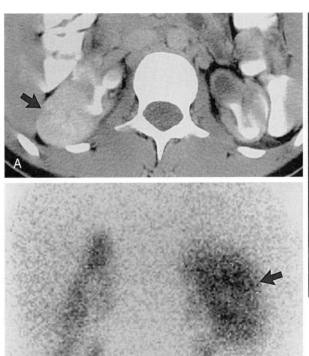

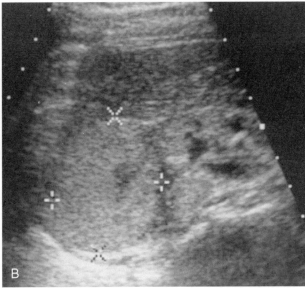

FIGURE 5–15. Reflux nephropathy, bilateral with a pseudotumor due to focal nodular compensatory hypertrophy in the right kidney.

A, Computed tomogram, contrast material–enhanced. Both kidneys demonstrate focal contour scars overlying dilated, retracted calyces. There is normal, homogeneous enhancement of the pseudotumor in the upper pole of the right kidney *(arrow).*

B, Ultrasonogram, right kidney, longitudinal projection. The dilated calyces and decreased renal parenchyma are noted in the lower portion of the kidney. The focal hypertrophied normal tissue constituting the pseudotumor is outlined by cursors.

C, Radionuclide scan, posterior projection. Radionuclide uptake by the pseudotumor is normal *(arrow).* Note small size and contour scars of the kidneys (same patient illustrated in Fig. 2–9).

assessed by excretory urography, ultrasonography, computed tomography, or radionuclide techniques. Each of these methods has specific advantages and disadvantages. The specific protocol chosen varies among institutions.

LOBAR INFARCTION

Definition

Each of the three diagnostic sets for small kidneys discussed in this and the following two chapters includes entities arising from abnormalities of blood flow. The specific diagnostic set to which each of these is assigned depends, first, on whether the interruption of blood supply is partial (ischemic) or complete (infarctive) and, second, on what amount of tissue is affected. Many combinations are possible. When the vascular abnormality is generalized in the small vessels, both kidneys are affected diffusely (see Chapter 7 on bilaterally small, smooth kidneys). On the other hand, when a major renal artery stenosis causes ischemia or when infarction of the entire kidney occurs, wasting is global but limited to one kidney (see Chapter 6 on unilaterally small, smooth kidneys).

The discussion in this chapter focuses on those circulatory abnormalities that follow thrombosis or embolization of one or a group of related interlobar or arcuate arteries. The infarction that results is limited to a portion of a lobe, a whole lobe, or neighboring parts of adjacent lobes, depending on the number and the size of arteries involved. If all the arteries perfusing a single lobe are occluded, the entire lobe will shrink, and a surface depression in the area of the centrilobar cortex and peripheral part of the medulla will be produced. Because each interlobar artery usually divides into arcuate arteries running to adjoining portions of two adjacent lobes, the surface depression is rarely limited to a single lobe. Instead, a depression bridging adjacent portions of each lobe is usually the minimal result of an interlobar artery occlusion (refer to Fig. 3–5 to better understand the anatomic basis for the contour deformities of lobar infarction).

The sequence of events that occurs following interruption of blood supply to a portion of the kidney has been studied most thoroughly in experimental animals; these parallel the changes that occur in humans. The earliest abnormality is venous and capillary hyperemia, seen within an hour after segmental arterial obstruction as a triangular reddish region, with its base in the subcapsular area and its apex pointing toward the medulla (Fig. 5–16). Owing to hyperemia, the area bulges above the surface of the rest of the kidney. Within 7 days the lesion begins to decrease in volume. After approximately 28 days, a pronounced surface depression

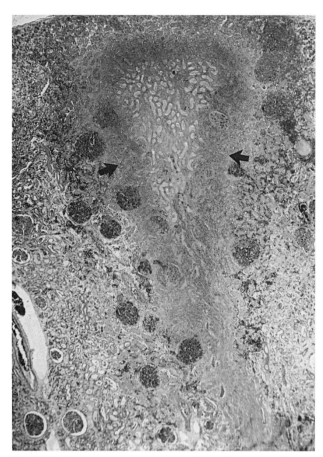

FIGURE 5–16. Acute lobar infarction. Photomicrograph. There is a triangular-shaped area of infarcted kidney surrounded by a zone of hyperemia at the interface between infarcted and viable tissue *(arrows)*. The base of the triangle is at the periphery of the kidney. At this stage, imaging studies demonstrate only the absence of perfusion and urine formation in the affected region and no contour defect.

forms as dead tubules and other cellular elements disappear (Fig. 5–17). Unlike reflux nephropathy, fibroblasts are not a prominent feature of this process, and the depression on the surface of the kidney is due to a "falling out" of dead tissue rather than retraction by fibrosis. The deformity is thereby limited to the area of actual tissue death, namely, the peripheral portion of the lobe. The papilla is usually not involved in lobar infarction because of the multiplicity of vessels, including the spiral arteries, that perfuse it. Even when infarcted, the papilla usually retains its normal shape. Thus, a cut section through a kidney with a mature lobar infarction reveals a deep surface depression limited to the area supplied by the interrupted vessel, obliteration of the corticomedullary junction, preservation of the papilla of the involved lobe, and normal adjacent tissue.

Clinical Setting

Lobar infarction is due either to embolism or to thrombosis at the site of arteriosclerotic plaque or aneurysm. Of these, embolism is by far the more common cause. Among patients with renal infarcts, 75 to 95 per cent have had embolic phenomena secondary to cardiac lesions, particularly rheumatic heart disease with arrhythmia. Other cardiac sources of renal arterial emboli are recent myocardial infarction, prosthetic valves, myocardial trauma, intracardiac catheters, and myocardial tumors. Renal infarcts secondary to emboli have been reported in as many as 25 per cent of patients with subacute bacterial endocarditis. Less common causes of lobar infarcts are arteriosclerosis, thromboangiitis obliterans, polyarteritis nodosa, syphilitic cardiovascular disease, aneurysm of the aorta or renal artery, and prolonged arterial catheterization.

Small renal infarcts often produce neither symptoms nor abnormal physical or laboratory findings. Diagnosis, therefore, is frequently based on incidental observations made during imaging studies or autopsy. Symptoms, when present, include the abrupt onset of abdominal or flank pain, fever, and nausea with vomiting. Albuminuria, often heavy, is present more frequently (approximately one-half of all patients) than hematuria (one-third of all patients). Hematuria is usually microscopic and only occasionally gross, but urinalysis is normal in one-third of the patients with renal infarction. Leukocytosis and elevation of serum lactic dehydrogenase level may occur within the first 24 hours after infarction and reflect responses to tissue death. In many patients with renal infarction, symptoms are vague and do not suggest the correct diagnosis. In sepsis, symptoms of cerebral and splenic infarction or mesenteric ischemia may overshadow those of renal infarcts. Laboratory evidence of functional impairment of the kidney is not a feature of small, focal renal infarcts unless these are numerous and bilateral or superimposed on kidneys already compromised by pre-existing disease.

Radiologic Findings

The radiologic findings in lobar or segmental infarction vary with the age of the lesion. Within the first week, renal size and contour remain normal because there is essentially no tissue loss during this period. Other abnormalities may be present early, however. Shortly after the onset of infarction, a nephrographic defect may be detected by contrast material–enhanced (computed tomography or magnetic resonance imaging) or radionuclide imaging techniques. This defect corresponds to the infarct itself and reflects the lack of perfusion of the involved area by blood containing contrast material. The defect is likely to be triangular, with the base situated on the outer margin of the kidney (Fig. 5–18). In some patients, a thin rim of outer cortex *(rim sign)* enhances with contrast material, representing collateral perfusion by way of the capsular artery (Fig. 5–19). The localized area of deficient perfusion may also be detectable at this stage by power Doppler ultrasonography. The depression on the kidney surface that forms later occurs at the

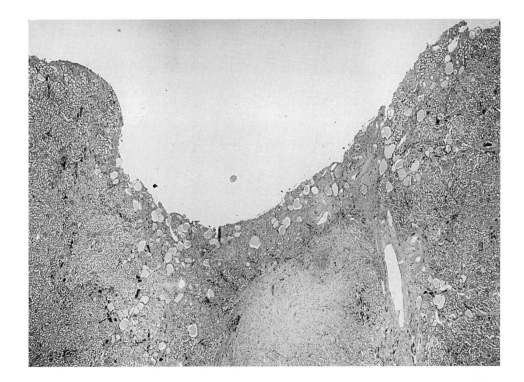

FIGURE 5–17. Mature lobar infarction. Photomicrograph. At this stage, the infarcted tissue has disappeared, leaving a broad-based defect on the surface of the kidney.

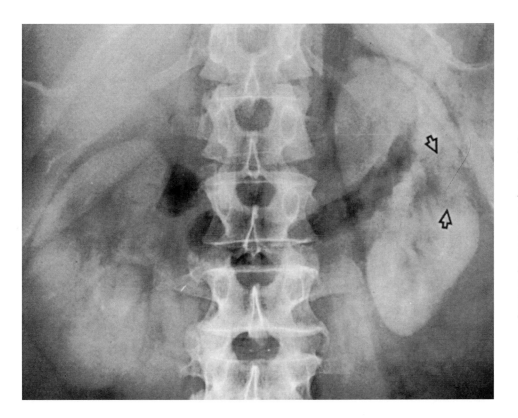

FIGURE 5–18. Lobar infarction in a 61-year-old man who experienced sudden left groin and flank pain accompanied by microscopic hematuria. Excretory urography was performed 3 days later. A triangular radiolucent nephrographic defect with its base on the renal margin is present in the interpolar region *(arrows)* (same patient illustrated in Figs. 5–20, 5–21, and 27–12.) Excretory urogram, early film. (Kindly provided by Ira Kanter, M.D., Peralta Hospital, Oakland, California.)

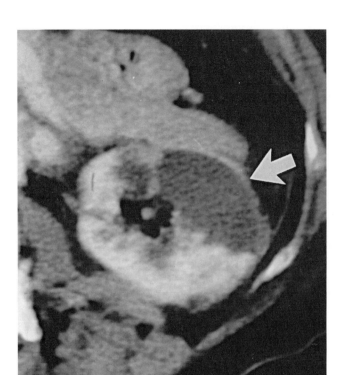

FIGURE 5–19. Lobar infarction, acute, left kidney. Computed tomogram, contrast material–enhanced. There is a thin rim of enhanced outer cortex *(arrow)* overlying the sharply defined nephrographic defect.

LOBAR INFARCTION TYPICAL FINDINGS

Early (within 4 weeks)

Primary Uroradiologic Elements

Size: normal
Contour: smooth
Lesion distribution: unilateral

Secondary Uroradiologic Elements

Collecting system: normal
Nephrogram: absent (focal); rim sign, occasional
Vascularity/perfusion: absent

Late (after 4 weeks)

Primary Uroradiologic Elements

Size: small
Contour: focal or multifocal depression
Lesion distribution: unilateral

Secondary Uroradiologic Elements

Parenchymal thickness: wasted (focal) with normal interpapillary line
Echogenicity: increased (focal)

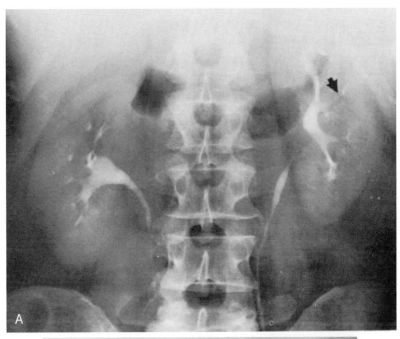

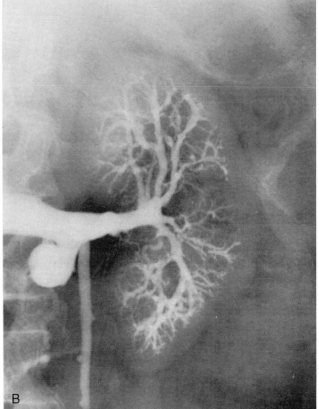

FIGURE 5–20. Lobar infarction (same patient illustrated in Figs. 5–18 and 5–21.)

A, The uppermost calyx and infundibulum *(arrow)* in the left interpolar region are attenuated, and the midportion of the pelvis is displaced medially.

B, Retrograde venogram. Marked attenuation of interlobar, arcuate, and interlobular veins in involved area illustrates the effect of localized hyperemic tissue swelling, which also produces the deformities in the pelvoinfundibulocalyceal system seen during excretory urography. (Kindly provided by Ira Kanter, M.D., Peralta Hospital, Oakland, California.)

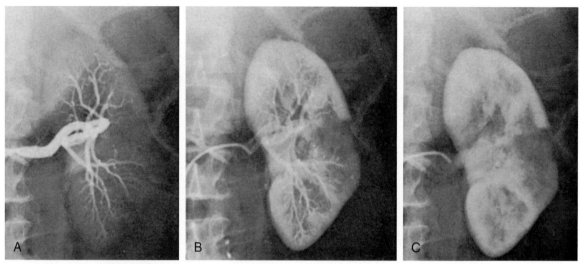

FIGURE 5–21. Lobar infarction (same patient illustrated in Figs. 5–18 and 5–20).
   A, Selective renal angiogram, arterial phase. There is an absence of arteries to the infarcted areas.
   B, Later arterial phase.
   C, Nephrographic phase. The nephrographic defect in the interpolar region representing nonperfused parenchyma is well illustrated. (Kindly provided by Ira Kanter, M.D., Peralta Hospital, Oakland, California.)

same site. The calyx and infundibulum may become attenuated or displaced by hyperemic tissue swelling (Fig. 5–20).

Selective renal angiography can provide important information in the early diagnosis of lobar renal infarction, although this is rarely required unless other imaging data or clinical findings are inconclusive. The embolus itself may be seen as an intraluminal filling defect or as an abrupt termination of an interlobar or arcuate artery. The involved vessels may not opacify, or they may retain contrast material longer than normal vessels of similar size in other parts of the kidney. This reflects downstream obstruction. A nephrographic defect is readily apparent in the nonperfused area (Figs. 5–21, 5–22).

With maturation of the infarct after approximately 4 weeks, the findings become quite specific: a wide-based depression in the renal contour at the site of infarction develops, whereas the underlying papillae remain normal (Figs. 5–23, 5–24). Abnormalities at this stage can be demonstrated best by contrast material–enhanced computed tomography, ultrasonography, or excretory urography. When viewing cross-sectional images, however, a focal surface depression in the polar region of the kidney may not be seen in profile and, thereby, may be overlooked.

The focal loss of renal parenchyma can be identified easily by drawing the interpapillary line, which remains normal, and an outline of the renal contour, which indents at the site of the infarct (Fig. 5–25). Occasionally, the amount of lobar tissue loss will be so extensive that some papillary distortion occurs. This is always minimal relative to the deformity that develops in the remainder of the lobe and does not approximate that seen in reflux nephropathy (Fig. 5–26). Sometimes, numerous small infarcts

cause multiple focal depressions in one or both kidneys without a detectable decrease in renal length or width (Fig. 5–27).

Selective renal angiography performed 3 to 4 weeks after lobar infarction may demonstrate irregular narrowing, prolonged retention of contrast material, or nonopacification of the affected vessel. The embolus itself will no longer be visible by this time. A surface depression on the margin of the kidney is usually well seen during the angiographic nephrogram (Fig. 5–28).

Gray-scale ultrasonography is not useful for the diagnosis of early lobar infarction. Power Doppler ultrasonography, on the other hand, may detect a zone of absent vascularity. As the infarct matures, increased echogenicity occurs at the site of the contour deformity. This is due to perirenal fat filling in the space left by the disappearance of the infarcted renal tissue (Fig. 5–29). This finding may be present whenever focal loss of renal tissue has occurred, including postsurgical scarring, and is not specific for lobar infarction.

DIFFERENTIAL DIAGNOSIS

When the lesions of **reflux nephropathy** and **lobar infarction** are fully developed, their radiologic patterns are quite specific. In the former, a focal contour scar overlies a smoothly dilated calyx, whereas in the latter a broadly based contour depression exists over a normal papilla. Both diseases, occurring as random events, may be multifocal, bilateral, or both.

Cases of minimal reflux nephropathy in which arrest of growth results in slight reduction in parenchymal thickness, usually in one pole, without contour or papillary deformity are radiologically indistinguishable from changes seen in ischemia or late

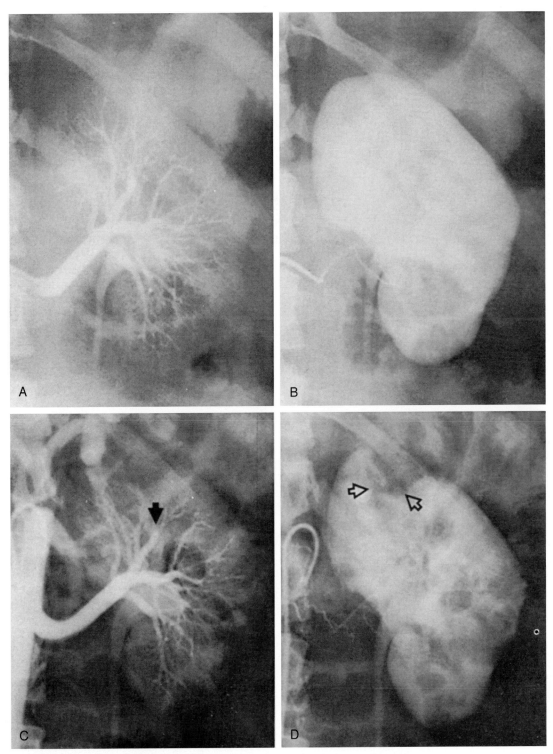

FIGURE 5–22. Lobar infarction. Iatrogenic embolization of arcuate arteries during angiography.

A and *B,* Initial selective renal arteriogram demonstrates normal arteries and angiographic nephrogram.

C, A few minutes later, a midstream aortogram reveals complete occlusion of some arcuate arteries to an upper pole lobe *(arrow),* presumably due to embolization during selective catheterization.

D, Prominent nephrographic defect *(arrows)* in area perfused by occluded vessels.

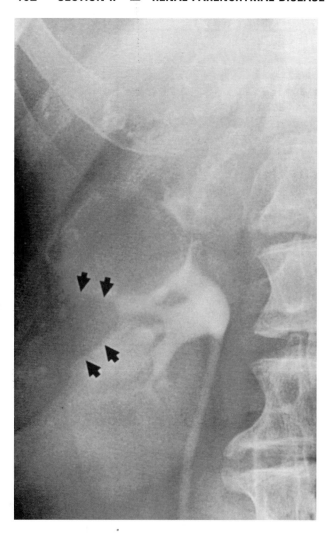

FIGURE 5–23. Mature lobar infarct seen as a deep focal depression of the renal contour in the interpolar region *(arrows)*. The underlying papillae remain normal. Simple renal cysts are present just above the infarct and in the lower pole.

FIGURE 5–24. Mature lobar infarct on the lateral aspect of the right kidney. The deep focal depression of the renal contour does not extend to the underlying calyx. Computed tomogram, contrast material–enhanced.

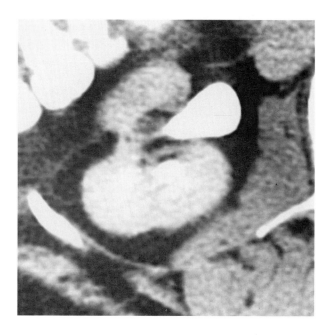

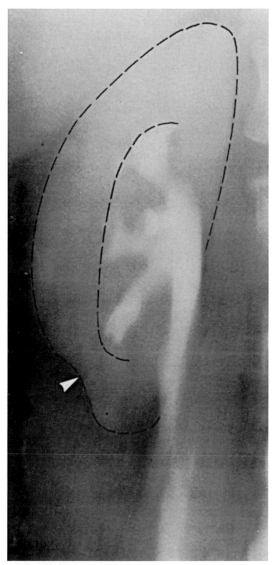

FIGURE 5–25. Mature lobar infarct. The interpapillary line remains normal, whereas the renal contour indents focally at the site of infarction *(arrow).*

infarction of a region of the kidney. Usually, the clinical history in these patients is not helpful in discriminating between these disorders, and a specific diagnosis cannot be made by the radiologist.

Diseases that produce radiologic abnormalities of the papillae or calyces must be considered in the differential diagnosis of reflux nephropathy. **Papillary necrosis** is one of these. Features of papillary necrosis not seen in reflux nephropathy include irregularity of the dilated calyx at the site of papillary slough, papillary calcification, and cavitation within attached papillae. In renal **tuberculosis,** focal papillary deformities and calyceal dilatation can be similar to those seen in reflux nephropathy, but cortical scarring tends to occur late in the course of the disease when other features characteristic of tuberculosis are also present. These include inflammatory parenchymal masses, calcification, and dilatation of all or part of the pelvoinfundibulocaly-

ceal system and ureter, which also have focal strictures. **Focal obstruction** confined to one calyx will cause papillary effacement and calyceal dilatation. A focal scar in the kidney contour overlying this site will not be present in this situation unless infection supervenes, in which case the lesion will take on the radiologic pattern of reflux nephropathy. Similarly, a **stone impacted in a papillary tip** may obstruct the related collecting ducts and cause infection and a focal scar in the overlying renal parenchyma.

Attenuation of a calyx or a group of related calyces occasionally present in early lobar infarction may also occur in inflammatory lesions such as **acute pyelonephritis,** in early **tuberculosis,** in small focal **abscess,** or in localized **hemorrhage.** Differentiation of these entities from lobar infarction is unlikely unless the nephrographic defect of early lobar infarction or absent vascularity is demonstrated by contrast material enhancement or Doppler imaging techniques. Infiltrating **uroepithelial carcinoma** can also obliterate a calyx. Retrograde pyelography may be useful in demonstrat-

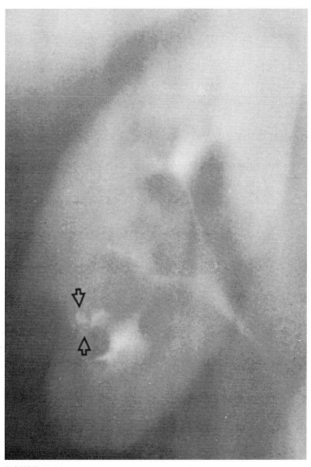

FIGURE 5–26. Mature lobar infarct in lateral aspect of lower pole extensive enough to cause slight papillary deformity *(arrows).* Papillary abnormalities are uncommon in lobar infarction and are always minimal compared with those seen in reflux nephropathy (same patient illustrated in Fig. 5–28). (Courtesy of Robert Clark, M.D., St. Francis Memorial Hospital, San Francisco, California.)

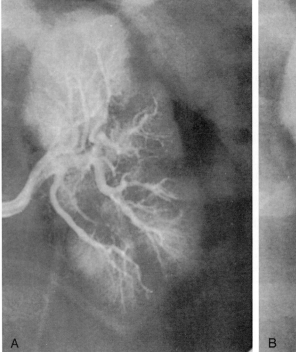

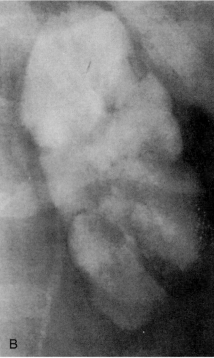

FIGURE 5–27. Multiple lobar infarcts in a 54-year-old man with hypertension.
A, Selective arteriogram. Arterial phase shows arteriosclerotic narrowing and dilatation of many arcuate arteries and absence of branching vessels.
B, Nephrographic phase. Several lobar infarcts are readily apparent.

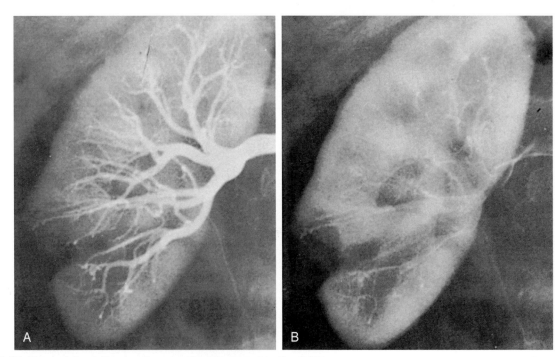

FIGURE 5–28. Mature lobar infarction (same patient illustrated in Fig. 5–26).
A, Selective arteriogram, early arterial phase. There is absence of arcuate arteries in the infarcted area and tortuosity of vessels adjacent to the infarct.
B, Late arterial phase. There is retention of contrast material in the tortuous vessels, indicating reduced flow. The broad-based contour defect is well demonstrated.

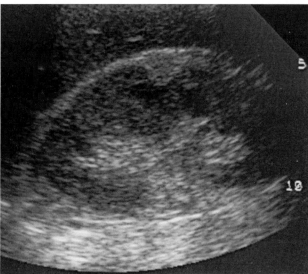

FIGURE 5–29. Mature lobar infarction (presumed diagnosis) in the right kidney of a 56-year old asymptomatic man. Ultrasonogram, longitudinal section. A triangular wedge of hyperechoic perirenal fat fills a defect on the ventral surface of the kidney. This appearance remained stable over time. (Kindly provided by Cynthia Caskey, M.D. and Ulrike Hamper, M.D., The Johns Hopkins University, Baltimore, Maryland.)

ing other features of tumor, such as mucosal irregularity or collecting system filling defects, in these cases.

BIBLIOGRAPHY

Reflux Nephropathy

Allen, T. D., Arant, B. S., and Roberts, J. A.: Commentary: Vesicoureteral reflux—1992. J. Urol. *148*:1758, 1992.

Alon, U., Berant, M., and Pery, M.: Intravenous pyelography in children with urinary tract infection and vesicoureteral reflux. Pediatrics *83*:332, 1989.

Angel, J. R., Smith, T. W., Jr., and Roberts, J. A.: The hydrodynamics of pyelorenal reflux. J. Urol. *122*:20, 1979.

Arant, B. S., Jr., Sotelo-Avila, C., and Bernstein, J.: Segmental "hypoplasia" of the kidney (Ask-Upmark). J. Pediatr. *95*:931, 1979.

Arima, M., Matsui, T., Ogino, T., Shimada, K., Hosokawa, S., Mori, Y., and Ikoma, F.: Vesicoureteral reflux in infants under one-year-old: Follow-up study and consideration on development of renal scarring. Urology *41*:372, 1993.

Arnold, A. J., Sunderland, D., Hart, C. A., and Rickwood, A. M. K.: Reconsideration of the roles of urinary infection and vesicoureteral reflux in the pathogenesis of renal scarring. Brit. J. Urol. *72*:554, 1993.

Bailey, R. R.: The relationship of vesico-ureteric reflux to urinary tract infection and chronic pyelonephritis. Clin. Nephrol. *1*:132, 1973.

Bailey, R. R., Lynn, K. L., Robson, R. A., Smith, A. H., Maling, T. M. J., and Turner, J. G.: DMSA renal scans in adults with acute pyelonephritis. Clin. Nephrol. *46*:99, 1996.

Benador, D., Benador, N., Nussle, D., Mermillod, B., and Giradin, E.: Cortical scintigraphy in the evaluation of renal parenchymal changes in children with pyelonephritis. J. Pediatr. *124*:17, 1994.

Benador, D., Benador, N., Slosman, D., Mermillod, B., and Girardin, E.: Are younger children at highest risk of renal sequelae after pyelonephritis? Lancet *349*:17, 1997.

Bernstein, J., and Arant, B. S.: Morphological characteristics of segmental renal scarring in vesicoureteral reflux. J. Urol. *148*:1712, 1992.

Cardiff-Oxford Bacteriuria Study Group: Sequelae of covert bacteriuria in schoolgirls: A four-year follow-up study. Lancet *1*:889, 1978.

Cardiff-Oxford Bacteriuria Study Group: Long-term effects of bacteriuria on the urinary tract in school girls. Radiology *132*:343, 1979.

Chapman, S. J., Chantler, C., Haycock, G. B., Maisey, M. N.,

and Saxton, H. M.: Radionuclide cystography in vesicoureteral reflux. Arch. Dis. Child. *63*:650, 1988.

Claësson, I., Jacobsson, B., Jodal, U., and Winberg, J.: Early detection of nephropathy in childhood urinary tract infection. Acta Radiol. (Diagn.) *22*:315, 1981.

Claësson, I., and Lindberg, U.: Asymptomatic bacteriuria in schoolgirls. Radiology *124*:179, 1977.

Connolly, L. P., Treves, S. T., Zurakowski, D., and Bauer, S. B.: Natural history of vesicoureteral reflux in siblings. J. Urol. *156*:1805, 1996.

Dacher, J. N., Pfister, C., Monroc, M., Eurin, D., and Ledosseur, P.: Power Doppler sonographic pattern of acute pyelonephritis in children: Comparison with CT. AJR *166*:1451, 1996.

Dalla Palma, L., Pozzi-Mucelli, R., and Pozzi-Mucelli, F.: Delayed CT in acute renal infection. Semin. Ultrasound CT MR *18*:122, 1997.

Ditchfield, M. R., De Campo, J. F., Cook, D. J., Nolan, T. M., Powell, H. R., Sloane, R., Grimwoos, K., and Cahill, S.: Vesicoureteric reflux: an accurate predictor of acute pyelonephritis in childhood urinary tract infection. Radiology *190*:413, 1994.

Elison, B. S., Taylor, D., Van der Wall, H., Pereira, J. K., Cahill, S., Rosenberg, A. R., Farnsworth, R. H., and Murray, I. P. C.: Comparison of DMSA scintigraphy with intravenous urography for the detection of renal scarring and its correlation with vesicoureteral reflux. Br. J. Urol. *69*:294, 1992.

Farnsworth, R. H., Rossleigh, M., Leighton, D. M., Bass, S. J., and Rosenberg, A. R.: The detection of reflux nephropathy in infants by [99m]technetium dimercaptosuccinic acid studies. J. Urol. *145*:542, 1991.

Fay, R., Winter, R., Cohen, A., Brosman, S. A., and Bennett, C.: Segmental renal hypoplasia and hypertension. J. Urol. *113*:561, 1975.

Fraser, I. R., Birch, D., Fairley, K. F., John, S., Lichtenstein, M., Tress, B., and Kincaid Smith, P. S.: A prospective study of cortical scarring in acute febrile pyelonephritis in adults: Clinical and bacteriological characteristics. Clin. Nephrol. *43*:159, 1995.

Freedman, L. R.: Chronic pyelonephritis at autopsy. Ann. Intern. Med. *66*:697, 1967.

Gillenwater, J. Y., Harrison, R. B., and Kunin, C. M.: Natural history of bacteriuria in schoolgirls: A long-term case-control study. N. Engl. J. Med. *301*:396, 1979.

Ginalski, J. M., Michaud, A., and Genton, N.: Renal growth retardation in children: Sign suggestive of vesicoureteral reflux? AJR *145*:617, 1985.

Goldraich, N. P., and Goldraich, I. H.: Update on dimercaptosuccinic acid renal scanning in children with urinary tract infection. Pediatr. Nephrol. *9*:221, 1995.

Hannerz, L., Wikstad, I., Johansson, L., Broberger, O., and Aperia, A.: Distribution of renal scars and intrarenal reflux in children with past history of urinary tract infection. Acta Radiol. 28:443, 1987.

Hellerstein, S.: Urinary tract infections: Old and new concepts. Pediatr. Clin. North Am. 42:1433, 1995.

Hellström, M., Jacobsson, B., Mårild, S., and Jodal, U.: Voiding cystourethrography as a predictor of reflux nephropathy in children with urinary tract infection. AJR 152:801, 1989.

Heptinstall, R. H.: Pathology of the Kidney, 4th ed. Boston, Little, Brown & Co., 1992.

Hill, G. S. (ed.): Uropathology. New York, Churchill Livingstone, 1989.

Himmelfarb, E., Rabinowitz, J. G., Parvey, L., Gammill, S., and Arant, B.: The Ask-Upmark kidney: Roentgenographic and pathological features. Am. J. Dis. Child. 129:1440, 1975.

Hodson, C. J.: The radiological diagnosis of pyelonephritis. Proc. R. Soc. Med. 52:669, 1959.

Hodson, C. J.: Coarse pyelonephritic scarring or atrophic pyelonephritis. Proc. R. Soc. Med. 58:785, 1965.

Hodson, C. J.: The radiological contribution toward the diagnosis of chronic pyelonephritis. Radiology 88:857, 1967.

Hodson, C. J.: Radiological diagnosis of renal involvement. In O'Grady, F., and Brumfitt, W. (eds.): Urinary Tract Infection. London, Oxford University Press, 1968, pp. 108–112.

Hodson, C. J.: The mechanism of scar formation in chronic pyelonephritis. In Kincaid-Smith, P., and Fairley, K. F. (eds.): Renal Infection and Renal Scarring. Proceedings of the International Symposium on Pyelonephritis, Vesicoureteral Reflux and Renal Papillary Necrosis. Melbourne, Mercedes Publishing Co., 1970.

Hodson, C. J., and Kincaid-Smith, P. (eds.): Reflux Nephropathy. New York, Masson Publishing USA, 1979.

Hodson, C. J., Mailing, T. M. J., McManamon, P. J., and Lewis, M. G.: The pathogenesis of reflux nephropathy (chronic atrophic pyelonephritis). Br. J. Radiol. (Suppl. 13), 1975.

Hodson, C. J. and Wilson, S.: Natural history of chronic pyelonephritic scarring. Br. Med J. 2:191, 1965.

Hugosson, C. O., Chrispin, A. R., and Wolverson, M. K.: The advent of the pyelonephritic scar. Ann. Radiol. 19:1, 1976.

Jakobsson, B., Berg, U., and Svensson, L.: Renal scarring after acute pyelonephritis. Arch. Dis. Child. 70:111, 1994.

Johnston, J. H., and Mix, L. W.: The Ask-Upmark kidney: A form of ascending pyelonephritis? Br. J. Urol. 48:393, 1976.

Kincaid-Smith, P.: Reflux nephropathy. Br. Med. J. 286:2002, 1983.

Lebowitz, R. L.: Neonatal vesicoureteral reflux: What do we know? Radiology 187:17, 1993.

Lebowitz, R. L., and Mandell, J.: Urinary tract infection in children: Putting radiology in its place. Radiology 165:1, 1987.

Longcope, W. T., and Winkenwerder, W. L.: Clinical features of the contracted kidney due to pyelonephritis. Bull. Johns Hopkins Hosp. 53:255, 1933.

Marra, G., Barbieri, G., Dell'agnola, C., Caccamo, M., Castellani, M., and Assael, B.: Congenital renal damage associated with primary vesicoureteral reflux detected prenatally in male infants. J. Pediatrics 124:726, 1994.

Martinell, J., Claesson, I., Lidinjanson, G., Jodal, U.: Urinary infection, reflux and renal scarring in females continuously followed for 13–38 years. Pediat. Nephrol. 9:131, 1995.

Newhouse, J. H., and Amis, E. S., Jr.: The relationship between renal scarring and stone disease. AJR 151:1153, 1988.

Olbing, H., Claësson, I., Ebel, K. D., Seppänen, U., Smellie, J. M., Tamminenmobius, T., and Wikstad, I.: Renal scars and parenchymal thinning in children with vesicoureteral reflux: A 5-year report of the International Reflux Study in Children (European branch). J. Urol. 148:1653, 1992.

Ransley, P. G.: Intrarenal reflux: Anatomical, dynamic and radiological studies: I. Urol. Res. 5:61, 1977.

Ransley, P. G., and Risdon, R. A.: Renal papillary morphology in infants and young children. Urol. Res. 3:111, 1975.

Ransley, P. G., and Risdon, R. A.: Reflux and renal scarring. Br. J. Radiol. (Suppl. 14), 1978.

Risdon, R. A.: The small scarred kidney in childhood. Pediatr. Nephrol. 7:361, 1993.

Roberts, J. A.: Factors predisposing to urinary tract infections in children. Pediatr. Nephrol. 10:517, 1996.

Rolleston, G. L., Maling, T. M. J., and Hodson, C. J.: Intrarenal reflux and the scarred kidney. Arch. Dis. Child. 49:531, 1974.

Rosenberg, A. R., Rossleigh, M. A., Brydon, M. P., Bass, S. J., Leighton, D. M., and Farnsworth, R. H.: Evaluation of acute urinary tract infection in children by dimercaptosuccinic acid scintigraphy: A prospective study. J. Urol. 148:1746, 1992.

Rubin, R. H., Cotran, R. S., and Tolkoff-Rubin, N. E.: Urinary tract infection, pyelonephritis and reflux nephropathy. In Brenner, B. M., and Rector, F. C., Jr. (eds.): The Kidney, 5th ed. Philadelphia, W. B. Saunders Co., 1996, p. 1597.

Rushton, H. G.: The evaluation of acute pyelonephritis and renal scarring with technetium ^{99m}dimercaptosuccinic acid renal scintigraphy: Evolving concepts and future directions. Pediatr. Nephrol. 11:108, 1997.

Saxton, H. M.: Computed tomography or intravenous urography for renal damage in childhood urinary infection? Pediatr. Nephrol. 9:256, 1995.

Shanon, A., Feldman, W., McDonald, P., Martin, D. J., Matzinger, M. A., Shillinger, J. F., McLaine, P. N., and Wolfish, N.: Evaluation of renal scars by technetium-labelled dimercaptosuccinic acid scan, intravenous urography and ultrasonography: A comparative study. J. Pediatr. 120:399, 1992.

Shimada, K., Matsui, T., Ogino, T., Arima, M., Mori, Y., and Ikoma, F.: Renal growth and progression of reflux nephropathy in children with vesicoureteral reflux. J. Urol. 140:1097, 1988.

Smellie, J. M.: The intravenous urogram in the detection and evaluation of renal damage following urinary tract infection. Pediatr. Nephrol. 9:213, 1995.

Stokland, E., Hellstrom, M., Jacobsson, B., Jodal, U., and Sixt, R.: Renal damage one year after first urinary tract infection: Role of dimercaptosuccinic acid scintigraphy. J. Pediatr. 129:815, 1996.

Strife, C. F., and Gelfand, M. J.: Renal cortical scintigraphy: Effect on medical decision making in childhood urinary tract infection. J. Pediatr. 129:785, 1996.

Sty, J. R., Wells, R. G., Starshak, R. J., and Schroeder, B. A.: Imaging in acute renal infection in children. AJR 148:471, 1987.

Tamminen, T. E., and Kaprio, E. A.: The relation of the shape of renal papillae and of collecting duct openings to intrarenal reflux. Br. J. Urol. 49:345, 1977.

Thomsen, H. S., Talner, L. B., and Higgins, C. B.: Intrarenal backflow during retrograde pyelography with graded intrapelvic pressure: A radiologic study. Invest. Radiol. 17:593, 1982.

Wallin, L., and Bajc, M.: Typical technetium dimercaptosuccinic acid distribution patterns in acute pyelonephritis. Acta Paediatr. 82:1061, 1993.

Wallin, L., and Bajc, M.: The significance of vesicoureteric reflux on kidney development assessed by dimercaptosuccinate scintigraphy. Brit. J. Urol. 73:607, 1994.

Wan, J. L., Greenfield, S. P., Ng, M. Y., Zerin, M., Ritchey, M. L., and Bloom, D.: Sibling reflux: A dual center retrospective study. J. Urol. 156:677, 1996.

Weiss, S., and Parker, F.: Pyelonephritis: Its relation to vascular lesions and to arterial hypertension. Medicine (Baltimore) 18:221, 1939.

White, R. H. R.: Vesicoureteral reflux and renal scarring. Arch. Dis. Child. 64:407, 1989.

Wikstad, I., Aperia, A., Broberger, O., and Löhr, G.: Long-time effect of large vesicoureteral reflux with or without urinary tract infection. Acta Radiol. (Diagn.) 22:325, 1981.

Winberg, J.: Progressive renal damage from infection with or without reflux: Commentary. J. Urol. 148:1733, 1992.

Wiswell, T. E., Smith, F. R., and Bass, J. W.: Decreased incidence of urinary tract infection in circumcised male infants. Pediatrics 75:901, 1985.

Woodard, J. R., and Rushton, H. G.: Reflux uropathy. Pediatr. Clin. North Am. 34:1349, 1987.

Zerin, J. M., Ritchey, M. L., and Chang, A. C. H.: Incidental vesicoureteral reflux in neonates with antenatally detected hydronephrosis and other renal abnormalities. Radiology 187:157, 1993.

Zuchelli, P., and Gaggi, R.: Reflux nephropathy in adults. Nephron 57:2, 1991.

Lobar Infarction

Barney, J. D., and Mintz, E. R.: Infarcts of the kidney. JAMA. *100*:1, 1933.

Belt, A. E., and Joelson, J. J.: The effect of ligation of branches of the renal artery. Arch. Surg. *10*:117, 1925.

Edwards, E.: Acute renal calcification: An experimental and clinicopathologic study. J. Urol. *80*:161, 1958.

Elkin, M.: Radiology of the urinary tract: Some physiological considerations. Radiology *116*:259, 1975.

Erwin, B. C., Carroll, B. A., Walter, J. F., and Sommer, F. G.: Renal infarction appearing as an echogenic mass. AJR *138*:759, 1982.

Halpern, M.: Acute renal artery embolus: A concept of diagnosis and treatment. J. Urol. *98*:552, 1967.

Heitzman, E. R., and Perchik, L.: Radiographic features of renal infarction: Review of 13 cases. Radiology *76*:39, 1961.

Hilton, S., Bosniak, M. A., Ragharendra, B. N., Subramanyam, B. R., Rothberg, M., and Megibow, A. J.: CT findings in acute renal infarction. Urol. Radiol. *6*:158, 1984.

Hodson, C. J.: The effects of disturbance of flow on the kidney. J. Infect. Dis. *120*:54, 1969.

Hodson, C. J.: The lobar structure of the kidney. Br. J. Urol. *44*:246, 1972.

Hoxie, H. J., and Coggin, C. B.: Renal infarction: Statistical study of 205 cases and detailed report of an unusual case. Arch. Intern. Med. *65*:587, 1940.

Janower, M. L., and Weber, A. L.: Radiologic evaluation of acute renal infarction. AJR *95*:309, 1965.

Karsner, H. T., and Austin, J. H.: Studies in infarction: Experimental bland infarction of the kidney and spleen. JAMA *57*:951, 1911.

Kelly, K. M., Craven, J. D., Jorgens, J., and Barenfus, M.: Experimental renal artery thromboembolism. Invest. Radiol. *11*:88, 1976.

Lang, E. K.: Arteriographic diagnosis of renal infarcts. Radiology *88*:1110, 1967.

Lang, E. K., Mertz, J. H. D., and Nourse, M.: Renal arteriography in the assessment of renal infarction. J. Urol. *99*:506, 1968.

MacNider, W. deB.: The pathological changes which develop in the kidney as a result of occlusion, by ligature, of one branch of the renal artery. J. Med. Res. *22*:91, 1910.

Naidich, J. B., Naidich, T. P., Pudlowski, R. M., Waldbaum, R. S., Hyman, R. A., and Stein, H. L.: Angiographic patterns of post-traumatic renal scarring. AJR *128*:729, 1977.

Papanicolaou, N., Habory, O. L., and Pfister, R. C.: Fat-filled postoperative renal cortical defects: Sonographic and CT appearance. AJR *151*:503, 1988.

Parker, J. M., and Lord, J. D.: Renal artery embolism: A case report with return of complete function of the involved kidney following anticoagulant therapy. J. Urol. *106*:339, 1971.

Regan, F. C., and Crabtree, E. G.: Renal infarction: Clinical and possible surgical entity. J. Urol. *59*:981, 1948.

Sheehan, H. L., and Davis, J. C.: Complete permanent renal ischaemia. J. Pathol. *76*:569, 1958.

Siegelman, S. S., and Caplan, L. H.: Acute segmental renal artery embolism: A distinctive urographic and arteriographic complex. Radiology *88*:509, 1967.

Solez, K.: Acute renal failure (acute tubular necrosis, infarction and cortical necrosis). In Heptinstall, R. H. (ed.): Pathology of the Kidney, 4th ed. Boston, Little, Brown & Co., 1992.

Wisoff, C. P., and Chambers, D. E.: Subtotal renal infarction. AJR *98*:63, 1966.

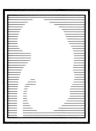

CHAPTER **6**

Diagnostic Set: Small, Smooth, Unilateral

ISCHEMIA DUE TO MAJOR ARTERIAL STENOSIS/
ANEURYSM
CHRONIC RENAL INFARCTION
RADIATION NEPHRITIS
CONGENITAL HYPOPLASIA

POSTOBSTRUCTIVE ATROPHY
POSTINFLAMMATORY ATROPHY
REFLUX ATROPHY
DIFFERENTIAL DIAGNOSIS

Generalized—that is, global—decrease in the size of one kidney with preservation of normal pelvocalyceal relationships characterizes the radiologic appearance of the entities discussed in this chapter. This pattern is the one common bond among these processes, which otherwise are widely dissimilar in their pathogenesis.

It will be noted that several of the entities included in the "small, smooth, unilateral" diagnostic set represent late stages of pathologic processes that initially produced unilateral enlargement of the kidney. Among these processes are infarction of all or large amounts of kidney tissue and obstructive uropathy. It is hoped that this order of presentation—late changes before acute ones—will not confuse the reader.

This is the first chapter to include diseases with "smallness" as the only radiologic abnormality. The reader should refer to Chapter 3 for a discussion on the assessment of renal size. Unfortunately, no accurate, practical, quantitative yardstick is available to establish "normal" renal size. In this subjective setting, one should keep in mind that apparent smallness may be erroneously suggested by abnormal enlargement of the contralateral kidney and that a kidney that may measure within normal limits actually was normally larger at an earlier time.

ISCHEMIA DUE TO MAJOR ARTERIAL STENOSIS/ANEURYSM

Definition

When renal blood flow is inadequate for normal cell metabolism, there is a global decrease in renal bulk, primarily due to tubule atrophy. The proximal convoluted segment, in particular, becomes smaller in diameter. This process is noted also in the glomeruli, which become crowded together, smaller in size, and hyalinized. These changes develop when stenosing lesions of the renal arterial tree become advanced. The number and size of the renal arteries involved determine the pattern of wasting. If arteriosclerosis is generalized in the interlobar and arcuate arteries, both kidneys will shrink uniformly (see discussion in Chapter 7). The pattern discussed in this chapter—global shrinkage of one kidney—occurs when a lesion in the main renal artery diminishes blood flow to the kidney.

Atherosclerosis. In the general population, focal narrowing of the main renal artery is usually due to an atheromatous lesion in the proximal 2 cm of the vessel. Less frequently, the distal main artery or its early branches are the site of stenosis, particularly at points of bifurcation. The atherosclerotic plaque is most often placed eccentrically in the arterial lumen. Narrowing results both from growth of the plaque and from intermittent bleeding into the plaque wall. Complete obstruction, aneurysm formation, and dissection are occasional complications of advanced atherosclerosis. With high-grade stenosis or complete obstruction, collateral vessels may develop. These vessels are derived variably from pre-existing lumbar, pelvic, ureteral, intercostal, adrenal, capsular, or other retroperitoneal arteries.

Arterial Dysplasia. Dysplastic lesions of the renal artery and its major branches also cause ischemia and renal wasting. These result from a variable mixture of collagen deposition, hyperplasia of smooth muscle and fibroblasts, and disruption or thinning of the elastica interna. Some authors group all forms of dysplasia under the single heading of *fibromuscular hyperplasia*. Others identify angiographic-pathologic subtypes. These include *intimal fibroplasia*, a symmetric, funnel-shaped band of narrowing; *medial fibroplasia*, multiple aneurysms larger in diameter than the renal artery itself; *subadventitial fibroplasia*, uneven stenosis that occurs singly or in a series, with bulges that do not exceed the diameter of the uninvolved parts of the artery; and *fibromuscular hyperplasia*, an uncommon form with a variable angiographic picture. Subtypes may differ to some degree in clinical features relating to sexual predilection, age distribution, and propensity for bilaterality. Any of these lesions can cause renovascular hypertension.

Miscellaneous Causes of Stenosis. Lesions other than atherosclerotic stenosis and dysplasia that can produce ischemia and a small kidney are quite uncommon. These include atherosclerotic renal artery aneurysm, renal arteriovenous fistula, Takayasu's disease, thromboangiitis obliterans, syphilitic arteritis, dissecting aortic aneurysm, postradiation renal artery stenosis, and extrinsic pressure on the renal artery from a lesion in the kidney hilus, such as tumor, fibrous bands, or parapelvic cyst.

Other aspects of renal arterial diseases are discussed in Chapter 16.

Clinical Setting

The development of ischemic atrophy becomes clinically important only when it is associated with hypertension. The focal arterial lesion that produces a small kidney in a person who remains normotensive is of no particular consequence except insofar as it may lead to renal insufficiency when it is bilateral or occurs in a solitary kidney or the normal, nonischemic kidney develops a tumor or becomes obstructed. Indeed, moderate-to-severe renal artery narrowing occurs often in older, normotensive patients and in patients with essential (i.e., nonrenovascular) hypertension.

The pathophysiology of the ischemic kidney centers on decreased perfusion pressure of the juxtaglomerular apparatus and the afferent arteriole, which, respectively, stimulates renin-angiotensin-aldosterone production and reduces the rate of glomerular filtration. The complex osmotic and humoral factors that follow lead to hyper-reninemic hypertension; an increase in the concentration of filtered, nonreabsorbable substances, including urographic contrast material; diminished urine volume; and decreased urine flow rate on the affected side as compared with the nonischemic contralateral kidney. Additionally, elevated angiotensin II levels stimulate constriction of efferent arterioles, which has the compensating effect of increasing glomerular filtration rate. Pharmacologic inhibition of angiotensin II production in patients with renovascular hypertension causes efferent arteriolar dilatation in the ischemic kidney and a precipitous drop in glomerular filtration rate. As discussed in Chapter 2, this technique is used to increase the

sensitivity of radionuclide renography for detecting renovascular hypertension by enhancing the difference in the transport of a radionuclide agent between the ischemic kidney and the contralateral, normal kidney.

The histologic nature of a stenosing lesion varies with age and sex. Males older than age 50 years are likely to have atherosclerotic stenoses or aneurysms, whereas females in younger age groups (mean age of 38 years) more frequently develop dysplastic arterial disease. Renal artery dysplasia may be a cause for hypertension in patients with neurofibromatosis. Both atherosclerotic and dysplastic lesions can be progressive and bilateral. This fact is of obvious importance in evaluating therapeutic choices for these patients.

One of the major clinical challenges in setting diagnostic strategies for the hypertensive population at large is to identify patients who have renovascular hypertension, that is, those with renal artery abnormalities that, if corrected, will mitigate or cure high blood pressure. These patients, who comprise less than 3 per cent of the hypertensive population, need to be distinguished from those whose hypertension is due to other causes or is essential. Historically, a modification of the excretory urogram, known as the "hypertensive" or "rapid sequence" urogram, was used as a primary screen of the hypertensive population to identify patients with curable hypertension. Critical assessment of the modified excretory urogram as a screening test of the general hypertensive population for a renovascular cause, however, has demonstrated its low positive predictive value, reflecting both the poor sensitivity of the test and the low prevalence of renovascular hypertension. The same considerations have limited the usefulness of traditional radionuclide renography. However, modified radionuclide renography performed before and after angiotensin II-converting enzyme inhibition has proven more successful. As a result, emphasis has shifted to using a combination of clinical features and modified renography as screening criteria for selecting the hypertensive patient who should be subjected to the definitive test of renal angiography. Clinical features include hypertension developing at extremes of age (i.e., before age 30 years and after age 55 years), a patient with stable hypertension that abruptly accelerates, and unexplained deterioration in renal function in a hypertensive patient. Other clinical features that increase the probability of a renovascular cause for hypertension include failure of moderate hypertension to respond to medical treatment and an abdominal bruit.

Patients whose clinical and renographic screening criteria point to a renovascular cause should be studied with an angiographic imaging modality, either film-screen or digital catheter angiography, computed tomographic angiography or magnetic resonance angiography. Angioplasty can be performed when a suitable renal artery stenosis is discovered. Sampling of renal veins for renin assay and duplex Doppler ultrasonography are additional diagnostic approaches whose efficacy is either disputed or yet to be proved. Angiotensin-converting enzyme inhibitor radionuclide renography is discussed in detail in Chapter 2.

Radiologic Findings

Calcification in a renal artery aneurysm or in the wall of a severely atheromatous renal artery may be detected in radiographic and computed tomographic images (Fig. 6–1; see Fig. 16–13). The reader should be familiar with the abnormalities that may be encountered in contrast material–enhanced imaging studies, such as excretory urography or computed tomography. These are briefly summarized in the following paragraphs. However, most abnormal findings are found in modified radionuclide renograms (discussed in Chapter 2) and angiographic imaging studies.

The ischemic kidney maintains a smooth contour despite a decrease in size (Fig. 6–2). Delay in appearance time of contrast material in the calyces on the involved side is the most direct functional radiologic sign of renovascular ischemia. This finding is present in a majority of patients with renovascular hypertension and in very few of those with essential hypertension (Fig. 6–3). This abnormality is a direct expression of the decrease in glomerular

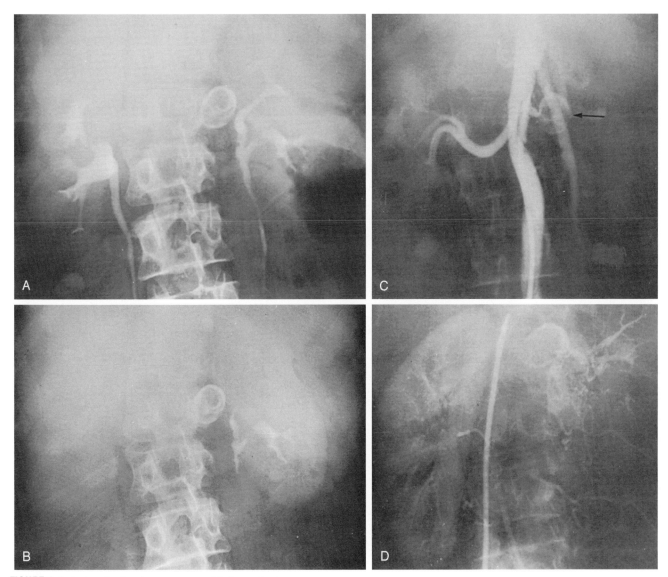

FIGURE 6–1. Ischemia due to aneurysm of left renal artery.

A, Five-minute film during excretory urography in a middle-aged hypertensive woman. The aneurysm is calcified. Diminished urine volume and pelviureteral notching due to arterial collaterals are present on the involved side. Renal length is within normal limits.

B, Delayed "washout" of contrast material from left kidney illustrates the diminished rate of urine flow in the ischemic kidney.

C, Aortogram, early arterial phase, anteroposterior projection. The occlusion is nearly complete *(arrow).*

D, Delayed film, right posterior oblique projection. Peripelvic and periureteric collaterals and intrarenal arteries are now opacified.

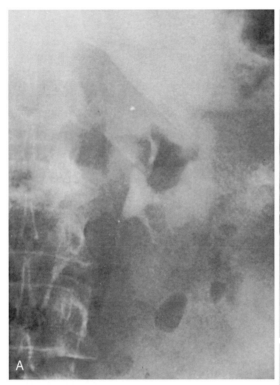

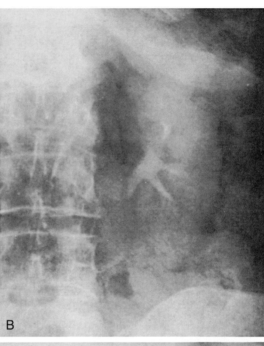

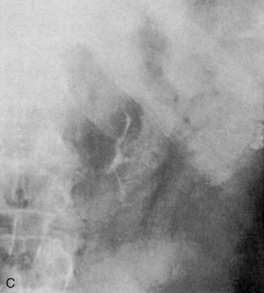

FIGURE 6–2. Ischemia due to major arterial stenosis. Progressive global decrease in left kidney length in a middle-aged hypertensive woman with angiographically proven left main renal artery stenosis.

   A, Baseline. Left kidney length = 10.5 cm.

   B, One year later. Left kidney length = 9.5 cm.

   C, Four years after baseline. Left kidney length = 8.0 cm. Note preservation of smooth margin. Patient was treated with antihypertensive medication.

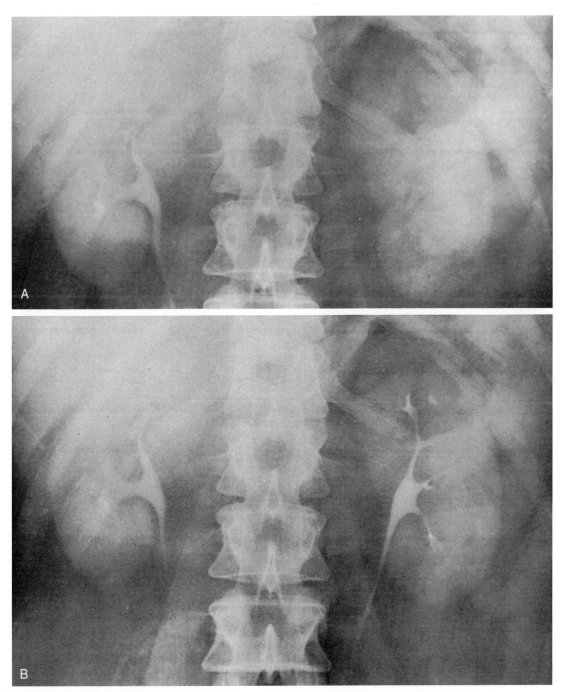

FIGURE 6–3. Bilateral renal artery dysplasia with predominant functional impairment on the left.
  A, Excretory urogram, 5-minute film. There is no calyceal opacification on the left, whereas the right system is opacified.
  B, Thirty-minute film, excretory urogram. There is diminished urine volume and increased urine density on the left side.
  (Courtesy of J. Shanser, M.D., St. Francis Memorial Hospital, San Francisco, California, and M. Korobkin, M.D., University of Michigan, Ann Arbor, Michigan.)

filtration rate that follows reduction in glomerular perfusion pressure. For each unit of time, fewer molecules of iodine-bearing contrast material are cleared from the plasma on the affected side than from the contralateral nonischemic kidney. As a result, there is a period of time after injection of contrast material when the number of atoms of iodine present in the calyces of the normal kidney allows radiographic detection, whereas the amount of iodine cleared on the ischemic side is insufficient for detection.

Because salt and water reabsorption is enhanced in the ischemic kidney, the volume of urine the ischemic kidney forms in any given time is less than the amount the normal side forms. This phenomenon is manifested as a lack of distention of the pelvocalyceal and ureteral structures on the involved side (see Figs. 6–1 and 6–3). Increased density of contrast material in the collecting structures is also due to increased water reabsorption, causing hyperconcentration in the urine of nonreabsorbable solutes (see Fig. 6–3).

Another physiologic consequence of reduced perfusion pressure and glomerular filtration rate is prolonged transit of urine through the tubules and down the ureter. This is detected in delayed images (usually after 30 minutes) by the persistent opacification of the pelvocalyceal system and ureter of the ischemic kidney at a time when the normal kidney shows "washing out" of contrast material (see Fig. 6–1B).

A classic urographic abnormality of ischemia is ureteral notching. This occurs as a result of enlargement of the collateral arteries that carry blood around the obstructing lesion (Fig. 6–4; see Fig. 6–1). Although there are many potential collateral arteries, the periureteric and peripelvic vessels are particularly important because they impress on structures visualized during urography and are seen as multiple mural notches in the proximal ureter and the pelvis.

Renal angiography precisely identifies the site, nature, and extent of the arterial lesion and is indispensable in establishing the diagnosis and planning a therapeutic approach, by either surgery or percutaneous transluminal angioplasty (Figs. 6–5, 6–6, 6–7; see Figs. 16–14, 16–15, 16–17, and 16–18 through 16–23). Film-screen angiography and digital subtraction angiography are most definitive. Neither computed tomographic nor magnetic resonance angiography are as precise as direct angiographic techniques, especially in detecting lesions

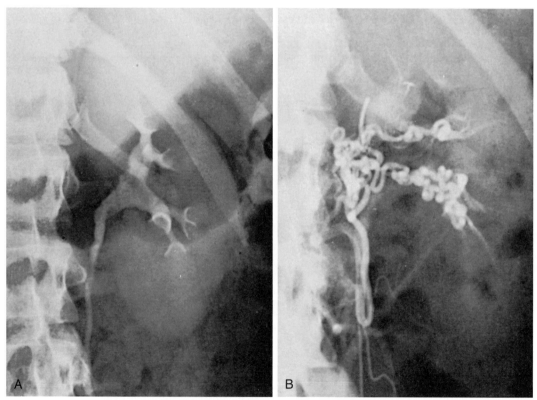

FIGURE 6–4. Ischemia due to major arterial disease. Ureteral and pelvic notching in a 16-year-old girl with severe hyper-reninemic hypertension due to surgically proven intimal fibroplasia of left renal artery.

A, Excretory urogram. Indentations on margin of pelvis and ureter are present.

B, Lumbar arteriogram. There are dilated tortuous periureteric and peripelvic collateral arteries that correspond to the abnormalities depicted in *A* (same patient illustrated in Figs. 16–18 and 16–22).

(Courtesy of Janet Dacie, M.B., St. Bartholomew's Hospital, London, England.)

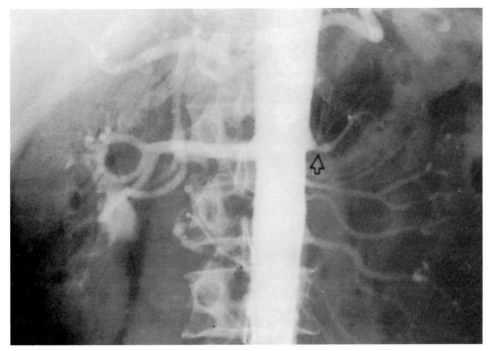

FIGURE 6–5. Atherosclerosis, proximal left renal artery. Aortogram. There is a high-grade stenosis of the left main renal artery *(arrow)* with post-stenotic dilatation (same patient illustrated in Fig. 27–7). (Courtesy of Department of Diagnostic Radiology, Hammersmith Hospital, Royal Postgraduate Medical School, London, England.)

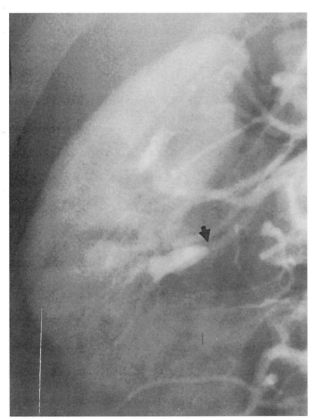

FIGURE 6–6. Renal artery dysplasia. Intimal fibroplasia subtype. Aortogram. There is post-stenotic dilatation immediately distal to a symmetric band of narrowing *(arrow)*.

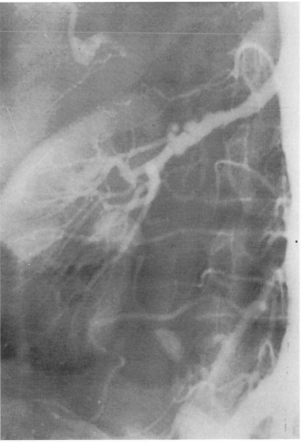

FIGURE 6–7. Renal artery dysplasia. Medial fibroplasia subtype. Aortogram. There are multiple aneurysms of the main renal artery, each larger than the renal artery itself (same patient illustrated in Fig. 16–19).

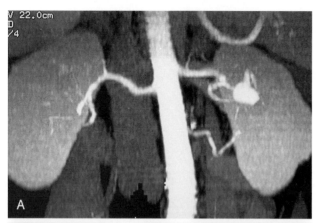

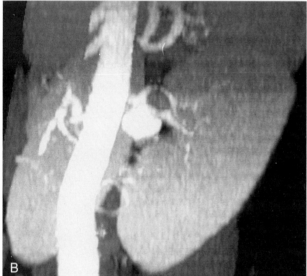

FIGURE 6–8. Renal artery aneurysm. Computed tomographic arteriogram (same patient illustrated in Figs. 1–9 and 16–21).
   A, Coronal reconstruction, frontal projection. An aneurysm is present at the bifurcation of the main renal artery.
   B, Coronal reconstruction, oblique projection.

ISCHEMIA DUE TO MAJOR ARTERIAL STENOSIS/ANEURYSM TYPICAL FINDINGS

Primary Uroradiologic Elements

Size: small
Contour: smooth
Lesion distribution: unilateral

Secondary Uroradiologic Elements

Collecting system: attenuated (global); notched (proximal ureter); delayed opacification
   time; increased density of contrast material; delayed washout of contrast material
Parenchymal thickness: wasted (global)
Calcification: linear (aneurysmal or atherosclerotic in renal hilus)

in branches of the main renal artery (Fig. 6–8). They are, however, useful for screening.

CHRONIC RENAL INFARCTION

Definition

The kidney that has undergone complete infarction eventually becomes globally small and is enhanced minimally or not at all during imaging procedures using contrast material. The sequence of histologic events is the same as described for lobar infarction in Chapter 5. All elements of the kidney atrophy, and interstitial fibrosis with obliteration of the vessels develops. Some perfusion of the renal tissue may persist through capsular, pelvic, and ureteric collateral arteries not affected by the occlusive process. This does not necessarily represent perfusion to functioning tissue, however.

There are times when infarction affects a major portion, but not all, of the kidney. In this situation an entire pole or the dorsal or ventral part of the organ becomes atrophic, whereas the noninvolved portion continues to function. Because infarction in these cases involves much more than the lobe, the pattern of wasting leaves a smooth margin.

Clinical Setting

Total or major segmental renal infarction is very uncommon when compared with the frequency of lobar infarction. Infarction may be due to embolization, thrombosis, or traumatic avulsion of the main renal artery or one of its major divisions. Blunt trauma to the kidney and renal venous thrombosis are two other situations that can produce major renal infarction leading to global atrophy.

The late stage of complete infarction is clinically silent. Total infarction rarely is associated with sustained hypertension or with any other renal symptoms if the contralateral kidney is adequate to maintain renal function. When infarction does not involve the whole kidney or when the process eventually resolves, the affected renal tissue may atrophy.

Radiologic Findings

The classic radiologic appearance of late total renal infarction includes global shrinkage of the kidney, absent contrast material enhancement, and a normal pelvocalyceal system shown on a retrograde pyelogram (Fig. 6–9). Decrease in renal size can be detected within 2 weeks after the onset of infarction and reaches maximal extent by 5 weeks. The contralateral kidney enlarges in individuals young enough to provide this reserve.

In cases of partial infarction, the involved area can be identified by regional thinning of the renal parenchyma (Figs. 6–10, 6–11). Although this find-

ing may be difficult to detect by excretory urography, computed tomography or other cross-sectional techniques clearly demonstrate these regions.

Global atrophy may follow a total infarction that resolves early enough to preserve organ viability (Fig. 6–12). In some cases, ischemia persists, and the same functional abnormalities seen in main renal artery stenosis are present.

The infarcted kidney produces greater than normal echogenicity. Ultrasonography also well demonstrates the wasting of renal parenchyma and the preservation of a smooth renal contour.

The angiographic findings in late renal infarction range from failure to demonstrate any arteries (see Fig. 6–9C) to the nonopacification of major regional branches (see Fig. 6–10B) or an accessory renal artery (see Fig. 6–11B). In kidneys that have undergone resolution of an infarctive process, the findings will vary and include normal to decreased numbers of vessels, diminished density of the nephrogram, and thinned parenchyma.

RADIATION NEPHRITIS

Definition

Radiation nephritis occurs as a result of the kidneys being included within a therapeutic field of radiation beyond 2300 R administered over a 5-week period.

Pathologically, all elements of renal tissue are affected. Interstitial fibrosis, tubule atrophy, glomerular sclerosis, sclerosis of arteries of all sizes, hyalinization of afferent arterioles, and thickening of the renal capsule are present in varying degrees.

Clinical Setting

Clinically, both acute and chronic forms have been described. The chronic form may follow a period of clinically apparent acute disease or appear *de novo* without any prior evidence of radiation-induced renal disease. This often occurs at a later time, perhaps 2 years or more after the initial exposure to radiation.

Radiation nephritis is associated with anemia, proteinuria, hyposthenuria, and azotemia. Granular epithelial and hyaline casts are seen in the urinary sediment. Moderate to malignant hypertension is present in half of the patients. This may be due to renin-angiotensin factors. In many respects the clinical picture is similar to that of chronic glomerulonephritis. However, radiation nephritis may be compatible with long life, even in the presence of progressive reduction in renal size.

Deterioration of renal function and clinical findings are most likely related to glomerular damage. The basic mediating factor in the pathogenesis of this disease, however, is radiation-induced damage to the small vessels of the kidney.

Text continued on page 122

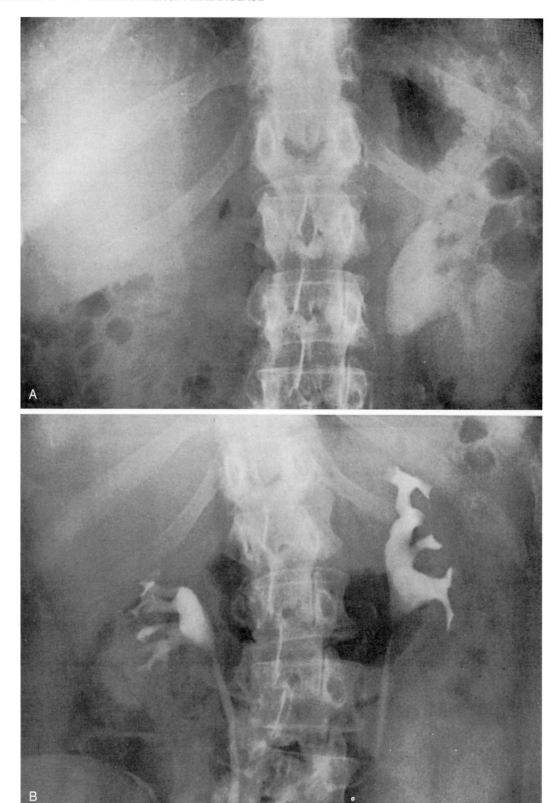

FIGURE 6–9. Chronic total infarction of the right kidney.
  A, No right renal substance is opacified at any time during excretory urography.
  B, Bilateral retrograde pyelography demonstrates normal papillae and calyces. Crowding of the right-sided structures suggests smallness of the kidney.

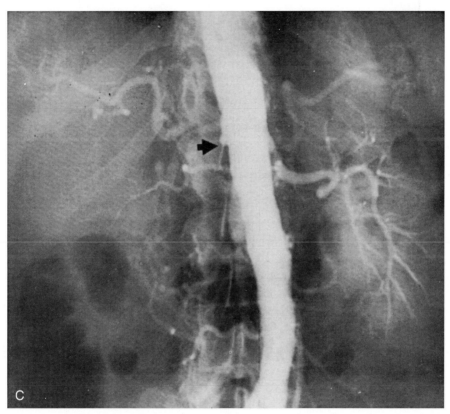

FIGURE 6–9 *Continued C,* Aortogram demonstrates complete occlusion of right renal artery *(arrow)* and no collateral flow. Autopsy revealed a small, smooth kidney due to old infarction from a thrombosis in the proximal main renal artery.

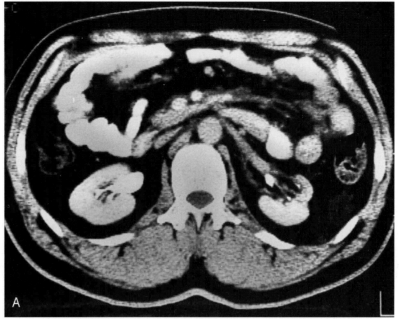

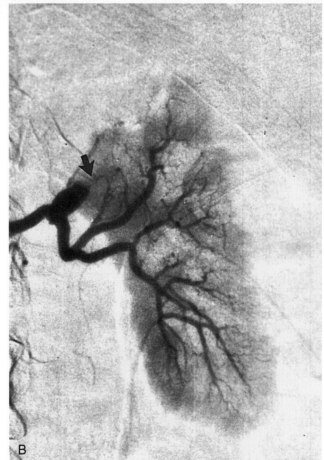

FIGURE 6–10. Chronic infarction of the ventral portion of the left kidney in a 41-year-old hypertensive woman. There has been occlusion of the major anterior branch of the renal artery caused by arterial dysplasia.

  A, Computed tomogram, contrast material–enhanced. Uniform wasting of the ventral portion of the left kidney parenchyma has occurred.

  B, Selective renal arteriogram. Subtraction technique. There is complete occlusion of the major branch of the renal artery to the ventral portion of the kidney *(arrow).*

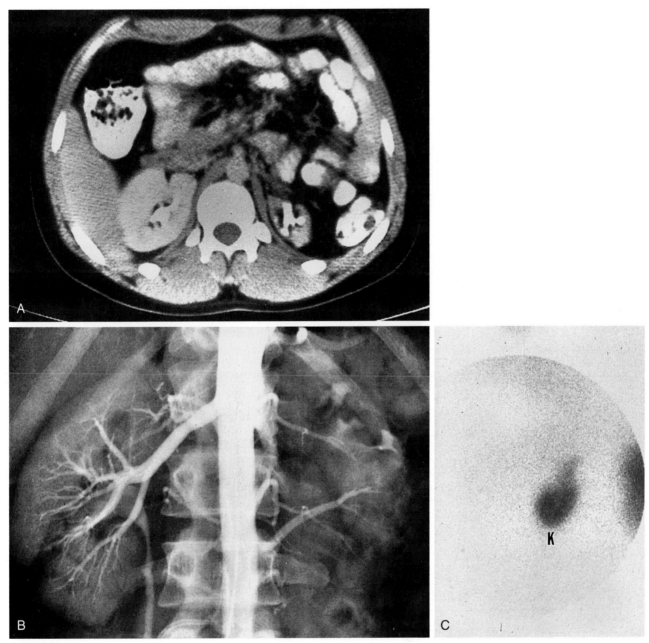

FIGURE 6–11. Chronic infarction of the upper half of a left kidney perfused by two renal arteries. The superior artery had been transected as a result of previous blunt abdominal trauma.

A, Computed tomogram, contrast material–enhanced. The global wasting of the upper pole is so marked that there is associated dilatation of underlying calyces.

B, Aortogram. The artery to the upper half of the left kidney is missing. The lower half of the kidney is perfused by a renal artery arising at the level of the superior end plate of the L-3 vertebral body.

C, Radionuclide scan. The upper half of the left kidney (K) is globally wasted.

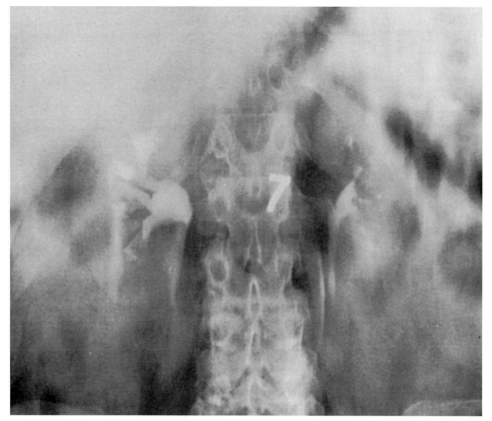

FIGURE 6–12. Chronic renal infarction. Unilateral global atrophy of left kidney with preservation of function 30 months after acute infarction complicating colon surgery. Infarction apparently resolved early enough to preserve organ viability. Despite atrophy, hypertension did not develop. Radiologic studies obtained in this patient during the acute episode are illustrated in Figure 9–11.

Radiologic Findings

There is nothing specific about the radiologic appearance of the kidney in radiation nephritis. In some patients, renal size remains normal; in others, the kidney becomes profoundly small. A smooth contour and a normal pelvocalyceal system are preserved. Atrophy is limited to those portions of the kidney included in the radiation field (Fig. 6–13).

In unilateral disease, the same radiologic abnormalities of ischemia seen in renal artery stenosis may also be present. The contralateral kidney is likely to undergo compensatory hypertrophy, particularly when radiation nephritis develops in younger patients. Depending on the size and shape of the radiation field, both kidneys may be involved.

CHRONIC RENAL INFARCTION TYPICAL FINDINGS

Primary Uroradiologic Elements

Size: small
Contour: smooth
Lesion distribution: unilateral

Secondary Uroradiologic Elements*

Parenchymal thickness: wasted (global, occasionally regional)
Nephrogram: diminished density
Echogenicity: increased

*Functional abnormalities seen in the ischemic kidney (see Radiologic Findings in the section on Ischemia Due to Major Arterial Stenosis/Aneurysm) may also be present in incomplete forms of chronic infarction.

RADIATION NEPHRITIS TYPICAL FINDINGS

Primary Uroradiologic Elements

Size: small
Contour: smooth
Lesion distribution: consistent with radiation field

Secondary Uroradiologic Elements*

Parenchymal thickness: wasted (global, related to radiation field)
Nephrogram: diminished density

*Functional abnormalities seen in the ischemic kidney (see Radiologic Findings in the section on Ischemia Due to Major Arterial Stenosis/Aneurysm) may also be present in unilateral cases of radiation nephritis.

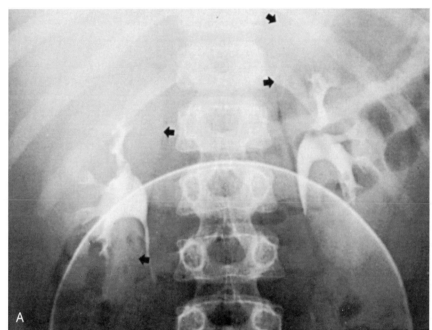

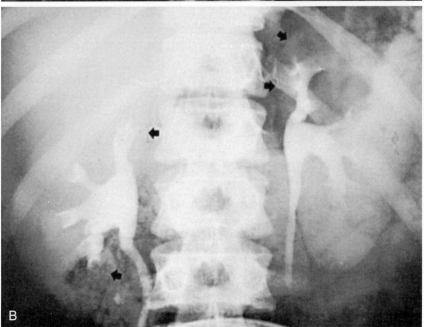

FIGURE 6–13. Radiation-induced atrophy.
A, Normal excretory urogram in an 11-year-old boy with Hodgkin's disease before para-aortic nodal radiation. Arrows point to the margin of the kidneys in those areas that eventually atrophied.
B, Excretory urogram 5 years later. Radiation field included medial aspect of the right kidney and upper pole of the left kidney. Arrows point to the margins of the kidney where atrophy can be detected by their proximity to adjacent calyces. Margins remain smooth. (Courtesy of the late A. J. Palubinskas, M.D., University of California, San Francisco.)

CONGENITAL HYPOPLASIA

Definition

A hypoplastic kidney is underdeveloped because of a quantitative deficiency in its ureteric and metanephric primordia. As a result, there is miniaturization of the kidney due to a reduction in both the number of renal lobes and the amount of nephrons contained in each lobe. The number of calyces and papillae are fewer than normal. Function persists in those nephrons that do develop. The microscopic anatomy of the hypoplastic kidney, uncomplicated by any superimposed process, is characterized by smallness of cell size and occasional hyaline degeneration of the glomeruli.

The *Ask-Upmark kidney* is considered by some to be an important variant of true renal hypoplasia, in which nephrogenesis is arrested in one or several adjacent lobes following the formation of juxtamedullary nephrons. The Ask-Upmark kidney is also referred to as *aglomerular focal hypoplasia* in the European literature. In terms of imaging, a focal area of renal wasting is associated with ectasia of the corresponding calyces. There are many who consider the Ask-Upmark kidney to be nothing more than a kidney with a single focus of reflux nephropathy. Certainly, the radiologic features are compatible with this diagnosis, and the absence of a history of urinary tract infection does not dissuade one from adopting this point of view. The issue is discussed in Chapter 5. The issue remains unresolved, however. The basis for the deep transverse groove on the cortical surface described in some case reports of Ask-Upmark kidney has not been established.

The diagnosis of renal hypoplasia is imprecise unless strict morphologic criteria are applied. The literature has been confused by the inclusion of many acquired diseases that produce small kidneys and because the true hypoplastic kidney often acquires disease, especially infection. If this diagnosis is to be made with accuracy, particular emphasis must be placed on finding five or fewer calyces in a small kidney, a very rare occurrence.

Clinical Setting

In unilateral renal hypoplasia, the contralateral kidney becomes hypertrophied, and normal renal

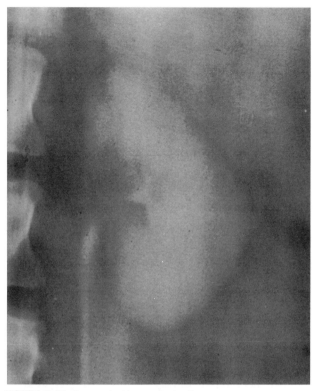

FIGURE 6–14. Congenital hypoplasia. Excretory urogram. Tomogram. The small, smooth left kidney has fewer than five identifiable calyces. (Courtesy of Professor L. Dalla Palma, University of Trieste, Trieste, Italy.)

function is maintained. Clinical concern in this situation is limited to the preservation of the dominant kidney. On the other hand, bilateral hypoplasia leads to renal failure, the intensity of which varies with the amount of tissue present. Failure to thrive, renal osteodystrophy, and other stigmata of impaired renal function appear during childhood, usually before the end of the 1st decade.

Radiologic Findings

The single, small, smooth kidney with five or fewer calyces and an enlarged contralateral kidney provides the basis for the radiologic diagnosis of renal hypoplasia (Fig. 6–14). Associated urogenital anomalies, such as ectopia and ureteral duplication, are common but of little value in distinguishing hypo-

---

CONGENITAL HYPOPLASIA TYPICAL FINDINGS

Primary Uroradiologic Elements

Size: small
Contour: smooth
Lesion distribution: unilateral

Secondary Uroradiologic Elements

Papillae: decreased number
Calyces: decreased number

plasia from other causes of the small kidney because of their common occurrence in general. The hypoplastic kidney usually has nephrons that function sufficiently for opacification of the pelvocalyceal system.

POSTOBSTRUCTIVE ATROPHY

Definition

Generalized papillary atrophy associated with a variable amount of caliectasis and global thinning of the renal parenchyma are changes that occasionally follow correction of urinary obstruction. Usually the kidney shrinks as well, but there are some cases in which renal length remains normal or even increases as the volume of the dilated pelvocalyceal system increases. Also included in this category are those unusual cases in which the kidney undergoes rather rapid parenchymal wasting, with little, if any, calyceal dilatation following relief of a limited period of urinary obstruction.

Clinical Setting

Atrophy of tissue due to urinary tract obstruction is thought to result from the direct effect of increased hydrostatic pressure on renal tissue and ischemia from compression of intrarenal arteries and veins. Presumably, progressive atrophy following relief of obstruction, particularly of a mild degree and moderate duration, is primarily due to ischemia. Experimental work in the pig indicates that direct pressure from obstruction causes tubule rupture, cell atrophy, and loss of bulk of the renal pyramids. This mechanism, rather than ischemia, may be dominant when the residual effect of relieved obstruction is clubbed calyces as well as global parenchymal atrophy.

Most patients with postobstructive atrophy have a proven history of obstruction or at least prior symptoms of renal colic. A significant number of the cases originally reported by Hodson and Craven (1966), however, had no such history, and the existence of previous obstruction was presumed by these authors.

Why some patients respond to relieved obstruction in this manner, whereas others in apparently identical circumstances do not, is not known.

Radiologic Findings

The postobstructive atrophic kidney is usually, but not invariably, a small kidney. Regardless of size,

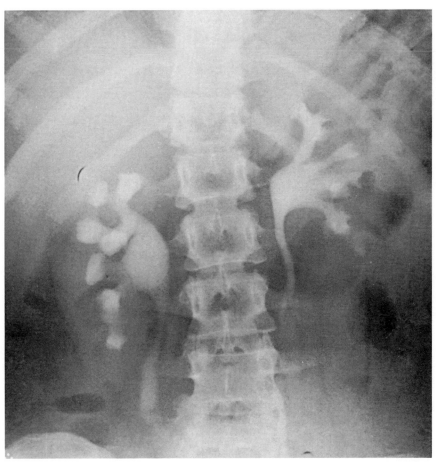

FIGURE 6–15. Nonobstructive caliectasis and global parenchymal atrophy involving the right kidney of a 26-year-old woman without a prior history of urinary tract disease. This pattern is associated either with previously reversed urinary tract obstruction or with vesicoureteral reflux. Kidney length may be normal, as in this case, reduced, or increased.

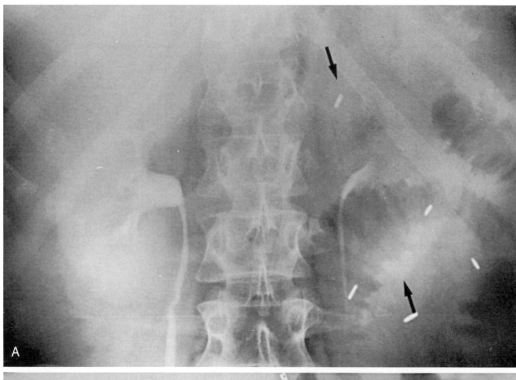

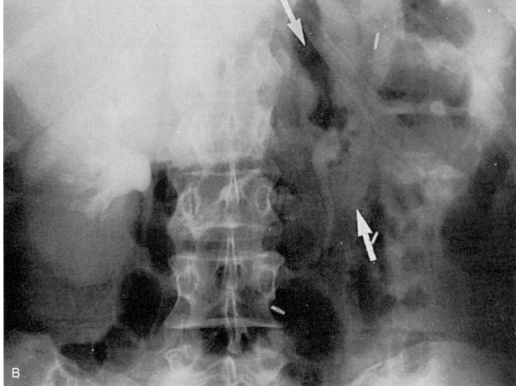

FIGURE 6–16. Postobstructive atrophy.

A, Normal baseline urogram in a patient with malignant lymphoma. Left kidney *(arrows)* measures 11.5 cm.

B, Excretory urogram 5 years later after an episode of treated left hydronephrosis. Kidney *(arrows)* now measures 7.4 cm and is smooth in outline. Papillary and calyceal architecture remain normal. No radiation therapy was given to the left kidney, and the patient was normotensive.

POSTOBSTRUCTIVE ATROPHY TYPICAL FINDINGS

Primary Uroradiologic Elements

Size: small
Contour: smooth
Lesion distribution: unilateral

Secondary Uroradiologic Elements

Papillae: effaced
Collecting system: calyces dilated
Parenchymal thickness: wasted

---

all kidneys with this condition are included in this diagnostic set because they all have undergone uniform loss of renal tissue. Dilatation of the collecting structures accounts for those situations in which renal size is preserved or increased (Fig. 6–15). Global atrophy with preservation of normal papillae and calyces is a rare presentation of postobstructive atrophy (Fig. 6–16). The progression of atrophy following relief of obstruction of moderate duration can be documented by serial urography, ultrasonography, or computed tomography and occurs rather rapidly over 6 to 12 weeks.

Compensatory hypertrophy of the contralateral kidney may be present, depending on the age of the patient, duration of the process, and severity of functional impairment in the involved kidney.

POSTINFLAMMATORY ATROPHY

An unusual form of severe acute pyelonephritis occurs in some adult patients who have altered host resistance due to diabetes mellitus or other underlying conditions. During the acute phase of this infection, the kidney becomes smoothly enlarged, with marked impairment of contrast material excretion. This condition is discussed in Chapter 9.

The rapid return of function following appropriate antibiotic therapy that characterizes severe acute pyelonephritis has been interpreted as evidence that the kidney is rendered ischemic by inflammatory infiltrate surrounding and occluding the interlobular arteries in the cortex. This concept is supported by laboratory investigations of acute infection in the rabbit kidney (Hill and Clark, 1972). Another possible cause of ischemia is effacement of medium-sized renal arteries by generalized swelling of the kidney or by vasospasm.

Generalized wasting of the renal parenchyma, a sequela to treated severe acute pyelonephritis, occurs within a few weeks after the initiation of appropriate antibiotic therapy. The loss of renal tissue is global, with preservation of a smooth or minimally irregular contour. Focal scars of the reflux nephropathy type do not occur in these patients.

Renal papillary necrosis is also a result of severe acute pyelonephritis, but it may go unrecognized during the acute phase because of the severely impaired excretion of contrast material. All of these changes may develop after only a single episode of infection.

Clinical Setting

No specific clinical abnormalities have been consistently associated with the late, treated stage of severe acute pyelonephritis. The possibility exists that hyper-reninemic hypertension may result from ischemic atrophy of the formerly infected kidney. The clinical manifestations of the acute phase are described in Chapter 9.

Radiologic Findings

In successfully treated severe acute pyelonephritis, global wasting of the kidney leads to a uniform decrease in renal size with a smooth or minimally

---

POSTINFLAMMATORY ATROPHY TYPICAL FINDINGS

Primary Uroradiologic Elements

Size: small
Contour: smooth
Lesion distribution: unilateral

Secondary Uroradiologic Elements

Papillae: disrupted
Parenchymal thickness: wasted

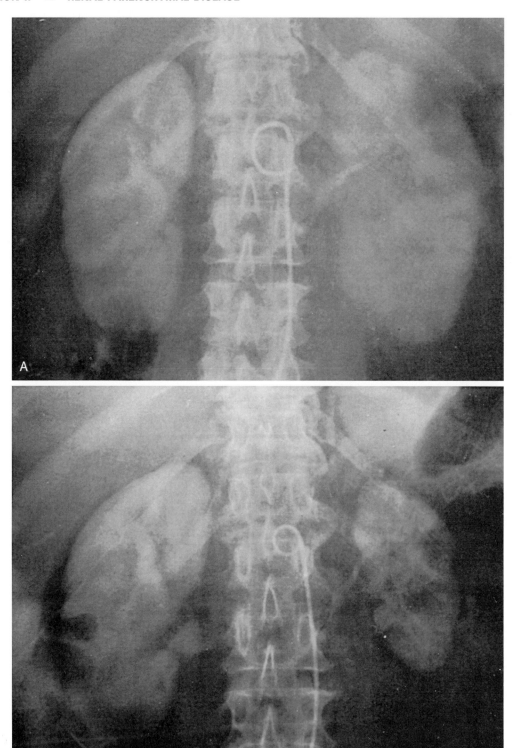

FIGURE 6–17. Postinflammatory atrophy developing in a 57-year-old woman with previously undiagnosed diabetes mellitus and severe acute pyelonephritis.

A, Nephrographic phase of aortogram performed during acute illness illustrates enlarged smooth left kidney (length = 15.7 cm) that did not excrete contrast material during urography.

B, Nephrographic phase of aortogram 12 months later shows global atrophy of left kidney (length = 10.3 cm). Faint pelvocalyceal opacification occurred during urography at this time.

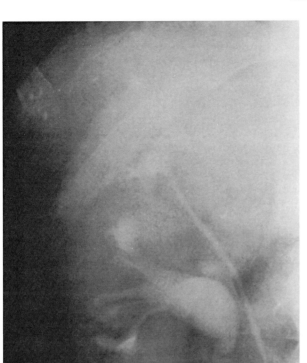

FIGURE 6–18. Postinflammatory atrophy with papillary necrosis. Excretory urogram. Uniform atrophy and papillary necrosis in the lower moiety of a completely duplicated system. Severe acute pyelonephritis was limited to this portion of the kidney. The superior moiety is normal.

irregular contour (Fig. 6–17). The change in renal size occurs over the few weeks after initiation of appropriate antibiotic therapy. Renal papillary necrosis is detected only after the kidney recovers its function and the pelvocalyceal system can once again be opacified (Fig. 6–18).

REFLUX ATROPHY

Definition

Vesicoureteral reflux severe enough to drive a large volume of urine under high pressure from the bladder to the pelvocalyceal system causes structural damage to the kidney characterized by generalized, uniform wasting of the renal parenchyma, with flattening of papillae and dilatation of the pelvocalyceal system.

This condition, known as reflux atrophy, differs fundamentally from that other form of renal damage associated with severe vesicoureteral reflux, namely, reflux nephropathy; neither infection nor intrarenal reflux need be present, and focal scars do not develop. (Reflux nephropathy is discussed in Chapter 5.)

The exact pathogenesis of reflux atrophy has not been elucidated. Undoubtedly, increased hydrostatic pressure of pelvocalyceal urine is a principal factor. Atrophy follows as a result of direct pressure on the nephrons and collecting ducts, impairment of the drainage of the nephrons, or, indirectly, through ischemia. In experimental animals, reflux atrophy evolves over a few weeks following the development of severe vesicoureteral reflux.

Clinical Setting

Reflux atrophy produces no clinical signs or symptoms. Symptom-producing urinary tract infection may develop incidentally. When reflux atrophy develops in both kidneys, loss of renal parenchyma can be severe enough to cause renal failure.

Reflux atrophy persists after the spontaneous or surgical resolution of vesicoureteral reflux. Thus, an exact cause may never be established in adult patients who are discovered to have global atrophy and a dilated pelvocalyceal system, as discussed in the section Differential Diagnosis.

Radiologic Findings

Overall reduction in renal size with preservation of a smooth contour, generalized flattening or retraction of papillae, and dilatation of the collecting system and ureter constitute the radiologic findings of reflux atrophy (Fig. 6–19). When the pelvocalyceal system is not fully distended, as in dehydration and other causes of oliguria, longitudinal striations may be seen as regular lucent bands in the pelvis or ureter (Fig. 6–20). These represent redundant mucosa and disappear when the collecting system is distended. This is discussed further in Chapter 15. Active vesicoureteral reflux is usually absent when this condition is discovered in the adult.

DIFFERENTIAL DIAGNOSIS

In the unilaterally small, smooth kidney, functional radiologic abnormalities such as delayed calyceal opacification time, diminished urine volume, increased urine opacity, and delayed washout of opacified urine (as compared with the normal contralateral kidney) indicate ischemia. These findings are usually due to **major arterial stenosis/aneurysm,** but **chronic incomplete infarction** and **radiation nephritis** also can cause identical abnormalities. Ureteral notching is not associated with the latter two and, when present, is evidence for renovascular ischemia. Vascular imaging, of course, leads to a definitive diagnosis.

When functional radiologic abnormalities are absent, using radiologic techniques to make a distinction among the several causes of unilaterally small, smooth kidney with normal calyces and papillae is difficult, if not impossible. This is true not only for major arterial disease, postinfarctive states, and radiation nephritis but also for the uncommon form of **postobstructive atrophy** (with normal papillae

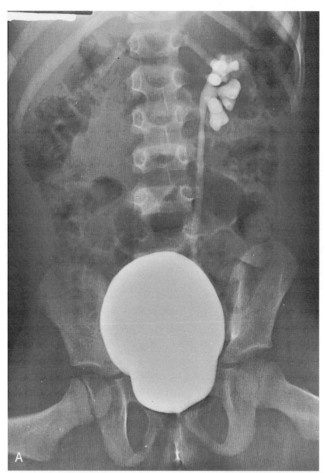

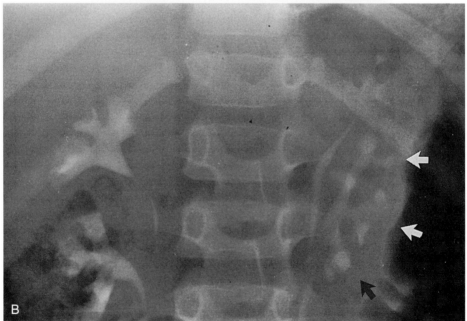

FIGURE 6–19. Reflux atrophy in the lower pole moiety of the left kidney with a completely duplicated collecting system.
A, Voiding cystourethrogram. Grade V vesicoureteral reflux into the lower pole moiety of the left kidney is present.
B, Excretory urogram. There is global wasting of that portion of the parenchyma affected by vesicoureteral reflux *(arrows).*

REFLUX ATROPHY TYPICAL FINDINGS

Primary Uroradiologic Elements

Size: small
Contour: smooth
Lesion distribution: unilateral

Secondary Uroradiologic Elements

Papillae: effaced
Collecting system: dilated; longitudinal striations may be seen when collapsed
Parenchymal thickness: wasted

---

and calyces) and **postinflammatory atrophy,** unless accompanied by papillary necrosis.

Postinflammatory atrophy causes both global atrophy and renal papillary necrosis. This combination of abnormalities is also found in advanced forms of **analgesic nephropathy** in which chronic interstitial fibrosis reduces kidney size. Analgesic nephropathy, however, is always bilateral, whereas postinflammatory atrophy is usually, although not invariably, unilateral.

Chronic renal infarction eventually produces

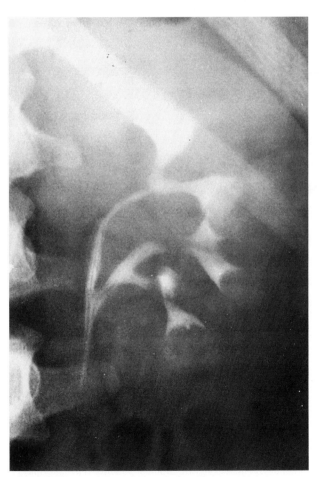

FIGURE 6–20. Longitudinal striations in the mucosa of the left renal pelvis in a patient with vesicoureteral reflux. Excretory urogram. The striations represent redundancy of the mucosa in a nondistended system.

a small, smooth kidney that does not opacify during contrast material–enhanced imaging. Retrograde pyelography is necessary to demonstrate the papillae and pelvocalyceal system, which are normal. This combination of imaging findings is unique to chronic renal infarction.

An appropriate clinical history of exposure to therapeutic radiation is often the only way to identify **radiation nephritis** as the cause of a small, smooth kidney. Abnormalities of the lumbar spine and pelvis, including disturbance of growth and maturation, are helpful observations when present.

A reduction in the number of calyces and papillae is basic to the diagnosis of **renal hypoplasia**. There is scant room for confusing this entity with others in the same diagnostic set if this criterion is strictly applied. Enlargement of the contralateral kidney should invariably be present because the process is lifelong. On the other hand, contralateral enlargement develops inconstantly as a function of age at onset when acquired disease results in a unilaterally small kidney.

Papillary effacement and calyceal dilatation in the absence of urinary tract infection are distinctive features of **postobstructive atrophy** and **reflux atrophy**. The global distribution of these findings and the preservation of a smooth outline distinguish these entities from **reflux nephropathy**, **tuberculosis**, and most forms of **renal papillary necrosis**. Postobstructive atrophy and reflux atrophy are radiologically indistinguishable. In fact, these entities probably have a common pathophysiologic basis, namely, increased hydrostatic pressure diffusely applied to the kidney parenchyma.

BIBLIOGRAPHY

Ischemia Secondary to Major Arterial Stenosis/ Aneurysm

Andersson, I.: Unilateral renal artery stenosis and hypertension: I. Angiography. Acta Radiol. (Diagn.) *20*:878, 1979.

Andersson, I., Bergentz, S.-E., Ericsson, B. F., Dymling, J. F., Hansson, B.-G., and Hökfelt, B.: Unilateral renal artery stenosis and hypertension: II. Angiographic findings correlated with blood pressure response after surgery. Acta Radiol. (Diagn.) *20*:895, 1979.

Bakker, J., Beek, F. J. A., Beutler, J. J., Hené, R. J., de Kort, G. A. P., de Lange, E. E., Moons, K. G. M., and Mali, W. P. T. M.:

Renal artery stenosis and accessory renal arteries: Accuracy of detection and visualization with gadolinium-enhanced breath-hold MR angiography. Radiology 207:497, 1998.

Beregi, J. P., Elkohen, M., Deklunder, G., Artaud, D., Coullet, J. M., and Wattinne, L.: Helical CT angiography compared with arteriography in the detection of renal artery stenosis. Am. J. Roentgenol. 167:495, 1996.

Berland, L. L., Koslin, D. B., Routh, W. O., and Keller, F. S.: Renal artery stenosis and prospective evaluation of diagnosis with color duplex US compared with angiography. Radiology 174:421, 1990.

Berman, L. B., and Vertes, V.: The pathophysiology of renin. Clin. Symp. 25:3, 1973.

Bourgoigne, J. J., Rubbert, K., and Sfakianakis, G. N.: Angiotensin-converting enzyme–inhibited renography for the diagnosis of ischemic kidneys. Am. J. Kidney Dis. 24:665, 1994.

Bude, R., and Rubin, J.: Detection of renal artery stenosis with Doppler sonography: It is more complicated than originally thought. Radiology 196:612, 1995.

Cragg, A. H., Smith, T. P., Thompson, B. H., Marone, T. P., Stanson, A. W., Shaw, G. T., Hunter, D. W., and Cochran, S. T.: Incidental fibromuscular dysplasia in potential renal changes: Long-term clinical follow-up. Radiology 172:145, 1989.

Davidson, R. A., Barry, Y. M., and Wilcox, C. S.: The simplified captopril test: an effective tool to diagnose renovascular hypertension. Am. J. Kidney Dis. 24:660, 1994.

Desberg, A. L., Paushter, D. M., Lammert, G. K., Hale, J. C., Troy, R. B., Novick, A. C., Nally, J. V., Jr., and Weltevreden, A. M.: Renal artery stenosis: Evaluation with color Doppler flow imaging. Radiology 177:749, 1990.

Dondi, M., Fanti, S., Defabritiis, A., Zuccala, A., Gaggi, R., Mirelli, M., Stella, A., Marengo, M., Losinno, F., and Monetti, N.: Prognostic value of captopril renal scintigraphy in renovascular hypertension. J. Nucl. Med. 33:11, 1992.

Dunnick, N. R., and Sfakianakis, G. N.: Screening for renovascular hypertension. Radiol. Clin. North Am. 29:497, 1991.

Dustan, H. P.: Renal artery disease and hypertension. Med. Clin. North Am. 81:1199, 1997.

Erbslöh-Möller, B., Dumas, A., Roth, D., Sfakianakis, G. N., and Bourgoignie, J. J.: Furosemide-131I-Hippuran renography after angiotensin-converting enzyme inhibition for the diagnosis of renovascular hypertension. Am. J. Med. 90:23, 1991.

Farres, M. T., Lammer, J., Schima, W., Wagner, B., Wildling, R., Winkelbauer, F., and Thurnher, S.: Spiral computed tomographic angiography of the renal arteries: A prospective comparison with intravenous and intraarterial digital subtraction angiography. Cardiovasc. Intervent. Radiol. 19:101, 1996.

Fine, E. J., and Sarkar, S.: Differential diagnosis and management of renovascular hypertension through nuclear medicine techniques. Semin. Nucl. Med. 19:101, 1989.

Gedroyc, W. M. W.: Magnetic resonance angiography of renal arteries. Urol. Clin. North Am. 21:201, 1994.

Goncharenko, V., Gerlock, A. J., Shaff, M. I., and Hollifield, J. W.: Progression of renal artery fibromuscular dysplasia in 42 patients as seen on angiography. Radiology 139:45, 1981.

Greco, B. A., and Breyer, J. A.: Atherosclerotic ischemic renal disease. Am. J. Kidney Dis. 29:167, 1997.

Grenier, N., Trillaud, H., Combe, C., Degreze, P., Jeandot, R., Gosse, P., Douws, C., and Palussiere, J.: Diagnosis of renovascular hypertension: Feasibility of captopril-sensitized dynamic MR imaging and comparison with captopril scintigraphy. Am. J. Roentgenol. 166:835, 1996.

Grist, T. M.: Magnetic resonance imaging of renal artery stenosis. Am. J. Kidney Dis. 24:700, 1994.

Halpern, E. J., Needleman, L., Nack, T. L., and East, S. A.: Renal artery stenosis: Should we study the main renal artery or segmental vessels? Radiology 195:799, 1995.

Halpern, M., and Evans, J. A.: Coarctation of the renal artery with "notching" of the ureter: A roentgenologic sign of unilateral renal disease as a cause of hypertension. AJR 88:159, 1962.

Heptinstall, R. H.: Hypertension II: Secondary forms. In Heptinstall, R. H. (ed.): Pathology of the Kidney, 4th ed. Boston, Little, Brown & Co., 1992, pp. 1029–1096.

Hill, S.: Renal vascular lesions. In Hill, G. S. (ed.): Uropathology. New York, Churchill Livingstone, 1989, pp. 189–234.

Hillman, B. J.: Imaging advances in the diagnosis of renovascular hypertension. AJR 153:5, 1989.

Kaatee, R., Beek, F. J. A., de Lange, E. E., van Leeuwen, M. S., Smits, H. F. M., van der Ven, P. J. G., Beutler, J. J., and Mali, W. P. T. M.: Renal artery stenosis: Detection and quantification with spiral CT angiography versus optimized digital subtraction angiography. Radiology 205:121, 1997.

Keogan, M. T., Kliewer, M. A., Hertzberg, B. S., DeLong, D. M., Tupler, R. H., and Carrol, B. A.: Renal resistive indexes: Variability in Doppler US measurement in a healthy population, Radiology, 199:165, 1996.

Khauli, R. D.: Defining the role of renal angiography in the diagnosis of renal artery disease. Am. J. Kidney Dis. 24:679, 1994.

King, B.F.: Diagnostic imaging evaluation of renovascular hypertension. Abdom. Imaging 20:395, 1995.

Loubeyre, P., Trolliet, P., Cahen, R., Grozel, F., Labeeuw, M., and Minh, V. A. T.: MR angiography of renal artery stenosis: Value of the combination of three-dimensional time-of-flight and three-dimensional phase-contrast MR angiography sequences. Am. J. Roentgenol. 167:489, 1996.

Luke, R. G.: Nephrosclerosis. In Schrier, R. W., and Gottschalk, C. W. (eds.): Diseases of the Kidney, 4th ed. Boston, Little, Brown & Co., 1988, pp. 1573–1596.

Mann, S. J., Pickering, T. G., Sos, T. A., Uzzo, R. G., Sarkar, S., Friend, K., Rackson, M. E., and Laragh, J. H.: Captopril renography in the diagnosis of renal artery stenosis: Accuracy and limitations. Am. J. Med. 90:30, 1991.

Mitty, H. A., Shapiro, R. S., Parsons, R. B., and Silberzweig, J. E.: Renovascular hypertension. Radiol. Clin. North Am. 34:1017, 1996.

Nally, J. V., Jr.: Provocative captopril testing in the diagnosis of renovascular hypertension. Urol. Clin. North Am. 21:227, 1994.

Olin, J. W.: Role of duplex ultrasonography in screening for significant renal artery disease. Urol. Clin. North Am. 21:215, 1994.

Oparil, S., and Harber, E.: The renin-angiotensin system. N. Engl. J. Med. 291:399, 446, 1974.

Paul, R. E., Ettinger, A., Faisinger, M. H., Callow, A. D., Kahn, P. C., and Inker, L. H.: Angiographic visualization of renal collateral circulation as a means of detecting and delineating renal ischemia. Radiology 84:1013, 1965.

Pickering, T. G.: Renovascular hypertension: Etiology and pathophysiology. Semin. Nucl. Med. 19:79, 1989.

Pohl, M. A.: Renal artery stenosis, renal vascular hypertension, and ischemic nephropathy. In Schrier, R. W., and Gottschalk, C. W. (eds.): Diseases of the Kidney, 6th ed. Boston, Little, Brown & Co., 1997, pp. 1367–1424.

Postma, C. T., Bijlstra, P. J., Rosenbusch, G., and Thien, T.: Pattern recognition of loss of early systolic peak by Doppler ultrasound has a low sensitivity for the detection of renal artery stenosis. J. Hum. Hypertens. 10:181, 1996.

Prince, M. R., Schoenberg, S. O., Ward, J. S., Londy, F. J., Wakefield, T. W., and Stanley, J. C.: Hemodynamically significant atherosclerotic renal artery stenosis: MR angiographic features. Radiology 205:128, 1997.

Romero, J. C., Feldstein, A. E., Rodriguez-Porcel, M. G., and Cases-Amenos, A.: New insights into the pathophysiology of renovascular hypertension. Mayo Clin. Proc. 72:251, 1997.

Schreiber, M. J., Pohl, M. A., and Novick, A. C.: The natural history of atherosclerotic and fibrous renal artery disease. Urol. Clin. North Am. 11:383, 1984.

Silverman, J. M., Friedman, M. I., and Vanallan, R. J.: Detection of main renal artery stenosis using phase-contrast cine MR angiography. AJR 166:1131, 1996.

Stewart, B. H., Dustan, H. P., Kiser, W. S., Meaney, T. F., Straffon, R. A., and McCormack, L. J.: Correlation of angiography and natural history in evaluation of patients with renovascular hypertension. J. Urol. 104:231, 1970.

Strandness, D. E., Jr.: Duplex imaging for the detection of renal artery stenosis. Am. J. Kidney Dis. 24:674, 1994.

Tack, C., and Sos, T. A.: Radiologic diagnosis of renovascular

hypertension and percutaneous transluminal renal angio-
plasty. Semin. Nucl. Med. *19*:89, 1989.
Taylor, A., Nally, J., Aurell, M., Blaufox, D., Dondi, M., Dubovsky,
E., Fine, E., Fommei, E., Geyskes, G., Granerus, G., et al.:
Consensus report on ACE inhibitor renography for detecting
renovascular hypertension. J. Nucl. Med. *37*:1876, 1996.
Textor, S. C.: Renovascular hypertension. Endocrinol. Metab.
Clin. North Am. *23*:235, 1994.
Verschuyl, E.-J., Kaatee, R., Beek, F. J. A., Patel, N. H., Fon-
taine, A. B., Daly, C. P., Coldwell, D. M., Bush, W. H., and
Mali, W. P. T. M.: Renal artery origins: Best angiographic
projection angles. Radiology *205*:115, 1997.
Wan, J. L., Greenfield, S. P., Ng, M. Y., Zerin, M., Ritchey, M. L.,
and Bloom, D.: Sibling reflux: A dual center retrospective
study. J. Urol. *156*:677, 1996.

Chronic Renal Infarction

Clark, R. E., Teplick, S. K., and Long, J. M.: Small atrophic
kidney secondary to renal vein thrombosis: Report of a case
diagnosed arteriographically. J. Urol. *114*:457, 1975.
Erwin, B. C., Carroll, B. A., Walter, J. F., and Sommer, F. G.:
Renal infarction appearing as an echogenic mass. AJR
138:759, 1982.
Glazer, G. M., Francis, I. R., Brady, T. M., and Teng, S. S.:
Computed tomography of renal infarction: Clinical and experi-
mental observations. AJR 139:721, 1983.
Heitzman, E. R., and Perchik, L.: Radiographic features of renal
infarction: Review of 13 cases. Radiology 76:39, 1961.
Hoxie, H. J., and Coggin, C. B.: Renal infarction: Statistical
study of 205 cases and detailed report of an unusual case.
Arch. Intern. Med. 65:587, 1940.
Janower, M. L., and Weber, A. L.: Radiologic evaluation of acute
renal infarction. AJR 95:309, 1965.
Lang, E. K.: Arteriographic diagnosis of renal infarcts. Radiology
88:1110, 1967.
Solez, K.: Acute renal failure (acute tubular necrosis, infarction
and cortical necrosis). In Heptinstall, R. H. (ed.): Pathology of
the Kidney, 4th ed. Boston, Little, Brown & Co., 1992, pp.
1235–1314.
Teplick, J. G., and Yarrow, M. W.: Arterial infarction of kidney.
Ann. Intern. Med. 42:1041, 1955.

Radiation Nephritis

Aron, B. S., and Schlesinger, A.: Complications of radiation ther-
apy: The genitourinary tract. Semin. Roentgenol. 9:65, 1974.
Crummy, A. B., Hellman, S., Stansel, H. C., Jr., and Hukill, P. B.:
Renal hypertension secondary to unilateral radiation damage
relieved by nephrectomy. Radiology 84:108, 1965.
Heptinstall, R. H.: Irradiation injury and effects of heavy metals.
In Heptinstall, R. H. (ed.): Pathology of the Kidney, 4th ed.
Boston, Little, Brown & Co., 1992, pp. 2085–2111.
Keane, W. F., Crosson, J. T., Staley, N. A., Anderson, W. R., and
Shapiro, F. L.: Radiation-induced renal disease: A clinicopatho-
logic study. Am. J. Med. 60:127, 1976.
Madrazo, A., Schwarz, G., and Churg, J.: Radiation nephritis: A
review. J. Urol. 114:822, 1975.
Moore, L., Curry, N. S., and Jenrette, J. M.: Computed tomogra-
phy of acute radiation nephritis. Urol. Radiol. 8:89, 1986.
Nolan, C. R., and Linas, S. L.: Malignant hypertension and other
hypertensive crises. In Schrier, R. W., and Gottschalk, C. W.

(eds.): Diseases of the Kidney, 6th ed. Boston, Little, Brown &
Co., 1997, pp. 1475–1555.
Shapiro, A. P., Cavallo, T., Cooper, W., Lapenas, D., Bron, K.,
and Berg, G.: Hypertension in radiation nephritis. Arch. In-
tern. Med. 137:848, 1977.
Vidt, D. G.: Hypertension induced by irradiation to the kidney.
Arch. Intern. Med. 137:840, 1977.

Congenital Hypoplasia

Boissant, P.: What to call the hypoplastic kidney? Arch. Dis.
Child. 37:142, 1962.
Risdon, R. A.: Development, developmental defects, and cystic
diseases of the kidney. In Heptinstall, R. H. (ed.): Pathology
of the Kidney, 4th ed. Boston, Little, Brown & Co., 1992,
pp. 93–168.
Risdon, R. A., Young, L. W., and Chrispin, A. R.: Renal hypoplasia and dysplasia: A radiological and pathological correlation.
Pediatr. Radiol. 3:213, 1975.
Templeton, A. W., and Thompson, I. M.: Aortographic differentiation of congenital and acquired small kidneys. Arch. Surg.
97:114, 1968.

Postobstructive Atrophy

Craven, J. D., Hodson, C. J., and Lecky, J. W.: An atypical
response on the kidney to a period of ureteric obstruction.
Radiology 105:39, 1972.
Craven, J. D., and Lecky, J. W.: The natural history of postob-
structive renal atrophy shown by sequential urograms. Radiol-
ogy 101:555, 1971.
Hodson, C. J.: Post-obstructive renal atrophy (nephropathy). Br.
Med. Bull. 28:237, 1972.
Hodson, C. J., and Craven, J. D.: The radiology of obstructive
atrophy of the kidney. Clin. Radiol. 17:305, 1966.
Hodson, C. J., Craven, J. D., Lewis, D. G., Matz, L. R., Clarke,
R. J., and Ross, E. J.: Experimental obstructive nephropathy
in the pig. Br. J. Urol. 41 (Suppl.):5, 1969.

Postinflammatory Atrophy

Bailey, R. R., Little, P. J., and Rolleston, G. L.: Renal damage
after acute pyelonephritis. Br. Med. J. 1:550, 1969.
Davidson, A. J., and Talner, L. B.: Urographic and angiographic
abnormalities in adult-onset acute bacterial nephritis. Radiology 106:249, 1973.
Davidson, A. J., and Talner, L. B.: Late sequelae of adult-onset
acute bacterial nephritis. Radiology 127:367, 1978.
Hill, G. S., and Clark, R. L.: A comparative angiographic, mi-
croangiographic, and histologic study of experimental pyelonephritis. Invest. Radiol. 7:33, 1972.
Lilienfield, R. M., and Lande, A.: Acute adult onset bacterial
nephritis: Long-term urographic and angiographic follow-up.
J. Urol. 114:14, 1975.

Reflux Atrophy

Hodson, C. J.: The diffuse form of reflux nephropathy. In Losse,
H., Asscher, A. W., and Lison, A. E. (eds.): Pyelonephritis, vol.
IV: Urinary Tract Infections. New York, Thieme-Stratton,
1980, pp. 84–90.
Wallin, L., and Bajc, M.: The significance of vesicoureteric reflux
on kidney development assessed by dimercaptosuccinate scintigraphy. Br. J. Urol. 73:607, 1994.

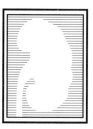

CHAPTER 7

Diagnostic Set: Small, Smooth, Bilateral

GENERALIZED ARTERIOSCLEROSIS
NEPHROSCLEROSIS (BENIGN AND
MALIGNANT)
ATHEROEMBOLIC RENAL DISEASE
CHRONIC GLOMERULONEPHRITIS
ACQUIRED CYSTIC KIDNEY DISEASE

HEREDITARY NEPHROPATHIES
   Hereditary Chronic Nephritis (Alport's Syndrome)
   Medullary Cystic Disease
AMYLOIDOSIS (LATE)
ARTERIAL HYPOTENSION
DIFFERENTIAL DIAGNOSIS

Bilaterally small, smooth kidneys are the result of diseases that affect all renal tissue either exclusively as a primary process or as part of a generalized, multisystem disorder. Chronic glomerulonephritis, acquired cystic kidney disease, hereditary chronic nephritis, and medullary cystic disease are examples of the former; and arteriosclerosis, nephrosclerosis, and the late stage of amyloidosis illustrate the latter group. Both kidneys can also become small and smooth when they are the target of an "upstream" shower of atheromatous emboli, an uncommon condition known as *atheroembolic renal disease*. Hypotension may cause the same change transiently by reducing the volume of intrarenal blood and urine that normally distends the kidneys.

Chronic interstitial nephritis is not treated as a separate category in this diagnostic set, even though kidneys with this histologic picture are uniformly wasted. Most authorities now believe that this term is simply a description of a histologic pattern reflecting a variety of etiologic factors, some yet to be defined, that can lead to small kidneys and renal failure.

The calyces and papillae remain normal in diseases included in this diagnostic set. The preservation of a smooth contour as the kidney shrinks reflects the generalized, or global, nature of tissue loss inherent in these abnormalities. A smooth contour, however, is not invariably maintained in arteriosclerosis, nephrosclerosis, or acquired cystic kidney disease, exceptions that will be discussed in detail in the following sections.

Abnormalities in the echogenicity of the renal parenchyma occur frequently in the varied chronic wasting disorders that cause both kidneys to become small and smooth. These abnormalities take several forms. A generalized increase in parenchy-

mal echoes, which often become greater in intensity than those of the liver, may be noted (Fig. 7–1). Additionally, an increased prominence of central sinus echoes, known as *sinus lipomatosis*, occurs when sinus fat proliferation accompanies parenchymal wasting (Fig. 7–2). Obliteration of differences in cortical and medullary echogenicity has been reported, but these differences are often not present even in normal kidneys. The presence of any of these abnormalities in ultrasonograms may denote parenchymal disease, but they are neither specific to any given entity or group of diseases nor indicative of particular prognoses.

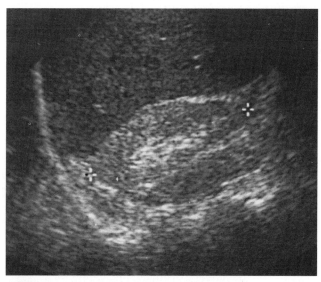

FIGURE 7–1. End-stage renal failure causing an increase in the echogenicity of kidney parenchyma relative to that of the liver. This pattern is not specific to any particular disease or group of diseases. Ultrasonography also demonstrates the small size and smooth contour of the kidneys. Ultrasonogram, longitudinal section.

135

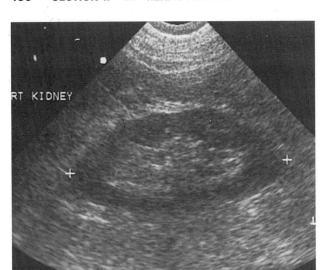

FIGURE 7–2. End-stage renal failure with increased prominence of central sinus echoes due to proliferation of sinus fat. Ultrasonogram, longitudinal section.

The entities discussed in this chapter, except for arterial hypotension, are associated with chronic renal failure. In some, renal failure is always present. In others, impaired renal function becomes apparent only as the disease progresses. In either situation, ultrasonography is most efficaciously employed to detect both the generalized loss of renal parenchyma and the bilateral involvement that characterizes the diseases included in this diagnostic set.

GENERALIZED ARTERIOSCLEROSIS

Definition

When arteriosclerosis involves most of the interlobar and arcuate arteries, the kidneys become wasted owing to insufficient nutrient blood flow for sustenance of the renal parenchyma. Unlike focal narrowing of the main renal artery, discussed in Chapter 6, the process is disseminated, and uniform shrinkage of both kidneys occurs.

Arteriosclerosis can reduce the kidney to one-half its normal weight. The degree of wasting is variable and depends on the extent of involvement of medium-sized arteries. Frequently, narrowing of vessels progresses to complete occlusion and focal infarction. As a result, the smooth surface of the arteriosclerotic kidney becomes punctuated with shallow scars, which are variable in number and random in distribution. The papillae and calyces remain normal. Occasionally, fat proliferates in the renal hilus and replaces the parenchyma lost in the central part of the kidney.

The histologic appearance of the arteriosclerotic kidney is nonspecific and difficult to distinguish from other entities that cause wasting of renal tissue. Medium-sized arteries develop multiple sites of atheromatous thickening, with fraying of the internal elastic lamina and calcification. The glomeruli vary from normal to sclerotic. The tubules, particularly proximal convoluted tubules, become atrophic and have thickened basement membranes. Interstitial fibrosis occurs, but it is finer than that seen in reflux nephropathy.

Small, smooth kidneys develop in patients with scleroderma or chronic tophaceous gout. It is generally held that this is due, at least in part, to premature or accelerated development of atherosclerosis in medium- and small-sized arteries. Other parenchymal changes seen in chronic gouty nephropathy are deposition of uric acid and urate in the tubules and interstitial tissue, interstitial fibrosis, and nephron atrophy.

Patients with the *classic form of polyarteritis nodosa* and *drug-abuse arteritis*, in whom necrotizing vascular lesions cause both aneurysms and occlusions of medium-sized renal arteries, also develop small, smooth kidneys as a result of diffuse ischemia.

Clinical Setting

Arteriosclerotic disease of the kidneys is a part of the generalized atherosclerosis associated with aging. Most authorities agree that ischemia resulting from vascular narrowing causes reduction of renal mass and a slowly progressive decrease in renal function. The possibility does exist, however, that these changes occur as part of an independent cellular involutional process unrelated to atherosclerosis.

By definition, arteriosclerosis of the kidney is as-

GENERALIZED ARTERIOSCLEROSIS TYPICAL FINDINGS

Primary Uroradiologic Elements

Size: small
Contour: smooth; may have random, shallow scars
Lesion distribution: bilateral

Secondary Uroradiologic Elements

Parenchymal thickness: wasted
Attenuation value: sinus fat increased
Echogenicity: increased parenchymal echogenicity

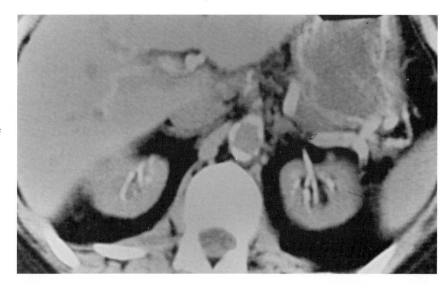

FIGURE 7–3. Arteriosclerotic calcification of both renal arteries in a diabetic patient. Computed tomogram, unenhanced.

sociated with normal arterial blood pressure and has little, if any, clinical importance. Renal plasma flow, glomerular filtration rate, and various tubule functions measurably deteriorate over a long time, but clinical manifestations are not seen. If hypertension develops, the situation is reclassified as benign or malignant nephrosclerosis.

The clinical features of scleroderma, chronic tophaceous gout, polyarteritis nodosa, and drug abuse arteritis obviously predominate when the accelerated atherosclerotic or necrotizing arterial lesions associated with these diseases produce small, smooth kidneys.

Radiologic Findings

Reduction in renal size due to uncomplicated arteriosclerosis is usually not detected before the 6th decade of life and becomes more apparent with advancing age. Both kidneys are affected more or less equally. Calcification of medium-sized intrarenal arteries may be noted on a preliminary film or computed tomogram (Fig. 7–3). Because wasting is global, the kidneys often have a smooth contour (Fig. 7–4). However, shallow focal scars may be present at sites where arterial narrowing has progressed to infarction (Fig. 7–5; see Fig. 7–10B). Uni-

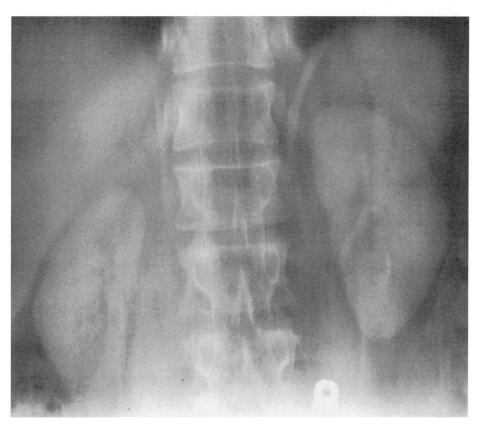

FIGURE 7–4. Arteriosclerosis. Global wasting of both kidneys with preservation of a smooth contour in an 80-year-old normotensive woman with normal blood urea nitrogen value. The pelvocalyceal system is normal. Tomogram. Right kidney length = 9.3 cm; left kidney length = 10.8 cm.

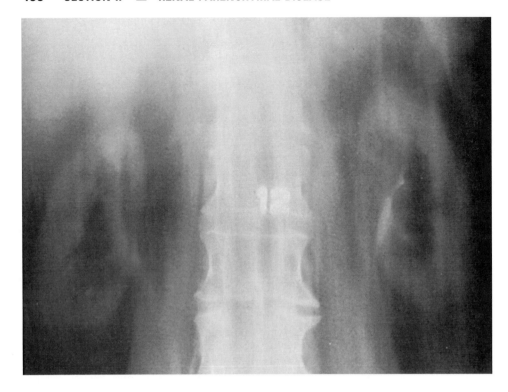

FIGURE 7–5. Arteriosclerosis. Shallow focal scars superimposed on globally wasted kidneys in an elderly normotensive woman without azotemia. Scars occur at random sites where arterial narrowing progresses to infarction. Uniform thinning of renal parenchyma is highlighted by marked renal sinus lipomatosis effacing the pelvocalyceal system. Tomogram. Right kidney length = 11.4 cm; left kidney length = 12.0 cm.

form narrowing of the distance between the interpapillary line and outer margin of the kidney reflects parenchymal loss (see Fig. 7–5). The nephrogram, papillae, and pelvocalyceal system are normal (see Fig. 7–4) or reflect renal sinus fat prolif-

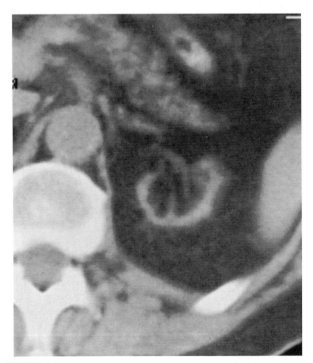

FIGURE 7–6. Renal sinus fat proliferation in global renal wasting is seen as increased sinus tissue with negative attenuation value. This often causes effacement of the pelvocalyceal system. Note general wasting of the parenchyma. Computed tomogram, contrast material–enhanced.

eration, which often accompanies diffuse parenchymal wasting. This is seen as a radiolucency in the central portion of the kidney that is accentuated during urography (see Fig. 7–5) or as sinus tissue of negative attenuation value in computed tomography (Fig. 7–6). An increase in the volume of echoes in the central sinus echo complex is seen ultrasonographically (see Fig. 7–2). Lack of distensibility of the pelvocalyceal system may occur when sinus fat proliferation is marked. Renal sinus lipomatosis, discussed in Chapter 16, may occur in any wasting process, in either one or both kidneys, and is thus nonspecific.

The imaging findings in scleroderma, chronic gouty nephropathy, the classic form of polyarteritis nodosa, and drug-abuse arteritis are the same as those seen in uncomplicated arteriosclerosis (Fig. 7–7). The angiographic abnormalities in polyarteritis nodosa and drug abuse result from focal areas of mural necrosis in intermediate-sized (arcuate) arteries. In polyarteritis nodosa, the aneurysms that result are multiple, sharply defined, and 2 to 3 mm wide (Fig. 7–8). These occur only in the "classic" form and are not seen in the "microscopic" form, in which the capillary bed, rather than larger vessels, is involved. The renal aneurysms of polyarteritis nodosa may heal with therapy. Thus, failure to demonstrate aneurysms does not exclude the diagnosis of polyarteritis nodosa. Unlike polyarteritis, angiitis associated with drug abuse has widespread irregularities of the arterial lumina. In addition, the aneurysms tend to be more irregular than those seen with polyarteritis (Fig. 7–9).

Renal angiography can clearly demonstrate arteriosclerotic disease of the interlobar- and arcuate-

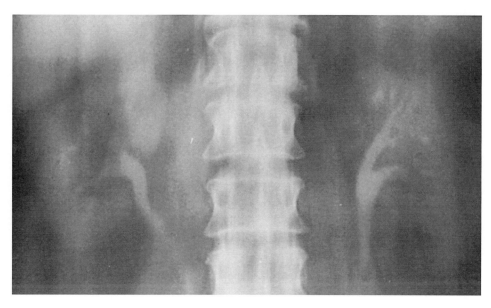

FIGURE 7–7. Gouty nephropathy. Bilaterally small kidneys in a 71-year-old normotensive man with severe chronic tophaceous gout and mild azotemia. Shallow focal scars are seen in several areas of the right kidney. Renal wasting in this situation is presumably due to severe arteriosclerosis and chronic interstitial fibrosis. Tomogram. Right kidney length = 10.4 cm; left kidney length = 9.9 cm.

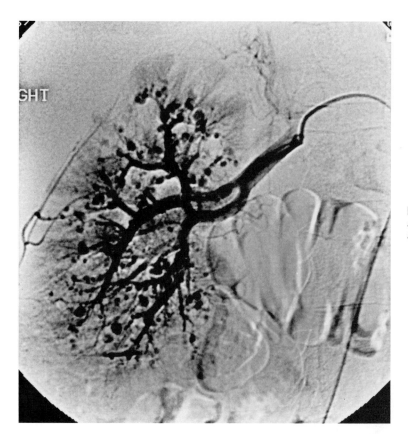

FIGURE 7–8. Polyarteritis nodosa, classic form. There are multiple, sharply defined aneurysms in the arcuate arteries. Selective renal arteriogram.

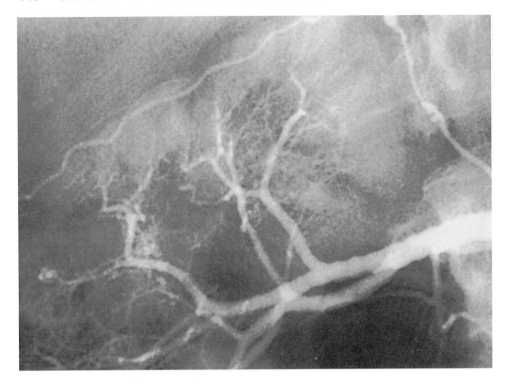

FIGURE 7–9. Drug-abuse arteritis. View of the superior portion of the right kidney. There are widespread irregularities of the medium-sized arteries in addition to small aneurysms. Selective renal arteriogram. (Courtesy of Robert Clark, M.D., St. Francis Memorial Hospital, San Francisco, California.)

sized vessels (Fig. 7–10). In addition to focal narrowing of these vessels, particularly at points of bifurcation, there is loss of normal arterial tapering, decrease in number of branching vessels, increased tortuosity, and abrupt change in the caliber of the distal arcuate arteries in advanced cases. These abnormalities are nonspecific and can be seen in most other forms of chronic renal disease. The similarity between normal patterns of vascular aging and patterns seen in chronic acquired diseases limits the usefulness of angiography in the diagnosis of parenchymal disease of the kidney (Fig. 7–11). Angiography is rarely indicated in the diagnosis of arteriosclerotic disease of the kidneys.

In advanced cases of arteriosclerotic wasting, the echogenicity of the renal parenchyma may be in-

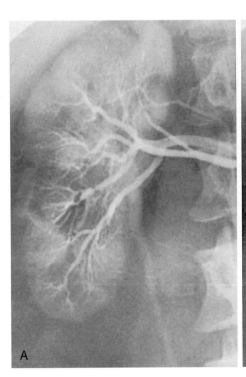

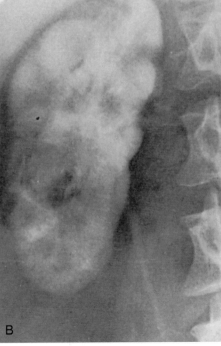

FIGURE 7–10. Arteriosclerosis of interlobar and arcuate arteries. *A,* Arterial phase of selective arteriogram. Note irregular narrowing and dilatation of arteries, especially at bifurcations. *B,* Shallow scars due to infarction are well illustrated during nephrographic phase.

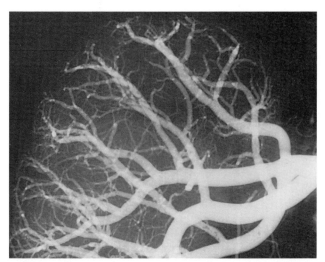

FIGURE 7–11. Radiograph of a barium-injected human kidney illustrating the effects of chronic parenchymal loss on the arterial tree. The interlobar arteries fail to taper normally and are tortuous distally. The arcuate arteries angle sharply and terminate abruptly. These changes follow a wide variety of chronic diseases but are also found in the aged although otherwise normal kidney, as in this illustration.

creased in a diffuse, but nonspecific, pattern. The central sinus echo complex may also become more prominent with sinus fat proliferation.

NEPHROSCLEROSIS (BENIGN AND MALIGNANT)

Definition

Patients with systemic hypertension develop thickening and subendothelial hyalinization of the afferent arterioles in addition to arteriosclerosis of the medium- and small-sized arteries. These changes constitute the histologic picture of benign nephrosclerosis.

The development of accelerated or malignant hypertension produces proliferative endarteritis of afferent arterioles and interlobular arteries, necrotizing arteriolitis, and necrotizing glomerulitis. Arteriolar rupture may occur as a result of these changes. Pronounced atrophy of tubules and fine interstitial fibrosis with chronic inflammatory cell infiltrate also contribute to the smallness of these kidneys.

Generalized reduction in kidney size, with smooth contour and normal pelvocalyceal and papillary structures, occurs in both benign and malignant nephrosclerosis. Superimposed scars of lobar infarction may be present. In malignant nephrosclerosis, intrarenal or subcapsular hemorrhage occasionally develops as a result of rupture of necrotic arterioles.

Clinical Setting

Hypertension is a basic clinical feature of nephrosclerosis. Whether elevated blood pressure is a cause or a result of the afferent arteriolar lesion is a historical controversy. The onset of hypertension usually occurs before 50 years of age. Even when hypertension exists for many years, serious renal functional impairment does not develop in the benign form of nephrosclerosis. Many patients do have some reduction in renal plasma flow and tubule function, slight proteinuria, and hyaline or granular casts in their urine, but these are rarely of clinical consequence.

The clinical situation in malignant hypertension is more serious than in benign hypertension. In the malignant form, rapid deterioration of renal function occurs in association with headache, weight loss, dizziness, and impaired vision. Papilledema with fundal hemorrhage and exudate develops. Gross hematuria and heavy proteinuria are common. Some patients die of renal failure or as a result of complications in other organ systems, particularly the heart and the brain.

Radiologic Findings

The radiologic findings in benign nephrosclerosis overlap those of arteriosclerotic kidney disease. The kidneys are symmetrically reduced in size, and their contour remains smooth except for occasional,

---

NEPHROSCLEROSIS (BENIGN AND MALIGNANT) TYPICAL FINDINGS

Primary Uroradiologic Elements

Size: small
Contour: smooth; may have random, shallow scars
Lesion distribution: bilateral

Secondary Uroradiologic Elements

Parenchymal thickness: wasted
Nephrogram: diminished density (malignant form)
Attenuation value: focal high values in parenchyma (malignant, nonenhanced scan)
Echogenicity: increased parenchymal echogenicity
Retroperitoneal space: subcapsular, perirenal blood (attenuation value, signal
   characteristics change with time)

random, shallow infarct scars in some patients. The pelvocalyceal and papillary structures are remarkable only for the surrounding fatty deposition sometimes present. The kidney opacifies normally (Fig. 7–12).

Malignant nephrosclerosis differs from renal arteriosclerosis and benign nephrosclerosis in that enhancement of the kidney by contrast material is invariably diminished, usually to a marked degree. In other respects, the radiologic findings are the same. It seems reasonable to expect small kidneys and sinus fat accumulation more often in patients whose malignant stage was preceded by a relatively long period of benign nephrosclerosis. When malignant nephrosclerosis arises *de novo*, as sometimes happens, the kidneys may be normal in size. This holds true only for a limited time before progressive reduction of renal mass occurs.

Parenchymal hemorrhage due to necrotizing arteriolitis is usually petechial and cannot be detected with the poor opacification achieved during urography, but it might be apparent as focal areas of high attenuation in computed tomograms performed without contrast material enhancement. Occasionally, bleeding extends to the subcapsular surface of the kidney or the perirenal space. This results in a concave, inward displacement of the nephrogram and adjacent calyces, occasional extension of blood into the perinephric space, and displacement of the capsular artery, seen during angiography (see discussion in Chapter 21.)

As stated earlier, renal parenchymal and central sinus echogenicity may be increased in chronic parenchymal disease such as nephrosclerosis. Subcapsular and perirenal hemorrhages are detectable by ultrasonography as hypoechoic or echo-free collections of fluid and as tissue with the attenuation value or signal characteristics of blood by computed tomography or magnetic resonance imaging, as described in further detail in Chapter 21.

ATHEROEMBOLIC RENAL DISEASE

Definition

Atheroembolic renal disease results from the dislodgement from the aorta of multiple atheromatous emboli that occlude intrarenal arteries, from arcuate-sized vessels down to the afferent arterioles. The appearance of the kidneys depends on the amount of time that has passed following such an event. Shortly after the embolic episode, the affected arteries are packed with cholesterol crystals and amorphous debris. Eventually, this leads to the production of foreign body giant cells. Finally, focal areas of concentric fibrosis develop at points where emboli initially were situated, usually at arterial bifurcations. The net result of these changes is diffuse patches of ischemia in which atrophy predominates over infarction.

Because this disorder occurs only when the aorta is severely atherosclerotic, the kidneys may already be somewhat reduced in size as a result of age or coexisting hypertension. Atheroembolic disease itself reduces renal mass, although this is not seen for some time following embolization. Infarct scars are often superimposed on the fine granular scars of ischemia. As is true in the other vascular disorders previously described in this chapter, papillary and pelvocalyceal structures retain their normal appearance.

Clinical Setting

Dislodgement of atheromatous debris from the aorta above the renal arteries may result from ex-

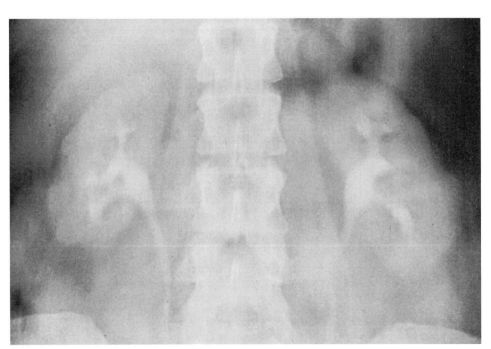

FIGURE 7–12. Benign nephrosclerosis. Excretory urogram in a 46-year-old woman with essential hypertension. Both kidneys are globally wasted and have several shallow infarct scars. The pelvocalyceal system and renal opacification are normal. (Courtesy of Department of Diagnostic Radiology, Hammersmith Hospital, Royal Postgraduate Medical School, London, England.)

ATHEROEMBOLIC RENAL DISEASE TYPICAL FINDINGS

Primary Uroradiologic Elements

Size: small
Contour: smooth; may have random, shallow scars
Lesion distribution: bilateral

Secondary Uroradiologic Elements

Parenchymal thickness: wasted
Nephrogram: diminished density (excretory urogram); patchy (computed tomogram)
Arteries: embolic occlusion (arteriogram)

---

ternal trauma or direct insult to the aorta during surgery or catheter manipulation. Spontaneous embolization also occurs, especially during thrombolytic therapy. As many as 15 to 30 per cent of patients with severe erosive atherosclerotic disease of the aorta have atherosclerotic emboli in the kidneys.

Massive embolization may lead to oliguria or anuria and uremia after a relatively short time. In most cases, however, the course is more indolent, although renal failure eventually ensues. Ischemic lesions in skin and muscle frequently dominate the clinical presentation. Hypertension is often present, occasionally in the accelerated form. Eosinophilia may be pronounced. Proteinuria is frequently present, but red blood cells and casts in the urine are rarely noted.

Radiologic Findings

No comprehensive study of the radiologic features of atheroembolic renal disease has been published. Nevertheless, pathologic and clinical evidence is abundant and suggests that the radiologic picture should show the kidneys to be normal to small, bilaterally involved, and smooth. Shallow infarct scars occur inconstantly. There is impaired opacification of the kidney, reflecting the deficiency in renal perfusion. This would be most readily apparent as a patchy nephrogram by computed tomography. Normal renal size in the early stage of this process is to be expected.

Cholesterol emboli large enough to occlude interlobar or arcuate-sized arteries have been demonstrated by angiography. These filling defects are indistinguishable from other types of emboli.

CHRONIC GLOMERULONEPHRITIS
Definition

When the many types of acute glomerulonephritis progress to the chronic stage, they assume a common final form in which loss of renal substance reflects the combined effects of both the nephritis and the secondary hypertension.

In chronic glomerulonephritis, reduction in kidney size is global, symmetric, and often profound. The lobular or idiopathic membranous forms of chronic glomerulonephritis may have normal-sized kidneys. A fine granularity of the subcapsular surface is noted on direct examination of the kidney, but this is not detectable radiologically. The cut surface of the chronic glomerulonephritic kidney reveals an evenly thinned parenchyma and normal papillae. Common to all situations in which wasting occurs over a long time, an excess of peripelvic fat is often present.

Clinical Setting

Chronic glomerulonephritis develops over weeks to months following an episode of acute glomerulonephritis. Not all cases result from acute post–

CHRONIC GLOMERULONEPHRITIS TYPICAL FINDINGS

Primary Uroradiologic Elements

Size: small
Contour: smooth
Lesion distribution: bilateral

Secondary Uroradiologic Elements

Parenchymal thickness: wasted
Nephrogram: diminished density
Calcification: cortical (uncommon)
Echogenicity: increased parenchymal echogenicity

streptococcal glomerulonephritis. Some may develop without a prior clinically apparent acute phase or from forms of acute glomerulonephritis unrelated to streptococcal infection. In any event, this disease occurs more frequently in the male than in the female and is most prevalent between the 2nd and 5th decade of life.

Patients with chronic glomerulonephritis usually present with insidious onset of peripheral edema associated with proteinuria. Occasionally, massive edema appears rapidly, along with other stigmata of the nephrotic syndrome. It is estimated that 50 per cent of patients with chronic glomerulonephritis eventually develop the nephrotic syndrome. Hypertension is present and progresses with advancing renal failure. Urinalysis reveals protein, red blood cells, leukocytes, renal epithelial cells, and hyaline and granular casts. Oval fat bodies are seen when the nephrotic syndrome is present.

Radiologic Findings

There is nothing unique about the radiologic picture of chronic glomerulonephritis. Both kidneys become globally small and have smooth contours, normal calyces and papillae, and occasional peripelvic fat proliferation (Fig. 7–13; see Fig. 7–2). Density of the nephrogram and pelvocalyceal system varies with severity of the disease. Calcification in the renal cortex is sometimes present (Fig. 7–14). Cysts in the cortex and medulla may be detected as early manifestations of acquired cystic kidney disease, which is discussed in the following section (see Fig. 7–13).

Increased echogenicity of the renal parenchyma and increased prominence of the central sinus complex are nonspecific findings in chronic glomerulonephritis.

Angiography in chronic glomerulonephritis reveals arterial tortuosity, loss of branches, and lack of normal tapering of the arteries. These changes are the same as those seen in both arteriosclerosis (aging) and nephrosclerosis; thus, angiography is of no value in the diagnosis of chronic glomerulonephritis.

ACQUIRED CYSTIC KIDNEY DISEASE

Definition

Multiple cyst formation occurs in kidneys that have failed for reasons other than a heritable cystic disorder. This condition, known as acquired cystic kidney disease, is noted particularly in patients whose life span has been extended by long-term hemodialysis or peritoneal dialysis. The affected kidneys usually remain small in size and smooth in contour. Sometimes, however, the kidneys enlarge. Some, indeed, may eventually approximate the large bulk usually associated with autosomal dominant (adult) polycystic kidney disease. The causes of this disorder have not been established, although a direct relationship between the prevalence of acquired cystic kidney disease and the duration of dialysis has been demonstrated. Some degree of remission of cysts following successful transplantation has been reported.

The cysts of uncomplicated acquired cystic kidney disease are filled with clear fluid and vary from microscopic to 3.0 cm in diameter. They may be as few as five but are most commonly multiple and bilateral. Bleeding into cysts is common. Most cysts are lined by a single layer of cuboidal or columnar epithelium and are in continuity with the tubule lumen. Commonly, however, atypical, hyperplastic, multilayered epithelium with papillary projections is present. This may represent a stage in the devel-

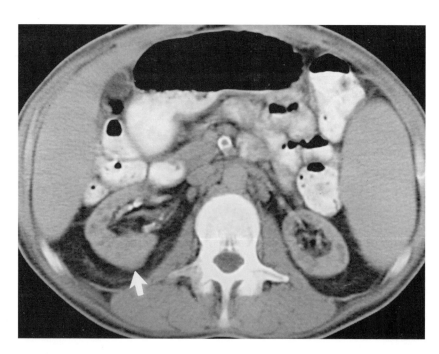

FIGURE 7–13. Chronic glomerulonephritis with early acquired cystic kidney disease in a patient maintained on hemodialysis. Computed tomogram, unenhanced. Both kidneys are small and smooth. The kidneys contain several small, low attenuation cysts. An adenocarcinoma is present on the dorsal aspect of the right kidney (arrow).

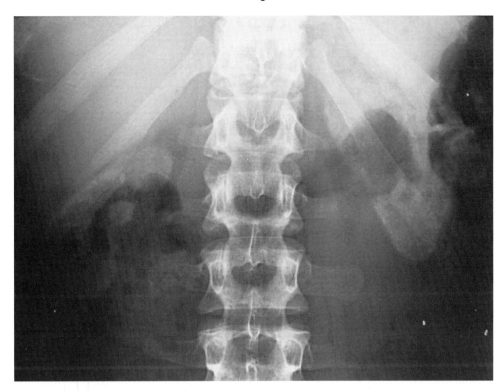

FIGURE 7–14. Diffuse cortical nephrocalcinosis associated with chronic glomerulo-nephritis is seen on a standard radiograph of the abdomen. Both kidneys are uniformly involved, and the medullae are spared. (Courtesy of the Department of Radiology, University of Ottawa, Ottawa, Canada.)

opment of small tubule epithelial neoplasms, of which most are adenomas and some carcinomas. Calcium may be found in the cyst wall.

Severe sclerosis occurs in the medium- and small-sized arteries of kidneys with acquired cystic disease. These vessels, which are unsupported by surrounding solid parenchyma, become markedly tortuous and project into the cavities of the cysts.

Clinical Setting

Acquired cystic kidney disease occurs during the course of long-term dialysis for the treatment of end-stage renal disease and, less frequently, in patients with chronic renal failure that does not require dialysis. Longitudinal studies have demonstrated that renal volume may diminish in the first 3 years after the start of treatment. Thereafter, cyst formation develops and progresses along with an increase in kidney bulk. As many as 90 per cent of end-stage renal disease patients are affected by acquired cystic disease after more than 5 years of dialysis.

Acquired cystic kidney disease by itself is clinically silent. Management concerns center on the development of potentially life-threatening renal adenocarcinoma or major hemorrhage from spontaneous arterial rupture. Small tubule epithelial neoplasms occur in approximately 7 per cent of dialysis patients. Most of these neoplasms are adenomas. Some, however, develop the malignant potential that accounts for an annual incidence of invasive or metastatic adenocarcinoma of the kidney that is up to six times greater in dialysis patients than in the general population in the United States. Hemorrhage due to spontaneous arterial rupture is often major and life-threatening when bleeding extends into the kidney tissue and perirenal space. Hypovo-

---

ACQUIRED CYSTIC KIDNEY DISEASE TYPICAL FINDINGS

Primary Uroradiologic Elements

Size: small; large (occasional)
Contour: smooth; multifocal masses (late)
Lesion distribution: bilateral

Secondary Uroradiologic Elements

Nephrogram: replaced (multiple masses with smooth margins; varying size; water characteristics and nonenhancing with computed tomography, magnetic resonance imaging)
Echogenicity: multiple, fluid-filled masses

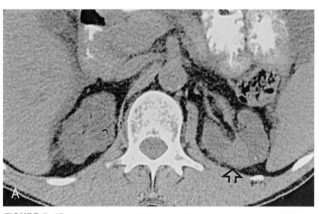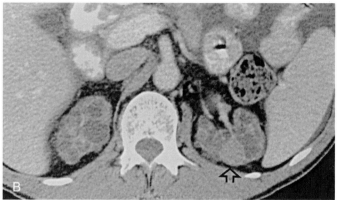

FIGURE 7–15. Acquired cystic kidney disease in patient with end-stage renal disease managed with peritoneal dialysis. The kidneys are small and smooth and contain multiple small cysts. A small adenocarcinoma is present in the dorsal aspect of the left kidney *(arrow)*.
A, Computed tomogram, unenhanced.
B, Computed tomogram, contrast material–enhanced.

lemic hypotension and severe pain may be the result. Minor bleeding into the cysts also occurs.

Radiologic Findings

Acquired cystic kidney disease is best detected and observed by computed tomography. Because of severe renal functional impairment and other limitations, excretory urography is of no value.

Renal size varies directly with the duration of hemodialysis. Early in the development of cysts, the kidneys remain small (Fig. 7–15; see Fig. 7–13). With time, kidney volume increases and may sometimes exceed normal. Cysts are sharply marginated and have attenuation values of water unless bleeding has caused an increase in this value. Contrast material can be effectively removed in dialysis patients, thus permitting contrast material–enhanced computed tomography despite severe renal failure. The residual renal parenchyma in acquired cystic kidney disease enhances slightly. Both adenomas and carcinomas demonstrate soft tissue attenuation values and are sharply defined (see Figs. 7–13 and 7–15). These solid masses, which may project into

the fluid-filled cysts, enhance in a homogeneous pattern after contrast material is administered. Carcinoma, however, cannot be distinguished from adenoma by computed tomography or any other imaging modality. With major hemorrhage due to a ruptured intrarenal artery aneurysm, computed tomography demonstrates fresh blood with a high attenuation value within and surrounding the kidney (Fig. 7–16).

The fluid-filled nature of the multiple cysts is well demonstrated by ultrasonography. The anechoic masses are surrounded by highly echogenic tissue representing the chronically diseased kidney. Carcinoma and adenoma can be detected by ultrasonography as echogenic masses, but computed tomography detects them more effectively. Ultrasonography and magnetic resonance imaging, however, are alternatives to contrast material–enhanced computed tomography in renal failure patients who are not managed with dialysis.

Angiography is used occasionally to evaluate the patient with major hemorrhage. Marked tortuosity of severely sclerotic vessels, aneurysmal dilatation, lack of tapering, and few branches are characteris-

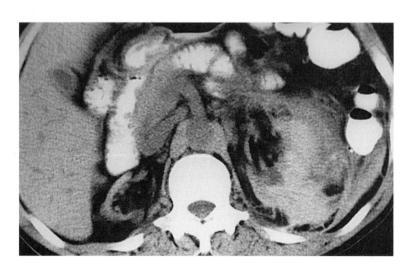

FIGURE 7–16. Acquired cystic kidney disease complicated by spontaneous hemorrhage into the left retroperitoneum. Computed tomogram, unenhanced. The right kidney is small and smooth and contains several small cysts as well as marked sinus lipomatosis. The left kidney is distorted by fresh hemorrhage that extends into the perirenal space (same patient illustrated in Fig. 21–15).

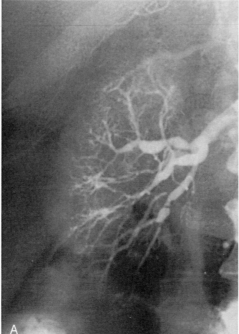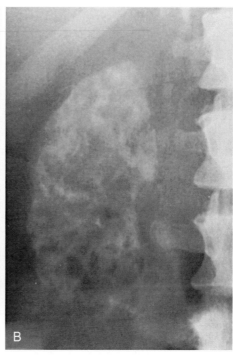

FIGURE 7-17. Acquired cystic kidney disease. The renal arteries are tortuous and lack normal tapering and branching. Aneurysmal dilatations in medium-sized vessels are common. Selective right renal arteriogram.
A, Arterial phase.
B, Nephrographic phase. Note the small size of the kidney and multiple radiolucencies due to cysts.

tic of this disorder (Fig. 7–17). With major bleeding, the nephrogram will be disordered, and the arteries will be displaced by blood in the perirenal space.

HEREDITARY NEPHROPATHIES

Hereditary chronic nephritis (Alport's syndrome) and medullary cystic disease are two hereditary diseases of the kidney that produce small kidneys and renal failure. These entities are dissimilar and are discussed separately in this section. Other radiologically detectable forms of hereditary disease produce large kidneys (autosomal dominant and recessive polycystic diseases), result in nephrocalcinosis (primary hyperoxaluria and renal tubular acidosis), or involve the kidneys secondarily (renal amyloidosis secondary to familial Mediterranean fever). These disorders are discussed in other chapters.

Hereditary Chronic Nephritis (Alport's Syndrome)

Definition

The kidneys in hereditary chronic nephritis are invariably decreased in size, often to a marked degree, but remain smooth.

The most distinctive histologic feature of hereditary chronic nephritis is the presence of fat-filled macrophages called "foam cells." Chronic interstitial inflammation, diffuse fibrosis, and chronic glomerulonephritis are also found.

Clinical Setting

The form of genetic transmission of hereditary chronic nephritis has yet to be precisely established. Males are affected with a more severe form of renal disease than females. Symptoms, usually episodic hematuria, begin in childhood. This is often preceded by upper respiratory tract infections. Renal insufficiency is progressive, with few males living

---

HEREDITARY CHRONIC NEPHRITIS TYPICAL FINDINGS

Primary Uroradiologic Elements

Size: small
Contour: smooth
Lesion distribution: bilateral

Secondary Uroradiologic Elements

Parenchymal thickness: wasted
Nephrogram: diminished density

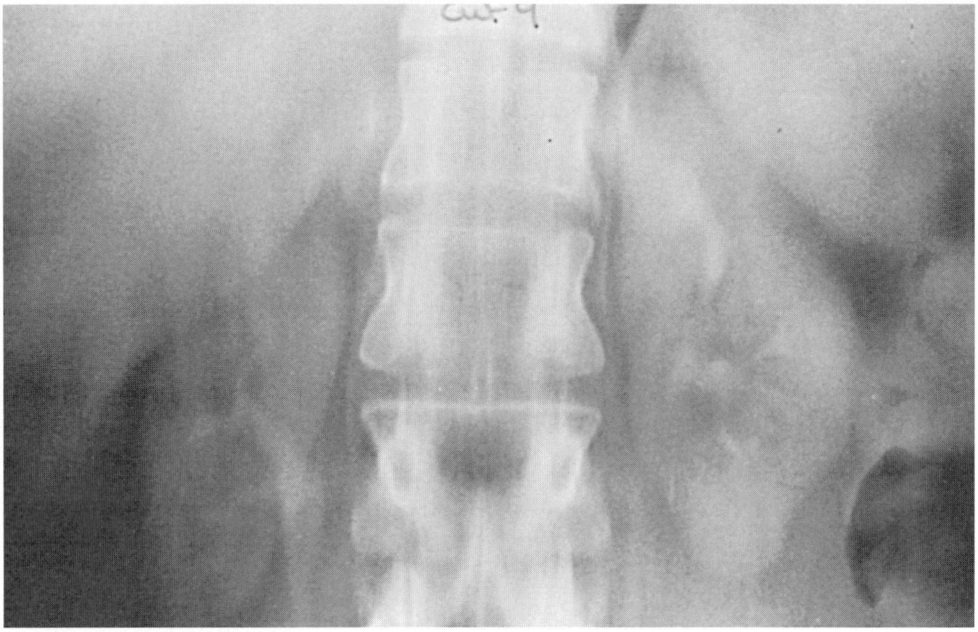

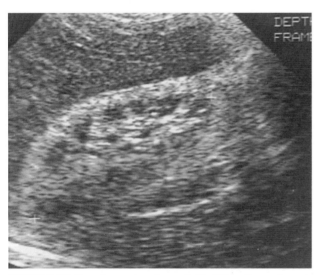

FIGURE 7–18. Hereditary chronic nephritis (Alport's syndrome). Bilaterally small, smooth kidneys with normal pelvocalyceal system in a 52-year-old woman with mild intermittent hypertension, proteinuria, and slight azotemia. One of her sons died of "nephritis," and another had renal function and auditory and ocular abnormalities. Tomogram. (Courtesy of Department of Diagnostic Radiology, Hammersmith Hospital, Royal Postgraduate Medical School, London, England.)

beyond the 5th decade without dialysis. In females, the disease is usually nonprogressive, and death due to chronic nephritis is uncommon. One striking feature in both sexes is the absence of hypertension as a prominent aspect of the disease.

In addition to renal abnormalities, most patients also have nerve deafness and a variety of ocular abnormalities.

Radiologic Findings

Small, smooth kidneys with impaired excretion of contrast material are the radiologic abnormalities

FIGURE 7–19. Hereditary chronic nephritis (Alport's syndrome). Right kidney, ultrasonogram, longitudinal section. The kidney was small and smooth, as was the left kidney. Cortical hyperechogenicity represents nephrocalcinosis of chronic glomerulonephritis and is not an inherent feature of hereditary chronic nephritis.

of hereditary chronic nephritis (Figs. 7–18, 7–19). Cortical hyperechoicity, if present, represents nephrocalcinosis of chronic glomerulonephritis and is not a feature inherent to hereditary chronic nephritis. Obviously, this diagnosis is dependent on clinical features in addition to radiologic findings.

Medullary Cystic Disease

Definition

Medullary cystic disease is the second of the heritable causes of renal failure associated with normal-sized to small kidneys with smooth outlines.

A variable number of cysts, found for the most part in the corticomedullary and medullary areas of the kidney, are seen in the cut section of these kidneys. The cysts range in size from less than 100 mm to 1 cm or more in diameter. The usual sharp demarcation between cortex and medulla is obliterated. Most cysts are too small to distort the pelvocalyceal system or the renal contour.

A flattened or low cuboidal tubule epithelium is seen on microscopy. Except for cysts, other findings are nonspecific. These include hyalinization of glomeruli, periglomerular fibrosis, fibrosis and chronic inflammatory cell infiltration of the interstitium, and tubule atrophy.

It is generally accepted that medullary cystic disease is the same as familial juvenile nephronophthisis. However, another point of view holds that nephronophthisis is distinguishable by age at onset and by pattern of inheritance.

Clinical Setting

Medullary cystic disease is inherited as either an autosomal dominant or an autosomal recessive

---

MEDULLARY CYSTIC DISEASE TYPICAL FINDINGS

Primary Uroradiologic Elements

Size: small
Contour: smooth
Lesion distribution: bilateral

Secondary Uroradiologic Elements

Parenchymal thickness: wasted
Nephrogram: diminished density; replaced (multiple masses with smooth margins; varying
    size; water characteristics and nonenhancing with computed tomography, magnetic
    resonance imaging); delayed
Echogenicity: increased; fluid-filled medullary or corticomedullary masses

---

trait. Disease presenting in the first 2 decades of life is usually transmitted as an autosomal recessive inheritance, whereas autosomal dominant patterns characterize those that appear in 3rd or subsequent decades.

The onset of symptoms (usually polydipsia, polyuria, and nocturia) is insidious. Hypertension is not a prominent feature of medullary cystic disease and may not appear at all until late in the course of the disease. A normochromic, normocytic anemia secondary to chronic uremia is a universal finding in symptomatic patients. Characteristically, these patients have hyposthenuria and are salt wasters. Apart from a loss of concentrating ability, abnormalities in the urine are usually absent. Death due to uremia usually occurs in the 3rd decade, although a few patients have been known to survive into the 7th decade of life.

Radiologic Findings

Normal-sized to small kidneys, smooth contour, and impaired excretion of contrast material are the common features of medullary cystic disease. In many patients, these are the only findings, and the radiologic examination is nonspecific. In some patients, sharply defined radiolucent nephrographic defects may be observed when the medullary cysts are large. A striated, late-appearing, and persistent nephrogram limited to the medullary portions of the parenchyma has also been described (Fig. 7–20). This corresponds to urine stasis in dilated tubules and collecting ducts. Because cysts are usually small, pelvocalyceal displacement and lobulation of the renal contour are uncommon.

Computed tomography and ultrasonography demonstrate kidneys that are small in size and smooth in contour. Both modalities are more sensitive than excretory urography in demonstrating numerous medullary cysts. Additionally, increased parenchymal echogenicity is seen by ultrasonography (Fig. 7–21).

AMYLOIDOSIS (LATE)

Amyloidosis of the kidneys causes smooth enlargement of both kidneys; this is discussed in Chapter 8.

With time, however, amyloid kidneys become small, with preservation of a normal contour and pelvocalyceal relationships. Presumably, this occurs as a result of ischemic atrophy of nephrons induced by involvement of the renal arteries by amyloid deposits. These changes occur consistently. Thus, amyloidosis must be considered in the differential diagnosis of bilaterally small, as well as large, smooth kidneys.

ARTERIAL HYPOTENSION

Definition

In normal circumstances, the kidney is distended by blood filling the vascular bed and by urine filling the tubules and pelvocalyceal system. When arterial hypotension occurs, intrarenal hypovolemia, primary vasoconstriction, and depletion of intratubular urine volume brought on by reduced glomerular filtration follow. The net consequence of these events can be seen radiologically as a reduction in renal size and an abnormal nephrogram.

Clinical Setting

Reduced renal size due to hypotension was first described in patients undergoing aortography under general anesthesia. In modern practice, hypotension is usually encountered as an adverse response to contrast material during the performance of an excretory urogram, computed tomogram, or arteriogram. The condition can go unsuspected because the patient may be free of pallor, diaphoresis, and lightheadedness. Sometimes the first indication of hypotension is the radiologist's observation that the kidneys are smaller on early films of the urogram than on the preliminary film and that the calyces fail to opacify despite the presence of a distinct nephrogram. With appropriate therapeutic measures, as discussed in Chapter 1, these abnormalities disappear.

Radiologic Findings

Because hypotension is systemic, shrinkage is global and bilateral. Because this finding is usually

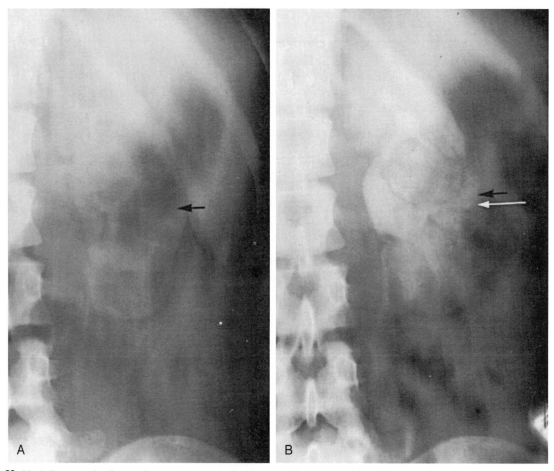

FIGURE 7–20. Medullary cystic disease in an asymptomatic 26-year-old woman with mild azotemia, salt-wasting, and normal blood pressure.

A, Excretory urogram, 15-second tomogram. Angiographic nephrogram demonstrates slight thinning of the cortex and a slightly enlarged medulla *(arrow)* that remains normally radiolucent.

B, Excretory urogram. Tomogram. A 30-minute delayed film reveals loss of opacification of the cortex and a persistent, dense nephrogram limited to the medulla *(large arrow),* representing stasis in tubules and collecting ducts. Small cysts are represented by round radiolucencies *(small arrow).*

(Courtesy of Daniel P. Link, M.D., University of California, Davis, and American Journal of Roentgenology *133*:303, 1979.)

seen as a reaction to contrast material, the acuteness of this process is often first noted by comparing renal size on post– and pre–contrast material images and then immediately observing the patient.

The nephrogram becomes progressively dense over time. This reflects reduced glomerular filtration and stasis of filtrate in the tubules as a result of reduced afferent arteriolar perfusion pressure. At the same time, increased sodium and water reabsorption promotes further filtration by depleting intratubular volume. An increased accumulation of contrast material in the tubules results in the nephrogram becoming increasingly dense.

Once hypotension is reversed, the nephrogram

ARTERIAL HYPOTENSION TYPICAL FINDINGS*

Primary Uroradiologic Elements

Size: small (compared with size on pre–contrast material image)
Contour: smooth
Lesion distribution: bilateral

Secondary Uroradiologic Elements

Collecting system: absent opacification
Nephrogram: increasingly dense (common); persistently dense (uncommon)

  *All findings revert to normal with correction of hypotension.

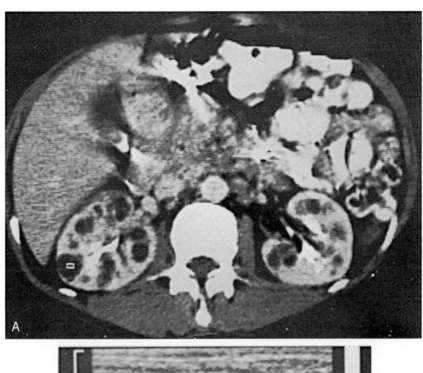

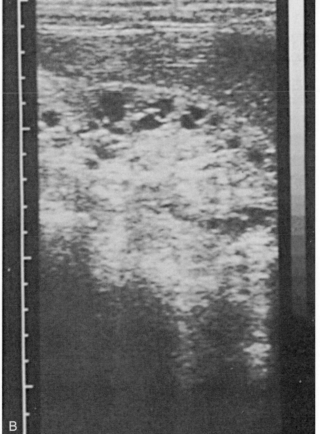

FIGURE 7–21. Medullary cystic disease in a 55-year-old man with salt-losing nephropathy.

A, Computed tomogram, contrast material–enhanced. Fluid-filled cysts of varying size are in the medulla and corticomedullary region. Characteristically, they are not of sufficient size to distort the contour or enlarge the size of the kidneys.

B, The same abnormalities demonstrated by computed tomography are seen by ultrasonography. Note also the nonspecific increase in renal parenchymal echogenicity.

(Courtesy of John D. Rego, M.D., et al., San Francisco General Hospital, San Francisco, California, and J. Ultrasound Med. *2*:433, 1983.)

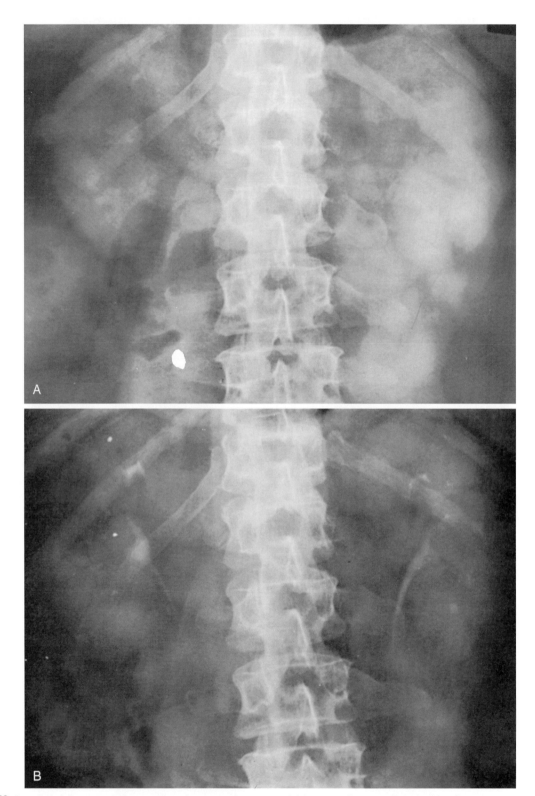

FIGURE 7–22. Renal shrinkage and abnormal nephrogram due to arterial hypotension associated with adverse response to contrast material (same patient illustrated in Fig. 27–16).

   A, 10-minute film. Right kidney length = 13.4 cm; left kidney length = 13.2 cm.

   B, 45-minute film following successful treatment of hypotension. Pelvocalyceal systems are now opacified, and the nephrogram is of normal density. Kidneys have increased 1 cm in length. Right kidney length = 14.4 cm; left kidney length = 14.2 cm.

characteristically reverts to normal, and there is progressive opacification of the collecting system (Fig. 7–22).

DIFFERENTIAL DIAGNOSIS

The radiologic pictures of **generalized arteriosclerosis** and **benign nephrosclerosis** are identical. Distinction between these two depends on clinical information; specifically, normal blood pressure and advanced age (6th decade and older) in the former and arterial hypertension and an onset before age 50 years in the latter. Renal opacification is normal in both disorders.

In **malignant nephrosclerosis, atheroembolic renal disease, chronic glomerulonephritis, acquired cystic kidney disease,** and the **hereditary nephropathies,** depressed renal function impairs contrast material enhancement, sometimes to a very marked degree. Systemic hypertension is a significant problem in all these disorders except the hereditary nephropathies. Hereditary nephropathy patients also have distinctive clinical features, such as a family history of renal disease, ocular and hearing disorders in hereditary chronic nephritis, or salt-wasting in medullary cystic disease.

Disorders that produce bilaterally small, smooth kidneys as a result of primary disease of the arterial bed occasionally demonstrate randomly placed, small infarct scars representing sites where the arterial lesion has progressed to complete occlusion. These are seen in **generalized arteriosclerosis, benign** and **malignant nephrosclerosis,** and **atheroembolic renal disease,** but not in the other entities of this diagnostic set.

The demonstration of medullary or corticomedullary cysts in bilaterally small, smooth kidneys is encountered in both **medullary cystic disease** and **acquired cystic kidney disease.** Their distinctive clinical setting serves to distinguish each from the other. Uncommonly, the kidneys of acquired cystic kidney disease become quite large and identical in appearance to kidneys in **autosomal dominant polycystic kidney disease.** A history of long-term dialysis serves to distinguish the former from the latter. Multiple renal cysts also are found in numerous syndromes that are known variably as **glomerulocystic, microcystic,** or **pluricystic disorders** of the kidney. Here, too, clinical findings help to clarify the diagnosis. These are discussed briefly in Chapter 8.

Uncommonly, the kidneys of **acquired cystic kidney disease** become enlarged by a combination of cysts, adenomas, and adenocarcinomas. In this circumstance, the radiologic findings will overlap with those of **von Hippel-Lindau disease** (cysts and adenocarcinomas) or **tuberous sclerosis** (cysts and angiomyolipomas). These two entities, however, have additional radiologic and clinical features that permit accurate diagnosis. These are described in Chapter 10.

Arterial hypotension as a cause of small, smooth kidneys is distinguishable by the transient nature of the abnormalities and by the abnormal time-density relationship of the nephrogram.

BIBLIOGRAPHY

General

Ambos, M. A., Bosniak, M. A., Gordon, R., and Madayag, M. D.: Replacement lipomatosis of the kidney. AJR *130*:1087, 1978.
Brenner, B. M. (ed.): Brenner and Rector's The Kidney, 5th ed. Philadelphia, W. B. Saunders, 1996.
Heptinstall, R. H. (ed.): Pathology of the Kidney, 4th ed. Boston, Little, Brown & Co., 1992.
Murray, T., and Goldberg, M.: Chronic interstitial nephritis: Etiologic factors. Ann. Intern. Med. *82*:453, 1975.
Page, J. E., Morgan, S. H., Eastwood, J. B., Smith, S. A., Webb, D. J., Dilly, S. A., Chow, J., Pottier, A., and Joseph, A. E. A.: Ultrasound findings in renal parenchymal disease: Comparison with histological appearances. Clin. Radiol. *49*:867, 1994.
Schrier, R. W., and Gottschalk, C. W. (eds.): Diseases of the Kidney, 6th ed. Boston, Little, Brown & Co., 1997.

Generalized Arteriosclerosis

Albers, F. J.: Clinical characteristics of atherosclerotic renovascular disease. Am. J. Kidney Dis. *24*:636, 1994.
Barlow, K. A., and Beilin, L. J.: Renal disease in primary gout. Q. J. Med. *37*:79, 1968.
Case records of the Massachusetts General Hospital: Case 34-1978: Scleroderma involving skin and kidneys. N. Engl. J. Med. *299*:466, 1978.
Greco, B. A., and Breyer, J. A.: Atherosclerotic ischemic renal disease. Am. J. Kidney Dis. *29*:167, 1997.
Griffiths, G. J., Robinson, K. B., Cartwright, G. O., and McLachlan, M. S. F.: Loss of renal tissue in the elderly. Br. J. Radiol. *49*:111, 1976.
Heptinstall, R. H. (ed.): Pathology of the Kidney, 4th ed. Boston, Little, Brown & Co., 1992.
Hill, G. S.: Renal vascular lesions. In Hill, G. S. (ed.): Uropathology. New York, Churchill Livingstone, 1989, pp. 189–234.
McLachlan, M., and Wasserman, P.: Changes in sizes and distensibility of the aging kidney. Br. J. Radiol. *54*:488, 1981.
Murray, T., and Goldberg, M.: Chronic interstitial nephritis: Etiologic factors. Ann. Intern. Med. *82*:453, 1975.
Novick, A. C.: Atherosclerotic ischemic nephropathy. Urol. Clin. North Am. *21*:195, 1994.
Oliver, J. A., and Cannon, P. J.: The kidney in scleroderma. Nephron *18*:141, 1977.
Pohl, M. A.: Renal artery stenosis, renal vascular hypertension, and ischemic nephropathy. In Schrier, R. W., and Gottschalk, C. W. (eds.): Diseases of the Kidney, 6th ed. Boston, Little, Brown & Co., 1997, pp. 1367–1424.
Siegel, C. L., Ellis, J. H., Korobkin, M., and Dunnick, N. R.: CT-detected renal arterial calcification: Correlation with renal artery stenosis on angiography. AJR *163*:867, 1994.
Talbott, J. H., and Terplan, K. L.: The kidney in gout. Medicine (Baltimore) *39*:405, 1960.

Nephrosclerosis (Benign and Malignant)

Heptinstall, R. H.: Hypertension I: Essential hypertension. In Heptinstall, R. H. (ed.): Pathology of the Kidney, 4th ed. Boston, Little, Brown & Co., 1992, pp. 951–1028.
Nolan, C. R., III, and Linas, S. L.: Accelerated and malignant hypertension. In Schrier, R. W., and Gottschalk, C. W. (eds.): Diseases of the Kidney, 4th ed. Boston, Little, Brown & Co., 1988, pp. 1703–1826.
Pohl, M. A.: Renal artery stenosis, renal vascular hypertension, and ischemic nephropathy. In Schrier, R. W., and Gottschalk, C. W. (eds.): Diseases of the Kidney, 6th ed. Boston, Little, Brown & Co., 1997, pp. 1367–1424.
Preston, R. A., Singer, I., and Epstein, M.: Renal parenchymal hypertension: Current concepts of pathogenesis and management. Arch. Intern. Med. *156*:602, 1996.

Raine, A. E. G.: Hypertension and the kidney. Brit. Med. Bull. *50*:322, 1994.

Atheroembolic Renal Disease

Case records of the Massachusetts General Hospital: Atheroembolic renal disease. N. Engl. J. Med. *329*:948, 1993.

Dahlberg, P. J., Frecentese, D. F., and Gobbill, T. H.: Cholesterol embolism: Experience with 22 histologically proven cases. Surgery *105*:737, 1989.

Fine, M. J., Kapoor, W., and Falonga, V.: Cholesterol crystal embolization: A review of 221 cases in the English literature. Angiology *38*:769, 1987.

Lie, J. T.: Cholesterol atheromatous embolism: The great masquerader revisited. In Rosen, P. P., and Fechner, R. E. (eds.): Series: Pathology Annual 27, Annual 1992, Pt. 2. Norwalk, Connecticut, Appleton & Lange, 1992, pp. 17–50.

Lye, W. C., Cheah, J. S., and Sinniah, R.: Renal cholesterol embolic disease. Am. J. Nephrol. *13*:489, 1993.

Palmer, F. J., and Warren, B. A.: Multiple cholesterol emboli syndrome complicating angiographic techniques. Clin. Radiol. *39*:519, 1988.

Saleem, S., Lakkis, F. G., and Martinez Maldonado, M.: Atheroembolic renal disease. Semin. Nephrol. *16*:309, 1996..

Scolari, F., Bracchi, M., Valzorio, B., Movilli, E., Costantino, E., Savoldi, S., Zorat, S., Bonardelli, S., Tardanico, R., and Maiorca, R.: Cholesterol atheromatous embolism: An increasingly recognized cause of acute renal failure. Nephrol. Dial. Transplant. *11*:1607, 1996.

Vidt, D. G.: Cholesterol emboli: A common cause of renal failure. Annu. Rev. Med. *48*:375, 1997

Chronic Glomerulonephritis

Arons, W. L., Christensen, W. G., and Sosman, M. C.: Nephrocalcinosis visible by x-ray associated with chronic glomerulonephritis. Ann. Intern. Med. *42*:260, 1955.

Cohen, H. L., Kassner, E. G., and Haller, J. D.: Nephrocalcinosis in chronic glomerulonephritis: Report of the youngest patient. Urol. Radiol. *2*:51, 1980.

Heptinstall, R. H.: Pathology of the Kidney, 4th ed. Boston, Little, Brown & Co., 1992.

Schrier, R. W., and Gottschalk, C. W. (eds.): Diseases of the Kidney, 6th ed. Boston, Little, Brown & Co., 1997.

Acquired Cystic Kidney Disease

Andersen, B. L., Curry, N. S., and Gobien, R. P.: Sonography of evolving renal cystic transformation associated with hemodialysis. AJR *141*:1003, 1983.

Basile, J. J., McCullough, D. L., Harrison, L. H., and Dyer, R. B.: End-stage renal disease associated with acquired cystic disease and neoplasia. J. Urol. *140*:938, 1988.

Brennan, J. F., Stilmant, M. M., Babayan, R. K., and Siroky, M. B.: Acquired renal cystic disease: Implications for the urologist. Br. J. Urol. *67*:342, 1991.

Chandhoke, P. S., Torrence, R. J., Clayman, R. V., and Rothstein, M.: Acquired cystic disease of the kidney: A management dilemma. J. Urol. *147*:969, 1992.

Chung-Park, M., Parveen, T., and Lam, M.: Acquired cystic disease of the kidneys and renal cell carcinoma in chronic renal insufficiency without dialysis treatment. Nephron *53*:157, 1989.

Dunnill, M. S., Millard, P. R., and Oliver, D.: Acquired cystic disease of the kidneys: A hazard of long-term intermittent maintenance haemodialysis. J. Clin. Pathol. *30*:868, 1977.

Grantham, J. J.: Acquired cystic kidney disease. Kidney Int. *40*:143, 1991.

Heinz-Peer, G., Schroder, M., Rand, T., Mayer, G., and Mostbeck, G. H.: Prevalence of acquired cystic kidney disease and tumors in native kidneys of renal transplant recipients: A prospective US study. Radiology *195*:667, 1995.

Heptinstall, R. H.: End-stage renal disease. In Heptinstall, R. H. (ed.): Pathology of the Kidney, 4th ed. Boston, Little, Brown & Co., 1992, pp. 749–753.

Hogg, R. J.: Acquired renal cystic disease in children prior to the start of dialysis. Pediatr. Nephrol. *6*:176, 1992.

Hughson, M. D., Schmidt, L., Zbar, B., Daugherty, S., Meloni, A. M., Silva, F. G., and Sandberg, A. A.: Renal cell carcinoma of end-stage renal disease: A histopathologic and molecular genetic study. J. Am. Soc. Nephrol. *7*:2461, 1996.

Ishikawa, I.: Acquired renal cystic disease. In Gardner, K. D., Jr., and Bernstein, J. (eds.): The Cystic Kidney. Dordrecht, Kluwer Academic Publishers, 1990, pp. 351–378.

Ishikawa, I.: Uremic acquired renal cystic disease: Natural history and complications. Nephron *58*:257, 1991.

Ishikawa, I., Shikura, N., and Shinoda, A.: Cystic transformation in native kidneys in renal allograft recipients with long-standing good function. Am. J. Nephrol. *11*:217, 1991.

Leichter, H. E., Dietrich, R., Salusky, I. B., et al.: Acquired cystic kidney disease in children undergoing long-term dialysis. Pediatr. Nephrol. *2*:8, 1988.

Levine, E.: Acquired cystic kidney disease. Radiol. Clin. North Am. *34*:947, 1996.

Levine, E., Grantham, J. J., and MacDougall, M. L.: Spontaneous subcapsular and perinephric hemorrhage in end-stage kidney disease: Clinical and CT findings. AJR *148*:755, 1987.

Levine, E., Hartman, D. S., and Smirniotopolous, J. G.: Renal cystic diseases associated with renal neoplasms. In Hartman, D. S. (ed.): Renal Cystic Disease. Philadelphia, W. B. Saunders, 1989, pp. 38–72.

Levine, E., Slusher, S. L., Grantham, J. J., and Wetzel, L. H.: Natural history of acquired renal cystic disease in dialysis patients: A prospective longitudinal CT study. AJR *156*:501, 1991.

Marple, J. T., Macdougall, M., and Chonko, A. M.: Renal cancer complicating acquired cystic kidney disease. J. Am. Soc. Nephrol. *4*:1951, 1994.

Matson, M. A., and Cohen, E. P.: Acquired cystic kidney disease: Occurrence, prevalence and renal cancers. Medicine *69*:217, 1990.

Port, F. K., Ragheb, N. E., and Schwartz, A. G.: Neoplasms in dialysis patients: A population-based study. Am. J. Kidney Dis. *14*:119, 1989.

Sarasin, F. P., Wong, J. B., and Levery, A. S.: Screening for acquired cystic kidney disease: A decision analytic perspective. Kidney Int. *48*:207, 1995.

Sasagawa, I., Terasawa, Y., Imai, K., Sekino, H., and Takahashi, H.: Acquired cystic disease of the kidney and renal carcinoma in hemodialysis patients: Ultrasonographic evaluation. Br. J. Urol. *70*:236, 1992.

Taylor, A. J., Cohen, E. P., Erickson, S. J., Olson, D. L., and Folley, W. D.: Renal imaging in long-term dialysis patients: A comparison of CT and sonography. AJR *153*:765, 1989.

Truong, L. D., Krishnan, B., Cao, J. T. H., Barrios, R., and Suki, W. N.: Renal neoplasm in acquired cystic kidney disease. Am. J. Kidney Dis. *26*:1, 1995.

Hereditary Chronic Nephritis

Choyke, P. L.: Inherited cystic diseases of the kidney. Radiol. Clin. North Am. *34*:925, 1996.

Chugh, K. S., Sakhuja, V., and Agarwal, A.: Hereditary nephritis (Alport's syndrome): Clinical profile and inheritance in 28 kindreds. Nephrol. Dial. Transplant. *8*:690, 1993.

Flinter, F.: Alport's syndrome. J. Med. Genet. *34*:326, 1997.

Gregory, M. C., and Atkin, C. L.: Alport's syndrome, Fabry's disease, and Nail-patella syndrome. In Schrier, R. W., and Gottschalk, C. W. (eds.): Diseases of the Kidney, 6th ed. Boston, Little, Brown & Co., 1997, pp. 561–590.

Gubler, M., Levy, M., and Broyer, M.: Alport's syndrome: A report of 58 cases and a review of the literature. Am. J. Med. *70*:493, 1981.

Kashtan, C. E., and Michael, A. F.: Alport syndrome. Kidney Int. *50*:1445, 1996.

Perkoff, G. T.: The hereditary renal diseases. N. Engl. J. Med. *277*:79, 1967.

Purriel, P., Drets, M., Cestau, R. S., Borras, A., Ferreira, W. A., De Lucca, A., and Fernandez, L.: Familial hereditary nephropathy (Alport's syndrome). Am. J. Med. *49*:753, 1970.

Medullary Cystic Disease

Burgener, F. A., and Spataro, R. F.: Early medullary cystic disease: A urographic diagnosis? Radiology *130*:321, 1979.

Cantani, A., Bamonte, G., Ceccoli, D., Biribicchi G., and Farinella, F.: Familial juvenile nephronophthisis: A review and differential diagnosis. Clin. Pediatr. 25:90, 1986.

Case records of the Massachusetts General Hospital: Case 15-1970. Medullary cystic disease. N. Engl. J. Med. 282:799, 1970.

Chuang, Y. F., and Tsai, T. C.: Sonographic findings in familial juvenile nephronopthisis—medullary cystic disease complex. J. Clin. Ultrasound 26:203, 1998.

Elzouki, A. Y., Alsuhaibani, H., Mirza, K., and Alsowailem, A. M.: Thin-section computed tomography scans detect medullary cysts in patients believed to have juvenile nephronophthisis. Am. J. Kidney Dis. 27:216, 1996.

Gardner, K. D., Jr., and Bernstein, J. (eds.): The Cystic Kidney. Boston, Kluwer Academic Publishers, 1990.

Giangiacomo, J., Monteleone, P. L., and Witzleben, C. L.: Medullary cystic disease vs. nephronophthisis: A valid distinction? JAMA 232:629, 1975.

Hildebrandt, F., Jungers, P., and Grunfeld, J-P.: Medullary cystic and medullary sponge renal disorders. In Schrier, R. W., and Gottschalk, C. W. (eds.): Diseases of the Kidney, 6th ed. Boston, Little, Brown & Co., 1997, pp. 499–520.

Link, D. P., Hansen, S., and Palmer, J.: High-dose excretory urography and medullary cystic disease of the kidney. AJR 133:303, 1979.

Olsen, A., Hojhus, J. H., and Steffensen, G.: Renal medullary cystic disease: Findings at urography and ultrasonography. Acta Radiol. 29:527, 1988.

Rego, J. D., Jr., Laing, F. C., and Jeffrey, R. B.: Ultrasonic diagnosis of medullary cystic disease. J. Ultrasound Med. 2:433, 1983.

Risdon, R. A.: Development, developmental defects, and cystic diseases of the kidney. In Heptinstall, R. H. (ed.): Pathology of the Kidney, 4th ed. Boston, Little, Brown & Co., 1992, pp. 93–168.

Rosenfield, A. T., Siegel, N. J., and Kappelman, N. B.: Gray scale ultrasonography in medullary cystic disease of the kidney and congenital hepatic fibrosis with tubular ectasia: New observations. AJR 129:297, 1977.

Steele, B. T., Lirenman, D. S., and Beattie, C. W.: Nephronophthisis. Am. J. Med. 68:531, 1980.

Swenson, R. S., Kempson, R. L., and Friedland, G. W.: Cystic disease of the renal medulla in the elderly. JAMA 228:1401, 1974.

Turner, A. N., and Rees, A. J.: Goodpasture's disease and Alport's syndromes. Ann. Rev. Med. 47:377, 1996.

Wood, B. P.: Renal cystic disease in infants and children. Urol. Radiol. 14:284, 1992.

Woolf, A. S., and Winyard, P. J. D.: Unraveling the pathogenesis of cystic kidney diseases. Arch. Dis. Child. 72:103, 1996.

Arterial Hypotension

Fry, I. K., and Cattell, W. R.: Nephrogram pattern during excretion urography. Br. Med. Bull. 28:227, 1972.

Haber, K.: Changes in renal size as related to blood pressure during an idiosyncratic reaction to radiographic contrast. J. Urol. 111:288, 1974.

Hodson, C. J.: Physiological changes in size of the human kidney. Clin. Radiol. 12:91, 1961.

Katzberg, R. W., and Schabel, S. T.: Bilaterally small kidneys in shock. JAMA 235:2213, 1976.

Korobkin, M.: The nephrogram of hemorrhagic hypotension. AJR 114:673, 1972.

Korobkin, M. T., Kirkwood, R., and Minagi, H.: The nephrogram of hypotension. Radiology 98:129, 1971.

Korobkin, M., Shanser, J. D., and Carlson, E. L.: The nephrogram of normovolemic, renal artery hypotension. Invest. Radiol. 11:71, 1976.

8

Diagnostic Set: Large, Smooth, Bilateral

Most of the diseases discussed in this chapter present as renal failure of recent onset. The value of performing imaging studies, usually ultrasonography or unenhanced computed tomography, on patients with these diseases lies in the demonstration of bilaterally enlarged, smooth, nonobstructed kidneys. The collecting structures are either normal or generally effaced by the swollen kidneys. When these findings are present, it can be surmised that the disease is parenchymal, of recent onset, and possibly reversible. Once this is established, the nephrologist usually turns to the study of needle biopsy tissue by light and electron microscopy and by immunologic techniques for a more specific diagnosis as clinical, laboratory, and radiologic features overlap and are nonspecific in acute renal failure.

On the other hand, there are some diseases or conditions in the diagnostic set, "large, smooth, bilateral," that are of long standing and are not associated with acute renal failure. In addition to autosomal recessive (infantile) polycystic kidney disease, these include a miscellaneous group that have clinical and/or radiologic features that distinguish them from the more commonly encountered causes of acute renal failure.

It is important for the radiologist to have some grasp of the varied diseases that cause global enlargement of both kidneys, even though most of these cannot be specifically diagnosed by radiologic techniques. The organization of this chapter is based for the most part on the pathologic mechanism of renal enlargement. With this approach, diseases are grouped under the following categories: proliferative/necrotizing disorders, abnormal protein deposition, abnormal fluid accumulation, neoplastic cell infiltration, and inflammatory cell infiltration. The final sections include autosomal recessive (infantile) polycystic kidney disease and a miscellaneous group of unrelated diseases and physiologic states in which both kidneys enlarge.

PROLIFERATIVE/NECROTIZING DISORDERS

Definition

In general, the proliferative and necrotizing diseases that cause smooth enlargement of the total renal mass fall into two groups: those that affect the kidneys alone and those that affect the kidneys as part of a multisystemic disorder. In both cases, the glomerulus is the principal site of abnormalities, which include proliferation or necrosis of cellular elements, increased lobulation, and enlargement of epithelial cells. Fibrinous and proteinaceous deposits may be found in the capsular space. The morphologic diagnosis of a specific disease within this group is dependent on integrating light, electron, and immunofluorescent microscopic patterns of glomerular involvement with other clinical or laboratory abnormalities.

These various disorders also affect other structural components of the kidney, particularly the blood vessels and the interstitium, but in a nonspecific way. The interlobular arteries may show collagenous intimal thickening, and in some of these diseases there are necrotizing cellular changes and thrombosis of small arteries, arterioles, and capillaries. Edema, scattered foci of round cells, and a fine fibrosis are frequently seen in the interstitial space.

The net effect of these abnormalities is an increase in renal bulk and an impairment of renal function, particularly glomerular filtration. Both of these features produce radiologic abnormalities.

Clinical Setting

The proliferative/necrotizing disorders that affect the kidney alone are those of the acute glomerulonephritides. These include *acute (post-streptococcal) glomerulonephritis, rapidly progressive glomerulonephritis, idiopathic membranous glomerulonephritis, membranoproliferative glomerulonephritis, immunoglobulin A (IgA) nephropathy glomerulosclerosis, glomerulosclerosis related to heroin abuse, and lobular glomerulonephritis*. All are characterized by enlargement of both kidneys during the early phase of the illness.

Patients with these diseases of the kidney have opalescent urine, periorbital and peripheral edema, and cardiovascular symptoms related to salt and water retention and hypertension. The nephrotic syndrome is often present. Red blood cell, granular, and leukocyte casts are found in the urine.

Proliferative and necrotizing abnormalities of the glomerulus also occur in multisystemic diseases. These include *polyarteritis nodosa* (microscopic form), *systemic lupus erythematosus, Wegener's granulomatosis, allergic angiitis, diabetic glomerulosclerosis, lung hemorrhage and glomerulonephritis (Goodpasture's syndrome), anaphylactoid purpura (Schönlein-Henoch syndrome), thrombotic thrombocytopenic purpura* in adults and *hemolytic-uremic syndrome* in infants and children, *focal glomerulonephritis associated with subacute bacterial endocarditis*, and *HIV-associated nephropathy*. In these diseases, clinical features that are more disease-specific are superimposed on features generally found in isolated acute glomerular disease.

Some multisystemic diseases have specific patterns. Granulomatous lesions with vascular necrosis are found in the kidney, lungs, and upper respiratory tract in Wegener's granulomatosis. Granulomatous foci occur in many organs in allergic angiitis, a syndrome that also includes asthma, fever, and eosinophilia in addition to the signs and symptoms produced by the renal lesion. Goodpasture's syndrome is a combination of glomerular disease and necrotizing alveolitis producing lung hemorrhage. Hemoptysis, dyspnea, and anemia appear during a rapidly progressive course of renal failure, which usually leads to death after a short time. In Schönlein-Henoch syndrome, purpuric skin lesions, intestinal colic, intussusception, joint pains, and gastrointestinal bleeding reflect involvement of the skin, gastrointestinal tract, and joints, whereas hematuria and proteinuria represent the glomerular disease seen in most of these patients. Thrombotic thrombocytopenic purpura is characterized by hemolytic anemia, hemorrhage, oliguric or anuric renal failure, gastrointestinal bleeding, splenomegaly, and central nervous system dysfunction in adults. This results from erythrocyte fragmentation, thrombocytopenia, and intravascular coagulation. The same condition is known as the hemolytic-uremic syndrome when it occurs in infants and children. Acute cortical necrosis may be a component of the hemolytic-uremic syndrome in which severe renal failure usually predominates.

Acute glomerular lesions and enlarged kidneys are present only in the "microscopic" form of polyarteritis nodosa. The other mode of presentation, bilaterally small kidneys, is seen in the "classic" form, which is discussed in Chapter 7.

Radiologic Findings

Invariably, both kidneys are involved in the proliferative and necrotizing disorders of the glomerulus, although asymmetry has been reported. Renal size varies from normal to markedly enlarged. Because involvement is global, parenchymal thickening is equal throughout, and the contour remains smooth.

Ultrasonography is the most efficacious test for

PROLIFERATIVE/NECROTIZING DISORDERS TYPICAL FINDINGS

Primary Uroradiologic Elements

Size: large
Contour: smooth
Lesion distribution: bilateral

Secondary Uroradiologic Elements

Collecting system: attenuated
Parenchymal thickness: expanded
Echogenicity: increased (diffuse); increased (cortex) in hemolytic-uremic syndrome

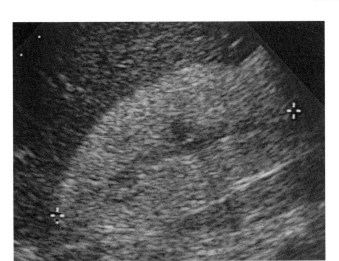

FIGURE 8–1. HIV-associated nephropathy in a 24-year-old woman. Ultrasonogram in a longitudinal section demonstrates a right kidney that is smooth in contour and enlarged for a person of small stature. There is diffuse hyperechoicity relative to the liver. The left kidney had similar characteristics. (Kindly provided by Cynthia Caskey, M.D., and Ulrike Hamper, M.D., Johns Hopkins University, Baltimore, Maryland.)

the demonstration of the radiologic findings that are characteristic of necrotizing and proliferative disorders of the glomerulus: bilaterally large, smooth kidneys; a homogeneous pattern of normal to increased echogenicity; and the absence of pelvocalyceal dilatation (Fig. 8–1). These findings indicate that the renal failure is acute and not due to obstruction of both kidneys ("postrenal failure") but give no indication of either the specific nature or the severity of the disease. Diagnostic evaluation thereafter is directed to renal biopsy. Unique within

this group of diseases, hemolytic-uremic syndrome characteristically produces selective hyperechoicity of the cortex relative to the medulla (Fig. 8–2). This pattern probably is due to platelet aggregation and fibrin thrombi within the microvasculature of the cortex in addition to swelling of endothelial and mesangial cells of the glomeruli (see the later section on acute cortical necrosis). The degree of cortical hyperechoicity correlates well with the severity of renal impairment in the hemolytic-uremic syndrome but does not predict outcome (Choyke et al., 1988).

Unenhanced computed tomography or contrast material–enhanced magnetic resonance imaging also demonstrate the findings of bilateral renal enlargement and the absence of urinary tract obstruction that are characteristic of proliferative and necrotizing disorders of the glomerulus. These modalities may substitute for ultrasonography.

ABNORMAL PROTEIN DEPOSITION

Amyloidosis

Definition

Amyloidosis is characterized by the accumulation of extracellular eosinophilic protein substances in various organs of the body. The kidneys are involved in more than 80 per cent of cases of amyloidosis secondary to chronic suppurative or inflammatory disease. Renal involvement is found in approximately 35 per cent of patients with primary amyloidosis in which the breast, alimentary tract, tongue, spleen, and connective tissue may also be affected.

The glomerulus is the principal site of amyloid

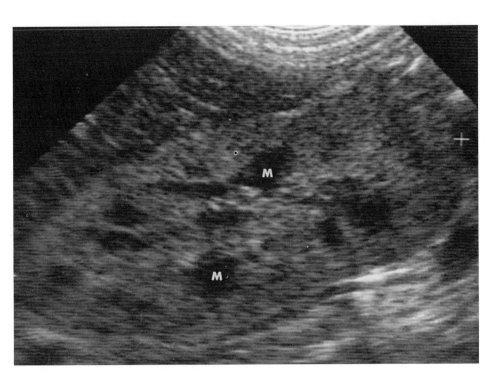

FIGURE 8–2. Hemolytic-uremic syndrome in a 5-year-old girl with azotemia, oliguria, diarrhea, and dehydration. Ultrasonogram of the enlarged right kidney demonstrates a hyperechoic cortex relative to the liver and hypoechoic medullae (M).

AMYLOIDOSIS TYPICAL FINDINGS

Primary Uroradiologic Elements

Size: large (becomes small with time)
Contour: smooth
Lesion distribution: bilateral

Secondary Uroradiologic Elements

Collecting system: attenuated (occasionally)
Parenchymal thickness: expanded; becomes wasted with time
Nephrogram: diminished density
Echogenicity: normal to increased
Renal vein: thrombus (occasionally)

---

deposition. The interstitium and the media and adventitia of the interlobular arteries are frequently also involved. Round-cell accumulation and a fine fibrosis develop in the interstitium, whereas the tubules become atrophic and actually may disappear in advanced disease.

Amyloid accumulation initially produces bilaterally enlarged, smooth kidneys. With time, however, the kidney in amyloidosis becomes diffusely wasted. This presumably reflects ischemic changes caused by amyloid involvement of arteries over a long time. Similarly, ischemia probably accounts for the tubule atrophy and interstitial fibrosis seen in this disease.

Clinical Setting

Renal amyloidosis occurs either in the primary form or in association with chronic suppurative or inflammatory diseases such as tuberculosis, osteomyelitis, bronchiectasis, ulcerative colitis, and rheumatoid arthritis. Amyloid deposition is also seen in the kidneys of patients with multiple myeloma and Waldenström's macroglobulinemia. In familial Mediterranean fever, amyloidosis is common and often severe enough to cause renal failure.

Although some patients may be asymptomatic and show no signs of renal impairment, proteinuria is present in most cases and may be part of the nephrotic syndrome. Nitrogen retention occurs but is usually not advanced until late in the disease.

Hypertension is either absent or not as severe as in other forms of chronic renal failure. Renal vein thrombosis is a well-recognized complication of renal amyloidosis and may transform a patient with mild chronic renal failure into one with acute oliguric failure.

Radiologic Findings

In the early stage of renal amyloidosis, the kidneys are enlarged and smooth in contour, with normal to impaired opacification and normal collecting systems (Fig. 8–3). With time, the kidneys decrease in size and eventually become small (Fig. 8–4). The echogenicity of the renal parenchyma is normal to increased in a nonspecific pattern. Ultrasonography effectively documents the change in renal size as well as the smooth contour. Renal vein thrombosis complicating amyloidosis can be demonstrated by ultrasonography, computed tomography, or magnetic resonance imaging.

Multiple Myeloma

Definition

Multiple myeloma causes renal insufficiency in 30 to 50 per cent of cases as a result of precipitation of abnormal proteins in the tubule lumina. Renal function may also be compromised by impaired re-

---

MULTIPLE MYELOMA TYPICAL FINDINGS

Primary Uroradiologic Elements

Size: large (may become small with time)
Contour: smooth
Lesion distribution: bilateral

Secondary Uroradiologic Elements

Collecting system: attenuated (occasionally)
Parenchymal thickness: expanded
Nephrogram: diminished density
Echogenicity: increased

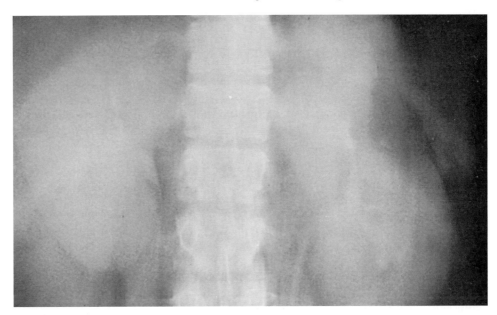

FIGURE 8–3. Amyloidosis in a 28-year-old man with proteinuria and a history of Still's disease that was diagnosed 23 years earlier. Bilateral global renal enlargement, impaired contrast material excretion, and normal pelvocalyceal systems are noted. Right kidney length = 14.2 cm; left kidney length = 14.3 cm. (Courtesy of Department of Diagnostic Radiology, Hammersmith Hospital, Royal Postgraduate Medical School, London, England.)

nal blood flow due to increased blood viscosity, by nephrocalcinosis resulting from hypercalcemia, by Bence Jones protein toxicity on the tubules, and by amyloidosis. Diffuse infiltration of plasma cells per se occurs uncommonly and is usually not associated with a clinically recognizable disturbance in renal function.

Most myelomatous kidneys are normal to enlarged in size. As in amyloidosis, some kidneys eventually become small. Because involvement is global, the pelvocalyceal relationships remain normal, and the kidney surface is smooth. Enlargement is most marked when acute renal failure supervenes.

Clinical Setting

Multiple myeloma is characterized by the presence of abnormal proteins in serum and urine. These are derived from the proliferation of abnormal plasma cells. Symptoms are insidious in onset and include progressive weakness, weight loss, anorexia, nausea and vomiting, and bone pain.

Proteinuria is present in more than 50 per cent of myeloma patients. Renal failure may be chronic or may present acutely as oliguria or anuria.

Radiologic Findings

Myelomatous kidneys are smooth and often markedly enlarged as demonstrated by ultrasonography, computed tomography, or magnetic resonance imaging. Ultrasonographic echo patterns vary from normal to increased. Nephrographic and collecting system opacification varies with the level of renal function. The distance between the interpapillary line and the outer margin of the kidney—the parenchymal thickness—is increased.

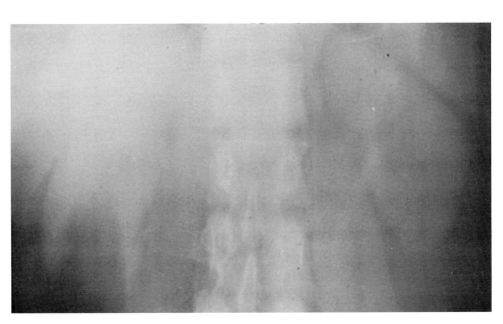

FIGURE 8–4. Amyloidosis presenting as bilaterally small, smooth kidneys and renal failure in a 34-year-old drug addict with chronic leg infection. Small kidneys may be the result of ischemia following amyloid involvement of the blood vessels. Right kidney length = 10.2 cm; left kidney length = 11.7 cm. (Courtesy of Department of Diagnostic Radiology, Hammersmith Hospital, Royal Postgraduate Medical School, London, England.)

The administration of contrast material in patients with multiple myeloma requires an awareness of potential hazards. It is essential that dehydration be avoided if the risk of complications is to be minimized. These concerns are dealt with in Chapter 1.

ABNORMAL FLUID ACCUMULATION

Acute Tubular Necrosis

Definition

Acute tubular necrosis is a state of reversible renal failure with or without oliguria that follows exposure of the kidney either to certain toxic agents or to a period of prolonged, severe ischemia.

Microscopically, the tubules vary from normal to dilated and are filled with cellular debris. Necrosis of the epithelium of the renal tubules occurs. In some situations, particularly when nephrotoxins are the cause, the basement membrane is spared. At other times, such as following ischemia, the basement membrane becomes fragmented. Acute tubular necrosis affects all portions of the nephron in a patchy distribution. Interstitial edema is pronounced and accompanied by infiltrates of lymphocytes, mononuclear cells, and plasma cells.

The kidneys are enlarged primarily as a result of interstitial edema. The surface remains smooth, and the parenchyma is uniformly increased in thickness.

The pathogenesis of acute tubular necrosis is the subject of considerable controversy. One theory holds that tubule damage is the primary event and causes tubule obstruction. In this scheme, the immediate cause of acute renal failure is passive backflow leakage of filtrate into the interstitium. Supporters of this theory continue to use the term *acute tubular necrosis*. An alternative name, *vasomotor nephropathy*, has been proposed by those who believe that the primary event is always preglomerular ischemia. In this concept, oliguria reflects failure of filtration at the glomerular level, not leakage of filtrate across damaged tubules. No final conclusion about the pathogenesis of acute tubular necrosis

has evolved. It is likely that both tubular and vascular mechanisms are interdependent.

Clinical Setting

Bichloride of mercury, ethylene glycol, carbon tetrachloride, bismuth, arsenic, and uranium can produce acute tubular necrosis. Urographic contrast material is also nephrotoxic, particularly when administered to a patient with pre-existing renal disease who has been dehydrated. Ischemic causes of acute tubular necrosis include shock from any cause, crush injuries, burns, transfusion reactions, and severe dehydration. Surgical procedures such as renal transplantation or aortic resection are associated with a high incidence of acute tubular necrosis as a result of temporary interruption of renal blood flow.

Oliguria (urine output of 500 mL or less per day) or anuria becomes evident shortly after the initiating incident and usually lasts for 10 to 20 days. During this time the urine darkens and contains protein. Isosthenuria is present. Dialysis during oliguria or anuria is often required. In some patients, urine volume is normal.

Recovery is signaled by the onset of the diuretic phase, characterized by an increase in urine output and a decrease in blood urea nitrogen. With time, tubule function returns, and the kidney once again regains its ability to concentrate the glomerular filtrate. Recovery is then complete.

The diagnosis of acute tubular necrosis is usually based on clinical history, urinalysis, ultrasonography to exclude obstruction, and renal biopsy.

Radiologic Findings

Contrast material–enhanced imaging studies should not be performed knowingly in patients with acute tubular necrosis. Sometimes, however, the diagnosis is not apparent, and contrast material is administered unwittingly. In other patients, the contrast material itself is the cause of acute tubular necrosis.

Usually, both kidneys are enlarged and smooth in outline. Most patients with acute tubular necrosis demonstrate a nephrogram that becomes dense immediately following contrast material injection and

---

ACUTE TUBULAR NECROSIS TYPICAL FINDINGS

Primary Uroradiologic Elements

Size: large
Contour: smooth
Lesion distribution: bilateral

Secondary Uroradiologic Elements

Collecting system: attenuated; opacification diminished or absent
Parenchymal thickness: expanded
Nephrogram: immediately and persistently dense (approximately 75 per cent of patients);
   increasingly dense and persistent (approximately 25 per cent of patients)
Echogenicity: normal to diminished (medulla); normal to increased (cortex)

remains so for a prolonged time (Fig. 8–5). A less common time-density pattern, seen in approximately 25 per cent of patients, is the nephrogram that becomes increasingly dense during the contrast material–enhanced study (Fig. 8–6). A feeble or absent nephrogram is very uncommon in acute tubular necrosis and should suggest a complicating perfusion problem, such as acute cortical necrosis.

Despite a large amount of contrast material in the kidney substance, seen as a dense nephrogram that may persist beyond 24 hours, the pelvocalyceal system may opacify faintly or not at all. This is not surprising because the tubules often are blocked by debris, and much of the contrast material may have leaked through damaged tubules into the interstitium. Opacification of the pelvocalyceal system might indicate a lesser degree of renal damage than in cases in which the pelvis and calyces do not opacify. Usually, the collecting systems are globally effaced by surrounding interstitial edema.

Following recovery from acute tubular necrosis due to mercury, uranium nitrite, or acetazolamide,

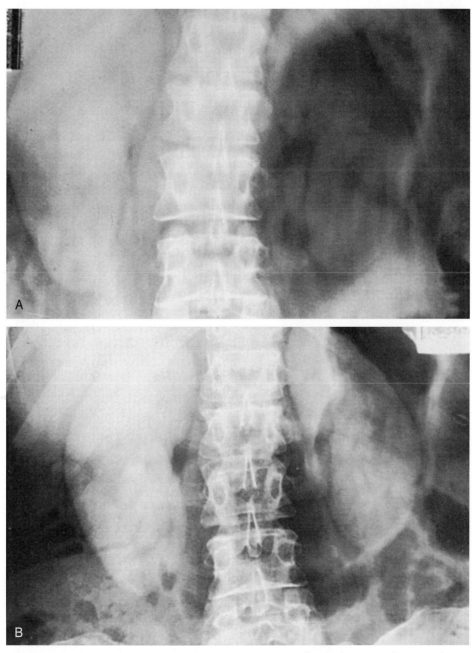

FIGURE 8–5. Acute tubular necrosis in a 30-year-old woman with anuria. Immediately dense, persistent nephrogram.

A, 2-minute tomogram reveals a nephrogram more dense than normal for this time period. Note global enlargement of both kidneys.

B, 16-hour film reveals persistent nephrographic density without substantial change from *A.* No collecting system opacification. Right kidney length = 15.8 cm; left kidney length = 15.2 cm (same patient illustrated in Fig. 27–18).

(Courtesy of Professor Thomas Sherwood, M.B., University of Cambridge, Cambridge, England.)

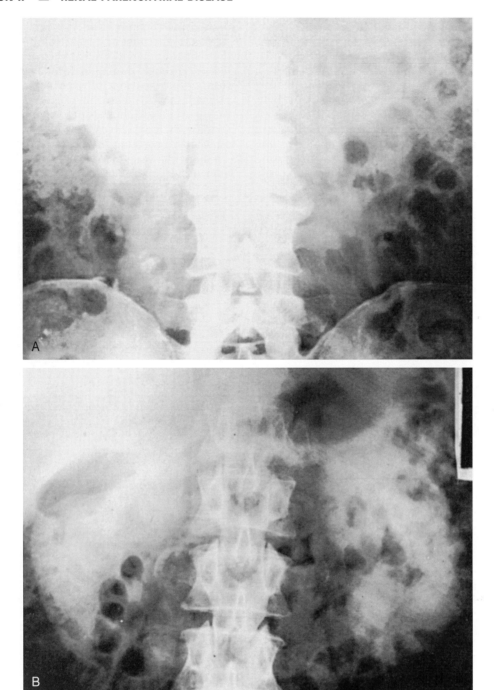

FIGURE 8–6. Acute tubular necrosis in a 60-year-old man who developed oliguric renal failure following severe trauma. Increasingly dense nephrogram.
  A, Preliminary film.
  B, 30 minutes after injection of contrast material.

calcium may be deposited in necrotic proximal convoluted tubules. This form of nephrocalcinosis is detected as increased density by radiography or computed tomography or as increased echogenicity and acoustic shadowing by ultrasonography.

Ultrasonography of the kidney is of primary value in acute tubular necrosis to document renal size and bilateral involvement and to eliminate obstruction as a cause of oliguria or anuria. The echogenicity of renal parenchyma has been reported as nor-

mal but might actually be hypoechoic (compared with a baseline study) because of interstitial edema in the medulla.

Acute Cortical Necrosis

Definition

Acute cortical necrosis is a very uncommon form of acute renal failure in which there is death of the

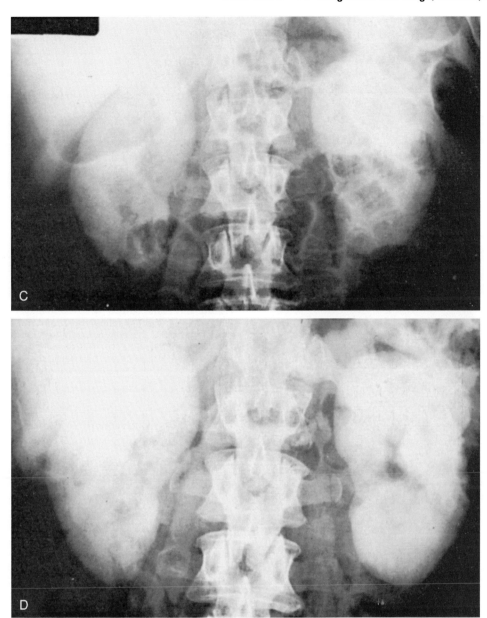

FIGURE 8–6 *Continued C,* Film at 5.5 hours.
D, Film at 18 hours. In addition, the kidneys are globally enlarged and smooth, and the pelvocalyceal system does not opacify. Right kidney length = 15.0 cm; left kidney length = 14.3 cm.
(Courtesy of Professor Thomas Sherwood, M.B., University of Cambridge, Cambridge, England.)

renal cortex and sparing of the medulla. When all cortical tissue is involved, renal failure is permanent, and life can be maintained only by dialysis or transplantation. Sometimes necrosis occurs in a patchy distribution, and enough viable cortex remains to support life, although with moderate renal failure.

The full extent of the microscopic changes of acute cortical necrosis is apparent between 36 and 72 hours after the process begins. Glomerular capillaries become distended with dehemoglobinized red blood cells. Tubule cells in the cortex undergo coagulation necrosis and are stripped away from the basement membrane. There is increased interstitial fluid in the area of necrosis and leuko-

cytic infiltrates along the margin of the infarct. The medulla is normal except for vascular congestion.

A thin rim of subcapsular tissue on the external surface of the cortex and a thin rim of juxtamedullary cortex are often preserved. Presumably, this occurs because these areas are perfused by arteries not involved in the process leading to infarction. These fine rims of viable cortex separate the necrotic cortex from the renal capsule externally and from the medulla internally. Dense calcification occurs at these interfaces, giving rise to the "tramline" calcification discussed in the section on radiologic findings. Calcium is deposited in tubules, glomeruli, and interstitium and can be detected microscopically as early as 6 days after the onset of acute cortical necrosis.

Grossly, the kidneys are large and smooth. On a cut section, the cortex forms a distinct pale band around the medulla. After 2 to 3 weeks, a generalized decrease in size occurs, eventually leaving small, smooth kidneys.

Clinical Setting

Acute cortical necrosis occurs most often in obstetric patients who have premature separation of the placenta with concealed hemorrhage, septic abortion, or placenta previa. Children with dehydration and fever, infections, and transfusion reactions also have an increased risk of developing acute cortical necrosis. In infants, the hemolytic-uremic syndrome combines features of acute cortical necrosis and an acute glomerulopathy and is described in a preceding section (see Fig. 8–2). In the adult, this condition is associated with sepsis, dehydration, shock, myocardial failure, burns, and snakebite and occurs as a complication of abdominal aortic surgery.

There is no agreement about what pathophysiologic mechanisms lead to acute cortical necrosis in these diverse clinical situations. Theories advanced to explain this condition have been based on concepts of ischemia due to vasospasm of small vessels, toxic damage to glomerular capillary endothelium, and primary intravascular thrombosis following excessive release of thromboplastin.

The onset of renal cortical necrosis is manifested by anuria, slight fever, leukocytosis, and few specific physical findings. When a sample of urine is available for analysis, protein and red blood cells are found. When all the renal cortex is involved, uremia develops rapidly and follows an unrelenting course to death, unless the situation is modified by dialysis or transplantation. With patchy cortical necrosis, survival is likely.

Radiologic Findings

At the earliest stage of acute cortical necrosis, the kidneys are diffusely enlarged and smooth. Enhanced computed tomography, if performed, demon-

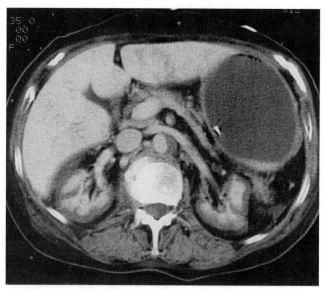

FIGURE 8–7. Acute cortical necrosis in a 74-year-old woman with anuria and shock following surgery for thoracic and abdominal aortic dissection. Computed tomogram with contrast material–enhancement demonstrates absence of enhancement of the cortex and selective enhancement of the medullae of both kidneys (same patient illustrated in Fig. 27–13).

strates a distinctive nephrographic pattern characterized by a thin zone of nonenhanced cortex between a rim of opacified outer cortex and enhanced medulla (Fig. 8–7). In patients with total cortical involvement, there is no opacification of the collecting system, whereas in patients with patchy cortical necrosis, some collecting system opacification may occur. Global shrinkage of the kidneys occurs within a few months, eventually leading to very small, smooth kidneys (Fig. 8–8).

The distinctive radiologic feature of acute cortical necrosis is the development of calcification in the cortex, including the septal cortex. Radiographically detectable calcification has been reported as early as 24 days after the onset of the disease at a time when the kidneys are still enlarged. The pattern of cortical nephrocalcinosis is either punctate or linear

---

ACUTE CORTICAL NECROSIS TYPICAL FINDINGS

Primary Uroradiologic Elements

Size: large (becomes small within a few months)
Contour: smooth
Lesion distribution: bilateral

Secondary Uroradiologic Elements

Collecting system: absent to faint opacification; effaced
Parenchymal thickness: expanded
Nephrogram: absent cortical nephrogram; selective enhancement of medulla
Calcification: cortical (diffuse or "tramline")
Echogenicity: cortex hypoechoic (early); hyperechoic with acoustic shadows after calcium
  deposition

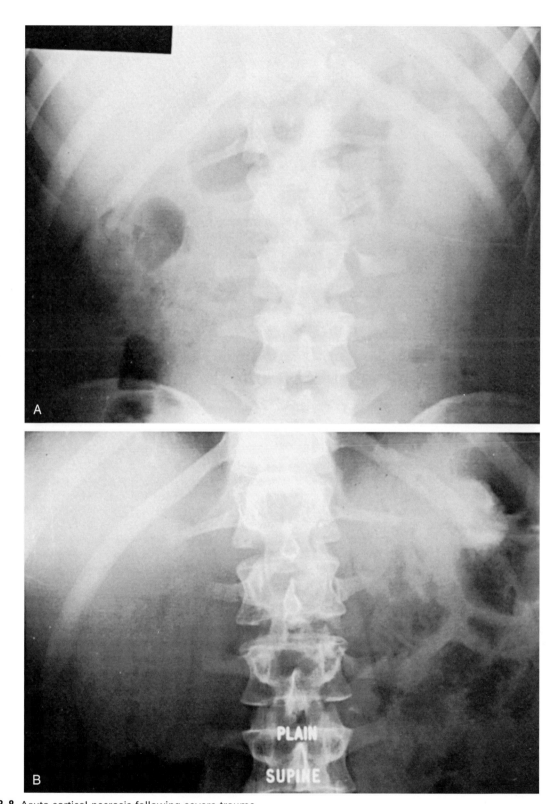

FIGURE 8–8. Acute cortical necrosis following severe trauma.

A, Film of abdomen at the time of injury. Multiple fractures. The kidney outlines are not well defined but appear to be diffusely enlarged.

B, Film taken 3 weeks after *A.* Kidneys are of normal size and smooth and contain faint calcification in a cortical distribution.

Illustration continued on following page

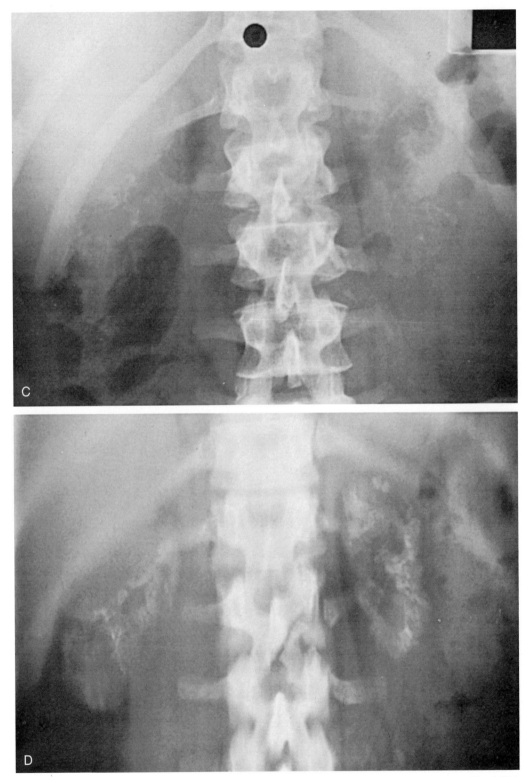

FIGURE 8–8 *Continued C,* Film taken 6 weeks after *A.* Extension of linear calcification throughout cortices of both kidneys. *D,* Tomogram, 1 year after *A.* Marked global wasting and cortical calcification of both kidneys. Patient was maintained by long-term dialysis. (Courtesy of Professor Thomas Sherwood, M.B., University of Cambridge, Cambridge, England.)

in the form of two thin, parallel tracks. The latter pattern, referred to as "tramline" calcification, reflects the interfaces made by the central zone of dead cortex with the viable subcapsular and juxtamedullary cortex on either side.

Ultrasonography of the patient with acute cortical necrosis demonstrates enlargement of both kidneys and documents the absence of obstruction. A circumferential hypoechoic zone corresponding to the necrotic cortex may be seen. Ultrasonography is particularly well suited for following the change in renal size from large to small. Deposition of cortical calcium causes dense cortical echoes and acoustic shadowing.

NEOPLASTIC CELL INFILTRATION

Leukemia

Definition

Leukemia is the most common malignant cause of bilateral global renal enlargement. Lymphoma occasionally produces this pattern but more commonly causes multifocal renal enlargement (see the discussion in Chapter 10).

The leukemic cells infiltrate the interstitial tissue and crowd out normal structures. All portions of the kidney parenchyma are involved. Rarely, leukemia causes a unifocal renal mass due to a chloroma, myeloblastoma, or a myeloblastic sarcoma.

The kidneys are often two to three times normal size but maintain smooth surfaces. At times, enlarged and smooth kidneys occur in leukemic patients without leukemic infiltration of the kidneys as a result of acute urate nephropathy, amphotericin-induced acute interstitial nephritis, or renal candidiasis associated with intensive chemotherapy.

Clinical Setting

Lymphocytic rather than granulocytic forms of leukemia are more frequently associated with renal enlargement. Children with acute leukemia are more likely to develop nephromegaly, but this occurrence is not uncommon in an adult patient with leukemia. Interestingly, renal leukemic infiltrate is unrelated to the peripheral white blood cell count, which can be normal or depleted at the time the kidneys are involved.

Varying degrees of renal failure accompany leukemic infiltration. Renal failure may be due to acute uric acid nephropathy, intrarenal hemorrhage, or obstructive uropathy from uric acid stone or blood clot, rather than due to cellular infiltration itself.

Radiologic Findings

The kidneys are symmetrically enlarged, and the contour is smooth with leukemic involvement. Nephrographic and pelvocalyceal density varies from normal to markedly depressed. Because of the added bulk produced by the abnormal white blood cells, the collecting systems may be attenuated and nondistensible.

Hemorrhage complicating leukemic kidney disease can appear as a focal mass or masses, subcapsular collections of blood, or obstructive or nonobstructive clots in the renal pelvis or ureters. The latter must be distinguished from uric acid stones, which also occur as a metabolic complication of high cell turnover in leukemic patients.

INFLAMMATORY CELL INFILTRATION

Acute Interstitial Nephritis

Definition

Acute interstitial nephritis is characterized histologically by infiltration of the interstitium by lymphocytes, plasma cells, eosinophils, and a few polymorphonuclear leukocytes. Interstitial edema is prominent. Fibrosis is absent, reflecting the transitory nature of this disorder.

Paradoxically, the type of cells found in this disease are those usually associated with chronic processes. The designation "acute" is based on clinical features, not on the nature of the cells.

The infiltrating inflammatory cells and interstitial edema produce bilateral global renal enlargement.

Clinical Setting

Acute interstitial nephritis is a complication of exposure to certain drugs. These most notably include

---

LEUKEMIA TYPICAL FINDINGS

Primary Uroradiologic Elements

Size: large
Contour: smooth
Lesion distribution: bilateral

Secondary Uroradiologic Elements

Collecting system: attenuated (occasionally)
Parenchymal thickness: expanded
Nephrogram: diminished density
Echogenicity: variable

ACUTE INTERSTITIAL NEPHRITIS TYPICAL FINDINGS

Primary Uroradiologic Elements

Size: large
Contour: smooth
Lesion distribution: bilateral

Secondary Uroradiologic Elements

Collecting system: attenuated
Parenchymal thickness: expanded
Nephrogram: diminished density
Echogenicity: increased

---

antibiotics (methicillin, ampicillin, cephalothin, penicillin, and amphotericin), sulfonamides, nonsteroidal anti-inflammatory drugs (fenoprofen, naproxen, ibuprofen), the anticonvulsive phenytoin, and the antihistamine cimetidine. Numerous other drugs have been reported in isolated cases. In general, it is held that acute interstitial nephritis is mediated through immunologic, rather than nephrotoxic, mechanisms.

Cases associated with drug reaction usually evolve between 5 days and 5 weeks of the exposure. Fever, eosinophilia, and a rash are associated with hematuria, proteinuria, and varying levels of azote-

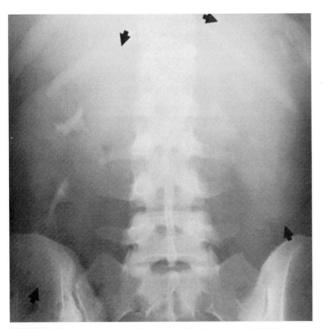

FIGURE 8–9. Acute interstitial nephritis due to methicillin toxicity in a 25-year-old heroin addict being treated for presumed subacute bacterial endocarditis that later was not substantiated. After 10 days of methicillin, there was development of flank pain, proteinuria, azotemia, and eosinophilia. Excretory urography at this time revealed smooth enlargement of both kidneys, with effacement of poorly opacified collecting structures. Abnormal findings were reversed by methicillin withdrawal. Right kidney length = 20.7 cm; left kidney length = 17.5 cm. Arrows depict upper and lower poles of both kidneys.

mia. Recovery occurs with withdrawal of the offending drug.

Radiologic Findings

Bilaterally enlarged, smooth kidneys with normal to diminished opacification are seen. In severe cases, effacement of the collecting systems can be expected (Fig. 8–9). Echogenicity is normal to increased.

AUTOSOMAL RECESSIVE (INFANTILE) POLYCYSTIC KIDNEY DISEASE

Definition

Autosomal recessive, or infantile, polycystic kidney disease is characterized pathologically by dilatation of renal collecting tubules, cystic dilatation of biliary radicles, and periportal fibrosis. Variable degrees of renal failure and portal hypertension are the clinical correlates of this heritable disorder, which occurs in between 1:6,000 and 1:14,000 births. In all respects, including the mode of genetic transmission, autosomal recessive polycystic kidney disease is distinct from autosomal dominant (adult) polycystic kidney disease.

Although the term *autosomal recessive polycystic kidney disease* is preferred, this condition has also been referred to as *infantile* or *Type I polycystic kidney disease, polycystic disease of the newborn, hamartomatous form of polycystic kidney disease, microcystic kidney, tubular gigantism,* and *sponge kidney.* The last term has been used almost exclusively in Europe.

The pathogenesis of autosomal recessive polycystic kidney disease has not been firmly established. Using microdissection techniques, Osathanondh and Potter (1964) found fusiform sacculation and cystic diverticula of the collecting tubules that communicated freely with functioning nephrons (Fig. 8–10). The earliest developing, most distal collecting tubules were more severely affected than were the later developing, more proximal collecting tubules. This finding suggested to these investigators that the pathologic alterations occurred after induction of the metanephric blastema and attachment of nephrons. They postulated that hyperplasia of the interstitial portion of the collecting tubule was the cause of this disease and that the hyperplasia began distally and progressed proximally. Within this concept, mild forms of medullary tubular ectasia seen in this disease presenting at a later age represent quantitatively lesser degrees of collecting tubule hyperplasia.

The etiologic factors of the hepatic disorder are, likewise, not clearly defined. Lieberman and colleagues (1971) demonstrated that the bile duct abnormality occurs at a specific level of the duct system, just as does the renal collecting duct abnormality. This suggests a developmental abnormality occurring between the 12th and 20th generation of branching of the biliary epithelial bud. It is likely that a common mechanism exists in both kidney and liver.

Autosomal recessive polycystic kidney disease is expressed within a spectrum that varies from predominant renal and minimal (subclinical) hepatic involvement that first becomes apparent in the newborn and infant to predominant hepatic and minimal (subclinical) renal involvement that is first encountered clinically in middle and late childhood. In the discussion that follows the two extremes are classified as "neonatal" and "juvenile," respectively. The reader, however, should understand that this entity may present at any point in a time continuum with clinical features that combine elements of both extremes.

Neonatal. In its most severe, neonatal form, this disease is characterized by massive enlargement of the kidneys, with each kidney weighing up to several hundred grams. The renal surface is smooth, and the kidneys maintain a reniform shape with fetal lobation. Small opalescent "cysts," which actually represent very dilated collecting tubules seen end-on, stud the subcapsular surface. These measure 1 to 8 mm, although a few are occasionally larger. The dilated, radially arranged collecting tubules that extend from papillary tips to renal cortex give the cut surface of the kidney the appearance of a sponge and obscure the corticomedullary junction. The fluid within the dilated tubules and cysts is clear, light-yellow urine; if hemorrhage has occurred, however, the color may be light brown. The collecting tubules open into the papillae through a normal number of dilated orifices or papillary ducts. Microscopically, the dilated tubules are lined by focal areas of hyperplastic low columnar or cuboidal epithelium. Microdissection of the dilated tubules demonstrates their communication with functioning, though compressed, nephrons. Interstitial tissue is moderately increased. Glomeruli are widely spaced but are normal in appearance and are probably normal in number.

Patients with the neonatal form of this disease have some form of associated hepatic pathology. The predominant findings are microscopic: a disordered proliferation and ectasia of bile ducts and an increase in portobiliary connective tissue. Both small and medium-sized interlobular bile ducts and septal bile ducts may be dilated. Bulbar protrusion of the duct wall occurs, apparently caused by an overgrowth of connective tissue into the lumen, and bridge formation occurs across duct walls. These findings create extensive irregularity along the course of the ectatic bile ducts. The hepatic lobular architecture is well preserved, and the parenchymal cells are normal.

Juvenile. When this disease presents in older children, hepatic disease predominates over renal impairment. Periportal fibrosis is marked and causes focal dilatation of the biliary tree. Portal hypertension, hepatofugal blood flow, splenomegaly, and gastric and esophageal varices often dominate the clinical picture. This form of autosomal recessive polycystic kidney disease has been termed *congenital hepatic fibrosis* by some investigators. It is not clear, however, whether all children with congenital hepatic fibrosis have autosomal recessive polycystic kidney disease. In an older child, cystic dilatation of renal tubules and associated renal enlargement is less pronounced than in an infant. In some patients, there is marked focal cystic dilatation of ducts and increased mature interstitial fibrosis. This advanced stage may be mistaken for autosomal dominant polycystic kidney disease.

Caroli's disease has been described as segmental

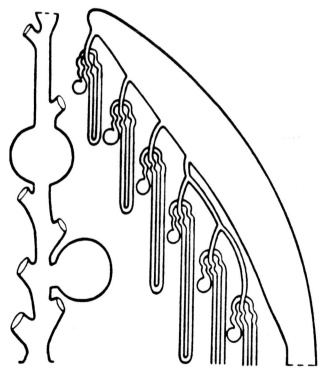

FIGURE 8–10. Schematic diagram of nephron dissection in autosomal recessive polycystic kidney disease. Fusiform dilatation of the terminal branch of a collecting duct with normal nephrons is illustrated on the right. Diverticular and saccular enlargements of a distal collecting duct from the medulla are represented on the left. (From Potter E. L.: Normal and Abnormal Development of the Kidney, 1972. Reproduced with kind permission of the author and Year Book Medical Publishers.)

saccular dilatation of hepatic bile ducts and periportal fibrosis. Caroli's disease may, in fact, be an expression of the same disorder as autosomal recessive polycystic kidney disease.

Clinical Setting

Neonatal. In the more common neonatal form of this disease, massive renal enlargement and severe renal failure dominate the clinical picture. Nephromegaly may be so severe as to cause dystocia. Diminished urine output *in utero* leads to marked oligohydramnios and development of Potter's facies. Secondary pulmonary hypoplasia develops due to oligohydramnios and compression of the thoracic contents by massive nephromegaly; the infant exhibits severe respiratory distress at birth. Recurrent pneumothoraces and pneumomediastinum may complicate efforts to ventilate the hypoplastic lungs. Death most frequently occurs from a combination of renal failure and pulmonary hypoplasia. The occasional infant who survives a neonatal presentation of this disease develops systemic hypertension and has persistent renal insufficiency with inability to concentrate urine.

Juvenile. Beyond the immediate period of birth, a more variable course is encountered in children with autosomal recessive polycystic kidney disease. In general, the earlier the presentation, the more severe the renal insufficiency and systemic arterial hypertension, whereas the older the infant or child is at the time of diagnosis, the more dominant are the hepatic manifestations. Children with intermediate forms of the disease present first with functionally impaired kidneys. With the passage of time, renal insufficiency persists, and portal hypertension from congenital hepatic fibrosis emerges as a major clinical problem. Portal hypertension should be anticipated as a complication of autosomal recessive polycystic kidney disease in all patients with long-term survival.

Congenital hepatic fibrosis with hepatosplenomegaly and variceal bleeding are the typical presentations of older children with the disease. In this type of patient, renal involvement is usually limited to mild nephromegaly and medullary tubular ectasia. Infrequently, patients who present with congenital hepatic fibrosis later develop renal insufficiency. Progression of portal hypertension is variable. In the majority of cases, a portocaval shunt will be necessary within several years.

Rarely, autosomal recessive polycystic kidney disease is first detected in adulthood in association with mild portal hypertension and renal failure.

Radiologic Findings

Neonatal. Abdominal enlargement due to large kidneys is evident on an abdominal film in the newborn with autosomal recessive polycystic kidney disease. A small, malformed thorax, pneumothorax, and pneumomediastinum are commonly seen on the chest radiograph (see Fig. 8–15). These findings represent pulmonary hypoplasia resulting from oligohydramnios.

Ultrasonography usually demonstrates enlarged, hyperechoic kidneys with obliteration of the distinction between cortex and medulla (Fig. 8–11). Reniform shape is preserved. The renal parenchyma may be as echogenic as the central sinus complex and more so than the liver. Increased echogenicity represents changes in acoustic impedance at the

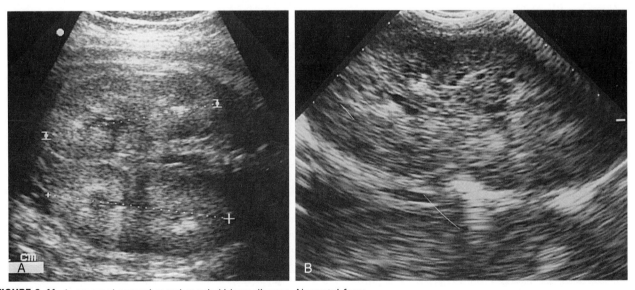

FIGURE 8–11. Autosomal recessive polycystic kidney disease. Neonatal form.

A, Obstetrical ultrasound at 30 weeks' gestation. The fetal kidneys, seen in a coronal projection, are markedly enlarged, smooth, and diffusely hyperechoic. Oligohydramnios is present.

B, Neonatal ultrasonography 2 weeks after birth. The right kidney is enlarged (8.7 cm in length), smooth, and diffusely hyperechoic.

The patient died at 4 weeks of age. (Kindly provided by Cynthia Caskey, M.D., and Ulrike Hamper, M.D., Johns Hopkins University, Baltimore, Maryland.)

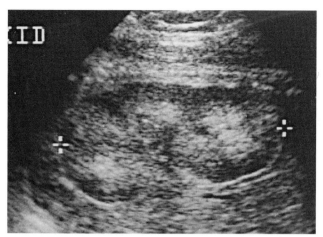

FIGURE 8–12. Autosomal recessive polycystic kidney disease. Neonatal form. Obstetrical ultrasonography at 33 weeks' gestation. The right fetal kidney, seen in sagittal projection, is enlarged (7.6 cm in length) and smooth. The cortex is hypoechoic relative to the medulla. Oligohydramnios is present. (Kindly provided by Cynthia Caskey, M.D., and Ulrike Hamper, M.D., Johns Hopkins University, Baltimore, Maryland.)

cyst lumen–cyst wall interface. In some cases, the cortex is hypoechoic relative to the medulla, which is the reversal of the normal neonatal pattern (Fig. 8–12). This reversal of the normal echo texture represents the fact that the peripheral collecting tubules in the cortex are more dilated and, thus, have a greater fluid volume than the collecting tubules of the medulla, which are more compressed. Occasionally, a few macroscopic cysts are present. In the newborn period, the liver may appear normal by ultrasonography or may show increased echogenicity and early bile duct ectasia or cysts. A presumptive prenatal diagnosis of autosomal recessive polycystic kidney disease can be made when bilateral large echogenic kidneys and oligohydramnios are demonstrated *in utero* (see Figs. 8–11 and 8–12). Although the ultrasonographic features of the disease can be detected as early as the late 2nd trimester, some affected fetuses appear normal well into the 3rd trimester. Serial ultrasonography in patients who survive the neonatal period may demonstrate some decrease in kidney size over time.

Unenhanced computed tomography demonstrates bilateral nephromegaly and attenuation values near those of water, representing the large proportion of the renal mass that is composed of urine in dilated tubules (Fig. 8–13A). Similar abnormalities are depicted by magnetic resonance imaging (Fig. 8–14). Contrast material–enhanced computed tomograms demonstrate delayed but prolonged renal opacification and a striated nephrogram that is especially prominent in the medulla (see Fig. 8–13B). The liver may demonstrate nonsegmental low-density linear bands that correspond to areas of either hepatic fibrosis or bile duct dilatation.

Excretory urography is rarely, if ever, performed in autosomal recessive polycystic kidney disease. Findings of historical interest were those of diminished renal enhancement, massively enlarged kidneys, and a striated nephrogram reflecting contrast material in dilated collecting tubules extending from the cortex through the medulla (Fig. 8–15). Retention of contrast material in the tubules was often documented for days.

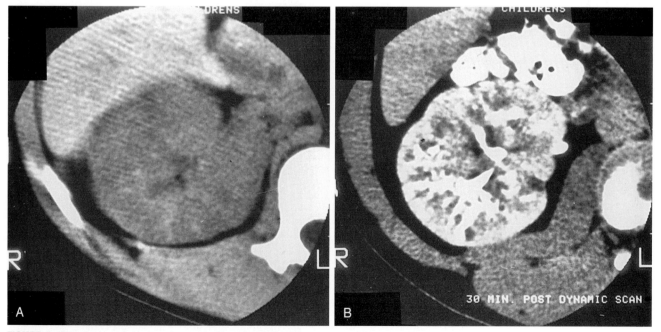

FIGURE 8–13. Autosomal recessive polycystic kidney disease. Neonatal form. Computed tomogram.
   A, Unenhanced scan. The kidneys are large but maintain their reniform shape. The overall attenuation value is less than soft tissue owing to the large volume of urine in the dilated tubules.
   B, Scan obtained 15 minutes after contrast material administration. Striations are prominent. There is persistent cortical enhancement.

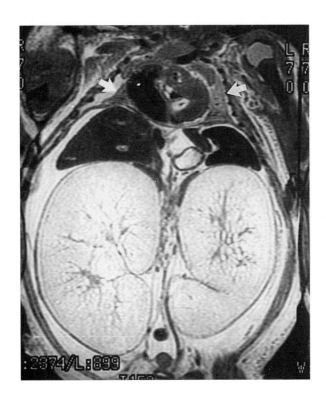

FIGURE 8–14. Autosomal recessive polycystic kidney disease. Neonatal form. Coronal T2-weighted fast spin echo magnetic resonance image obtained post mortem. Both kidneys are markedly enlarged and the lungs *(arrows)* are hypoplastic. (Kindly provided by Paula J. Woodward, M.D., University of Utah, Salt Lake City, Utah.)

FIGURE 8–15. Autosomal recessive polycystic kidney disease. Neonatal form. Excretory urogram. A film obtained 2 hours after contrast material administration demonstrates large, smooth kidneys with delayed excretion and a striated nephrogram representing accumulation of contrast material in dilated collecting ducts. Air along the aorta *(arrow)* is secondary to pneumothorax and pneumomediastinum caused by mechanical ventilation necessitated by pulmonary hypoplasia.

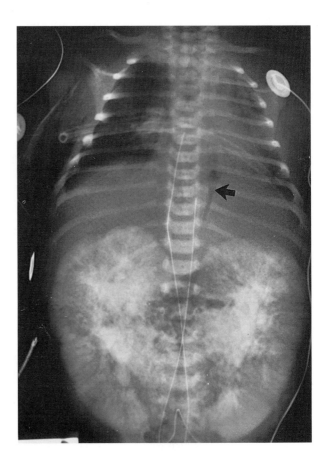

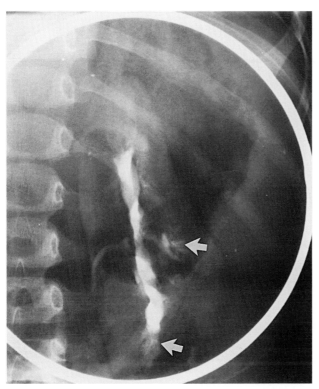

FIGURE 8–16. Autosomal recessive polycystic kidney disease. Juvenile form. Excretory urogram. There are linear collections of contrast material within papillae *(arrows)* in a pattern that is indistinguishable from medullary sponge kidney. The kidney is enlarged.

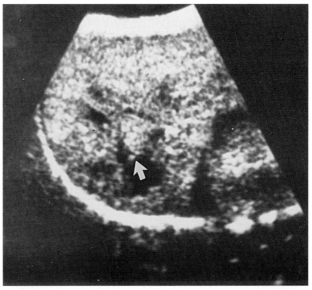

FIGURE 8–17. Autosomal recessive polycystic kidney disease. Juvenile form. Ultrasonogram of the liver. Focal dilatations of the biliary tract with intraluminal wall protrusion *(arrow)* are present. These bridges occasionally contain branches of the portal vein and its surrounding connective tissue core. The echogenicity of the hepatic parenchyma is increased.

Juvenile. An abdominal radiograph in the older child with autosomal recessive polycystic kidney disease may be normal or may demonstrate hepatosplenomegaly, nephromegaly with or without nephrocalcinosis, or both. Esophageal varices due to portal hypertension may be seen on upper gastrointestinal studies. Excretory urography usually demonstrates normal opacification of the kidneys. A striated accumulation of contrast material in the papillae corresponding to slightly dilated distal collecting ducts has the same appearance as medullary sponge kidney (Fig. 8–16) (see Chapter 13).

Abdominal ultrasonographic findings include hepatomegaly, splenomegaly, increased hepatic echogenicity, and biliary ectasia (Fig. 8–17). Intraluminal bulbar protrusions, bridge formations across dilated lumina, and portal radicles partially or completely surrounded by bile ducts may also be seen. When liver disease is complicated by cholangitis, ultrasonography may detect associated choledocholithiasis. Ultrasonography of the kidney may be normal in the juvenile form, although moderate nephromegaly, increased parenchymal echogenicity (especially in the medullary pyramid), and loss of corticomedullary differentiation are sometimes present. Discrete cysts corresponding to dilated collecting ducts may also be identified within the medulla.

Computed tomography of the abdomen in the juvenile form of the disease frequently demonstrates

hepatosplenomegaly (Fig. 8–18). Discrete cysts in the liver corresponding to focal bile duct dilatation may be identified. The portal and splenic veins may be enlarged as a result of portal hypertension and hepatofugal flow. Computed tomography of the kidney may demonstrate renal enlargement; the nephrocalcinosis pattern of medullary sponge kidney; multiple, discrete, cortical, and medullary cysts; and a striated nephrogram in papillary tips (see Fig. 8–18).

Liver-spleen radionuclide scans demonstrate hepatosplenomegaly and numerous well-circumscribed

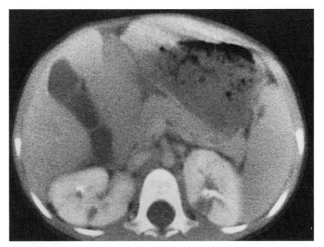

FIGURE 8–18. Autosomal recessive polycystic kidney disease. Juvenile form. Contrast material–enhanced computed tomogram demonstrates hepatosplenomegaly and slight nephromegaly. Several low-density areas in the kidney represent dilated collecting ducts. The kidneys are, however, minimally involved.

AUTOSOMAL RECESSIVE (INFANTILE) POLYCYSTIC KIDNEY DISEASE TYPICAL FINDINGS

Primary Uroradiologic Elements

Size: large
Contour: smooth
Lesion distribution: bilateral

Secondary Uroradiologic Elements

Neonatal Form:

Collecting system: attenuated
Parenchymal thickness: expanded
Nephrogram: diminished density; striated
Attenuation value: less than soft tissue (unenhanced)
Echogenicity: increased (diffuse); loss of corticomedullary differentiation

Juvenile Form:

Nephrogram: striated (papillae, common; diffuse, rare)
Calcification: nephrocalcinosis (papillae)
Echogenicity: increased (papillae)
Miscellaneous: hepatosplenomegaly, varices, dilated bile ducts, increased hepatic
    echogenicity

---

photopenic regions in the liver when technetium 99m sulfur colloid is utilized. These same photopenic areas will accumulate radioactivity when a technetium 99m–labeled hepatobiliary agent is used. Transhepatic, intravenous, or retrograde cholangiography also demonstrates focal biliary dilatation.

MISCELLANEOUS CONDITIONS

Acute Urate Nephropathy

When nephrons are flooded with large amounts of uric acid, minute biurate crystals form and become deposited in the collecting tubules and interstitium. Acute oliguric renal failure follows from intratubular obstruction. Although this may occur in any patient with a very high serum uric acid level, it is seen most commonly during therapy for cancer, particularly leukemia, Hodgkin's disease and malignant lymphoma, myeloproliferative disorders, and polycythemia vera. In these patients, the cytotoxic agents release large amounts of nucleoprotein, which are metabolized to uric acid.

There is scant radiologic literature on acute urate nephropathy. From what is known about pathologic factors, the kidneys are globally enlarged and have normal collecting systems. The nephrographic pattern shows increasing density with time. This relationship reflects continued glomerular filtration and retention of filtered contrast material in the obstructed tubules. Delayed opacification of the pelvocalyceal system does not occur because of the tubule blockage (Fig. 8–19). In this setting, contrast material is eliminated by alternate pathways of excretion in the gastrointestinal tract.

The radiologist must undertake excretory urogra-

phy or computed tomography with considerable caution in the severely hyperuricemic patient because of the uricosuric effect of contrast material. Alkaline diuresis, a large fluid intake, and the use of allopurinol should be instituted before the administration of contrast material if the risk of causing acute urate nephropathy is to be minimized.

Glycogen Storage Disease, Type I (von Gierke's Disease)

Nephromegaly to a marked degree occurs in children and young adults with glycogen storage disease, Type I, because of accumulation of glycogen in the epithelium of proximal convoluted tubules. Renal failure is not invariably present but develops mainly in older patients who have not had optimal therapy. Kidneys may be normal in size when patients are under good metabolic control. Other features of this genetically transmitted disorder that may produce radiologic abnormalities are growth retardation, hepatomegaly, hepatic adenoma and adenocarcinoma, gouty arthritis, and uric acid stones.

Physiologic Response to Urographic Contrast Material and Diuretics

Agents that cause vasodilatation and/or diuresis may increase renal size, presumably because of volume expansion of the vascular tree, the tubule lumina, and the interstitial fluid space. Increases of up to 35 per cent of the renal area have been reported. The mean increase, however, is close to 5 per cent. This degree of enlargement does not produce kidney images that necessarily fall into the category

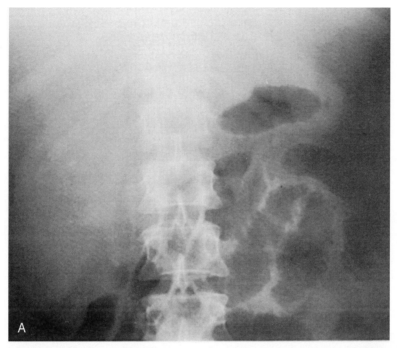

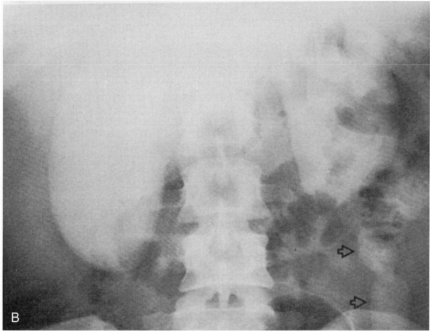

FIGURE 8–19. Acute urate nephropathy in a 31-year-old woman with extensive hepatic metastases from a poorly differentiated carcinoma thought to be gastrointestinal in origin. Serum uric acid = 25 mg/dL. Patient developed oliguria while dehydrated. Anuria ensued, despite correction of fluid balance. Excretory urogram performed at this time demonstrates globally enlarged kidneys with a progressive increase in density of the nephrogram over 2 days. Excretory urography should be avoided in a situation such as this.

A, 10-minute film. Homogeneous nephrogram.

B, 64-hour film. Persistent nephrogram. Extrarenal excretion of contrast material opacifies descending sigmoid colon *(arrows).* Right kidney length = 16.0 cm; left kidney length = 15.2 cm.

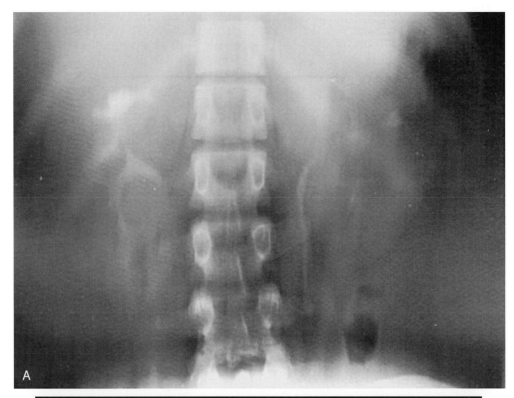

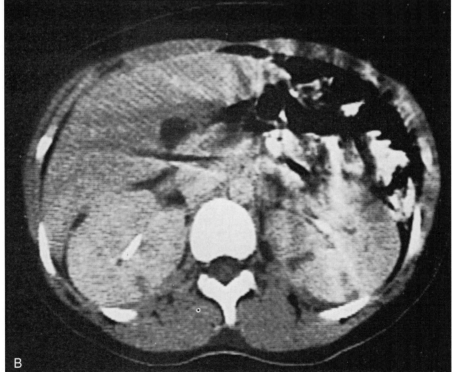

FIGURE 8–20. Homozygous S disease with bilateral, smooth renal enlargement.
A, Excretory urogram. Tomogram. Note findings of papillary necrosis at several sites.
B, Computed tomogram, contrast material–enhanced. Focal areas of nonenhanced parenchyma represent small lobar infarcts.
(Courtesy of M. Federle, M.D., University of Pittsburgh, Pittsburgh, Pennsylvania.)

of abnormally large. In addition to urographic contrast material, this phenomenon is also seen with urea, glucose, furosemide, acetylcholine, and prostaglandins.

Homozygous S Disease

Both kidneys may enlarge in homozygous S (sickle cell) disease, owing to vascular dilatation, engorgement of vessels, glomerular enlargement, and interstitial edema (Fig. 8–20). Increased renal blood flow may also be a factor. Other radiologic abnormalities in homozygous S disease are lobar infarction, impaired density of contrast material, and dilated pelvocalyceal systems and ureters. The latter reflect defective water-concentrating ability. Papillary necrosis may also be seen in homozygous S disease but is more common in heterozygous S states (see Chapter 13). Decreased cortical signal intensity, most evident on T2-weighted magnetic resonance images, has been reported. Because of the sharply reduced life expectancy of patients with sickle cell disease, these changes usually are seen only in young persons.

Paroxysmal Nocturnal Hemoglobinuria

This rare, acquired hemolytic disorder results from complement-mediated membrane damage to erythrocytes, granulocytes, and platelets that have been derived from an abnormal clone of stem cells. Young adults are most frequently affected with clinical manifestations of fever, abdominal and back pain, and the effects of venous thrombosis of both peripheral and viscera-draining veins (portal and hepatic, cerebral, mesenteric, and renal). Chronic hemolysis causes anemia, hemoglobinuria, and hemosiderinuria. Repeated microvascular thromboses in the kidney produce nephromegaly, lobar infarcts, and papillary necrosis. These findings are similar to those of homozygous S disease described in the preceding section. In addition, massive deposition of ferric iron–containing hemosiderin in proximal convoluted tubules causes markedly decreased magnetic resonance signal intensity of the renal cortex, most notably on gradient-echo and T2-weighted sequences (Fig. 8–21). This is a reversal of the normal signal relationship of cortex to medulla.

Hemophilia

In a series of 12 patients with hemophilia, four had global enlargement of both kidneys that otherwise were normal (Dalinka et al., 1975). All of the patients were adults, and none had obstruction of the urinary tract. Apart from enlargement of the glomeruli seen in biopsy specimens of two of these patients, no explanation is available for the nephromegaly associated with this disorder. Papillary necrosis in hemophilia has also been described, as discussed in Chapter 13.

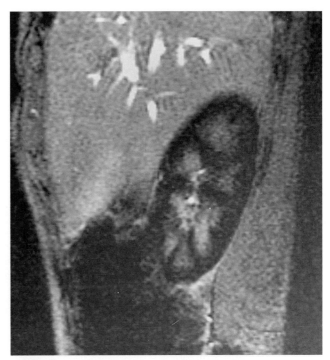

FIGURE 8–21. Paroxysmal nocturnal hemoglobinuria in a 16-year-old male with three episodes of fever, abdominal pain, brown urine, and jaundice over a 3-year period. Gradient-echo sequence magnetic resonance image in the sagittal plane. There is marked decrease in the signal intensity in the cortex and normal signal intensity in the medullae. (Kindly provided by the Department of Radiology and Radiological Sciences, Johns Hopkins University, Baltimore, Maryland.)

Nephromegaly Associated with Cirrhosis, Hyperalimentation, and Diabetes Mellitus

Nephromegaly has been reported in cases of hepatic cirrhosis, regardless of the cause. Renal enlargement is particularly prominent in patients with marked fatty changes in the liver. The basis for this relationship is unknown. Renal tissue fluid, proteins, lipids, and carbohydrates are normal. Hyperplasia and hypertrophy of renal cells are believed to account for the increased kidney bulk.

Smooth enlargement of both kidneys as a response to hyperalimentation (total parenteral nutrition) has been well documented. This is most likely due to an increase in the fluid compartments of the kidney related to hyperosmolality of the administered solutions. Renal enlargement reverses promptly following cessation of this form of nutritional therapy.

Bilateral nephromegaly also occurs in some patients with both non–insulin dependent and insulin-dependent diabetes mellitus early in the course of their illness and in the absence of diabetic glomerulosclerosis. This is often associated with an increase in glomerular filtration rate as well as renal plasma flow. Possible explanations for this well-documented occurrence include a growth hormone effect, nephron hypertrophy, and glycosuric osmotic diuresis. Transient nephromegaly in newborns born of diabetic mothers also occurs.

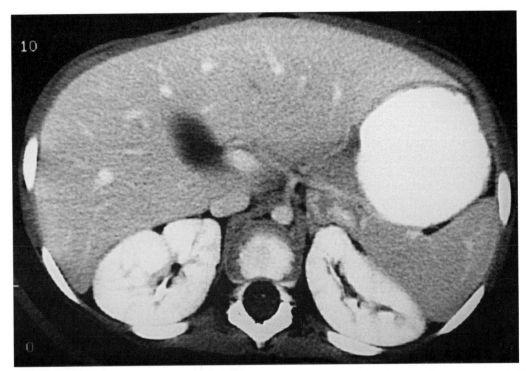

FIGURE 8–22. Beckwith-Wiedemann syndrome. Computed tomogram, contrast material–enhanced. Both kidneys are enlarged and smooth. Hepatosplenomegaly is present. (Courtesy of the Department of Radiology, University of Virginia, Charlottesville, Virginia.)

Acromegaly

The kidneys are part of the generalized organomegaly seen in acromegaly. Renal function and structure are otherwise normal.

Fabry's Disease

Smooth enlargement of both kidneys has been reported in young adults with Fabry's disease, or angiokeratoma corporis diffusum universale. Nephromegaly develops in the stage of the disease before the onset of renal failure. Thereafter, the kidneys become small. Presumably, renal enlargement is due to lipid deposition in the parenchyma.

Bartter's Syndrome

Bartter's syndrome is a metabolic disorder that leads to growth retardation, distinctive craniofacial features, and muscle weakness. Hypercalciuria, hypokalemia, hyperaldosteronism, and increased plasma renin levels are also present. Paradoxically, blood pressure is normal despite elevated plasma

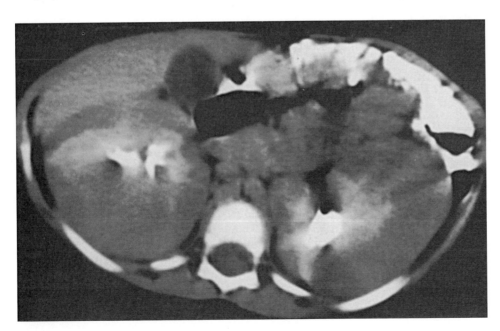

FIGURE 8–23. Nephroblastomatosis involving both kidneys, which are diffusely enlarged by extensive, lobulated peripheral masses that enhance minimally.

renin. Children and young adults are most often affected, but there are variants of the syndrome that present in the neonatal period. Kidney enlargement, when present, probably reflects either hyperplasia of the juxtaglomerular apparatus, which is the principal morphologic abnormality found in the kidney, or polyuria, or both. Radiologic findings that may be present in Bartter's syndrome, in addition to nephromegaly, include dilatation of the pelvocalyceal system and ureter from polyuria, hyperechoicity of the renal medulla due to nephrocalcinosis, and diffuse increase in renal parenchymal echo intensity with loss of corticomedullary distinction—a nonspecific finding.

Beckwith-Wiedemann Syndrome

Bilateral global enlargement of the kidneys is one feature of Beckwith-Wiedemann syndrome, an uncommonly encountered set of abnormalities in infants (Fig. 8–22). In addition to nephromegaly, other findings include large body size, macroglossia, hemihypertrophy (including unilateral renal enlargement), advanced skeletal maturation, omphalocele, diastasis recti or umbilical hernia, hepatomegaly, mild microcephaly, earlobe deformities, and facial nevi. Neonatal hypoglycemia may dominate the clinical presentation, and polycythemia may be present. Macroglossia and macrosomia become less apparent with age.

As many as 10 per cent of patients with Beckwith-Wiedemann syndrome develop an abdominal malignancy involving the liver (hepatoblastoma), kidney (Wilms' tumor), gonad (gonadoblastoma), or adrenal (carcinoma and neuroblastoma). Other kidney abnormalities associated with Beckwith-Wiedemann syndrome include medullary sponge kidney, medullary dysplasia, and pyelocalyceal diverticulum.

Nephroblastomatosis

Microscopic foci of nephrogenic blastema are present as incidental findings in 1:400 kidneys of autopsied infants. Neoplastic or hyperplastic growth of these foci causes bilateral renal enlargement with preservation of a smooth contour, a condition known as nephroblastomatosis. Only uncommonly does nephroblastomatosis appear as a unifocal mass.

Nephroblastomatosis is discovered in the newborn, infant, or child as a unilateral or bilateral abdominal mass. Small foci of persistent metanephric blastema, also part of the nephroblastomatosis complex, are asymptomatic. Nephroblastomatosis is a precursor of Wilms' tumor, being present in all patients with bilateral Wilms' tumors and in approximately 30 per cent of those with a solitary tumor. Like Wilms' tumor, which is discussed in Chapter 12, nephroblastomatosis is associated with hemihypertrophy, sporadic aniridia, pseudohermaphroditism, and Beckwith-Wiedemann syndrome. Although not malignant in and of itself,

chemotherapy and radiation are used as treatment modalities in recognition of the malignant potential of nephroblastomatosis.

The computed tomographic findings of nephroblastomatosis are characteristic (Figs. 8–23, 8–24). Multiple nodules of varying size are situated in the peripheral portions of the kidneys, causing their enlargement. The surface contour of the kidney remains smooth, although the nodules themselves might be somewhat lobulated. Enhancement of the nephroblastomatous tissue following contrast material is absent to minimal. Sometimes, one or more expansive, exophytic Wilms' tumors coexist and dominate the findings (see Fig. 8–24).

Ultrasonography is less sensitive than computed tomography in detecting nephroblastomatosis, probably because the involved cortical tissue is sometimes isoechoic to normal renal parenchyma. Occasionally, the nephroblastomatosis nodules are hypoechoic. Ultrasonography does document well the smooth, contoured renal enlargement that is a feature of the nephroblastomatosis complex as well as the development of Wilms' tumor (see Fig. 8–24).

DIFFERENTIAL DIAGNOSIS

Except for **autosomal recessive (infantile) polycystic kidney disease**, **hemolytic-uremic syndrome**, and **paroxysmal nocturnal hemoglobinuria**, there are no radiologic findings that specifically distinguish any one of the disorders from another in the diagnostic set "large, smooth, bilateral." Clinical and laboratory findings, histologic and immunologic studies, and clinical course must be relied on for establishing a diagnosis in most cases.

Some of the diseases that produce enlarged, smooth kidneys can be distinguished from each other by their association with abnormalities in other organs. **Goodpasture's syndrome, Wegener's granulomatosis, Schönlein-Henoch syndrome, thrombotic thrombocytopenic purpura** and **hemolytic-uremic syndrome, amyloidosis, multiple myeloma, leukemia, glycogen storage disease Type I**, and **Beckwith-Wiedemann syndrome** are in this category.

The radiologic findings in **acute cortical necrosis** are not specific early in the course of the illness except when a cortical rim nephrographic defect or hypoechoic zone is identified. The appearance of calcification in a cortical distribution and rapid global wasting of the kidneys are features unique to acute cortical necrosis, but these findings require a few weeks' lapse of time before they become detectable.

Hemolytic-uremic syndrome characteristically causes intense hyperechoicity of the cortex relative to the medulla. Likewise, reversal of the normal signal relationship between cortex and medulla on magnetic resonance images of the kidney is a hallmark of **paroxysmal nocturnal hemoglobinuria**.

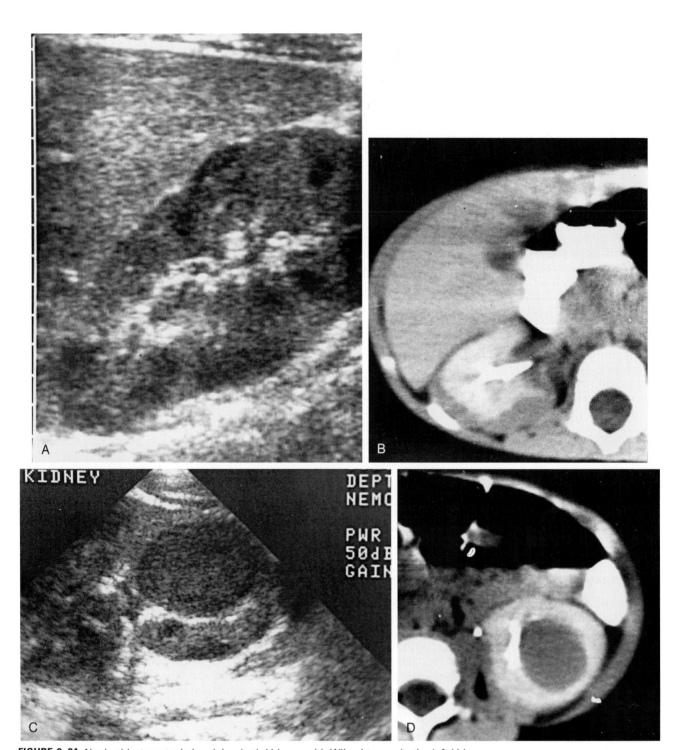

FIGURE 8–24. Nephroblastomatosis involving both kidneys with Wilms' tumor in the left kidney.

A, Ultrasonogram, right kidney, longitudinal section. The kidney is enlarged by peripheral, slightly hypoechoic, masses.

B, Computed tomogram with contrast material enhancement demonstrates the poorly enhancing, peripheral, lobulated tissue of nephroblastomatosis.

C, Ultrasonogram, lower pole, left kidney demonstrates expansile solid intrarenal Wilms' tumor.

D, Computed tomogram, contrast material–enhanced, of lower pole of the left kidney depicts a homogeneous, poorly enhancing tumor in addition to some peripheral nephroblastomatosis.

In the newborn and infant, the ultrasonographic findings of hyperechoic, enlarged, smooth kidneys leave little doubt about the diagnosis of **autosomal recessive (infantile) polycystic kidney disease**, especially if the cortex is selectively hyperechoic. However, hyperechoicity and smooth enlargement may also be present in the uncommon case of **autosomal dominant (adult) polycystic kidney disease** that presents in the newborn or infant. Here, an accurate diagnosis requires pathologic examination of tissue. The juvenile form of autosomal recessive polycystic kidney disease may be confused with **medullary sponge kidney** (see Chapter 13). The latter, however, is uncommon in childhood and is not associated with nephromegaly or liver disease.

Occasionally, **autosomal dominant (adult) polycystic kidney disease** discovered in adulthood is associated with smooth renal enlargement, normal opacification, and nondisplaced collecting structures. This is discussed and illustrated in Chapter 10. Careful evaluation of the nephrogram in these patients will always reveal sharply defined radiolucent defects quite unlike the homogeneous nephrogram found in the disorders presented in this chapter. Both ultrasonography and computed tomography invariably yield a specific pattern in these patients.

BIBLIOGRAPHY

General

Brenbridge, A. N., Cheralier, R. L., El-Dahr, S., and Kaiser, D. L.: Pathologic significance of nephromegaly in pediatric disease. Am. J. Dis. Child. 141:652, 1987.
Brady, H. R., Brenner, B. M., and Lieberthal, W.: Acute renal failure. In Brenner, B. M. (ed.): The Kidney, 5th ed. Philadelphia, W. B. Saunders, 1996, pp. 1200–1252.
Heptinstall, R. H. (ed.): Pathology of the Kidney, 4th ed. Boston, Little, Brown & Co., 1992.
Platt, J. F., Rubin, J. M., Bowerman, R. A., and Marn, C. S.: The inability to detect kidney diseases on the basis of echogenicity. AJR 151:317, 1988.

Proliferative/Necrotizing Disorders

Adler, S. G., Cohen, A. H., and Glassock, R. J.: Secondary glomerular diseases. In Brenner, B. M. (ed.): The Kidney, 5th ed. Philadelphia, W. B. Saunders, 1996, pp. 1498–1596.
Amorosi, E. L., and Ultmann, J. E.: Thrombotic thrombocytopenic purpura: Report of 16 cases and review of the literature. Medicine (Baltimore) 45:139, 1966.
Bell, D. S. H.: Diabetic nephropathy: Changing concepts of pathogenesis and treatment. Am. J. Med. Sci. 301:195, 1991.
Benoit, F. L., Rulon, D. B., Theil, G. B., Doolan, P. D., and Watten, R. H.: Goodpasture's syndrome: A clinicopathologic entity. Am. J. Med. 37:424, 1964.
Boyd, R. M., Warren, L., and Garrow, D. G.: Renal size in various nephropathies. AJR 119:723, 1973.
Case records of the Massachusetts General Hospital: Goodpasture's syndrome. N. Engl. J. Med. 329:2019, 1993.
Chesney, R. W., O'Regan, S., Kaplan, B. S., and Nogrady, M. B.: Asymmetric renal enlargement in acute glomerulonephritis. Radiology 122:431, 1977.
Choyke, P. L., Grant, E. G., Hoffer, F. A., Tina, L., and Korec, S.: Cortical echogenicity in the hemolytic-uremic syndrome: Clinical correlation. J. Ultrasound Med. 7:439, 1988.
Connor, E., Gupta, S., and Joshi, V.: Acquired immunodeficiency syndrome: Associated renal disease in children. J. Pediatr. 113:39, 1988.
Cunningham, E. E., Brentjens, J. R., Zielezny, M. A., Andres, G. A., and Venuto, R. C.: Heroin nephropathy: A clinicopathologic and epidemiologic study. Am. J. Med. 68:47, 1980.
Davson, J., Ball, J., and Platt, R.: Kidney in periarteritis nodosa. Q. J. Med. 17:175, 1948.
Duncan, D. A., Drummond, K. N., Midrach, A. F., and Vermier, R. L.: Pulmonary hemorrhage and glomerulonephritis. Ann. Intern. Med. 62:920, 1965.
Falkoff, G. E., Rigsby, C. M., and Rosenfield, A. T.: Partial, combined cortical and medullary nephrocalcinosis: US and CT patterns in AIDS-associated MAI infection. Radiology 162:343, 1987.
Glassock, R. J., Cohen, A. H., and Adler, S. G.: Primary glomerular diseases. In Brenner, B. M. (ed.): The Kidney, 5th ed. Philadelphia, W. B. Saunders, 1996, pp. 1392–1497.
Graif, M., Shohet, I., Strauss, S., Yahar, J., and Itzchok, Y.: Hemolytic-uremic syndrome: Sonographic-clinical correlation. J. Ultrasound Med. 3:563, 1984.
Hamper, U. M., Golblum, L. E., and Hutchins, G. M.: Renal involvement in AIDS: Sonographic-pathologic correlation. AJR 150:1321, 1988.
Heptinstall, R. H.: Classification of glomerulonephritis; focal and mesangial proliferative forms of glomerulonephritis; recurrent hematuria. In Heptinstall, R. H. (ed.): Pathology of the Kidney, 4th ed. Boston, Little, Brown & Co., 1992, pp. 261–296.
Heptinstall, R. H.: Hemolytic-uremic syndrome, thrombotic thrombocytopenic purpura, and systemic sclerosis (systemic scleroderma). In Heptinstall, R. H. (ed.): Pathology of the Kidney, 4th ed. Boston, Little, Brown & Co., 1992, pp. 1163–1234.
Heptinstall, R. H.: Polyarteritis (periarteritis) nodosa, Wegener's syndrome, and other forms of vasculitis. In Heptinstall, R. H. (ed.): Pathology of the Kidney, 4th ed. Boston, Little, Brown & Co., 1992, pp. 1097–1162.
Kenney, P. J., Brinsko, R. E., Patel, D. V., Spitzer, R. E., and Farrar, F. M.: Sonography of the kidneys in hemolytic-uremic syndrome. Invest. Radiol. 21:547, 1986.
Lakkis, F. G., Campbell, O. C., and Badr, K. F.: Microvascular diseases of the kidney. In Brenner, B. M. (ed.): The Kidney, 5th ed. Philadelphia, W. B. Saunders, 1996, pp. 1712–1730.
Llach, F., Descoeudres, C., and Massry, S. G.: Heroin-associated nephropathy: Clinical and histological studies in 19 patients. Clin. Nephrol. 11:7, 1979.
McCluskey, R. T.: Immunologic aspects of renal disease. In Heptinstall, R. H. (ed.): Pathology of the Kidney, 4th ed. Boston, Little, Brown & Co., 1992.
Miller, F. H., Parikh, S., Gore, R. M., Nemcek, A. A. J., Fitzgerald, S. W., and Vogelzand, R. L.: Renal manifestations of AIDS. Radiographics 13:587, 1993.
Neild, G. H.: Haemolytic uraemic syndrome: Nephrology grand rounds: Clinical issues in nephrology. Nephron 59:194, 1991.
Parvinger, H.-H., Österby, R., Anderson, P. W., and Hsueh, W. A.: Diabetic nephropathy. In Brenner, B. M. (ed.): The Kidney, 5th ed. Philadelphia, W. B. Saunders, 1996, pp. 1864–1892.
Rao, T. K. S.: Renal complications in HIV disease. Med. Clin. North Am. 80:1437, 1996.
Rao, T. K. S., Friedman, E. A., and Nicastri, A. D.: The types of renal disease in acquired immunodeficiency syndrome. N. Engl. J. Med. 316:1062, 1987.
Rousseau, E., Russo, P., and Lapointe, N.: Renal complications of acquired immunodeficiency syndrome in children. Am. J. Kidney Dis. 11:48, 1988.
Ruggenenti, P., Schieppati, A., Bertani, T., and Remuzzi, G.: Thrombotic thrombocytopenic purpura, hemolytic-uremic syndrome, and acute cortical necrosis. In Schrier, R. W., and Gottschalk, C. W. (eds.): Diseases of the Kidney, 6th ed. Boston, Little, Brown & Co., 1997, pp. 1823–1850.
Schrier, R. W., and Gottschalk, C. W. (eds.): Disease of the Kidney, 6th ed. Boston, Little, Brown & Co., 1997.
Schwartz, E. E., Teplick, J. G., Onesti, G., and Schwartz, A. B.: Pulmonary hemorrhage in renal disease: Goodpasture's syndrome and other causes. Radiology 122:39, 1977.
Siegler, R. L., Pavia, A. T., and Cook, J. B.: Hemolytic-uremic syndrome in adolescents. Arch. Pediatr. Adolesc. Med. 151:165, 1997.

Slovis, T. L., Sty, J. R., and Haller, J. O.: Imaging of the Pediatric Urinary Tract. Philadelphia, W. B. Saunders, 1989.

Strauss, J., Abitol, C., Zillervelo, G., Scott, G., Parades, A., Malaga, S., Montane, B., Mitchell, C., Parks, W., and Pardo, V.: Renal disease in children with acquired immunodeficiency syndrome. N. Engl. J. Med. *321*:625, 1989.

Teague, C. A., Doak, P. B., Simpson, I. J., Rainer, S. P., and Herdson, P. B.: Goodpasture's syndrome: An analysis of 29 cases. Kidney Int. *13*:492, 1978.

Turner, A. N., and Rees, A. J.: Goodpasture's disease and Alport's syndromes. Annu. Rev. Med. *47*:377, 1996.

Abnormal Protein Deposition

Auerbach, O., and Stemmerman, M. G.: Renal amyloidosis. Arch. Intern. Med. *74*:244, 1944.

Brandt, K., Catcart, E. S., and Cohen, A. S.: A clinical analysis of the course prognosis of forty-two patients with amyloidosis. Am. J. Med. *44*:955, 1968.

Dixon, H. M.: Renal amyloidosis in relation to renal insufficiency. Am. J. Med. Sci. *187*:401, 1934.

Ekelund, L.: Radiologic findings in renal amyloidosis. AJR *129*:851, 1977.

Kyle, R. A., and Bayrd, E. D.: Amyloidosis: Review of 236 cases. Medicine (Baltimore) *54*:271, 1975.

Pear, B. L.: Radiographic manifestations of amyloidosis. AJR *111*:821, 1971.

Ronco, P. M., Aucouturier, P., and Mougenot, B.: Monoclonal gammopathies: Multiple myeloma, amyloidosis, and related disorders. In Schrier, R. W., and Gottschalk, C. W. (eds.): Diseases of the Kidney, 6th ed. Boston, Little, Brown & Co., 1997, pp. 2129–2174.

Subramanyam, B. R.: Renal amyloidosis in juvenile rheumatoid arthritis: Sonographic features. AJR *136*:411, 1981.

Wang, C. C., and Robbins, L. L.: Amyloid disease: Its roentgen manifestations. Radiology *66*:489, 1956.

Abnormal Fluid Accumulation

Anderson, R. J., and Schrier, R. W.: Acute renal failure. In Schrier, R. W., and Gottschalk, C. W. (eds.): Diseases of the Kidney, 6th ed. Boston, Little, Brown & Co., 1997, pp. 1069–1114.

Berman, L. B.: Vasomotor nephropathy. JAMA *231*:1067, 1975.

Bowley, N. B.: Renal opacification during intravenous urography in acute cortical necrosis (the nephrogram in cortical necrosis). Br. J. Radiol. *54*:524, 1981.

Chugh, K. S., Jha, V., Sakhuja, V., and Joshi, K.: Acute cortical necrosis: A study of 113 patients. Ren. Fail. *16*:37, 1994.

Goergen, T. G., Lindstrom, R. R., Tan, H., and Lilley, J. J.: CT appearance of acute renal cortical necrosis. AJR *137*:176, 1981.

Lloyd-Thomas, H. G., Balme, R. H., and Key, J. J.: Tramline calcification in renal cortical necrosis. Br. Med. J. *1*:909, 1962.

McAlister, W. H., and Nedelman, S. H.: The roentgen manifestations of bilateral renal cortical necrosis. AJR *86*:129, 1961.

Mertens, P.R., Duquerina, D., Ittel, T.H., Keulers, P., and Sieberth, H.G.: Contrast-enhanced computed tomography for demonstration of bilateral renal cortical necrosis. Clin. Invest. *72*:499, 1994.

Möell, H.: Gross bilateral renal cortical necrosis during long periods of oliguria-anuria: Roentgenologic observations in two cases. Acta Radiol. (Diagn.) *48*:355, 1957.

Nomura, G., Kinoshita, E., Yamagata, Y., and Koga, N.: Usefulness of ultrasonography for assessment of severity and course of acute tubular necrosis. J. Clin. Ultrasound *12*:135, 1984.

Older, R. A., Korobkin, M., Cleeve, D. M., Schaaf, R., and Thompson, W.: Contrast-induced acute renal failure: Persistent nephrogram as clue to early detection. AJR *134*:339, 1980.

Rosenberg, H. K., Gefter, W. B., Lebowitz, R. L., Mahboubi, S., and Rosenberg, H.: Prolonged dense nephrograms in battered children. Urology *221*:325, 1983.

Ruggenenti, P., Schieppati, A., Bertani, T., and Remuzzi, G.: Thrombotic thrombocytopenic purpura, hemolytic-uremic syndrome, and acute cortical necrosis. In Schrier, R. W., and Gottschalk, C. W. (eds.): Diseases of the Kidney, 6th ed. Boston, Little, Brown & Co., 1997, pp. 1823–1850.

Sefczek, R. J., Beckman, I., Lupetin, A. R., and Dash, N.: Sonography of acute cortical necrosis. AJR *142*:553, 1984.

Sty, J. R., Starshak, R. J., and Hubbard, A. M.: Acute renal cortical necrosis in hemolytic uremic syndrome. J Clin Ultrasound *11*:175, 1983.

Whelan, J. G., Jr., Ling, J. T., and Davis, L. A.: Antemortem roentgen manifestations of bilateral renal cortical necrosis. Radiology *89*:682, 1967.

Neoplastic Cell Infiltration

Amromin, G. O.: Pathology of Leukemia. New York, Hoeber, 1968, p. 251.

Besse, B. E., Jr., Lieberman, J. E., and Lusted, L. B.: Kidney size in acute leukemia. AJR *80*:611, 1958.

Wewerka-Lutz, Y.: Renal involvement in malignant lymphoma. Schweiz. Med. Wochenschr. *102*:689, 1972.

Inflammatory Cell Infiltration

Appel, G. B.: A decade of penicillin-related acute interstitial nephritis: More questions than answers. Clin. Nephrol. *13*:151, 1980.

Eknoyan, G.: Acute tubulointerstitial nephritis. In Schrier, R. W., and Gottschalk, C. W. (eds.): Diseases of the Kidney, 6th ed. Boston, Little, Brown & Co., 1997, pp. 1249–1273.

Heptinstall, R. H.: Interstitial nephritis. In Heptinstall, R. H. (ed.): Pathology of the Kidney, 4th ed. Boston, Little, Brown & Co., 1992, pp. 1315–1368.

Kelly, C. J., and Neilson, E. G.: Tubulointerstitial diseases. In Brenner, B. M. (ed.): The Kidney, 5th ed. Philadelphia, W. B. Saunders, 1996, pp. 1655–1679.

Autosomal Recessive (Infantile) Polycystic Kidney Disease

Alvarez, F., Bernard, O., Brunelle, F., and Hadchuoel, M.: Congenital hepatic fibrosis in children. J. Pediatr. *99*:370, 1981.

Argubright, K. F., and Wicks, J. D.: Third trimester ultrasonic presentation of infantile polycystic kidney disease. Am. J. Perinatol. *4*:1, 1987.

Boal, D., and Teele, R.: Sonography of infantile polycystic kidney disease. AJR *135*:575, 1980.

Cuarrarino, G., Stannard, M. W., and Rutledge, J. C.: The sonolucent cortical rim in infantile polycystic kidneys: Histologic correlation. J. Ultrasound Med. *8*:571, 1989.

Davies, C. H., Stringer, D. A., Whyte, H., Daneman, A., and Mancer, K.: Congenital hepatic fibrosis with saccular dilatation of intrahepatic bile ducts and infantile polycystic kidneys. Pediatr. Radiol. *16*:302, 1986.

Eggli, K. H., and Hartman, D. S.: Autosomal recessive polycystic kidney disease. In Hartman, D. S. (ed.): Renal Cystic Disease, fascicle I of the Atlas of Radiologic Pathologic Correlation. Washington, D.C., Armed Forces Institute of Pathology, 1989.

Fitch, S. J., and Stapleton, F. B.: Ultrasonographic features of glomerulocystic disease in infancy: Similarity to infantile polycystic kidney disease. Pediatr. Radiol. *16*:400, 1986.

Fredericks, B. J., de Campo, M., Chow, C. W., and Powell, H. R.: Glomerulocystic disease: Ultrasound appearances. Pediatr. Radiol. *19*:184, 1989.

Glassberg, K. I., and Filmer, R. B.: Renal dysplasia, renal hypoplasia, and cystic disease of the kidney. In Kelalis, P., King, L., and Belman, A. B. (eds.): Clinical Pediatric Urology, 2nd ed. Philadelphia, W. B. Saunders, 1985, p. 922.

Hayden, C. K., Swischuk, L. E., Smith, T. H., and Armstrong, E. A.: Renal cystic disease in childhood. Radiographics *6*:97, 1986.

Howie, J. L., and Nicholson, R. L.: CT evaluation of infantile polycystic disease. J. Can. Assoc. Radiol. *31*:202, 1980.

Hussman, K. L., Friedwald, J. P., Gollub, M. J., and Melamed, J.: Caroli's disease associated with infantile polycystic kidney disease. J. Ultrasound Med. *10*:235, 1991.

Jorgensen, M. J.: The ductal plate malformation. Acta Pathol. Microbiol. Immunol. Scand. (Suppl.) *257*:1, 1977.

Kääriäinen, H., Jääskeläinen, J., Kivisaan, L., Koskimies, O., and Norio, R.: Dominant and recessive polycystic kidney disease in children: Classification by intravenous pyelography, ultrasound, and computed tomography. Pediatr. Radiol. *18*:45, 1988.

Kaiser, J. A., Mall, J. C., Salmen, B. J., and Parker, J. J.: Diagnosis of Caroli's disease by computed tomography: Report of two cases. Radiology *132*:661, 1979.

Kogutt, M. S., Robichaux, W. H., Boineau, F. G., Drake, G. K., and Simonton, S. C.: Asymmetric renal size in autosomal recessive polycystic kidney disease: A unique presentation. AJR *160*:835, 1993.

Lieberman, E., Salinas-Madrigal, L., Gwinn, J., Brennan, L. P., Fine, R. N., and Landing, B. H.: Infantile polycystic disease of the kidneys and liver: Clinical, pathological and radiological correlations and comparison with congenital hepatic fibrosis. Medicine *50*:277, 1971.

Luthy, D. A., and Hirsch, J. H.: Infantile polycystic kidney disease: Observations from attempts at prenatal diagnosis. Am. J. Med. Genet. *20*:505, 1985.

Madewell, J. E., Hartman, D. S., and Lichtenstein, J. E.: Radiologic-pathologic correlations in cystic disease of the kidney. Radiol. Clin. North Am. *17*:261, 1979.

Mall, J. C., Ghahremani, G. G., and Bayer, J. L.: Caroli's disease associated with congenital hepatic fibrosis and renal tubular ectasia. Gastroenterology *66*:1029, 1974.

Marchal, G. J., Desmet, V. J., Proesmans, W. C., et al.: Caroli's disease: High-frequency US and pathologic findings. Radiology *158*:507, 1986.

Melson, G. L., Shackelford, G. D., Cole, B. R., et al.: The spectrum of sonographic findings in infantile polycystic kidney disease with urographic and clinical correlations. J Clin Ultrasound *13*:113, 1985.

Mittelstaedt, C. A., Volberg, F. M., Fischer, G. J., and McArtney, W. H.: Caroli's disease: Sonographic findings. AJR *134*:585, 1980.

Moreno, A. J., Parker, A. L., Spicer, M. J., et al.: Scintigraphic and radiographic findings in Caroli's disease. Am. J. Gastroenterol *79*:299, 1984.

Mujahed, Z., Glenn, F., and Evans, J. A.: Communicating cavernous ectasia of the intrahepatic ducts (Caroli's disease). AJR *113*:21, 1971.

Nakanuma, Y., Terada, T., Ohta, G., Kurachi, M., and Matsubara, F.: Caroli's disease in congenital hepatic fibrosis and infantile polycystic disease. Liver *2*:346, 1982.

Osathanondh, V., and Potter, E. L.: Pathogenesis of polycystic kidneys. Arch. Pathol. *77*:461, 1964.

Patriquin, H. B., and O'Regan, S.: Medullary sponge kidney in childhood. AJR *145*:315, 1985.

Potter, E. L.: Normal and Abnormal Development of the Kidney. Chicago, Year Book Medical Publishers, 1972.

Premkumar, A., Berdon, W. E., Levy, J., Amondio, J., Abramson, S. J., and Newhouse, J. H.: The emergence of hepatic fibrosis and portal hypertension in infants and children with autosomal polycystic kidney disease. Pediatr. Radiol. *18*:123, 1988.

Rosenfield, A. T., Siegel, N. J., Kappelman, N. B., and Taylor, K. J. W.: Gray scale ultrasonography in medullary cystic disease of the kidney and congenital hepatic fibrosis with tubular ectasia: New observations. AJR *129*:297, 1977.

Six, R., Oliphant, M., and Grossman, H.: A spectrum of renal tubular ectasia and hepatic fibrosis. Radiology *117*:117, 1975.

Stapleton, F. B., Magill, H. L., and Kelly, D. R.: Infantile polycystic kidney disease: An imaging dilemma. Urol. Radiol. *5*:89, 1983.

Sztriha, L., Gyurkovits, K., Ormos, J., and Monus, Z.: Congenital hepatic fibrosis with polycystic disease of the kidneys. Hepatogastroenterology *29*:259, 1982.

Taxy, J. B., and Filmer, R. B.: Glomerulocystic kidney. Arch. Pathol. Lab. Med. *100*:186, 1976.

Unite, I., Maitem, A., Bagnasco, F., and Irwin, G. A.: Congenital hepatic fibrosis associated with renal tubular ectasia. Radiology *109*:565, 1973.

Weese-Mayer, D. E., Smith, K. M., Reddy, J. K., Salafsky, I., Poznanski, A. K.: Computerized tomography and ultrasound in the diagnosis of cerebro-hepato-renal syndrome of Zellinger. Pediatr. Radiol. *17*:170, 1987.

Welling, L. W., and Grantham, J. J.: Cystic and developmental diseases of the kidney. In Brenner, B. M. (ed.): The Kidney, 5th ed. Philadelphia, W. B. Saunders, 1996, pp. 1828–1863.

Wernecke, K., Heckemann, R., Bachmann, H., and Peters, P. E.: Sonography of infantile polycystic kidney disease. Urol. Radiol. *7*:138, 1985.

Wood, B. P.: Renal cystic disease in infants and children. Urol. Radiol. *14*:284, 1992.

Woodward, P. J., Sohaey, R., Harris, D. P., Jackson, G. M., Klatt, E. C., Alexander, A. L., and Kennedy, A.: Postmortem fetal MR imaging: Comparison with findings at autopsy. *AJR* 168:41, 1997.

Acute Urate Nephropathy

Kelley, W. M.: Uricosuria and x-ray contrast agents. N. Engl. J. Med. *284*:975, 1971.

Martin, D. J., and Jaffe, N.: Prolonged nephrogram due to hyperuricaemia. Br. J. Radiol. *44*:806, 1971.

Postlethwaite, A. E., and Kelley, W. M.: Uricosuric effect of radiocontrast agents: A study in man of four commonly used preparations. Ann. Intern. Med. *74*:845, 1971.

Robinson, R. R., and Yarger, W. E.: Acute uric acid nephropathy. Arch. Intern. Med. *137*:839, 1977.

Glycogen Storage Disease, Type I

Chen, Y.-T.: Type I glycogen storage disease: Kidney involvement, pathogenesis and its treatment. Pediatr. Nephrol. *5*:71, 1991.

Chen, Y.-T., Coleman, R. A., Sheinman, J. L., Kolbeck, P. C., and Sidury, J. B.: Renal disease in type I glycogen storage disease. N. Engl. J. Med. *318*:7, 1988.

Chen, Y.-T., Feinstein, K. A., Coleman, R. A., and Effmann, E. L.: Variability of renal length in type I glycogen storage disease. J. Inherit. Metab. Dis. *13*:259, 1990.

Miller, J. H., Stanley, P., and Gates, G. F.: Radiography of glycogen storage disease. AJR *132*:379, 1979.

Slovis, T. L., Sty, J. R., and Haller, J. O.: Imaging of the Pediatric Urinary Tract. Philadelphia, W. B. Saunders, 1989.

Verani, R., and Bernstein, J.: Renal glomerular and tubular abnormalities in glycogen storage disease type I. Arch. Pathol. Lab. Med. *112*:271, 1988.

Physiologic Response to Urographic Contrast Material and Diuretics

Dorph, S., and Øigaard, A.: Variations in size of the normal kidney following intravenous administration of water-soluble contrast medium and urea. Br. J. Radiol. *46*:183, 1973.

Dorph, S., and Øigaard, A.: Renal distention in response to water-soluble contrast medium and various diuretics: A comparative study. Scand. J. Urol. Nephrol. *9*:114, 1975.

Vuorinen, P., and Wegelius, U.: Changes of renal size after drinking and intravenous glucose infusion. Br. J. Radiol. *38*:673, 1965.

Wolpert, S. M.: Variation in kidney length during intravenous pyelography. Br. J. Radiol. *38*:100, 1965.

Homozygous-S Disease

Addae, S. K.: The kidney in sickle cell disease: V. Clinical manifestations. Ghana Med. J. *12*:352, 1973.

Berman, L. B.: Sickle cell nephropathy. JAMA *228*:1279, 1974.

Buckalew, V. M., and Someren, A.: Renal manifestations of sickle cell disease. Arch. Intern. Med. *133*:660, 1974.

Karayalcin, G., Dorfman, J., Rosner, F., and Aballi, A. J.: Radiological changes in 127 patients with sickle cell anemia. Am. J. Med. Sci. *271*:132, 1976.

Lakkis, F. G., Campbell, O. C., and Badr, K. F.: Microvascular diseases of the kidney. In Brenner, B. M. (ed.): The Kidney, 5th ed. Philadelphia, W. B. Saunders, 1996, pp. 1712–1730.

Lande, J. M., Glazer, G. M., Sarnaik, S., Aisen, A., Rucknagle, D., and Martel, W.: Sickle cell nephropathy: MR imaging. Radiology *158*:379, 1986.

McCall, I. W., Moule, N., Desai, P., and Serjeant, G. R.: Urographic findings in homozygous sickle cell disease. Radiology *126*:99, 1978.

Mostofi, F. K., Bruegge, C. F. V., and Diggs, L. W.: Lesions in kidneys removed for unilateral hematuria in sickle cell disease. Arch. Pathol. *63*:336, 1957.

van Eps, L. W. S., and de Jong, P. E.: Sickle cell disease. In Schrier, R. W., and Gottschalk, C. W. (eds.): Diseases of the Kidney, 6th ed. Boston, Little, Brown & Co., 1997, pp. 2201–2220.

Paroxysmal Nocturnal Hemoglobinuria

Braren, V., Butler, S. A., Hartmann, R. C., and Jenkins, D. E., Jr.: Urologic manifestations of paroxysmal nocturnal hemoglobinuria. J. Urol. *114*:430, 1975.

Clark, D. A., Butler, S. A., Braren, V., Hartmann, R. C., and Jenkins, D. E.: The kidneys in paroxysmal nocturnal hemoglobinuria. Blood *57*:83, 1981.

Kaplan, M. E.: Acquired hemolytic disorders. In Wyngaarden, J. B., and Smith, L. H., Jr. (eds.): Cecil's Textbook of Medicine. Philadelphia, W. B. Saunders, 1988, p. 922.

Lupetin, A. R.: Magnetic resonance appearance of the kidneys in paroxysmal nocturnal hemoglobinuria. Urol. Radiol. *8*:101, 1986.

Hemophilia

Dalinka, M. K., Lally, J. F., Rancier, L. F., and Mata, J.: Nephromegaly in hemophilia. Radiology *115*:337, 1975.

Roberts, G. M., Evans, K. T., Bloom, A. L., and Al-Gailani, F.: Renal papillary necrosis in haemophilia and Christmas disease. Clin. Radiol. *34*:201, 1983.

Cirrhosis, Hyperalimentation, and Diabetes Mellitus

Bos, A. F., Aalders, A. L., Vandoormaal, J. J., Martijn, A., and Okken, A.: Kidney size in infants of tightly controlled insulin-dependent diabetic mothers. J. Clin. Ultrasound *22*:443, 1994.

Christiansen, J. S., Gammelgaard, J., Tronier, B., Svendsen, P. A., and Parving, H.-H.: Kidney function and size in diabetes before and during initial insulin treatment. Kidney Int. *21*:638, 1982.

Cochran, S. T., Pagani, J. J., and Barbaric, Z. L.: Nephromegaly in hyperalimentation. Radiology *130*:603, 1979.

Derchi, L. E., Martinoli, C., Saffioto, S., Pontermoli, R., Demicheli, A., and Bordone, C.: Ultrasonographic imaging and Doppler analysis of renal changes in non–insulin dependent diabetes mellitus. Acad. Radiol. *1*:100, 1994.

Ginès, P., and Schrier, R. W.: Hepatorenal syndrome and renal dysfunction associated with liver disease. In Schrier, R. W., and Gottschalk, C. W. (eds.): Diseases of the Kidney, 6th ed. Boston, Little, Brown & Co., 1997, pp. 2099–2128.

Laube, H., Norris, H. T., and Robbins, S. L.: The nephromegaly of chronic alcoholics with liver disease. Arch. Pathol. Lab. Med. *84*:290, 1967.

Mauer, M., Mogensen, C. E., and Friedman, E. A.: Diabetic nephropathy. In Schrier, R. W., and Gottschalk, C. W. (eds.): Diseases of the Kidney, 6th ed. Boston, Little, Brown & Co., 1997, pp. 2019–2062.

Mogensen, C. E., and Andersen, M. J. F.: Increased kidney size and glomerular filtration rate in early juvenile diabetes. Diabetes *22*:706, 1973.

Osterby, R., and Gundersen, H. J. G.: Glomerular size and structure in diabetes mellitus: I. Early abnormalities. Diabetologia *11*:225, 1975.

Rabkin, R., and Fervenza, F. C.: Renal hypertrophy and kidney disease in diabetes. Diabetes Metab. Rev. *12*:217, 1996.

Wirta, O., Pasternack, A., Laippala, P., and Turjanmaa, V.: Glomerular filtration rate and kidney size after six years' disease duration in non–insulin-dependent diabetic subjects. Clin. Nephrol. *45*:10, 1996.

Fabry's Disease

Case records of the Massachusetts General Hospital: Case 2-1984. Fabry's disease. N. Engl. J. Med. *310*:106, 1984.

Gregory, M. C., and Atkin, C. L.: Alport's syndrome, Fabry's disease, and nail-patella syndrome. In Schrier, R. W., and Gottschalk, C. W. (eds.): Diseases of the Kidney, 6th ed. Boston, Little, Brown & Co., 1997, pp. 561–590.

Novello, A. C., and Bennett, W. M.: Fabry's disease and nail-patella syndrome. In Schrier, R. W., and Gottschalk, C. W. (eds.): Diseases of the Kidney, 4th ed. Boston, Little, Brown & Co., 1988, pp. 643–662.

Stiennon, M., and Goldberg, M. E.: Renal size in Fabry's Disease. Urol. Radiol. *2*:17, 1980.

Bartter's Syndrome

Cogan, M. G., and Rector, F. C., Jr.: Acid base disorders. In Brenner, B. M., and Rector, F. C. (eds.): The Kidney, 4th ed. Philadelphia, W. B. Saunders, 1991, pp. 737–804.

Garel, L., Filiatrault, D., and Robitaille, P.: Nephrocalcinosis in Bartter's syndrome. Pediatr. Nephrol. *2*:315, 1988.

Matsumoto, J., Han, B. K., Rovetto, C. R., and Welch, T. R.: Hypercalciuric Bartter syndrome: Resolution of nephrocalcinosis with indomethacin. AJR *152*:1251, 1989.

Strause, S., Robinson, G., Lotan, D., and Itzechak, Y.: Renal sonography in Bartter syndrome. J. Ultrasound Med. *6*:205, 1987.

Taybi, H.: Radiology of Syndromes and Metabolic Disorders, 2nd ed. Chicago, Year Book Medical Publishers, 1983, p. 32.

Beckwith-Wiedemann Syndrome

Beckwith, J. B.: Macroglossia, omphalocele, adrenal cytomegaly, gigantism and hyperplastic visceromegaly. Birth Defects *5*:188, 1969.

Bronk, J. B., and Parker, B. R.: Pyelocalyceal diverticula in the Beckwith-Wiedemann syndrome. Pediatr. Radiol. *17*:80, 1987.

Chesney, R. W., Kaufman, R., Stapleton, F. B., and Rivas, M. L.: Association of medullary sponge kidney and medullary dysplasia in Beckwith-Wiedemann syndrome. J. Pediatr. *115*:761, 1989.

Lee, F. A.: Radiology of the Beckwith-Wiedemann syndrome. Radiol. Clin. North Am. *10*:261, 1972.

McCarten, K. M., Cleveland, R. H., Simeone, J. F., and Aretz, T.: Renal ultrasonography in Beckwith-Wiedemann syndrome. Pediatr. Radiol. *11*:46, 1981.

Nephroblastomatosis

Fernbach, S. K., Feinstein, K. A., Donaldson, J. S., and Baum, E. S.: Nephroblastomosis: Comparison of CT with US and urography. Radiology *166*:153, 1988.

Hartman, D.S., Taveras, J., Ferucci, J. (eds.): Radiology Diagnosis, Imaging, Intervention. Philadelphia: J. B. Lippincott Co., 1986, pp. 1–9.

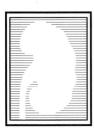

CHAPTER

9

Diagnostic Set: Large, Smooth, Unilateral

RENAL VEIN THROMBOSIS/STENOSIS
ACUTE ARTERIAL INFARCTION
OBSTRUCTIVE UROPATHY
ACUTE PYELONEPHRITIS
XANTHOGRANULOMATOUS PYELONEPHRITIS

MISCELLANEOUS CONDITIONS
  Compensatory Hypertrophy
  Duplicated Pelvocalyceal System
DIFFERENTIAL DIAGNOSIS

Diseases discussed in this chapter classically involve one kidney only. This is not to say that both kidneys are never involved in renal vein thrombosis/stenosis, acute hemorrhagic infarction, obstructive uropathy, acute pyelonephritis, or duplication of the pelvocalyceal system. When bilateral involvement does occur, however, it is a chance phenomenon, not a natural feature of the disease process itself.

RENAL VEIN THROMBOSIS/STENOSIS

Definition

The rapidity with which renal vein occlusion occurs partially determines the pattern of response in the kidney. At one extreme, sudden, total occlusion produces hemorrhagic infarction, permanent loss of function, and eventual shrinkage of the kidney. At the other extreme, gradual onset of venous occlusion or a partial obstruction allows time for collateral channels to develop, leaving renal anatomy and function undisturbed. The appearance of the kidney depends not only on the rapidity with which occlusion occurs but also on the completeness of the occlusion, the amount of collateral channel development, and the degree to which the thrombosis eventually recanalizes. In addition, venous thrombosis in the adult is usually a complication of a primary renal disease that itself will alter the appearance of the kidney.

When renal vein occlusion is sudden, there is no time for effective development of collateral pathways. The interstices of the kidney swell with blood from ruptured venules and capillaries. The organ becomes generally enlarged and tense, and urine formation ceases. Eventually, fibrous tissue replaces necrotic nephrons, resulting in a globally wasted, nonfunctioning kidney. The pattern is the same as

that seen in acute infarction due to main renal artery occlusion or severe trauma to the kidney.

There are times when venous occlusion develops rapidly and extensively, yet irreversible changes leading to renal atrophy do not follow because collateral drainage develops to some degree. In this circumstance, interstitial edema and congested intrarenal vessels cause global enlargement of the kidney. Function, although impaired, continues. Either these changes persist in a steady state or complete resolution occurs as recanalization of the thrombus or further expansion of collateral venous pathways provides adequate venous drainage. In these cases, there is thickening of basement membranes, interstitial edema, and polymorphonuclear leukocyte margination in capillaries. Mild tubule atrophy and interstitial fibrosis may eventually develop.

Finally, the process of venous obstruction, either complete or partial, can be so indolent as to alter gross renal morphologic features minimally or not at all. Cases of this type may present as the nephrotic syndrome even when the process is unilateral. A glomerular lesion similar to that of membranous glomerulonephritis has been described in these patients.

Clinical Setting

Renal vein thrombosis in the newborn is usually associated with dehydration, birth asphyxia, hypotension, sepsis, or maternal diabetes mellitus. In the older child, severe dehydration is sometimes complicated by renal vein thrombosis. In the adult, thrombosis is most often a complication of another renal disease, such as amyloidosis, membranous glomerulonephritis, lupus glomerulonephritis, or other conditions that cause the nephrotic syndrome. Thrombosis of the inferior vena cava with retrograde propagation of clot into the renal vein, extrinsic pressure by tumor on the inferior vena cava or renal vein, extension of a kidney tumor into the renal vein, and trauma are other conditions that predispose to renal vein thrombosis. A narrow space between the aorta and the superior mesenteric artery may compress the left renal vein, a condition known as the *nutcracker syndrome.*

A sudden, major occlusion causes sharp flank pain and tenderness, and the kidney often becomes palpable. Fever and leukocytosis develop. Gross or microscopic hematuria may be present, but a normal urinalysis result is not uncommon when urine formation ceases on the involved side.

When the degree of occlusion is less acute, unilateral global renal enlargement will be accompanied by deteriorating function of the involved kidney. This may progress or may reverse, depending on the extent of recanalization of the thrombus, the lysis of clot by therapy, or the opening up of collateral venous drainage.

Patients with a slowly developing occlusion or partial obstruction may have some increase in renal size with a clinical presentation that varies along a spectrum from asymptomatic through slight proteinuria or hematuria to a fully developed nephrotic syndrome (edema, hyperlipidemia, hypoproteinemia, and massive proteinuria) when a predisposing condition is present.

Radiologic Findings

Kidney enlargement can be striking in acute renal vein thrombosis. Experimental and clinical studies have shown that the flow of contrast material into the kidney is very much reduced or even absent. When this occurs, a very large, smooth renal mass with little or no opacification is seen during contrast material–enhanced studies such as excretory urography or computed tomography (Fig. 9–1). If unresolved, this form of venous occlusion produces renal infarction and eventually causes a small, smooth, nonfunctioning renal outline on late follow-up studies. This transition may occur over 2 months. Deposition of calcium in a fine reticular pattern within the renal substance has been reported as a late sequela of renal vein thrombosis in infants. This is believed to represent calcium deposition in intrarenal veins and might also occur in adults.

Adequate collateral formation may develop in response to complete or partial renal vein obstruction. Still, the kidney may be large and smooth and contrast material excretion may vary from normal to impaired (see Fig. 9–7). The collecting system has a normal distribution within the renal substance but is usually attenuated by the surrounding swollen parenchyma (Fig. 9–2A and B). In a few cases, the nephrogram has been described as increasingly dense with time. This undoubtedly represents con-

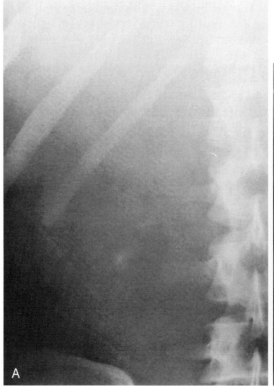
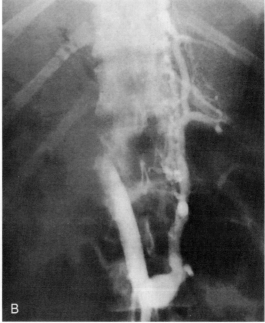

FIGURE 9–1. Acute right renal vein occlusion following trauma in a young man with congenital absence of the left kidney.
  A, Excretory urogram. The kidney is enlarged and poorly outlined. A small collection of contrast material is present in a lower pole calyx. The remainder of the collecting system is effaced.
  B, Inferior vena cavogram. Renal vein obstruction is secondary to a large retroperitoneal hematoma displacing and occluding the inferior vena cava. Collateral drainage is through the azygous system.

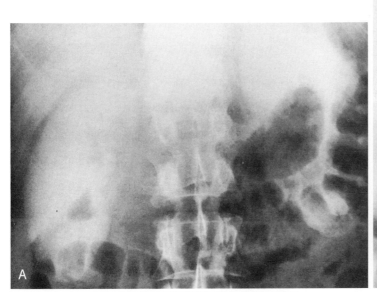

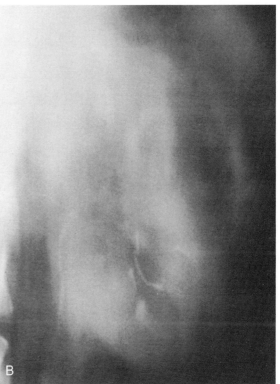

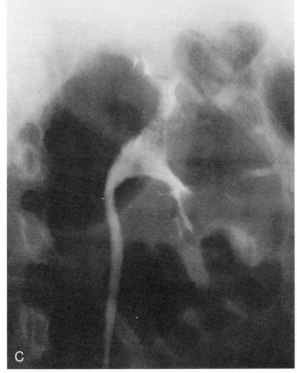

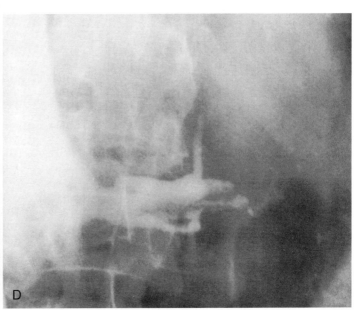

FIGURE 9–2. Left renal vein thrombosis in a 60-year-old man with nephrotic syndrome.

A, Film taken 1 minute after contrast material injection demonstrates a large left kidney (length = 16.9 cm).

B, Tomogram during excretory urography. The collecting system is normally distributed within the kidney substance but is effaced by surrounding interstitial edema.

C, Retrograde pyelogram. Nodular defects and a feathery mucosal pattern are seen in the pelvis, presumably reflecting distended submucosal veins, mural edema, or hemorrhage.

D, Left retrograde renal venogram. The proximal part of the renal vein contains a large thrombus.

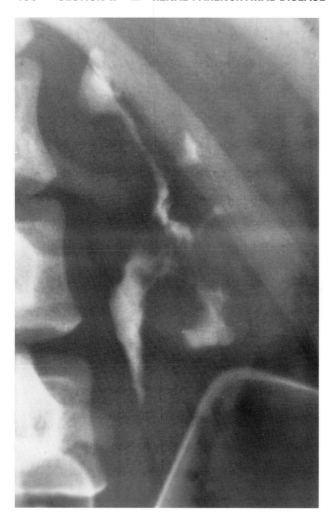

FIGURE 9–3. Renal vein thrombosis, left kidney. Excretory urogram with compression. There are multiple mural notches deforming the pelvis, which does not distend normally. The notches represent distended collateral veins.

tinued arterial perfusion to a kidney unable to eliminate the accumulating contrast material through usual venous or urinary pathways. Alternating radiolucent and radiopaque nephrographic striations, believed to represent contrast material in dilated tubules in the medullary rays, have been described in excretory urograms and computed tomograms as well as in angiograms. A cortical rim sign, usually associated with acute arterial infarction, has also been associated with renal vein thrombosis.

Enlargement of collateral pathways for renal venous outflow, known as *varices*, is an important sequel to partial or complete obstruction of the renal vein. Gonadal, ureteric, lumbar, adrenal, and capsular veins participate. Varices produce easily identified, sharply defined indentations on a well-distended, opacified pelvis and ureter. These may resemble ureteritis or pyelitis cystica (Fig. 9–3). Sometimes, a feathery or nodular mucosal pattern is seen in the pelvis and the proximal ureter. This appearance, representing distended submucosal veins, mural edema, and occasionally hemorrhage, may resemble transitional cell carcinoma (Fig. 9–2C). These abnormal patterns often disappear when the pelvis is distended during retrograde pyelogra-

phy or following effective ureteral compression (Fig. 9–4).

Patients with renal vein thrombosis, including cases associated with the nephrotic syndrome, may have entirely normal radiologic studies. This suggests an incomplete occlusion from the onset, the recanalization or lysis of an earlier thrombus, or the presence of collaterals adequate in volume to carry the renal venous efflux.

Computed tomographic findings include those described for excretory urography. Additional features may include prolonged corticomedullary differentiation, distended collateral veins in the renal sinus, focal zones of nonenhanced parenchyma in areas of infarction, retroperitoneal hemorrhage, and enlargement of the renal vein in which there is low attenuation thrombus (Figs. 9–5, 9–6, 9–7). Fine linear densities radiating from the kidney into the perirenal space have been described as characteristic, although not pathognomonic, of renal vein thrombus. These structures, which enhance with contrast material, most likely represent collateral renal veins traversing the perirenal space. In the nutcracker syndrome, computed tomography identifies the narrowness of the space between the aorta

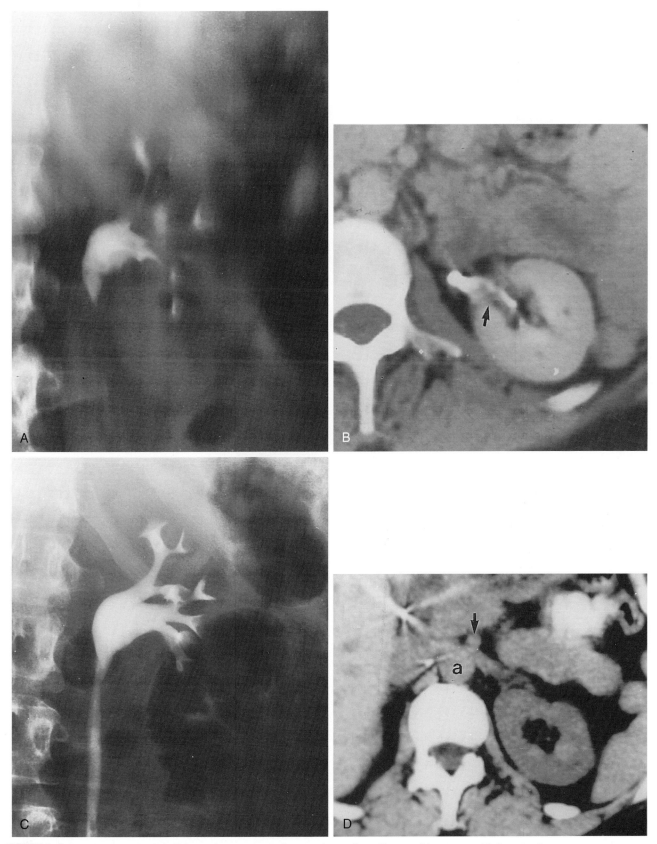

FIGURE 9–4. Renal vein varix, left kidney, due to nutcracker syndrome in a 45-year-old woman with hematuria.

A, Excretory urogram; *B*, Computed tomogram, contrast material–enhanced. A nodular, mural-based filling defect *(arrow)* is present in the pelvis of the left kidney on both studies.

C, Retrograde pyelogram. With the pelvis distended during retrograde injection of contrast material, the pelvic filling defect disappears.

D, Computed tomogram, unenhanced. The space between the superior mesenteric artery *(arrow)* and the aorta (a) is narrow and compresses the left renal vein.

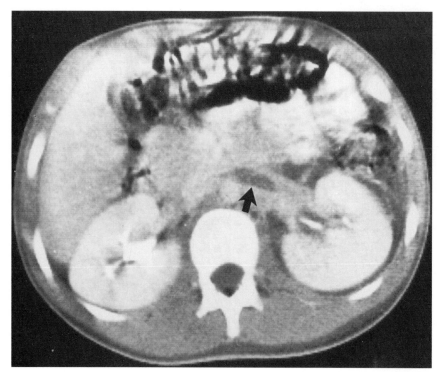

FIGURE 9–5. Renal vein thrombosis, left kidney. Computed tomogram, contrast material–enhanced. The left kidney is enlarged and smooth, and the pelvocalyceal system is attenuated. Enhancing soft tissue representing venous collateral pathways surrounds the thrombosed left renal vein, which is unenhanced *(arrow).*

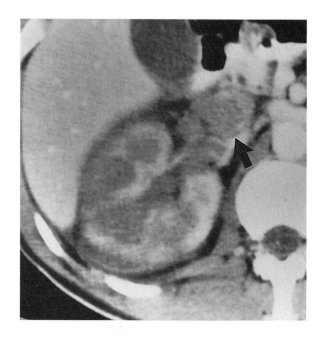

FIGURE 9–6. Renal vein thrombosis, right kidney, in a young male with sepsis. Computed tomogram, contrast material–enhanced. The right kidney is large and smooth and has prolonged corticomedullary differentiation. A small perinephric fluid collection is present. Thrombus distends renal veins and inferior vena cava *(arrow).*

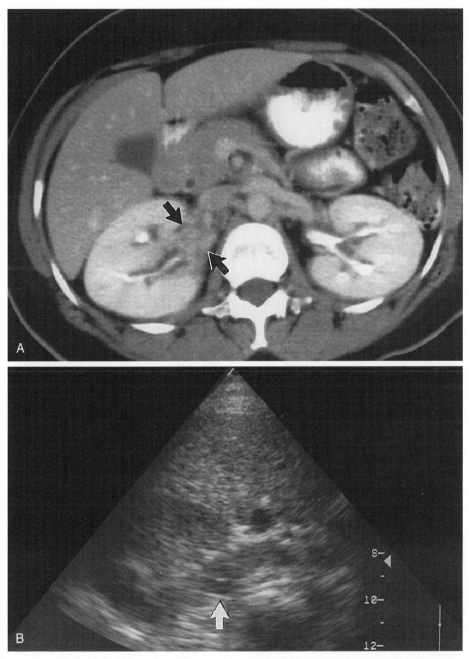

FIGURE 9–7. Renal vein thrombosis, right kidney, in a 26-year-old woman with systemic lupus erythematosus.

A, Computed tomogram, contrast material–enhanced. Abnormal soft-tissue structures in the right renal sinus *(arrows)* represent collateral veins. Normal kidney size and nephrographic density indicate compensated renal venous outflow through collateral veins.

B, Ultrasonogram, transverse section. There is increased soft tissue in the right renal sinus *(arrow)* and an absence of a normal renal vein. The echo pattern of the kidney is normal.

(Kindly supplied by Wendelin Hayes, D.O., Georgetown University, Washington, D.C.)

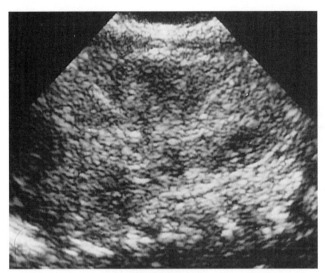

FIGURE 9–8. Renal vein thrombosis, left kidney, in a neonate born of a mother with diabetes mellitus. Ultrasonogram, sagittal projection. The kidney is large and smooth and exhibits a generalized pattern of increased echogenicity.

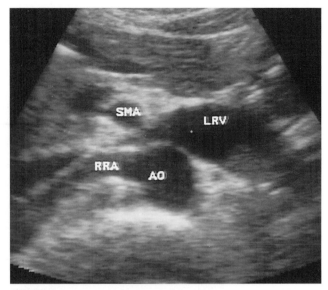

FIGURE 9–9. Tumor thrombus in left renal vein. Ultrasonogram, transverse section. The left renal vein (LRV) is dilated and contains echogenic tumor. AO = aorta; SMA = superior mesenteric artery; RRA = right renal artery.

and the superior mesenteric artery that is traversed by the left renal vein.

Ultrasonography demonstrates smooth enlargement of the kidney, with increased parenchymal thickness and a variable echo pattern (Fig. 9–8; see also Fig. 9–7). Within the first 2 to 3 weeks of the onset of thrombosis, the echogenicity of the kidney diminishes, presumably owing to interstitial fluid accumulation. Thereafter, echogenicity increases as fibrosis causes global wasting of the kidney. Hyperechoic areas may be present at the site of intrarenal hemorrhage. The renal vein is enlarged, and thrombus may be demonstrated as intraluminal echogenic tissue that extends into the inferior vena cava (Figs. 9–9, 9–10). The same findings are seen with bland thrombus as well as tumor thrombus arising in an adenocarcinoma of the kidney. Doppler ultrasound scanning detects reduction or absence of venous

blood flow. Diminished or reversed diastolic flow is seen during spectral Doppler ultrasonography of the renal arteries. Ultrasonography also detects perirenal hemorrhage when acute renal vein thrombosis causes rupture of the kidney.

Magnetic resonance imaging of the inferior vena cava, main renal vein, and intrarenal branches provides a means for directly confirming the presence of thrombus. Magnetic resonance imaging is particularly helpful when the renal vein cannot be visualized by ultrasonography and the patient is not a candidate for contrast material–enhanced computed tomography.

Venography provides information similar to that obtained from magnetic resonance images or ultrasonography (Fig. 9–2D). It is prudent first to perform an inferior vena cavogram with a catheter

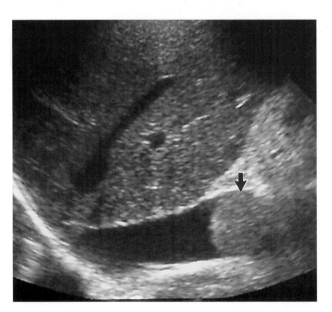

FIGURE 9–10. Thrombus from a renal adenocarcinoma extending into the inferior vena cava. Ultrasonogram, sagittal projection. The tumor *(arrow)* is echogenic.

RENAL VEIN THROMBOSIS/STENOSIS TYPICAL FINDINGS

Primary Uroradiologic Elements

Size: normal to large
Contour: smooth
Lesion distribution: unilateral

Secondary Uroradiologic Elements

Collecting system: attenuated; mucosal irregularity, nodularity; notching; abnormalities
    disappear on retrograde pyelography
Parenchymal thickness: expanded
Nephrogram: density varies from absent to normal; prolonged corticomedullary
    differentiation
Echogenicity: variable
Renal veins: dilated; intraluminal thrombus; diminished to absent flow
Retroperitoneum: dilated collaterals; hemorrhage

---

placed well below the renal veins to evaluate the inferior vena cava for diseases that might be the cause of secondary renal venous occlusion. Clots extending into the vena cava from the renal veins can also be identified during cavography. Cautious selective catheterization of the renal vein can then follow if caval disease is absent. Retrograde injection of contrast material into interlobar and arcuate veins is necessary to detect thrombi limited to these vessels. Careful interpretation is necessary to avoid confusing normal renal vein valves with thrombotic occlusion.

Renal arteriography in renal vein thrombosis is usually not required, but when it is performed it shows stretching of intrarenal arteries, increased circulation time, and diminished or absent venous opacification. The angiographic nephrogram may stain more intensely than normal, and the corticomedullary border is disrupted. A striated nephrogram has been reported. These findings are not specific, however. Occasionally, venous collaterals will opacify.

ACUTE ARTERIAL INFARCTION

Definition

Acute hemorrhagic infarction of the kidney follows embolic or thrombotic renal artery occlusion, blunt abdominal trauma, or sudden, complete renal venous occlusion. In this section, the early changes of infarction following arterial occlusion or blunt trauma are discussed; renal vein occlusion is presented in the preceding section, and a comprehensive discussion of renal trauma is presented in Chapter 29.

When infarction involves most or all of the kidney, there is marked hyperemia of the glomeruli and capillaries. The interstitial spaces, too, become filled with blood, owing to altered capillary permeability.

The source of the blood is subsidiary arterial channels, such as capsular arteries, retrograde flow from veins, or continued main arterial perfusion in the case of renal vein occlusion. With time, the hemorrhage and necrotic tissue become surrounded with leukocytes, and the cellular elements lose their identifying features.

The infarcted kidney is large and tense, with red discoloration. After 2 to 3 weeks the kidney begins to shrink as a result of autolysis of cells, resorption of free hemoglobin, and development of interstitial fibrosis.

Clinical Setting

Only a small number of cases of renal infarction involve the whole (or even a major segment of) kidney. The majority are either lobar or regional and are discussed in Chapters 5 and 6. Main renal artery occlusion is usually due to an embolus from the heart with rheumatic valvular disease and arrhythmia, subacute bacterial endocarditis, left atrial mural thrombus or tumor, myocardial trauma, or prosthetic valves. In only a minority of cases is the occlusion due to primary arterial disease, such as atherosclerotic plaque or aneurysm or dissection of the aorta and/or renal artery.

The kidney commonly suffers damage in blunt abdominal trauma, usually in the form of parenchymal contusion. Renal artery occlusion or avulsion leads to infarction of the kidney. Fracture of the renal capsule and parenchyma, subcapsular or perirenal hematoma, and laceration of the pelvocalyceal system and ureter also occur. Trauma to the kidney is discussed further in Chapter 29.

Signs and symptoms of acute renal infarction vary from none to abrupt onset of severe abdominal or flank pain, with nausea, vomiting, hematuria, and albuminuria. Fever and leukocytosis may be present. An enlarged, tender renal mass can occa-

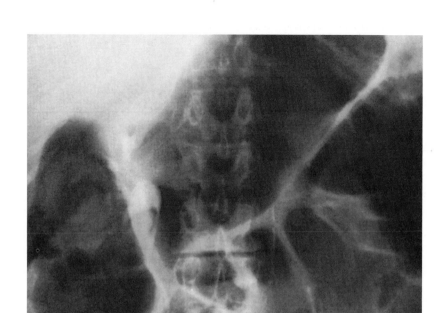

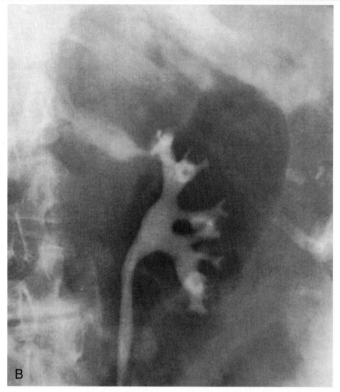

FIGURE 9–11. Acute left renal infarction in a 78-year-old woman who developed left-flank pain and slight leukocytosis following colon surgery. Urinalysis results were normal. Radionuclide scan revealed markedly diminished left-kidney flow.

A, Excretory urogram. The left kidney did not opacify over a 24-hour period. The right kidney is normal.

B, Left retrograde pyelogram performed to exclude obstructive uropathy. The pelvocalyceal system is normal. Thirty months later, excretory urography showed that function had returned and that global atrophy had developed (see Fig. 6–12).

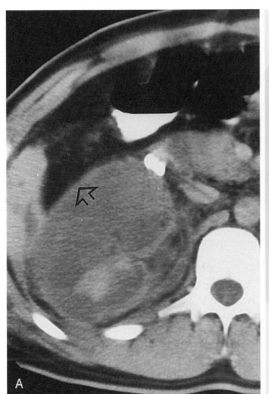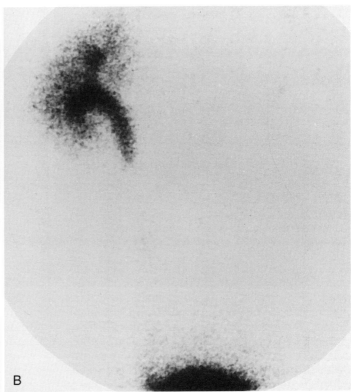

FIGURE 9–12. Acute infarction, right kidney, secondary to blunt abdominal trauma.
  A, Computed tomogram, contrast material–enhanced. The right kidney is markedly enlarged and smooth. The nephrogram does not develop except for a very faint cortical rim sign *(arrow).* An area of increased attenuation in the dorsal portion of the kidney represents fresh hemorrhage.
  B, ⁹⁹ᵐTc Mag₃ radionuclide renogram. No function is demonstrated in the right kidney.

sionally be palpated. It is important to note that urinalysis may be completely normal when damage to the kidney is severe enough to prevent urine formation. In traumatic infarction due to avulsion of the renal artery, shock may be the dominant clinical finding.

Radiologic Findings

A nonopacified kidney of normal to enlarged size with a normal pelvocalyceal system demonstrated by retrograde pyelography is characteristic of renal artery occlusion due to embolus or thrombosis (Fig. 9–11). The same finding is seen in avulsion of the renal artery, in which case other evidence of trauma, such as fractures or retroperitoneal hematoma, will be noted on the plain film examination of the abdomen. When renal trauma or venous occlusion is the cause of renal infarction, interstitial hemorrhage is the dominant feature. In any of these circumstances, the kidney is enlarged, and the nephrogram, if it develops at all, will be diminished and sometimes patchy (Figs. 9–12, 9–13, 9–14*A*). The pelvocalyceal system, when opacified, is effaced and attenuated by the surrounding swollen interstitial fluid. Blood clots may form filling defects in the collecting system.

A *cortical rim nephrographic* sign is a distinctive abnormality that occurs in nearly one-half of pa-

tients with infarction of either the entire kidney or of the major ventral or dorsal segments (see Figs. 9–12, 9–13). This thin rim of contrast material–enhanced tissue represents peripheral cortex that continues to be perfused by capsular collateral

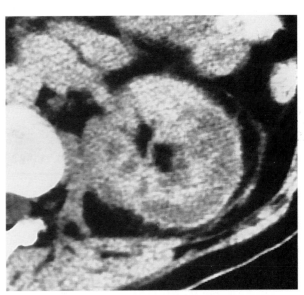

FIGURE 9–13. Acute infarction, left kidney, secondary to embolus. Computed tomogram, contrast material–enhanced. The kidney is enlarged and smooth, and the nephrogram is patchy. A cortical rim nephrogram is present.

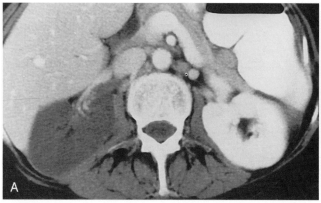 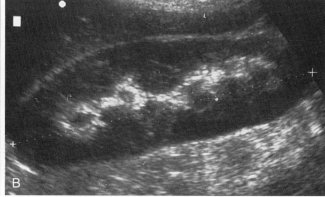

FIGURE 9–14. Acute infarct, right kidney due to septic embolus.
  A, Computed tomogram, contrast material–enhanced. The right kidney is large and smooth and does not enhance.
  B, Ultrasonogram, sagittal projection. The parenchymal echogenicity is normal, and the central sinus structures are compressed.

arteries. Following administration of contrast material, this region is distinguishable from the nonperfused, and thus nonenhanced, underlying parenchyma. A cortical rim sign is best identified by computed tomography, but it can also be demonstrated by excretory urography with tomography (see Fig. 9–16*C*). The same finding has also been described in renal vein thrombosis, probably due to renal ischemia or infarction. Nephrographic striations are another abnormality that has been described in renal contusion due to blunt trauma. Subcapsular collections of blood and thickening of the renal fascia are additional abnormalities that are well demonstrated by computed tomography.

Ultrasonography in acute renal infarction may document the global increase in renal size, but it is more useful in eliminating obstructive uropathy as a cause of unilateral, smooth renal enlargement. The echogenicity of the acutely infarcted kidney may be diminished as a reflection of interstitial fluid accumulation (Fig. 9–14*B*). With time, this pattern will reverse, as fibrosis develops and causes renal wasting. Doppler ultrasonography demonstrates markedly diminished to absent renal arterial and venous blood flow.

Angiography provides specific diagnostic information in renal infarction by identifying traumatic avulsion or occlusion of the renal artery or an embo-

lus or thrombus in the main renal artery or its major branches (Figs. 9–15, 9–16). When infarction is due to blunt trauma or venous thrombosis, the findings are nonspecific and reflect swelling of the interstitium. This is seen as attenuation of arteries, decreased number of branches, increased circulation time, and a disrupted corticomedullary junction. With severe trauma, extravasation may occur within renal parenchyma or into the perirenal space. Other angiographic findings that follow blunt injury to the kidney are arteriovenous fistulas, pseudoaneurysms, and the development of collateral veins.

The magnetic resonance appearance of acute renal infarction has not been studied thoroughly. Limited experience suggests prolongation of T1 relaxation time, low signal intensity, and a loss of corticomedullary differentiation. Enhanced magnetic resonance T1-weighted images may demonstrate wedge-shaped defects that correspond to renal infarcts.

Partial or complete recovery of renal infarction from any cause is always possible. The severity of the initiating event will determine the speed of resolution, which is usually in the range of a few weeks to a few months. If recovery is not complete, the kidney eventually atrophies, as discussed in Chapter 6.

ACUTE ARTERIAL INFARCTION TYPICAL FINDINGS

Primary Uroradiologic Elements

Size: large
Contour: smooth
Lesion distribution: unilateral

Secondary Uroradiologic Elements

Collecting system: attenuated
Nephrogram: absent to diminished density; cortical rim enhancement
Echogenicity: normal

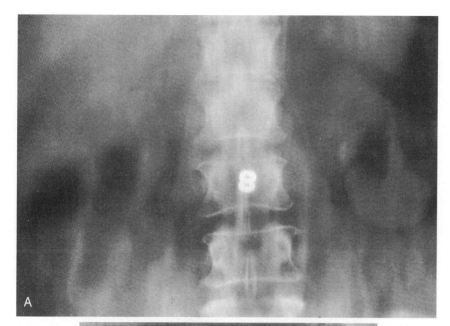

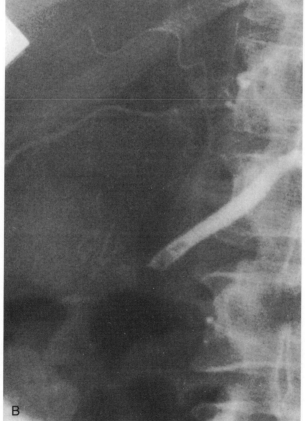

FIGURE 9–15. Acute embolus to main right renal artery in a woman with rheumatic heart disease and atrial fibrillation.
A, Excretory urogram. Tomogram obtained at 30 minutes. The right kidney is enlarged (length = 14.5 cm) and has a faint nephrogram. The left kidney has evidence of old and recent lobar infarctions.
B, Selective right renal arteriogram demonstrates complete occlusion of the main renal artery.

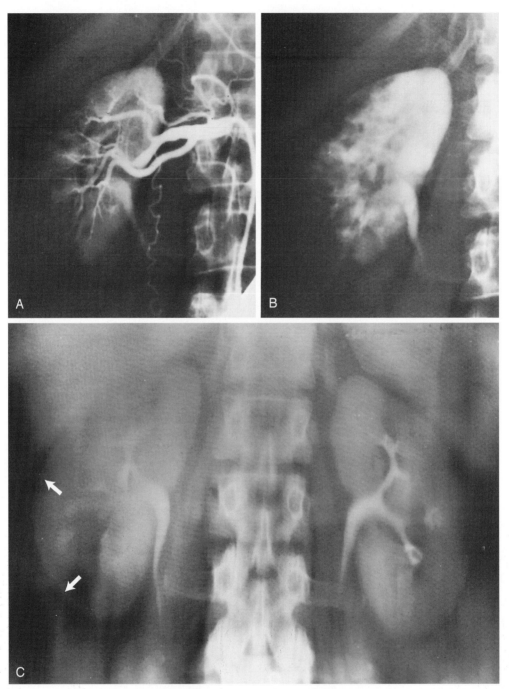

FIGURE 9–16. Segmental renal artery occlusion. Multiple emboli have occluded both interlobar and arcuate arteries. The nephrogram is absent in those portions of the kidney served by the occluded vessels. Collateral blood flow causes a rim of nephrographic density in the cortex.

A, Selective right renal arteriogram, arterial phase. There are numerous points of occlusion.

B, Selective right renal arteriogram, nephrographic phase. The distribution of the perfusion abnormality is well visualized.

C, Excretory urogram. Tomogram. The nephrogram is absent in the lateral portion of the right kidney, except at the rim of the cortex *(arrows)* (same patient illustrated in Fig. 27–10).

(Courtesy of Professor César Pedrosa and E. Ramirez, M.D., Hospital Clinico de San Carlos, Madrid, Spain.)

OBSTRUCTIVE UROPATHY

Obstruction of the urinary tract is discussed in this section in the context of the diagnostic set "large, smooth, unilateral." Other aspects of the subject are presented in Chapter 11, in which the relationship between *in utero* urinary tract obstruction and multicystic dysplastic kidney disease is presented; in Chapter 15, in which congenital ureteropelvic junction obstruction is discussed in detail; and in Chapter 17, in which obstruction is considered as one of several causes of dilatation of the pelvocalyceal system.

Definition

Urinary tract obstruction produces anatomic and functional changes that vary with the rapidity of onset, the degree of occlusion, and the distance between the kidney and the obstructing lesion. The anatomy of the involved renal pelvis, particularly whether its location is intrarenal or extrarenal, is an important additional variable. Some authorities distinguish between an obstruction that produces dilatation of the collecting structures without functional deficit, terming this *hydronephrosis* or *obstructive uropathy,* and an obstruction in which renal functional impairment accompanies dilatation of the urinary conduit, calling this *obstructive nephropathy.*

Urinary tract obstruction has a broad range of characteristics. When obstruction is acute, it is usually due to an easily reversible condition, and only transient functional abnormalities without major structural change develop. Ureteral stone is the prototypical example of this form, in which slight global enlargement of the kidney occurs as a result of interstitial edema and dilatation of renal tubules, principally the distal tubules and the collecting ducts. At the other end of the range, obstruction develops insidiously and silently. By the time of discovery there may be marked structural damage and profound functional derangement. This form of obstruction is seen with congenital narrowing of the ureter, slow-growing ureteral tumors, and retroperitoneal disease. In these cases, the kidney is globally enlarged, often extremely so, owing to marked dilatation of the pelvis and infundibulocalyceal system. Atrophy and fibrosis of the surrounding renal parenchyma occur as a result of pressure from the dilated collecting system and ischemia from a decrease in the size and number of arteries and arterioles.

Clinical Setting

Acute urinary obstruction is most commonly associated with the passage of a calculus or a blood clot. Ureteral colic dominates the clinical picture. Hematuria is usually microscopic in calculus disease and macroscopic when a blood clot is present. With gross hematuria, carcinoma, renal arteriovenous malfor-

mation, trauma, or excessive anticoagulant therapy must be considered as possible alternative causes arising in the upper urinary tract. Surgical trauma, either an inadvertent suture on the ureter or ureteral edema following instrumentation, is a cause of acute obstruction that may be clinically silent.

Urinary tract obstruction can develop insidiously with few, if any, clinical symptoms in a variety of conditions. These include benign and malignant tumors of the ureter and inflammatory strictures and retroperitoneal diseases, usually tumor or fibrosis. Ureteropelvic junction obstruction and ureteral valves are congenital disorders that produce obstructive uropathy. When any of these conditions are bilateral, the ensuing obstructive nephropathy causes azotemic renal failure, which is categorized as *postrenal.*

Regardless of the cause, hydrostatic pressure is increased proximal to an obstruction as long as the kidney produces a normal volume of urine. Rather quickly, however, the increased pressure in the tubule lumina approaches filtration pressure in the glomerular capillaries, and glomerular filtration and urine volume diminish. However, complete cessation of urine formation does not occur because a number of factors operate to partially compensate for the elevated hydrostatic pressure, thereby favoring continued glomerular filtration. These factors include continued urine flow beyond the site of obstruction, continued water reabsorption by the tubules, distention of the pelvis and ureters (whose muscular contractions eventually diminish when a certain degree of dilatation is reached), increased lymphatic uptake of urine, and leakage of urine into interstitial and vascular spaces following spontaneous rupture of the collecting system at the calyceal fornices. Despite these compensating factors, hydrostatic pressure remains elevated throughout the nephrons, collecting tubules, and the extrarenal collecting system to the point of obstruction. This is reversible if the obstruction is relieved. Over time, however, the increased hydrostatic pressure of persistent obstruction causes atrophy of nephrons and an irreversible decrease in the volume of urine formed by the kidney. At this point the thickness of renal parenchyma decreases uniformly while dilatation of the collecting system causes progressive overall enlargement of the kidney. When nephron atrophy reduces the volume of urine formed by the obstructed kidney to an amount equal to that which can pass through the obstruction, the pressure proximal to the obstruction becomes normal, and parenchymal atrophy ceases. Input-output equilibrium may occur at any point along a continuum of severity. Thus, patients with intermediate degrees of obstruction develop moderate parenchymal atrophy and collecting system dilatation that does not progress beyond a certain point, whereas patients with severe obstruction develop nearly total atrophy of nephrons, loss of function, and striking dilatation of the pelvocalyceal system.

Infection is a particularly serious complication

of a chronically obstructed collecting system that requires early recognition and treatment. *Pyonephrosis,* as this condition is known, presents as sepsis in an individual whose urinary tract obstruction has often gone undiagnosed. Purulent exudate collects in the dilated pelvocalyceal system, giving rise to characteristic ultrasonographic features. Renal function, if previously present at all, deteriorates rapidly. Without prompt intervention, the kidney will be destroyed.

Radiologic Findings

The predominant radiologic findings in acute urinary tract obstruction reveal diminished filtration of contrast material rather than the structural effect of obstruction. Compared with the nonobstructed kidney, there is delayed but progressive increase in the density of the nephrogram with time and delayed opacification of the collecting system. These abnormalities are sometimes recognized more easily than subtle dilatation of the calyces, pelvis, or ureter (Fig. 9–17). The nephrogram reflects continued accumulation of iodine-bearing molecules in the tubule lumina and the sluggish or absent forward flow of urine. As obstruction becomes chronic, the radiologic picture is dominated by ureteral and/or pelvic dilatation and renal parenchymal loss in addition to delayed opacification. The nephrogram, no longer progressively dense, becomes faint as the number of nephrons is reduced through pressure atrophy. Global enlargement of the kidney occurs in both acute and chronic obstruction (Fig. 9–18). In some cases of long-standing, unrelieved obstruction, however, the kidney eventually shrinks (Fig. 9–19).

Rupture of the calyceal fornix as a result of rapid calyceal dilatation provides one of the more dramatic imaging findings in acute obstructive uropathy (Figs. 9–20, 9–21). When this occurs, opacified urine can be seen in the renal sinus extending around the renal pelvis and ureters or in the lymphatics or veins. Forniceal rupture may occur spontaneously. Sometimes it is associated with the radiologic procedure itself when the contrast material–induced diuresis produces a sudden increase in urine volume or when abdominal compression is used. Forniceal rupture is more likely to occur in the kidney whose pelvis is surrounded by parenchymal tissue ("intrarenal" pelvis) than in the one whose pelvis is predominantly external to the kidney tissue ("extrarenal" pelvis). The lack of distensibility of the intrarenal pelvis in the face of increased hydrostatic pressure makes the fornix of each calyx more susceptible to rupture. Decompression of the obstructed collecting system follows forniceal rupture. This, in turn, may lead to forward movement of an obstructing calculus on resumption of peristalsis, which had been inhibited by the elevated pressures within the obstructed upper urinary tract. Chronic leakage into the perirenal space leads to the formation of a uriniferous perirenal

pseudocyst or urinoma, which is discussed in Chapter 21.

Acute urinary tract obstruction is associated with two additional findings. The first is alternating radiolucent and radiopaque striae in the nephrogram seen commonly during computed tomography and less often with excretory urography (Fig. 9–22). The striae are oriented perpendicular to the surface of the kidney and are seen in some cases of acute obstruction due to ureteral calculus. Striae are believed to represent contrast material in dilated tubules and collecting ducts in the medullary rays. The second urographic finding, which is uncommon, is opacification of the gallbladder late in the course of the urographic examination in patients with acute unilateral obstruction due to ureteral stone and a normal contralateral kidney (Fig. 9–23). This phenomenon is related to increased hepatic excretion of contrast material due to prolonged plasma disappearance time. Gallbladder opacification in this circumstance is detected on radiographs of the abdomen obtained 8 to 24 hours after administration of contrast material.

When urinary tract obstruction has been present for an extended time, the radiologic findings are dominated by dilatation of the pelvocalyceal system and ureter proximal to the obstruction (Fig. 9–24). The silhouette of the calyces usually produces a multilobulated sac, but in extreme cases only a single dilated structure is all that remains of the entire pelvoinfundibulocalyceal system. Contrast material enhancement of the compressed and atrophic renal parenchyma surrounding dilated calyces produces the *rim sign of chronic obstruction* (Fig. 9–25). This sign must be kept separate from the *cortical rim* sign of complete or major segmental acute arterial infarction that was discussed in the previous section. Opacification of this tissue is slower and less dense than that of tissue on the contralateral side. The pattern of increasing nephrographic density over time that is seen in acute obstructive uropathy is absent, representing nephron loss through atrophy, a reduction in the volume of urine being formed, and the resulting normalization of hydrostatic pressure in the collecting system (Fig. 9–26). On early urographic films, the nephrogram of the compressed parenchyma outlines the nonopacified dilated collecting systems, producing a *negative pyelogram* (Fig. 9–27; see Fig. 9–25). Delayed films will eventually demonstrate opacification of the dilated collecting system itself as contrast material passes downward from nephrons into the large reservoir of nonopacified urine. The demonstration of the pelvocalyceal system may require films as late as 24 hours after injection of contrast material. Upright films in which contrast material accumulates in dependent portions of the dilated system may facilitate earlier visualization (Fig. 9–28). In chronic obstruction of intermediate severity, a narrow, semilunar band of marked radiodensity at the interface between renal parenchyma and a dilated calyx may be seen during contrast material–

Text continued on page 208

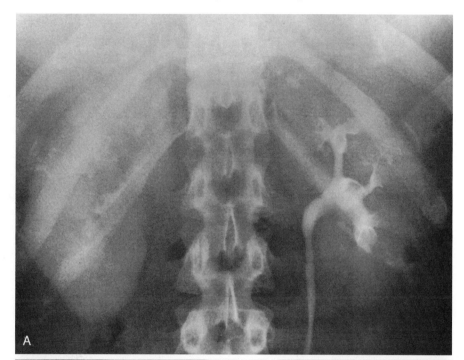

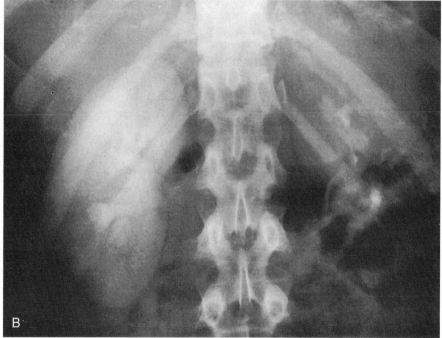

FIGURE 9–17. Acute obstructive uropathy in a young woman with right distal ureteral obstruction due to stone (same patient illustrated in Fig. 27–15).

A, Excretory urogram, 10-minute film. There is delayed parenchymal and collecting system opacification as compared with that of the normal left kidney.

B, Excretory urogram, 4-hour film. The nephrogram has become increasingly dense, and the slightly dilated collecting system is opacified.

C, Delayed upright film of pelvis demonstrates distal ureteral obstruction secondary to stone. The calculus itself is not identified.

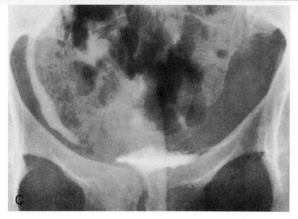

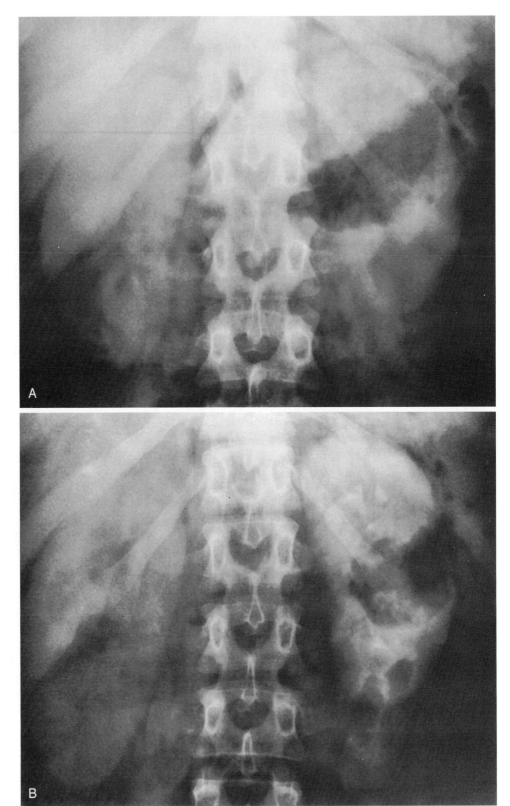

FIGURE 9–18. Obstructive uropathy causing renal enlargement in a 36-year-old woman who developed a vesicovaginal fistula following radiation therapy for carcinoma of the cervix. Bilateral ureteral obstruction, more severe on the right side, developed after a ureteroileostomy was performed because of the fistula.

A, Excretory urogram, 1-minute film before radiation therapy. Right kidney length = 12.0 cm; left kidney length = 11.0 cm.

B, Excretory urogram, 1-minute film, 2 years after ureteroileostomy. Obstruction is present bilaterally, and both kidneys have enlarged. A negative pyelogram is present on the more severely obstructed right side. Right kidney length = 14.3 cm; left kidney length = 12.3 cm.

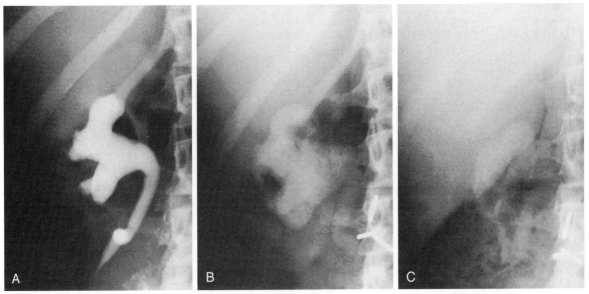

FIGURE 9–19. Obstructive uropathy leading to atrophy in an 18-year-old woman with choriosarcoma of the ovary metastatic to the right periaortic lymph nodes.

A, Initial excretory urogram. Metastatic nodes, opacified following lymphangiography, displace and obstruct the proximal ureter. Kidney length = 12.4 cm.

B, Excretory urogram 5 months later. Obstruction has not been relieved by intervening surgery. Kidney length = 12.1 cm.

C, Excretory urogram 2 years after initial study. Right kidney function is severely impaired. Kidney length = 5.8 cm.

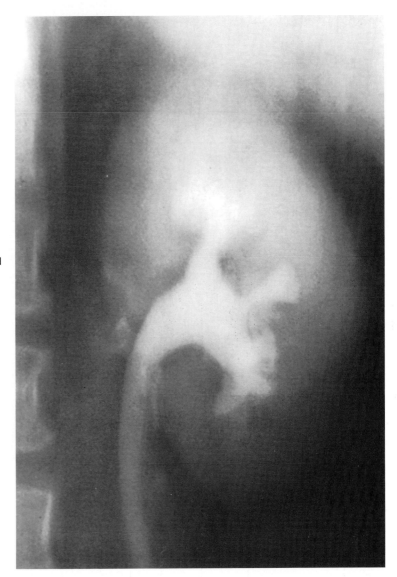

FIGURE 9–20. Acute obstructive uropathy complicated by forniceal rupture and by leakage of contrast material into the renal sinus. Contrast material is seen in tissue between the calyces and outside the pelvis and the proximal ureter. This complication occurs more frequently in kidneys with "intrarenal" location of the pelvis, as illustrated in this patient.

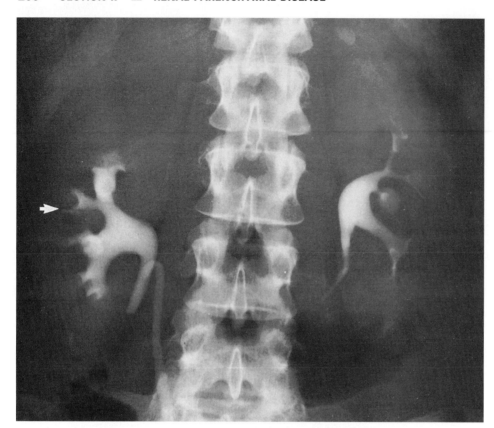

FIGURE 9–21. Acute obstructive uropathy due to stone in the right distal ureter. There is minimal enlargement of the pelvocalyceal system. Dilatation of the forniceal angles and leakage of contrast material into the sinus *(arrow)* through a ruptured fornix reflect elevated hydrostatic pressure in the pelvis of the kidney. Excretory urogram, 20-minute film (same patient illustrated in Fig. 17–4).

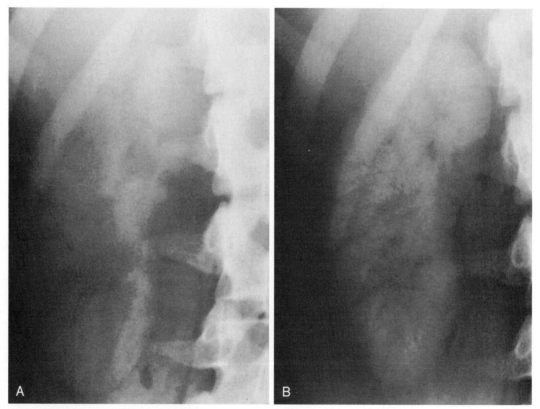

FIGURE 9–22. Acute obstructive uropathy associated with a striated nephrogram believed to represent contrast material in dilated tubules in the medullary rays (same patient illustrated in Fig. 27–19).
   A, Excretory urogram, 5-minute film. Delayed opacification.
   B, Excretory urogram, 45-minute film. Striae are well illustrated.

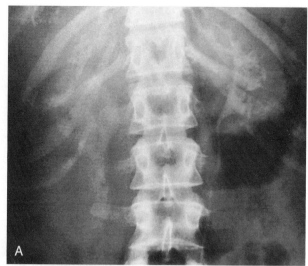

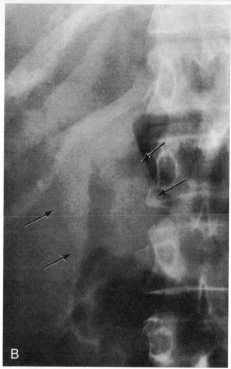

FIGURE 9–23. Gallbladder opacification following excretory urography in a 33-year-old woman with acute obstructive uropathy due to right ureteral stone.

 A, Excretory urogram, 5-minute film. Delayed right-sided opacification. Normal left kidney.

 B, 24-hour film of the abdomen. The faintly opacified gallbladder is to the right of the first and second lumbar vertebrae *(arrows).*

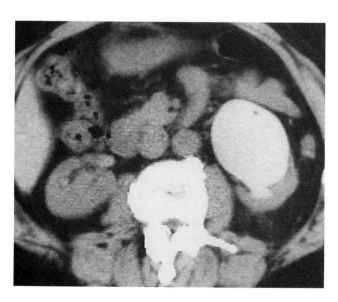

FIGURE 9–24. Chronic obstructive uropathy of the left kidney. Computed tomogram, contrast material–enhanced. There is marked dilatation of the collecting system and thinning of the renal parenchyma. The nephrogram no longer demonstrates the increasingly dense pattern of acute obstruction (same patient illustrated in Fig. 17–12).

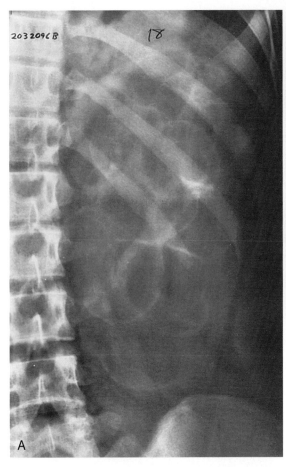

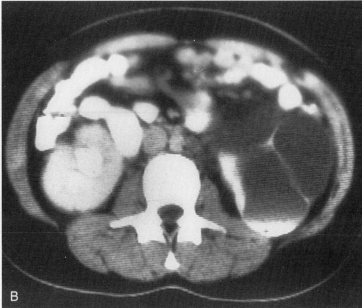

FIGURE 9–25. Chronic obstructive uropathy of the left kidney. The kidney is enlarged and smooth and composed of very thin bands of atrophic renal parenchyma surrounding dilated calyces. Opacification of the atrophied bands of parenchyma constitute the *rim sign of chronic obstruction.* The nonopacified, dilated collecting structures are called the *negative pyelogram.*

A, Excretory urogram.

B, Computed tomogram, contrast material–enhanced. Layering of contrast material in the dilated collecting system is also demonstrated.

enhanced studies of the kidney (see Fig. 9–28A). This observation—the *calyceal crescent* sign—represents concentrated contrast material in the distal collecting ducts that have become oriented perpendicular rather than parallel to the normal axis of their calyx and infundibulum.

The radiologist should attempt to demonstrate the point of obstruction and thereby eliminate the need for retrograde instrumentation. This can be achieved in many obstructed patients by using an appropriately large dose of contrast material and by obtaining delayed films supplemented by fluoroscopy (see Fig. 9–17C). Positioning the patient upright or prone encourages the high-specific-gravity–contrast material to settle into the distal portions of the urinary collecting system. Antegrade pyelography performed through a catheter or a needle placed percutaneously through the flank and into the dilated system is a valuable technique in the demonstration of the point of obstruction.

A balanced state between the volume of urine formed and the volume of urine that passes beyond an incomplete obstruction produces urographic findings of moderate parenchymal thinning and collecting system dilatation with variable degrees of renal enlargement (Fig. 9–29; see also Fig. 9–24). The nephrogram may be diminished in peak density compared with that of the nonobstructed contralateral kidney, but the time-density curve follows a normal rather than an increasingly dense pattern (see Chapter 27). These abnormalities do not progress unless the severity of the obstruction progresses.

Unenhanced helical computed tomography using 5-mm collimation with image reconstruction as needed is an efficacious method for the diagnosis of acute ureteral obstruction, especially when the obstruction is caused by a stone (Fig. 9–30). In addition to the direct identification of an obstructing calculus, other findings include slight dilatation of the collecting system and ureter to the point of obstruction, linear strands of soft-tissue density coursing through the perinephric fat, increased thickness of the parenchyma of the obstructed kidney, and edema of the ureter at the site of the impacted calculus. The presence of this latter finding, called the *tissue-rim* sign, serves to distinguish an obstructing stone from a pelvic phlebolith in close proximity to the ureter. The urine-filled, dilated pelvocalyceal system has an attenuation value close to that of water and is readily distinguished from the higher values of the unenhanced renal parenchyma. Parapelvic cysts (discussed in Chapter 16) have an appearance on unenhanced computed tomograms that may be identical to that of hydronephrosis. Distinction between these two entities requires the use of contrast material to demonstrate enhancement of the obstructed system or the ab-

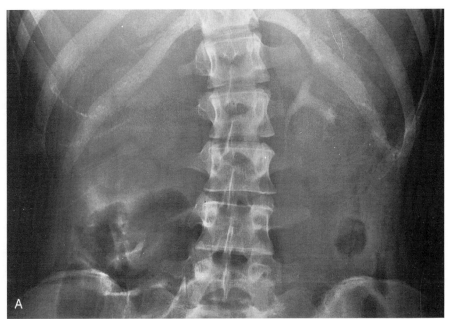

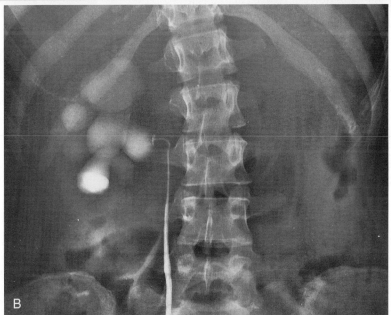

FIGURE 9–26. Chronic obstructive uropathy of the right kidney due to lymphoma of the retroperitoneum infiltrating the proximal ureter.

A, Excretory urogram, 10-minute film. The nephrogram is barely perceived even at its maximum. There is faint opacification of dilated calyces.

B, Retrograde pyelogram. A narrowed proximal ureter and the dilated collecting system are identified.

C, Ultrasonogram, longitudinal section. The anechoic, dilated collecting system confirms the diagnosis.

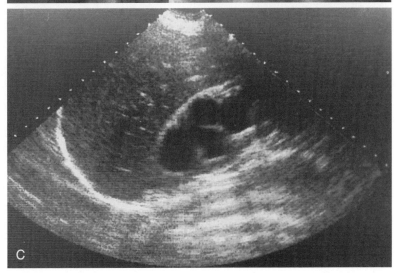

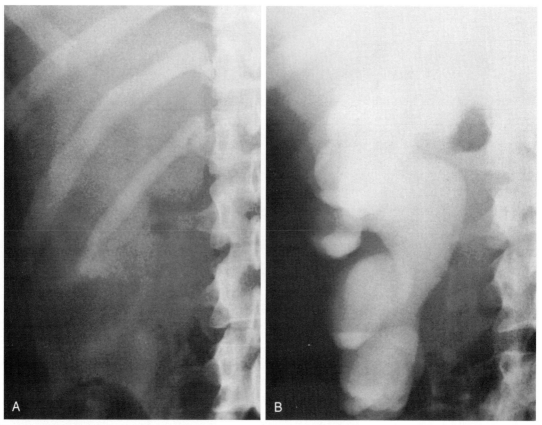

FIGURE 9–27. Chronic obstructive uropathy in a 27-year-old woman with long-standing ureteropelvic junction obstruction. Kidney length = 16.3 cm (same patient illustrated in Fig. 17–8).

A, Excretory urogram. Early film demonstrates the nephrogram of compressed parenchyma (the "rim" sign) surrounding the nonopacified dilated calyces: the *negative pyelogram.*

B, Excretory urogram. The previously radiolucent dilated calyces are opacified on a delayed upright film.

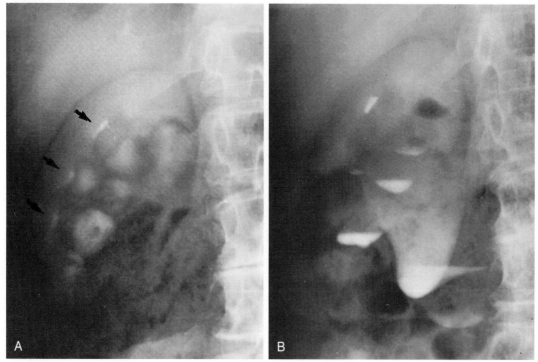

FIGURE 9–28. Chronic obstructive uropathy. Early demonstration of dilated collecting system on an upright film.

A, Excretory urogram, supine film. Narrow, semilunar bands of contrast material *(arrows)* called *calyceal crescents* are present at the interface between renal parenchyma and the faintly opacified dilated calyces.

B, Excretory urogram, upright film. Layering of contrast material facilitates visualization of dilated calyces.

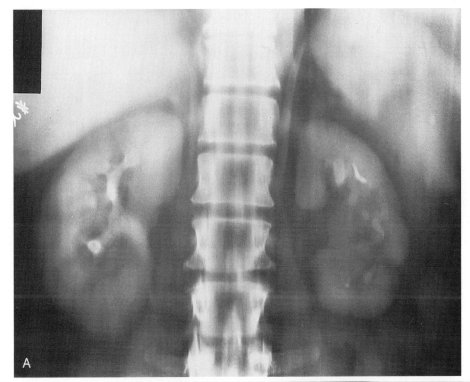

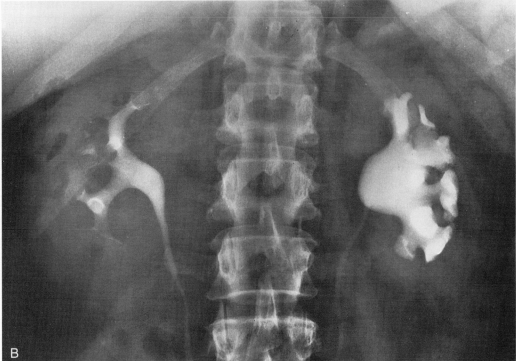

FIGURE 9–29. Chronic obstructive uropathy of the left kidney, intermediate grade. There is moderate parenchymal thinning and collecting system dilatation, but the time-density pattern of the nephrogram is normal, indicating a stable state.

    A, Excretory urogram, 3-minute tomogram.

    B, Excretory urogram, 10-minute film.

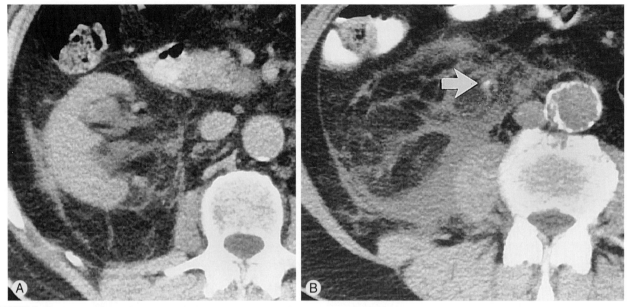

FIGURE 9–30. Acute obstruction due to right ureteral stone. Helical computed tomography, unenhanced.

A, Section at level of the right renal hilum demonstrates slight dilatation of the collecting system, global enlargement of the kidney, and thickening of the renal fascia and perirenal septa.

B, Section at level of a dense obstructing ureteral calculus *(arrow).* The ureteral tissue surrounding the calculus is thickened: the *tissue rim* sign. There are numerous soft-tissue densities throughout the perirenal space.

sence of enhancement in the case of the parapelvic cyst (see Fig. 16–4). In pyonephrosis, the attenuation value of the pus-filled hydronephrotic collecting system is greater than that of water. In the absence of an obstructing stone to explain acute colic, unenhanced helical computed tomography is likely to define another cause.

The contrast material-enhanced computed tomographic findings of acute and chronic obstruction parallel those of excretory urography. In addition, computed tomography demonstrates prolonged selective enhancement of the cortex relative to the medulla in acute obstruction, an observation not seen during excretory urography because of the superimposition of cortex and medulla on standard radiography of the kidney.

The sensitivity of ultrasonography in the diagnosis of obstructive uropathy is dependent on the degree of dilatation of the pelvocalyceal system. Because dilatation of the collecting system is not a major early feature of acute obstructive uropathy, ultrasonography is of limited value in establishing this diagnosis. Here, unenhanced helical computed tomography, as described previously, is the most sensitive test. The period for the progression of collecting system dilatation has not been established precisely. Nevertheless, within a few days following the onset of symptoms, dilatation becomes detectable as a central, fluid-filled, branching structure (see Fig. 9–26C). Consequently, the sensitivity of ultrasonography is approximately 98 per cent in the diagnosis of obstruction beyond the immediate stage of acute obstruction. This subject, including causes of false-positive and false-negative results, is discussed in detail in Chapter 17. Ultrasonogra-

phy is particularly valuable in suggesting the diagnosis of pyonephrosis. In this condition, the dilated, fluid-filled collecting system will also contain echogenic material representing pus, stones, and cellular debris (Fig. 9–31). This echo pattern may be limited to the dependent part of the pelvis and form a fluid-debris level that shifts with changes in the position of the patient. Other ultrasonographic patterns of pyonephrosis are dense peripheral echoes

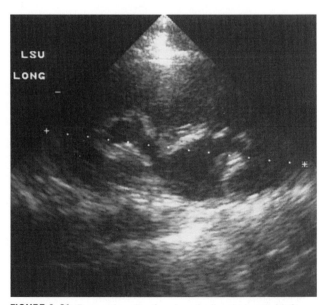

FIGURE 9–31. Pyonephrosis of a chronically obstructed left kidney. Ultrasonogram, longitudinal section. The dilated pelvocalyceal system separates the central sinus complex and contains diffuse faint echoes caused by inflammatory debris. (Kindly provided by Sheila Sheth, M. D., and Ulrike Hamper, M.D., Johns Hopkins University, Baltimore, Maryland).

OBSTRUCTIVE UROPATHY TYPICAL FINDINGS

Acute Obstructive Uropathy

Primary Uroradiologic Elements

Size: large
Contour: smooth
Lesion distribution: unilateral

Secondary Uroradiologic Elements

Collecting system: opacification time delayed; dilated (minimal); disrupted (occasional focal forniceal tear)
Nephrogram: delayed; increasingly dense
Perirenal space: stranding
Ureter: *tissue-rim* sign
Parenchymal Doppler: variable elevation resistive index

Chronic Obstructive Uropathy

Primary Uroradiologic Elements

Size: large
Contour: smooth
Lesion distribution: unilateral

Secondary Uroradiologic Elements

Collecting system: opacification time delayed *(negative pyelogram)*; dilated (moderate to marked); attenuation value equal to water
Parenchymal thickness: wasted
Nephrogram: diminished density; thick walls (*rim* sign); *calyceal crescent* sign
Echogenicity: anechoic, dilated collecting system

---

caused by bubbles of gas and diminished sound transmission with diffuse echoes throughout the collecting system. Stones are strongly echogenic and cause acoustic shadows.

The radiologic findings in obstructive uropathy are not always straightforward, particularly in cases in which the severity or the duration of the abnormality is intermediate or the obstruction is intermittent. Provocative tests, such as diuresis urography or diuresis renography, have been developed for these problems. Further discussion of these as well as of direct pressure-flow studies of the pelvocalyceal system are included in Chapters 2, 15, and 17.

Doppler ultrasonography has been suggested for the evaluation of patients with suspected acute obstructive uropathy (Platt, 1994, 1996). The potential value of this technique has been based on the concept that an elevated resistive index in acute obstruction provides greater diagnostic accuracy than gray-scale ultrasonography, in which accuracy is diminished by both false-negative findings (patients imaged at a time before dilatation of the collecting system is detectable by ultrasonography) and false-positive diagnoses (patients with dilatation that is not caused by obstruction). The potential value of Doppler ultrasonography has not been realized, however, because of the considerable overlap in resistive index values in patients with and without disease. Presumably, this represents both wide vari-

ation of normal values and the operator-dependent nature of Doppler ultrasonography.

Magnetic resonance urography is another technique that has been proposed for imaging the acutely obstructed urinary tract. This technique takes advantage of the very long T2 relaxation time of urine within a dilated collecting system and ureter in comparison with other tissues. T2-weighted images obtained in the coronal plane to encompass the kidneys, ureters, and bladder are obtained during suspended respiration to decrease motion artifact. A variety of techniques have been used. The advantages of this form of urography over existing techniques are that it avoids both ionizing radiation and exposure to contrast material and, thus, may be of particular value in children and pregnant women. Disadvantages, on the other hand, include the failure to discern the normal ureter in most cases, obscuring of the ureter by bowel and other high-signal structures in the retroperitoneum, and the inability to distinguish stone from tumor as the cause of the obstruction. The ultimate role of magnetic resonance urography remains to be determined.

ACUTE PYELONEPHRITIS

Definition

Acute upper urinary tract infection, characterized by fever, flank pain, bacteriuria, and pyuria, is a cause of unilateral global renal enlargement. Acute pyelonephritis develops from pathogenic coliform bacteria that initially enter the bladder from perineal or vaginal colonies by way of the urethra. A short urethra explains the prevalence of urinary tract infections in females, whereas both the greater length of the urethra and antibacterial properties of prostatic secretions have a protective effect against urinary tract infection from coliform bacteria in males. Pathogenic bacteria move from the bladder into the upper tract by either of two mechanisms: vesicoureteral reflux (most commonly in newborns and infants) or moving against urine flow while adhering to ureteral epithelium (more commonly in children and adults).

Acute pyelonephritis develops when bacteria pass from pelvocalyceal urine through papillary duct orifices and provoke an acute tubulointerstitial nephritis along the course of the medullary rays (see Chapter 3). From a gross morphologic view, this inflammatory response involves the full thickness of a renal lobe or a part of a lobe, extending from the tip of the papilla to the surface of the kidney. There is a sharp line of demarcation between the area of inflammation and the adjacent portions of normal parenchyma. Inflammatory exudate fills and obstructs collecting tubules and ducts, and the acute inflammatory cell infiltrate diminishes urine formation in the affected nephrons by obliterating the microvasculature of the affected tissue.

Lobar or sublobar acute tubulointerstitial nephritis involving the medullary rays, then, is the elemental pathologic process present in the earliest stages of reflux nephropathy (see Chapter 5); in all degrees of severity of acute pyelonephritis, including emphysematous pyelonephritis (discussed in this section); and in the evolution of renal abscess secondary to ascending infections (see Chapter 12). These entities differ from each other by virtue of differences in the cellular, humoral, or immunologic factors that constitute the host response of any given individual. Thus, scarring in the newborn *(reflux nephropathy)*, early resolution without structural damage to the kidney in the older child or adult *(uncomplicated acute pyelonephritis)*, overwhelming involvement of the kidney with eventual structural damage *(severe acute pyelonephritis or emphysematous pyelonephritis)*, and liquefaction and encapsulation *(abscess)* represent different tissue responses to the common element of acute tubulointerstitial nephritis. Patient age, use of anti-inflammatory or immunosuppressive drugs, or coexistent diseases (diabetes mellitus, autoimmune deficiency syndrome, drug abuse) determine host response.

Renal parenchymal involvement may not be present in all cases of uncomplicated acute pyelonephritis. The limited nature of the clinical syndrome and the lack of structural or functional damage to the kidney over time suggest that the clinical syndrome may sometimes be due to pyelitis rather than to pyelonephritis. However, there is a substantial anecdotal radiologic experience that suggests parenchymal involvement in at least some, if not most, patients.

Clinical Setting

Acute pyelonephritis, thus defined, predominantly affects girls and women to approximately age 40 years. The infecting organism is most commonly *Escherichia coli.* Recurrent episodes may involve different serotypes of the same genus or other gram-negative bacteria, such as *Enterobacter* species, *Klebsiella* species, *Pseudomonas aeruginosa,* or *Proteus mirabilis.* It is generally accepted that these organisms ascend to the upper urinary tract by way of the ureter rather than by following lymphatic or hematogenous routes.

The sudden onset of fever, chills, flank pain, frequency, and dysuria is the usual clinical pattern of acute pyelonephritis. Leukocytosis is present. Urinalysis reveals bacteria, leukocytes, leukocyte casts, and red blood cells. Bacteriuria is considered "significant" if quantitative culture of a cleanly voided urine specimen reveals more than 100,000 bacteria per milliliter of urine.

This disorder may be limited to a single episode or may follow a pattern of recurrent attacks. In the interval between acute symptomatic episodes, some patients have sterile urine; others have bacteriuria without symptoms. In some individuals, especially infants and very young children, structural damage in the form of focal kidney scars overlying dilated calyces evolve, as discussed in the section on reflux nephropathy in Chapter 5. In others, particularly older children and adults, scarring of this nature does not occur even with recurrent episodes of uncomplicated acute pyelonephritis unless there is underlying obstruction or neuropathic bladder disease leading to vesicoureteral reflux.

There is a severe form of acute pyelonephritis that causes both functional and structural damage to the affected kidney with distinctive radiologic abnormalities. This form of acute pyelonephritis occurs in patients with compromised host resistance, most often due to diabetes mellitus but also associated with immunosuppression, long-term corticosteroid therapy, intravenous drug abuse, or acquired immunodeficiency syndrome. Cases of women with diabetes mellitus, often previously undiagnosed, and without a prior history of urinary tract infection have been the predominant ones reported. The acute infection of the parenchyma may be diffuse and generalized or may have a patchy or multifocal distribution. In some patients, a regional pattern of involvement is demonstrated by radiologic studies, principally computed tomography. Involvement of both kidneys leading to acute renal failure has been reported. Patients with severe acute pyelonephritis present with fever or septicemia and often do not have localized physical findings. *E. coli* is the most common pathogen. Appropriate antibiotic therapy usually produces favorable results when the infection is recognized promptly. Unlike uncomplicated acute pyelonephritis in older children and adults, severe acute pyelonephritis may lead to global renal atrophy and papillary necrosis. Other terms used to describe this condition are *acute bacterial nephritis, acute suppurative pyelonephritis, adult-onset acute bacterial nephritis, acute focal bacterial nephritis, segmental bacterial nephritis,* and *lobar nephronia.* It has been recommended that none of these terms be used as a substitute for the term acute pyelonephritis (Talner et al., 1994).

Emphysematous pyelonephritis is the most severe form of acute pyelonephritis, representing a stage of infection that includes the formation of gas in the pelvocalyceal system, in the interstices of renal parenchyma, and in the subcapsular and perirenal space. This develops in patients with compromised host response, most commonly due to diabetes mellitus. Septicemia and shock dominate the clinical picture. Mortality in this condition, which also has distinctive radiologic features, is greater than 50 per cent.

Radiologic investigations are usually not performed in older girls and adult women who develop acute pyelonephritis that responds rapidly to treatment. Imaging studies are performed in those patients who either fail to respond to therapy or who have relapses involving the same serotype organism. Here, a careful assessment is required to exclude underlying papillary necrosis, congenital anomalies, obstruction, urolithiasis, medullary sponge kidney, or evidence of vesicoureteral reflux.

On the other hand, urinary tract imaging is usually indicated in males who develop acute pyelonephritis for the first time, even when response to therapy is rapid.

Radiologic Findings

The likelihood of detecting radiologic abnormalities in uncomplicated acute pyelonephritis depends on how soon after the onset of symptoms the examination is performed. Abnormal excretory urographic findings can be expected in nearly one-half of the patients who are examined within the first 24 hours of the onset of symptoms. This number diminishes rapidly following successful antibiotic therapy.

Global enlargement of the kidney is the most frequent abnormal finding. Decreased density of contrast material, delayed calyceal opacification, pelviectasis and caliectasis, focal polar swelling, and focal calyceal compression are additional excretory urographic abnormalities found in these patients (Figs. 9–32, 9–33). The same abnormalities are demonstrable by computed tomography, whose greater contrast resolution and cross-sectional anatomic display result in more readily detectable nephrographic abnormalities. These are characterized by sharply defined wedge-shaped zones of diminished enhancement that radiate from the collecting system to the renal surface and enhance only slightly after contrast material is administered. These features reflect lobar or sublobar acute tubulointerstitial nephritis in the distribution of medullary rays. Striations within these wedge-shaped, low-density zones may be present (Figs.

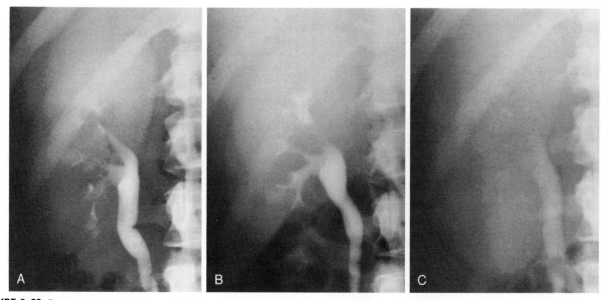

FIGURE 9–32. Recurrent acute pyelonephritis in a 29-year-old woman.
A, Excretory urogram during an acute episode of pyelonephritis. There is some enlargement of the kidney and calycealinfundibular effacement. Kidney length = 13.3 cm.
B, Normal excretory urogram 2 years after the initial examination, taken when the patient was asymptomatic. Kidney length = 12.9 cm.
C, Excretory urogram during another acute episode of pyelonephritis 3 years after the first study. There is impaired excretion of contrast material, smooth enlargement of the kidney, and an effaced pelvocalyceal system. Note the absence of focal scars. Kidney length = 13.9 cm.

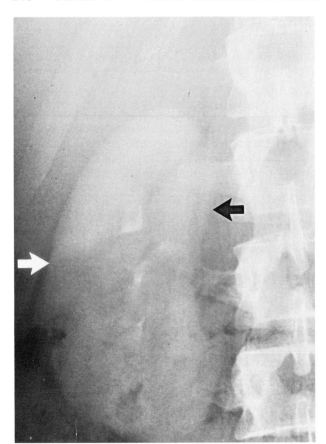

FIGURE 9–33. Acute pyelonephritis of the lower two-thirds of the right kidney. Excretory urogram, 2-minute film. There is a sharp demarcation in nephrographic density between the normal upper one-third and the involved lowered portion of the kidney (arrows) where the nephrogram is less dense. The acutely infected portion of the kidney is enlarged and smooth, and its collecting system is effaced.

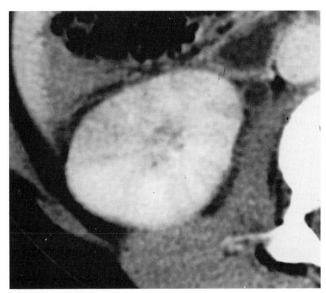

FIGURE 9–35. Acute pyelonephritis, right kidney. A striated nephrogram in the dorsomedial kidney represents sublobar areas of involvement. There is also an unenhanced area in the ventrolateral kidney that conforms to a lobar distribution (same patient illustrated in Fig. 5–5). (Kindly provided by Massoud Majd, M.D., Children's National Medical Center, Washington, D.C.)

9–34, 9–35, 9–36). In some patients, the nephrographic defects are patchy and less sharply defined. All of these areas are isodense with normal parenchyma before contrast material is administered. If delayed computed tomographic scans are obtained, the sites of nephrographic deficiency may become abnormally dense and persistent as contrast material slowly accumulates in tubules and collecting ducts that are plugged with inflammatory cells (see Fig. 9–36).

Radionuclide images of acute pyelonephritis using parenchymal agents, such as ^{99m}Tc-DMSA, demonstrate the areas of lobar or sublobar tubulointerstitial nephritis as striated, wedge-shaped or regional areas of diminished uptake (Fig. 9–37).

Ultrasonography results in uncomplicated acute pyelonephritis are generally normal, but ultrasonography is often performed to exclude processes

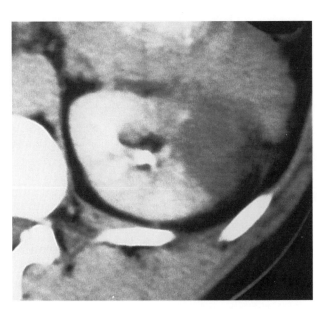

FIGURE 9–34. Acute pyelonephritis in a lobar distribution, left kidney. Computed tomography, contrast material–enhanced. A sharply defined, full-thickness, wedge-shaped unenhanced region representing lobar acute infection. There is some perinephric involvement.

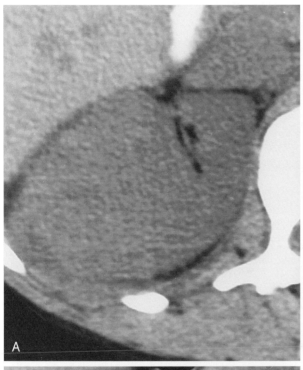

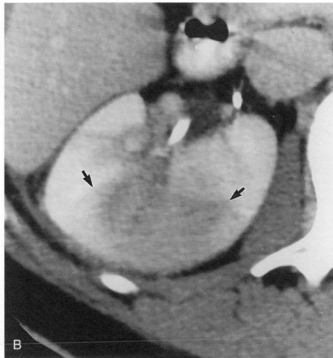

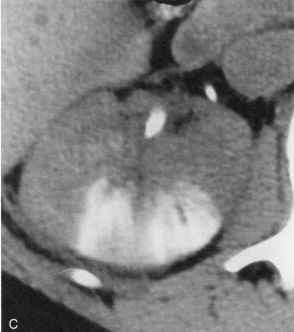

FIGURE 9–36. Acute pyelonephritis, upper pole, right kidney. Computed tomography.

A, Unenhanced scan demonstrates smooth enlargement of the kidney. The area of acute infection has the same attenuation value as uninvolved areas.

B, Scan obtained soon after contrast material administration demonstrates a wedge-shaped area of decreased attenuation *(arrows).*

C, Delayed scan. There is accumulation of contrast material in the area of acute infection, which was previously unenhanced.

(Kindly provided by Professor Ludovico Dalla Palma, M.D., Roberto Pozzi-Mucelli, M.D., and Fabio Pozzi-Mucelli, M.D., University of Trieste, Italy. Reproduced from Semin Ultrasound CT MRI *18*:122, 1997, with permission of the authors and publisher.)

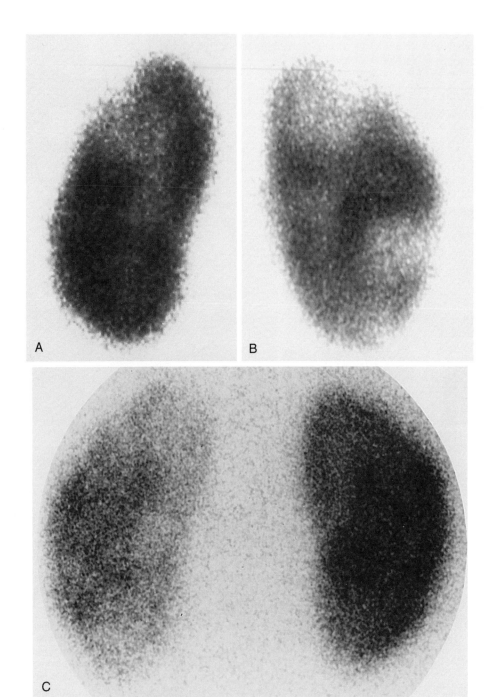

FIGURE 9–37. Acute pyelonephritis in three different individuals. ^{99m}Tc-DMSA posterior scans demonstrate decrease in radionuclide uptake at sites of involvement.
  A, Single focus, upper pole, left kidney.
  B, Multifocal involvement, right kidney.
  C, Severe acute pyelonephritis, left kidney, in a diabetic patient with diffuse involvement.
  (Kindly provided by Massoud Majd, M.D., Children's National Medical Center, Washington, D.C.)

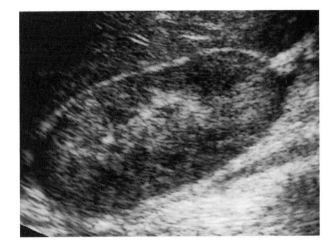

FIGURE 9–38. Acute pyelonephritis, right kidney. Ultrasonogram, sagittal projection. The kidney is enlarged with a smooth contour. There are some areas of borderline decrease in echogenicity. (Kindly provided by Lee Talner, M.D., University of Washington, Seattle, Washington.)

such as obstruction, pyonephrosis, or abscess. Enlargement of the kidney and diminished parenchymal echogenicity may be either generalized or regional (Fig. 9–38). A smooth renal margin is preserved. The focal decreased perfusion characteristic of acute pyelonephritis can be documented by power Doppler ultrasonography (Fig. 9–39).

The radiologic findings of severe acute pyelonephritis that occur in patients with a compromised immune status reflect an extreme expression of the spectrum of abnormalities of acute pyelonephritis. In these patients, there is a marked reduction in renal function seen on contrast material–enhanced images as a diminished to absent nephrogram and collecting system opacification (see Fig. 9–42). The kidney is markedly enlarged and smooth in outline. Computed tomography and radionuclide scans demonstrate the nephrographic defects particularly well, and they may be patchy or involve the entire kidney uniformly (Fig. 9–40). Severe acute pyelonephritis may be associated with multifocal areas of suppuration and liquefaction (Fig. 9–41). These abscesses cause mass effects on the collecting structures and produce the same radiologic findings as a simple, unifocal abscess, which is described in Chapter 12. The abscesses may rupture through the subcapsular space into the perinephric space.

Severe acute pyelonephritis appears as a large,

smooth kidney with diminished echogenicity in ultrasonographic studies. Anechoic focal masses in areas where abscess formation has developed may be seen.

Characteristically, the radiologic and functional abnormalities of severe acute pyelonephritis return to normal shortly after the start of the appropriate antibiotic therapy (Fig. 9–42). However, unlike resolved, uncomplicated acute pyelonephritis, permanent structural damage is often present. Papillary necrosis is apparent as soon as the kidney is able to excrete enough contrast material to opacify the collecting system. In fact, it is likely that papillary necrosis is present in the earliest stage of severe acute pyelonephritis but goes undetected because visualization of the calyces is not possible. Within a few weeks to months, global wasting of the recovered kidney will become apparent (see Figs. 6–17, 6–18). Thus, postinflammatory atrophy enters the differential diagnosis of the unilateral, small, smooth kidney (see the discussion in Chapter 6).

Radiolucent gas in and around an enlarged, non-opacified kidney characterizes the radiologic findings in a gas-forming infection of the kidney, known as emphysematous pyelonephritis (Figs. 9–43, 9–44, 9–45). In this serious condition, gas is present in the pelvocalyceal system, interstitial tissue, and perirenal space and is best demonstrated by com-

Text continued on page 224

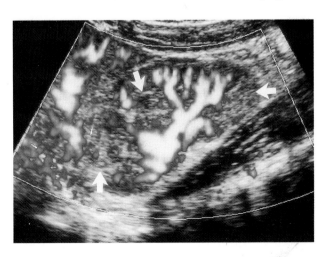

FIGURE 9–39. Acute pyelonephritis, multifocal, right kidney. Power Doppler ultrasonogram, sagittal projection. There are three areas of hypoperfusion *(arrows)*. (Kindly provided by Massoud Majd, M.D., Children's National Medical Center, Washington, D.C.)

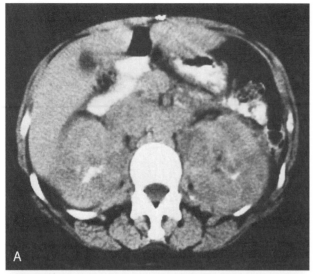

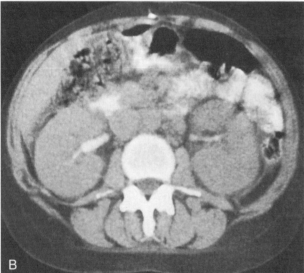

FIGURE 9–40. Acute bacterial nephritis involving both kidneys in a drug addict with acute renal failure. Computed tomogram, contrast material–enhanced.

A, Section through the superior part of the kidneys demonstrates smooth, global enlargement and patchy nephrograms.

B, Section obtained through the lower parts of the kidneys demonstrates homogeneous, although diminished, nephrograms and effaced collecting systems.

(Courtesy of H. Hricak, M.D., University of California, San Francisco.)

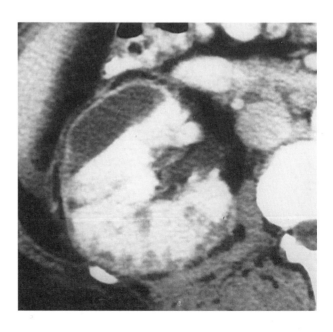

FIGURE 9–41. Severe acute pyelonephritis, right kidney, evolving into multiple abscesses and a subcapsular fluid collection. Computed tomography, contrast material–enhanced.

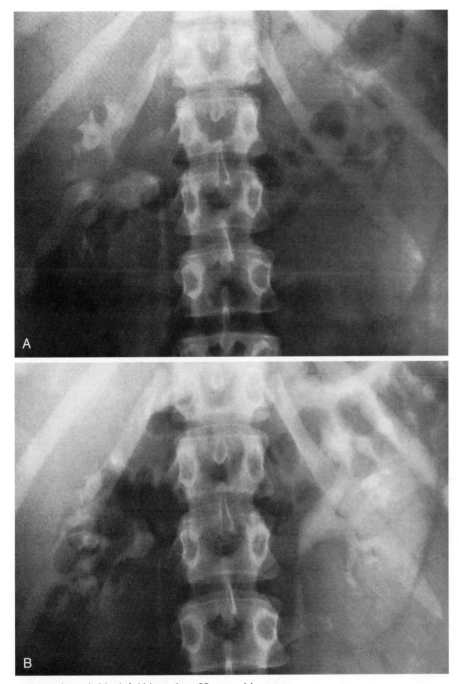

FIGURE 9–42. Severe acute pyelonephritis, left kidney, in a 23-year-old woman.

A, Excretory urogram reveals enlarged left kidney, persistent nephrogram of diminished density, and faint opacification of nondilated calyces.

B, Excretory urogram 7 days after initial examination during the course of appropriate antibiotic therapy. Kidney size is smaller. The calyces opacify promptly and are no longer effaced. (Reproduced from Radiology *106:*249, 1973, with permission).

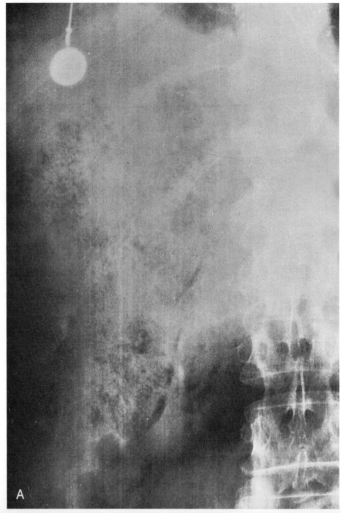

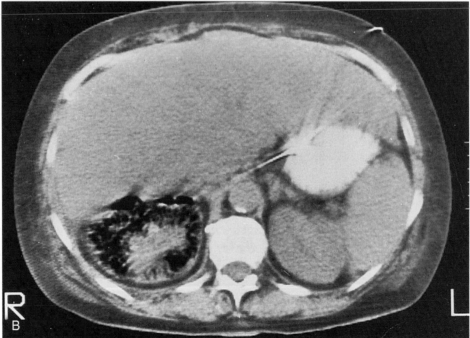

FIGURE 9–43. Emphysematous pyelonephritis of the right kidney. Gas is present in the interstitium of the kidney and the medial and ventral perirenal space.

   A, Radiograph of the abdomen.

   B, Computed tomogram, unenhanced.

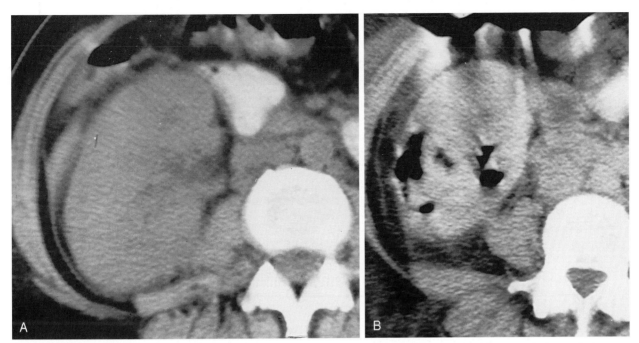

FIGURE 9–44. Severe acute pyelonephritis, right kidney, evolving into emphysematous pyelonephritis over a 2–day period.
   A, Computed tomogram, unenhanced. The right kidney is large and has a smooth contour.
   B, Computed tomogram, contrast material–enhanced. Collections of gas have formed within the kidney.

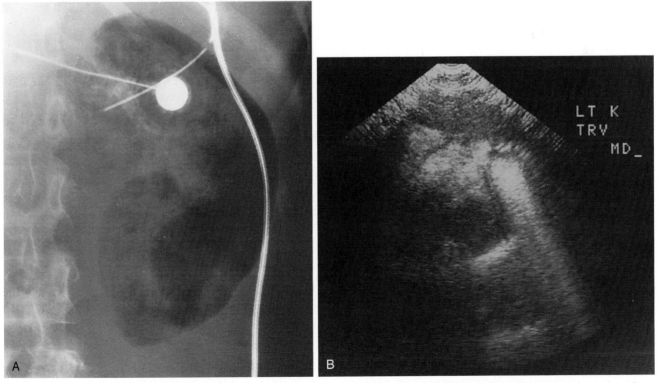

FIGURE 9–45. Emphysematous pyelonephritis of the left kidney. Gas is present in the interstitium of the kidney and the perirenal space.
   A, Radiograph of the abdomen.
   B, Ultrasonogram, longitudinal section. The gas reflects sound transmission, resulting in a hyperechoic appearance with acoustic shadowing.

ACUTE PYELONEPHRITIS* TYPICAL FINDINGS

Primary Uroradiologic Elements

Size: large
Contour: smooth
Lesion distribution: unilateral

Secondary Uroradiologic Elements

Collecting system: opacification time delayed; attenuated
Nephrogram: diminished (striated or wedge-shaped; focal, multifocal, diffuse); delayed
    enhancement
Echogenicity: normal to decreased (focal, regional, or global)

*Note: Abnormalities vary with severity of infection and host response from none to intermediate
(uncomplicated acute pyelonephritis) to severe (severe acute pyelonephritis) to extreme (emphysematous pyelonephritis)

EMPHYSEMATOUS PYELONEPHRITIS TYPICAL FINDINGS

Primary Uroradiologic Elements

Size: large
Contour: smooth
Lesion distribution: unilateral

Secondary Uroradiologic Elements

Collecting system: contains gas
Nephrogram: interstitial gas; does not enhance
Echogenicity: increased; heterogeneous; attenuates sound

---

puted tomography. Gas-attenuated sound causes ill-defined increased echogenicity associated with acoustic shadowing on ultrasonography.

XANTHOGRANULOMATOUS PYELONEPHRITIS

Definition

Xanthogranulomatous pyelonephritis is a chronic renal infection that in its most common form leads to a scarred, contracted renal pelvis, dilated calyces, and diffuse infiltration of the renal parenchyma by plasma cells and lipid-laden macrophages that may form multiple yellow-colored masses. Less often, this disease process is unifocal and affects a single infundibulum and calyx and the corresponding parenchyma. The term "xanthogranulomatous" describes the yellow color imparted to the renal parenchyma and inflammatory masses by the high lipid content of the macrophages. Calculus in the pelvis of xanthogranulomatous kidneys occurs in over 90 per cent of cases. Calculus usually assumes a stag-horn shape and is composed of struvite. The dilated calyces, whose walls are thickened by inflammation, are filled with pus. Extension of the inflammatory process into the psoas muscle and perirenal and

pararenal spaces occurs frequently. Parenchymal calcification is uncommon.

It is generally held that xanthogranulomatous pyelonephritis develops as a complication of chronic infection in a collecting system that has a long-standing partial obstruction caused by stones, stricture, or, uncommonly, uroepithelial tumor. The characteristic histologic response is thought to result from the liberation of lipid from tissue destroyed through bacterial action. The possibility that an undefined metabolic defect plays a role in the genesis of this unusual disorder has also been proposed.

Clinical Setting

Xanthogranulomatous pyelonephritis occurs predominantly in females and affects all age groups from children to the elderly. Chronic, undiagnosed illness for several months usually precedes the diagnosis. Signs and symptoms include abdominal and flank pain, low-grade fever, weight loss, and malaise. Many patients have no lower urinary tract symptoms. A renal mass may be palpable. Anemia, leukocytosis, pyuria, and albuminuria may be present. *Proteus mirabilis* and *Escherichia coli* are the organisms most likely to be found in the urine.

Pseudomonas aeruginosa and *Enterobacter aerogenes* are isolated less frequently.

Radiologic Findings

Xanthogranulomatous pyelonephritis is most commonly encountered in its diffuse form. In this situation, a radiopaque calculus is present in the renal pelvis of a smooth-contoured, enlarged kidney that fails to opacify or has diminished opacification during contrast material–enhanced imaging studies. Thickening of the renal fascia may be identified with standard or computed tomograms. On retrograde pyelography, irregular filling defects in a contracted pelvis and marked caliectasis are demonstrated (Fig. 9–46).

In the diffuse form of xanthogranulomatous pyelonephritis, ultrasonography well demonstrates the enlargement of the kidney with preservation of a smooth outline. The dominant finding reflects the markedly dilated calyces that are filled with the products of inflammation and are seen as hypoechoic structures with an internal pattern of fine echoes. The calyces may be surrounded by a thin zone of increased echogenicity that probably represents the surrounding inflammatory reaction. The frequently present pelvic calculus causes a highly reflective image with acoustic shadowing (Fig. 9–47). Additional calculi may be found in the dilated calyces or even extruded into a perirenal abscess (see Fig. 9–48A). These calculi might be broken remnants of a larger central staghorn calculus. Parenchymal xanthogranulomatous masses cause focal zones of echogenicity similar to that of the renal parenchyma.

Computed tomography demonstrates the generalized nature of renal enlargement in diffuse xanthogranulomatous pyelonephritis (Fig. 9–48; see Fig. 9–47A, B). With this modality, the calyces appear as dilated structures with attenuation values that are in the range of those of water. Calculi in the pelvis, calyx, or perirenal space are readily identified as radiopaque structures. Characteristically, there is intense enhancement of tissue surrounding the dilated calyces (see Fig. 9–47B). This presumably reflects the inflammatory tissue in the calyceal wall and renal parenchyma. Computed tomography is particularly valuable in identifying extension of the xanthogranulomatous infection into the psoas muscle and perirenal and pararenal spaces, where it appears as a soft-tissue mass, sometimes containing gas, in continuity with the affected kidney (see Fig. 9–48).

Angiography in xanthogranulomatous pyelonephritis reveals a lack of normal arborization of the intrarenal arteries, displacement of vessels around dilated calyces or granulomatous masses, and attenuation of arterial caliber. Neovascularity indistinguishable from that of neoplastic processes, nephrographic defects, and enlargement of capsular arteries have been described. None of these angiographic findings are specific.

The radiologic findings in the focal form of xanthogranulomatous pyelonephritis are similar to those for the diffuse type but are limited to the calyces and the parenchyma of a portion of the kidney, often in association with an obstructive calyceal stone or an obstructed duplicated pelvocalyceal system (Figs. 9–49, 9–50). In focal forms, the renal pelvis may be involved only to the extent of being displaced by the limited inflammatory mass. Here, the uninvolved portion of the kidney is functionally and structurally normal. Xanthogranulomatous pyelonephritis of a duplicated collecting system involves the entire hemipelvis.

MISCELLANEOUS CONDITIONS

Compensatory hypertrophy and duplication of the pelvocalyceal system are two situations in which a normal kidney becomes globally enlarged. Both of these conditions must be considered in the differential diagnosis of the unilaterally large, smooth kidney.

Compensatory Hypertrophy

When a kidney is congenitally absent, is surgically removed, or becomes diseased to the point that its excretory workload falls below a certain point, the functional capabilities and size of the normal contralateral kidney increase by virtue of an increase in the size of individual nephrons (Fig. 9–51). In cases of renal aplasia, severe hypoplasia, or unilateral multicystic dysplasia, the functioning kidney will be large from birth, whereas growth occurs slowly over years when function of the diseased kidney deteriorates gradually. Even though compensatory hypertrophy following surgical removal of the opposite kidney has been shown to begin within a few days in experimental animals, it is not detectable by clinical tests of renal function in humans for several weeks. Maximum increase in size is reached in approximately 6 months.

It is known that renal function and size decrease gradually as a function of age. It therefore might be expected that the ability of the kidney to undergo compensatory hypertrophy would also diminish with age. In fact, it has been claimed by some that compensatory hypertrophy does not occur at all after contralateral nephrectomy in patients older than 30 years. This is clearly not accurate, as evidenced by other studies that have shown that enlargement may occur at any age, although a greater degree of hypertrophy occurs in children than in adults (Fig. 9–52).

Radiologically, the hypertrophied kidney is normal in all respects except for its size and the thickness of the renal parenchyma. Because the urine flow rate from this kidney is twice normal, the pelvocalyceal system and ureter may appear more distended than usual.

Text continued on page 231

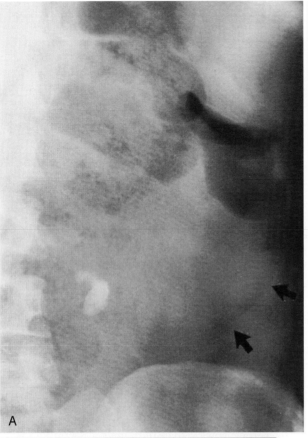

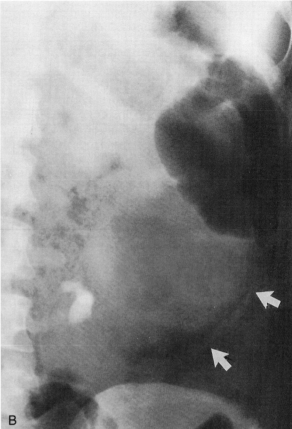

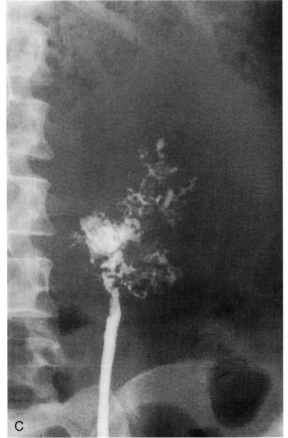

FIGURE 9–46. Xanthogranulomatous pyelonephritis (diffuse form) in a 40-year-old woman with a 6-year history of urinary tract infection, 6 months of left flank pain, and a tender left-flank mass palpable for 2 weeks. Hematuria and pyuria were present, and the urine was infected with *Escherichia coli.* A large radiopaque calculus is present in the region of the renal pelvis. The kidney outline is enlarged, and the renal fascia is thickened *(arrows).*

A, Preliminary film.

B, Excretory urogram, 10-minute film. There is no apparent accumulation of contrast material.

C, Retrograde pyelogram. There is obstruction of the ureteropelvic junction. The multiple filling defects seen in the collecting system are caused by debris and xanthogranulomas projecting into the lumen.

(Courtesy of Lee Talner, M.D., University of Washington, Seattle).

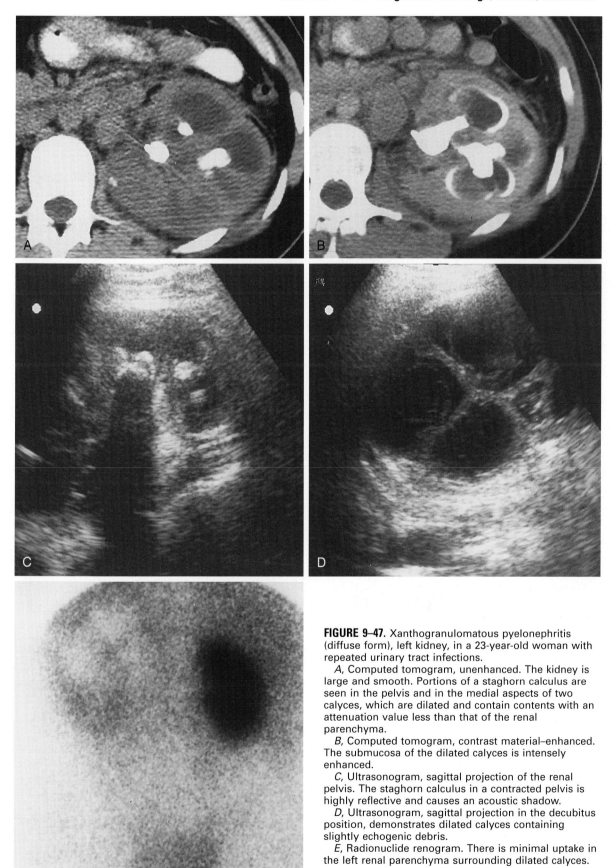

FIGURE 9–47. Xanthogranulomatous pyelonephritis (diffuse form), left kidney, in a 23-year-old woman with repeated urinary tract infections.

A, Computed tomogram, unenhanced. The kidney is large and smooth. Portions of a staghorn calculus are seen in the pelvis and in the medial aspects of two calyces, which are dilated and contain contents with an attenuation value less than that of the renal parenchyma.

B, Computed tomogram, contrast material–enhanced. The submucosa of the dilated calyces is intensely enhanced.

C, Ultrasonogram, sagittal projection of the renal pelvis. The staghorn calculus in a contracted pelvis is highly reflective and causes an acoustic shadow.

D, Ultrasonogram, sagittal projection in the decubitus position, demonstrates dilated calyces containing slightly echogenic debris.

E, Radionuclide renogram. There is minimal uptake in the left renal parenchyma surrounding dilated calyces.

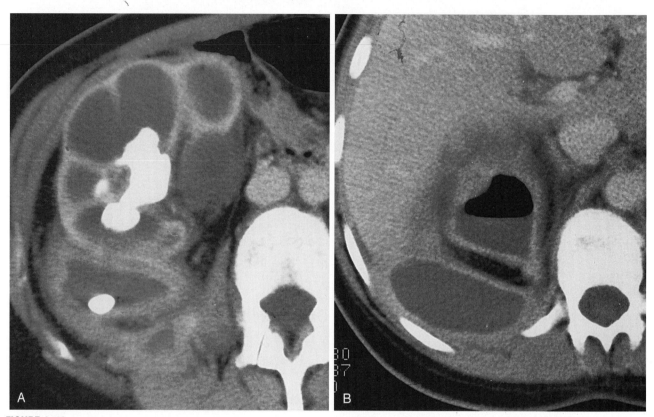

FIGURE 9–48. Xanthogranulomatous pyelonephritis (diffuse form) in the right kidney of a 45-year-old woman with night sweats and intermittent fever. Computed tomography, contrast material–enhanced.

A, Scan through the right kidney demonstrates a staghorn calculus in a contracted renal pelvis. The kidney is large and smooth. A thin rim of enhancing parenchyma surrounds nonenhanced, dilated calyces. There is a collection of fluid containing an extruded fragment of the staghorn calculus in the posterior aspect of the perirenal space. The adjoining renal fascia is thickened.

B, Scan through the right suprarenal area demonstrates loculated fluid and gas in the perirenal space, which communicates with loculated fluid in the posterior pleural space.

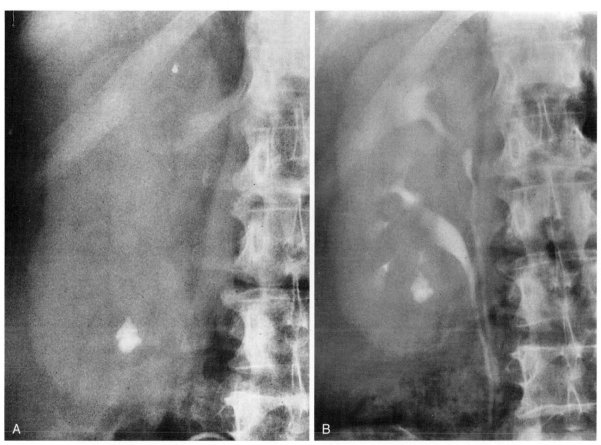

FIGURE 9–49. Xanthogranulomatous pyelonephritis, focal form, right kidney. Excretory urogram.
A, Preliminary radiograph. There is a mass and a calyceal calculus in the lower pole.
B, 10-minute radiograph. The calculus is located at the apex of the mass.

FIGURE 9–50. Xanthogranulomatous pyelonephritis, focal form, right kidney. Computed tomogram, contrast material–enhanced. The characteristic abnormality is limited to the dorsal portion of the kidney.

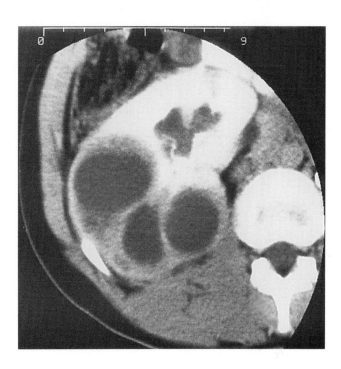

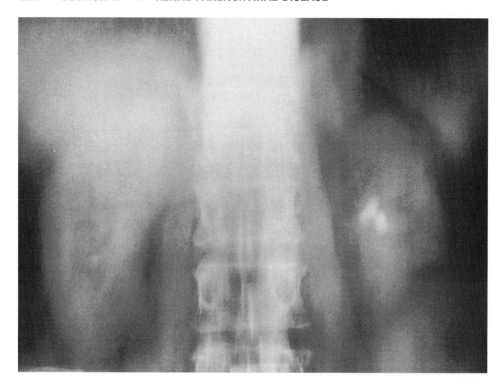

FIGURE 9–51. Compensatory hypertrophy of the right kidney in a middle-aged woman with severe reflux nephropathy of the left kidney. The right kidney is large but otherwise normal. Right kidney length = 14.2 cm; left kidney length = 10.3 cm.

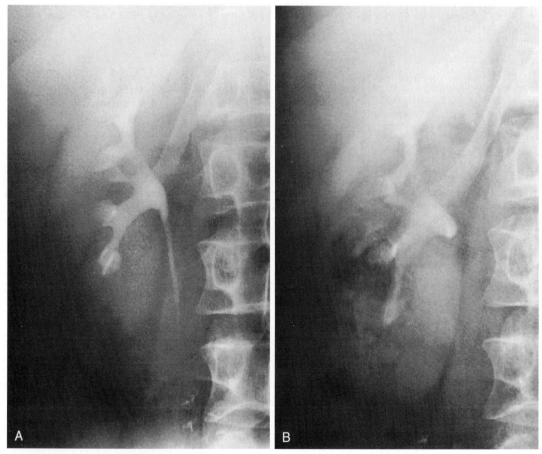

FIGURE 9–52. Compensatory hypertrophy of the right kidney following left nephrectomy in a 76-year-old man.
   A, Excretory urogram at age 70 years. Normal examination results. Kidney length = 14.8 cm.
   B, Excretory urogram at age 76 years. Contralateral nephrectomy had been performed 2 years earlier. The right kidney has enlarged but is otherwise normal. Kidney length = 18.0 cm.

XANTHOGRANULOMATOUS PYELONEPHRITIS TYPICAL FINDINGS

Primary Uroradiologic Elements

Size: large
Contour: smooth
Lesion distribution: unilateral

Secondary Uroradiologic Elements

Collecting system: pelvis contracted and calyces dilated; attenuation values slightly less to
    slightly greater than those of water; rim enhancement
Nephrogram: absent (diffuse form); focal replacement (focal form)
Echogenicity: calyces (hypoechoic with echogenic rim)
Calcification: calculus in pelvis
Retroperitoneum: loculated fluid/gas

Duplicated Pelvocalyceal System

In Chapter 3 it was noted that the metanephric blastema differentiates into nephrons under the inductive influence of the advancing point of the ureteric bud, which itself contributes collecting tubules to the renal parenchyma. Duplication of the renal pelvis represents earlier-than-normal dichotomous branching of the ureteral bud. The two branches encounter a greater mass of metanephric blastema than would otherwise have occurred. This is the basis for the larger-than-normal amount of renal parenchyma associated with a duplex collecting system (Fig. 9–53).

Of the two pelvocalyceal systems, the larger is usually the inferior one, which combines both interpolar and lower polar calyces. The renal lobes draining into the two systems do not assimilate with each other to the degree that occurs in a single system. As a result, an excessive amount of renal parenchyma, including cortex, may lie between the two sets of collecting structures and cause a mass-like effect on adjacent calyces and infundibula. This commonly occurs both in complete and partial forms of duplications and is described as *lobar dysmorphism* in the section on anomalies in Chapter 3.

DIFFERENTIAL DIAGNOSIS

The radiologic features of the diseases discussed in this chapter overlap to a great extent. All produce enlargement of one kidney and are often associated with diminished opacification.

Obstructive uropathy is the only abnormality in this diagnostic set in which the collecting struc-

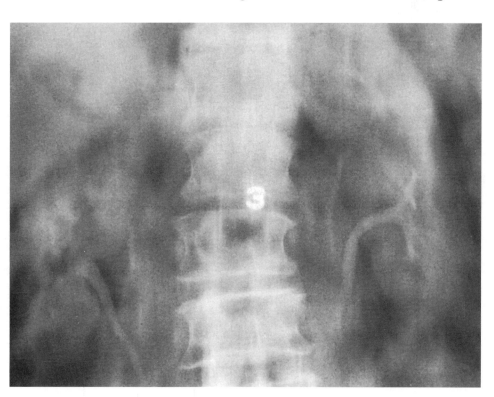

FIGURE 9–53. Duplicated collecting system causing smooth enlargement of the left kidney. Tomogram during excretory urography. Right kidney length = 13.9 cm; left kidney length = 17.8 cm.

ture dilates. This finding, particularly when coupled with an increasingly dense nephrogram, firmly establishes the diagnosis. The specific diagnosis of diseases in this diagnostic set, other than obstructive uropathy, often requires information derived from such procedures as Doppler ultrasonography, computed tomography, magnetic resonance imaging, or angiography to define **renal vein thrombosis/obstruction** or to confirm renal artery occlusion as a cause of **kidney infarction**. Acute pyelonephritis has no specific radiologic abnormality, except in the severe form in which computed tomographic findings and the clinical setting are characteristic. A large, smooth kidney containing calculi, especially staghorn in form, and opacifying poorly or not at all suggests the diagnosis of **xanthogranulomatous pyelonephritis**. However, staghorn calculus may lead to squamous cell carcinoma of the pelvis with the same radiologic appearance.

BIBLIOGRAPHY

Renal Vein Thrombosis/Stenosis

Beckmann, C. F., and Abrams, H. L.: Renal venography: Anatomy, technique, application, analysis of 132 venograms, and a review of the literature. Cardiovasc. Intervent. Radiol. 3:45, 1980.

Beckmann, C. F., and Abrams, H. L.: Idiopathic renal vein varices: Incidence and significance. Radiology 143:649, 1982.

Beinart, C., Sniderman, K. W., Saddekhi, S., Weiner, M., Vaughan, E. D., Jr., and Sos, T. A.: Left renal vein hypertension: A cause of occult hematuria. Radiology 145:647, 1982.

Bigongiari, L. R., Patel, S. K., Appelman, H., and Thornbury, J. R.: Medullary rays: Visualization during excretory urography. AJR 125:795, 1975.

Braun, B., Wellemann, L. S., and Weigand, W.: Ultrasonographic demonstration of renal vein thrombosis. Radiology 138:157, 1981.

Coel, M. N., and Talner, L. B.: Obstructive nephrogram due to renal vein thrombosis. Radiology 101:573, 1971.

DeTroyer, A., Paduart, P., Shockert, J., and Parmentier, R.: Unilateral renal vein thrombosis and nephrotic syndrome. Br. Med. J. 4:730, 1975.

Gatewood, O. M. B., Fishman, E. K., Burrow, C. R., Walker, W. G., Goldman, S. M., and Siegelman, S. S.: Renal vein thrombosis in patients with nephrotic syndrome: CT diagnosis. Radiology 159:117, 1986.

Glazer, G. M., Francis, I. R., Gross, B. H., and Amendola, M. A.: Computed tomography of renal vein thrombosis. J. Comput. Assist. Tomogr. 8:288, 1984.

Habboub, H. K., Abu-Yousef, M. M., Williams, R. D., See, W. A., and Schweiger, G. D.: Accuracy of color Doppler sonography in assessing venous thrombus extension in renal cell carcinoma. Am. J. Roentgenol. 168:267, 1997.

Hibbert, J., Howlett, K. L., MacDonald, L. M., and Saunders, A. J. S.: The ultrasound appearances of neonatal renal vein thrombosis. Br. J. Radiol. 70:1191–1194, 1997.

Keating, M. A., and Althausen, A. F.: The clinical spectrum of renal vein thrombosis. J. Urol. 133:938, 1985.

Kim, S. H., Cho, S. W., Kim, H. D., Chung, J. W., Park, J. H., and Han, M. C.: Nutcracker syndrome: Diagnosis with Doppler US. Radiology 198:93, 1996.

Llach, F., and Nikakhtar, B.: Renal thromboembolism, atheroembolism and renal vein thrombosis. In Schrier, R. W., and Gottschalk, C. W. (eds.): Diseases of the Kidney, 6th ed. Boston, Little, Brown & Co., 1997, pp. 1893–1918.

McDonald, P. T., and Hutton, J. E., Jr.: Renal vein valve. JAMA 238:2303, 1977.

Rosenberg, E. R., Trought, W. S., Kirks, D. R., Sumner, T. E., and Grossman, H.: Ultrasonic diagnosis of renal vein thrombosis in neonates. AJR 134:35, 1980.

Rosenfield, A. T., Zeman, R. K., Cronan, J. J., and Taylor, K. J. W.: Ultrasound in experimental and clinical renal vein thrombosis. Radiology 137:735, 1980.

Shaper, K. R. L., Jackson, J. E., and Williams, G.: The nutcracker syndrome: An uncommon cause of haematuria. Br. J. Urol. 74:144, 1994.

Sutton, T. J., Leblanc, A., Gauthier, N., and Hassan, M.: Radiological manifestations of neonatal renal vein thrombosis on follow-up examinations. Radiology 122:435. 1977.

Trew, P. A., Biava, D. G., Jacobs, R. P., and Hopper, J., Fr.: Renal vein thrombosis in membranous glomerulopathy: Incidence and association. Medicine (Baltimore) 57:69, 1978.

Wicks, J. D., Bigongiari, L. R., Foley, W. D., and Walter, J.: Parenchymal striations in renal vein thrombosis: Arteriographic demonstration. AJR 129:95, 1977.

Winfield, A. C., Gerlock, A. J., Jr., and Shaff, M. I.: Perirenal cobwebs: A CT sign of renal vein thrombosis. J. Comput. Assist. Tomogr. 5:405, 1981.

Witz, M., Kantarovsky, A., Morag, B., and Shifrin, E. G.: Renal vein occlusion: A review. J. Urol. 155:1173, 1996.

Acute Arterial Infarction

Cass, A. S., and Luxenberg, M.: Accuracy of computed tomography in diagnosing renal artery injuries. Urology 34:249, 1989.

Fishman, M. C., Naidich, J. B., and Stein, H. L.: Vascular magnetic resonance imaging. Radiol. Clin. North Am. 24:485, 1986.

Gasparini, M., Hofmann, R., and Stoller, M.: Renal artery embolism: Clinical features and therapeutic options. J. Urol. 147:567, 1992.

Glazer, G. M., Francis, I. R., Brady, T. M., and Teng, S. S.: Computed tomography of renal infarction: Clinical and experimental observations. AJR 140:721, 1983.

Glazer, G. M., and London, S. S.: CT appearance of global renal infarction. J. Comput. Assist. Tomogr. 5:847, 1981.

Hann, L., and Pfister, R. C.: Renal subcapsular rim sign: New etiologies and pathogenesis. AJR 138:51, 1982.

Ishikawa, I., Masuzaki, S., Saito, T., Yuri, T., Shinoda, A., and Tsujigiwa, M.: Magnetic resonance imaging in renal infarction and ischemia. Nephron 51:99, 1989.

Lessman, R. K., Johnson, S. F., Coburn, J. W., and Kaufman, J. J.: Renal artery embolism: Clinical features and long-term follow-up of 17 cases. Ann. Intern. Med. 89:477, 1978.

Llach, F., and Nikakhtar, B.: Renal thromboembolism, atheroembolism and renal vein thrombosis. In Schrier, R. W., and Gottschalk, C. W. (eds.): Diseases of the Kidney, 6th ed. Boston, Little, Brown & Co., 1997, pp. 1893–1918.

Martin, K. W., McAlister, W. H., and Schakelford, G. O.: Acute renal infarction: Diagnosis by Doppler ultrasound. Pediatr. Radiol. 18:373, 1988.

Nunez, D., Becerra, J. L., Fuentes, D., and Pagson, S.: Traumatic occlusion of the renal artery: Helical CT diagnosis. Am. J. Roentgenol. 167:777, 1996.

Paul, G. J., and Stephenson, T. F.: The cortical rim sign in renal infarction. Radiology 122:338, 1977.

Rubin, B. E., and Schliftman, R.: The striated nephrogram in renal contusion. Urol. Radiol. 1:119, 1979.

Sheehan, H. L., and Davis, J. C.: Complete permanent renal ischaemia. J. Pathol. 76:569, 1958.

Solez, K.: Acute renal failure (acute tubular necrosis, infarction, and cortical necrosis). In Heptinstall, R. H. (ed.): Pathology of the Kidney, 4th ed. Boston, Little, Brown & Co., 1992, pp. 1235–1314.

Teplick, J. G., and Yarrow, M. W.: Arterial infarction of kidney. Ann. Intern. Med. 42:1041, 1955.

Wong, W., Moss, A. A., Federle, M. P., Cochran, S. T., and London, S. S.: Renal infarction: CT diagnosis and correlation between CT findings and etiologies. Radiology 150:201, 1984.

Obstructive Uropathy

Amis, E. S., Jr., Cronan, J. J., and Pfister, R. C.: Pseudohydronephrosis on non-contrast computed tomography. J. Comput. Assist. Tomogr. 6:511, 1982.

Bell, T. V., Fenlon, H. M., Davison, B. D., Ahari, H. K., and Hussain, S.: Unenhanced helical CT criteria to differentiate distal ureteral calculi from pelvic phleboliths. Radiology 207:363, 1998.

Bigongiari, L. R., Davis, R. M., Novak, W. G., Wicks, J. D., Kass, E., and Thornbury, J. R.: Visualization of medullary rays on excretory urography in experimental ureteric obstruction. AJR 129:89, 1977.

Bigongiari, L. R., Patel, S. K., Appelman, H., and Thornbury, J. R.: Medullary rays: Visualization during excretory urography. AJR 125:795, 1975.

Choyke, P. L.: The urogram: Are rumors of its death premature? Radiology 184:33, 1992.

Coleman, B. G., Arger, P. H., Mulhern, C. B., Jr., Pollack, H. M., and Banner, M. P.: Pyelonephrosis: Sonography in the diagnosis and management. AJR 137:939, 1981.

Coley, B. D., Arellano, R. S., Talner, L. B., Baker, K. B., Peterson. T., and Mattrey, R. F.: Renal resistive index in experimental partial and complete ureteral obstruction. Acad. Radiology 2:373, 1995.

Cooke, G. M., and Bartucz, J. P.: Spontaneous extravasation of contrast medium during intravenous urography: Report of fourteen cases and a review of the literature. Clin. Radiol. 25:87, 1974.

Cremin, B. J.: Urinary ascites and obstructive uropathy. Br. J. Radiol. 48:113, 1975.

Cronan, J. J.: Contemporary concepts in imaging urinary tract obstruction. Radiol. Clin. North Am. 29:527, 1991.

Cronan, J. J., and Tublin, M. E.: Role of the resistive index in the evaluation of acute renal obstruction. Am. J. Roentgenol. 164:377, 1995.

Curhan, G. C., and Zeidel, M. L.: Urinary tract obstruction. In Brenner, B. M. (ed.): The Kidney, 5th ed. Philadelphia, W. B. Saunders, 1996, pp. 1936–1958.

Dalla Palma, L., Bazzocchi, M., Pozzi-Mucelli, R. S., Stacul, F., Rossi, M., and Agostini, R.: Ultrasonography in the diagnosis of hydronephrosis in patients with normal renal function. Urol. Radiol. 5:221, 1983.

Dalrymple, N. C., Verga, M., Anderson, K. R., Bove, P., Covey, A. M., Rosenfield, A. T., and Smith, R. C.: The value of unenhanced helical computerized tomography in the management of acute flank pain. J. Urol. 159:735–740, 1998.

Deyoe, L. A., Cronan, J. J., Breslaw, B. H., and Ridlen, M. S.: New techniques of ultrasound and color Doppler in the prospective evaluation of acute renal obstruction: Do they replace the intravenous urogram? Abdom. Imaging 20:58, 1995.

Dyer, R. B., Gilpin, J. W., Zagona, R. J., Chen, M. Y. M., and Case, L. D.: Vicarious contrast material excretion in patients with acute unilateral ureteral obstruction. Radiology 177:739, 1990.

Ellenbogen, P. H., Scheible, F. W., Talner, L. B., and Leopold, G. R.: Sensitivity of grey scale ultrasound in detecting urinary tract obstruction. AJR 130:731, 1978.

Erwin, B. C., Carroll, B. A., and Sommer, F. G.: Renal colic: The role of ultrasound in initial evaluation. Radiology 152:147, 1984.

Fernbach, S. K.: The dilated urinary tract in children. Urol. Radiol. 14:34, 1992.

Fielding, J. R., Steele, G., Fox, L. A., Heller, H., and Loughlin, K. R.: Spiral computerized tomography in the evaluation of acute flank pain: A replacement for excretory urography. J. Urol. 157:2071, 1997.

Haddad, M. C., Sharif, H. S., Abomelha, M. S., Riley, P. J., Sammak, B. M., and Shahed, M. S.: Management of renal colic: Redefining the role of the urogram? Radiology 184:35, 1992.

Haddad, M. C., Sharif, H. S., Shahed, M. S., Mutaiery, M. A., Samihan, A. M., Sammak, B. M., Southcombe, L. A., and Crawford, A. D.: Renal colic: Diagnosis and outcome. Radiology 184:83, 1992.

Heneghan, J. P., Dalrymple, N. C., Verga, M., Rosenfield, A. T., and Smith, R. C.: Soft-tissue "rim" sign in the diagnosis of ureteral calculi with use of unenhanced helical CT. Radiology 202:709, 1997.

Hill, G. S.: Basic physiology and morphology of hydronephrosis. In Hill, G. S. (ed.): Uropathology. New York, Churchill Livingstone, 1989, pp. 467–516.

Katz, D. S., Lane, M. J., and Sommer, F. G.: Unenhanced helical CT of ureteral stones: Incidence of associated urinary tract findings. Am. J. Roentgenol. 166:1319, 1996.

Kawashima, A., Sandler, C. M., Boridy, I. C., Takahashi, N., Benson, G. S., and Goldman, S. M.: Unenhanced helical CT of ureterolithiasis: Value of the tissue rim sign. AJR 168:997, 1997.

Keogan, M. T., Kliewer, M. A., Hertzberg, B. S., DeLong, D. M., Tupler, R. H., and Carroll, B. A.: Renal resistive indexes: Variability in Doppler US measurement in a healthy population. Radiology 199:165, 1996.

Klahr, S.: Urinary tract obstruction. In Schrier, R. W., and Gottschalk, C. W. (eds.): Diseases of the Kidney, 6th ed. Boston, Little, Brown & Co., 1997, pp. 709–738.

Levine, J. A., Neitlich, J., Verga, M., Dalrymple, N., and Smith, R. C.: Ureteral calculi in patients with flank pain: Correlation of plain radiography with unenhanced helical CT. Radiology 204:27, 1997.

O'Malley, M. E., Soto, J. A., Yucel, E. K., and Hussain, S.: MR urography: Evaluation of a three-dimensional fast spin-echo technique in patients with hydronephrosis. AJR 168:387, 1997.

Parkhouse, H. F., and Barratt, T. M.: Investigation of the dilated urinary tract. Pediatr. Nephrol. 2:43, 1988.

Peters, C. A.: Urinary tract obstruction in children. J. Urol. 154:1874, 1995.

Platt, J. F.: Looking for renal obstruction: The view from renal Doppler US. Radiology 193:610, 1994.

Platt, J. F.: Urinary obstruction. Radiol. Clin. North Am. 34:1113, 1996.

Preminger, G. M., Vieweg, J., Leden, R. A., and Nelson, R. C.: Urolithiasis: Detection and management with unenhanced spiral CT—a urologic perspective. Radiology 207:308, 1998.

Ramsey, E. W., Jarzylo, S. V., and Bruce, A. W.: Spontaneous extravasation of urine from the renal pelvis and ureter. J. Urol. 110:507, 1973.

Regan, F., Bohlman, M. E., Khazan, R., Rodriguez, R., and Schultze-Haakh, H.: MR urography using HASTE imaging in the assessment of ureteric obstruction. Am. J. Roentgenol. 167:1115, 1996.

Smith, R. C., Rosenfield, A. T., Choe, K. A., Essenmacher, K. R., Verga, M., Glickman, M. G., and Lange, R. C.: Acute flank pain: Comparison of non-contrast enhanced CT and intravenous urography. Radiology 194:789, 1995.

Smith, R. C., Verga, M., Dalrymple, N., McCarthy, S., and Rosenfield, A. T.: Acute ureteral obstruction: Value of secondary signs on helical unenhanced CT. Am. J. Roentgenol. 167:1109, 1996.

Smith, R. C., Verga, M., McCarthy, S., and Rosenfield, A. T.: Diagnosis of acute flank pain: value of unenhanced helical CT. Am. J. Roentgenol. 166:97, 1996.

Subramanyam, B. R., Raghavendra, N. G., Bosniak, M. A., Lefleur, R. S., Rosen, R. J., and Horii, S. C.: Sonography of pyelonephrosis: A prospective study. AJR 140:991, 1983.

Talner, L. B.: Urinary obstruction. In Pollack, H. M. (ed.): Clinical Urography. Philadelphia, W. B. Saunders, 1990, pp. 1535–1629.

Talner, L. B., Scheible, W., Ellenbogen, P. H., Beck, C. H., and Gosink, B. B.: How accurate is ultrasonography in detecting hydronephrosis in uremic patients? Urol. Radiol. 3:1, 1981.

Tanagho, E. A.: Mechanics of ureteral dilatation. Can. J. Surg. 15:4, 1972.

Tublin, M. E., Dodd, G. D., III, and Verdile, V. P.: Acute renal colic: Diagnosis with duplex Doppler US. Radiology 193:697, 1994.

Yilmaz, S., Sindel, T., Arslan, G., Ozkaynak, C., Karaali, K., Kabaalioglu, A., and Luleci, E.: Renal colic: Comparison of spiral CT, US and IVU in the detection of ureteral calculi. Eur. Radiol. 8:212–217, 1998.

Acute Pyelonephritis

Adler, S. N.: Nonobstructive pyelonephritis initially seen as acute renal failure. Arch. Intern. Med. 138:816, 1978.

Bailey, R. R., Little, P. J., and Rolleston, G. L.: Renal damage after acute pyelonephritis. Br. Med. J. 1:550, 1969.

Bailey, R. R., Lynn, K. L., Robson, R. A., Smith, A. H., Maling,

T. M. J., and Turner, J. G.: DMSA renal scans in adults with acute pyelonephritis. Clin. Nephrol. *46*:99, 1996.

Benador, D., Benador, N., Slosman, D., Mermillod, B., and Girardin, E.: Are younger children at highest risk of renal sequelae after pyelonephritis? Lancet *349*:17, 1997.

Berliner, L., and Bosniak, M. A.: The striated nephrogram in acute pyelonephritis. Urol. Radiol. *4*:41, 1982.

Björgivinsson, E., Majd, M., and Eggli, K. D.: Diagnosis of acute pyelonephritis in children: Comparison of sonography and Tc-DMSA scintigraphy. AJR *157*:539, 1991.

Dacher, J. N., Pfister, C., Monroc, M., Eurin, D., and Ledosseur, P.: Power Doppler sonographic pattern of acute pyelonephritis in children: Comparison with CT. Am. J. Roentgenol. *166*:1451, 1996.

Dalla Palma, L., Pozzi-Mucelli, R., and Pozzi-Mucelli, F.: Delayed CT in acute renal infection. Semin. Ultrasound CT MR *18*:122, 1997.

Davidson, A. J., and Talner, L. B.: Urographic and angiographic abnormalities in adult-onset acute bacterial nephritis. Radiology *106*:249, 1973.

Davidson, A. J., and Talner, L. B.: Late sequelae of adult-onset acute bacterial nephritis. Radiology *127*:367, 1978.

Eggli, D. F., and Tulchinsky, M.: Scintigraph evaluation of pediatric urinary tract infection. Semin. Nucl. Med. *23*:199, 1993.

Evanhoff, G. V., Thompson, C. S., Foley, R., and Weinman, E. J.: Spectrum of gas within the kidney. Am. J. Med. *83*:149, 1987.

Fierer, J.: Acute pyelonephitis. Urol. Clin. North Am. *14*:251, 1987.

Fraser, I. R., Birch, D., Fairley, K. F., John, S., Lichtenstein, M., Tress, B., and Kincaid-Smith, P. S.: A prospective study of cortical scarring in acute febrile pyelonephritis in adults: Clinical and bacteriological characteristics. Clin. Nephrol. *43*:159, 1995.

Gold, R. P., McClennan, B. L., and Rottenberg, R. R.: CT appearance of acute inflammatory disease of the renal interstitium. AJR *141*:343, 1983.

Greenhill, A. H., Norman, M. E., Cornfield, D., Chatten, J., Buck, B., and Witzleben, C. L.: Acute renal failure secondary to acute pyelonephritis. Clin. Nephrol. *8*:400, 1977.

Hansen, A., Wagner, A. A., Lavard, L. D., and Nielsen, J. T.: Diagnostic imaging in children with urinary tract infection: The role of intravenous urography. Acta Paediat. *84*:84, 1995.

Hellerstein, S.: Evolving concepts in the evaluation of the child with a urinary tract infection. J. Pediatr. *124*:589, 1994.

Hellerstein, S.: Urinary tract infections: Old and new concepts. Pediatr. Clin. North Am. *42*:1433, 1995.

Heptinstall, R. H.: Pyelonephritis: Pathologic features. In Heptinstall, R. H. (ed.): Pathology of the Kidney, 4th ed. Boston, Little, Brown & Co., 1992, pp. 1489–1562.

Heptinstall, R. H.: Urinary tract infection and clinical features of pyelonephritis. In Heptinstall, R. H. (ed.): Pathology of the Kidney, 4th ed. Boston, Little, Brown and Co., 1992, pp. 1433–1488.

Hill, G. S.: Renal infection. In Hill, G. S. (ed.): Uropathology. New York, Churchill Livingstone, 1989, pp. 333–430.

Hill, G. S.: Urinary tract infections: General considerations. In Hill, G. S. (ed.): Uropathology. New York, Churchill Livingstone, 1989, pp. 279–332.

Hoddick, W., Jeffrey, R. B., Goldberg, H. I., Federle, M. P., and Laing, F. C.: CT and sonography of severe renal and perirenal infections. AJR *140*:517, 1983.

Hoffman, E. P., Mindelzun, R. E., and Anderson, R. V.: Computed tomography in acute pyelonephritis associated with diabetes. Radiology *135*:691, 1980.

Huang, J. J., Sung, J. M., Chen, K. W., Ruaan, M. K., Shu, G. H. F., and Chuang, Y. C.: Acute bacterial nephritis: A clinicoradiologic correlation based on computed tomography. Am. J. Med. *93*:289, 1992.

Huland, H., Busch, R., and Riebel, T.: Renal scanning after symptomatic and asymptomatic upper urinary tract infection: A prospective study. J. Urol. *128*:682, 1982.

Ishikawa, I., Saito, Y., Onouchi, Z., Matsura, H., Saito, T., Suzuki, M., and Futyu, Y.: Delayed contrast enhancement in acute focal bacterial nephritis: CT features. J. Comput. Assist. Tomogr. *9*:894, 1985.

Jakobsson, B., and Svenson, L.: Transient pyelonephritic changes on (99m)technetium-dimercaptosuccinic acid scan for at least five months after infection. Acta Paediatr. *86*:803, 1997.

Johnson, J. R., Vincent, L. M., Wang, K., Roberts, P. L., and Stamm, W. E.: Renal ultrasonographic correlates of acute pyelonephritis. Clin. Infect. Dis. *14*:15, 1992.

June, C. H., Browning, M. D., Smith, P., Wenzel, D. J., Pyatt, R. S., Checchio, L. M., and Amis, E. S., Jr.: Ultrasonography and computed tomography in severe urinary tract infection. Arch. Intern. Med. *145*:841, 1985.

Kanel, K. T., Kroboth, F. J., Schwentker, F. N., and Lecky, J. W.: The intravenous pyelogram in acute pyelonephritis. Arch. Intern. Med. *148*:2144, 1988.

Lebowitz, R. L., and Mandell, J.: Urinary tract infection in children: Putting radiology in its place. Radiology *165*: 1, 1987.

Lee, S. E., Yoon, D. K., and Kim, Y. K.: Emphysematous pyelonephritis. J. Urol. *118*:916, 1977.

Lonergan, G. J., Pennington, D. J., Morrison, J. C., Haws, R. M., Grimley, M. S., and Kao, T-C.: Childhood pyelonephritis: Comparison of gadolinium-enhanced MR imaging and renal cortical scintigraphy for diagnosis. Radiology *207*:377, 1998.

Mackenzie, J. R., Fowler, K., Hollman, A. S., Tappin, D., Murphy, A. V., Beattie, T. J., and Azmy, A. F.: The value of ultrasound in the child with an acute urinary tract infection. Br. J. Urol. *74*:240, 1994.

Majd, M., and Rushton, H. G.: Renal cortical scintigraphy in the diagnosis of acute pyelonephritis. Semin. Nucl. Med. *22*:98, 1992.

Measley, R. E., Jr., and Levison, M. E.: Host defense mechanisms in the pathogenesis of urinary tract infection. Med. Clin. North Am. *75*:275, 1991.

Papanicolaou, N., and Pfister, R. C.: Acute renal infections. Radiol. Clin. North Am. *34*:965, 1996.

Parsons, C. L.: Pathogenesis of urinary tract infection: Bacterial adherence, bladder defense mechanisms. Urol. Clin. North Am. *13*:563, 1986.

Rauschkolb, E. N., Sandler, C. M., Patel, S., and Childs, T. L.: Computed tomography of renal inflammatory disease. J. Comput. Assist. Tomogr. *6*:502, 1982.

Roberts, J. A.: Etiology and pathophysiology of pyelonephritis. Am. J. Kidney Dis. *17*:1, 1991.

Roberts, J. A.: Factors predisposing to urinary tract infections in children. Pediat. Nephrol. *10*:517, 1996.

Rosenfeld, D. L., Fleischer, M., Yudd, A., and Makowsky, T.: Current recommendations for children with urinary tract infections. Clin. Pediatr. *34*:261, 1995.

Rubin, R. H., Cotran, R. S., and Tolkoff-Rubin, N. E.: Urinary tract infection, pyelonephritis and reflux nephropathy. In Brenner, B. M. (ed.): The Kidney, 5th ed. Philadelphia, W.B. Saunders, 1996, pp. 1597–1654.

Rushton, H. G.: Pyelonephritis: Pathogenesis and management update. Dialogues in Pediatr. Urol. *13*:1, 1990.

Rushton, H. G.: The evaluation of acute pyelonephritis and renal scarring with technetium 99m-dimercaptosuccinic acid renal scintigraphy: Evolving concepts and future directions. Pediat. Nephrol. *11*:108, 1997.

Rushton, H. G., Majd, M., Jantausch, B., Wiedermann, B. L., and Belman, A. B.: Renal scarring following reflux and nonreflux pyelonephritis in children: Evaluation with technetium-99m-dimercaptosuccinic acid scintigraphy. J. Urol. *147*:1327, 1992.

Sakarya, M. E., Arslan, H., Erkoc, R., Bozkurt, M., and Atilla, M. K.: The role of power Doppler ultrasonography in the diagnosis of acute pyelonephritis. Br. J. Urol. *81*:360–363, 1998.

Shortliffe, L. M. D.: Urinary tract infections in infants and children. In Walsh, P. C., Retik, A. B., Vaughan, E. D., Jr., and Wein, A. J. (eds.): Campbell's Urology, 7th ed. Philadelphia, W. B. Saunders, 1998, pp. 1681–1707.

Sobel, J. D.: Bacterial etiologic agents in the pathogenesis of urinary tract infection. Med. Clin. North Am. *75*:253, 1991.

Svanborg, C., deMan, P., and Sandberg, T.: Renal involvement in urinary tract infection. Kidney Int. *39*:541, 1991.

Talner, L. B., Davidson, A. J., Lebowitz, R. L., Dalla Palma, L. and Goldman, S. M.: Acute pyelonephritis: Can we agree on terminology? Radiology *192*:297, 1994.

Tsugaya, M., Hirao, N., Sakagami, H., Ontagurao, K., and Washida, H.: Renal cortical scarring in acute pyelonephritis. Br. J. Urol. *69*:245, 1992.

Wallin, L., and Bajc, M.: Typical technitium dimercaptosuccinic acid distribution patterns in acute pyelonephritis. Acta Paediatr. *82*:1061, 1993.

Wan, Y. L., Lee, T. Y., Bullard, M. J., and Tsai, C. C.: Acute gas-producing bacterial renal infection: Correlation between imaging findings and clinical outcome. Radiology *198*:433, 1996.

Webb, J. A.: The role of imaging in adult acute urinary tract infection. Eur. Radiol. 7:837:1997.

Xanthogranulomatous Pyelonephritis

Antonakopoulos, G. N., Chapple, C. R., Newman, J., Crocker, J., Tudway, D. C., O'Brien, J. M., and Considine, J.: Xanthogranulomatous pyelonephritis: A reappraisal and immunohistochemical study. Arch. Pathol. Lab. Med. *112*:275, 1988.

Cohen, M. S.: Granulomatous nephritis. Urol. Clin. North Am. *13*:647, 1986.

Goldman, S. M., Hartman, D. S., Fishman, E. K., Finizio, J., Gatewood, O. M. B., and Siegelman, S. S.: CT of xanthogranulomatous pyelonephritis: Radiologic-pathologic correlation. AJR *141*:963, 1984.

Goodman, M., Curry, T., and Russell, T.: Xanthogranulomatous pyelonephritis (XGP): A local disease with systemic manifestations: Report of 23 patients and review of the literature. Medicine *58*:171, 1979.

Grainger, R. G., and Longstaff, A. J.: Xanthogranulomatous pyelonephritis: A reappraisal. Lancet *1*:1398, 1982.

Hartman, D. S., Davis, C. J., Jr., Goldman, S. M., Isbister, S. S., and Sanders, R. C.: Xanthogranulomatous pyelonephritis: Sonographic-pathologic correlation of 16 cases. J. Ultrasound Med. *3*:481, 1984.

Hayes, W. S., Hartman, D. S., and Sesterhenn, I.: Xanthogranulomatous pyelonephritis. Radiographics *11*:485, 1991.

Kenney, P. J.: Imaging of chronic renal infections. AJR *155*:485, 1990.

Levin, D. C., Gordon, D., Kinkhabwala, M., and Becker, J. A.: Reticular neovascularity in malignant and inflammatory renal masses. Radiology *120*:61, 1976.

Parker, M. D., and Clark, R. L.: Evolving concepts in the diagnosis of xanthogranulomatous pyelonephritis. Urol. Radiol. *11*:7, 1989.

Saeed, S. M., and Fine, G.: Xanthogranulomatous pyelonephritis. Am. J. Clin. Pathol. *39*:616, 1963.

Tolia, B. M., Iloreta, A., Freed, S. Z., Fruchtman, B., Bennett, B., and Newman, H. R.: Xanthogranulomatous pyelonephritis: Detailed analysis of 29 cases and a brief discussion of atypical presentations. J. Urol. *126*:437, 1981.

Van Kirk, O. C., Go, R. T., and Wedel, V. J.: Sonographic features of xanthogranulomatous pyelonephritis. AJR *134*:1035, 1980.

Compensatory Hypertrophy

Boner, G., Sherry, J., and Rieselbach, R. E.: Hypertrophy of the normal human kidney following contralateral nephrectomy. Nephron *9*:364, 1972.

Dossetor, R. S.: Renal compensatory hypertrophy in the adult. Br. J. Radiol. *48*:993, 1975.

Ekelund, L., and Gothlin, J.: Compensatory renal enlargement in older patients. AJR *127*:713, 1976.

Glazebrook, K. N., McGrath, F. P., and Steele, B. T.: Prenatal compensatory renal growth: Documentation with US. Radiology *189*:733, 1993.

Heideman, H. D., and Rosenbaum, H. D.: A study of renal size after contralateral nephrectomy. Radiology *94*:599, 1970.

Malt, R. A.: Compensatory growth of the kidney. N. Engl. J. Med. *280*:1446, 1969.

Ogden, D. A.: Donor and recipient function 2 to 4 years after renal homotransplantation: A paired study of 28 cases. Ann. Intern. Med. *67*:998, 1967.

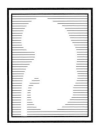

10

Diagnostic Set: Large, Multifocal, Bilateral

AUTOSOMAL DOMINANT (ADULT) POLYCYSTIC
KIDNEY DISEASE
TUBEROUS SCLEROSIS COMPLEX

VON HIPPEL-LINDAU DISEASE
LYMPHOMA
DIFFERENTIAL DIAGNOSIS

Autosomal dominant polycystic kidney disease, tuberous sclerosis complex, and von Hippel-Lindau disease are three major inherited cystic diseases that cause enlargement of both kidneys, multifocal nephrographic defects, and distortion of the renal contour by multiple mass lesions. The same pattern is commonly, but not invariably, present when lymphoma involves the kidney. Together, these diseases constitute the diagnostic set "large, multifocal, bilateral."

AUTOSOMAL DOMINANT (ADULT) POLYCYSTIC KIDNEY DISEASE

Definition

Approximately 85 to 95 per cent of patients with autosomal dominant polycystic kidney disease have a genetic abnormality in chromosome 16p; this gene has been termed PKD1. A second genetic locus has been identified in chromosome 4q and has been termed PKD2. Additional loci for this disease may also exist. These differences influence clinical severity, as discussed subsequently.

Although this disease is commonly associated with severely impaired renal function, only 2 to 5 per cent of the nephrons of affected kidneys are directly involved with cystic changes. The earliest manifestation of the disease, found in fetal kidneys, is fusiform dilatation of a limited number of nephrons. All segments of the nephron, from the glomerulus to the distal convoluted tubule, as well as the collecting ducts are involved. As the involved nephrons and collecting ducts continue to dilate, they acquire a corkscrew-like appearance, become tortuous, and eventually closure occurs between the nascent cyst and the lumen of the tubule or collecting duct. Thereafter, cysts accumulate fluid, enlarge, and compress other, uninvolved, nephrons. Thickening of the basement membrane, interstitial inflammation, and fibrosis throughout the kidney with impairment of renal function follow. These

events are illustrated schematically in Figure 10–1, which is based on the early microdissection studies of Osathanondh and Potter (1964), who classified autosomal dominant polycystic kidney disease as Type III in the Potter classification of cystic disease of the kidney. The abnormalities illustrated are in

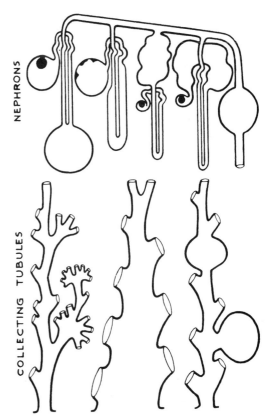

FIGURE 10–1. Schematic diagram of nephron dissection in autosomal dominant polycystic kidney disease. Localized or diffuse saccular and fusiform dilatations of any segment of nephrons and collecting ducts are illustrated. (From Potter, E. L.: Normal and Abnormal Development of the Kidney, 1972. Reproduced with kind permission of the author and Year Book Medical Publishers.)

237

contradistinction to autosomal recessive (infantile) polycystic kidney disease, in which the cystic dilatation is limited to the collecting ducts, and the nephrons are not primarily involved (see Chapter 8 and Fig. 8–10).

Flattened or cuboidal epithelium characterizes the lining of cysts in autosomal dominant polycystic kidney disease. Parenchymal changes are those of end-stage kidney disease, with tubule atrophy and vascular and glomerular sclerosis. Dystrophic calcification is common.

Cyst size varies from barely visible to several centimeters in diameter. Involvement may be quite asymmetric between the two kidneys. The cysts of this disease presenting in the newborn or infant may be macroscopic but are usually so small as to be microscopic or just barely visible to the unaided eye. As the size and number of cysts increase, the kidneys enlarge, and the renal contours become bosselated. Although the pelves and calyces are intrinsically normal, they are usually deformed by the expanding cysts. In some patients with minimal disease, the kidneys are only slightly enlarged, and the contours remain smooth, yet the presence of multiple cysts can be detected as nephrographic defects on contrast material–enhanced images.

Uncomplicated cysts contain clear, yellow fluid with electrolyte and urea levels similar to those of urine. This is in contrast to simple renal cyst fluid, which is chemically similar to plasma. Hemorrhage, however, is common. Cysts may also contain purulent material as a result of infection.

Although reports of unilateral "polycystic kidney disease" exist, it is unlikely that these actually represent the disorder described here because the genetic nature of autosomal dominant polycystic kidney disease implies involvement of both organs. Cases of so-called unilateral polycystic kidney disease probably are examples either of multiple simple cysts involving only one kidney or, in fact, are cases of autosomal dominant polycystic kidney disease with marked asymmetry and with the "normal" kidney containing cysts too small for radiologic detection. For similar reasons, multiple simple cysts localized to one portion of the kidney, known as localized cystic disease, are neither genetically transmitted nor associated with renal failure and should not be considered a form of autosomal dominant polycystic kidney disease.

Liver cysts of biliary origin are found in up to 75 per cent of patients with this disease. These cysts are usually spherical, unilocular, and occasionally large enough to cause hepatomegaly and/or biliary obstruction. Pancreatic cysts are found in approximately 10 per cent and splenic cysts are found in up to 5 per cent of patients. Cysts of thyroid, ovary, endometrium, seminal vesicles, lung, brain, pituitary gland, breasts, peritoneum, parathyroid, pineal, and epididymis have also been reported.

Cerebral aneurysms are estimated to occur in up to 26 per cent of patients with the disease. Valvular abnormalities of the heart (mitral, tricuspid, or aortic insufficiency or mitral valve prolapse), aortic dissection or aneurysm, inguinal hernia, and colonic diverticula are additional abnormalities that occur with this disease.

There is no increased prevalence of renal adenocarcinoma in patients with the disease. Some of the cases cited in support of such a relationship have been of cystic kidneys that were part of von Hippel-Lindau disease or have occurred in patients already on dialysis for end-stage renal disease. Certainly, there is no justification for routine screening for renal adenocarcinoma in patients with autosomal dominant polycystic kidney disease.

Clinical Setting

Autosomal dominant polycystic kidney disease is the most common of the hereditary renal diseases, accounting for up to 15 per cent of all patients on long-term hemodialysis in the United States. Because the disease may be clinically silent, the reported prevalence in autopsy series is somewhat higher than in clinical series. There is no sex predilection.

The disease is transmitted as an autosomal dominant trait with nearly 100 per cent penetrance, if the carrier lives long enough. Most families have a similar intensity of disease between generations. However, considerable variability in the severity of the disease may occur among individuals from the same family with presumably the same genetic mutation. Because the disease is characterized by variable expressivity, and because some cases may represent spontaneous mutation, many affected patients have no family history of renal disease. PKD2 patients have a milder form of disease than those with PKD1, as manifested by an older age of clinical presentation and less likelihood of requiring dialysis or transplantation.

The morphologic changes of the disease probably begin *in utero* in most patients but go undetected. Only rarely is the severity of the disease sufficient to cause renal failure *in utero*, in which case the pregnancy is complicated by oligohydramnios, and the infant demonstrates the findings of Potter's syndrome and abnormal ultrasonographic findings. Otherwise, clinical manifestations are very uncommon in children. Most patients become symptomatic with cyst pain or uremia in the 4th or 5th decade of life. Rarely, the disease is uncovered as late as the 9th decade. As ultrasonographic or computed tomographic screening of patients at risk increases, the mean age of discovery will surely decrease.

Palpable mass, hypertension, abdominal pain, hematuria, and urinary tract infection are common. Hypertension may antedate renal impairment. The absence of hypertension at the time of diagnosis may be a favorable prognostic sign. Proteinuria and hematuria are often present. Polycythemia occurs secondary to erythropoietin production by the affected kidneys. As the cysts enlarge, more renal parenchyma is compromised, and azotemia worsens. Those patients who develop renal failure usually do so by the age of 60 years.

Infection, hemorrhage, stone formation, cyst rupture, and obstruction are complications of this disease. Infected cysts may be asymptomatic and detected only through aspiration or as an incidental finding at surgery or autopsy. Hemorrhage is intracystic, retroperitoneal, or into the collecting system with resultant hematuria. Occasionally, bleeding is massive and requires nephrectomy. Calculi form presumably as a result of urine stasis in partially obstructed collecting structures in up to 35 per cent of patients. Urate stones are more common than oxalate stones.

Extrarenal cysts seldom cause symptoms. There is no correlation between the severity of renal cystic disease and severity of hepatic cysts. Hepatic function and portal pressure are usually normal, although prolonged survival may lead to morbidity and mortality from impaired hepatic function or biliary obstruction.

Death due to rupture of a cerebral aneurysm into the brain and subarachnoid space occurs in approximately 10 per cent of patients with the disease. This complication of cerebral aneurysm rupture may increase as survival is prolonged by dialysis and transplantation.

It is generally held that if cysts are not identified by age 30 years in a screening ultrasonogram of a patient with a positive family history for this disease, there is little likelihood that the patient has the disease. Age-related screening criteria (Ravine et al., 1994) for the diagnosis of autosomal dominant polycystic kidney disease in patients with a positive family history include two unilateral or bilateral cysts (patients younger than 30 years of age), two cysts in each kidney (patients between 30 and 59 years of age), and more than four cysts in each kidney (patients older than 60 years of age).

Radiologic Findings

The abdominal film is normal in the early stage of autosomal dominant polycystic kidney disease. As the disease progresses, the enlarged kidneys may become recognizable as retroperitoneal soft-tissue masses. Enlargement is frequently asymmetric and may result in displacement of the duodenum, the flexures of the colon, and other intraperitoneal and extraperitoneal structures. Extrinsic scalloping of the posterior wall of the stomach may be seen on upper gastrointestinal studies. The psoas muscles may be obscured. Dystrophic calcification has variable patterns, including thin or thick curvilinear densities or scattered amorphous plaques (Fig. 10–2). Renal calculi may signify superimposed infection.

The nephrogram is characterized by numerous sharply marginated radiolucencies throughout the parenchyma of both kidneys. This is best demonstrated by computed tomography, although tomograms during excretory urography will also docu-

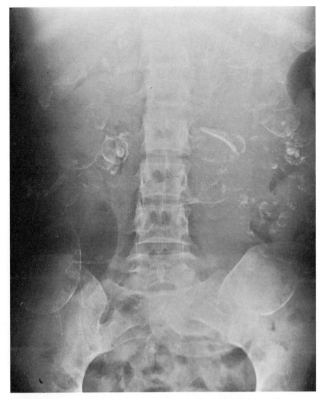

FIGURE 10–2. Autosomal dominant polycystic kidney disease. Abdominal radiograph. The kidneys fill the upper abdomen and midabdomen and displace intestine into the pelvis. Psoas margins are obscure. Calcium is deposited in a curvilinear pattern in the walls of a large number of cysts. (Courtesy of Stanford M. Goldman, M.D., University of Texas, Houston, Texas.)

ment this abnormality. Young, asymptomatic patients frequently have enlarged kidneys with smooth outlines and normal collecting structures, although the nephrogram will be abnormal even at this stage (Fig. 10–3). As the disease progresses, however, the contour becomes bosselated. The larger cysts will elongate, efface, and displace the calyces (Fig. 10–4). Occasionally, a large cyst will obstruct one or more calyces.

Ultrasonography may detect minimal disease as small echo-free masses in slightly large but otherwise normal kidneys. As the disease progresses, the kidneys enlarge, their contour becomes bosselated, and numerous cysts are visualized as masses containing uncomplicated fluid (Figs. 10–5, 10–6). Marked variation in the size of the cysts is common. The central sinus echo complex is distorted by the larger cysts. Cysts complicated by hemorrhage or infection have internal echoes, fluid-debris levels, and thick walls. Differentiation between hemorrhage and infection is impossible by ultrasonography alone. Calcification (dystrophic or nephrolithiasis) is very echogenic and causes acoustic shadows.

Ultrasonography may detect the disease *in utero* as enlarged kidneys, ascites, hepatomegaly, and renal cysts. In the newborn, the ultrasonographic features of the disease may be indistinguishable from

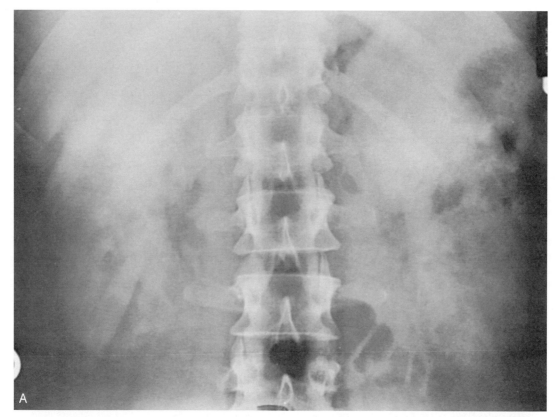

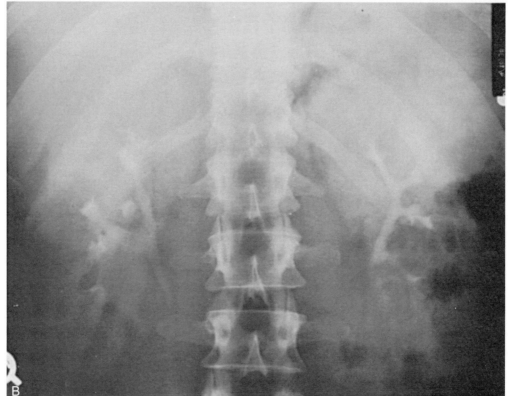

FIGURE 10–3. Autosomal dominant polycystic kidney disease in a 38-year-old man with hypertension and bilaterally large, smooth kidneys.

A, Excretory urogram, 2-minute film. Characteristic multiple radiolucencies of varying size are present in the nephrogram. Right kidney length = 17.5 cm; left kidney length = 18.0 cm.

B, Excretory urogram, 5-minute film. There is no distortion of the pelvocalyceal system.

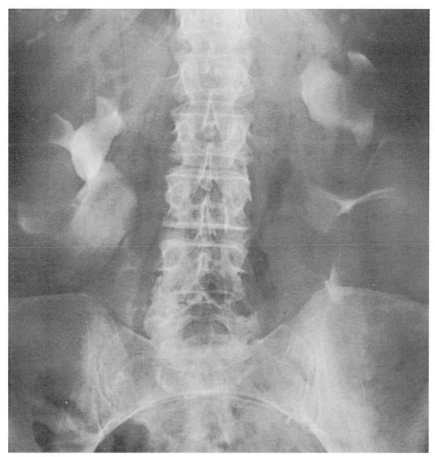

FIGURE 10–4. Autosomal dominant polycystic kidney disease in a 74-year-old woman. Marked multifocal enlargement of both kidneys, focal displacement of the collecting structures, and normal opacification are common urographic features of this disease.

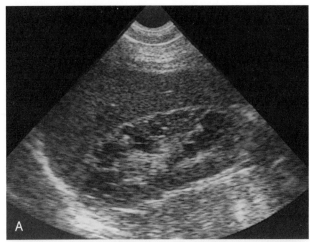

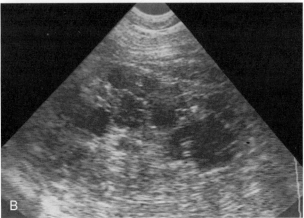

FIGURE 10–5. Autosomal dominant polycystic kidney disease increasing in size over a 4-year interval. The kidney also changes from a smooth to a bosselated contour in the same interval. Ultrasonograms of the right kidney in longitudinal section.

    A, 1983. Length = 9 cm.

    B, 1987. Length = 13 cm. (Kindly provided by Brian Garra, M.D., Georgetown University, Washington, D.C.)

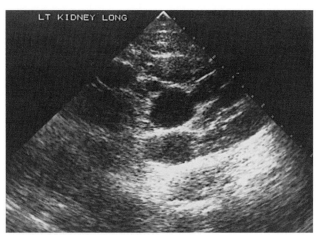

FIGURE 10–6. Autosomal dominant polycystic kidney disease. Ultrasonogram of the left kidney in a longitudinal section. The kidney is enlarged and bosselated by numerous, varying-sized cysts containing uncomplicated fluid.

the nephromegaly and diffuse increased echogenicity of autosomal recessive polycystic kidney disease, although in some instances small cysts are visible as well (Fig. 10–7). In older children, the pattern is similar to that seen in adults. Ultraso-

nography may reveal nephromegaly and cysts in asymptomatic children of parents with known disease and, thus, is an excellent modality for screening (Fig. 10–8).

Cysts of the liver, pancreas, or spleen appear as echo-free masses with increased through-sound transmission. Their detection helps confirm the diagnosis of the disease. When these extrarenal cysts are prominent, it is often difficult to assess the boundaries of contiguous organs.

Computed tomography demonstrates multiple round-to-oval cysts that are variable in size and scattered throughout the cortex and medulla (Fig. 10–9). Uncomplicated cysts have attenuation values near those of water and do not enhance. Because of the dense parenchymal blush of uninvolved surrounding renal parenchyma, cysts are accentuated on contrast material–enhanced scans. With advanced disease, unenhanced scans often demonstrate curvilinear or amorphous dystrophic calcifications within cyst walls or compressed atrophic parenchyma and acute hemorrhage into cysts recognized as a well-defined hyperdense mass on an unenhanced scan (Fig. 10–10). These high-density

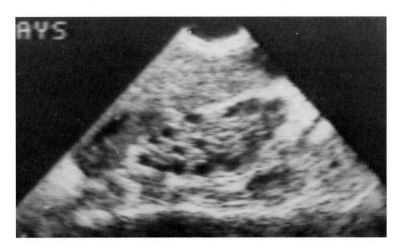

FIGURE 10–7. Autosomal dominant polycystic kidney disease in a newborn. Ultrasonogram of the right kidney, longitudinal section. The kidney is smooth and hyperechoic and contains a small number of detectable cysts.

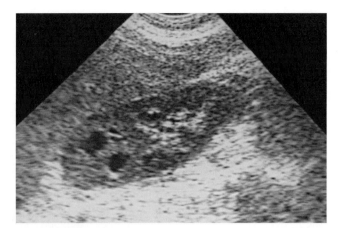

FIGURE 10–8. Autosomal dominant polycystic kidney disease in an asymptomatic 14-year-old boy with a positive family history. Ultrasonogram of the right kidney in a longitudinal section. Hyperechoicity and several cysts indicate a carrier state. (Kindly provided by Brian Garra, M.D., Georgetown University, Washington, D.C.)

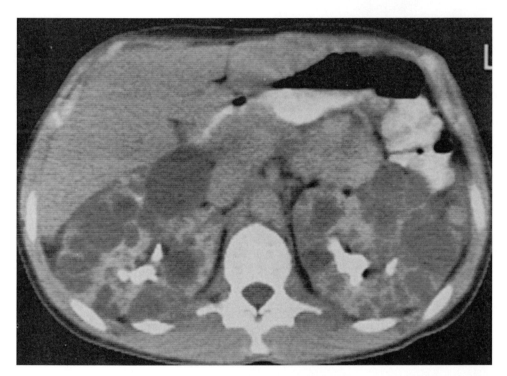

FIGURE 10–9. Autosomal dominant polycystic kidney disease. Computed tomogram, contrast material–enhanced. The large kidneys, with multiple masses of varying size, are well demonstrated in this 35-year-old hypertensive man with mild azotemia. The masses have a water attenuation value and do not enhance after contrast material is injected. Note distorted and compressed collecting structures.

FIGURE 10–10. Autosomal dominant polycystic kidney disease in a 56-year-old man. Computed tomogram, unenhanced. Multiple foci of calcification are present in the cyst walls. There are two cysts in the right kidney that have an increased attenuation representative of cyst hemorrhage *(arrows).*

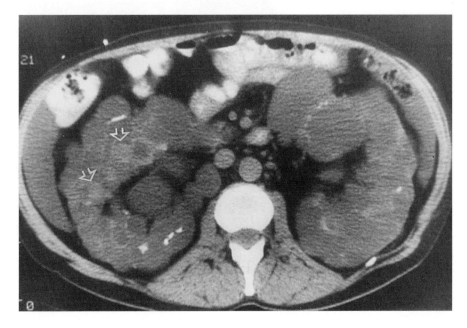

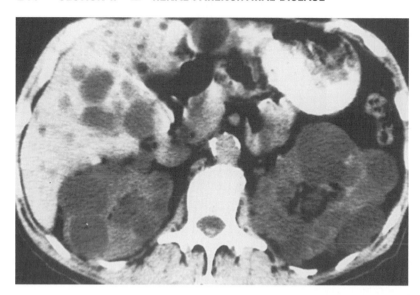

FIGURE 10–11. Autosomal dominant polycystic kidney disease. Computed tomogram, unenhanced. Multiple hepatic cysts of varying size are present. Note the asymmetry of renal involvement.

cysts are common especially in patients with marked renal enlargement and flank pain. They are often multiple and subcapsular or perirenal. With time, the computed tomographic density of a hemorrhagic cyst may diminish. Both urate and oxalate stones appear as densities in the collecting systems.

An infected cyst may also have a thick, irregular wall that calcifies. The attenuation value of an infected cyst is slightly higher than that of water and may be variable within a single cyst. Localized thickening of Gerota's fascia is a nonspecific finding sometimes seen with infection. Gas within an infected cyst is easily detected with computed tomography. A perinephric abscess may also develop in conjunction with infection of the cystic kidney.

Cysts are frequently identified in the liver and, occasionally, in the pancreas and spleen (Figs. 10–11, 10–12). There is no relationship between the number of cysts recognized in the liver and their frequency in the kidney.

Magnetic resonance imaging demonstrates uncomplicated cysts as homogeneous and low-intensity on T1-weighted images and homogeneous and high-intensity on T2-weighted images (Fig. 10–12). Cysts complicated by hemorrhage are usually hyperintense, but their appearance varies with the amount of time since the bleeding episode. Layering may be present in cysts with recent hemorrhage. Infected cysts and cysts with high protein content are intermediate between the two extremes of uncomplicated and complicated cysts. Screening magnetic resonance angiography should be used in patients whose family history includes rupture of an intracranial aneurysm and in those patients who have already experienced a spontaneous rupture of an intracranial aneurysm.

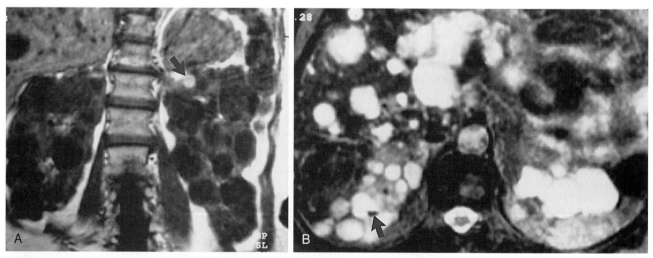

FIGURE 10–12. Autosomal dominant polycystic kidney disease. Magnetic resonance images.
A, T1-weighted scan, coronal projection. The kidneys are enlarged by multiple cysts of low-signal intensity. A small hemorrhagic cyst in the upper pole of the left kidney *(arrow)* is of high-signal intensity. Several liver cysts are present.
B, T2-weighted image, transverse plane. High-signal intensity cysts are present in the kidneys, liver, and head of pancreas. Low-signal area in right kidney *(arrow)* probably represents cyst hemorrhage.

AUTOSOMAL DOMINANT (ADULT) POLYCYSTIC KIDNEY DISEASE TYPICAL FINDINGS

Primary Uroradiologic Elements

Size: large
Contour: multifocal masses
Lesion distribution: bilateral (may be asymmetric)

Secondary Uroradiologic Elements

Collecting system: displaced and attenuated
Nephrogram: replaced (multiple masses with smooth margins, varying size; radiolucent
    with urography or angiography; water density/intensity and nonenhancing with
    computed tomography/magnetic resonance imaging)
Echogenicity: multiple, fluid-filled masses

Angiography demonstrates well the multiple, sharply defined, variably sized nephrographic defects caused by the cysts, which also stretch and displace intrarenal arteries. Cysts complicated by hemorrhage or infection may have abnormal vessels that simulate those usually associated with neoplasia. Hepatic and splenic cysts appear as avascular masses on selective visceral injections. Angiography, however, is generally not required in the evaluation of autosomal dominant polycystic kidney disease except, perhaps, in the evaluation of a possible adenocarcinoma.

TUBEROUS SCLEROSIS COMPLEX

Definition

Tuberous sclerosis complex is an autosomal dominant genetic disorder characterized by hamartomatous growths in the central nervous system, eyes, skin, heart, liver, kidney, and adrenal glands. A seizure disorder is the major clinical problem in these patients. In the kidney, multiple angiomyolipomas and cysts dominate.

The predominant gene, TSC2, in this complex is located on chromosome 16p, immediately adjacent to PKD1, described in the previous section. Another locus on chromosome 9q, designated TSC1, is implicated in approximately one-third of cases. New mutations account for up to 80 per cent of patients with this complex. Virtually all patients with the genetic disorder have clinical manifestations.

The primary criteria for the diagnosis of tuberous sclerosis complex is the presence of any one of the following: cerebral cortical tubers, subependymal nodules, retinal hamartomas, facial angiofibromas, periungual fibromas, fibromas or fibrous plaques on the forehead or scalp, and multiple angiomyolipomas of the kidney.

Dominant renal manifestations of the complex include multiple angiomyolipomas and/or cysts and, much less commonly, perirenal lymphangioma. Renal involvement, usually with multiple angiomyolipomas, occurs in approximately 50 per cent of patients. These patients have typical fatty hamarto-matous lesions that, by virtue of their multiplicity and bilaterality, cause renal enlargement and a bosselated contour in both kidneys. Abnormal blood vessels within the angiomyolipomas are prone to rupture. A variant form of simple fluid-filled cyst is frequently found in kidneys of patients with tuberous sclerosis in addition to angiomyolipomas. These cysts are lined with hyperplastic columnar cells that resemble the epithelial cells of the proximal tubule. In both macroscopic and radiologic appearance, however, the cyst of tuberous sclerosis is indistinguishable from the common form of simple nephrogenic cyst. Cysts may develop before other stigmata of the disease and are thus more likely to be encountered in youthful patients. They are not, however, a principal diagnostic feature of the tuberous sclerosis complex.

Renal adenocarcinoma occurs in 1 to 2 per cent of patients with the complex. The fact that these lesions tend to occur in patients of a younger age than spontaneous renal adenocarcinoma in the general population and are often bilateral suggest that they reflect a hereditary predisposition rather than a sporadic occurrence.

Clinical Setting

The clinical manifestations of renal involvement in tuberous sclerosis complex patients include vague chronic abdominal or flank pain, hematuria, and uremia. Major hemorrhage of an angiomyolipoma can result in perinephric hematoma, massive hematuria, renal obstruction, and worsening of renal failure. In these cases, renal arterial embolization is often employed to spare renal function, although in some cases nephrectomy may be required. End-stage renal disease develops in up to 15 per cent of cases and is the result of renal parenchymal compression and fibrosis induced by multiple, large angiomyolipomas and/or cysts compressing adjacent parenchyma.

Other features of the complex reflect hamartomas of the brain, skin, eyes, bones, heart, and lungs. These include seizure disorders, various skin lesions, mental retardation, visual disturbance, di-

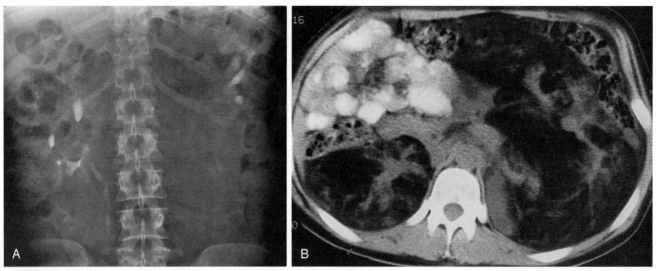

FIGURE 10–13. Tuberous sclerosis complex in a 37-year-old woman.

A, Excretory urogram. The kidneys are markedly enlarged, and the pelvocalyceal systems are deformed by multiple fatty masses that impart a mottled lucency to the radiograph.

B, Computed tomogram, unenhanced. The kidneys are enlarged by multiple masses of fat attenuation. The renal parenchyma is replaced by the angiomyolipomas.

minished air exchange, spontaneous pneumothorax, cardiac outflow obstruction, and arrhythmia.

Radiologic Findings

Abdominal radiographs and excretory urograms demonstrate marked increase in renal size and may also exhibit the radiolucency associated with the fatty component of the multiple angiomyolipomas (Fig. 10–13). Focal densities in the spine or pelvis representing osseous hamartomas may be present.

Computed tomography or magnetic resonance imaging best define the abnormalities in the kidneys of patients with this complex (Fig. 10–14; see Fig. 10–13*B*). Multiplicity and bilaterality of angiomyolipomas and cysts, the contents of which have the imaging characteristics of uncomplicated fluid, are the hallmarks of this abnormality. In many pa-

tients, only angiomyolipomas are present. These are expansive masses of fatty and nonfatty soft tissue that cause nephrographic defects in contrast material–enhanced images as they displace nephrons. Although all angiomyolipomas arise in the kidneys, some have most of their bulk in the perirenal space, where they may simulate the appearance of a liposarcoma. Fresh hemorrhage, either intratumoral, intrarenal, or perirenal in location, creates characteristic attenuation values or signal intensities relative to those of normal renal parenchyma. Occasionally, intratumoral hemorrhage is extensive enough to obliterate the imaging characteristics of fat and thereby obscures the diagnosis of angiomyolipoma. Cysts, when present, will be interspersed with characteristic angiomyolipomas. Uncommonly, and especially in children, multiple bilateral cysts will be the only lesions accounting for the enlarged and

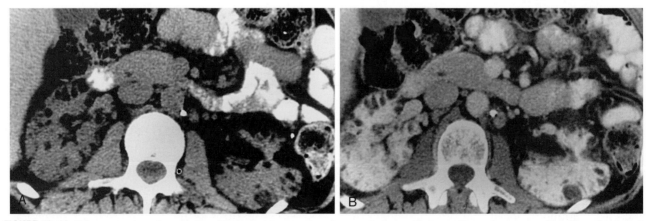

FIGURE 10–14. Tuberous sclerosis complex. Computed tomograms demonstrate multiple small renal masses with either dominant fat- or mixed fat- and soft-tissue attenuation values.

A, Unenhanced scan.

B, Contrast material–enhanced scan.

TUBEROUS SCLEROSIS COMPLEX TYPICAL FINDINGS

Primary Uroradiologic Elements

Size: large
Contour: multifocal masses
Lesion distribution: bilateral

Secondary Uroradiologic Elements

Collecting system: displaced and attenuated
Nephrogram: replaced (multiple masses, varying size; **cysts**: water density/intensity and nonenhancing with computed tomography/magnetic resonance imaging; **angiomyolipomas**: mixed fat/soft-tissue density/intensity and enhancing with computed tomography/magnetic resonance imaging)
Echogenicity: multiple, fluid-filled masses; multiple solid masses

---

bosselated kidneys (Fig. 10–15). Rarely, imaging evidence of a lymphangioma is present as a multiloculated collection of uncomplicated, waterlike fluid distributed along the periphery of the kidney in a capsular or subcapsular configuration. Also rare are periaortic lymphadenopathy representing hamartomatous change in lymph nodes, liver hamartomas, and pulmonary lymphangiomyomatosis.

Ultrasonography characterizes the kidneys of tuberous sclerosis complex as large and bosselated by multiple fluid-filled and/or solid masses. The fatty component of angiomyolipomas is hyperechoic but no more so than the echogenicity that may be encountered in some adenocarcinomas of the kidney. Therefore, ultrasonography does not have the diagnostic accuracy inherent in either computed tomography or magnetic resonance imaging.

Angiographic findings in the tuberous sclerosis complex kidney are dominated by the vascular component of the angiomyolipomas. These angiomyolipomas are seen as tortuous, large vessels with aneurysmal dilatations. Blood flow to the angiomyolipoma is usually through a single, enlarged artery.

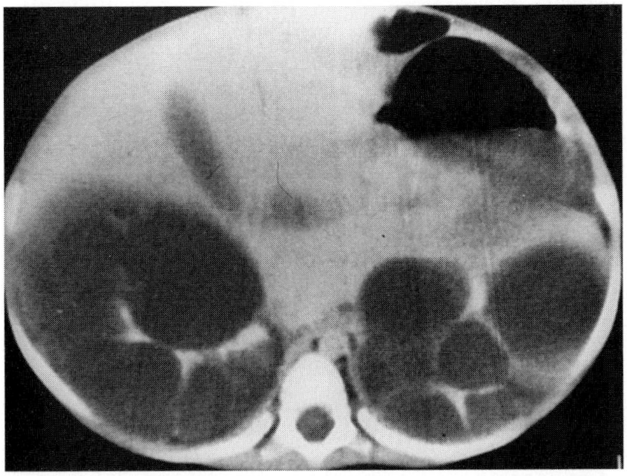

FIGURE 10–15. Tuberous sclerosis complex in a 14-year-old female. Computed tomogram, contrast material–enhanced. The kidneys are enlarged by multiple fluid-filled cysts. There are no apparent angiomyolipomas.

Arteriovenous shunting is not a feature of angiomyolipoma of the kidney. Angiography not only demonstrates active bleeding from an angiomyolipoma but also can serve as the means for therapeutic embolization.

VON HIPPEL-LINDAU DISEASE

Definition

Von Hippel-Lindau disease is a multisystem disorder that involves the kidneys, central nervous system, spinal cord, retina, adrenal glands, and pancreas. The gene for von Hippel-Lindau disease, which is transmitted as an autosomal dominant trait, has been localized to chromosome 3. The expressivity of the disease is quite varied among families and between individuals. Some patients have a form of the disease that is not associated with pheochromocytoma, whereas others have a particular mutation that is associated with pheochromocytoma and paraganglioma.

Renal lesions in von Hippel-Lindau disease are characterized by multiple bilateral cysts as well as by cystic and solid adenocarcinomas. These abnormalities become detectable in patients' late teenage years and are generally progressive thereafter. Metastases usually do not occur until after the age of 35 years. The cysts found in von Hippel-Lindau disease are benign, but they are histologically distinctive from simple nephrogenic cysts by their epithelial lining of hyperplastic or metaplastic clear cells, which may give rise to adenocarcinoma. Those cysts that remain benign grow slowly or not at all and contain uncomplicated fluid. Adenocarcinomas arise either *de novo* from microscopic foci in renal tubule cells or from cysts whose epithelial lining has become neoplastic. Those that arise from originally benign cysts are transformed by atypical characteristics that suggest their malignant nature. As adenocarcinomas increase in size, they assume a higher histologic grade of malignancy. A common cause of death in von Hippel-Lindau patients is metastatic adenocarcinoma of the kidney.

Extrarenal sites of abnormalities in von Hippel-

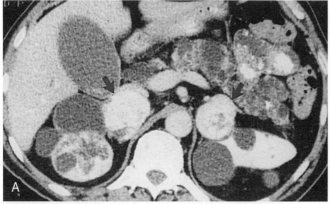

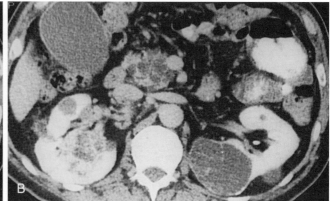

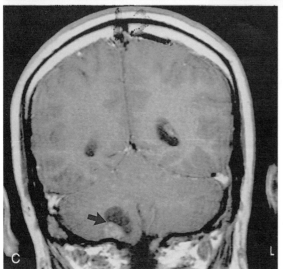

FIGURE 10–16. von Hippel-Lindau disease.

A, Computed tomogram with contrast material enhancement in the region of the upper poles of the kidneys. There are bilateral solid and complex cystic renal masses and bilateral solid pheochromocytomas *(arrows).* The pancreas is replaced by multiple cysts.

B, Computed tomogram at the level of the renal hila. There are bilateral, multiple solid and complex cystic adenocarcinomas.

C, Postgadolinium T1-weighted magnetic resonance image, coronal plane. A cystic hemangioblastoma appears as an enhancing nodule in the right cerebellum *(arrow).*

Lindau disease include the cerebellum, brain stem, and spinal cord (hemangioblastomas); the retina (angiomas); the pancreas (cysts, cystadenomas, and neuroendocrine tumors); the adrenal gland (pheochromocytoma); the sympathetic ganglia throughout the body (paragangliomas); and the epididymis (cystadenomas).

Clinical Setting

The clinical manifestations of renal involvement in von Hippel-Lindau disease are predominantly re-

lated to the growth of malignant tumors. These include abdominal or flank pain, increasing abdominal girth, gross or microscopic hematuria, and retroperitoneal hemorrhage. Symptoms related to metastases to other organs appear in the course of the disease.

Clinical findings related to central nervous system involvement include gait disturbance, loss of balance, headache, and disorientation. Pancreatic lesions may cause symptoms owing to mass effect. These include abdominal pain, early satiety, and

---

VON HIPPEL-LINDAU DISEASE TYPICAL FINDINGS

Primary Uroradiologic Elements

Size: large
Contour: multifocal masses
Lesion distribution: bilateral

Secondary Uroradiologic Elements

Collecting system: displaced and attenuated
Nephrogram: replaced (multiple masses, varying size; **cysts:** water density/intensity and nonenhancing with computed tomography/magnetic resonance imaging; **adenocarcinomas:** soft-tissue density/intensity and enhancing with computed tomography/magnetic resonance imaging; cystic components)
Echogenicity: multiple, fluid-filled masses; multiple solid masses

partial gastric outlet obstruction. Diabetes mellitus or malabsorption may occur with extensive replacement of the pancreas by cysts. Neuroendocrine tumors of the pancreas may metastasize. Pheochromocytoma and paraganglioma tend to arise at an earlier age and are more commonly bilateral than are their sporadic counterparts. Pheochromocytoma and paraganglioma usually produce hypertension, tachycardia, and anxiety, although they may be asymptomatic. Epididymal cystadenomas are usually asymptomatic but may obstruct the rete testis.

Radiologic Findings

Renal involvement in von Hippel-Lindau disease is best documented by contrast material–enhanced computed tomography or magnetic resonance imaging (Fig. 10–16). The renal cyst of von Hippel-Lindau disease is unicameral and contains waterlike, uncomplicated fluid. This is the same appearance as a sporadic nephrogenic cyst despite the presence of hyperplastic or metaplastic epithelial lining. The cyst is usually multiple and bilateral. Mixed cystic and solid tumors, and completely solid tumors, enlarge both kidneys and bosselate their contours. Tumors of solid tissue usually enhance with contrast material and represent malignancy. Hemorrhage and necrosis are often present in those adenocarcinomas that are predominantly solid. Ultrasonography may demonstrate many of these findings but is generally not as efficacious as computed tomography or magnetic resonance imaging, both of which may also demonstrate metastases to regional lymph nodes and distant organs.

Computed tomography and magnetic resonance imaging also demonstrate well the extrarenal manifestations of von Hippel-Lindau disease (see Fig. 10–16A, C). Adrenal pheochromocytomas, paragangliomas, and pancreatic cysts or tumors often are documented during kidney imaging. Gadolinium-enhanced magnetic resonance images effectively detect hemangioblastomas in the central nervous system and spinal cord.

LYMPHOMA

Definition

All forms of lymphoma have similar patterns of renal involvement, although each has distinctive pathologic, clinical, and prognostic features. In the largest published autopsy series of patients with lymphoma, renal involvement occurred in one-third (Richmond et al., 1962). Bilateral involvement occurred three times more often than unilateral disease. Of all the cases, multiple nodules were present in 61 per cent, although some were too small for detection on the radiographic techniques in use at the time of the study. Eleven per cent had invasion from perirenal disease, 7 per cent had a single, bulky tumor, and 7 per cent had a small, solitary nodule. Diffuse infiltration occurred in 6 per cent,

and microscopic disease was found in only 7 per cent. Most subsequent, smaller series reporting renal involvement in lymphoma confirm this pattern of lesion distribution.

Renal involvement occurs most frequently with non-Hodgkin's lymphoma and less often with Hodgkin's disease. Leukemia, which is quite separate from malignant lymphoma, causes bilateral, diffuse infiltration of the kidneys and is discussed in Chapter 8.

Lymphoid tissue is not native to the kidney. Renal lymphoma, therefore, always represents either bloodborne metastases or direct invasion by tumor growing in the perirenal space. Hematogenous metastases most commonly produce multiple, bilateral nodules. Because lymphoma grows by infiltration, the interface between lymphomatous deposits in the kidney and normal surrounding parenchyma is not sharp. As the kidney enlarges, the reniform or bean shape is preserved, at least initially. Eventually, the lymphomatous masses become so large that they appear expansive or ball-shaped (see discussion of patterns of tumor growth in Chapter 12). Direct invasion of the kidney by lymphoma in the perirenal space occurs either through the renal sinus from tumor medial to the kidney (trans-sinus spread) or across the renal capsule from tumor in the perirenal space lateral to the kidney (transcapular spread). Trans-sinus spread is often associated with obstructive uropathy as a result of involvement of the ureter or renal pelvis. When tumor surrounds the pelvis, caliectasis without pelviectasis is seen.

Clinical Setting

Lymphoma does not commonly produce clinical findings referable to the urinary tract. Uremia is rare. Renal parenchymal nodules may produce flank pain or tenderness, a palpable mass, or hematuria. Masses in the region of the renal hilus can produce hypertension or renal vein occlusion as a result of pressure on the renal pedicle. Obstructive uropathy may follow directly from retroperitoneal involvement of ureters or indirectly from retroperitoneal fibrosis.

Proteinuria, cylindruria, elevated blood urea nitrogen levels, and hypercalcemia are often present. Hypercalcemia may be severe enough to cause nephropathy. Complications of irradiation or chemotherapy that may be manifest in the urinary tract are acute urate nephropathy (see Chapter 8) and radiation nephritis (see Chapter 6).

Radiologic Findings

The earliest stages of lymphoma in the kidneys are represented by metastatic nodules detected as nephrographic defects on contrast material–enhanced imaging studies at a time when the kidneys may be normal in size and contour. Eventually, however, lymphoma produces bilaterally enlarged kidneys, multifocal bulges of the renal contour, and

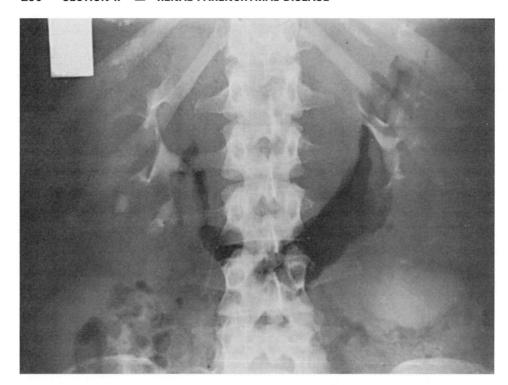

FIGURE 10–17. Non-Hodgkin's lymphoma producing bilateral renal enlargement due to multifocal masses. The collecting systems are displaced at several sites. Excretory urogram.

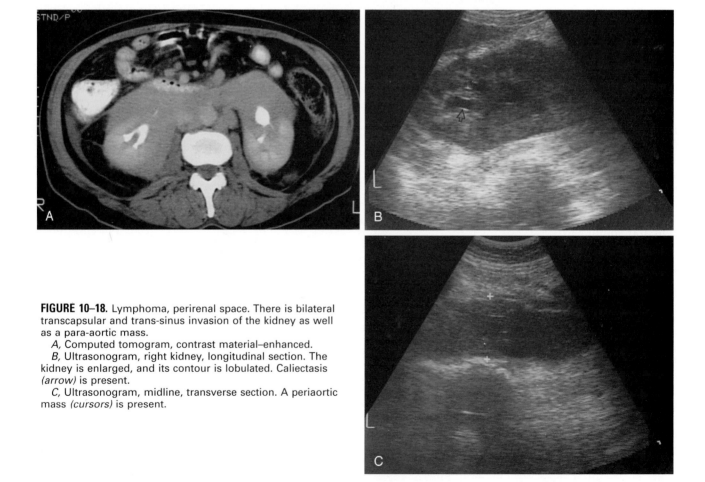

FIGURE 10–18. Lymphoma, perirenal space. There is bilateral transcapsular and trans-sinus invasion of the kidney as well as a para-aortic mass.

    A, Computed tomogram, contrast material–enhanced.

    B, Ultrasonogram, right kidney, longitudinal section. The kidney is enlarged, and its contour is lobulated. Caliectasis *(arrow)* is present.

    C, Ultrasonogram, midline, transverse section. A periaortic mass *(cursors)* is present.

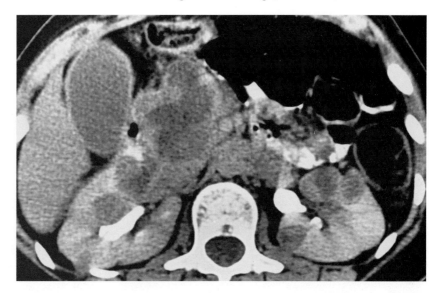

FIGURE 10–19. Non-Hodgkin's lymphoma with multiple bilateral renal masses and marked retroperitoneal adenopathy. Computed tomogram, contrast material–enhanced.

displacement of the collecting system (Fig. 10–17). At times, a single mass in one kidney will be the only finding. Opacification of the kidney progressively diminishes as lymphomatous masses grow, coalesce, and replace nephrons. Lymphoma invading the kidney from the perirenal space, either by a trans-sinus or a transcapular route, produces a large, retroperitoneal soft-tissue mass and displacement of the kidney. The nephrogram is deficient and poorly marginated wherever the parenchyma has been invaded. With trans-sinus invasion, the kidney may be displaced laterally, and the pelvis may be surrounded by tumor. In this situation, the pelvis is obstructed but not necessarily dilated. Caliectasis, however, is usually present (Fig. 10–18). Obstructive uropathy may also result from ureteral encasement by lymphomatous tissue more caudal in the retroperitoneum.

Computed tomography identifies the lympho-matous mass or masses more often than excretory urography or ultrasonography (Fig. 10–19). These masses are nonencapsulated and may have irregular margins. Before contrast material administration, the attenuation value of lymphomatous tissue is slightly less than that of normal parenchyma; rarely, the lymphoma tissue is hyperdense. Contrast material enhancement is minimal, always less than that of the renal parenchyma, and usually homogeneous. Trans-sinus and transcapular invasion of lymphoma from the perirenal space and from ureteral, lymph node, and other organ involvement are well demonstrated by computed tomography (Fig. 10–20; see also Figs. 10–18 and 10–19).

Lymphomatous kidney and perirenal space masses are identified by ultrasonography as hypoechoic structures, with poor sound transmission and fine internal echoes (Fig. 10–21; see also Fig. 10–18B and C). The central sinus echoes of the kidney

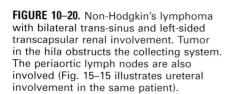

FIGURE 10–20. Non-Hodgkin's lymphoma with bilateral trans-sinus and left-sided transcapsular renal involvement. Tumor in the hila obstructs the collecting system. The periaortic lymph nodes are also involved (Fig. 15–15 illustrates ureteral involvement in the same patient).

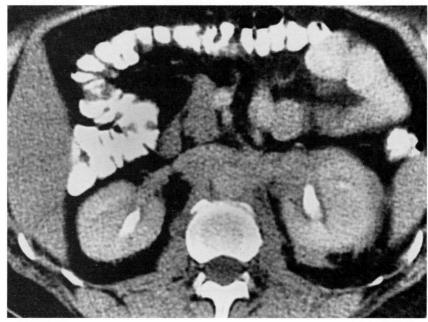

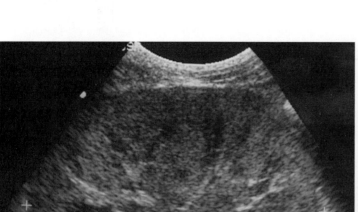

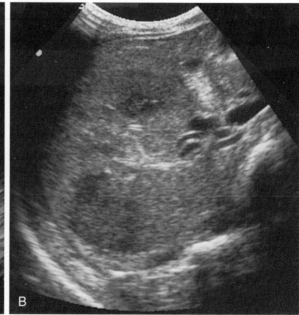

FIGURE 10–21. Lymphoma in both kidneys of a 30-year-old male with autoimmune deficiency syndrome. Ultrasonogram. Both kidneys are enlarged by multiple hypoechic masses.
  A, Left kidney, sagittal projection.
  B, Right kidney, transverse projection.
  (Kindly contributed by Cynthia Caskey, M.D., and Ulrike Hamper, M.D., Johns Hopkins University, Baltimore, Maryland.)

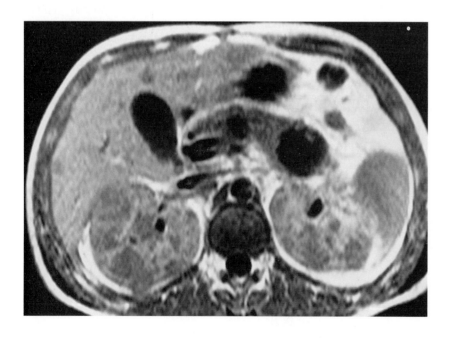

FIGURE 10–22. Non-Hodgkin's lymphoma. There are multiple focal nodules of intermediate-signal intensity in both kidneys. Magnetic resonance image, T1-weighted, contrast material–enhanced.

LYMPHOMA TYPICAL FINDINGS

Primary Uroradiologic Elements

Size: large
Contour: normal to multifocal masses
Lesion distribution: bilateral

Secondary Uroradiologic Elements

Collecting system: displaced; caliectasis without pelviectasis (trans-sinus invasion)
Parenchymal thickness: expanded (focal)
Nephrogram: multifocal masses (attenuation value less than that of normal tissue; minimal enhancement with contrast material)
Echogenicity: multifocal hypoechoic solid masses

---

may be diminished or disappear when sinus fat is replaced by lymphomatous tissue.

Magnetic resonance images of renal and perirenal lymphoma demonstrate low to intermediate signal intensity on T1- and T2-weighted images (Fig. 10–22). The pattern of contrast material enhancement is heterogeneous and less than that of renal parenchyma.

Other radiologic findings in renal lymphoma include occasional global enlargement of both kidneys with smooth contours and ureteral displacement. Renal vein occlusion may be associated with renal sinus tumor.

Most lymphomatous renal masses are hypovascular. The angiographic findings of lymphoma in the kidney overlap those of renal carcinoma and of other solid tumors and inflammatory masses. Angiography offers no useful information in the assessment of this disease.

DIFFERENTIAL DIAGNOSIS

The differential diagnosis of diseases within this diagnostic set is guided by the determination of whether the lesions are fluid-filled cysts or solid tumors or a combination of the two and by the clinical setting. The distinction between fluid-filled and solid masses is best accomplished by ultrasonography, computed tomography, or magnetic resonance imaging.

If the lesions producing bilateral, multifocal enlargement of the kidneys are filled with fluid, the differential diagnosis strongly favors **autosomal dominant polycystic kidney disease.** Less likely possibilities include **multiple simple cysts of both kidneys; chronic, severe, bilateral obstructive uropathy with marked caliectasis; von Hippel-Lindau disease; tuberous sclerosis complex;** or those instances of **acquired cystic kidney disease** with large kidneys. Multiple simple cysts are fewer and more uniform than those seen in polycystic kidney disease. Further, they occur in patients who do not necessarily have hypertension, renal failure, or a family history of renal disease. The demonstration of communication

among multiple dilated fluid-filled spaces by ultrasonography or computed tomography distinguishes chronic obstructive uropathy from cystic disease of the kidney. This distinction can also be made by the conversion of radiolucent areas to radiodense ones on late films during contrast material-enhanced studies. In von Hippel-Lindau disease, tuberous sclerosis complex, and acquired cystic kidney disease, other distinguishing clinical and radiologic features are usually present. Finally, multiple fluid-filled renal cysts are found in numerous syndromes that are known variably as **glomerulocystic, microcystic,** or **pluricystic disorders** of the kidney. Here, too, clinical findings help to clarify the diagnosis. These are discussed briefly in Chapter 8.

The combination of both solid tumors and cysts as a cause of bilateral kidney enlargement strongly suggests **von Hippel-Lindau disease** (cysts and adenocarcinomas) or **tuberous sclerosis** (cysts and angiomyolipomas) as the most likely diagnosis. The presence of fat as one of the soft-tissue components distinguishes the latter from the former. The combination of solid tumors and cysts may be also seen in **acquired cystic kidney disease** (cysts, adenomas, and adenocarcinomas), although uncommonly in enlarged kidneys. As discussed earlier, each of these diseases has additional radiologic and clinical features that permit accurate diagnosis.

When masses in both kidneys are solid, **lymphoma** is the most likely diagnosis. Rarely, masses composed of erythroid and myeloid cells in **agnogenic myeloid metaplasia** and **extramedullary hematopoiesis** can cause identical radiologic abnormalities. Occasionally, **metastases** are bilateral and multiple and must be included in this differential diagnosis. In patients with **tuberous sclerosis complex** or **von Hippel-Lindau disease** multiple, exclusively solid bilateral masses representing either angiomyolipomas in the former or adenocarcinoma in the latter may dominate the appearance of the kidneys. These masses may occur without the usual accompanying cystic masses. In patients with tuberous sclerosis, the correct diagnosis is established by the demonstration of fat as one of the soft-tissue components of the renal masses, by the stigmata of tuberous sclerosis in other organs, and by a characteristic clinical history. Likewise, in von Hippel-Lindau disease, the solid masses are usually suggestive of adenocarcinoma, which in combination with other characteristic imaging and clinical data indicate the correct diagnosis. In infants and children, large kidneys with multifocal and bilateral solid masses suggest the diagnosis of **Wilms' tumor in association with nephroblastomatosis** or other predisposing conditions. This is discussed in Chapter 8.

BIBLIOGRAPHY

General

Choyke, P. L.: Inherited cystic diseases of the kidney. Radiol. Clin. North Am. *34*:925, 1996.
Grantham, J. J., Davidow, C., Foo, I., and Dirks, J. H.: Forefronts in nephrology: The molecular basis of renal cystic disease. Kidney Int. *47*:715, 1995.
Levine, E., Hartman, D. S., Meilstrup, J. W., Van Slyke, M. A., Edgar, K. A., and Barth, J. C.: Current concepts and controversies in imaging of renal cystic disease. Urol. Clin. North Am. *24*:523, 1997.
Ravine, D., Gibson, R. N., Donlan, J., and Sheffield, L. J.: An ultrasound renal cyst prevalence survey: Specificity data for inherited renal cystic diseases. Am. J. Kidney Dis. *22*:803, 1993.
Woolf, A. S., and Winyard, P. J. D.: Unravelling the pathogenesis of cystic kidney diseases. Arch. Dis. Child. *72*:103, 1995.

Autosomal Dominant (Adult) Polycystic Kidney Disease

Barbaric, Z. L., Spataro, R. F., and Segal, A. J.: Urinary tract obstruction in polycystic renal disease. Radiology *125*:627, 1977.
Bennett, W. M.: Diagnostic considerations in autosomal dominant polycystic kidney disease. Semin. Nephrol. *10*:552, 1990.
Black, W. C.: Intracranial aneurysms in adult polycystic kidney disease: Is screening with MR angiography indicated? Radiology *191*:18, 1994.
Chapman, A. B., Johnson, A. M., and Gabow, P. A.: Intracranial aneurysms in patients with autosomal dominant polycystic kidney disease: How to diagnose and who to screen. Am. J. Kidney Dis. *22*:526, 1993.
Elles, R. G., Hodgkinson, K. A., Mallick, N. P., O'Donoghue, D. J., Read, A. P., Rimmer, S., Watters, E. A., and Harris, R.: Diagnosis of adult polycystic kidney disease by genetic markers and ultrasonographic imaging in a voluntary family register. J. Med. Genet. *31*:115, 1994.
Everson, G. T.: Hepatic cysts in autosomal dominant polycystic kidney disease. Am. J. Kidney Dis. *22*:520, 1993.
Fick, G. M., Duley, I. T., Strain, J. C., Manco-Johnson, M. L., and Gabow, P. A.: The spectrum of autosomal dominant polycsytic kidney disease in children. J. Am. Soc. Nephrol. *4*:1654, 1994.
Fick, G. M., and Gabow, P. A.: Natural history of autosomal dominant polycystic kidney disease. Annu. Rev. Med. *45*:23, 1994.
Fick, G. M., Johnson, A. M., Strain, J. D., Kimberling, W. J., Kumar, S., Manco-Johnson, M. L., Duley, I. T., and Gabow, P. A.: Characteristics of very early onset autosomal dominant polycystic kidney disease. J. Am. Soc. Nephrol. *3*:1863, 1993.
Gabow, P. A.: Autosomal dominant polycystic kidney disease. Am. J. Kidney Dis. *22*:511, 1993.
Gabow, P. A.: Medical progress: Autosomal dominant polycystic kidney disease. N. Engl. J. Med. *329*:332, 1993.
Goldman, S. M., and Hartman, D. S.: Autosomal dominant polycystic kidney disease. In Hartman, D. S. (ed.): Renal Cystic Disease. Philadelphia, W. B. Saunders, 1989, pp. 88–107.
Gonzalo, A., Rivera, M., Quereda, C., and Ortuno, J.: Clinical

features and prognosis of adult polycystic kidney disease. Am. J. Nephrol. *10*:470, 1990.
Grantham, J. J.: Polycystic kidney disease: There goes the neighborhood. N. Engl. J. Med. *333*:56, 1995.
Gregoire, J. R., Torres, V. E., Holley, K. E., and Farrow, G. M.: Renal epithelial hyperplastic and neoplastic proliferation in autosomal dominant polycystic kidney disease. Am. J. Kidney Dis. *9*:27, 1987.
Huston, J., Torres, V. E., Sullivan, P. P., et al.: Value of magnetic resonance angiography for the detection of intracranial aneurysm in autosomal dominant polycystic kidney disease. J. Am. Soc. Nephrol. *3*:1871, 1993.
Keith, D. S., Torres, V. E., King, B. F., Zincki, H., and Farrow, G. M.: Renal cell carcinoma in autosomal dominant polycystic kidney disease. J. Am. Soc. Nephrol. *4*:1661, 1994.
Kutcher, R., Schneider, M., and Gordon, D. H.: Calcification in polycystic disease. Radiology *122*:77, 1977.
Levine, E., and Grantham, J. J.: Perinephric hemorrhage in autosomal dominant polycystic kidney disease: CT and MR findings. J. Comput. Assist. Tomogr. *11*:108, 1987.
Lieske, J. C., and Toback, F. G.: Autosomal dominant polycystic kidney disease. J. Am. Soc. Nephrol. *3*:1442, 1993.
McHugo, J. M., Shafi, M. I., Rowlands, D., and Weaver, J. B.: Prenatal diagnosis of adult polycystic kidney disease. Br. J. Radiol. *61*:1072, 1988.
Osathanondh, V., and Potter, E. L.: Pathogenesis of polycystic kidneys: Type 3 due to multiple abnormalities of development. Lab. Med. Arch. Pathol. *77*:485, 1964.
Parfrey, P. S., Bear, J. C., Morgan, J., et al.: The diagnosis and prognosis of autosomal dominant polycystic kidney disease. N. Engl. J. Med. *323*:1085, 1990.
Potter, E. L.: Normal and Abnormal Development of the Kidney. Chicago, Year Book Medical Publishers, 1972.
Ravine, D., Gibson, R. N., Sheffield, L. J., Kincaid-Smith, P., and Danks, D. M.: Evaluation of ultrasonographic diagnostic criteria for autosomal dominant polycystic kidney disease. Lancet *343*:824, 1994.
Risdon, R. A.: Development, developmental defects, and cystic diseases of the kidney. In Heptinstall, R. H. (ed.): Pathology of the Kidney, 4th ed. Boston, Little, Brown & Co., 1992, pp. 93–167.
Ruggieri, P. M., Poulos, N., Masaryk, T. J., Ross, J. S., Obuchowski, N. A., Awad, I. A., Braun, W. E., Nally, J., Lewin, J. S., and Modic, M. T.: Occult intracranial aneurysms in polycystic kidney disease: Screening with MR angiography. Radiology *191*:33, 1994.
Strand, W. R., Rushton, H. G., Markle, B. M., and Kapur, S.: Autosomal dominant polycystic kidney disease in infants: Asymmetric disease mimicking a unilateral renal mass. J. Urol. *141*:1151, 1989.
Wakabayashi, T., Fujita, S., Ohbora, Y., Suyama, T., Tamuki, N., and Matsumoto, S.: Polycystic kidney disease and intracranial aneurysms. J. Neurosurg. *58*:488, 1983.
Welling, L. W., and Granthan, J. J.: Cystic and developmental diseases of the kidney. In Brenner, B. M. (ed.): The Kidney, 5th ed. Philadelphia, W. B. Saunders, 1996, pp. 1828–1863.

Tuberous Sclerosis Complex

Bernstein, J.: Renal cystic disease in the tuberous sclerosis complex. Pediatr. Nephrol. *7*:490, 1993.
Bjornsson, J., Short, M. P., Kwiatkowski, D. J., and Henske, E. P.: Tuberous sclerosis–associated renal cell carcinoma: Clinical, pathological, and genetic features. Am. J. Pathol. *149*:1201, 1996.
Chonko, A. M., Weiss, S. M., Stein, J. H., and Ferris, T. F.: Renal involvement in tuberous sclerosis. Am. J. Med. *56*:124, 1974.
Compton, W. R., Lester, P. D., Kyaw, M. M., and Madsen, J.: The abdominal angiographic spectrum of tuberous sclerosis. AJR *126*:807, 1976.
Kerr, L. A., Blute, M. L., Ryu, J. H., Swensen, S. J., and Malek, R. S.: Renal angiomyolipoma in association with pulmonary lymphangioleiomyomatosis: Forme fruste of tuberous sclerosis. Urology *41*:440, 1993.
O'Hagan, A. R., Ellsworth, R., Secic, M., Rothner, A. D., and

Brouhard, B. H.: Renal manifestations of tuberous sclerosis complex. Clin. Pediat. *35*:483, 1996.

Pickering, S. P., Fletcher, B. D., Bryan, P. J., and Abramowsky, C. R.: Renal lymphangioma: A cause of neonatal nephromegaly. Pediatr Radiol *14*:445, 1984.

Savin, H., Jutrin, I., and Ravid, M.: Reversible renal hypertension due to renal hygroma. Urology *33*:317, 1989.

Sampson, J. R.: The kidney in tuberous sclerosis: Manifestations and molecular genetic mechanisms. Nephrol. Dial. Transplant 11(Suppl. 6):34, 1996.

Sampson, J. R., Patel, A., and Mee, A. D.: Multifocal renal carcinoma in sibs from a chromosome 9 linked (TSC1) tuberous sclerosis family. J. Med. Genet. *32*:848, 1995.

Torres, V. E., Bjornsson, J., King, B. F., Kumar, R., Zincke, H., Edell, E. S., Wilson, T. O., Hattery, R. R., and Gomez, M. R.: Extrapulmonary lymphangioleiomyomatosis and lymphangiomatous cysts in tuberous sclerosis complex. Mayo Clin. Proc. *70*:641, 1995.

Van Baal, J. G., Smits, N. J., Keman, J. N., Lindhout, D., and Verhoef, S.: The evolution of renal angiomyolipomas in patients with tuberous sclerosis. J. Urol. *152*:35, 1994.

Webb, D. W., Kabala, J., and Osborne, J. P.: A population study of renal disease in patients with tuberous sclerosis. Br. J. Urol. *74*:151, 1994.

Younathan, C. M., and Kaude, J. V.: Renal peripelvic lymphatic cysts (lymphangiomas) associated with generalized lymphangiomatosis. Urol. Radiol. *14*:161, 1992.

Zimmerhackl, L. B., Rehm, M., Kaufmehl, K., Kurlemann, G., and Brandis, M.: Renal involvement in tuberous sclerosis complex: A retrospective survey. Pediatr. Nephrol. *8*:451, 1994.

Von Hippel-Lindau Disease

Choyke, P. L., Filling-Katz, M. R., Shawker, T. H., Gorin, M. B., Travis, W. D., Chang, R., Seizinger, B. R., Dwyer, A. J., and Linehan, W. M.: von Hippel-Lindau Disease: Radiologic screening for visceral manifestations. Radiology *174*:815, 1990.

Choyke, P. L., Glenn, G. M., Walther, M. M., Patronas, N. J., Linehan, W. M., and Zbar, B.: von Hippel-Lindau disease: Genetic, clinical and imaging features. Radiology *194*:629, 1995.

Choyke, P. L., Glenn, G. M., Walther, M. M., Zbar, B., Weiss, G. H., Alexander, R. B., Hayes, W. S., Long, J. P., Thakore, K. N., and Linehan, K. N.: The natural history of renal lesions in von Hippel-Lindau disease: A serial CT study in 28 patients. AJR *159*:1229, 1992.

Hough, D. M., Stephens, D. H., Johnson, C. D., and Binkowitz, L. A.: Pancreatic lesions in von Hippel-Lindau disease: Prevalence, clinical significance and CT findings. AJR *162*:1091, 1994.

Linehan, W. M., Lerman, M. I., and Zbar, B.: Identification of the von Hippel-Lindau (VHL) gene: Its role in renal cancer. JAMA *273*:564, 1995.

Neumann, H. P. H., Berger, D. P., Sigmund, G., Blum, U., Schmidt, D., Parmer R. J., Volk, B., and Kirste, G.: Pheochromocytomas, multiple endocrine neoplasia type 2 and von Hippel-Lindau disease. N. Engl. J. Med. 329:1531, 1993.

Lymphoma

Cohan, R. H., Dunnick, N. R., Leder, R. A., and Baker, M. E.: Computed tomography of renal lymphoma. J. Comput. Assist. Tomogr. *14*:933, 1990.

Ellman, L., Davis, J., and Lichtenstein, N. S.: Uremia due to occult lymphomatous infiltration of the kidneys. Cancer *33*:203, 1974.

Eisenberg, P. J., Papanicolaou, N., Lee, M. J., and Yoder, I. C.: Diagnostic imaging in the evaluation of renal lymphoma. Leuk. Lymph. 7:195, 1997.

Ferry, J. A., Harris, N. L., Papanicolaou, N., and Young, R. H.: Lymphoma of the kidney: A report of 11 cases. Am. J. Surg. Pathol. *19*:134, 1995.

Hartman, D. S., Davis, C. J., Jr., Goldman, S. M., Friedman, A. C., and Fritzsche, P.: Renal lymphoma: Radiologic-pathologic correlation of 21 cases. Radiology *144*:759, 1982.

Heiken, J. P., Gold, R. P., Schnur, M. J., King, D. L., Bashist, B., and Glazer, H. S.: Computed tomography of renal lymphoma with ultrasound correlation. J. Comput. Assist. Tomogr. 7:245, 1983.

Horii, S. C., Bosniak, M. A., Megibow, A. J., et al.: Correlation of CT and ultrasound in the evaluation of renal lymphoma. Urol. Radiol. *5*:69, 1983.

Ng, Y. Y., Healy, J. C., Vincent, J. M., Kingston, J. E., Armstrong, P., and Reznek, R. H.: The radiology of non-Hodgkin's lymphoma in childhood: A review of 80 cases. Clin. Radiol. *49*:594, 1994.

Reznek, R. H., Mootoosamy, I., Webb, J. A. W., and Richards, M. A.: CT in renal and perirenal lymphoma: A further look. Clin. Radiol. *42*:233, 1990.

Richmond, J., Sherman, R. S., Diamond, N. D., and Craver, L. F.: Renal lesions associated with malignant lymphomas. Am. J. Med. *32*:184, 1962.

Ruchman, R. B., Yeh, H. C., Mitty, H. A., et al.: Ultrasonographic and computed tomographic features of renal sinus lymphoma. J. Clin. Ultrasound *16*:35, 1988.

Salem, Y. H., and Miller, H. C.: Lymphoma of the genitourinary tract. J. Urol. *151*:1162, 1994.

Semelka, R. C., Kelekis, N. L., Burdeny, D. A., Mitchell, D. G., Brown, J. J., and Siegelman, S.: Renal lymphoma: Demonstration by MR imaging. Am. J. Roentgenol. *166*:823, 1996.

Townsend, R. R., Laing, F. C., Jeffrey, R. B., and Bottles, K.: Abdominal lymphoma in AIDS: Evaluation with US. Radiology *171*:719, 1989.

Weinberger, E., Rosenbaum, D. M., and Pendergrass, T. W.: Renal involvement in children with lymphoma: Comparison of CT with sonography. AJR *155*:347, 1990.

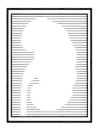

11

Diagnostic Set: Large, Multifocal, Unilateral

MALAKOPLAKIA
MULTICYSTIC DYSPLASTIC KIDNEY DISEASE
DIFFERENTIAL DIAGNOSIS

Two diseases characteristically appear as a multi-lobulated enlargement of a single kidney. The first, malakoplakia, is a chronic infection associated with multiple inflammatory masses. The other, multicystic dysplastic kidney disease, is a congenital disorder leading to multiple cystic masses.

MALAKOPLAKIA

Definition

Malakoplakia of the renal parenchyma is a very uncommon inflammation that is characterized by cortical and medullary granulomatous masses that contain large mononuclear cells with abundant cytoplasm. These cells, called Hansemann's macrophages, contain large intracytoplasmic inclusion bodies composed of calcium and iron-laden lysosomal material. Known as Michaelis-Gutmann bodies, these inclusions are probably phagocytized bacilli in various stages of defective digestion. Michaelis-Gutmann bodies can also be found in an extracellular location. Ultrastructural studies suggest the likely cause of malakoplakia: namely, an intracellular abnormality of the macrophage, probably occurring at the level of the phagolysosomes. Malakoplakia is usually associated with *Escherichia coli* infections, although *Klebsiella* species have also been involved.

The granulomas of renal parenchymal malakoplakia are sharply demarcated, soft, yellow-brown masses situated in the cortex and the medulla. Approximately 75 per cent of reported cases have been multifocal, and 50 per cent have been bilateral. Unifocal masses occur in about 25 per cent of cases. Extension of the inflammatory process into the renal sinus and perirenal space and renal vein thrombosis have been noted in many instances. *Megalocytic interstitial nephritis* is a term that has been used to describe a pathologic process that differs from malakoplakia only in that the granulomas are limited to the renal cortex. In all other respects, this process is identical to malakoplakia, and the two terms should probably be considered synonymous.

Malakoplakia of the urinary tract most commonly affects the bladder. Involvement of the prostate, testes, ureter, and renal pelvis and parenchyma is much less frequent. The radiologic appearance of malakoplakia of the pelvocalyceal system and ureter is described in Chapter 15; that of the bladder is described in Chapter 19.

Clinical Setting

Middle-aged women with a history of urinary tract infection and patients with altered host resistance are the usual groups affected by renal parenchymal malakoplakia. Infants and children are rarely affected. Clinical features include dysuria, fever, anemia, leukocytosis, pyuria, and bacteriuria. A renal mass may be palpable, especially with retroperitoneal extension. Malakoplakia may cause renal failure either by bilateral renal parenchymal involvement or by obstructive uropathy due to bladder or bilateral ureteropelvocalyceal involvement.

Radiologic Findings

Malakoplakia of the renal parenchyma causes multifocal enlargement of the kidney without pelvocalyceal obstruction or calcification (Fig. 11–1). Contrast material excretion is diminished to absent. The multiple granulomas cause a mass effect on the pelvocalyceal system and a lobulated contour. Uncommonly, the radiologic findings are those of a unifocal mass indistinguishable from those discussed in Chapter 12.

Ultrasonography defines well the multifocal enlargement of the kidney and the absence of obstruction. Malakoplakia granulomas distort the central sinus echoes by their mass effect, contain low-amplitude internal echoes, and have poorly defined margins.

MALAKOPLAKIA TYPICAL FINDINGS

Primary Uroradiologic Elements

Size: large
Contour: multifocal masses
Lesion distribution: unilateral (bilateral in up to 50 per cent of cases)

Secondary Uroradiologic Elements

Collecting system: displaced (multifocal)
Nephrogram: diminished to absent opacification; replaced (multifocal)
Echogenicity: hypoechoic masses; distorted central sinus complex

---

Computed tomography of this rare form of renal infection shows multiple soft-tissue masses that enhance less than do the renal parenchyma following contrast material administration. Computed tomography is particularly valuable in detecting extension of the inflammatory process into the retroperitoneum.

Angiographic findings in renal malakoplakia include hypovascular masses, displacement, and stretching of intrarenal arteries around the granulomas, and occasional encasement of arteries. Lack of normal branching and the presence of neovascularity have been described. The angiographic nephrogram is inhomogeneous, owing to replacement of the nephrons by multiple granulomas. Renal vein thrombosis may be present.

MULTICYSTIC DYSPLASTIC KIDNEY DISEASE

Definition

Multicystic dysplastic kidney disease is a nonhereditary developmental anomaly characterized by cysts and varying amounts of dysplastic tissue with little or no discernible renal parenchyma. Common synonyms include *renal dysplasia, renal dysgenesis, multicystic kidney, and Potter Type II renal cystic disease.* Commonly, multicystic dysplastic kidney disease is unilateral and involves the entire kidney. Uncommonly, it is bilateral and fatal or limited to just one region of the kidney.

This disease has two forms: the *pelvoinfundibular*

atretic form and the *hydronephrotic* form. Each form represents a disorder in the interaction between the ampullary tips of ureteral buds and the metanephric blastema during formation of the renal parenchyma (see Chapter 3 for a discussion of the normal embryonic development of the kidney). The two forms differ as to the point during embryogenesis of the kidney that the disorder begins. Further, it is likely that the renal dysplasia of the hydronephrotic form is only one component of a generalized maldevelopment of the ureter, bladder, and urethra.

In the *pelvoinfundibular atretic* form, the failure of the ureteral bud branches to induce metanephric blastema occurs early in fetal life. Very few nephrons develop, no urine is formed, and the ureter and renal artery are atretic. The few branches of the ureteral bud that do develop terminate in cysts. Thus, the "kidney" lacks a reniform shape and is composed of only a cluster of thin-walled cysts of varying size and number (Fig. 11–2). These cysts are held together by connective tissue. Microscopically, a few widely scattered glomeruli with or without aggregates of tubules can be identified. The dominant tissue is dysplastic and consists of collagen, vascular channels, nerve trunks, cartilage, and, most characteristically, primitive ducts derived from ureteral buds. These ducts are lined by cuboidal or low columnar epithelium and are circumscribed by undifferentiated spindle cells. Large cysts have a flattened or destroyed epithelium and an acellular, collagenous wall. With time, these cyst walls may calcify or, alternatively, the entire con-

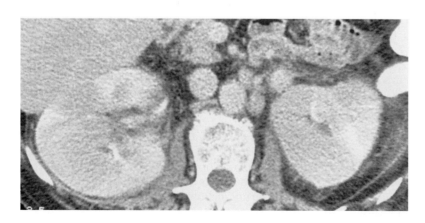

FIGURE 11–1. Malakoplakia involving both kidneys of a 58-year-old woman. The kidneys are enlarged by multiple focal granulomas that are seen as nephrographic defects. Computed tomogram, contrast material–enhanced.

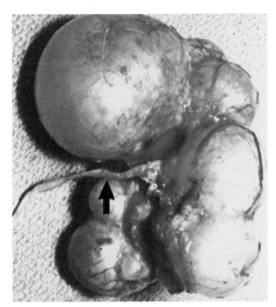

FIGURE 11–2. Multicystic dysplastic kidney, pelvoinfundibular atretic type. Gross specimen. The lesion is a grapelike aggregate of cysts with no renal pelvis. The ureter *(arrow)* is atretic.

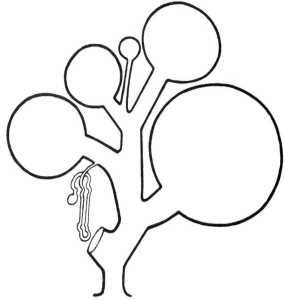

FIGURE 11–3. Multicystic dysplastic kidney, pelvoinfundibular atretic type. Schematic nephron demonstrates enlarged collecting ducts that are sparsely branched and terminate in cysts. Only one abnormal nephron connected to a collecting duct is present. (From Potter, E. L.: Normal and Abnormal Development of the Kidney, 1972. Reproduced with kind permission of the author and Year Book Medical Publishers.)

glomerate of cysts may regress, leaving a mass of solid dysplastic tissue. Uncommonly, the pelvoinfundibular atretic form occurs bilaterally or is segmental and limited to one portion of an otherwise normal kidney. The pelvoinfundibular atretic form is classified as Type II in the Potter classification of renal cystic disease. The characteristic abnormality as seen in nephron dissection is schematized in Figure 11–3.

In the *hydronephrotic* form, severe urinary tract obstruction develops at some point in fetal life *after* an initial period of normal organogenesis. This congenital obstruction is usually at the ureteropelvic or the ureterovesical junction or due to posterior urethral valves. The effect of obstruction on the kidney is twofold: both hydronephrosis and dysplasia are superimposed on a kidney that has already undergone a period of normal differentiation before the onset of the obstruction. In the hydronephrotic form, the kidney retains its reniform shape. Dilatation of the pelvis or of the pelvis and ureter proximal to the site of obstruction is present. This may be bilateral in cases of posterior urethral valve. The cysts that form are peripheral in the renal parenchyma and project from the surface of the kidney (Fig. 11–4). These communicate with the dilated pelvocalyceal system. Microscopically, normal nephrons are numerous and coexist with dysplastic tissue composed of primitive ducts with mesenchymal collars arranged in aggregates resembling renal medullary tissue. Islands of cartilage are occasionally present. The hydronephrotic form thus represents a combination of normal organogenesis, hydronephrosis, and cystic dysplasia. The severity of the hydronephrotic form of cystic dysplasia correlates with the degree of obstruction and the stage at which it occurs. A severe obstruction oc-

curring very early in fetal life results in a pathologic appearance similar to the multicystic dysplastic kidney of the pelvoinfundibular atretic form with the added unique feature of dilatation of the pelvis. In the mildest form, partial urinary tract obstruction develops late in gestation after formation of most of the renal parenchyma has been completed. On this mild end, only small cysts involving the last one to two generations of nephrons adjacent to the

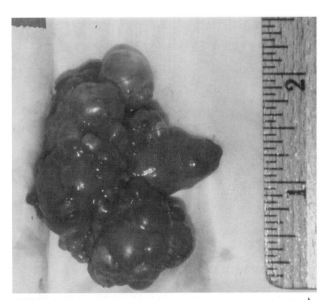

FIGURE 11–4. Multicystic dysplastic kidney, hydronephrotic type. Gross specimen. The kidney is grossly distorted by cysts aggregated on the surface of the kidney but retains its reniform shape. The renal pelvis is dilated as a result of a congenital ureteropelvic junction obstruction.

renal capsule are found. This corresponds to the Potter Type IV cystic kidney. Hydronephrotic cystic dysplasia as seen in nephron dissection is schematized in Figure 11–5. Hydronephrotic cystic dysplasia may be segmental in association with a completely duplicated, obstructed ureter, or it may be bilateral as a result of a posterior urethral valve or prune-belly syndrome. When cysts are microscopic or barely macroscopic, the gross pathology and corresponding radiologic images are dominated by the findings of hydronephrosis and dysplastic solid tissue with a diminished cystic component.

Clinical Setting

The clinical features of pelvoinfundibular atretic and severe hydronephrotic multicystic dysplastic kidney disease are similar. It is commonly stated that males and females are equally affected and that there is no predilection for one side of involvement over the other. However, an extensive review of the literature reveals a preponderance of males and left-sided lesions (Piel, 1990). The pelvoinfun-

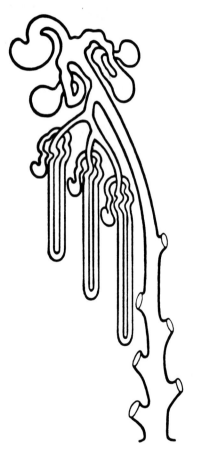

FIGURE 11–5. Multicystic dysplastic kidney, hydronephrotic type. Schematized diagram demonstrates three early generations of normal nephrons, cystic dilatation and dysplasia of more peripheral, later-forming generations of nephrons, and the terminal portions of the collecting ducts into which they drain. (From Potter, E. L.: Normal and Abnormal Development of the Kidney, 1972. Reproduced with kind permission of the author and Year Book Medical Publishers.)

dibular atretic form of the disease is usually encountered as a large abdominal mass in an otherwise asymptomatic newborn. Once the disorder is discovered, the most important clinical consideration is the search for a coexistent anomaly that might pose a risk of damage to the contralateral kidney. This occurs in 30 to 40 per cent of cases, usually in the form of a ureteropelvic junction obstruction, renal agenesis, or hypoplasia.

The pelvoinfundibular atretic form of the disease is sometimes discovered in the older child or in an adult. In most of these cases, the malformed kidney is small or normal in size and is detected as an incidental radiologic finding, usually in the form of ring calcification or a mass of nonenhancing solid or cystic tissue in the renal fossa. Because the risk of malignant change in the pelvoinfundibular atretic form is exceedingly low, the need for removal is usually limited to those infants in whom symptoms develop as a result of the large size of the mass. In many instances, however, a large cystic mass regresses into a smaller mass of predominant solid tissue during the first few months of life.

The clinical features of the hydronephrotic form reflect the underlying hydronephrosis rather than the cystic dysplastic component of the abnormality. These features include a hydronephrotic mass and urinary tract infection. The recognition of marked hydronephrosis in a fetus raises the likelihood of renal dysplasia. This should prompt postnatal studies to detect obstruction, vesicoureteral reflux, or urethral abnormalities in males, especially if urinary tract infection develops.

Neither the pelvoinfundibular atretic nor the severe hydronephrotic form is compatible with life when both kidneys are involved. In this circumstance the fetus or newborn demonstrates the stigmata of Potter's syndrome reflecting anuria or severe oliguria *in utero*. These include oligohydramnios, pulmonary hypoplasia, thoracic underdevelopment, wide-set eyes, low-set ears, a beaked nose, and a deep palmar crease.

Radiologic Findings

The radiologic findings of multicystic dysplastic kidney disease vary with the age of the patient, the form (pelvoinfundibular atretic or hydronephrotic), and whether involvement is unilateral or bilateral and segmental or total.

In the newborn, abdominal radiography demonstrates a large, noncalcified abdominal mass that displaces bowel gas and frequently crosses the midline (Fig. 11–6). Contrast enhancement does not occur in the pelvoinfundibular atretic form, whereas demonstrable enhancement of compressed parenchyma and delayed accumulation of contrast material in cysts is seen in the hydronephrotic form. Bilateral involvement is detected as abdominal distention and pulmonary hypoplasia (Fig. 11–7).

Multicystic dysplastic kidney disease discovered in the older child or in the adult may have one or

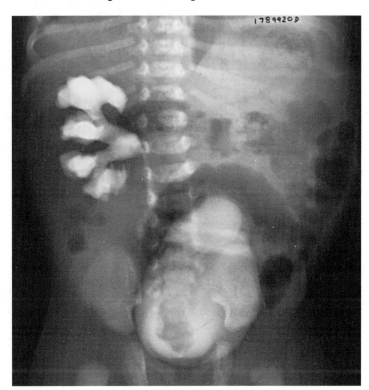

FIGURE 11–6. Multicystic dysplastic kidney, pelvoinfundibular atretic type, left kidney in a male newborn. Excretory urogram. The left kidney is not seen. There is a ureteropelvic junction obstruction on the right side.

more ring calcifications and no evidence of function (Fig. 11–8). Compensatory hypertrophy of the contralateral kidney is present.

Segmental multicystic dysplasia is most commonly the result of obstruction of the upper pole of a duplicated collecting system. This segmental form of dysplasia appears as a focal mass with some degree of delayed enhancement and dilatation of the collecting system and ureter to the point of obstruction, usually an ectopic ureterocele. In the rare instance of segmental atretic form of this disease, the nonfunctioning mass of cysts and/or dysplastic tissue is limited to a portion of the kidney.

The ultrasonographic findings of multicystic dysplastic kidney disease with pelvoinfundibular atresia include cysts that vary in size and shape, with the largest cyst being peripheral in location; absent communication between adjacent cysts; absent re-

---

MULTICYSTIC DYSPLASTIC KIDNEY DISEASE TYPICAL FINDINGS

Primary Uroradiologic Elements

Size: large (may be small in adults)
Contour: multifocal masses
Lesion distribution: unilateral

Secondary Uroradiologic Elements

Collecting System

Atretic form: absent (including absent or atretic proximal ureter)
Hydronephrotic form: dilated (including ureter) to level of obstruction

Nephrogram

Atretic form: enhancement absent
Hydronephrotic form: faint, delayed rims

Calcification: curvilinear (occasional)

Echogenicity

Atretic form: nonreniform, anechoic masses; echogenic septa; largest cyst not medial; no communications; central sinus complex absent
Hydronephrotic form: reniform, dilated pelvis, cysts peripheral and may communicate

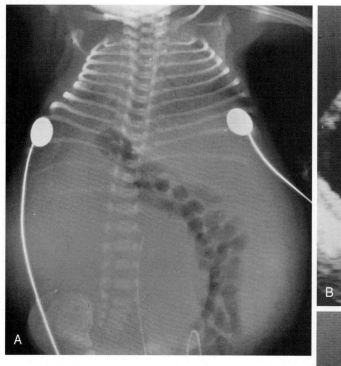

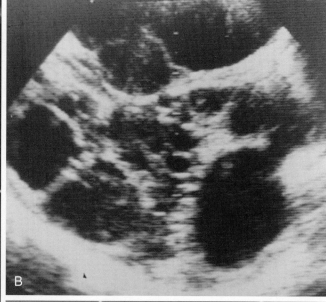

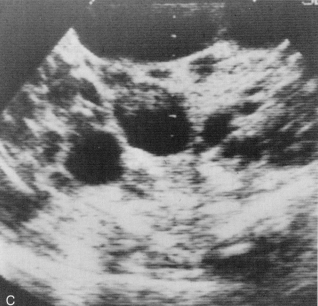

FIGURE 11–7. Multicystic dysplastic kidney, pelvoinfundibular atretic type, involving both kidneys in a neonate.
A, Radiograph of thorax and abdomen. There is a large abdominal mass displacing gas-filled bowel. The thorax is deformed, and the lungs are atretic.
B, C, Ultrasonograms, sagittal projection of the right and left kidneys, respectively. Multiple noncommunicating fluid-filled masses of varying size comprise both kidneys.

nal parenchyma between cysts; absent central sono-lucency corresponding to a renal pelvis; and echogenic areas representing primitive mesenchyme or tiny cysts in an eccentric location. The proportion of cysts to dysplastic tissue may be quite variable (Fig. 11–9). The hydronephrotic kidney demonstrates numerous peripheral cysts and a large medial fluid-filled structure corresponding to the dilated renal pelvis. The peripheral cysts may communicate with each other or with the renal pelvis. A reniform shape is preserved to some extent.

In many cases there may be considerable difficulty in distinguishing by ultrasonography severe hydronephrosis without renal dysplasia from the hydronephrotic form of multicystic dysplastic kidney disease.

Ultrasonography is useful in detecting bilateral

disease and contralateral anomalies, especially hydronephrosis. Serial ultrasonographic examinations have demonstrated marked reduction in the size of cysts and the eventual complete disappearance of cysts in multicystic dysplastic kidney disease within the first months of life (Fig. 11–10). When this process is complete, differentiation from renal agenesis may be impossible without documentation by serial examination. Surgical findings in such cases show no trace of a kidney, artery, or ureter or a very small multicystic dysplastic kidney.

In the adult, ultrasonography usually reveals one or more cystic masses in the renal fossa. The multicystic kidney is often not large, and cyst-wall calcification is easily recognized by acoustic shadowing.

Segmental multicystic dysplastic kidney disease

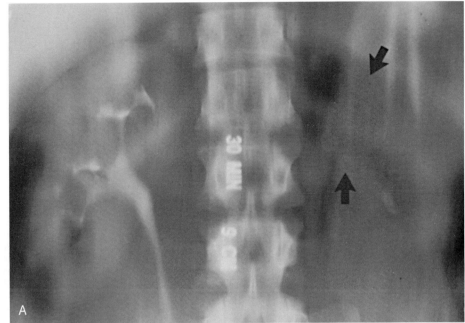

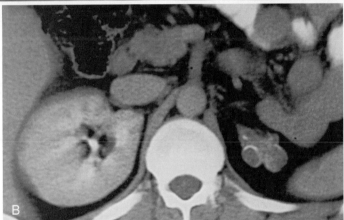

FIGURE 11–8. Multicystic dysplastic kidney, pelvoinfundibular type, left kidney, incidentally discovered in a 23-year-old male. A small soft-tissue mass with curvilinear calcification *(arrows in A)* occupies the left renal fossa. There is compensatory hypertrophy of the right kidney.
  A, Excretory urogram with tomography.
  B, Computed tomogram, contrast material–enhanced.

may present as a focal multiloculated mass. When the cysts are very small, the multicystic segment may be echogenic. Reniform shape is preserved in this disease.

Multicystic dysplastic kidney disease is often detected prenatally by maternal ultrasonography. Precise differentiation among the pelvoinfundibular atretic form, the hydronephrotic form, and uncomplicated hydronephrosis may, however, be extremely difficult *in utero.* Maternal ultrasonography is also helpful in detecting contralateral renal anomalies, which can be detected in about 30 per cent of fetuses with unilateral multicystic kidney (see Fig. 11–6). Contralateral, mild fetal pyelectasis is found in about 15 per cent of fetuses with multicystic dysplastic kidney disease and is not clinically significant.

By computed tomography, multicystic dysplastic kidney disease appears as a nonreniform mass that replaces the normal kidney. The aggregate is made up of numerous, variably sized, smaller masses of water density. Septa may be visible and enhance with contrast medium. Less commonly, only one

cystic mass is present. No function is seen in the pelvoinfundibular atresia form. In the hydronephrotic form, computed tomography is more sensitive than urography in demonstrating calyceal crescents and contrast medium puddling in cysts and the collecting system. In the adult, cyst-wall calcification or a small amount of residual dysplastic tissue may be seen. Abnormalities of the vascular pedicle in adults with sufficient retroperitoneal fat may also be demonstrated.

Radionuclide imaging provides functional and morphologic information about the multicystic kidney. Visualization depends on the presence of normal glomeruli and tubules within the cystic kidney and is, thus, limited to the hydronephrotic form. In cases of pelvoinfundibular atresia, radionuclide studies demonstrate a photon-deficient mass in the renal fossa, reflecting absent perfusion. With segmental multicystic dysplastic kidney disease, activity will be decreased or absent in the involved portion of the kidney.

Angiography demonstrates absence or hyperplasia of the ipsilateral renal artery in the pelvoinfun-

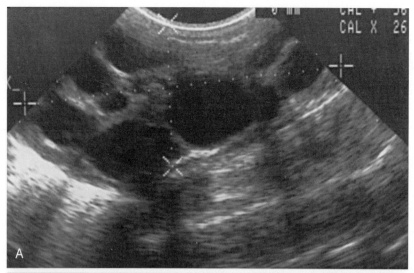

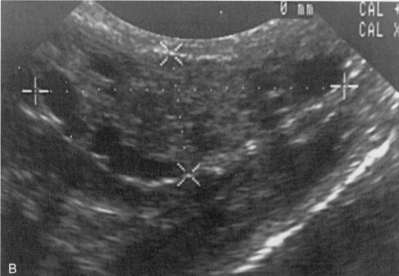

FIGURE 11–9. Multicystic dysplastic kidney, pelvoinfundibular atretic type, involving both kidneys in a newborn. Ultrasonograms, longitudinal sections, demonstrate asymmetric findings.

A, Left kidney. Multiple cysts of varying size are the prominent finding. Dysplastic tissue is represented by thick septa between cysts.

B, Right kidney. The dominant finding is the echogenic mass of dysplastic tissue, with a few small scattered cysts.

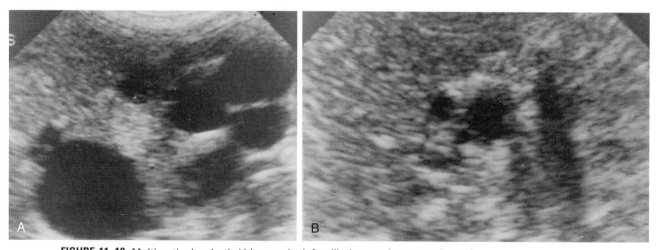

FIGURE 11–10. Multicystic dysplastic kidney, pelvoinfundibular atretic type, unilateral.

A, Neonatal ultrasonogram demonstrates a large renal mass composed of multiple cysts of varying size.

B, Ultrasonogram at 6 months of age. The mass has decreased in size as most of the cysts have involuted.

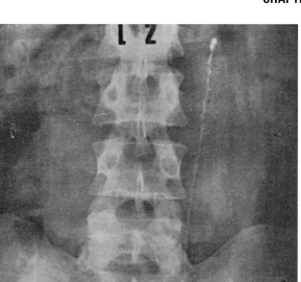

FIGURE 11–11. Multicystic dysplastic kidney. Retrograde pyelogram demonstrates atresia of the proximal ureter.

dibular atresia form. A nephrogram is absent, and no renal vein is seen during the venous phase of the study. A focal avascular or hypovascular mass without neovascularity is found in segmental involvement.

In cases of pelvoinfundibular atresia, retrograde pyelography demonstrates a small-caliber ureter that ends blindly (Fig. 11–11). Sacculations or pseudodiverticula are frequently present. Retrograde studies performed on a hydronephrotic multicystic kidney demonstrate communication of the collecting system with dysplastic ducts and cysts.

Cyst puncture in pelvoinfundibular atresia usually demonstrates noncommunication of the punctured cyst with the other cysts. The hydronephrotic form often shows communication of the cysts with dilated calyces and pelvis.

DIFFERENTIAL DIAGNOSIS

A large kidney with multiple masses and poor to absent contrast material enhancement suggests the diagnosis of **malakoplakia**. The absence of pelvic calculi serves to distinguish malakoplakia from **xanthogranulomatous pyelonephritis**, which usually is associated with a staghorn calculus. Un-

usual presentations of other diseases, such as **multiple angiomyolipomas** with or without tuberous sclerosis, **adenocarcinomas**, **metastatic deposits**, **lymphoma,** and **multiple simple cysts,** must be considered. Of these, the feature of uncomplicated fluid comprising multiple simple cysts is unique.

The **pelvoinfundibular atretic** form of **multicystic dysplastic kidney disease** in the neonate and young child can be distinguished from **obstructive hydronephrosis** by the ultrasonographic demonstration of a centrally placed, fluid-filled renal pelvis communicating with branching, dilated infundibula and calyces. Of course, the neonate or child with obstructive hydronephrosis may have a co-existing dysplastic component as well. **Multicystic dysplastic kidney disease** in the adult must be distinguished from **chronic obstructive uropathy** and **tuberculous autonephrectomy**, especially when the latter contains curvilinear calcifications. This distinction is easily made by ultrasonography, with the demonstration of characteristic fluid-filled masses. Similarly, ultrasonography also distinguishes the fluid-filled nature of the masses in multicystic dysplastic kidney disease from other causes of multifocal enlargement of one kidney, such as **xanthogranulomatous pyelonephritis**, **malakoplakia**, **multiple angiomyolipomas**, **multiple metastatic deposits**, and **cystic degeneration of a large carcinoma** in which the masses are either solid or solid and cystic. Demonstration of an atretic ureter and of absence or hypoplasia of the renal artery firmly establishes the diagnosis of multicystic dysplastic kidney disease.

BIBLIOGRAPHY

Malakoplakia

Abdou, N. I., Na Pombejara, C., Sagawa, A., Ragland, C., Stechschulte, D. J., Nilsson, U., Gourley, W., Watanabe, I., Lindsey, N. J., and Allen, M. S.: Malakoplakia: Evidence for monocyte lysosomal abnormality correctable by cholinergic agonist in vitro and in vivo. N. Engl. J. Med. *297*:1413, 1977.

Al-Sulaiman, M., Al-Khader, A. A., Mousa, D. H., Al-Swailem, R. Y., Dhar, J., and Haleen, A.: Renal parenchymal malacoplakia and megalocystic interstitial nephritis: Clinical and histological features. Am. J. Nephrol. *13*:483, 1993.

Dobyan, D. C., Truong, L. D., and Eknoyan, G.: Renal malacoplakia revisited. Am. J. Kidney Dis. *22*:243, 1993.

Esparza, A. R., McKay, D. B., Cronan, J. J., and Chazan, J. A.: Renal parenchymal malakoplakia: Histologic spectrum and its relationship to megalocytic interstitial nephritis and xanthogranulomatous pyelonephritis. Am. J. Surg. Pathol. *13*:225, 1989.

Gonzalez, A. C., Karcioglu, Z., Waters, B. B., and Weens, H. S.: Megalocytic interstitial nephritis: Ultrasonic and radiographic changes. Radiology *133*:449, 1979.

Hartman, D. S., Davis, C. J., Jr., Lichtenstein, J. E., and Goldman, S. M.: Renal parenchymal malakoplakia. Radiology *136*:33, 1980.

Kenney, P. J.: Imaging of chronic renal infections. AJR *155*:485, 1990.

Long, J. P., Jr., and Althausen, A. F.: Malakoplakia: A 25-year experience with a review of the literature. J. Urol. *141*:1328, 1989.

Mitchell, M. A., Markowitz, D. M., Killen, P., and Braun, D. K.:

Bilateral renal parenchymal malakoplakia presenting as fever of unknown origin: Case report and review. Clin. Infect. Dis. *18*:704, 1994.

Pamilo, M., and Kulatunga, A.: Renal parenchymal malakoplakia: A report of two cases—the radiological and ultrasound images. Br. J. Radiol. *57*:751, 1984.

Schaeffer, A. J.: Infections of the urinary tract. In Walsh, P. C., Retik, A. B., Vaughan, E. D., Jr., and Wein, A. J. (eds.): Campbell's Urology, 7th ed. Philadelphia, W. B. Saunders, 1998, pp. 533–614.

Multicystic Dysplastic Kidney Disease

Al-Khaldi, N., Watson, A. R., Zuccollo, J., Twinning, P., and Rose, D. H.: Outcome of antenatally detected cystic dysplastic disease. Arch. Dis. Child. *70*:520, 1994.

Atiyeh, B., Husmann, D., and Baum, M.: Contralateral renal abnormalities in multicystic dysplastic kidney disease. J. Pediatr. *121*:65, 1992.

Bernstein, J.: The multicystic kidney and hereditary renal adysplasia. Am. J. Kidney Dis. *18*:495, 1991.

Blane, C. E., Barr, M., DiPietro, M. A., Sedman, A. B., and Bloom, D. A.: Renal obstruction dysplasia: Ultrasound diagnosis and therapeutic implications. Pediatr. Radiol. *21*:274, 1991.

Cooperman, L. R.: Delayed opacification in congenital multicystic dysplastic kidney: An important roentgen sign. Radiology *121*:703, 1976.

Dewan, P. A., and Goh, D. W.: A study of the radiological anatomy of the multicystic kidney. Pediatr. Surg. Int. *9*:368, 1994.

Dungan, J. S., Fernandez, M. T., Abbitt, P. L., Thiagarajah, S., Howards, S. S., and Hogge, W. A.: Multicystic dysplastic kidney: Natural history of prenatally detected cases. Prenat. Diagn. *10*:175, 1990.

Elkin, M.: Renal cysts and abscesses. Curr. Probl. Diagn. *5*:11, 1975.

Flack, C. E., and Bellinger, M. F.: The multicystic dysplastic kidney and contralateral vesicoureteral reflux: Protection of the solitary kidney. J. Urol. *150*:1873, 1993.

Glassberg, K. I.: Renal dysplasia and cystic disease of the kidney. In Walsh, P. C., Retik, A. B., Vaughan, E. D., Jr., and Wein, A. J. (eds.): Campbell's Urology, 7th ed. Philadelphia, W. B. Saunders, 1998, pp. 1757–1813.

Gordon, A. C., Thomas, D. F. M., Arthur, R. J., and Irving, H. C.: Multicystic dysplastic kidney: Is nephrectomy still appropriate? J. Urol. *140*:1231, 1988.

Griscom, N. T., Vanter, G. F., and Fellers, F. X.: Pelvoinfundibular atresia: The usual form of multicystic kidney: 44 unilateral and two bilateral cases. Semin. Roentgenol. *10*:125, 1975.

Grossman, H., Rosenberg, E. R., Bowie, J. D., Ram, P., and Merten, D. F.: Sonographic diagnosis of renal cystic disease. AJR *140*:81, 1983.

Hartman, D. S., and Davis, C. J.: Multicystic dysplastic kidney. In Hartman, D. S. (ed.): Renal Cystic Disease. Philadelphia, W. B. Saunders, 1989, pp. 127–142.

Hashimoto, B. E., Filly, R. A., and Callen, P. W.: Multicystic dysplastic kidney in utero: Changing appearance on US. Radiology *159*:107, 1986.

Hellerstein, S.: Urinary tract infections: Old and new concepts. Pediatr. Clin. North Am. *42*:1433, 1995.

Homsy, Y. L., Anderson, J. H., Oudjhane, K., and Russo, P.: Wilms' tumor and multicystic dysplastic kidney disease. J. Urol. *158*:2256, 1997.

Karmazyn, B., and Zerin, J. M.: Lower urinary tract abnormalities in children with multicystic dysplastic kidney. Radiology *203*:223, 1997.

Kleiner, B., Filly, R. A., Mack, L., and Callen, P. W.: Multicystic dysplastic kidney: Observations of contralateral disease in the fetal population. Radiology *161*:27, 1986.

Levine, E., Hartman, D. S., Meilstrup, J. W., Van Slyke, M. A., Edgar, K. A., and Barth, J. C.: Current concepts and controversies in imaging of renal cystic diseases. Urol. Clin. North Am. *24*:523, 1997.

Marra, G., Barbieri, G., Dell'Agnola, C. A., Caccamo, M. L., Casstellani, M. R., and Assael, B.: Congenital renal damage associated with primary vesicoureteral reflux detected prenatally in male infants. J. Pediatr. *124*:726, 1994.

Murugasu, B., Cole, B. R., Hawkins, E. P., Blanton, S. H., Conley, S. B., and Portman, R. J.: Familial renal adysplasia. Am. J. Kidney Dis. *18*:490, 1991.

Osathanondh, V., and Potter, E. L.: Pathogenesis of polycystic kidneys: Type 2 due to inhibition of ampullary activity. Arch. Pathol. Lab. Med. *77*:474, 1964.

Pedicelli, G., Jequier, S., Bowen, A., and Boisvert, J.: Multicystic dysplastic kidneys: Spontaneous regression demonstrated with US. Radiology *160*:23, 1986.

Piel, C. F.: Congenital multicystic kidney. In Gardner, K. D., and Bernstein, J. (eds.): The Cystic Kidney. Dordrecht, Kluwer Academic Publishers, 1990, pp. 393–407.

Rackley, R. R., Angermeier, K. W., Levin, H., Pontes, J. E., and Kay, R.: Renal cell carcinoma arising in a regressed multicystic dysplastic kidney. J. Urol. *152*:1543, 1994.

Risdon, R. A.: The small scarred kidney in childhood. Pediatr. Nephrol. *7*:361, 1993.

Robson, W. L. M., Leung, A. K. C., and Thomason, M. A.: Multicystic dysplasia of the kidney. Clin. Pediatr. *34*:32, 1995.

Sanders, R. C., Nussbaum, A. R., and Solez, K.: Renal dysplasia: Sonographic findings. Radiology *167*:623, 1988.

Saxton, H. M., Golding, S. J., Chartler, C., and Haycock, G. D.: Diagnostic puncture in renal cystic dysplasia (multicystic kidney): Evidence on the etiology of the cysts. Br. J. Radiol. *54*:555, 1981.

Vinocur, L., Slovis, T. L., Perimutter, A. D., Watts, F. B., Jr., and Chang, C. H.: Follow-up studies of multicystic dysplastic kidneys. Radiology *167*:311, 1988.

Wacksman, J., and Phipps, L.: Report of the multicystic kidney register: Preliminary findings. J. Urol. *150*:1870, 1993.

Wood, B. P.: Renal cystic disease in infants and children. Urol. Radiol. *14*:284, 1992.

Woodward, P. J., Sohaey, R., Harris, D. P., Jackson, G. M., Klatt, E. C., Alexander, A. L., and Kennedy, A.: Postmortem fetal MR imaging: Comparison with finding at autopsy. AJR *168*:41, 1997.

Woolf, A. S., and Winyard, P. J. D.: Unravelling the pathogenesis of cystic kidney diseases. Arch. Dis. Child. *72*:103, 1995.

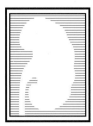

12

Diagnostic Set: Large, Unifocal, Unilateral

MALIGNANT NEOPLASMS
  Adenocarcinoma
  Invasive Transitional Cell Carcinoma
  Wilms' Tumor
  Miscellaneous
BENIGN NEOPLASMS
  Oncocytoma
  Angiomyolipoma
  Multilocular Cystic Nephroma
  Mesoblastic Nephroma
  Mesenchymal/Juxtaglomerular Cell Tumor

NON-NEOPLASTIC MASSES
  Simple Cyst/Localized Cystic Disease
  Focal Hydronephrosis
  Focal Pyelonephritis/Abscess
  Arteriovenous Malformation
DIFFERENTIAL DIAGNOSIS

The entities discussed in this chapter include a wide variety of pathologic lesions not usually grouped together. In the organizational format used in this text, they are unified under the diagnostic set *large, unifocal, unilateral* because each usually causes enlargement of the kidney by formation of a single, focal mass. Included in this category are malignant and benign tumors and non-neoplastic processes, such as simple cyst or localized cystic disease, focal hydronephrosis, focal pyelonephritis or abscess, and arteriovenous malformation.

The radiologist performs two functions in regard to the unifocal renal mass. The first is *discovery* of the mass using an imaging study initiated either because of clinical abnormalities referable to the urinary tract or by incidental and unexpected findings noted in radiologic studies undertaken for unrelated reasons. The second, and most challenging, function is *characterization of the nature* of a renal mass once it is discovered. Here, the goal of the radiologist is to separate masses that usually have little or no clinical consequence, such as a simple cyst, from those that have great potential importance, such as a malignant neoplasm. This chapter emphasizes radiologic interpretation of a unifocal mass using two criteria: the geometry of renal enlargement and the solid, cystic, or combined solid-cystic composition of the mass. The pathologic characteristics of specific diseases and their radiologic analogues are emphasized. In the Essays section of this book, Chapter 28 approaches the radiologic assessment of renal masses in the context of differential diagnosis and implications for patient care.

Chapter 28 also presents related topics, such as renal masses that are small and incidentally discovered, those that are hyperdense, and those that are too small to characterize.

There are two general patterns by which neoplastic and non-neoplastic masses of the kidney grow: *expansion* and *infiltration*. Each usually alters the gross morphology of the kidney in a characteristic manner that can be detected radiologically. Expansive growth occurs when neoplasia develops or fluid accumulates at an epicenter and enlargement occurs in all directions, pushing adjacent normal renal tissue away as the process progresses. This form of growth by apposition of cells or accumulation of fluid occurs in all directions and yields a mass whose geometry is roughly ball-shaped and often surrounded by a pseudocapsule of compressed renal parenchyma that becomes fibrotic as a result of ischemia (Fig. 12–1). Infiltrative growth, on the other hand, represents enlargement of the kidney as a result of the accumulation of abnormal cells or fluid in the interstitial spaces of the kidney. Here, the cells use the nephrons and collecting ducts as scaffolding that guides their spread diffusely throughout the kidney. The normal microscopic elements of the kidney are thereby *surrounded* rather than *displaced* in this growth pattern. The reniform shape of the enlarged kidney is thus preserved (Fig. 12–2). Although interstitial infiltrative processes are often neoplastic, they may also be inflammatory, as in acute pyelonephritis, or simply caused by interstitial accumulation of blood or edema, as in acute renal infarction, contusion, or tubular necro-

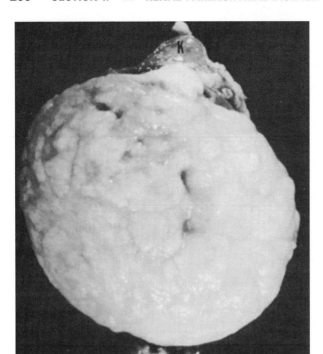

FIGURE 12–1. Expansive growth that creates a tumor with a ball-shaped geometry. A small amount of kidney (K) remains in the upper pole. Gross specimen, bivalved, Wilms' tumor.

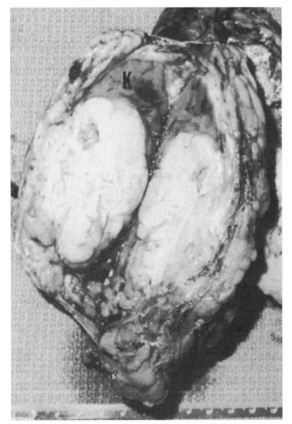

FIGURE 12–2. Infiltrative pattern of growth that enlarges the kidney with preservation of the reniform, or bean-shaped, geometry. A small amount of uninvolved kidney (K) remains in the upper pole. Gross specimen, bivalved, transitional cell carcinoma of the renal pelvis invading the kidney.

sis. These are discussed in previous chapters. Radiologically, a kidney that enlarges by virtue of an infiltrative process retains its reniform, or bean, shape.

Specific diseases characteristically become manifest either as ball-shaped, expansive enlargement of the kidney or as bean-shaped, infiltrative enlargement. Others may evolve from one pattern to the other, as is seen when focal, acute pyelonephritis transforms from an infiltrative "bean" into a liquefied, ball-shaped abscess. Table 12–1 lists the usual geometric patterns associated with specific entities. Using this approach, the radiologic assessment of the geometry of an enlarged kidney can yield useful clues as to the underlying disease. This concept is used in this and other chapters in attributing patterns of growth to specific diseases.

MALIGNANT NEOPLASMS

Definition

Malignant primary neoplasms of the kidney arise from epithelial cells, mature mesodermal elements, or primitive tissues. Adenocarcinoma, originating in the tubule epithelium, accounts for over 90 per cent of malignant neoplasms in the adult kidney. Transitional cell carcinoma arises in the uroepithelium-lined structures of the collecting system and may invade the renal parenchyma as one mode of

TABLE 12–1. Characteristic Patterns of Renal Enlargement for Various Neoplastic and Non-Neoplastic Processes

	INFILTRATION	EXPANSION
Malignant Tumor	Transitional cell (invasive)* Medullary carcinoma Sarcoma Metastasis† Lymphoma‡ Leukemia§ Sarcoma/ Sarcomatoid adenocarcinoma	Adenocarcinoma Wilms' tumor Metastasis† Mesenchymal Clear cell sarcoma Malignant rhabdoid sarcoma
Benign Tumor	Mesoblastic nephroma	Oncocytoma Angiomyolipoma Multilocular cystic nephroma Juxtaglomerular cell tumor Mesenchymal
Non-Neoplastic Processes	Focal pyelonephritis¶ Contusion¶ Infarction¶	Abscess Simple cyst Focal hydronephrosis Arteriovenous malformation

*See discussion Chapter 15
†Growth pattern varies according to tissue type.
‡See discussion Chapter 10.
§See discussion Chapter 8.
¶See discussion Chapter 9.

spread, as discussed in Chapter 15. Wilms' tumor (nephroblastoma) accounts for most of the primary malignant neoplasms in the kidneys of children.

Adenocarcinoma

Microscopically, adenocarcinoma is characterized by cellular appearance (granular/clear cell, chromophobe or sarcomatoid) and by the pattern by which the cells are arranged (medullary, tubular, or papillary). Several cytologic and architectural features may coexist. Adenocarcinoma with a papillary architecture is thought to be associated with less aggressive biologic behavior than other forms of this tumor and thus may have a favorable prognosis. Only extremely rarely does an adenocarcinoma contain radiologically detectable intratumoral fat.

A ball-shaped focal enlargement of the kidney represents growth of an adenocarcinoma by expansion in all directions from an epicenter at its origin in an epithelial cell of the proximal convoluted tubule. A fibrous, poorly vascularized pseudocapsule surrounds the tumor as a result of compression and ischemia of nephrons at the interface between the tumor and normal renal parenchyma. Additional pathologic features that influence the radiologic appearance of these tumors are their tendency to undergo necrosis or hemorrhage, or both, with secondary deposition of dystrophic calcification, the rich supply of arterial and venous channels that may develop with the cancer, and a tendency to extend into the draining renal vein and inferior vena cava.

Not all adenocarcinomas are solid. Some have intermixed areas of fluid representative of hemorrhage or necrosis. Others, particularly those with a papillary architecture, develop de novo as either an inherently unilocular cystic mass that may simulate some of the imaging features of a simple cyst or as multilocular cysts with tumor cells lining the walls of the fluid-filled mass. This latter form of adenocarcinoma may have gross morphologic and imaging features that are identical to a benign multilocular cystic nephroma. These possibilities must always be considered in the radiologic assessment of a unilocular or multilocular fluid-filled mass, as discussed subsequently in this chapter and also in Chapter 28. Only with extreme rarity does an adenocarcinoma arise in the wall of an otherwise benign, simple cyst.

A renal adenoma arises from tubule epithelial cells and is the subject of controversy regarding its benign or malignant nature. Some pathologists take the position that an adenoma is always benign regardless of size if all cytologic and histologic criteria for benignancy are present. Others classify adenomas that have grown larger than 3 cm in diameter as adenocarcinoma, even though the cells are benign and identical in all respects to smaller lesions. Support for this practice is based on occasional cases that demonstrate a transition from benignancy to malignancy in the same lesion. From yet another point of view, the broad range of biologic behavior seen in lesions with the microscopic diagnosis of adenoma leads many pathologists to classify all as low-grade adenocarcinoma. These controversies over classification aside, adenomas of the kidney almost always remain small, usually do not produce symptoms, and are for the most part discovered incidentally.

Sarcomatoid adenocarcinoma is an undifferentiated form of renal adenocarcinoma. This uncommon and aggressive tumor may exhibit an invasive, rather than expansive, pattern of growth and thus cause reniform enlargement of the kidney.

Anatomic landmarks used to determine the stage of spread of an adenocarcinoma are the renal capsule, perirenal fat, Gerota's fascia, renal vein, inferior vena cava, and lymph nodes. Blood-borne metastases to distant organs, notably lung, brain, bone, liver, and adrenal gland, are common. Two commonly used schemes for staging are given in Table 12-2.

Invasive Transitional Cell Carcinoma

Transitional cell carcinoma that has invaded the renal parenchyma causes unifocal enlargement of the kidney with preservation of reniform shape. See Chapter 15 for a complete discussion of transitional cell carcinoma.

Wilms' Tumor

Wilms' tumor is derived from primitive nephrogenic blastema. The microscopic appearance of a typical case is that of a triphasic tumor composed of epithelial (glomerular and tubular), blastemal, and stromal elements. The stromal components may variably differentiate into fibroblasts, smooth or striated muscle, cartilage, osteoid, or fat. The last two account for the occasional radiologic detection of bone or fat in a Wilms' tumor. Wilms' tumor grows by expansion into a large ball-like mass, which frequently exhibits hemorrhage and necrosis but uncommonly contains calcium. Local venous spread and distant metastases, especially to lung and liver, are common. Wilms' tumor may take the form of a multiloculated cystic mass with the triphasic histologic features of malignancy present in the septa. In this circumstance, the gross morpho-

TABLE 12–2. Two Commonly Used Schemes for Staging Adenocarcinoma of the Kidney

ROBSON	EXTENT OF TUMOR	TNM
I	Tumor confined to kidney (small) intrarenal	T1
	Tumor confined to kidney (large)	T2
II	Tumor spread to perinephric fat, but within Gerota's fascia	T3a
III	Tumor spread to renal vein	T3b
	Tumor spread to inferior vena cava	T3c
	Tumor spread to regional lymph nodes	N1–N3
IV	Tumor invasion of neighboring structures	T4
	Distant metastases	M1

logic and imaging features may be the same as those of benign multilocular cystic nephroma or a malignant multiloculated cystic adenocarcinoma, as discussed in other sections of this chapter.

Wilms' tumor may develop either as a sporadic event or in association with persistent nephrogenic blastoma, a condition known as *nephroblastomatosis*, in which both kidneys are usually enlarged. This is discussed in Chapter 8. Only rarely does nephroblastomatosis appear as a unifocal mass.

Miscellaneous Malignant Tumors

Malignant renal neoplasms other than adenocarcinoma, invasive transitional cell carcinoma, and Wilms' tumor are very uncommon and usually manifest a pattern of invasive growth. These include *clear cell sarcoma* and *malignant rhabdoid tumor* of the kidney in children and, at any age, malignant tumors of mesodermal elements, such as *fibrosarcoma, myosarcoma, liposarcoma,* and *angioendothelioma. Chloroma, myeloblastoma,* and *myeloblastic sarcoma* are focal masses that may develop in the kidney of patients with leukemia.

Medullary carcinoma is an infiltrative neoplasm that originates in the renal medulla of patients with sickle cell trait. This aggressive tumor preserves the reniform shape as it enlarges the kidney. Because of its central location, the renal pelvis is usually obliterated, leading to caliectasis without pelviectasis.

Another uncommon cause of unifocal renal enlargement is *metastatic disease* to the kidney. This is somewhat paradoxical, since secondary deposits in the kidney occur twice as often as primary neoplasms in autopsy series. At autopsy, however, the majority of metastases are multiple but only a few millimeters across or are seen only microscopically. Metastases usually do not grow large enough to become radiologically demonstrable because of the very brief survival period of these patients. Nevertheless, antemortem radiologic abnormalities due to a large unifocal metastatic deposit may occur in lymphoma, melanoma, carcinoma of the lung or breast, osteogenic sarcoma, choriocarcinoma, and muscle sarcoma. The geometric pattern of renal enlargement in metastatic disease varies with the type of primary tumor. With the advantage of the greater sensitivity of computed tomography over excretory urography, it is also apparent that metastases now are more often detected as bilateral and multiple masses than heretofore. Lymphoma is an exception to these generalizations in that it may produce large renal masses that tend to be both multiple and bilateral. These are discussed separately in Chapter 10.

Clinical Setting

Adenocarcinoma

Adenocarcinoma of the kidney occurs more than twice as frequently in males as in females and has a peak prevalence in the sixth decade of life. Uncommonly, adenocarcinoma is encountered in early adulthood and rarely in infancy and childhood. Clinical symptoms may be due to the local effect of the tumor (hematuria, pain, or palpable mass) or to distant metastases (bone pain or central nervous system dysfunction). Adenocarcinoma of the kidney is a well-known cause of constitutional or hormonal paraneoplastic syndromes, which may obscure the correct diagnosis. These syndromes include fever, erythrocytosis, hypercalcemia and constipation, anorexia, nausea, polyuria, and weight loss. Hepatic dysfunction in the absence of liver metastases also occurs and is reversible when the primary tumor is resected. Arteriovenous fistulae associated with tumor neovascularity can produce abdominal or flank bruit, high-output cardiac failure, or renal ischemia and hypertension. In a male, the sudden appearance of a varicocele, almost always left-sided, signals impairment of venous drainage from the testicular vein into a renal vein occluded by a tumor. With the widespread use of computed tomography and ultrasonography, many adenocarcinomas are discovered in asymptomatic patients, as discussed in Chapter 28. Bilateral adenocarcinomas have been described in less than 2 per cent of patients. Of these, approximately one-half are bilateral at the time of initial diagnosis and the remainder develop in the contralateral kidney after initial diagnosis. Multicentricity of adenocarcinoma in the same kidney, on the other hand, occurs in as many as 15 per cent of patients. Bilaterality and multicentricity are, however, the rule when adenocarcinomas develop in patients with von Hippel-Lindau disease, in patients on dialysis with acquired cystic disease of the kidney, and in the rare cohorts of individuals with a familial form of adenocarcinoma.

Wilms' Tumor

Approximately 50 per cent of Wilms' tumors are diagnosed between the first and third years of life and more than 75 per cent by the fifth birthday. Wilms' tumor is uncommon in the first year of life. Those tumors that are related to heritable disorders or that are bilateral are usually diagnosed at a somewhat younger age than are those that are sporadic. The prevalence curves for adenocarcinoma and Wilms' tumor cross in the second decade of life, with Wilms' tumor rarely occurring beyond young adulthood. Several heritable and nonheritable congenital malformations are associated with Wilms' tumor, some in association with an anomaly on the short arm of chromosome 11. These include sporadic aniridia, trisomies 8 and 18, Turner's syndrome, pseudohermaphroditism with glomerulonephritis and nephrotic syndrome (Drash syndrome), other genitourinary anomalies, hemihypertrophy, Beckwith-Wiedemann syndrome, and musculoskeletal anomalies. Approximately one-third of patients with sporadic aniridia develop Wilms' tumor.

A large abdominal mass is the most common presentation for Wilms' tumor. In 5 to 10 per cent of patients, the tumor is bilateral. In these cases, nephroblastomatosis is always present, as discussed in Chapter 8. Other clinical manifestations of Wilms' tumor include abdominal pain, anorexia, nausea, vomiting, fever, and gross hematuria. Venous obstruction can cause leg edema, varicocele, or the Budd-Chiari syndrome. Signs and symptoms of distant metastases are often present.

Miscellaneous Malignant Tumors

The miscellaneous tumors listed in the preceding section cause many of the clinical findings associated with adenocarcinoma or Wilms' tumor. Clear cell sarcoma in childhood is frequently associated with bone metastases, while rhabdoid tumor of the kidney, also in children, has a predilection for metastatic spread to the central nervous system. Medullary carcinoma of the kidney is unique to patients with sickle cell trait and characteristically first becomes apparent at an advanced stage of local and distant spread. Metastatic disease to the kidney is usually silent unless the lesion invades the collecting system and causes hematuria. Rarely, abdominal mass or symptoms of urinary tract infection may be the result of renal metastases.

Radiologic Findings

Excretory Urography

Most malignant neoplasms produce a ball-shaped expansion of the kidney that is seen as increased length or width or, simply, as a localized bulge (Figs. 12–3 through 12–5). A centrally located mass, however, may cause only enlargement of renal thickness, a dimension not readily measured on standard urographic projections. In this situation, both size and contour may be normal, and detection of the neoplasm will depend on infundibular, calyceal, or pelvic displacement or obliteration (Fig. 12–6). Some tumors eventually destroy the entire kidney, leaving only a large nonfunctioning mass (Fig. 12–7). Uncommon malignant tumors of the kidney, for example medullary carcinoma or certain metastases, grow by infiltration and thereby preserve the reniform shape of the kidney even as the organ enlarges.

Tilting of the renal axis may occur if the mass grows in an exophytic manner, particularly medially. With an upper pole medial mass, the axis becomes vertical, whereas a lower pole medial mass will shift the axis toward the horizontal plane. Particularly large tumors, as is often the case in Wilms' tumor and some carcinomas, may markedly displace the entire kidney in one direction or another (Fig. 12–8). Marked ventral displacement enlarges the image of the kidney on anteroposterior radiographs owing to increase in the distance of the kidney to the film.

The collecting system is frequently abnormal in the presence of a malignant neoplasm. There may be marked displacement of adjacent portions of the

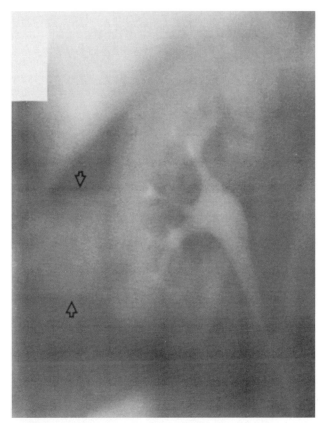

FIGURE 12–3. Adenocarcinoma of the kidney producing a localized bulge on the lateral contour of the kidney (arrows). The interpapillary line is normal. Tomogram during excretory urography.

pelvis, infundibulum, or calyx around the tumor (see Figs. 12–4 and 12–5). Ureteral compression, a large dose of contrast material, or prone films are often necessary to distend the collecting structures well enough to visualize these abnormalities (see Fig. 12–6). Sometimes only minor splaying of a single calyx is present. Filling defects within the calyces, representing growth of tumor into the collecting system, are either smooth or irregular. One sensitive sign of a tumor is a focal increase in the distance between the calyx (interpapillary line) and the overlying outer margin of the kidney compared with the remainder of the renal substance. This is schematized in Figure 4–4. Compression or invasion of a draining infundibulum by a malignant tumor can lead to focal dilatation of a group of calyces (Fig. 12–9). Advanced hydronephrosis of the obstructed region may develop in some patients (see Fig. 12–27).

Solid, non-necrotic neoplasms of the kidney, regardless of the degree of vascularization, enhance during the early nephrographic phase of urography but over time do not retain their initial intensity of enhancement relative to the surrounding normal parenchyma. Enhancement reflects perfusion of the lesion with contrast material–laden blood. If perfusion of all or part of the tumor is disrupted, as occurs with hemorrhage or necrosis or in cystic neo-

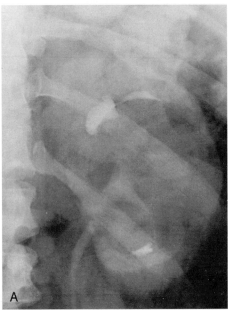

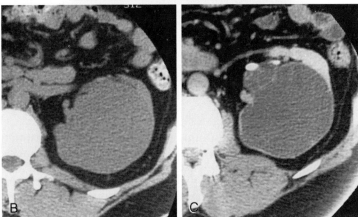

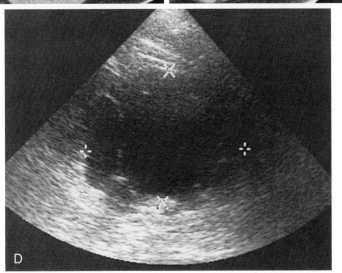

FIGURE 12–4. Cystic adenocarcinoma, left kidney, causing mass effect in the central portion of the kidney without increase in overall length.

A, Excretory urogram. There is marked displacement of the infundibula and calyces and effacement of the pelvis by the tumor.

B, Computed tomogram, unenhanced. The attenuation value of the tumor is slightly less than that of the normal kidney.

C, Computed tomogram, contrast material–enhanced. There is increased density of a thickened and slightly nodular rim of tissue on the periphery of the tumor. The bulk of the tumor enhances minimally.

D, Ultrasonogram, longitudinal section. The tumor is hypoechoic, but the far wall is poorly defined and there is no increased through-transmission of sound.

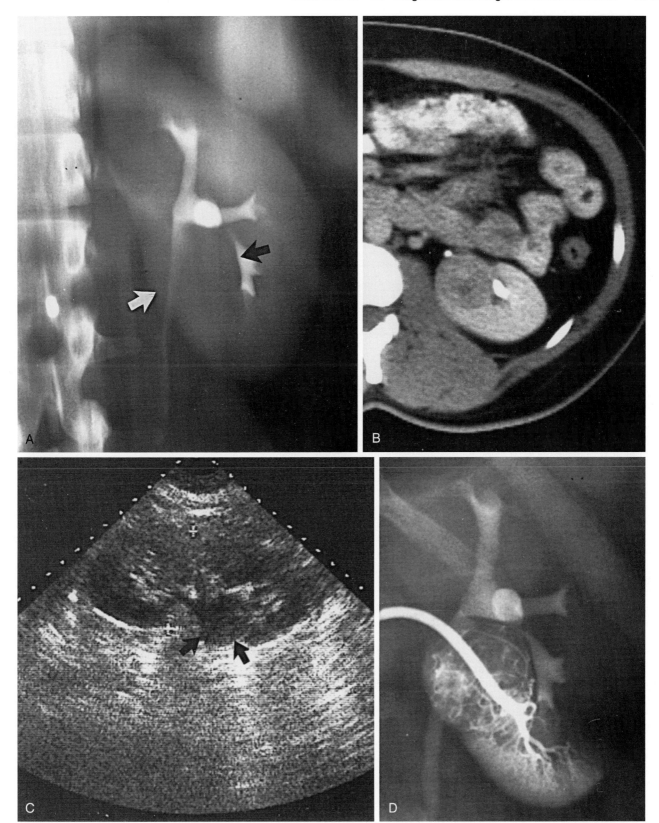

FIGURE 12–5. Adenocarcinoma, inferior hilar lip, left kidney.

A, Excretory urogram. The tumor causes a focal bulge of the contour of the kidney, a slightly diminished nephrogram, as well as effacement and lateral displacement of the infundibulum and calyx of the lower pole *(arrows)*.

B, Computed tomogram, contrast material–enhanced. The small tumor, which is more easily visualized than on excretory urography, does not enhance as much as the normal renal parenchyma. A small focus of decreased central density represents hemorrhage or necrosis.

C, Ultrasonogram, coronal section. The tumor *(arrows)* is isoechoic with renal parenchyma.

D, Selective arteriogram, accessory renal artery. There is moderate neovascularity.

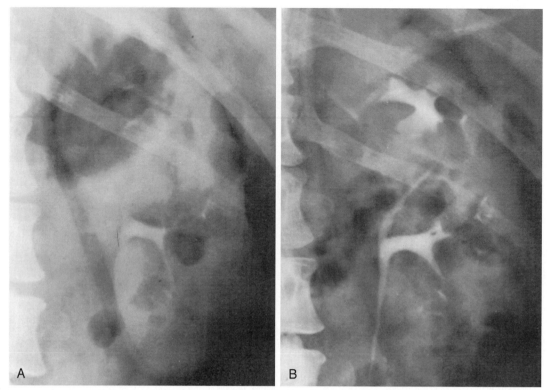

FIGURE 12–6. Adenocarcinoma of the kidney causing focal displacement of the collecting structures of the upper pole.
A, Standard excretory urogram without ureteral compression. The upper pole calyces are seen faintly.
B, Excretory urogram with effective ureteral compression results in visualization of the entire upper pole collecting system and identification of the mass lesion in the medial aspect of the upper pole.
(Courtesy of Janet Dacie, M.B., St. Bartholomew's Hospital, London, England.)

plasms, the affected area remains relatively unenhanced throughout the urographic examination. The area of diminished enhancement may be small and centrally located, may be eccentric, or may involve the whole mass. The perfused, peripheral portion of a cystic or necrotic lesion is sometimes seen as a radiodense, thick wall with an irregular inner margin surrounding the relatively radiolucent center. This finding, schematized in Figure 4–4, is a feature of malignant disease.

Detecting calcium in a focal renal mass is quite useful in predicting the nature of the lesion. Based on detection by computed tomography, approximately 30 per cent of carcinomas are calcified. Only one-third of these are detected by film radiography, however. In differentiating a fluid-filled simple cyst from a solid tumor, the *location* (peripheral or nonperipheral) of calcification within the mass is a more important factor than the *pattern* of calcification (amorphous, mottled, punctate, wavy, or curvilinear). Approximately 90 per cent of all masses containing calcium in a nonperipheral location are carcinoma (see Figs. 12–7 and 12–8). Non-neoplastic conditions, such as xanthogranulomatous pyelonephritis and tuberculosis, as well as uncommon tumors account for the remainder. It is important to remember, however, that peripheral, curvilinear calcification, while suggestive of simple cyst, may

also occur in carcinoma, although never as the only radiologic sign of malignancy (Fig. 12–10). Calcification occurs in approximately 5 per cent of Wilms' tumors (see Fig. 12–7).

Other urographic findings are associated with malignant masses. Ureteral notching in the presence of a focal renal mass reflects periureteric collateral veins that develop following invasion of the main renal vein by tumor or by propagation of bland thrombus from the tumor (Fig. 12–11). Occasionally, faint, serpentine opacities may be seen in the perirenal fat. These are enlarged arteries and veins associated with a vascular tumor and are best imaged by computed tomography. Although dilated capsular vessels are usually a sign of carcinoma, they may be seen in benign conditions, such as arteriovenous fistula with a high-flow state (Fig. 12–12).

Computed Tomography

Most of the characteristics of malignant tumors described in the section on excretory urography apply to their appearance on computed tomographic images. Because of the cross-sectional anatomic display and enhanced contrast discrimination, computed tomography has a sensitivity that far exceeds excretory urography in detecting solid mass lesions in the kidney. This advantage is particularly appar-

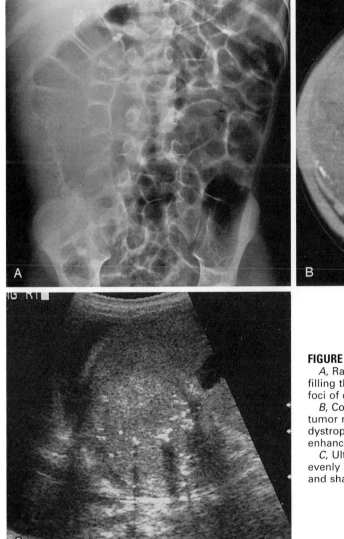

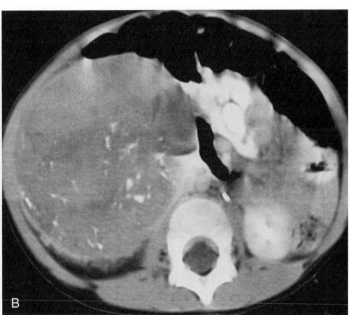

FIGURE 12–7. Wilms' tumor, right kidney, in a 4-year-old boy.

A, Radiograph of abdomen. There is a large soft tissue mass filling the right mid-abdomen and displacing bowel. Fine, stippled foci of calcium are visible within the tumor.

B, Computed tomogram, contrast material–enhanced. The large tumor replaces the kidney, contains numerous foci of nonperipheral dystrophic calcification, and is heterogeneous in its pattern of enhancement.

C, Ultrasonogram, longitudinal section. The tumor is diffusely and evenly echogenic. The foci of calcification cause specular echoes and shadowing.

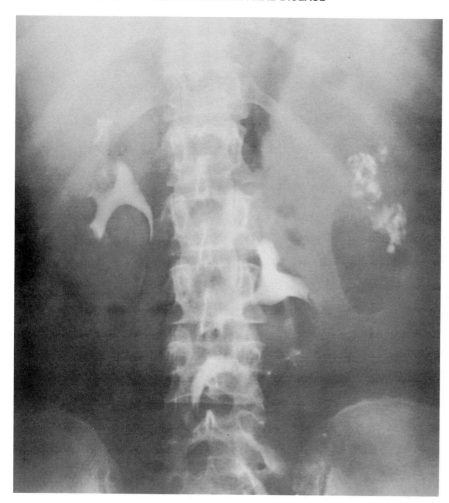

FIGURE 12–8. Adenocarcinoma of the left kidney. Lateral growth of the tumor causes marked medial displacement of the collecting structures. Note "nonperipheral" calcification characteristic of adenocarcinoma of the kidney. Excretory urogram.

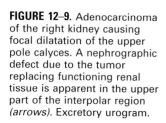

FIGURE 12–9. Adenocarcinoma of the right kidney causing focal dilatation of the upper pole calyces. A nephrographic defect due to the tumor replacing functioning renal tissue is apparent in the upper part of the interpolar region (arrows). Excretory urogram.

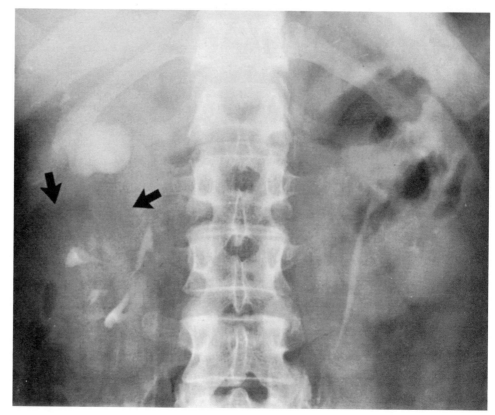

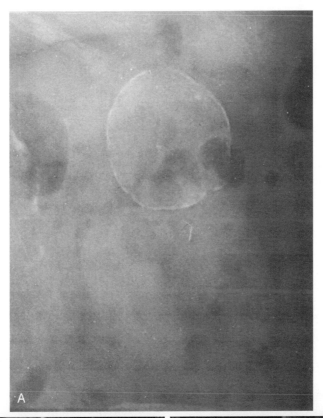

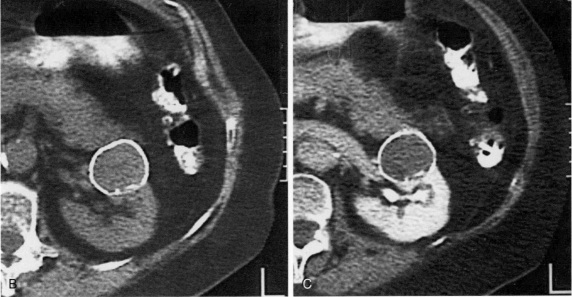

FIGURE 12–10. Adenocarcinoma, left kidney, with a thick rim of peripheral calcification.
 A, Excretory urogram.
 B, Computed tomogram without contrast material enhancement demonstrates a thick rim of calcium and an attenuation value of the tumor that approximates that of the renal parenchyma.
 C, Computed tomogram with contrast material demonstrates less tumor enhancement than the surrounding normal renal parenchyma.

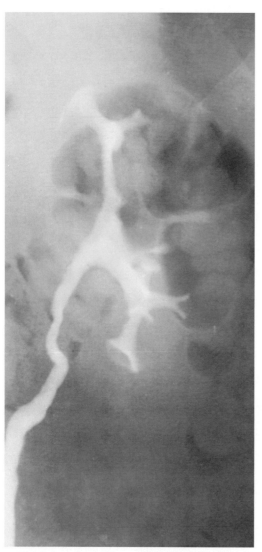

FIGURE 12–11. Adenocarcinoma of the kidney associated with pelvic and ureteral notching due to periureteric and peripelvic venous collaterals forming in response to renal vein obstruction by the tumor. Retrograde pyelogram. (Courtesy of Janet Dacie, M.B., St. Bartholomew's Hospital, London, England.)

ent for tumors that grow on the anterior or posterior surface of the kidney, that are deeply embedded within the parenchyma, or that are less than 3 cm in diameter (see Fig. 12–5). The attenuation value of unenhanced malignant tissue varies from slightly less than to slightly more than that of normal kidney tissue and from homogeneous to heterogeneous (Figs. 12–13 and 12–14; see also Figs. 12–4B and 12–10B). Foci of decreased attenuation within the mass correspond to areas of necrosis, old hemorrhage, or cystic change. Areas of recent hemorrhage are slightly hyperdense compared with normal renal tissue. There are two potential sources of error in assessing tumor enhancement patterns using helical computed tomography. Both are associated with very early dynamic scans obtained at a time when only the cortical nephrogram has developed. First, a small, solid malignant tumor may not be conspicuous during the cortical or vascular nephrographic phase if it enhances to the same degree as surrounding normal renal cortex. Second, a tumor within medullary tissue may not be apparent until contrast material moves into the medulla (Fig. 12–15). In either of these circumstances, error is avoided by obtaining delayed scans at a time when the tumor in either of these circumstances is of less density than surrounding renal tissue. The anatomic and functional aspects of the nephrogram are discussed in Chapters 3 and 27. Low-attenuation foci of old hemorrhage, necrosis, or cyst formation do not enhance.

A zone of relative radiolucency surrounding a tumor that has grown by expansion represents a fibrous pseudocapsule that has formed in response to ischemia of compressed nephrons at the interface between the neoplasm and adjacent renal parenchyma (Fig. 12–16). This finding, which has been called the *halo* sign, may also be observed by excretory urography or ultrasonography and is encountered in benign as well as malignant masses. Tumors that have an infiltrative pattern of growth, on the other hand, cause regional enlargement without a mass circumscribed by a pseudocapsule.

Computed tomography is particularly valuable in the assessment of malignant tumors that are partially or predominantly cystic (Figs. 12–17 and 12–18; see also Figs. 12–4 and 12–10). Uncommonly, the attenuation value of the tumor contents may be equal to or only slightly higher than water and may be nonenhancing (Fig. 12–19). Usually, however, the attenuation value is sufficiently above that of water as to raise the suspicion that the lesion is not an ordinary simple cyst. When a diagnosis of a cystic malignancy is suggested, additional clues derived from computed tomography are thickened walls or septations, mural nodules, and inhomogeneous attenuation values of the contents of the mass. Lesions other than a cystic malignancy that may simulate these findings include simple cyst or pyelocalyceal diverticulum with infection or hemorrhage, abscess, hematoma, multilocular cystic nephroma, and congenital arteriovenous malformation.

The significance of the pattern and distribution of calcification in a focal mass is included in the discussion of excretory urographic findings in the preceding section. Computed tomography is the standard for detecting calcium and for characterizing its location (see Figs. 12–7 and 12–10). Calcium within a mass that has an attenuation value greater than the range for water is strong evidence of malignancy, whereas a thin rim of calcification in the periphery of a mass whose contents uniformly have the attenuation value of water militates for a diagnosis of simple cyst.

Staging of malignant tumors of the kidney is accomplished by computed tomography as well as magnetic resonance imaging. These modalities are particularly accurate for detecting spread into the perirenal or pararenal spaces, extension into the renal vein or inferior vena cava, and involvement of

Text continued on page 285

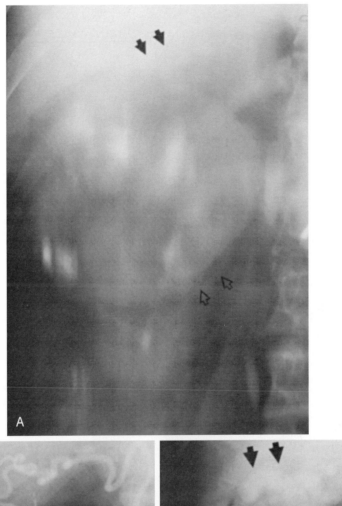

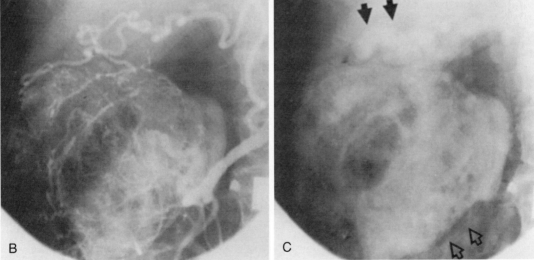

FIGURE 12–12. Adenocarcinoma of the kidney. Enlarged vessels are seen both inferior *(open arrows)* and superior *(solid arrows)* to the mass. The superior vessels represent parasitized adrenal arteries and veins. The inferior vessels reflect dilated renal arteries and veins.

A, Tomogram during excretory urography.

B, Arterial phase of selective renal arteriogram. The large parasitized inferior adrenal artery is seen feeding the vascular tumor.

C, Venous phase of selective renal arteriogram. Large, tortuous veins in the upper part of the tumor *(solid arrows)* drain into the inferior vena cava. Other venous structures embedded in perirenal fat drain inferior to the tumor *(open arrows).*

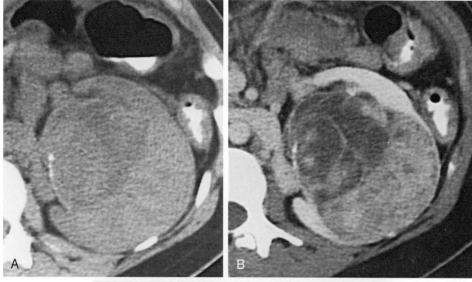

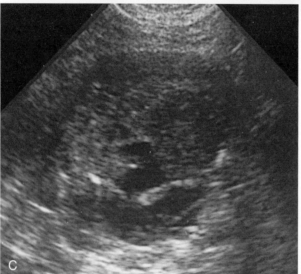

FIGURE 12–13. Adenocarcinoma, left kidney, in a 24-year-old female. Computed tomograms.

A, Unenhanced scan. The large tumor is composed of tissue with heterogeneous attenuation values that are equal to or less than that of normal renal parenchyma.

B, Contrast material–enhanced scan. The heterogeneous nature of the tumor is characterized by areas that vary from no enhancement to enhancement.

C, Ultrasonogram. The tumor is composed of both solid and cystic elements.

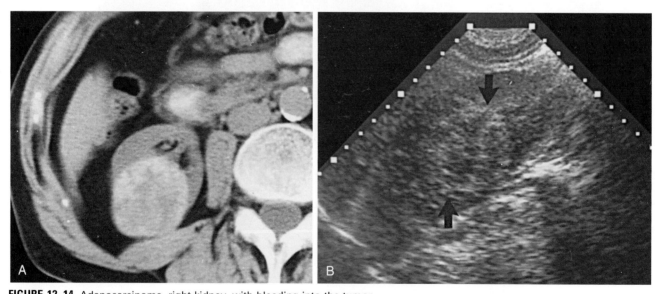

FIGURE 12–14. Adenocarcinoma, right kidney, with bleeding into the tumor.

A, Computed tomogram, unenhanced. The high attenuation value of the tumor represents fresh hemorrhage.

B, Ultrasonogram, longitudinal section. Most of the tumor is slightly more echogenic than the surrounding normal kidney *(arrows).* Some central areas of diminished echogenicity are present as well.

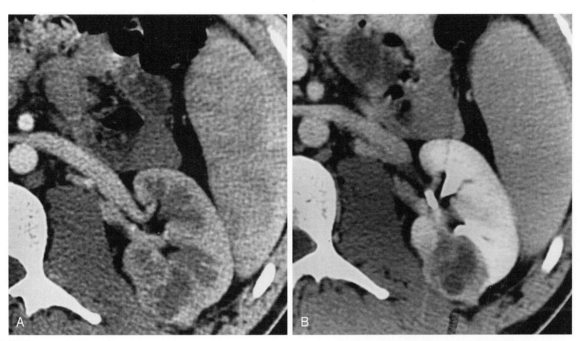

FIGURE 12–15. Adenocarcinoma, left kidney. Dynamic helical computed tomogram, contrast material–enhanced.

A, Early scan during cortical nephrogram. The carcinoma is indistinguishable from either the enhanced cortex or the unenhanced medulla.

B, Delayed scan during the parenchymal or urographic nephrographic phase. The tumor enhances less than surrounding parenchyma and is readily visualized.

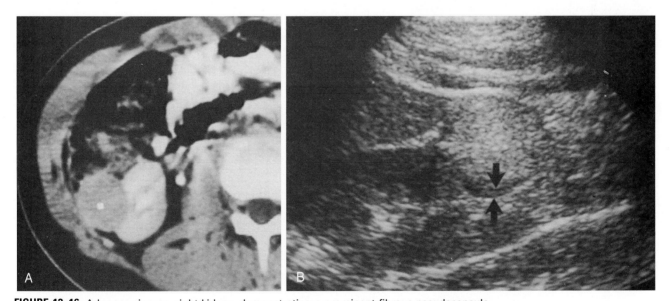

FIGURE 12–16. Adenocarcinoma, right kidney, demonstrating a prominent fibrous pseudocapsule.

A, Computed tomogram, contrast material–enhanced. There is a faint area of relatively diminished attenuation between the tumor and the underlying renal tissue.

B, Ultrasonogram, longitudinal section. The tumor is hyperechoic relative to renal tissue. The pseudocapsule is represented by a narrow hypoechoic band at the interface between the tumor margin and adjacent kidney parenchyma *(arrows)*.

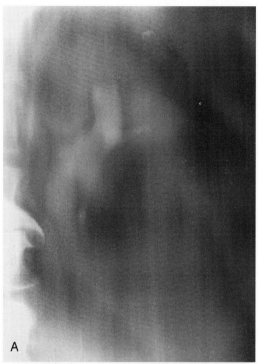

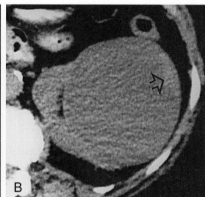

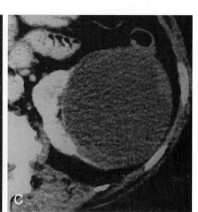

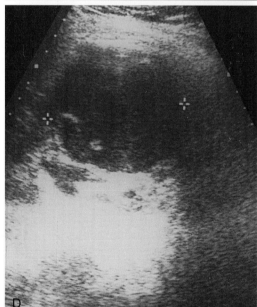

FIGURE 12–17. Cystic adenocarcinoma, left kidney.

A, Excretory urogram with tomography. The lower pole tumor does not enhance and displaces the lower and interpolar portions of the collecting system.

B, Computed tomogram, unenhanced. The tumor has a very slightly lower attenuation value than the renal parenchyma, except in an area of mural thickening *(arrow).*

C, Computed tomogram, contrast material–enhanced. The thick wall of the tumor enhances slightly in comparison to the unenhanced bulk of the tumor.

D, Ultrasonogram. The cystic tumor exhibits through-transmission of sound. Intratumoral echoes represent necrotic debris within the tumor.

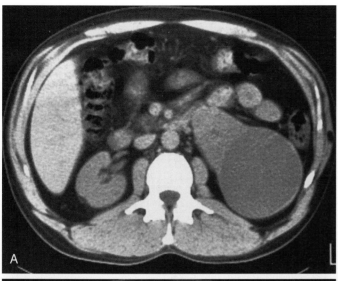

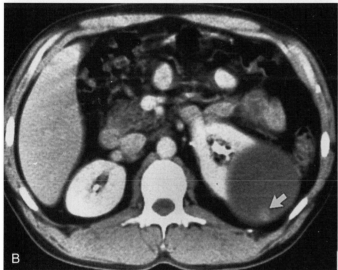

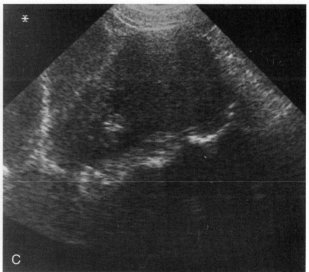

FIGURE 12–18. Cystic adenocarcinoma, left kidney.

A, Computed tomogram without contrast material enhancement demonstrates an attenuation value lower than that of the renal parenchyma with a thick, slightly nodular rim.

B, Computed tomogram with contrast material enhances the feature noted in part *A* and also reveals an enhancing mural nodule *(arrow)*.

C, Ultrasonogram, longitudinal section. Despite the "cystic" nature of the tumor, there are diffuse, low-level echoes throughout its contents.

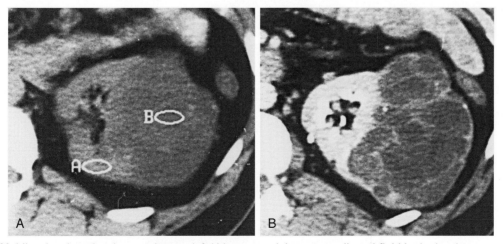

FIGURE 12–19. Multiloculated cystic adenocarcinoma, left kidney, containing uncomplicated fluid in the locules.

A, Computed tomogram, unenhanced. The attenuation value of the loculated fluid content is in the range of water (1.2 Hounsfield units).

B, Computed tomogram, contrast material–enhanced. The rim and septa enhance while the contents of the locules remain unenhanced.

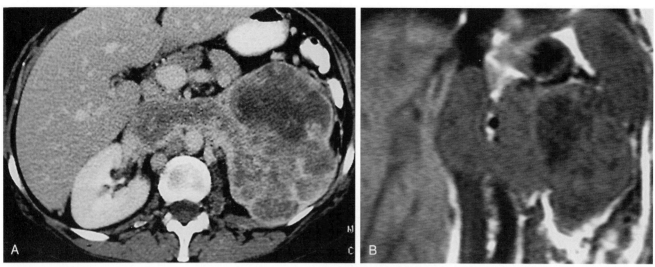

FIGURE 12–20. Adenocarcinoma, left kidney, with extension into renal vein and inferior vena cava.
 A, Computed tomogram, contrast material–enhanced. The renal vein and vena cava are enlarged and contain tumor.
 B, The same finding is demonstrated on a coronal section T1-weighted magnetic resonance image.

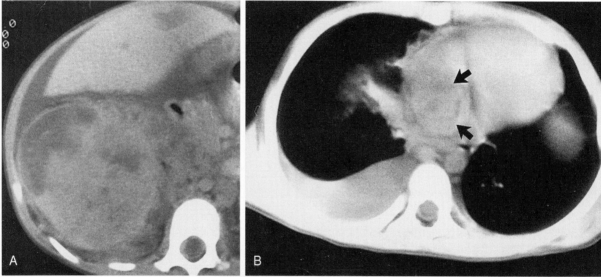

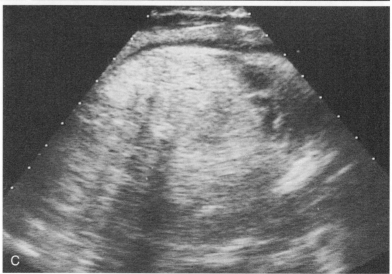

FIGURE 12–21. Wilms' tumor, right kidney, in a 4-year-old girl with Budd-Chiari syndrome secondary to spread of tumor to hepatic veins and the right atrium.
 A, Computed tomogram with contrast material enhancement demonstrates a large tumor of mixed attenuation values with ascites.
 B, Computed tomogram demonstrates tumor within the right atrium (arrows) as well as pleural effusion.
 C, Ultrasonogram, longitudinal section, demonstrates a hyperechoic pattern throughout most of the tumor.

the contralateral kidney or regional lymph nodes (Figs. 12–20 and 12–21; see Fig. 12–24*B*). A filling defect within the renal vein, inferior vena cava, or right atrium can be detected by computed tomography, as well as by ultrasonography and magnetic resonance imaging. However, the characterization of a filling defect as tumor rather than bland thrombus requires demonstration that the filling defect is vascularized. This can be documented either by enhancement after contrast material administration or, more directly, by use of power Doppler ultrasonography or phase-contrast magnetic resonance imaging.

Occasionally, malignant tumors of the kidney bleed spontaneously into the subcapsular and the perirenal space. This may be the first clinical manifestation of tumor in some patients. In this situation, computed tomography readily detects the hematoma as a high-density fluid collection and usually identifies the underlying tumor, which is often small and has a cortical location.

Computed tomography is a highly reliable technique for establishing the solid or complex solid and cystic nature of a focal renal tumor and for demonstrating characteristics that suggest malignancy. There are no specific computed tomographic features that routinely permit distinction of any one particular histologic form of malignancy from another. Exceptions may occur, however, as in the rare demonstration of fat in a Wilms' tumor in a child. Similarly, distinction between benign and malignant tumors by computed tomographic characteristics is not feasible, except in the diagnosis of angiomyolipoma, as described in the section Benign Neoplasms, which follows.

Ultrasonography

The characteristics of malignant tumors of the kidney as viewed by ultrasonography are based principally on their solid echogenic nature. The tumor margin may or may not be defined. The density of echoes produced by a solid renal mass may vary from hyperechoic to anechoic, as compared with renal parenchyma. Most, however, are echogenic to some degree (see Figs. 12–4*D*, 12–5*C*, 12–14*B*, 12–16*B*, 12–17*D*, 12–18*C*, and 12–21*C*). A solid malignant tumor that is anechoic requires distinction from a simple cyst, whereas one that is as echogenic as renal sinus fat simulates the appearance of angiomyolipoma.

Regardless of the echo pattern of a malignant tumor, sound transmission through a malignant tumor is usually impaired relative to water. As a result, malignant tumors almost always fail to demonstrate either the far wall of the tumor well or acoustic enhancement beyond the lesion. Calcification within a tumor produces specular echoes and acoustic shadowing (see Fig. 12–7*C*).

Malignant tumors that are intrinsically cystic produce ultrasonographic images that suggest their fluid-filled nature (Fig. 12–22; see Fig. 12–4*D*). In this circumstance, however, either the fluid content is not completely anechoic or the wall of the mass is not completely smooth (Fig. 12–23). Therefore, it is essential for the radiologist to keep in mind that a mass that fails to meet *all* of the criteria for a simple cyst (anechogenicity, enhanced through-transmission, a smooth, well-defined far wall, and a few thin septa) usually requires a tissue diagnosis, as discussed in Chapter 28.

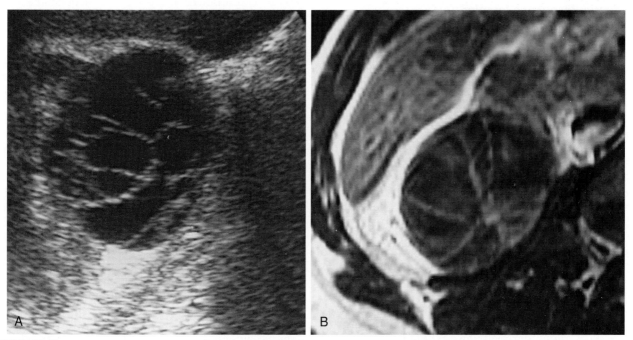

FIGURE 12–22. Multilocular cystic adenocarcinoma, right kidney. The imaging characteristics are of multiple, water-filled locules with thick, smooth, enhancing septa. These findings are identical to those of multilocular cystic nephroma.
   A, Ultrasonogram.
   B, Contrast material–enhanced magnetic resonance image.

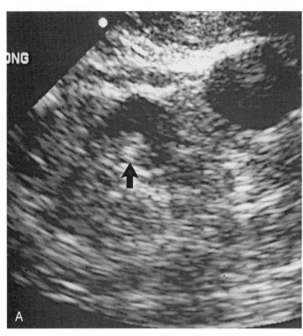 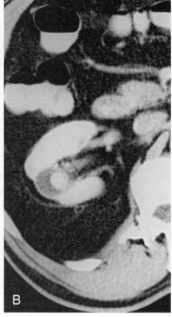

FIGURE 12–23. Cystic adenocarcinoma, right kidney. *A,* Ultrasonogram. An echogenic nodule *(arrow)* is in the wall of a unicameral cyst. *B,* Computed tomogram, contrast material–enhanced. The mural nodule is enhanced. The cystic component measures 17.1 Hounsfield units.

Gray-scale or color Doppler ultrasonography is useful in detecting renal vein enlargement, collateral venous channels in the renal hilum, and tumor or bland thrombus within renal veins or the inferior vena cava (Fig. 12–24). Enlargement of the renal vein may result from either occlusion or increased blood flow caused by vascular tumor. Echogenicity within the renal veins or inferior vena cava or absence of flow on color Doppler ultrasonography indicates tumor or bland thrombus in these structures.

Magnetic Resonance Imaging

The information derived from magnetic resonance imaging of malignant tumors of the kidney is similar to that of computed tomography. Patterns of enhancement with gadolinium contrast material parallel those of iodinated contrast material. Magnetic resonance imaging is preferred in patients with sensitivity to iodinated contrast material or renal insufficiency. It is also of advantage in cases of very large tumors in which coronal or sagittal planes better define involvement of adjacent organs. Often, magnetic resonance imaging is reserved for those cases in which venous involvement is not conclusively demonstrated by computed tomography or ultrasonography. This is especially so when the extent of venous involvement, which can be of importance in surgical planning, is clearly depicted by coronal or sagittal imaging of the inferior vena cava and through the use of flow-sensitive magnetic angiography sequences (Fig. 12–25).

Most adenocarcinomas are of low signal intensity on T1-weighted images and are thus nearly isointense with renal parenchyma. When hemorrhage has occurred, high signal may be seen on T1-weighted images (Fig. 12–26). Although an adenocarcinoma is somewhat more conspicuous on T2-weighted images as a lesion of slightly higher signal than renal parenchyma, this sequence is still of limited benefit. A low signal rim, which correlates with the pseudocapsule seen on contrast-enhanced computed tomography, is occasionally seen on T2-weighted images, especially in smaller tumors. Owing to high lesion conspicuity, and capitalizing on the fact that nearly all renal adenocarcinomas enhance less than normal renal parenchyma, dynamic gadolinium-enhanced T1-weighted images are most useful. Unenhanced images are still needed for assessing lymphadenopathy.

Angiography

Angiography is rarely used to characterize a renal mass, but may be useful as an adjunct to preoperative planning or for tumor embolization. Most renal adenocarcinomas are very vascular. Common features include an enlarged renal artery, chaotically distributed intrarenal vessels of irregular size, small aneurysms, arteriovenous communications, and "lakes" of contrast material that clear slowly (Fig. 12–27). Necrosis appears as radiolucent areas within the mass. The main renal vein may opacify earlier than normal because of arteriovenous shunts. Dilated capsular veins may drain from the tumor into the main renal vein or into other vessels such as the intercostal, lumbar, adrenal, inferior phrenic, and gonadal veins (see Fig. 12–12). Arteries from these locations may also supply the tumor. Branches of the inferior or superior mesenteric arteries can be parasitized as tumor spreads into the mesentery vessel.

Some adenocarcinomas are of moderate vascularity, whereas others are hypovascular, enhance minimally during the nephrographic phase of the angiogram, and exhibit a sharp interface between

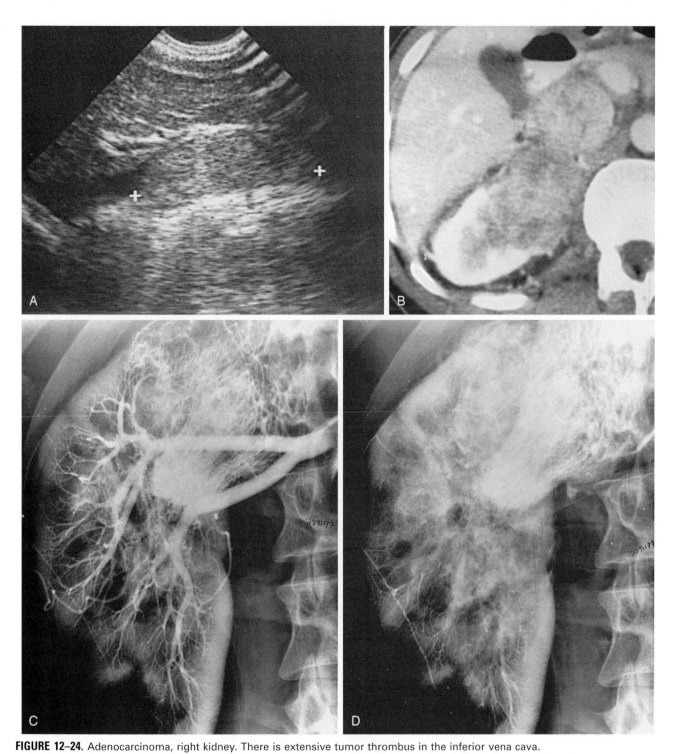

FIGURE 12–24. Adenocarcinoma, right kidney. There is extensive tumor thrombus in the inferior vena cava.
 A, Ultrasonogram, sagittal section. The echogenic tumor *(cursors)* is within the lumen of the inferior vena cava.
 B, Computed tomogram, contrast material–enhanced. Enhanced tumor fills the renal sinus and enlarges the inferior vena cava.
 C and *D*, Selective renal arteriogram. The tumor in the medial upper pole is moderately vascular. Neovascularity extends into the tumor thrombus in the renal vein, causing a striated pattern of enhancement.

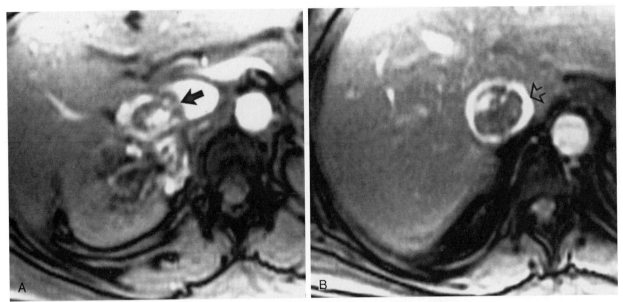

FIGURE 12–25. Adenocarcinoma with extension into the inferior vena cava. Axial gradient echo magnetic resonance images.
A, Scan at level of renal vein. The thrombus *(arrow)* contains high signal indicative of blood flow.
B, Scan at hepatic level of inferior vena cava. There is flow within the residual lumen *(arrow)*.

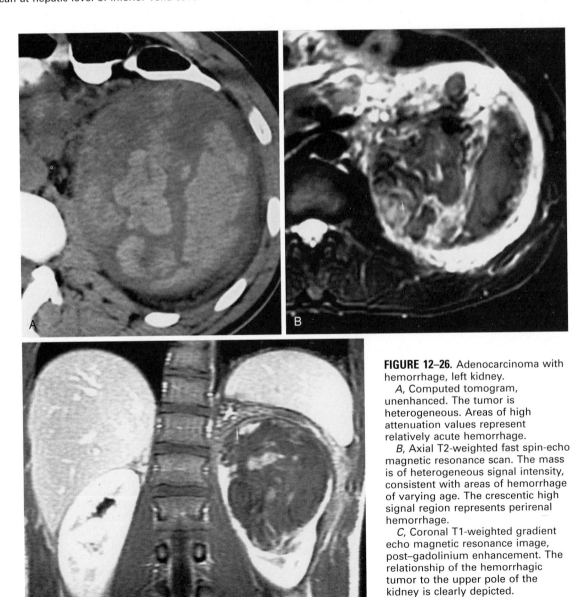

FIGURE 12–26. Adenocarcinoma with hemorrhage, left kidney.

A, Computed tomogram, unenhanced. The tumor is heterogeneous. Areas of high attenuation values represent relatively acute hemorrhage.

B, Axial T2-weighted fast spin-echo magnetic resonance scan. The mass is of heterogeneous signal intensity, consistent with areas of hemorrhage of varying age. The crescentic high signal region represents perirenal hemorrhage.

C, Coronal T1-weighted gradient echo magnetic resonance image, post–gadolinium enhancement. The relationship of the hemorrhagic tumor to the upper pole of the kidney is clearly depicted.

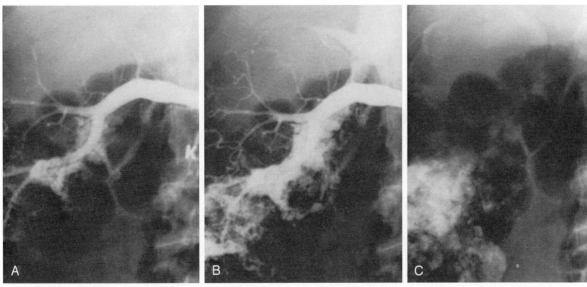

FIGURE 12–27. Adenocarcinoma involving the lower pole of the right kidney and causing marked hydronephrosis of the upper pole.
A and *B*, Arterial phase of selective renal arteriogram. The main renal artery is enlarged. There is rapid arteriovenous shunting into the renal veins and the inferior vena cava. The arteries to the hydronephrotic upper pole are stretched.
C, Late phase of selective renal arteriogram. "Lakes" of contrast material persist in the tumor. Thick nephrographic rims remain in the hydronephrotic upper pole.

tumor and adjacent normally enhanced renal parenchyma (Fig. 12–28; see also Fig. 12–5). Hypovascularity usually indicates a tumor composed of cells arranged in a papillary pattern.

Invasion of the main renal vein and inferior vena cava is common with renal adenocarcinoma and Wilms' tumor and can be established by the demonstration of a nest of arterial tumor vessels leading into the renal vein or inferior vena cava. Sometimes, linear striated capillary staining of tumor in the renal vein is seen (see Fig. 12–24*C, D*). Venous involvement is well demonstrated by inferior vena cavography. However, noninvasive modalities are usually employed for this purpose (see Figs. 12–20 and 12–24). Filling defects alone in the renal vein

or inferior vena cava should not be considered conclusive evidence of venous spread of tumor, however, since propagated bland thrombus can produce this appearance.

Small amounts of epinephrine (5 to 10 μg) rapidly injected into the artery of a cancer-bearing kidney cause transient contraction of normal intrarenal arteries but do not similarly affect tumor neovascularity. Contrast material injection immediately following epinephrine permits radiographic recording of this phenomenon. Failure of neovascular contraction after epinephrine is not a specific sign of cancer, however, since similar results occur in inflammatory lesions and angiomyolipoma of the kidney as well.

MALIGNANT NEOPLASMS TYPICAL FINDINGS

Primary Uroradiologic Elements

Size: large
Contour: unifocal mass (ball- or bean-shaped geometry)
Lesion distribution: unilateral

Secondary Uroradiologic Elements

Collecting system: attenuated (focal); displaced (focal); dilated (focal); replaced (focal)
Nephrogram: replaced (focal); irregular margin; thick wall; mottled density
Attenuation value: diminished before contrast material; enhanced less-than-normal
  parenchyma
Calcification: nonperipheral (common); peripheral (uncommon)
Echogenicity: variable
Magnetic resonance: signal intensity similar to parenchyma on unenhanced T1- and T2-
  weighted scans; enhances with gadolinium; flow-sensitive sequences detect venous
  thrombus
Vascularity: neovascularity; venous thrombus

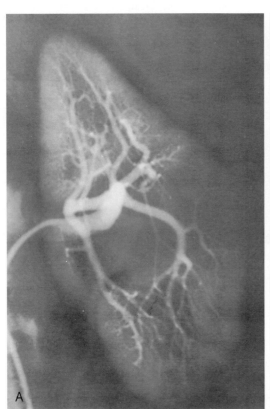

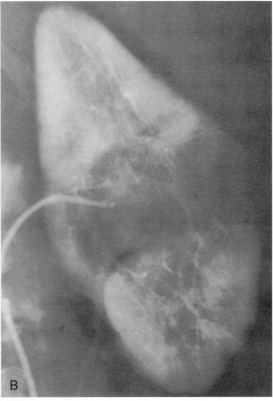

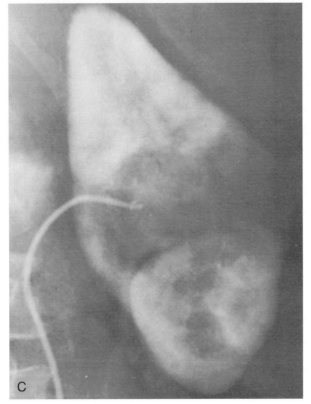

FIGURE 12–28. Adenocarcinoma involving the interpolar area of the left kidney. This hypovascular form is usually associated with a tumor composed of cells arranged in a papillary pattern.

A, Arterial phase of selective renal arteriogram. Note the paucity of arteries to the tumor.

B, Late arterial phase. Some abnormal vessels are present along the upper margin of the tumor.

C, Venous phase. Note the radiolucent area of the tumor and the sharp interface between the tumor and adjacent normal tissue.

(Reproduced from Weiss, R. M., Becker, J. A., Davidson, A. J., et al.: Angiographic appearance of renal papillary-tubular adenocarcinomas. J. Urol. *102*:661, 1969, with permission. Copyright by Williams & Wilkins, 1969.)

BENIGN NEOPLASMS

Oncocytoma

Definition

Oncocytoma, or adenoma with oncocytic features, is a benign renal neoplasm that has received much attention in the radiologic literature. This tumor is characterized by large cells with small, uniform, round nuclei and abundant eosinophilic cytoplasm. The ultrastructural characteristic of these cells is the presence of a large number of mitochondria. Oncocytomas tend to grow to a large size and are usually, but not invariably, homogeneous in consistency. Calcification may occur.

Clinical Setting

Oncocytomas tend to grow to a size large enough to cause a palpable abdominal mass, pain, and hematuria, and these findings lead to an investigation for malignancy of the urinary tract.

Radiologic Findings

Excretory Urography. Urographic features of oncocytoma are the same as those of any other solid tumor, either benign or malignant, and are related to the mass effect of the lesion. These include a contour bulge, focal collecting system attenuation, and displacement or focal caliectasis due to local pressure on a draining infundibulum. Irregular obliteration of the calyces or infundibula, tumor calcification, and other signs of malignant disease, such as capsular vessels and ureteric notching, are usually not present.

Computed Tomography. An oncocytoma appears as a focal, ball-shaped, homogeneous mass that, when large enough, is sharply marginated by a relatively low attenuating pseudocapsule. Many of these are isodense or very slightly less dense than normal renal tissue. Contrast enhancement is usually homogeneous and less than that of the surrounding kidney parenchyma. Adenomas tend to be much smaller than oncocytomas. These features are nonspecific and overlap with other benign and malignant tumors. A central, clearly defined stellate area of low attenuation, representative of ischemic fibrosis, is sometimes present in oncocytoma (Fig. 12–29). This pattern overlaps the appearance of some adenocarcinomas, however, and cannot be used as a reliable indicator for the diagnosis of oncocytoma (Fig. 12–30).

Ultrasonography. Ultrasonography in oncocytoma shows a solid mass composed of homogeneous tissue (see Fig. 12–29). Low-level echoes similar to those of renal tissue, a poorly defined far wall, and sound attenuation indicate only the presence of a solid mass that is indistinguishable from a malignant tumor.

Magnetic Resonance Imaging. The magnetic resonance imaging characteristics of oncocytoma are variable. The central scar, if present, has been described as both hyperintense and hypointense. The absence of tumoral hemorrhage or necrosis, adenopathy, and venous tumor thrombus are noteworthy but do not distinguish an oncocytoma from an adenocarcinoma.

Angiography. Oncocytoma is usually a vascular,

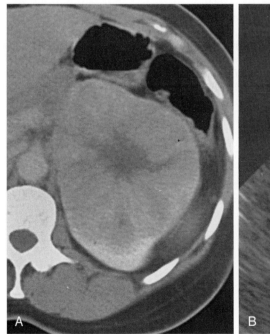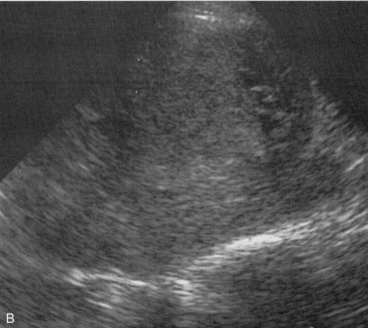

FIGURE 12–29. Oncocytoma, left kidney.
   A, Computed tomogram, contrast material–enhanced. The tumor is a ball-shaped, expansile mass of homogeneous density except for a central stellate pattern of low attenuation representing ischemic and fibrotic portions of the tumor.
   B, Ultrasonogram, longitudinal section. The oncocytoma produces an image of an expansile, ball-shaped mass of uniform echogenicity.

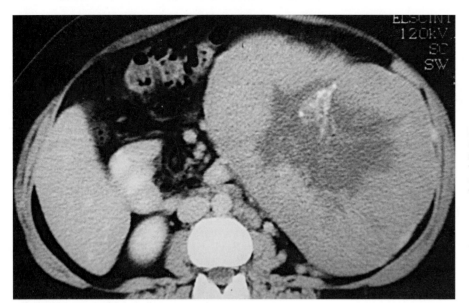

FIGURE 12–30. Adenocarcinoma, left kidney. The centrally placed, calcified scar simulates the computed tomographic findings associated with oncocytoma. Computed tomogram with contrast material enhancement.

encapsulated mass that often has a homogeneous nephrogram and occasional neovascularity. There is no characteristic arrangement of the feeding arteries that distinguishes this tumor from other benign or malignant histologic types. However, in common with other benign tumors, arterial encasement and venous shunting are usually absent.

Angiomyolipoma

Definition

Radiologically, the most commonly diagnosed benign kidney neoplasm is angiomyolipoma. This tumor is a hamartoma rather than a true neoplasm in that it represents excessive growth of mature fat, smooth muscle, and arteries normally present in the kidney. A clinically apparent renal angiomyolipoma usually appears as a large tumor mass situated in one portion of the kidney. These lesions are expansive rather than invasive. Often, a large portion of the mass projects into the perirenal space with only a small point of attachment to the kidney at its site of origin. At the other extreme, very small, fat-containing tumors are a common finding in the kidney at autopsy and an incidental finding on computed tomography, ultrasonography, and magnetic resonance imaging of the abdomen. These, too, are angiomyolipomas, but their small size causes neither symptoms nor distortion of the kidney.

Muscle and fat vary in relative amounts from one tumor to another, although most angiomyolipomas have an abundance of both tissues. Approximately 5 per cent have a fatty component that is detectable only by microscopy and not by imaging studies. Arteries found in an angiomyolipoma are characterized by an absent internal elastic membrane and a disordered adventitial cuff of smooth muscle. This is the basis for the aneurysms frequently demon-

---

ONCOCYTOMA TYPICAL FINDINGS

Primary Uroradiologic Elements

Size: large
Contour: unifocal mass
Lesion distribution: unilateral

Secondary Uroradiologic Elements

Collecting system: attenuated (focal); displaced (focal)
Nephrogram: replaced (focal)
Attenuation values: soft tissue, homogeneous, central "scar"
Echogenicity: soft tissue echogenicity, homogeneous
Magnetic resonance: enhances less than parenchyma; variable signal intensity of central
    scar

strated by arteriography. The cut surface of the tumor varies in appearance and texture, with the predominant tissue component being yellow and soft when fat is in abundance and pearl-colored and firm when muscle elements are the major component. Most angiomyolipomas are very vascular. Cytologic changes of malignancy are absent.

Clinical Setting

Most angiomyolipomas are clinically silent. Discovery is usually unexpected and occurs during the investigation of the urinary tract for unrelated symptoms. Some patients present with a palpable renal mass. In others, intrarenal, subcapsular, and perirenal hemorrhage occurs and produces flank pain, hypotension, and hematuria. Angiomyolipoma is diagnosed in women more often than in men over a wide age range, from young adulthood through the eighth decade. Most symptomatic angiomyolipomas occur as isolated, unifocal, unilateral kidney lesions in otherwise normal individuals. Lesions larger than 4 cm in diameter tend to hemorrhage more frequently than smaller tumors and should be removed. Up to 80 per cent of patients with tuberous sclerosis develop multiple angiomyolipomas of the kidneys, as discussed in Chapter 10.

Radiologic Findings

Excretory Urography. Renal angiomyolipoma causes unifocal enlargement of one kidney in uncomplicated cases and bilateral, multifocal enlarge-

ment when associated with tuberous sclerosis (see Fig. 10–13). One distinctive radiologic feature of this lesion is radiolucency within the mass when there is a large component of fat in the tumor (Fig. 12–31). This finding can be observed with certainty only on films obtained before administration of contrast material, since any radiolucency seen within the tumor following injection of contrast material might represent necrosis or diminished perfusion in a nonhamartomatous tumor that has no fatty component. Unfortunately, fat-related radiolucency within the tumor is an infrequent radiographic observation, being reported in less than 10 per cent of patients. Other urographic features of angiomyolipoma are the same as those of any other solid tumor, either benign or malignant, and are related to the mass effect of the lesion.

Computed Tomography. Fat in a renal tumor in an adult is a finding that is virtually specific to angiomyolipoma. The demonstration of tissue with fat-equivalent negative attenuation values is the basis for the unique specificity of computed tomography in the detection of angiomyolipoma of the kidney (Figs. 12–32 and 12–33; see also Figs. 12–34 and 12–36). The fat of an angiomyolipoma is sometimes largely extrarenal and easily confused with a primary retroperitoneal tumor such as liposarcoma. Computed tomography is valuable in this situation for detecting the nephrographic defect that indicates the true renal origin of the mass (see Fig. 12–33). Intermixed with the fat are muscle and

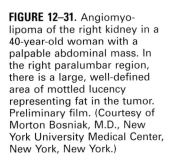

FIGURE 12–31. Angiomyolipoma of the right kidney in a 40-year-old woman with a palpable abdominal mass. In the right paralumbar region, there is a large, well-defined area of mottled lucency representing fat in the tumor. Preliminary film. (Courtesy of Morton Bosniak, M.D., New York University Medical Center, New York, New York.)

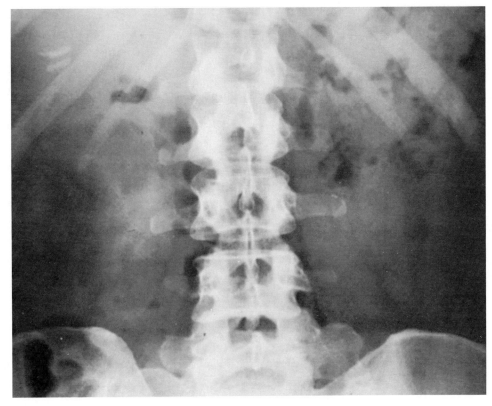

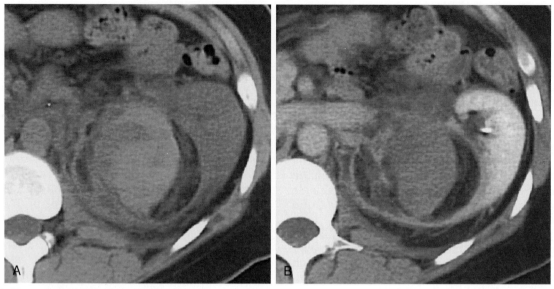

FIGURE 12–32. Angiomyolipoma, left kidney. Computed tomograms.
A, Unenhanced scan. The tumor is composed of tissue that is of both negative attenuation value (fat) and attenuation values greater than normal renal parenchyma (hemorrhage).
B, Contrast material–enhanced scan. The tumor capsule and the nonfat components of the angiomyolipoma enhance slightly.

blood vessels, which yield attenuation values similar to those of renal parenchyma; fresh hemorrhage, if present, is represented by higher attenuation values (Fig. 12–34; see also Fig. 12–32). Computed tomography is also of value in documenting perinephric blood in symptomatic patients (see Fig. 12–34B). If fat is not detectable in an angiomyolipoma, as is estimated to occur in 5 per cent of cases, the computed tomographic findings are those of other solid tumors, either benign or malignant (Fig. 12–35). Calcification, however, is very rare in angiomyolipoma.

Ultrasonography. An angiomyolipoma exhibits an ultrasonographic image of a mass whose echo intensity is equal to or greater than that of perirenal fat (Fig. 12–36). This pattern may be diffuse within a large mass or appear as isolated foci of echogenicity in an otherwise normal kidney in which there are one or more tiny asymptomatic angiomyolipomas. However, this finding does not apply to all angiomyolipomas. When the fatty component is minimal, or when hemorrhage has occurred, the echo pattern has a mixed or diminished intensity. The ultrasonographic finding of a highly echogenic renal mass is not specific to angiomyolipoma, since adenocarcinoma may yield an identical image. In other respects, the ultrasonographic image of an angiomyolipoma reveals a solid mass that attenuates sound and prevents both far-wall enhancement and through-transmission of sound. As described previously, most of the mass may be extrarenal and give the impression of a retroperitoneal soft tissue origin rather than a renal origin.

Magnetic Resonance Imaging. Magnetic reso-

ANGIOMYOLIPOMA TYPICAL FINDINGS

Primary Uroradiologic Elements

Size: large
Contour: unifocal mass
Lesion distribution: unilateral

Secondary Uroradiologic Elements

Collecting system: attenuated (focal); displaced (focal)
Nephrogram: replaced (focal)
Attenuation values: mixed (negative and positive values)
Echogenicity: heterogeneous; often hyperechoic
Magnetic resonance: signal intensity follows fat on T1-weighted, T2-weighted, and fat-suppressed images.

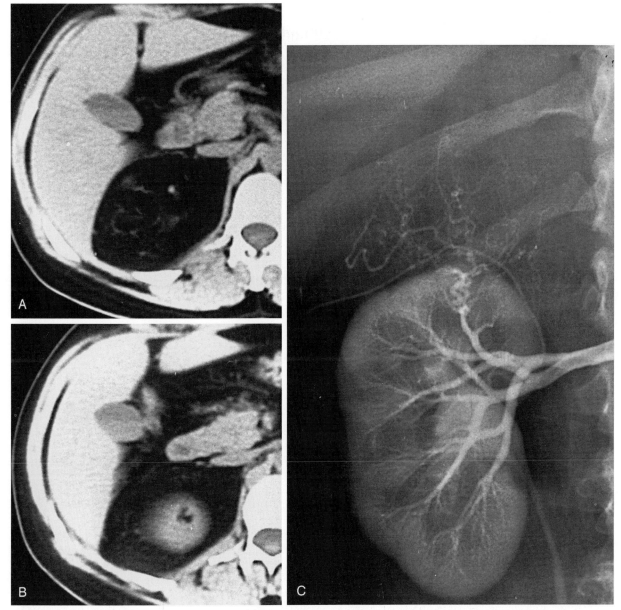

FIGURE 12-33. Angiomyolipoma arising in the superior pole of the right kidney. Almost all of the mass *is* extrarenal.

A, Computed tomogram with contrast material enhancement of right suprarenal area. A fat-containing tumor fills the perirenal space.

B, Computed tomogram with contrast material enhancement at level of most superior tip of the upper pole of the kidney. The nephrogram is disrupted by fatty tissue representing the site of origin of the angiomyolipoma within the renal parenchyma.

C, Selective renal arteriogram demonstrates the artery to the upper pole that supplies the angiomyolipoma.

nance imaging rarely offers an advantage over computed tomography in the diagnosis of angiomyolipoma (Fig. 12–37). In large, exophytic tumors, coronal or sagittal plane images may be of value in differentiating an angiomyolipoma from a retroperitoneal liposarcoma by identifying the site where the angiomyolipoma arises from renal parenchyma.

Hemorrhage, as well as fat, may be present within an angiomyolipoma, just as an adenocarcinoma may have fresh intratumoral hemorrhage. This gives rise to a potential for diagnostic error when hemorrhage mimics the high signal intensity of fat on T1-weighted images. Fat-suppressed im-

ages serve to demonstrate signal loss within the mass in the case of angiomyolipoma (see Fig. 12–37C). If fat cannot be identified with certainty, a presumptive diagnosis of adenocarcinoma should be made.

Angiography. There are no angiographic features of angiomyolipoma that permit a specific diagnosis. As might be expected from their histology, these tumors are quite vascular. Distinctive features include one dominant feeding artery with a circumferential arrangement of vessels around the tumor and multiple small aneurysms of medium-sized arteries that pool contrast material (see Figs.

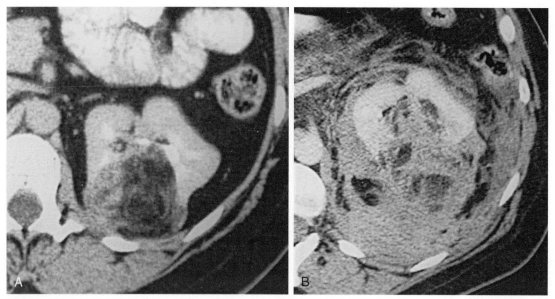

FIGURE 12–34. Angiomyolipoma, left kidney, with interval hemorrhage.

A, Initial contrast material–enhanced computed tomogram demonstrates an angiomyolipoma in the dorsal portion of the kidney. The diameter of the mass exceeds 4 cm.

B, Spontaneous hemorrhage one year later. Blood fills the perirenal space and obliterates some, but not all, of the computed tomographic features of fat.

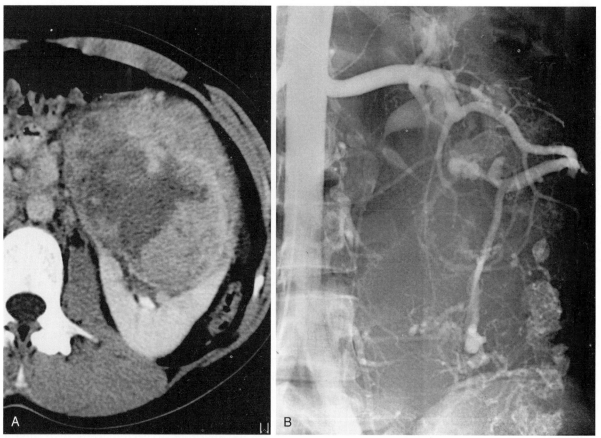

FIGURE 12–35. Angiomyolipoma of the left kidney with no fat detected by computed tomography.

A, Computed tomogram, contrast material–enhanced. Representative section. The mass is of mixed attenuation values, but no fat was detected on contiguous thin slices throughout the lesion. The "beak" sign indicates an intrarenal origin.

B, Aortogram. A single large artery with focal aneurysms perfuses the angiomyolipoma.

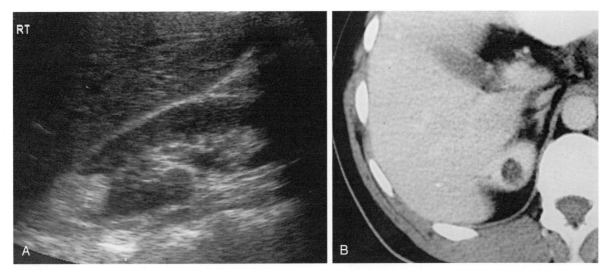

FIGURE 12–36. Angiomyolipoma, right kidney.

A, Ultrasonogram, longitudinal section. The lesion occupies the upper pole and is seen as a round, sharply marginated mass with echogenicity equal to or slightly more than that of the adjacent perirenal fat.

B, Computed tomogram, contrast material–enhanced. A small fatty mass is present in the upper pole of the kidney.

12–33 and 12–35). Arteriovenous shunts are very uncommon. Any of these angiographic features may be seen in renal adenocarcinoma as well as in angiomyolipoma. Similarly, the abnormal arteries of angiomyolipoma may fail to contract following injection of epinephrine.

Multilocular Cystic Nephroma

Definition

Multilocular cystic nephroma is an uncommon neoplasm composed of multiple, variably sized cysts with prominent septa. The cysts contain clear, yellow, turbid, or gelatinous fluid and do not communicate with each other. Calcification uncommonly is present in cyst walls. Hemorrhage, however, is rare. Characteristically, although not invariably, one or more of the cysts herniate into the renal pelvis to form a nonopaque filling defect that may at times obstruct portions of the collecting system and ulcerate the uroepithelium. Multilocular cystic nephroma arises as a unifocal mass, with the remaining portion of the kidney uninvolved or compressed by the tumor.

Multilocular cystic nephroma grows by expansion and has a dense fibrous capsule. The cysts most commonly are lined by cuboidal epithelial cells that

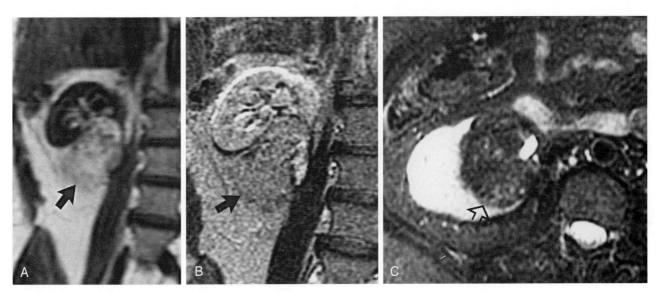

FIGURE 12–37. Angiomyolipoma, right kidney. Magnetic resonance images.

A, Coronal T1-weighted image. There is a mass on the medial aspect of the kidney *(arrow)* that is of slightly heterogeneous signal intensity.

B, Coronal T2-weighted image. The signal characteristics of the mass *(arrow)* approximate the signal intensity of fat.

C, Fat-suppressed axial T2-weighted image. Fat is confirmed by the marked decrease in the signal intensity of the mass *(arrow).*

project into the cyst lumen. Septal stroma is usually composed of loose connective tissue with sparse cellularity, indicating the benign nature of this tumor.

There is a form of Wilms' tumor and of adenocarcinoma that has gross morphologic and imaging features identical to those of benign multilocular

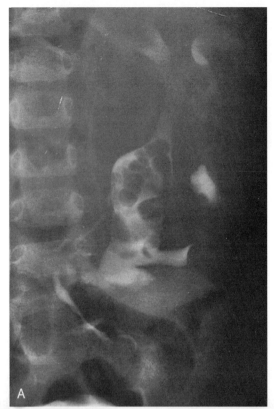

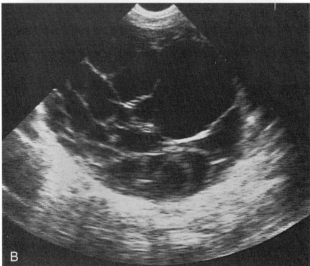

FIGURE 12–38. Multilocular cystic nephroma, left kidney, in a 7-year-old boy.

A, Excretory urogram. The mass distorts and displaces the central portion of the kidney. Multiple filling defects in the pelvocalyceal system represent herniated cysts.

B, Ultrasonogram, longitudinal section. The tumor is composed of numerous locules of varying size with thick septa and uncomplicated fluid. (Kindly provided by the Department of Radiology, Alberta Children's Hospital, Calgary, Alberta, Canada.)

cystic nephroma. These features are discussed in previous sections on malignant tumors in the chapter.

Multilocular cystic nephroma is sometimes confused with multicystic dysplastic kidney. Multilocular cystic nephroma is a unifocal mass involving only a portion of an otherwise normal kidney. Multicystic dysplastic kidney, on the other hand, usually, but not invariably, involves an entire kidney. When multicystic dysplastic kidney is segmental, it lacks a fibrous capsule, a finding that is always present in multilocular cystic nephroma. Additional aspects of multicystic dysplastic kidney are discussed in Chapter 11.

Clinical Setting

Multilocular cystic nephroma has a biphasic age and sex distribution. One peak in prevalence occurs in infants and young children with a male bias, and a second peak occurs in middle-aged adults with a predominance among females. This lesion may be detected as a palpable mass, particularly in infants. Some cases present with hematuria, but many are discovered incidentally.

Radiologic Findings

Excretory Urography. In multilocular cystic nephroma, the kidney is enlarged by a unifocal mass that distorts the collecting system (Fig. 12–38). Calcium may be detectable in the walls of the locules (Fig. 12–39). With careful radiographic technique, faint opacification of septa may be detectable. Otherwise, the urographic nephrogram is absent in the area of involvement. The interface between the lesion and the adjacent normally opacified renal tissue is sharply defined. Herniation of one or more cysts into the pelvis presents as a sharply defined, rounded filling defect in the opacified renal pelvis (Fig. 12–40; see also Fig. 12–38). If the prolapsed cysts are large enough or are located in a critical position, obstruction of the collecting system draining the normal portions of the kidney may occur.

Computed Tomography. Multilocular cystic nephroma is a well-marginated, expansive mass on computed tomographic images (Fig. 12–41). The cysts vary greatly in size, and there may be variation in attenuation values from that of water to slightly higher. The portion of the tumor that has prolapsed into the pelvis is readily identified (see Fig. 12–40). The thick septa that characterize this lesion enhance after contrast material is administered. Computed tomography detects calcium in the septa much more often than does standard radiography (see Fig. 12–39). The pattern of calcium deposition varies from linear to flocculent.

Ultrasonography. A sharply defined multiloculated mass characterizes the ultrasonographic appearance of multilocular cystic nephroma (Fig. 12–42; see also Figs. 12–38, 12–40, and 12–41). A collection of tiny cysts, each too small to be individually resolved, may be imaged as an echogenic focus. Echoes may also originate in locules filled with the gelatinous material found in some cysts.

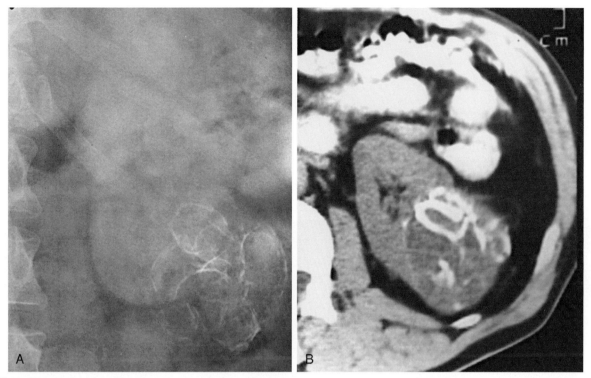

FIGURE 12–39. Multilocular cystic nephroma with dense calcification in the walls of involuted cysts.
  A, Excretory urogram.
  B, Computed tomogram, unenhanced.

Magnetic Resonance Imaging. Magnetic resonance imaging of multilocular cystic nephroma produces findings similar to those of computed tomography (see Fig. 12–42*B*). Signal intensity within the locules typically parallels that of water, being hypointense on T1-weighted images and hyperintense on T2-weighted images. The smooth septations enhance after gadolinium administration. Uncommonly, increased signal intensity within one or more locules is noted, presumably representing increased protein content of the locule fluid. No specific magnetic resonance imaging features allow confident differentiation of multilocular cystic nephroma from adenocarcinoma.

Angiography. Angiography may reveal neovascularity in the form of irregular vessels coursing through the septa and around the lesion (Fig. 12–43). These are indistinguishable from neovascularity in other tumors. The septa can be seen during the angiographic nephrogram as relatively thick bands of radiodensity curving around radiolucent, fluid-filled areas.

Mesoblastic Nephroma

Definition

A mesoblastic nephroma is a neoplasm of considerable clinical importance because it is the most com-

---

MULTILOCULAR CYSTIC NEPHROMA TYPICAL FINDINGS

Primary Uroradiologic Elements

Size: large
Contour: unifocal mass
Lesion distribution: unilateral

Secondary Uroradiologic Elements

Collecting system: attenuated (focal); displaced (focal); filling defects
Nephrogram: replaced (focal)
Attenuation value: variable, water or slightly higher; enhancing, thick, smooth septa
Calcification: uncommon
Echogenicity: multilocular cystic mass
Magnetic resonance: cyst fluid generally follows signal intensity of water

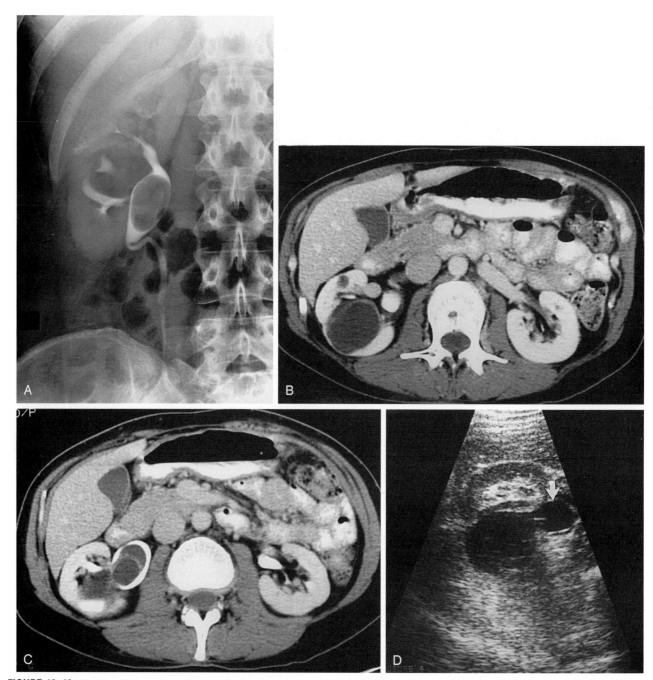

FIGURE 12–40. Multilocular cystic nephroma in the right kidney of a middle-aged woman. The tumor is in the central portion of the kidney. Herniation of locules produces a filling defect in the renal pelvis.

A, Excretory urogram. The mass displaces and partially obstructs infundibula and calyces.

B and *C,* Computed tomogram, contrast material–enhanced. The tumor is sharply defined and composed of locules of water attenuation, some of which are herniated into the renal pelvis.

D, Ultrasonogram, transverse section. The locules are anechoic with faint septa. The *arrow* indicates the locule in the pelvis.

(Kindly provided by Marge Stahl, M.D., and Wendelin Hayes, D.O., Georgetown University, Washington, D.C.)

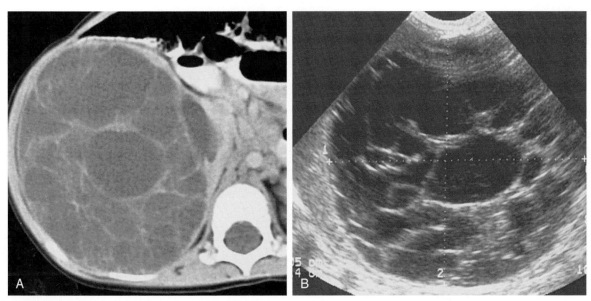

FIGURE 12–41. Multilocular cystic nephroma, right kidney, in an 18-month-old female with a palpable mass.
   A, Computed tomogram, contrast material–enhanced. The tumor is composed of multiple locules containing water-density fluid and demarcated by thick, smooth septa.
   B, Ultrasonogram. Multiple cysts with thick, smooth septa are present.

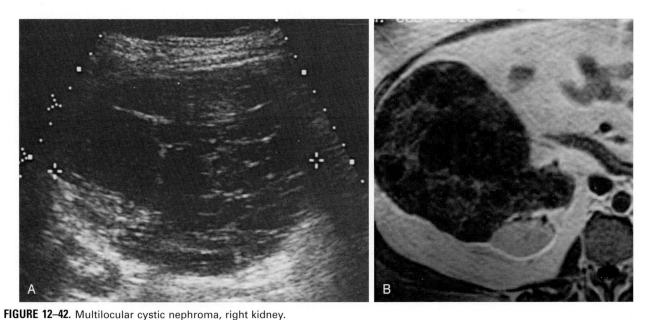

FIGURE 12–42. Multilocular cystic nephroma, right kidney.
   A, Ultrasonogram, longitudinal section. The multiple locules of the cystic mass are defined by thick septations.
   B, Magnetic resonance image. T1-weighted axial scan. The mass is well circumscribed and composed of locules of approximately fluid signal intensity separated by faint septations.

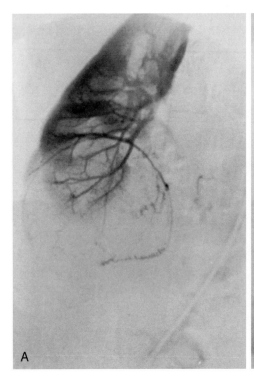

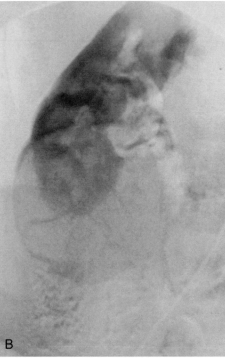

A

B

FIGURE 12–43. Multilocular cystic nephroma. Subtraction films of an angiogram demonstrate displaced major arteries, fine arterial supply to the septa, and the staining of the septa during the angiographic nephrogram. *A*, Arterial phase. *B*, Nephrographic phase.

mon solid renal mass discovered in the newborn or infant in the first few months of life. Mesoblastic nephroma is uncommonly discovered in older children and only rarely in the adult. While of mesenchymal origin and usually benign, the demography and imaging features of mesoblastic nephroma are distinctive from the other entities discussed in this section. The typical tumor is a solid, yellow-tan, unencapsulated mass that often grows large enough to replace most of the kidney parenchyma. Because the growth pattern is infiltrative, there is preservation of a reniform shape until the tumor becomes quite large. Hemorrhage and necrosis are uncommon and suggest a malignant form of this usually benign tumor.

Clinical Findings

Mesoblastic nephroma is usually discovered either *in utero* during an obstetric ultrasonographic examination or in the newborn as a large, nontender abdominal mass. Polyhydramnios is a well-recognized complication of mesoblastic nephroma developing during fetal life. This may be acute and give rise to premature labor. The size of the mass in the fetus may also cause dystocia.

Radiologic Findings

Excretory Urography. The urographic features of mesoblastic nephroma include a large, noncalcified mass that preserves to some extent the reniform shape of the kidney until a very large size is reached. Even with very large tumors, excretion of contrast material is preserved to some extent, as evidenced by opacification of dilated calyces that have been "trapped" by tumor as it infiltrates the central portions of the collecting system. This pat-

tern of caliectasis without pelviectasis is characteristic of any tumor that spreads by infiltration rather than expansion.

Computed Tomography. Mesoblastic nephroma is characteristically large and of homogeneous attenuation both before and after contrast material enhancement (Fig. 12–44). Low-density areas of hemorrhage, necrosis or cyst formation, and calcification are uncommon. The infiltrating nature of mesoblastic nephroma is suggested both by a lack

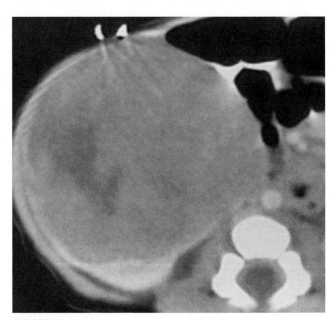

FIGURE 12–44. Mesoblastic nephroma, right kidney, in a newborn male. Computed tomogram, contrast material–enhanced. A large, relatively homogeneous mass expands the kidney.

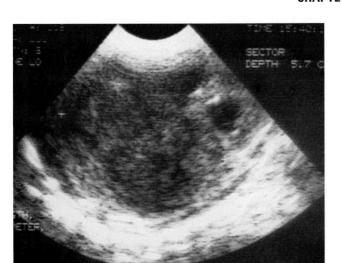

FIGURE 12–45. Mesoblastic nephroma, left kidney. Ultrasonogram, longitudinal section. The tumor produces a uniform pattern of echoes.

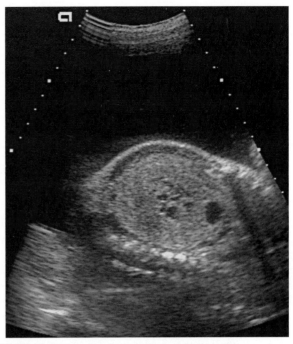

FIGURE 12–46. Mesoblastic nephroma. Maternal ultrasonogram, 38 weeks. There is a large echogenic paraspinal abdominal mass with several foci of anechoicity. Polyhydramnios is prominent.

of sharp margination between tumor and renal parenchyma and by a tendency toward preservation of the reniform shape at least until the tumor grows to a very large size.

Ultrasonography. Mesoblastic nephroma is usually evenly echogenic with low-level echoes (Fig. 12–45). The reniform shape of the enlarged kidney is best demonstrated by longitudinal scans, but this feature may not be apparent in very large tumors. "Trapped" calyces, often associated with tumors that infiltrate rather than expand, may be identified as small, dilated, fluid-filled structures. Hemorrhage, necrosis, and cyst formation are seen as focal hypoechoic areas with a larger echogenic mass. *In utero*, the tumor is readily detected in the fetal abdomen and is sometimes associated with polyhydramnios (Fig. 12–46).

Mesenchymal/Juxtaglomerular Cell Tumor

Definition

Mesenchymal tissue gives rise to *fibroma, lipoma, myoma, angioma*, and *juxtaglomerular cell tumor.*

The juxtaglomerular cell tumor usually arises near the surface of the kidney, distorts renal contour, and causes unique symptoms. Contrariwise, the other benign tumors of mesenchymal origin are usually small and do not distort either the internal architecture or the contour of the kidney. Thus, they usually escape detection during life.

Clinical Setting

Benign mesenchymal tumors of the adult kidney become symptomatic only when they grow large enough to cause pain or hematuria, or both. Juxtaglomerular cell tumors are different in this regard. As a metabolically active tumor, there is an excess production of renin, causing hypertension and secondary aldosteronism leading to severe headache

---

MESOBLASTIC NEPHROMA TYPICAL FINDINGS

Primary Uroradiologic Elements

Size: large
Contour: infiltrative, bean-shaped mass
Lesion distribution: unilateral

Secondary Uroradiologic Elements

Collecting system: attenuated; caliectasis without pelviectasis
Nephrogram: replaced
Attenuation values: soft tissue, homogeneous (common); heterogeneous with focal cysts (uncommon)
Echogenicity: soft tissue echogenicity, homogeneous (common); hypoechoic foci (occasional)
Other: polyhydramnios *(in utero)*

MESENCHYMAL/JUXTAGLOMERULAR CELL TUMOR TYPICAL FINDINGS

Primary Uroradiologic Elements

Size: large
Contour: unifocal mass
Lesion distribution: unilateral

Secondary Uroradiologic Elements

Collecting system: attenuated (focal); displaced (focal)
Nephrogram: replaced (focal)
Attenuation values: soft tissue, homogeneous
Echogenicity: soft tissue echogenicity, homogeneous

---

and muscle weakness. Women are predominantly affected.

Radiologic Findings

Excretory Urography. Urographic features of mesenchymal and juxtaglomerular cell tumors are the same as those of any other solid tumor, either benign or malignant, and are related to the mass effect of the lesion. These include focal collecting system attenuation and displacement or focal caliectasis due to local pressure on a draining infundibulum. Juxtaglomerular cell tumors are apt to project off the surface of the kidney as a ball-shaped, expansive mass. This reflects their origin in the periphery of the renal parenchyma.

Computed Tomography. Mesenchymal tumors and juxtaglomerular cell tumor usually are homogeneous expansive masses that uniformly enhance following administration of contrast material, but to a lesser degree than surrounding normal renal parenchyma. Their computed tomographic features are nonspecific.

Ultrasonography. The solid nature of mesenchymal and juxtaglomerular cell tumors is well documented in the ultrasonographic demonstration of echogenic, expansive masses situated either deep within the parenchyma or on the surface of the kidney.

Angiography. Mesenchymal neoplasms of the kidney are usually hypovascular. This characterization applies to juxtaglomerular cell tumor as well. Angiography contributes little specific information in the diagnosis of these lesions other than confirming their solid nature, which is information that is more readily derived from ultrasonography or computed tomography.

NON-NEOPLASTIC MASSES

Simple Cyst/Localized Cystic Disease

Definition

Simple parenchymal, or nephrogenic, cyst is the most common focal mass of the kidney. Although included in this chapter as an inherently unifocal and unilateral mass, cysts frequently occur at mul-

tiple sites in one or both kidneys. With modern cross-sectional imaging, it is likely that radiologic detection approaches the true prevalence of simple cyst, which is certainly much higher than the historical estimate of 3 to 5 per cent based on autopsy studies.

The pathogenesis of renal cysts has not been conclusively established. Their rarity below the age of 30 years, as discussed subsequently, points to an acquired nature. Obstruction of a renal tubule has been the generally accepted explanation, but the possibility that these develop as a result of blockage and expansion of a calyceal diverticulum has also been considered.

Simple cysts are lined with low cuboidal or flattened epithelium. The wall is composed of fibrous tissue and compressed nephrons and is only 1 to 2 mm thick in those portions that do not abut normal parenchyma.

Simple renal cysts occur most often in the renal cortex and usually expand outward, causing a bulge on the kidney surface. When observed directly, a bluish coloration underlies the thin, glistening membrane, which is the cyst wall. This appearance explains the description of these lesions as "blue domed." The majority are reported to occur in the polar regions, particularly in the lower pole. In most cases, a cyst contains a single cavity. In some instances, thin septa divide the cyst into chambers. Calcification may deposit as a thin layer within either the wall or the septum of a cyst. Cysts vary in size from microscopic to very large and symptomatic.

The fluid within a cyst is serous, not urine, clear, and slightly yellow and has a specific gravity of 1.002 to 1.010. Small amounts of protein, urea, chlorides, and sugar are present. Lactic dehydrogenase content is considerably lower than that of serum, a finding of potential importance in the chemical evaluation of cyst aspirate. Fluid from a simple cyst should be cell free and contain little or no fat or cholesterol. If a cyst becomes infected, or if bleeding into the cyst occurs, the nature of the fluid changes accordingly. In this circumstance, the wall thickens and may develop dense calcification.

Rarely, numerous simple cysts completely replace

the parenchyma of either the entire kidney or, sometimes, only a portion of one kidney, while the contralateral kidney remains free of cysts. This condition is referred to as *localized cystic disease*. Here, microscopic examination reveals cysts that have formed from dilatation of ducts and tubules. The cysts vary in size from millimeters to several centimeters and compress intervening normal renal parenchyma. When an entire kidney is replaced, a misdiagnosis of unilateral autosomal dominant polycystic kidney disease is sometimes made. This diagnosis is a contradiction of terms, because by definition autosomal dominant polycystic kidney disease is always bilateral, although sometimes asymmetric. Localized cystic disease that is limited to only a portion of one kidney must be distinguished from the usually benign, but sometime malignant, multiloculated cystic neoplasms. These tumors, which are discussed in previous sections of this chapter, characteristically grow by expansion and appear as a ball-shaped, encapsulated mass. Focal localized cystic disease, on the other hand, is composed of a cluster of simple cysts that lacks a capsule and preserves the reniform shape of the enlarged kidney.

The occurrence of adenocarcinoma within the wall of a simple renal cyst has been the subject of a few isolated case reports. Adenocarcinoma within a cyst wall is very rare but, nevertheless, is always of concern. Much more common, on the other hand, is the coexistence of adenocarcinoma and cyst in the same kidney. This occurred in approximately 0.1 per cent of patients with carcinoma of the kidney in one large series (Emmett et al., 1963), but this figure is probably too conservative. Although the occurrence of adenocarcinoma and simple cyst in the same kidney is undoubtedly a chance relationship, these data emphasize the need for caution in ascribing a given set of urinary tract symptoms to a simple cyst discovered during an imaging procedure.

Variant forms of simple fluid-filled cyst are frequently found in kidneys of patients with tuberous sclerosis and von Hippel-Lindau disease, as discussed in Chapter 10. Multiple simple cysts also occur in a wide variety of congenital and other conditions, known variably as glomerulocystic, microcystic, and pluricystic disorders. These are discussed briefly in Chapters 8 and 10.

Clinical Setting

Development of simple renal cyst is rare in individuals younger than the age of 30 years. Thereafter, cysts form with increasing frequency. Both sexes are affected equally. Most cysts grow slowly over a few years, although occasionally rapid growth can be noted. Cysts usually do not cause symptoms. If numerous or large, they may decrease renal function or produce pain. Rarely, simple cysts have caused hypertension, presumably from ischemia of compressed adjacent tissue. Cysts may rupture into the pelvocalyceal system and cause flank pain and hematuria. When this occurs, the cyst is converted into a smooth-walled cavity that communicates with the collecting system.

In patients with multiple cysts in both kidneys, careful recording of family history, evaluation of renal function, and search for cysts in other organs are sometimes required to differentiate simple parenchymal cysts from autosomal dominant polycystic kidney disease.

Radiologic Findings

Excretory Urography. Because renal cysts are usually cortical, they commonly produce focal contour expansion of the kidney outline. Calcification occurs in only 3 per cent of all cysts (Fig. 12–47). When present, it is curvilinear and thin and is deposited only along the periphery of the lesion. In one series based on film radiography (Daniel et al., 1972), 80 per cent of all kidney masses with peripheral, curvilinear calcification were simple cysts. The remaining 20 per cent were adenocarcinomas (see Fig. 12–10). These data emphasize the need for extreme caution in relying too much on a pattern of peripheral curvilinear calcification alone as a sign of benign status.

Several urographic features are characteristic of simple cyst. The nephrogram is always absent because the cyst is avascular and its fluid content, uninfluenced by glomerular filtration, does not accumulate contrast material. The interface between the cyst and the adjacent renal parenchyma is sharply defined and smooth. A 1 mm to 2 mm rim of tissue is opacified where the cyst protrudes beyond the confines of the kidney (Fig. 12–48). This finding, the *thin rim* sign, is caused by the accumulation of contrast material in compressed nephrons and in the small vessels of the fibrous tissue portion of the capsule. The normal cortex at the margin of a slowly expanding and protruding cyst is deflected outward. This is seen in profile as an angular-shaped extension of normally dense renal tissue at the point where the cyst extends beyond the renal surface (see Fig. 12–48). This urographic finding, the *beak* or *claw* sign, reflects slow expansion of an intrarenal mass, and it may be seen in any slow-growing lesion, including adenocarcinoma.

When a simple cyst is completely embedded in the kidney parenchyma, the thin rim and beak signs are absent. Renal size and contour are normal. In addition, the nephrographic radiolucency of the cyst may be obscured by contrast material in parenchyma surrounding the cyst. Here, the diagnosis of simple cyst can only be suggested by smooth displacement of the collecting system and by tomographic definition of sharply marginated nephrographic radiolucency.

A renal cyst causes focal displacement of adjacent portions of the pelvoinfundibulocalyceal system. The displaced, attenuated collecting structure remains smooth in contradistinction to the shagginess and obliteration that often occur when focal displacement is caused by a malignant neoplasm.

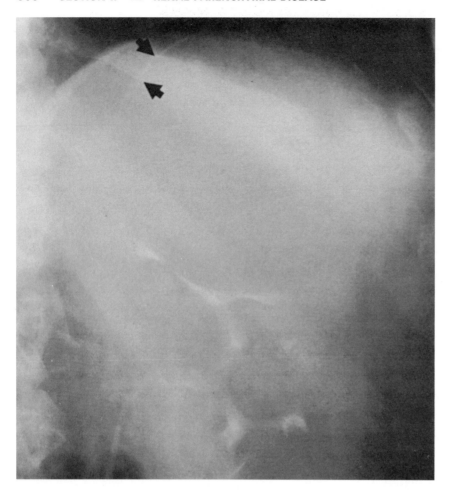

FIGURE 12–47. Simple cyst. Curvilinear, peripheral calcification outlines part of the cyst wall *(arrows).* There is smooth splaying of the upper pole calyces. Excretory urogram.

A confident diagnosis of simple cyst is not possible by excretory urography. Typical urographic features require confirmation, usually by ultrasonography rather than computed tomography.

Computed Tomography. A simple cyst has a homogeneous water density and a sharply demarcated margin (Fig. 12–49). The wall is either imperceptible or just barely perceptible where the cyst projects beyond the confines of the kidney. Thin septations with or without fine linear deposits of calcium may be identified within the cyst (Figs. 12–50 and 12–51). Contrast material does not alter the attenuation value of a simple cyst by more than 15 Hounsfield units, assuming constancy of all technical factors.

Errors in the computed tomographic diagnosis of simple cyst are usually associated with partial volume averaging in very small cysts (less than 1 cm diameter), cysts that are both small and completely intrarenal, or failure to maintain technical factor constant between scans obtained before and after contrast material enhancement. Another cause for error is the misleading impression of a thick wall that occurs when the parenchymal beak is included in the transverse cross section of the cyst (Fig. 12–52). Another source of potential error is confusion with a pyelocalyceal diverticulum that has become noncommunicating, as discussed in Chapter 15.

The contents of a cyst that becomes infected or hemorrhagic produce attenuation values higher than those of water (Fig. 12–53). The density of a hemorrhagic cyst, in fact, may be the same as or greater than that of renal parenchyma on unenhanced scans. The hyperdense cyst, therefore, may be inapparent on contrast material–enhanced scans or misinterpreted as a solid mass (Fig. 12–54). Thickening, and sometimes calcification, of the wall of an infected or hemorrhagic cyst is also seen with computed tomography (see Fig. 12–53).

Computed tomography provides a precise display of the anatomy of a simple cyst. A conclusive computed tomographic diagnosis of simple cyst demands adherence to strict criteria. Variants such as thick mural calcification, mural nodule, thickened or irregular septation or wall, an attenuation value greater than water, and enhancement after administration of contrast material demand special considerations, which are discussed in Chapter 28.

Ultrasonography. The ultrasonographic characteristics of a simple cyst are a well-defined, smooth, anechoic mass with far-wall enhancement and increased through-transmission of sound (Fig. 12–55). Each of these criteria must be fulfilled to establish a confident diagnosis by ultrasonography. Thin septa may be present (see Fig. 12–55). Small-sized cysts, cysts located in the upper pole of the left kidney,

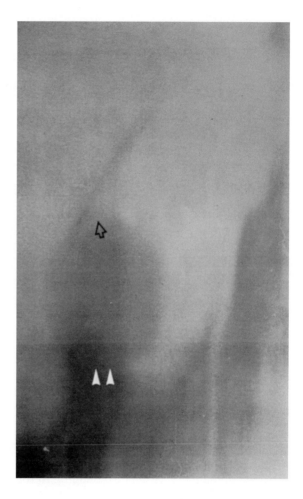

FIGURE 12–48. Simple cyst in the lateral portion of the lower pole. The cyst does not enhance, and there is a sharp interface between the cyst and the adjacent renal parenchyma. A *thin rim* sign is present along the inferior free margin of the cyst *(closed arrows)*. A *beak* sign is noted at the superior interface between the cyst and the parenchyma *(open arrow)*.

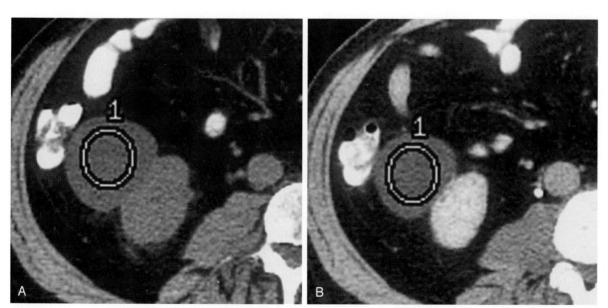

FIGURE 12–49. Simple cyst of the right kidney projecting into the perirenal space. Computed tomograms.
A, Unenhanced. The contents have the same attenuation value as water.
B, Contrast material–enhanced. The attenuation value of the cyst does not change. The level of the sections, size and location of the cursors, and other technical factors are held constant for both studies.

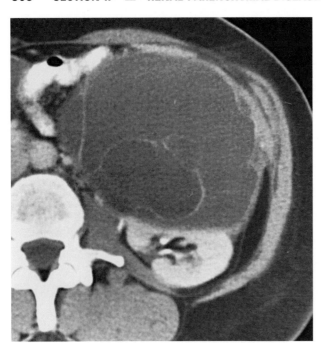

FIGURE 12–50. Simple cyst with septations. Computed tomogram, contrast material–enhanced. A few filamentous, undulating septa are present.

mural calcification, improper technical settings, and internal septa are factors that may degrade the ultrasonographic image and lead to a misdiagnosis. Infection and hemorrhage within a simple cyst usually cause internal echoes, fluid-debris level, or impaired sound through-transmission (Figs. 12–56 and 12–57). The implications of these results in terms of management are discussed in Chapter 28.

Magnetic Resonance. There is no unique value intrinsic to magnetic resonance imaging in the evaluation of a cyst. A simple cyst is of homogeneous low signal intensity on T1-weighted images and of high signal intensity on T2-weighted images. The cyst wall is smooth and sharply defined from adjacent renal parenchyma. Occasionally, high signal intensity on T1-weighted images is seen, reflecting prior hemorrhage or infection, or altered cyst fluid.

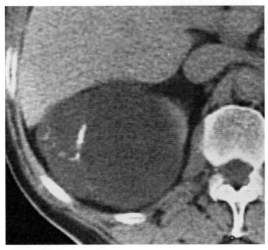

FIGURE 12–51. Simple cyst with calcified septations. Computed tomogram, contrast material–enhanced. Thin, linear calcification is present along portions of the septa.

This is the magnetic resonance analogue of the hyperdense cyst detected by computed tomography. The interpretation that such a lesion is most likely a simple cyst should be based on the lack of enhancement on dynamic post-gadolinium T1-weighted images. This issue is discussed further in Chapter 28.

Cystography. Cyst contents can be removed by percutaneous needle aspiration and replaced with radiopaque contrast material or air, or both, to further define radiologic anatomy. Complete cystography requires the study of all aspects of the cyst, either by serial computed tomographic images or by multiple radiographic projections, including horizontal beam films. All walls should be smooth and the septations thin. Aspiration of the contents of a fluid-filled mass may be a valuable diagnostic adjunct, especially when a fluid-filled mass is discovered in the clinical context of infection. Here, the aspiration of pus militates for a diagnosis of infected cyst, abscess, or focal hydronephrosis. Aspirate from an uncomplicated simple cyst is clear, yellow, and free of abnormal cells.

Angiography. Angiography demonstrates the avascular nature of simple cysts. The nephrographic defect and beak and thin rim signs are shown to better advantage than with urography because of the higher dose of contrast material administered to the kidney in a short time span. Angiography also demonstrates smooth displacement of arteries around cysts embedded deep within the kidney substance. Neovascularity, abnormal stains within the mass, early venous opacification, and pericapsular draining veins are not features of simple cysts.

The angiographic study of an infected cyst may demonstrate a hypervascular rim, neovascularity, an indistinct interface between the cyst and the

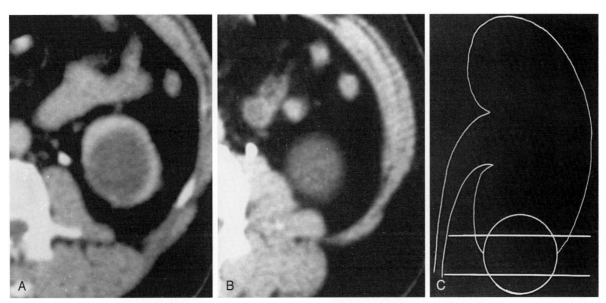

FIGURE 12–52. Spurious finding of a thick wall in an uncomplicated simple cyst. Computed tomograms, contrast material–enhanced.
  A, The normally enhanced parenchyma surrounding the cyst simulates a thick wall.
  B, Section at a more caudal level than in part *A* demonstrates no visible wall surrounding the unenhanced cyst.
  C, Diagram of the level of the sections shown in parts *A* and *B*.

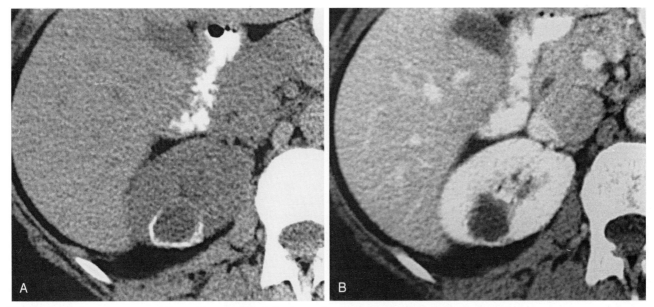

FIGURE 12–53. Simple cyst complicated by previous infection or hemorrhage. Computed tomograms.
  A, Unenhanced scan. The attenuation value of the cyst contents approaches that of renal parenchyma. The wall of the cyst is densely calcified.
  B, Contrast material–enhanced scan. The cyst does not enhance, but exhibits an irregular wall.

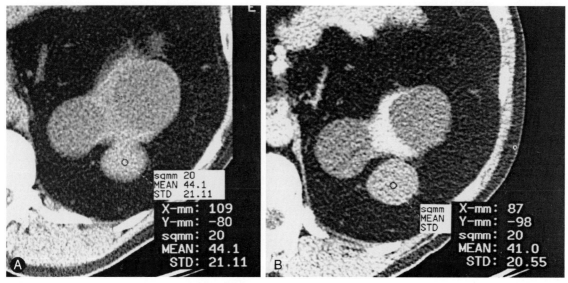

FIGURE 12–54. Hyperdense simple cyst. Computed tomograms.

A, Unenhanced scan. The cyst *(cursor)* has an attenutation value of 44.1 Hounsfield units and is visually of greater density than two other cysts in the same region.

B, Contrast material–enhanced scan. The attenuation value of the hyperdense cyst remains essentially unchanged (41.0 Hounsfield units).

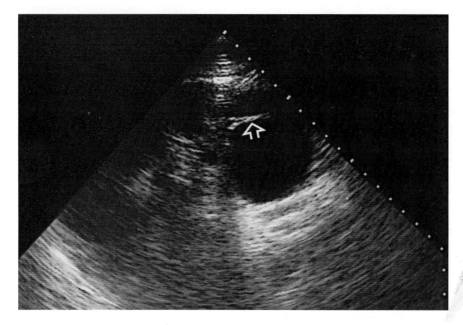

FIGURE 12–55. Simple cyst of the kidney demonstrating anechoicity, a well-defined far-wall, and increased through-sound transmission. A thin septum is also present *(arrow).*

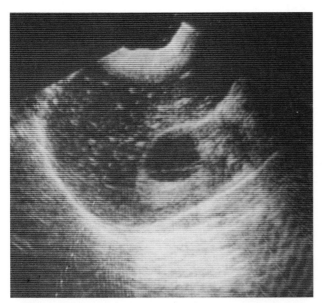

FIGURE 12–56. Simple cyst of the right kidney with infection causing a fluid-debris level. Enhanced transmission of sound is preserved. Ultrasonogram, longitudinal section.

adjacent renal parenchyma, or a prominent capsular artery. These findings are indistinguishable from those associated with malignant neoplasm or other forms of inflammatory disease of the kidney.

Focal Hydronephrosis

Definition

When the drainage of one portion of the kidney is obstructed, regional hydronephrosis and focal renal enlargement may develop. Overall, focal hydronephrosis is most commonly found in children with complete ureteropelvic duplication and an ectopic insertion of the ureter with or without a complicating ureterocele. In the adult, as well as in the child, obstruction may be from a congenital cause or the

result of infection, particularly tuberculosis with infundibular stenosis. Calculus and tumor obstructing an infundibulum are additional causes. Less frequent, but still worth mentioning, is congenital ureteropelvic junction obstruction of the lower moiety of a duplicated collecting system.

Clinical Setting

Focal hydronephrosis is usually asymptomatic. Symptoms, if present, may be limited to vague abdominal or flank pain or be due to infection complicating the obstruction. A renal mass might be palpable, but this is more likely to be found in children. Focal hydronephrosis is often detected *in utero* during the course of obstetric ultrasonographic examination.

Radiologic Findings

Excretory Urography. Increased renal length and a localized bulge in contour are produced by focal hydronephrosis. A sharply marginated radiolucency corresponding to dilated calyces filled with nonopacified urine is seen during the nephrographic phase. This is also apparent as increased distance between the margin of the upper pole and the interpapillary line on later films. During the course of the urogram, the obstructed area will slowly opacify as contrast material passes into the dilated, urine-filled system. Detection of this transition from radiolucent to radiopaque may require filming as late as 24 to 36 hours after injection of contrast material. The wall of tissue around the dilated collecting structure is several millimeters or more in thickness and enhances in normal fashion during the urographic nephrogram. The nonobstructed calyces draining the remainder of the kidney opacify normally but may be displaced by the mass effect of the hydronephrotic segment (Fig. 12–58). Figure 4–4 illustrates these features schematically.

Pyelography. Retrograde or antegrade pyelography is sometimes valuable for precise visualization

---

SIMPLE CYST TYPICAL FINDINGS

Primary Uroradiologic Elements

Size: variable
Contour: unifocal mass
Lesion distribution: variable

Secondary Uroradiologic Elements

Collecting system: attenuated (focal); displaced (focal)
Nephrogram: replaced (focal); smooth margin; *thin rim* sign when peripheral; *beak* sign when peripheral
Calcification: uncommon; curvilinear; peripheral
Attenuation value: water
Echogenicity: anechoic; well-defined far-wall; enhanced through-sound transmission
Magnetic resonance: signal intensity parallels water; does not enhance after gadolinium
Cystography: smooth internal walls; clear aspirate

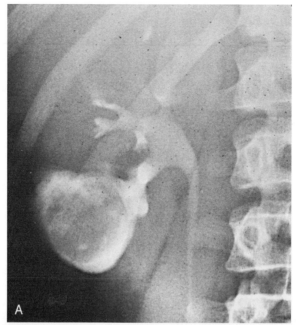

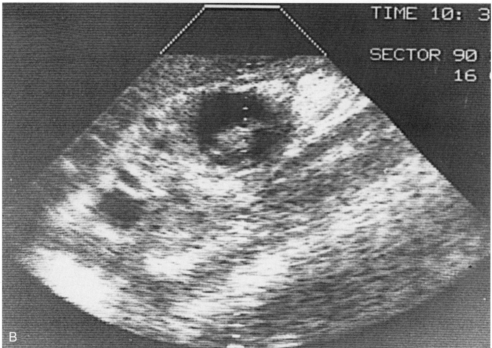

FIGURE 12–57. Chronic hemorrhagic cyst communicating with the pelvocalyceal system.

A, Excretory urogram. Opacification of the cyst during the course of the study reveals a large filling defect that represents an organized blood clot.

B, Ultrasonogram, longitudinal section. The echogenic clot within the anechoic cyst is in a dependent position.

of the point of obstruction, although delayed films during urography may provide the same information.

Computed Tomography. Focal hydronephrosis is seen in cross-sectional images as a smooth-walled mass usually in the superior and medial part of the kidney. The homogeneous content has the attenuation characteristics of water, and enhances slowly after administration of contrast material. Com-

pressed renal tissue that comprises the wall of this mass enhances following contrast material administration (Fig. 12–59). A duplicated, obstructed ureter might also be demonstrated by computed tomography as a dilated tubular structure filled with urine having the density of water. This can usually be traced directly into the bladder, where a ureterocele is frequently present.

Ultrasonography. Ultrasonographic findings in

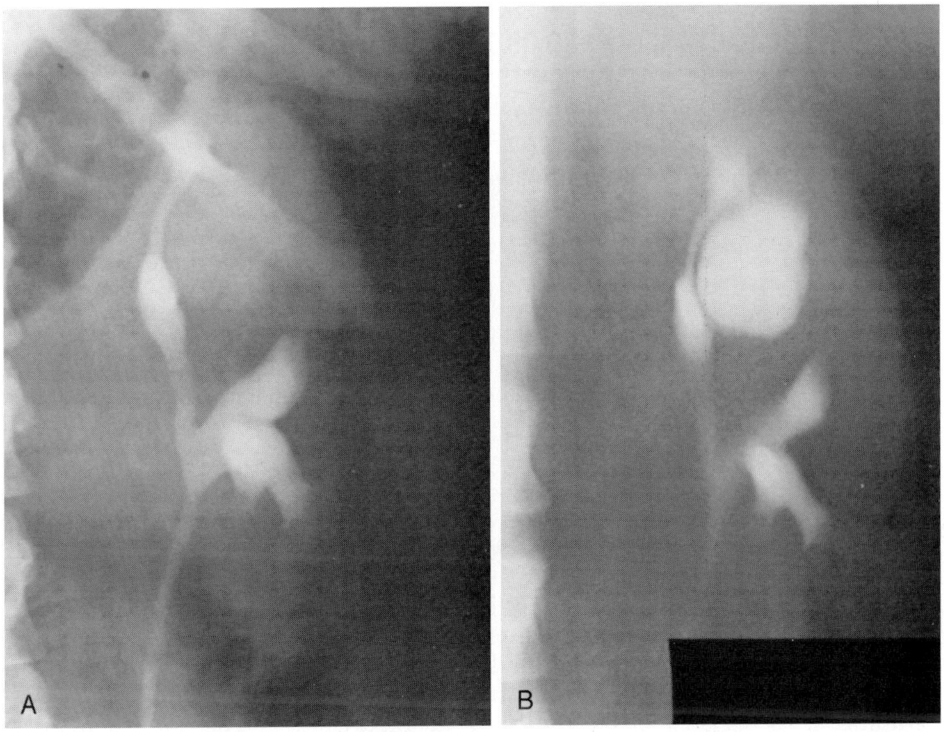

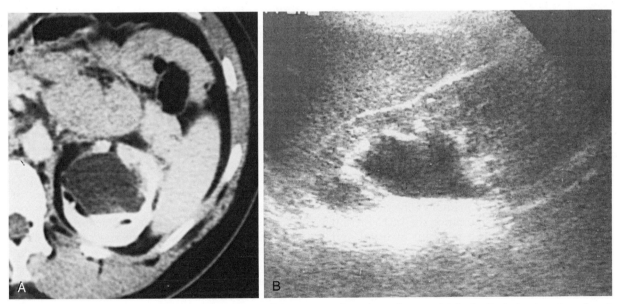

FIGURE 12–58. Focal hydronephrosis. Displacement of nonobstructed collecting system by an upper pole calyx dilated because of infundibular obstruction.

A, Excretory urogram, 10-minute film. There is only faint density over the dilated calyx.

B, Excretory urogram. Delayed tomogram. Late filling of the dilated calyx and the area of infundibular narrowing (possibly due to crossing vessel) are well identified.

focal hydronephrosis are those of a thick-walled anechoic upper pole mass with an enhanced far-wall and through-sound transmission (see Fig. 12–59). Ultrasonography also identifies the dilated ureter to the point of obstruction and a ureterocele, if present.

Arteriography. Arteriography in focal hydronephrosis reveals displacement and attenuation of the arteries serving the affected portion of the kidney.

None of the angiographic stigmata of neoplasm are seen with this condition.

Focal Pyelonephritis/Abscess

Definition

Ascending bacterial invasion of the renal parenchyma causes a full-thickness, lobar or sublobar

FIGURE 12–59. Focal hydronephrosis due to obstruction of the upper pole moiety of a completely duplicated pelvocalyceal system and ureter. Left kidney.

A, Computed tomogram, contrast material–enhanced. The focal hydronephrosis appears as a water density mass with dependent layering of contrast material. The wall of the mass is compressed renal parenchyma.

B, Ultrasonogram, longitudinal section. In this projection, the dilated, fluid-filled structure has the configuration of an upper pole pelvis.

FOCAL HYDRONEPHROSIS TYPICAL FINDINGS

Primary Uroradiologic Elements

Size: large
Contour: unifocal mass (usually upper pole)
Lesion distribution: unilateral

Secondary Uroradiologic Elements

Collecting system: absent polar group (early); delayed enhancement of dilated polar group (late)
Nephrogram: replaced (focal); smooth margin; thick wall
Attenuation value: water
Echogenicity: anechoic; well-defined far-wall; enhanced through-sound transmission

---

interstitial inflammation that begins in the distribution of the medullary rays, a process called *acute pyelonephritis*. Unifocal enlargement of the kidney occurs when acute pyelonephritis is limited to one portion of the kidney. In this circumstance, renal enlargement and other radiologic findings initially follow patterns common to all infiltrative processes, including a bean-shaped or reniform geometry. These concepts are discussed generally elsewhere in this chapter and specifically in terms of acute pyelonephritis in Chapter 9. If, in some individuals, the infiltrative inflammatory process does not resolve spontaneously or in response to therapy in the acute phase, multiple, small foci of neutrophilic white blood cells accumulate, coalesce, and begin to form a central necrotic core. As this process progresses, a thick capsule of highly vascularized connective tissue forms around the central liquefying collection of necrotic renal parenchyma, neutrophils, and bacteria, and a mature abscess is formed.

The abscess may drain through the renal capsule, causing perinephritis and perinephric abscess. Sometimes cavitation and drainage into the collecting system occur.

The same process may begin with a blood-borne infection. In this circumstance, the initial tubulointerstitial infiltrate is miliary and cortical rather than a full-thickness involvement of all or part of a lobe, as is seen in ascending infections.

Clinical Setting

In the preantibiotic era, renal abscess was usually the result of blood-borne metastatic seeding of *Staphylococcus aureus* from primary infection of the skin, teeth, lungs, or tonsils. Since the introduction of antibiotics, more than 80 per cent of renal and perirenal abscesses in the general population are the result of an ascending infection from the lower urinary tract. Most kidney abscesses are associated with calculous obstruction of the ureter or the pelvis. Other lesions, such as ureteropelvic junction or distal ureteral obstruction, also increase the risk for abscess. In these cases, gram-negative bacteria, particularly *Escherichia coli, Enterobacter aerogenes,* and *Proteus mirabilis,* predominate. Overall,

males are afflicted twice as frequently as females. Immunocompromised patients are a subpopulation that is at particular risk for both blood-borne and ascending infections of the kidney leading to abscess. In this group, a variety of organisms that are not usually urinary tract pathogens may be involved.

The clinical picture may be quite nonspecific. In the acute phase, fever, chills, malaise, and signs of sepsis are present. Flank or abdominal pain may accompany a palpable renal mass. Urinalysis, including urine culture, may be normal if the infection is behind an obstructing lesion that prevents urine flow from the involved kidney. In chronic abscess, fever and leukocytosis may be minimal or absent, and localizing signs are rare. Pyuria and bacteriuria may be absent. Obviously, diagnosis on clinical grounds alone is exceedingly difficult in these patients.

Radiologic Findings

Radiologic findings of focal acute pyelonephritis are described in Chapter 9.

Excretory Urography. Since renal and perirenal abscesses often coexist, partial or complete obscuration of the renal outline, loss of the psoas margin, immobility of the kidney with respiration, and lumbar scoliosis concave to the side of involvement are often seen. These abnormalities may be absent if the abscess is confined solely to the kidney parenchyma.

The involved kidney is enlarged by a unifocal, usually polar, mass. The mass may displace or efface adjacent portions of the collecting system. A nephrographic radiolucent defect within the well-defined mass corresponds to the central collection of necrotic tissue. The wall of the mass is thick, and its inner margin is irregular (Fig. 12–60). It is not uncommon to see multiple rounded nephrographic radiolucencies representing several abscesses. Opacification of the collecting structures on the involved side is sometimes less than that seen in the contralateral kidney. Calcification is not a feature of acute or chronic renal abscess.

Computed Tomography. The appearance of a

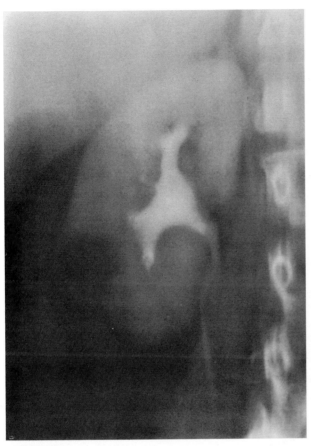

FIGURE 12–60. Abscess of the right kidney demonstrating contour bulge due to mass, radiolucent nephrographic defect with irregular margins, and a thick wall. Tomogram during excretory urography. (Courtesy of Robert R. Hattery, M.D., Mayo Clinic, Rochester, Minnesota.)

renal abscess on computed tomography varies with the evolution of the inflammatory process from early necrosis within an area of acute interstitial nephritis to an encapsulated, fluid-filled mass (Figs. 12–61 through 12–63). On unenhanced scans, the early abscess may not be discernible because it has a density equal to or slightly less than that of the adjacent normal parenchyma and is not circumscribed. Following contrast material administration, however, the early abscess enhances less than the remainder of the kidney and is readily identified. With time, the liquefied abscess yields attenuation values substantially below those of normal renal tissue but greater than those of water. Enhancement does not occur at this stage.

Computed tomography is highly sensitive in detecting rupture of the abscess into the subcapsular and perinephric spaces. Thickening of the renal fascia is common, especially with extension of the abscess beyond the kidney itself.

Ultrasonography. The localized area of acute interstitial nephritis in an early abscess has an echo pattern that is indistinguishable from a solid neoplasm (see Fig. 12–62C). As liquefaction develops, there is progressive decrease of echogenicity. Eventually, the abscess becomes anechoic or demon-

strates only faint internal echoes, depending on the amount of tissue debris within the cavity (Fig. 12–64). Although the margins of the mass may be irregular, its extent is well defined by ultrasonography. At the mature, fluid-filled stage, through-sound transmission is always less than that of water but

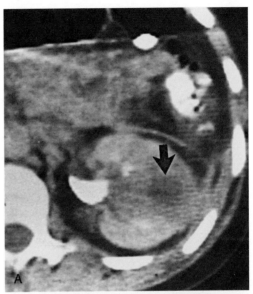

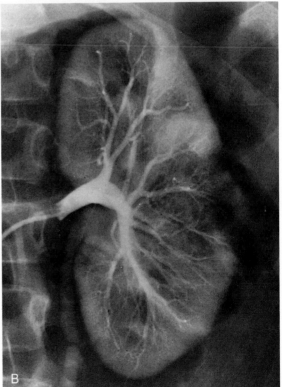

FIGURE 12–61. Evolving abscess, left kidney.
A, Computed tomogram, contrast material–enhanced. A central low density *(arrow)* represents liquefaction within an area of tubulointerstitial nephritis seen as a well-defined larger region of diminished enhancement.
B, Selective renal arteriogram. The number of small arteries in the affected area is decreased, but the vessels are not yet displaced around the early abscess.

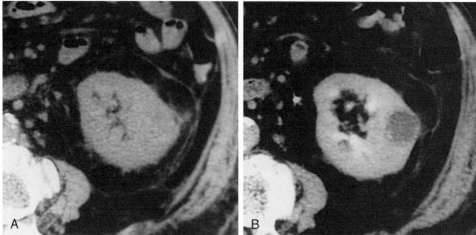

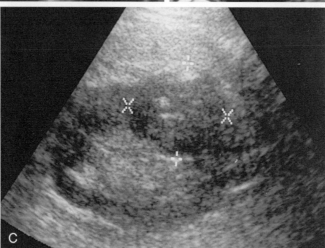

FIGURE 12–62. Early abscess, left kidney in an elderly male with febrile urinary tract infection. Diagnosis established by needle aspiration with positive culture.

A, Computed tomogram, unenhanced. The abscess, which causes a focal bulge on the lateral surface of the kidney, is isodense with normal renal parenchyma.

B, Computed tomogram, contrast material–enhanced. The abscess does not enhance to the same degree as does the renal parenchyma.

C, Ultrasonogram, transverse plane. The abscess *(cursors)* is as echogenic as surrounding renal tissue.

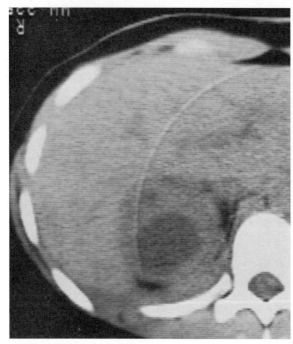

FIGURE 12–63. Mature (liquefied) abscess in the upper pole of the right kidney. Computed tomogram, unenhanced. The contents of the abscess have an attenuation value lower than that of the kidney tissue but greater than that of water.

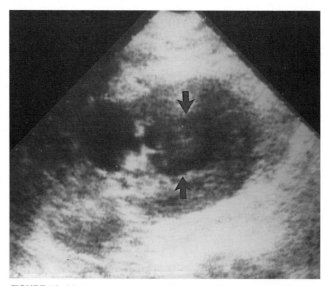

FIGURE 12–64. Abscess, lower pole of left kidney, extending into perirenal space. Ultrasonogram, longitudinal section. The abscess *(arrows)* exhibits slight echogenicity and impaired through-sound transmission. A simple cyst is situated superior to the abscess. (Kindly provided by Sheila Sheth, M.D., and Ulrike Hamper, M.D., The Johns Hopkins University, Baltimore, Maryland.)

ABSCESS TYPICAL FINDINGS

Primary Uroradiologic Elements

Size: large
Contour: unifocal mass
Lesion distribution: unilateral

Secondary Uroradiologic Elements

Collecting system: attenuated (focal); displaced (focal)
Nephrogram: normal (early phase); replaced (focal); irregular, thick wall (late phase)
Attenuation value: normal to slightly diminished before contrast material administration;
    enhances less than normal parenchyma (early); decreased and nonenhancing (late)
Echogenicity: variable, hypoechoic (early) to anechoic (late)

---

varies as a function of the amount of sound-absorbing material in the cavity of the abscess.

Angiography. Early in the development of an abscess, blood vessels are diminished in the area of involvement, but are not yet displaced (see Fig. 12–61B). As an abscess ages and a thick capsule forms, displacement of medium-sized arteries around the mass occurs. The capsule may stain intensely, and a fine, uniform set of small arteries, similar to those seen in some neoplasms, may be present. The central radiolucency of the abscess and its thick wall with irregular borders are apparent during the capillary phase of angiography (Fig. 12–65). With perinephritis or perinephric abscess, the

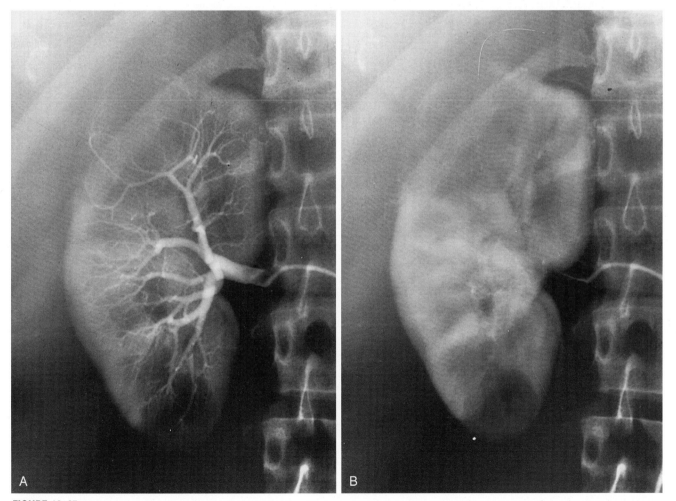

FIGURE 12–65. Mature abscess, upper pole of right kidney with an incidental simple cyst in the lower pole. Selective renal arteriogram.
  A, Arterial phase. Small arteries are displaced around the liquefied, encapsulated abscess.
  B, Nephrographic phase. The thick, irregular margins of the abscess are defined.

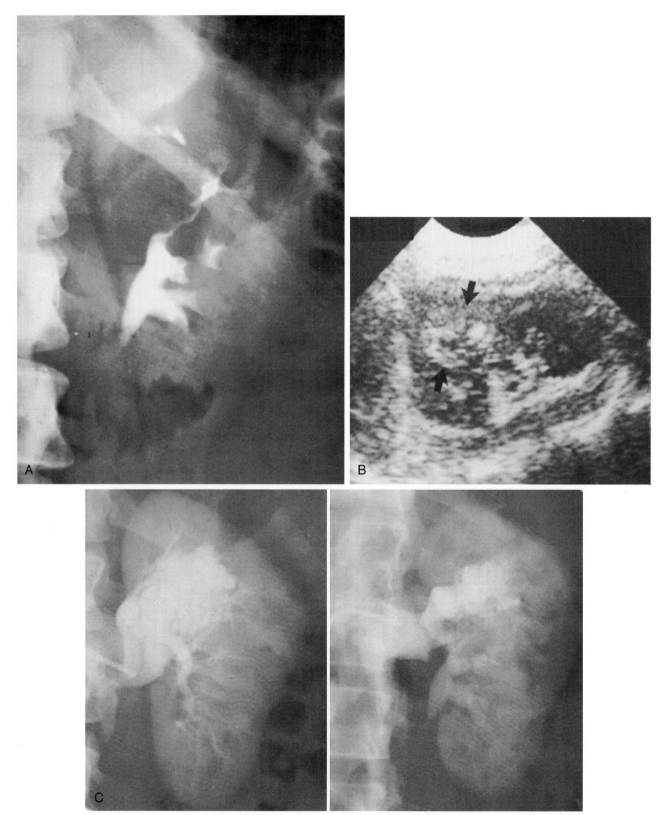

FIGURE 12–66. Congenital arteriovenous malformation of the left kidney. Cirsoid type.
   A, Excretory urogram. A mass lesion on the medial part of the upper pole creates nodular impressions on the pelvocalyceal system.
   B, Ultrasonogram, longitudinal section. The cirsoid malformation appears as an echogenic mass in the upper pole of the left kidney *(arrows).*
   C, Selective left angiogram, arterial and venous phases. Note cirsoid channels.
   (Courtesy of Jalil Farah, M.D., and Robert Ellwood, M.D., William Beaumont Hospital, Royal Oak, Michigan.)

capsular arteries are usually pushed outward from the kidney. None of these angiographic findings is specific to focal inflammatory disease. All of them overlap those seen in neoplastic disorders. Even early venous filling and noncontractility of feeding vessels after intra-arterial epinephrine injection have been reported.

Congenital Arteriovenous Malformation

Definition

Congenital arteriovenous malformation, also known as hemangioma, is classified as either *cirsoid* or *cavernous*. The cirsoid form is more common and is composed of multiple coiled vascular channels grouped in a cluster. This vascular mass is supplied by one or more arteries that arise at the segmental or interlobar level. Drainage of the mass is into one or more veins. The arterial feeders and the draining veins may or may not be enlarged. The much less common cavernous form is composed of a single well-defined artery feeding into a single large chamber that is drained by a single vein. The artery and vein are often dilated. Curvilinear calcification may form in the wall of the cavernous malformation.

Congenital arteriovenous malformation is distinguished from an arteriovenous communication that results from trauma or spontaneous rupture of an aneurysm into a vein, a condition classified as *acquired arteriovenous aneurysm* or *fistula*. Here, the dominant abnormality is an arterial to venous shunt rather than a mass. This is discussed further in the section on Vascular Abnormalities in Chapter 16 and in Chapter 29 on Trauma.

Clinical Setting

Congenital arteriovenous malformation occurs in all age groups. No sex predilection has been established conclusively, although a female predominance has been suggested. These malformations usually have a submucosal or mucosal relationship to the collecting system. Thus, hematuria, which may be major, is a common clinical presentation. Increased blood flow to the affected kidney is not a common feature of congenital arteriovenous malformation, unlike arteriovenous aneurysm or fistula. Thus, wide pulse pressure and high-output heart failure are absent in most cases.

Radiologic Findings

Excretory Urography. Because congenital arteriovenous malformation is usually located in the medulla, a mass effect on the collecting system may be present (Figs. 12–66 and 12–67). On the other hand, the excretory urogram may be normal in a patient with a small malformation and minimal to absent bleeding. Sometimes, blood clot is the only abnormality noted. Curvilinear, peripheral calcification is sometimes present in the cavernous form of congenital arteriovenous malformation (see Fig. 12–67).

Computed Tomography. Computed tomography effectively documents the vascular nature of a congenital arteriovenous malformation by demonstrating enhancement of the entire mass with contrast material. This is best documented by using a spiral scanning technique with early acquisition of images. An enlarged feeding artery and draining vein may be identified. In other respects, the computed tomographic manifestations are the same as those noted in the preceding section on excretory urography, obstructive uropathy due to a large blood clot in the renal pelvis (Fig. 12–68).

Ultrasonography. The ultrasonographic image of congenital arteriovenous malformation varies with the type. In the cirsoid form, the cluster of small vessels appears as an echoic mass, indistinguishable from a solid neoplasm (see Fig. 12–66). The cavernous form, on the other hand, yields an image of an anechoic fluid-filled mass (see Fig. 12–67). The enlarged feeding and draining vessels may also be identified. The vascular nature of an arteriovenous malformation can be established by color Doppler ultrasonography.

Angiography. Arteriovenous shunts with early venous opacification are not a prominent feature of congenital arteriovenous malformation and often are not present at all. The malformation, either

---

CONGENITAL ARTERIOVENOUS MALFORMATION TYPICAL FINDINGS

Primary Uroradiologic Elements

Size: large (may be normal)
Contour: unifocal mass (may be normal)
Lesion distribution: unilateral

Secondary Uroradiologic Elements

Collecting system: attenuated (focal); displaced (focal)
Nephrogram: replaced
Calcification: curvilinear, peripheral
Attenuation value: Rapid rise (arterial phase), enhanced soft tissue (late)
Echogenicity: echoic mass (cirsoid); anechoic mass (cavernous)
Vascularity: Single feeding artery/draining vein; shunt absent to minimal

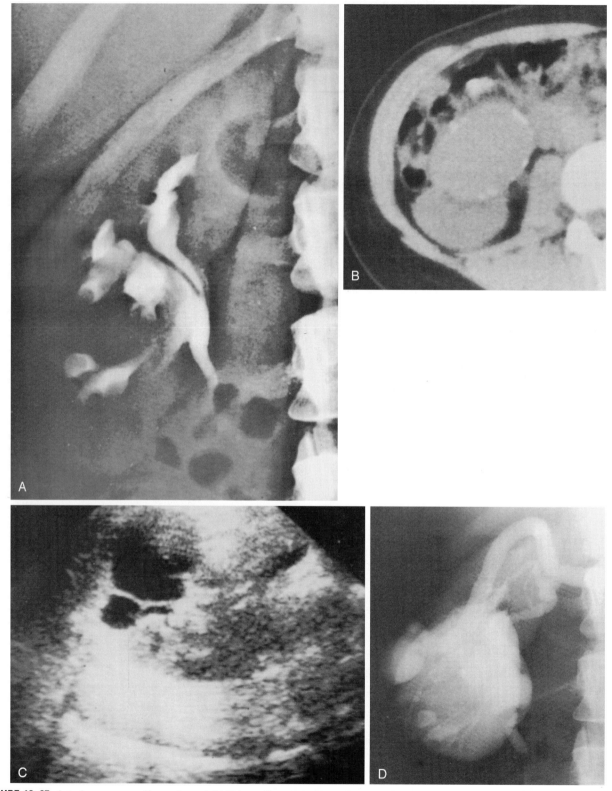

FIGURE 12–67. Arteriovenous malformation, right kidney. Cavernous type.

A, Excretory urogram. The malformation causes a focal displacement of the collecting system.

B, Computed tomogram, unenhanced. The malformation is of soft tissue attenuation and contains some mural calcification.

C, Ultrasonogram, longitudinal section. The cavernous malformation has fluid characteristics and a thick septum.

D, Selective renal arteriogram, late arterial phase. There is a single large artery supplying a large vascular chamber. Early venous filling is absent.

(Courtesy of Jalil Farah, M.D., and Robert Ellwood, M.D., William Beaumont Hospital, Royal Oak, Michigan.)

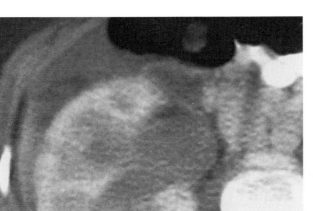

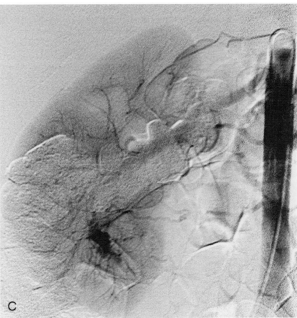

FIGURE 12–68. Arteriovenous malformation, right kidney, cirsoid type in a 25-year-old woman with massive hematuria.
A, Computed tomogram, contrast material–enhanced. The delayed nephrogram indicates obstructive uropathy due to the large blood clot dilating the renal pelvis.
B, Selective renal arteriogram, arterial phase. There is a small cluster of abnormal vessels in the lower pole. Note the characteristic central location.
C, Selective renal arteriogram, late phase. There is slow blood flow through the malformation.

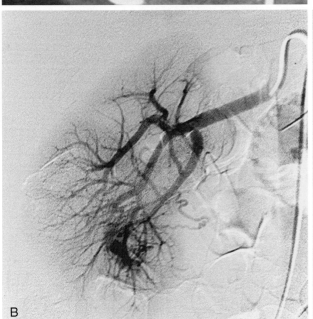

cirsoid or cavernous, opacifies directly from the feeding artery, which is usually single and enlarged. The draining vein may be single or multiple and also enlarged (see Figs. 12–66 and 12–67). A small cirsoid malformation is sometimes seen only as a small cluster of abnormal vessels or, yet more obscure, as a poorly defined homogeneous blush during the nephrographic phase of an angiogram (see Fig. 12–68*B, C*). In some patients, the arteriovenous malformation is too small for angiographic detection.

DIFFERENTIAL DIAGNOSIS

Some of the entities discussed in this chapter have radiologic features characteristic enough to support a confident diagnosis based solely on imaging, rather than histologic, data. Some **malignant re-** **nal tumors, simple cyst, angiomyolipoma**, and **arteriovenous malformations** are examples. A radiologic diagnosis of one of these entities, carrying as it does high confidence levels, leads to a clinical strategy that varies from no further intervention (simple cyst) to therapeutic interventions that may include limited surgical excision based on lesion size or symptoms (angiomyolipoma, arteriovenous malformation) or radical surgical excision (malignant renal tumor). The other unifocal masses described in this chapter, on the other hand, have radiologic features that overlap. Even when clinical, demographic, and prevalence factors are taken into account, the radiologic interpretation is uncertain enough to require tissue for a final diagnosis. Cases of **malignant renal tumor, oncocytoma, multilocular cystic nephroma, mesoblastic nephroma, mesenchymal tumors/juxtaglomer-**

ular cell tumor, and **complicated cyst** or **abscess** often cannot be distinguished one from the other with enough confidence to obviate the need for a tissue diagnosis.

Chapter 28 discusses the differential diagnosis of a unifocal renal mass in the context of implications for patient care. The small, asymptomatic renal mass, the small hyperdense mass, and masses that are too small to characterize are additional topics that are also presented in Chapter 28. A careful review of both chapters is essential to a comprehensive understanding of the complex issues associated with unifocal renal masses.

BIBLIOGRAPHY

General

Bennington, J. L., and Beckwith, J. B.: Tumors of the upper urinary tract. In Tumors of the Kidney, Renal Pelvis, and Ureter. Washington, D.C., Armed Forces Institute of Pathology, 1975, pp. 25–192.

Birnbaum, B. A., Jacobs, J. E., and Ramchandani, P.: Multiphasic renal CT: Comparison of renal mass enhancement during the corticomedullary and nephrographic phases. Radiology 200:753, 1996.

Bosniak, M. A.: Difficulties in classifying cystic lesions of the kidney. Urol. Radiol. 13:91, 1991.

Bosniak, M. A., Birnbaum, B. A., Krinsky, G. A., and Waisman, J.: Small renal parenchymal neoplasms: Further observations on growth. Radiology 197:589, 1995.

Bosniak, M. A., and Rofsky, N. M.: Problems in the detection and characterization of small renal masses. Radiology 198:638, 1996.

Curry, N. S.: Small renal masses (lesions smaller than 3 cm): Imaging evaluation and management. AJR 164:355, 1995.

Curry, N. S., and Bissada, N. K.: Radiologic evaluation of small and indeterminant renal masses. Urol. Clin. North Am. 24:493, 1997.

Curry, N. S.: Atypical cystic renal masses. Abdom. Imaging 23:230, 1998.

Davidson, A. J., Hartman, D. S., Choyke, P. L., and Wagner, B. J.: Radiologic assessment of renal masses: Implications for patient care. Radiology 202:297, 1997.

Eble, J. N., and Bonsib, S. M.: Extensively cystic renal neoplasms: Cystic nephroma, cystic partially differentiated nephroblastoma, multilocular cystic renal cell carcinoma, and cystic hamartoma of renal pelvis. Semin. Diagn. Pathol. 15:2, 1998.

Einstein, D. M., Herts, B. R., Weaver, R., Obuchowski, N., Zepp, R., and Singer, A.: Evaluation of renal masses detected by excretory urography: Cost-effectiveness of sonography versus CT. AJR 164:371, 1995.

Hartman, D. S.: Pediatric renal tumors. In Taveras, J., and Ferucci, J. (eds.): Radiology Diagnosis, Imaging, Intervention, vol. 4. Philadelphia, J. B. Lippincott Co., 1986, pp. 1–9.

Jamis-Dow, C. A., Choyke, P. L., Jennings, S. B., Linehan, W. M., Thakore, K. N., and Walther, M. M.: Small (≤3-cm) renal masses: Detection with CT versus US and pathologic correlation. Radiology 198:785, 1996.

Marshall, F. F.: Renal tumors—editorial. J. Urol. 152:1992, 1994.

Millan, J. C.: Tumors of the kidney. In Hill, G. S. (ed.): Uropathology. New York, Churchill Livingstone, 1989, pp. 623–702.

Montie, J. E.: The incidental renal mass: Management alternatives. Urol. Clin. North Am. 18:427, 1991.

Siegel, C. L., McFarland, E. G., Brink, J. A., Fisher, A. J., Humphrey, P., and Heiken, J. P.: CT of cystic renal masses: Analysis of diagnostic performance and interobserver variation. Am. J. Roentgenol. 169:813, 1997.

Silverman, S. G., Lee, B. Y., Seltzer, S. E., Bloom, D. A., Corless, C. L., and Adams, D. F.: Small (< or = 3 cm) renal masses: Correlation of spiral CT features and pathologic findings. AJR 163:597, 1994.

Warshauer, D. M., McCarthy, S. M., Street, L., Bookbinder, M. J., Clicleman, M. G., Richter, J., Hammers, L., Taylor, C., and Rosenfield, A. T.: Detection of renal masses: Sensitivities and specificities of excretory urography/linear tomography, US and CT. Radiology 169:363, 1988.

Wills, J. S.: The diagnosis and management of small (<3 cm) renal neoplasms: A commentary. Seminars in Ultrasound, CT, and MRI 18:75, 1997.

Wilson, T. E., Doelle, E. A., Cohan, R. H., Wojno, K., and Korobkin, M.: Cystic renal masses: A reevaluation of the usefulness of the Bosniak classification system. Acad. Radiol. 3:564, 1996.

Yuh, B. I., and Cohan, R. H.: Helical CT for detection and characterization of renal masses. Semin. Ultrasound CT MR 18:82, 1997.

Zagoria, R. J., and Dyer, R. B.: The small renal mass: Detection, characterization and management. Abdom. Imaging 23:256, 1998.

Zeman, R. K., Zeiberg, A., Hayes, W. S., Silverman, P. M., Cooper, C., and Garra, B. S.: Helical CT of renal masses: The value of delayed scans. Am. J. Roentgenol. 167:771, 1996.

Malignant Neoplasms

Agrons, G. A., Kingsman, K. D., Wagner, B. J., and Sotelo-Avila, C.: Rhabdoid tumor of the kidney in children: A comparative study of 21 cases. Am. J. Roentgenol. 168:447, 1997.

Agrons, G. A., Wagner, B. J., Davidson, A. J., and Suarez, E. S.: Multilocular cystic renal tumor in children: Radiologic-pathologic correlation. Radiographics 15:653, 1995.

Avery, R. A., Harris, J. E., Davis, C. J., Borgaonkar, D. S., Byrd, J. C., and Weiss, R. B.: Renal medullary carcinoma: Clinical and therapeutic aspects of a newly described tumor. Cancer 78:128, 1996.

Babyn, P., Owens, C., Gyepes, M., and Dangio, G. J.: Imaging patients with Wilms' tumor. Hematol. Oncol. Clin. North Am. 9:1217, 1995.

Beckwith, J. B.: Precursor lesions of Wilms' tumor: Clinical and biological implications. Med. Pediatr. Oncol. 21:158, 1993.

Bielsa, O., Anrango, O., Corominas, J. M., Llado, C., and Gelabert-Mas, A.: Collecting duct carcinoma of the kidney. Br. J. Urol. 74:127, 1994.

Buckley, J. A., Urban, B. A., Soyer, P., Scherrer, A., and Fishman, E. K.: Transitional cell carcinoma of the renal pelvis: A retrospective look at CT staging with pathologic correlation. Radiology 201:194, 1996.

Campbell, S. C., Fichtner, J., Novick, A. C., Steinbach, F., Stockle, M., Klein, E. A., Filipas, D., Levin, H. S., Storkel, S., Schweden, F., et al.: Intraoperative evaluation of renal cell carcinoma: A prospective study of the role of ultrasonography and histopathological frozen sections. J. Urol. 155:1191, 1996.

Cheng, W. S., Farrow, G. M., and Zincke, H.: The incidence of multicentricity in renal cell carcinoma. J. Urol. 146:1221, 1991.

Choyke, P. L.: MR imaging in renal cell carcinoma. Radiology 169:572, 1988.

Choyke, P. L., Walther, M. M., Glenn, G. M., Wagner, J. R., Venzon, D. J., Lubensky, I. A., Zbar, B., and Linehan, W. M.: Imaging features of hereditary papillary renal cancers. J. Comput. Assist. Tomogr. 21:737, 1997.

Choyke, P. L., White, E. M., Zeman, R. K., Jaffe, M. H., and Clark, L. R.: Renal metastases: Clinicopathologic and radiologic correlation. Radiology 162:359, 1987.

Chung, C. J., Lorenzo, R., Rayder, S., Schemankewitz, E., Gup, C. D., Cutting, J., and Mundem, M.: Rhabdoid tumors of the kidney in children: CT findings. AJR 164:697, 1995.

Coleman, B. G., Arger, P. H., Mintz, M. C., Pollack, H. M., and Banner, M. P.: Hyperdense renal masses: A computed tomographic dilemma. AJR 143:291, 1994.

Cremin, B. J.: Wilms' tumor: Ultrasound and changing concepts. Clin. Radiol. 38:465, 1987.

Daniel, W. W., Hartman, G. W., Witten, D. M., Farrow, G. M., and Kelalis, P. P.: Calcified renal masses: A review of ten years experience at the Mayo Clinic. Radiology 103:503, 1972.

Davidson, A. J., Choyke, P. L., Hartman, D. S., and Davis, C. J.: Renal medullary carcinoma associated with sickle cell trait: Radiologic findings. Radiology 195:83, 1995.

Davidson, A. J., and Davis, C. J.: Fat in renal adenocarcinoma: Never say never. Radiology 188:316, 1993.

Davidson, A. J., Hayes, W. S., Hartman, D. S., McCarthy, W. F., and Davis, C. J., Jr.: Renal oncocytoma and carcinoma: Failure of differentiation with CT. Radiology 186:693, 1993.

Davis, C. J., Jr., Mostofi, F. K., and Sesterhenn, I. A.: Renal medullary carcinoma. The seventh sickle cell nephropathy. Am. J. Surg. Pathol. 1:1, 1995.

Eschwege, P., Saussine, C., Steiche, G., Delepaul, B., Drelon, L., and Jacqmin, D.: Radical nephrectomy for renal cell carcinoma 30 mm or less: Long-term followup results. J. Urol. 155:1196, 1996.

Exelby, P. R.: Wilms' tumor 1991: Clinical evaluation and treatment. Urol. Clin. North Am. 18:589, 1991.

Feldberg, M. A. M., and van Waes, F. G. M.: Multilocular cystic renal cell carcinoma. AJR 138:953, 1982.

Fernbach, S. K., Donaldson, J. S., Gonzalez-Crussi, F., and Sherman, J. O.: Fatty Wilms' tumor simulating teratoma: Occurrence in a child with horseshoe kidney. Pediatr. Radiol. 18:424, 1988.

Fernbach, S. K., Feinstein, K. A., Donaldson, J. S., and Baum, E. S.: Nephroblastomosis: Comparison of CT with US and urography. Radiology 166:153, 1988.

Ferrozzi, F., Bova, D., and Campodonico, F.: Computed tomography of renal metastases. Semin. Ultrasound CT MR 18:115, 1997.

Figenshau, R. S., Basler, J. W., Ritter, J. H., Siegel, C. L., Simon, J. A., and Dierks, S. M.: Renal medullary carcinoma. J. Urol. 159:711, 1998.

Fishman, E. K., Hartman, D. S., Goldman, S. M., and Siegelman, S. S.: The CT appearance of Wilms' tumor. J. Comput. Assist. Tomogr. 7:659, 1983.

Forman, H. P., Middleton, W. D., Melson, G. L., and McClennan, B. L.: Hyperechoic renal cell carcinoma: Increase in detection at US. Radiology 188:431, 1993.

Frank, W., Guinan, P., Stuhldreher, D., Saffrin, R., Ray, P., and Rubenstein, M.: Renal cell carcinoma: The size variable. J. Surg. Oncol. 54:163, 1993.

Fujimoto, H., Tobisu, K., Sakamoto, M., Kamiya, M., and Kakizoe, T.: Intraductal tumor involvement and renal parenchymal invasion of transitional cell carcinoma in the renal pelvis. J. Urol. 153:57, 1995.

Gash, J. R., Zagoria, R. J., Dyer, R. B., and Assimos, D. G.: Imaging features of infiltrating renal lesions. Crit. Rev. Diagn. Imag. 33:4, 1992.

Glass, R. B. J., Davidson, A. J., and Fernbach, S. K.: Clear cell sarcoma of the kidney: CT sonographic and pathologic correlation. Radiology 180:715, 1991.

Guinan, P. D., Vogelzang, N. J., Fremgen, A. M., Chmiel, J. S., Sylvester, J. L., Sener, S. F., Imperato, J. P., Barrera, E., Berk, R., Flanigan, R., et al.: Renal cell carcinoma: Tumor size, stage and survival. J. Urol. 153:901, 1995.

Hammadeh, M. Y., Thomas, K., Philp, T., and Singh, M.: Renal cell carcinoma containing fat mimicking angiomyolipoma: Demonstration with CT scan and histopathology. Eur. Radiol. 8:228, 1998.

Hartman, D. S., Weatherby, E., Laskin, W. B., Brody, J. M., Corse, W., and Baluch, J. D.: Cystic renal cell carcinoma: CT findings simulating a benign hyperdense cyst: Case report. AJR 159:1235, 1992.

Hélénon, O., Chrétien, Y., Paraf, F., Melki, P., Denys, A., and Moreau, J.-F.: Renal cell carcinoma containing fat: Demonstration with CT. Radiology 188:429, 1993.

Herring, J. C., Schmetz, M. A., Digan, A. B., Young, S. T., and Kalloo, N. B.: Renal medullary carcinoma: A recently described highly aggressive renal tumor in young black patients. J. Urol. 157:2246, 1997.

Hietala, S.-O., and Wahlqvist, L.: Metastatic tumors to the kidney: A post-mortem radiologic and clinical investigation. Acta Radiol. (Diagn.) 23:585, 1982.

Hohenfellner, M., Schultz-Lampbel, D., Lampel, A., Steinbach, F., Cramer, B. M., and Thuroff, J. W.: Tumor in the horseshoe kidney: Clinical implications and review of embryogenesis. J. Urol. 147:1098, 1992.

Holland, J. M.: Cancer of the kidney—Natural history and staging. Cancer 32:1030, 1973.

Holland, J. M.: Certain subsets of renal neoplasms behave differently, but why? Editorial. J. Urol. 156:40, 1996.

Honda, H., Coffman, C. E., Berbaum, K. S., Barloon, T. J., and Masuda, K.: CT analysis of metastatic neoplasms of the kidney: Comparison with primary renal cell carcinoma. Acta Radiol. 33:39, 1992.

Kallman, D. A., King, B. F., Hattery, R. R., Charboneau, J. W., Ehman, R. L., Gothman, D. A., and Blute, M. L.: Renal vein and inferior vena cava tumor thrombosis in renal cell carcinoma: CT, US, MRI and venacavography. J. Comput. Assist. Tomogr. 16:240, 1992.

Kissane, J. M., and Dehner, L. P.: Renal tumors and tumor-like lesions in pediatric patients. Pediatr. Nephrol. 6:4, 1992.

Ljungberg, B., Stenling, R., Osterdahl, B., Farrelly, E., Aberg, T., and Roos, G.: Vein invasion in renal cell carcinoma: Impact on metastatic behavior and survival. J. Urol. 154:1681, 1995.

Mesrobian, H.-G. J.: Wilms' tumor: Past, present, future. J. Urol. 140:231, 1988.

Mostofi, F. K., and Davis, C. J., Jr.: Histologic typing of kidney tumors. In WHO International Histological Classification of Tumours. Heidelberg, Springer-Verlag, 1997.

Nissenkorn, I., and Bernheim, J.: Multicentricity in renal cell carcinoma. J. Urol. 153:620, 1995.

Ooi, G. C., Sagar, G., Lynch, D., Arkell, D. G., and Ryan, P. G.: Cystic renal cell carcinoma: Radiological features and clinicopathological correlation. Clin. Radiol. 51:791, 1996.

Polascik, T. J., Meng, M. V., Epstein, J. I., and Marshall, F. F.: Intraoperative sonography for the evaluation and management of renal tumors: Experience with 100 patients. J. Urol. 154:1676, 1995.

Prati, G. F., Saggin, P., Boschiero, L., Martini, P. T., Montemezzi, S., and Muolo, A.: Small renal-cell carcinomas: Clinical and imaging features. Urol. Int. 51:19, 1993.

Reiman, T. A. H., Siegel, M. J., and Shackelford, G. D.: Wilms' tumor in children: Abdominal CT and US evaluation. Radiology 160:501, 1986.

Rodriguez-Rubio, F. I., Diez-Caballero, F., Martin-Marquina, A., Abad, J. I., and Berian, J. M.: Incidentally detected renal cell carcinoma. Br. J. Urol. 78:29, 1996.

Roosen, J. U., Engel, U., Jensen, R. H., Kvist, E., and Schou, G.: Renal cell carcinoma prognostic factors. Br. J. Urol. 74:160, 1994.

Roubidoux, M. A., Dunnick, N. R., Sostman, H. D., and Leder, R. A.: Renal carcinoma: Detection of venous extension with gradient-echo MR imaging. Radiology 182:269, 1992.

Schmidt, D., and Beckwith, J. B.: Histopathology of childhood renal tumors. Hematol. Oncol. Clin. North Am. 9:1179, 1995.

Siegel, C. L., Middleton, W. D., Teefey, S. A., and McClennan, B. L.: Angiomyolipoma and renal cell carcinoma: US differentiation. Radiology 198:789, 1996.

Sisler, C. L., and Siegel, M. J.: Malignant rhabdoid tumor of the kidney: Radiologic features. Radiology 172:211, 1989.

Srigley, J. R., and Eble, J. N.: Collecting duct carcinoma of kidney. Semin. Diagn. Pathol. 15:54, 1998.

Strotzer, M., Lehner, K. B., and Becker, K.: Detection of fat in a renal cell carcinoma mimicking angiomyolipoma. Radiology 188:427, 1993.

Sufrin, G.: Biological and therapeutic challenges of renal carcinoma—editorial. J. Urol. 153:917, 1995.

Sweeney, J. P., Thornhill, J. A., Grainger, R., McDermott, T. E. D., and Butler, M. R.: Incidentally detected renal cell carcinoma: Pathological features, survival trends and implications for treatment. Br. J. Urol. 78:351, 1996.

Volpe, J. P., and Choyke, P. L.: The radiologic evaluation of renal metastases. Crit. Rev. Diagn. Imag. 30:219, 1990.

Vujanic, G. M., Sandstedt, B., Harms, D., Boccongibod, L., and Delemarre, J. F. M.: Rhabdoid tumour of the kidney: A clinicopathological study of 22 patients from the International Society of Paediatric Oncology (SIOP) nephroblastoma file. Histopathology 28:333, 1996.

Welch, T. J., and Leroy, A. J.: Helical and electron beam CT scanning in the evaluation of renal vein involvement in patients with renal cell carcinoma. J. Comput. Assist. Tomogr. 21:467, 1997.

White, K. S., Kirks, D. R., and Bove, K. E.: Imaging of nephroblastomatosis: An overview. Radiology 182:1, 1992.

Yamashita, Y., Honda, S., Nishiharu, T., Urata, J., and Taka-hashi, M.: Detection of pseudocapsule of renal cell carcinoma with MRI and CT. AJR 166:1151, 1996.

Yamashita, Y., Takahashi, M., Watanabe, O., Yoshimatsu, S., Ueno, S., Ishimaru, S., Kan, M., Takano, S., and Ninomiya, N.: Small renal cell carcinoma: Pathologic and radiologic corre-lation. Radiology 184:493, 1992.

Yamashita, Y., Veno, S., Makita, O., Ogata, I., Hatanaka, Y., Watanabe, O., and Takahashi, M.: Hyperechoic renal tumors: Anechoic rim and intratumoral cysts in US differentiation of renal cell carcinoma from angiomyolipoma. Radiology 188:179, 1993.

Yip, K. H., Peh, W. C. G., and Tam, P. C.: Spontaneous rupture of renal tumours: The role of imaging in diagnosis and man-agement. Br. J. Radiol. 71:146, 1998.

Zagoria, R. J., and Bechtold, R. E.: The role of imaging in staging renal adenocarcinoma. Semin. Ultrasound CT MR 18:91, 1997.

Zbar, B., Glenn, G., Lubensky, I., Choyke, P., Walther, M. M., Magnusson, G., Bergerheim, U. S. R., Pettersson, S., Amin, M., Hurley, K., et al.: Hereditary papillary renal cell carci-noma: Clinical studies in 10 families. J. Urol. 153:907, 1995.

Zbar, B., and Linehan, M.: Hereditary papillary renal cell carci-noma: Clinical studies in 10 families. J. Urol. 156:1781, 1996.

Benign Neoplasms

Agrons, G. A., Wagner, B. J., Davidson, A. J., and Suarez, E. S.: Multilocular cystic renal tumor in children: Radiologic-pathologic correlation. Radiographics 15:653, 1995.

Ambos, M. A., Bosniak, M. A., Valensi, Q. J., Madayag, M. A., and Lefleur, R. S.: Angiographic patterns in renal oncocyto-mas. Radiology 129:615, 1978.

Beckwith, J. B., and Kiviat, N. B.: Multilocular renal cysts and cystic renal tumors. AJR 136:435, 1981.

Bennington, J. L., and Beckwith, J. B.: Mesenchymal tumors of the kidney. In Tumors of the Kidney, Renal Pelvis, and Ureter. Washington, D.C., Armed Forces Institute of Pathology, 1975, pp. 201–242.

Blute, M. L., Malek, R. S., and Segura, J. W.: Angiomyolipoma: Clinical metamorphosis and concepts for management. J. Urol. 139:20, 1988.

Bosniak, M. A., Megibow, A. J., Hulnick, D. H., Horii, S., and Raghavendra, B. N.: CT diagnosis of renal angiomyolipoma: The importance of detecting small amounts of fat. AJR 151:497, 1988.

Castiolo, O. A., Boyle, E. T., Jr., and Kramer, S. A.: Multilocular cysts of the kidney: A study of 29 patients and review of literature. Urology 37:156, 1991.

Cohan, R. H., Dunnick, N. R., Degesys, G. E., and Korobkin, M.: Computed tomography of renal oncocytoma. J. Comput. Assist. Tomogr. 8:284, 1984.

Conn, J. W., Bookstein, J. J., and Cohen, E. L.: Renin-secreting juxtaglomerular-cell adenoma: Preoperative clinical and angio-graphic diagnosis. Radiology 106:543, 1973.

Corvol, P., Pinet, F., Plouin, P. F., Bruneval, P., and Menard, J.: Renin-secreting tumors. Endo. Metab. Clin. North Am. 23:255, 1994.

Daniel, W. W., Hartman, G. W., Witten, D. W., Farrow, G. M., and Kelalis, P. P.: Calcified renal masses: A review of ten years experience at the Mayo Clinic. Radiology 103:503, 1972.

Davidson, A. J., Hayes, W. S., Hartman, D. S., McCarthy, W. F., and Davis, C. J., Jr.: Renal oncocytoma and carcinoma: Failure of differentiation with CT. Radiology 186:693, 1993.

Davidson, J. K., and Clark, D. C.: Renin-secreting juxtaglomeru-lar-cell tumor. Br. J. Radiol. 47:594, 1974.

Davis, C. J., Sesterhenn, I. A., Mostofi, F. K., and Ho, C. K.: Renal oncocytoma: Clinicopathology study of 166 patients. J. Urogen. Pathol. 1:41, 1991.

Defossez, S. M., Yoder, I. C., Papanicolaou, N., Rosen, B. R., and McGovern, F.: Nonspecific magnetic resonance appearance of renal oncocytoma: Report of three cases and review of litera-ture. J. Urol. 145:552, 1991.

Dickinson, M., Ruckle, H., Beaghler, M., and Hadley, H. R.: Renal angiomyolipoma: Optimal treatment based on size and symptoms. Clin. Nephrol. 49:281, 1998.

Dunnick, N. R., Hartman, D. S., Ford, K. K., Davis, C. J., Jr.,

and Amis, E. S., Jr.: The radiology of juxtaglomerular tumors. Radiology 147:321, 1983.

Durham, J. R., Bostwick, D. G., Farrow, G. M., and Ohorodnik, J. M.: Mesoblastic nephroma of adulthood — report of 3 cases. Am. J. Surg. Pathol. 17:1029, 1993.

Eble, J. N.: Angiomyolipoma of kidney. Semin. Diagn. Pathol. 15:21, 1998.

Gonzalez-Crussi, F., Sotelo-Avila, C., and Kidd, J. M.: Mesenchy-mal renal tumors in infancy: A reappraisal. Hum. Pathol. 12:78, 1981.

Grossman, H., Rosenberg, E. R., Bowie, J. D., Ram, P., and Merten, D. F.: Sonographic diagnosis of renal cystic diseases. AJR 140:81, 1983.

Hartman, D. S.: Pediatric renal tumors. In Taveras, J., and Ferucci, J. (eds.): Radiology Diagnosis, Imaging, Intervention, vol. 4. Philadelphia, J. B. Lippincott Co., 1986, pp. 1–9.

Hartman, D. S.: Cysts and cystic neoplasms. Urol. Radiol. 12:7, 1990.

Hartman, D. S., Lesar, M. S. C., Madewell, J. E., and Davis, C. J.: Mesoblastic nephroma: Radiologic-pathologic correlation of 20 cases. AJR 136:69, 1981.

Javadpour, N., Dellon, A. L., and Kumpe, D. A.: Multilocular cystic disease in adults: Imitator of renal cell carcinoma. Urol-ogy 1:596, 1973.

Katz, D. S., Gharagozloo, A. M., Peebles, T. R., and Oliphant, M.: Renal oncocytomatosis. Am. J. Kidney Dis. 27:579, 1996.

Kennelly, M. J., Grossman, H. B., and Cho, K. J.: Outcome analysis of 42 cases of renal angiomyolipoma. J. Urol. 152:1988, 1994.

Klein, M. J., and Valensi, Q. J.: Proximal tubular adenomas of kidney with so-called oncocytic features: A clinicopathologic study of 13 cases of a rarely reported neoplasm. Cancer 38:906, 1976.

Kurosaki, Y., Tanaka, Y., Kuromoto, K., and Itai, Y.: Improved CT fat detection in small kidney angiomyolipomas using thin sections and single voxel measurements. J. Comput. Assist. Tomogr. 17:745, 1993.

Larcos, G., Mullan, B. P., and Forstrom L. A.: Scintigraphic findings of renal oncocytoma. Clin. Nucl. Med. 18:884, 1993.

Lemaitre, L., Claudon, M., Bubrulle, F., and Mazeman, E.: Im-aging of angiomyolipomas. Semin. Ultrasound CT MR 18:100, 1997.

Lemaitre, L., Robert, Y., Dubrulle, F., Claudon, M., Duhamel, A., Danjou, P., and Mazeman, E.: Renal angiomyolipoma: Growth followed up with CT and/or US. Radiology 197:598, 1995.

Levine, E., and Huntrakoon, M.: Computed tomography of renal oncocytoma. AJR 141:741, 1983.

Madewell, J. E., Goldman, S. M., Davis, C. J., Jr., Hartman, D. S., Feigin, D., and Lichtenstein, J. E.: Multilocular cystic nephroma: A radiographic-pathologic correlation of 58 pa-tients. Radiology 146:309, 1983.

Morra, M. N., and Das, S.: Renal oncocytoma: A review of histo-genesis, histopathology, diagnosis and treatment. J. Urol. 150:295, 1993.

Neisius, D., Braedel, H. U., Schridler, E., Hoene, E., and Allooss, S.: Computed tomographic and angiographic findings in renal oncocytoma. Br. J. Radiol. 61:1019, 1988.

Oesterling, J. E., Fishman, E. K., Goldman, G. M., and Marshall, F. F.: The management of renal angiomyolipoma. J. Urol. 135:1121, 1986.

Parienty, R. A., Pradel, J., Imbert, M.-C., Picard, J.-D., and Savart, P.: Computed tomography of multilocular cystic nephroma. Radiology 140:135, 1981.

Perez Ordonez, B., Hamed, G., Campbell, S., Erlandson, R. A., Russo, P., Gaudin, P. B., and Reuter, V. E.: Renal oncocytoma: A clinicopathologic study of 70 cases. Am. J. Surg. Pathol. 21:871, 1997.

Redman, J. F., and Harper, D. L.: Nephroblastoma occurring in a multilocular cystic kidney. J. Urol. 120:356, 1978.

Siegel, C. L., Middleton, W. D., Teefey, S. A., and McClennan, B. L.: Angiomyolipoma and renal cell carcinoma: US differentia-tion. Radiology 198:789, 1996.

Silverman, S. G., Pearson, G. D. N., Seltzer, S. E., Polger, M., Tempany, C. M. C., Adams, D. F., Brown, D. L., and Judy, P. F.: Small (≤ 3 cm) hyperechoic renal masses: Comparison of helical and conventional CT for diagnosing angiomyolipoma. AJR 167:877, 1996.

Steiner, M. S., Goldman, S. M., Fishman, E. K., and Marshall, F. F.: The natural history of renal angiomyolipoma. J. Urol. 150:1782, 1993.

Thijssen, A. M., Carpenter, B., Jiminez, C., and Schillinger, J.: Multilocular cyst (multilocular cystic nephroma) of the kidney: A report of 2 cases with an unusual mode of presentation. J. Urol. 142:346, 1989.

Tong, Y. C., Chieng, P. U., Tsai, T. C., and Lin, S. N.: Renal angiomyolipoma: Report of 24 cases. Br. J. Urol. 66:585, 1990.

Udsom, S. V., and Melicow, M. M.: Multilocular cysts of the kidney with intrapelvic herniation of a "daughter" cyst: Report of 4 cases. J. Urol. 89:341, 1963.

Wagner, B. J., Wong You Cheong, J. J., and Davis, C. J.: Adult renal hamartomas. Radiographics 17:155, 1997.

Wills, J. S.: Management of small renal neoplasms and angiomyolipoma: A growing problem. Radiology 197:583, 1995.

Simple Cyst/Localized Cystic Disease

Bosniak, M. A.: The current radiological approach to renal cysts. Radiology 158:1, 1986.

Cloix, P., Martin, X., Pangaud, C., Marechal, J. M., Bouvier, R., Barat, D., and Dubernard, J. M.: Surgical management of complex renal cysts: A series of 32 cases. J. Urol. 156:28, 1996.

Coleman, B. G., Arger, P. H., Mintz, M. C., Pollack, H. M., and Banner, M. P.: Hyperdense renal masses: A computed tomographic dilemma. AJR 143:291, 1984.

Daniel, W. W., Hartman, G. W., Witten, D. M., Farrow, G. M., and Kelalis, P. P.: Calcified renal masses: A review of ten years experience at the Mayo Clinic. Radiology 103:503, 1972.

Dunnick, N. R., Korobkin, M., and Clark, W. M.: CT demonstration of hyperdense renal carcinoma. J. Comput. Assist. Tomogr. 8:1023, 1984.

Dunnick, N. R., Korobkin, M., Silverman, P. H., and Foster, W. L., Jr.: Computed tomography of high density renal cysts. J. Comput. Assist. Tomogr. 8:458, 1984.

Emmett, J. L., Levine, S. R., and Woolner, L. B.: Coexistence of renal cyst and tumor: Incidence in 1007 cases. Br. J. Urol. 35:403, 1963.

Frishman, E., Orron, D. E., Heiman, Z., Kessler, A., Kaver, I., and Graif, M.: Infected Renal Cysts: Sonographic diagnosis and management. J. Ultrasound Med. 13:7, 1994.

Goldman, S. M., and Hartman, D. S.: The simple cyst. In Hartman, D. S. (ed.): Renal Cystic Disease, fascicle I. AFIP Atlas of Radiologic-Pathologic Correlation. Philadelphia, W. B. Saunders, 1989, pp. 6–37.

Hartman, D. S.: Cysts and cystic neoplasms. Urol. Radiol. 12:7, 1990.

Kleist, H., Jonsson, O., Lundstam, S., Naucler, J., Nilson, A. E., and Petterson, S.: Quantitative lipid analysis in the differential diagnosis of cystic renal lesions. Br. J. Urol. 54:441, 1982.

Ljungberg, B., Holmberg, G., Sjodin, J. G., Hietala, S. O., and Stenling, R.: Renal cell carcinoma in a renal cyst: A case report and review of the literature. J. Urol. 143:797, 1990.

McHugh, K., Stringer, D. A., Hebert, D., and Babiak, C. A.: Simple renal cysts in children: Diagnosis and followup with US. Radiology 178:383, 1991.

Pearlstein, A. E.: Hyperdense renal cysts. J. Comput. Assist. Tomogr. 7:1029, 1983.

Pedersen, J. F., Emamian, S. A., and Nielsen, M. B.: Simple renal cyst (relations to age and arterial blood pressure. Br. J. Radiol. 66:581, 1993.

Rosenberg, E. R., Korobkin, M., Foster, W., Silverman, P. M., Bowie, J. D., and Dunnick, N. R.: The significance of septations in a renal cyst. AJR 144:593, 1985.

Silverman, J. F., and Kilhenny, C.: Tumor in the wall of a simple renal cyst: Report of a case. Radiology 93:95, 1969.

Sussman, S., Cochran, S. T., Pagani, J. J., McArdle, C., Wong, W., Austin, R., Curry, N., and Kelly, K. M.: Hyperdense renal masses: A CT manifestation of hemorrhagic renal cysts. Radiology 150:207, 1984.

Zirinsky, K., Auh, Y. H., Rubenstein, W. A., Williams, J. J., Pasmantier, M. W., and Kazam, E.: CT of the hyperdense renal cyst: Sonographic correlation. AJR 143:151, 1984.

Focal Hydronephrosis

Cramer, B. C., Twomey, B. P., and Katz, D.: CT findings in obstructed upper moieties of duplex kidneys. J. Comput. Assist. Tomogr. 7:251, 1983.

Cronan, J. J., Amis, E. S., Zeman, R. K., and Dorfman, G. S.: Obstruction of the upper-pole moiety in renal duplication in adults: CT evaluation. Radiology 161:17, 1986.

Nusbacher, N., and Bryk, D.: Hydronephrosis of the lower pole of the duplex kidney. AJR 130:967, 1978.

Winters, W. D., and Lebowitz, R. L.: Importance of prenatal detection of hydronephrosis of the upper pole. AJR 155:125, 1990.

Focal Pyelonephritis/Abscess

Anderson, K. A., and McAninch, J. W.: Renal abscesses: Classification and review of 40 cases. Urology 16:333, 1980.

Brown, E. D., Brown, J. J., Kettritz, U., Shoenut, J. P., and Semelka, R. C.: Renal abscesses: Appearance on gadolinium-enhanced magnetic resonance images. Abdom. Imaging 21:172, 1996.

Daniel, W. W., Hartman, G. W., Witten, D. M., Farrow, G. M., and Kelalis, P. P.: Calcified renal masses: A review of ten years experience at the Mayo Clinic. Radiology 103:503, 1972.

Fowler, J. E., and Perkins, T.: Presentation, diagnosis and treatment of renal abscess: 1972–1988. J. Urol. 151:847, 1994.

Funston, M. R., Fisher, K. S., van Blerk, P. J. P., and Borte, J. H.: Acute focal bacterial nephritis or renal abscess? A sonographic diagnosis. Br. J. Urol. 54:461, 1982.

Hoddick, W., Jeffrey, R. B., Goldberg, H. I., Federle, M. P., and Laing, F. C.: CT and sonography of severe renal and perirenal infections. AJR 140:517, 1983.

Malgieri, J. J., Kursh, E. D., and Persky, L.: The changing clinicopathological pattern of abscesses in or adjacent to the kidney. J. Urol. 118:230, 1977.

Salvatierra, O., Jr., Bucklew, W. B., and Morrow, J. W.: Perinephric abscess: A report of 71 cases. J. Urol. 98:296, 1967.

Talner, L. B., Davidson, A. J., Lebowitz, R. L., Dalla Palma, L., and Goldman, S. M.: Acute pyelonephritis: Can we agree on terminology? Radiology 192:297, 1994.

Congenital Arteriovenous Malformation

Cho, K. J., and Stanley, J. C.: Non-neoplastic congenital and acquired renal arteriovenous malformations and fistulas. Radiology 129:333, 1978.

Crotty, K. L., Orihuela, E., and Warren, N. M. M.: Recent advances in the diagnosis and treatment of renal arteriovenous malformations and fistulas. J. Urol. 150:1355, 1993.

Ekelund, L., and Göthlin, J.: Renal hemangiomas: An analysis of 13 cases diagnosed by angiography. AJR 125:788, 1975.

Honda, H., Onitsuka, H., Naitov, S., Hasoo, K., Kamoi, I., Hanada, K., Kumazoma, J., and Masuda, K.: Renal arteriovenous malformations: CT features. J. Comput. Assist. Tomogr. 15:261, 1991.

Kopchick, J. H., Bourne, N. K., Fine, S. W., Jacoshoh, H., Jacobs, S. C., and Lawson, R. K.: Congenital renal arteriovenous malformations. Urology 17:13, 1981.

Regan, J. B., and Benson, R. C., Jr.: Congenital renal arteriovenous malformations. J. Urol. 136:1184, 1986.

Subramanyam, B. R., Lefleur, R. S., and Bosniak, M. A.: Renal arteriovenous fistulas and aneurysm: Sonographic findings. Radiology 149:261, 1983.

Takaha, M., Matsumoto, A., Ochi, K., Takeuchi, M., Takemoto, M., and Sonoda, T.: Intrarenal arteriovenous malformation. J. Urol. 124:315, 1980.

Takebayashi, S., Aida, N., and Matsui, K.: Arteriovenous malformations of the kidneys: Diagnosis and followup with color Doppler sonography in six patients. AJR 157:991, 1991.

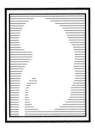
13

Parenchymal Disease with Normal Size and Contour

NEPHROCALCINOSIS
PAPILLARY NECROSIS

TUBERCULOSIS
DIFFERENTIAL DIAGNOSIS

In the preceding chapters, the discussion focused on diseases that produce either abnormal kidney size or abnormal contour. However, when those diseases are excluded, there remain three important groups of abnormalities in which the kidney retains normal size and contour. One group is characterized by generalized calcification of the renal substance, nephrocalcinosis, as the dominant abnormality. A second group, papillary necrosis, is also associated with nephrocalcinosis. Here, however, papillary and calyceal abnormalities are the principal findings and only in exceptional and advanced cases do the kidneys become globally small. Tuberculosis and brucellosis constitute a third group in which collecting system abnormalities are either the earliest or the only manifestations of parenchymal disease.

NEPHROCALCINOSIS

Definition

When sought by careful light or electron microscopic techniques, calcium deposits are present in virtually all kidneys whether they are diseased or not. The term *nephrocalcinosis* is reserved for radiologically detectable diffuse calcium deposition within the renal substance and implies a metabolic or renal abnormality. Histologically, calcium is deposited in the interstitium, in tubule epithelial cells, or along basement membranes of the collecting ducts, distal convoluted tubules, or ascending limb of the loop of Henle. Concretions occur within the tubule lumina as well. In medullary sponge kidney specifically, calcium is found in communicating cystic dilatations of the distal collecting tubules. Usually, nephrocalcinosis is limited to the medulla, or is dominant in the medulla with some involvement of cortex. Only in limited circumstances, such as chronic glomerulonephritis (see Chapter 7) or acute

cortical necrosis (see Chapter 8) is the cortex exclusively involved.

The mechanisms of calcium deposition are (1) metastatic, (2) dystrophic and (3) urine stasis.

Metastatic nephrocalcinosis usually occurs in kidneys that are morphologically normal (including normal size) but that have been subjected to metabolic disorders that promote tissue deposition of calcium, often as a result of hypercalcemia or increased tissue alkalinity. Metastatic calcification is diffuse, involves both kidneys, and is predominantly found in the medullae of the renal parenchyma.

Dystrophic calcification refers to the deposition of calcium in renal tissue that has been injured by hemorrhage, ischemia, or infarction or by suppuration or necrosis. Uncommonly, dystrophic calcification is seen as generalized, bilateral nephrocalcinosis, as in acute cortical necrosis or chronic glomerulonephritis or as a consequence of nephrotoxins. More commonly, dystrophic calcification is focal or unilateral and is not considered to fall within the definition of nephrocalcinosis. Examples of this type include calcification in an adenocarcinoma, the wall of a simple cyst, xanthogranulomatous pyelonephritis, or tuberculosis.

Urine stasis is the probable mechanism for nephrocalcinosis in medullary sponge kidney. In this concept, small stones form in previously formed cystic spaces that contain static urine because they communicate with collecting ducts. An alternative mechanism, that obstructive microlithiasis is initially present and causes secondary ductal dilatation, has also been proposed.

Some diseases in which nephrocalcinosis does occur are not discussed in this chapter because in addition to radiologically detectable calcium in the renal substance, abnormalities of renal size or contour also occur. Acute cortical necrosis, multiple myeloma, acute tubular necrosis following intake of nephrotoxins, and chronic glomerulonephritis are examples that are covered in other chapters.

Some functional abnormalities may result from nephrocalcinosis. Much of the depression in renal function found in association with nephrocalcinosis, however, is related to an elevated serum calcium level *per se*. Improvement in function may occur by lowering this value even when the extent of nephrocalcinosis remains unchanged.

Clinical Setting

Conditions associated with nephrocalcinosis and normal renal size and contour can be classified as follows:

Some forms of skeletal deossification

> **Primary and secondary hyperparathyroidism**
> **Metastatic carcinoma to bone**
> **Humoral hypercalcemia of malignancy**
> **Prolonged immobilization**

Increased intestinal absorption of calcium

> **Sarcoidosis**
> **Milk-alkali syndrome**
> **Hypervitaminosis D**

Miscellaneous

> **Renal tubular acidosis**
> **Medullary sponge kidney**
> **Hyperoxaluria**
> **Bartter's syndrome**
> **Prolonged furosemide administration in premature newborns**
> **Nephrotoxic drugs**
> **Papillary necrosis**

The clinical aspects of each of these are considered briefly.

Primary Hyperparathyroidism. Primary hyperparathyroidism is caused by an adenoma or carcinoma of a single parathyroid gland or by diffuse hyperplasia of all parathyroid glands. High serum calcium and decreased serum phosphate levels are the biochemical features of this disease. Primary hyperparathyroidism has signs that are common to hypercalcemia, regardless of its cause. These include muscular weakness, myocardial failure, ulcer disease, impaired renal function, and urolithiasis. Polyuria and polydipsia reflect hypercalcemia-induced impairment of urine-concentrating ability. Normochromic, normocytic anemia, pruritus, bone pain and resorption, and tenderness may also be present in primary hyperparathyroidism.

Metastatic Carcinoma to Bone. Hypercalcemia and nephrocalcinosis occur occasionally in cases of metastatic cancer in which considerable bone destruction leads to a release of excessive amounts of calcium.

Humoral Hypercalcemia of Malignancy. In primary carcinoma, particularly of the lung or kid-

ney, a syndrome with hypercalcemia and nephrocalcinosis sometimes occurs. Inappropriate secretion of parathyroid-like humoral factors by the tumor presumably underlies this phenomenon.

Prolonged Immobilization. Individuals subject to prolonged immobilization may develop hypercalcemia or hypercalciuria and subsequent nephrocalcinosis. Increased bone turnover, as might be seen in children, adolescents, or patients with Paget's disease, is an increased risk factor.

Sarcoidosis. Patients with sarcoidosis develop hypercalcemia owing to increased intestinal sensitivity to vitamin D, which results in excessive absorption of dietary calcium. Renal disease in sarcoidosis is related principally to hypercalcemia and is not dependent on the development of nephrocalcinosis.

Milk-Alkali Syndrome. Patients with the milk-alkali syndrome have a long history of excessive calcium ingestion, usually in the form of milk and antacids containing calcium carbonate. Positive calcium balance and alkalosis follow, although measurable hypercalcemia may be transitory. Nephrocalcinosis occurs as a result of large tubule loads of calcium and phosphate in the presence of alkaline urine and interstitial fluid. Not all individuals who ingest milk and antacids develop the syndrome, suggesting a predisposition in some people who cannot handle the increased load of calcium and phosphate.

Hypervitaminosis D. Hypervitaminosis D results from excessive intake of this vitamin. Hypercalcemia occurs from increased absorption of calcium through the intestine, just as in sarcoidosis. Excessive vitamin D also promotes dissolution of calcium salts from bone, a second mechanism for producing hypercalcemia.

Renal Tubular Acidosis. Renal tubular acidosis is a form of tubule insufficiency in which there is impairment of the ability of the distal nephron to secrete hydrogen ion against a concentration gradient. As a result, the kidney is unable to excrete an acid urine (below pH 5.4) during metabolic acidosis or even under stimulus of ammonium chloride ingestion. Renal tubular acidosis associated with nephrocalcinosis and urolithiasis is known as *classic* or *distal* and takes two forms. In the *complete* form, the patient experiences states of metabolic acidosis with hyperchloremia, hypokalemia, hypercalciuria, and a high urine pH. This form may be idiopathic or may be associated with a variety of genetically transmitted, autoimmune, or toxin-induced diseases of the kidney. Nephrocalcinosis caused by other disorders may itself produce the metabolic abnormality of distal renal tubular acidosis. In the *incomplete* form of distal renal tubular acidosis, electrolytes are normal, but stone formation occurs because of an insufficient amount of citrate excreted to keep calcium soluble in the urine. Patients with distal renal tubular acidosis experience muscle weakness and paralysis and rickets or osteomalacia or both; in children, growth retardation occurs. Symptoms of stone passage are common. Azotemia may develop. Another type of renal tubular acidosis is known as the *proximal* form. Nephrocalcinosis is not a feature of this disorder.

Medullary Sponge Kidney. Patients with medullary sponge kidney may be entirely free of urinary tract symptoms and have a normal life expectancy. When problems do occur, they are related to stone formation, urinary tract infection, and hematuria. A familial incidence has been reported rarely. Although usually seen in adults, medullary sponge kidney has been described in childhood. There is a well-established, but infrequently seen, relationship between medullary sponge kidney and congenital hemihypertrophy. Coexistence of medullary sponge kidney and primary hyperparathyroidism, reported in numerous instances, raises the possibility of a causal relationship between these two entities.

Hyperoxaluria. Hyperoxaluria produces nephrocalcinosis through interstitial deposition of calcium oxalate. The primary form is inherited as an autosomal recessive trait and represents enzymatic defects in the metabolic pathway of glyoxylic acid. Symptoms of calculous disease of the urinary tract occur early in childhood. Infection, hypertension, and obstructive uropathy lead to death (usually before 20 years of age). Acquired forms of hyperoxaluria follow ingestion of oxalate precursors, occur in association with intestinal disease (particularly regional enteritis), or are secondary to gastric bypass surgery for morbid obesity. This leads to calcium oxalate stone formation and is discussed in Chapter 14.

Bartter's Syndrome. Bartter's syndrome is characterized by hypokalemia, metabolic alkalosis, hyperreninemia, hypoaldosteronism, and normal blood pressure. Hyperplasia of the juxtaglomerular apparatus is seen histologically. For the most part, children and adolescents are affected, although young adults have been reported with this syndrome. These abnormalities occur either sporadically or as an autosomal recessive inheritance. Individuals with Bartter's syndrome experience muscle weakness and cramps, polyuria, abdominal pain, growth failure, and mental retardation.

Furosemide-Induced Nephrocalcinosis. Furosemide-induced nephrocalcinosis occurs in premature and low-birth-weight infants who have been treated for a prolonged period (usually 2 to 3 weeks) for congestive heart failure secondary to either patent ductus arteriosus or bronchopulmonary dysplasia. These patients develop hypercalciuria and alkaline urine. Calcium oxalate and calcium phosphate deposition occurs both in the renal parenchyma and as stones in the pelvocalyceal system. These abnormalities tend to resolve over time.

Nephrotoxic Drugs. Some drugs that cause nephrotoxicity uncommonly cause nephrocalcinosis, presumably due to damage to nephrons, collecting ducts or the interstitium. Triampterene and amphotericin B are two such examples.

Papillary Necrosis. Nephrocalcinosis occurs as dystrophic calcification in papillary necrosis. This subject is discussed in detail in the following section of this chapter.

Radiologic Findings

Radiographic detection of calcium in the renal substance is facilitated by low kilovoltage technique and careful collimation of the x-ray beam. Films of the kidneys must be obtained before injection of contrast material, which otherwise might obscure small calcific deposits as it passes through the renal tubules. Preliminary films should be obtained in frontal and oblique projections to localize calcifications accurately within the renal substance. Tomographic cuts accomplish the same purpose. Sometimes it is difficult to determine whether a calcification is in a papilla or is lying free in the immediately adjacent calyx. This distinction can usually be resolved by careful comparison of the preliminary films with those taken after the calyces are opacified. Unless very small, the calcium deposit usually remains faintly visible when it is within the papilla but becomes obscured when it is calyceal in location (see Fig. 13–4).

The extent of renal parenchymal calcification is highly variable (Figs. 13–1 through 13–3). In most cases of nephrocalcinosis due to deossification of the skeleton (primary hyperparathyroidism, primary or metastatic cancer, Cushing's syndrome, or adrenal corticosteroid medication) or increased absorption of calcium (sarcoidosis, milk-alkali syndrome, and hypervitaminosis D), only a few scattered punctate densities in the medullary portion of each kidney are seen. The pattern of calcium deposition in renal tubular acidosis may be similar in some cases, but more often there is very dense and extensive calcification of the medullary portions of the renal lobes (Figs. 13–4 and 13–5). This pattern is quite characteristic of renal tubular acidosis.

Medullary sponge kidney is different from other entities in this section because a confident diagnosis can be made by detecting urographic abnormalities other than nephrocalcinosis. Because the cystic dilatations that characterize this disorder communicate with the distal collecting ducts, they fill with contrast material during urography. Therefore, those cystic spaces that do not contain stones become apparent only during urography as clusters of small, rounded opacities grouped together in the papillary tip of the renal pyramid. These vary in number from a few to many and may involve one, several, or all papillae. On the other hand, those cystic spaces that do contain stones are detected as nephrocalcinosis on the preliminary film. With contrast enhancement, however, these baseline calcific densities become obscured as contrast material flows into the cystic spaces in which they reside and surrounds the individual calculi. This unique feature, in which baseline densities become obscured after contrast enhancement, serves to distinguish medullary sponge kidney from other causes

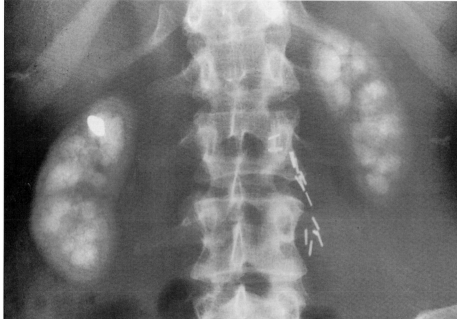

FIGURE 13–1. Nephrocalcinosis due to primary oxalosis in a 38-year-old woman complicated by end-stage renal disease. The diffuse calcification is most prominent in the medullae but is also present in the cortex. Abdominal radiograph.

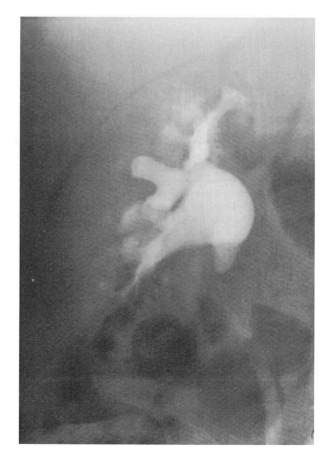

FIGURE 13–2. Nephrocalcinosis secondary to hypercalcemia associated with sarcoidosis. Calcifications are most apparent in the medullary portions of the upper pole. Excretory urogram. (Courtesy of Department of Diagnostic Radiology, Hammersmith Hospital, Royal Postgraduate Medical School, London, England.)

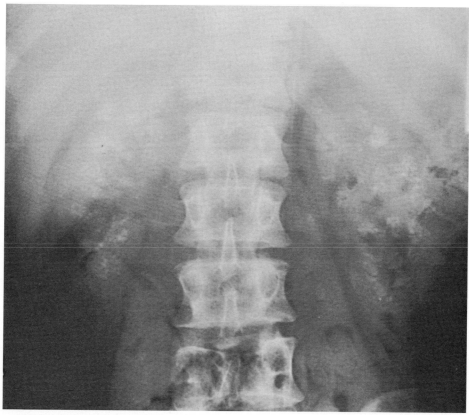

FIGURE 13–3. Nephrocalcinosis associated with primary hyperparathyroidism. Extensive medullary calcification is present in both kidneys. A brown tumor can be seen in the body of L-4. Preliminary film. (Courtesy of Janet Dacie, M.B., St. Bartholomew's Hospital, London, England.)

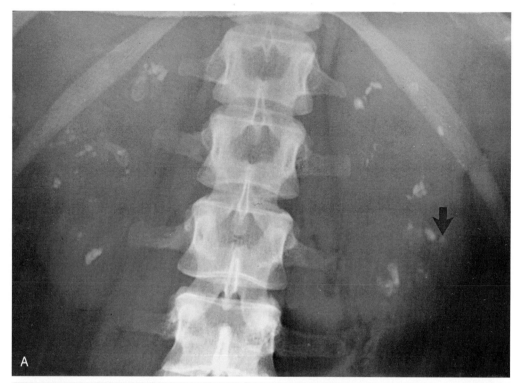

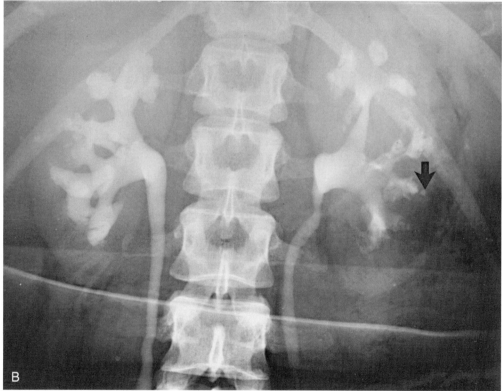

FIGURE 13–4. Nephrocalcinosis due to renal tubular acidosis in a 25-year-old woman. Extensive deposits of calcium are present. Evidence that the calcification is in the renal parenchyma (nephrocalcinosis) rather than in the collecting system (nephrolithiasis) is derived from the fact that individual foci can still be identified after contrast material fills the collecting system *(arrows)*.

  A, Preliminary film.

  B, Excretory urogram with compression. (Compare with Fig. 13–7.)

  Same patient is illustrated in Fig. 14–8.

  (Courtesy of the Department of Diagnostic Radiology, Hammersmith Hospital, Royal Postgraduate Medical School, London, England.)

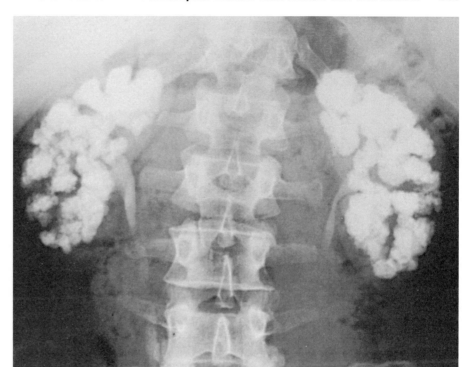

FIGURE 13–5. Nephrocalcinosis due to renal tubular acidosis in a 34-year-old man with skeletal deformity, first noted at age 2. Nephrocalcinosis was first detected at age 8. Dense confluent deposition of calcium in the medullae is characteristic of renal tubular acidosis. Excretory urogram. (Courtesy of Janet Dacie, M.B., St. Bartholomew's Hospital, London, England.)

of nephrocalcinosis (Figs. 13–6 and 13–7; see also Fig. 13–4).

In patients with medullary sponge kidneys, many of the affected collecting ducts are ectatic rather than cystic. In these cases, numerous radiodense linear striae appear in the papillae during urography (Figs. 13–8 and 13–9). This appearance may be confused with the intense, homogeneous enhancement of the pyramids that is sometimes seen when urography is performed without ureteral compression and in the absence of ureteral obstruction. This "papillary blush" occurs in normal kidneys owing to a high dose of contrast material, normal renal function, and a state of antidiuresis induced by

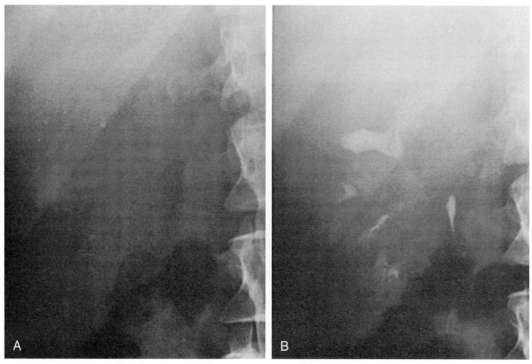

FIGURE 13–6. Medullary sponge kidney in a 50-year-old man. The preliminary film *(A)* demonstrates a few scattered punctate densities. During excretory urography *(B)*, additional round densities become apparent, particularly in the lower pole, as contrast material fills cystic dilatations of the collecting ducts.

334 SECTION II ☰ RENAL PARENCHYMAL DISEASE

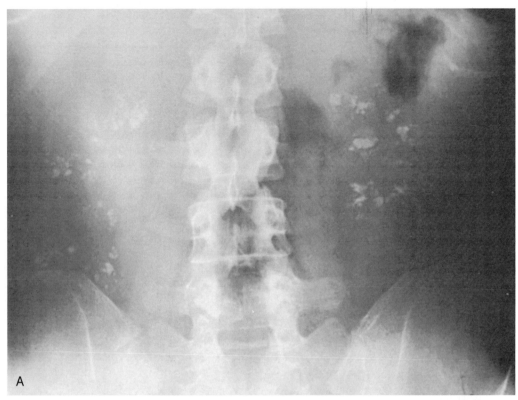

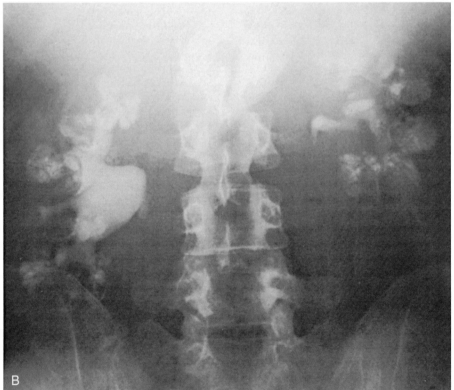

FIGURE 13–7. Medullary sponge kidney with advanced radiographic abnormalities in a 45-year-old woman. The preliminary film *(A)* demonstrates extensive small and large densities in the papillae. This pattern is indistinguishable from that resulting from other causes of nephrocalcinosis. The 10-minute urogram *(B)*, however, demonstrates added density accumulating in the papillae as contrast material fills those cystic spaces that do not already contain stones. At the same time, discrete foci of calcification identified on the preliminary film become obscure as contrast material flows into the cystic spaces in which they are located. These features are characteristic of medullary sponge kidney. (Compare with Fig. 13–4.)

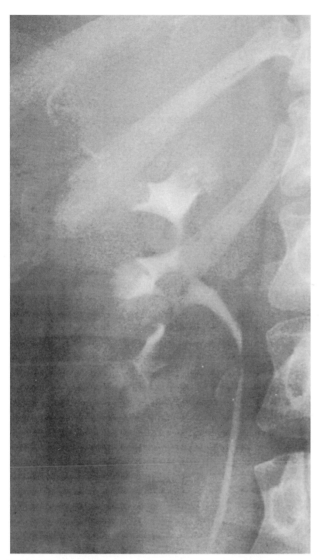

FIGURE 13–8. Medullary sponge kidney in a 48-year-old woman. Preliminary film revealed no nephrocalcinosis. Fine linear striations, particularly in the lower pole, represents the minimal changes of medullary sponge kidney. This diagnosis could not be made, however, without the cystic dilatations that were present in the papillae of the opposite kidney.

dehydration. Even when the papillary blush can be shown to be composed of separate, fine linear striations (the collecting tubules), it is generally held that these are normal collecting tubules that have become very dense during excretory urography. This normal, brushlike appearance is more frequently seen with low osmolality than with high osmolality contrast material. *Therefore, the diagnosis of medullary sponge kidney requires, in addition to linear striations in the papillae, the demonstration of nephrocalcinosis either by radiography or ultrasonography and/or cystic dilatations in the papillae following contrast material enhancement.*

Medullary sponge kidney has been reported with smooth enlargement of the kidneys and with congenital hemihypertrophy. In the latter circumstance, the sponge kidney may be bilateral or either ipsilateral or contralateral to the side of hypertrophy. Additionally, medullary sponge kidney may coexist with Caroli's disease and congenital hepatic fibrosis. Medullary sponge kidney has been reported in children as well as in adults (see Fig. 13–9).

Unilateral medullary sponge kidney without hemihypertrophy also occurs, as does a unifocal form. However, the radiologic abnormalities of medullary sponge kidney limited to one part of a kidney may represent obstruction of papillary duct orifices by a slowly growing transitional cell carcinoma or other neoplasm (Fig. 13–10).

Nephrocalcinosis, regardless of cause, is more readily detectable by computed tomography than film radiography owing to the greater contrast resolution of the former technique (Fig. 13–11). The search for nephrocalcinosis should include computed tomographic scanning without contrast material enhancement when standard radiographs, including tomograms, of the kidneys are normal. A ringlike pattern of medullary nephrocalcinosis has been described on computed tomograms, suggesting a predilection for crystal deposition in the corticomedullary area of the medullae.

Medullary nephrocalcinosis causes increased echo-

NEPHROCALCINOSIS TYPICAL FINDINGS

Primary Uroradiologic Elements

Size: normal
Contour: normal
Lesion distribution: bilateral

Secondary Uroradiologic Elements

Papillae: linear tracts or cystic dilatation (medullary sponge kidney)
Calcification: papilla (medullary sponge kidney); papilla and medulla (increased calcium absorption, renal tubular acidosis, and hyperoxaluria)
Echogenicity: medullary echogenicity with or without acoustic shadowing

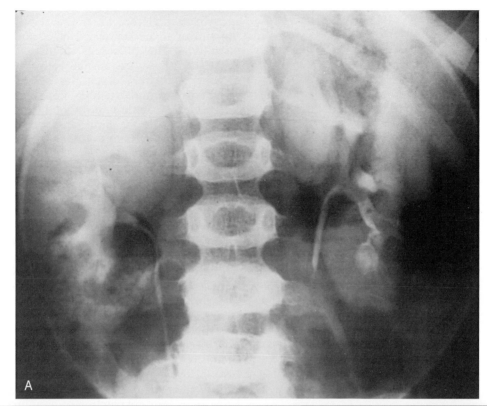

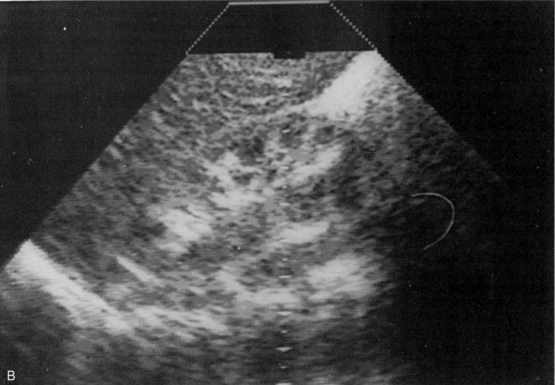

FIGURE 13–9. Medullary sponge kidney in a 6-year-old boy with polydipsia in whom similar findings had been present since the age of 5 months.

A, Excretory urogram. No calcification was identified on the preliminary radiograph. The collecting ducts in the papillae are distinctly ectatic. Both kidneys are enlarged.

B, Ultrasonogram, longitudinal section, right kidney. There is medullary hyperechoicity.

(Courtesy of Heidi B. Patriquin, M.D., University of Montreal, Montreal, Quebec, Canada, and American Journal of Roentgenology *145*:315, 1985.)

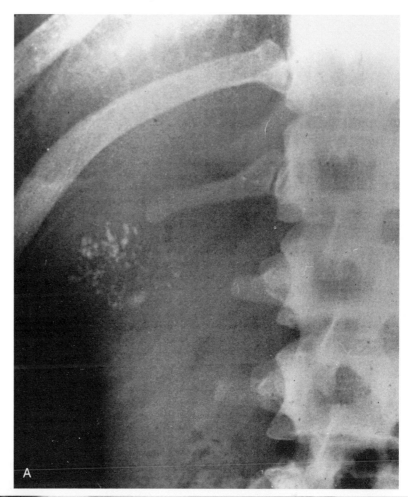

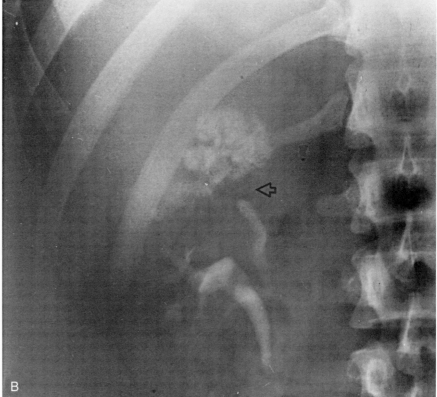

FIGURE 13–10. Focal medullary sponge kidney, upper pole, right kidney, at the site of a transitional cell carcinoma *(arrow).* The preliminary film *(A)* and excretory urographic *(B)* findings are those of medullary sponge kidney. The finding of focal medullary sponge kidney requires careful evaluation of the adjacent calyx for an obstructing lesion *(arrow),* as illustrated in this example.

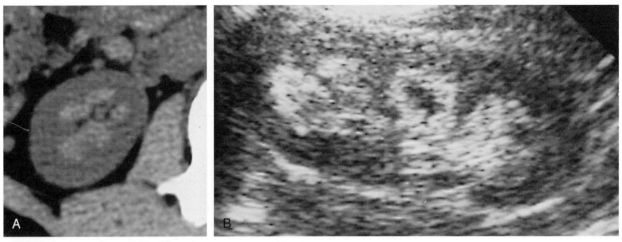

FIGURE 13–11. Nephrocalcinosis in renal tubular acidosis.
A, Computed tomogram, unenhanced. There is diffuse increase in attenuation values in the medullary pyramids compared with other portions of the renal parenchyma.
B, Ultrasonogram, sagittal plane. The medullae are hyperechoic.

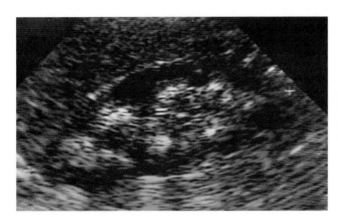

FIGURE 13–12. Nephrocalcinosis in medullary sponge kidney. Ultrasonogram, longitudinal section. There is increased echogenicity in the medullary pyramids, some of which also exhibit shadowing.

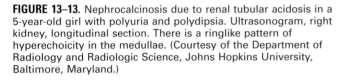

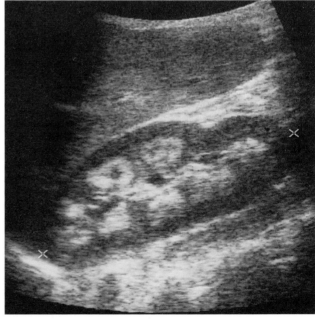

FIGURE 13–13. Nephrocalcinosis due to renal tubular acidosis in a 5-year-old girl with polyuria and polydipsia. Ultrasonogram, right kidney, longitudinal section. There is a ringlike pattern of hyperechoicity in the medullae. (Courtesy of the Department of Radiology and Radiologic Science, Johns Hopkins University, Baltimore, Maryland.)

genicity in the medullae, usually sparing the cortex (Fig. 13–12; see also Fig. 13–11*B*). As in computed tomography, a ringlike pattern had been described on ultrasonograms as well (Fig. 13–13). Acoustic shadowing depends on the extent of crystal deposition. This finding may be absent, as is frequently so in furosemide-induced nephrocalcinosis. Increased medullary echogenicity without acoustic shadowing in nephrocalcinosis, therefore, may simulate other forms of renal parenchymal disease, as discussed in the differential diagnosis section at the end of this chapter. Ultrasonography, like computed tomography, is more sensitive than film radiography in the detection of nephrocalcinosis.

PAPILLARY NECROSIS

Definition

Necrosis of the renal papilla has several causes and a number of clinical, pathologic, and radiologic forms. In mild to moderate cases, renal size and function are normal and structural changes are limited to one, several, or all papillae. In advanced states, however, especially with analgesic nephropathy, the kidneys become globally shrunken and have impaired function.

This discussion is focused on renal papillary necrosis associated with analgesic use, since this form has been most comprehensively studied and is most prevalent in North America, Europe, and Australia. Differences between analgesic nephropathy and other causes of papillary necrosis, such as diabetes mellitus, urinary tract infection, renal vein thrombosis, prolonged hypotension, urinary tract obstruction, dehydration, S hemoglobinopathy, hemophilia, and Christmas disease are commented on in each section.

Medullary ischemia is the central finding in experimental analgesic nephropathy. Necrobiosis of the loops of Henle and of the vasa recta in the papillary tip are early abnormalities. Patchy necrosis of the papilla with overall survival of the collecting tubules occurs at an intermediate stage of severity. Frank necrosis of all elements of the papilla and formation of a clear line of demarcation between the necrotic and the viable portions of the papillary tissue characterize the most advanced stage. These observations suggest that initial damage occurs at the loop of Henle and the vasa recta.

In humans, severity of pathologic change varies directly with the amount of analgesic drugs ingested and closely parallels the sequence of events seen in the experimental animal. The precise pathogenesis of papillary necrosis is unknown. A combination of direct tubule toxicity by metabolites of phenacetin and medullary ischemia due to prostaglandin synthetase inhibition is a likely explanation. In any case, a high concentration of the toxic material occurs in the loop of Henle region of the papilla where the initial and maximal damage occurs. Early change is represented by a yellowish-

appearing papilla, with necrosis of the epithelium of the loops of Henle and occasional foci of calcification but no disruption of papillary integrity. As damage progresses, there may be total loss of the loops of Henle, while the collecting duct epithelium remains intact. At this stage, the endothelium of the vasa recta is also destroyed and calcium accumulates in many areas of the papilla. In the most advanced form, there is diffuse fibrosis and chronic inflammatory cell infiltration in the interstitium as well as tubule atrophy and glomerular hyalinization. These changes, representing chronic interstitial fibrosis, are "end stage" and account for a decrease in renal size and function. In general, the collecting ducts draining the nephrons of the septal cortex at the margin of the lobe better maintain their viability than the ducts located centrally in the lobe, probably because they are not obstructed by necrosis at the papillary tip. As a result, tubule atrophy is predominantly centrilobar and is associated with an increased prominence (either relative or due to true hypertrophy) of the septal cortex drained by the more intact peripheral collecting tubules. These changes produce an uneven pattern of atrophy on the surface of the kidney in which broad, flat, depressed areas of centrilobar cortex are bordered by raised ridges of preserved or hypertrophic septal cortex.

Most investigators interested in this disorder take the position that chronic interstitial inflammation is caused by obstruction of the collecting tubules by necrosis of the papilla. Some, however, believe that global shrinkage and renal failure are the result of a direct effect of toxic material on the renal parenchyma. Infection does not appear to be a major factor in causing papillary necrosis in analgesic nephropathy.

Changes in the gross appearance of the papilla parallel the severity of the histologic damage. Initially, the papilla enlarges slightly. Patchy disruption of the integrity of the papilla follows, with the development of tracts communicating with the calyceal system. Cavitation of the papillary substance, with or without complete separation of the papilla from the remainder of the medulla, is a late finding. Occasionally, the necrotic papilla remains *in situ*, where it may calcify or ossify.

It is not uncommon to observe marked papillary necrosis in kidneys that are normal in size and smooth in contour. This simply reflects the very important point that shrinkage of size occurs only in the advanced state, when chronic interstitial fibrosis and tubule atrophy occur. Wasting may occur rapidly, however, once it begins.

Other etiologies may produce patterns that are different from those seen with analgesic abuse. Fulminant papillary necrosis is produced by urinary tract obstruction and infection, with or without diabetes mellitus, and was the first type of papillary necrosis to be described. Acute inflammation, extensive papillary sloughing, and enlarged kidneys are seen in these cases. At the other extreme, papillary necrosis associated with heterozygous-S hemoglobinopathy is very minimal, and progression to small kidneys and renal failure has not been noted. In some circumstances, papillary necrosis affects only one kidney, as may be seen in ureteral obstruction, severe acute pyelonephritis, tuberculosis, and renal vein thrombosis. It should be apparent, therefore, that the presentation of papillary necrosis depends on the clinical setting in which it occurs.

Clinical Setting

The diagnosis of analgesic nephropathy is made most often in middle-aged and elderly women who give a history, sometimes difficult to elicit, of ingestion of large amounts of nonsteroidal anti-inflammatory drugs over a long period of time. This disorder can be particularly severe in hot, dry climates, suggesting that dehydration enhances the effect of the toxic material, presumably by increasing its concentration in the interstitium of the papilla. Symptoms closely resemble those of acute urinary tract infection and include recurrent attacks of fever, dysuria, headache, and malaise. Passage of necrotic papillae or stones produces urinary tract obstruction and colic. Heavy pyuria and fragments of papillae are seen on microscopic examination of the urine. Eventually, sometimes over a short period, these changes may lead to small kidneys with the clinical findings of chronic renal failure. Rarely, analgesic nephropathy presents as acute oliguric renal failure with large kidneys and intact papillae. Transitional cell carcinoma of the kidney is more common in patients with analgesic nephropathy than in the general population. It is important for the radiologist to assess the urograms of these individuals with this complication in mind (see discussion in Chapter 15.)

The association of renal papillary necrosis with *diabetes mellitus* has not been investigated as thoroughly as analgesic nephropathy has. A combination of ischemia and infection is considered the basis for this relationship. Fulminating disease with severe infection and azotemia frequently leading to death was once the most common presentation of renal papillary necrosis in the diabetic patient. This is rarely encountered now because of advances in the management of both diabetes and urinary tract infection. Papillary necrosis is also found in some diabetic patients with chronic or recurrent infection of the urinary tract and moderate impairment of renal function. These patients have hematuria, pyuria, bacteriuria, and proteinuria in addition to glycosuria. Papillary necrosis developing in patients with diabetes mellitus uncomplicated by urinary tract infection or obstruction is alluded to in the literature but remains undocumented.

Patients with *S hemoglobinopathy* also develop papillary necrosis. When the affected red blood cells enter the hypertonic and hypoxic area of the medulla, sickling occurs and causes blockage of the vasa recta perfusing the papillary region. In the homozygous-S state, papillary necrosis can be part of a more complex disorder of the kidneys, which includes glomerular microinfarcts, glomerulopathy, lobar infarcts, obliteration of tubules, and fibrosis.

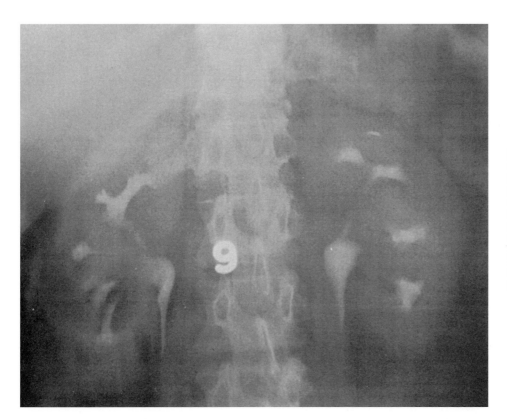

FIGURE 13–14. Renal papillary necrosis with normal-sized kidneys in a 54-year-old alcoholic, diabetic, and analgesic-abusing woman. Uniform thinning of renal parenchyma has occurred, with multiple papillary abnormalities. Tomogram. Same patient is illustrated in Fig. 13–22. Right kidney length is 13.8 cm; left kidney length is 13.3 cm.

Because symptoms from other organ systems usually predominate in sickle cell disease (homozygous-S), contrast material–enhanced studies of the kidneys are not often performed on these patients. In patients with heterozygous-S hemoglobinopathy, particularly those with SA hemoglobin, minimal papillary necrosis develops without specific signs or symptoms. This abnormality is not progressive and not associated with renal failure.

Rarely, papillary necrosis is associated with noninfected *urinary tract obstruction, renal vein thrombosis,* or *trauma.* Here, papillary necrosis would likely be unilateral, and the clinical findings would be dominated by the underlying disease. Similarly, *renal tuberculosis* often includes a necrotizing papillitis as one of its many manifestations, and this is sometimes limited to one kidney or a part of one kidney. Papillary necrosis also occurs in infants in association with *shock* from a variety of disorders and has been reported in *hemophilia* and *Christmas disease.* Finally, a relationship between *hepatic cirrhosis* and renal papillary necrosis has been proposed but, because of the sparse available evidence, must be considered tentative.

Radiologic Findings

The radiologic appearance of papillary necrosis has been studied extensively and is best demonstrated by excretory urography. Renal size is normal in most cases of analgesic nephropathy, although in some patients both kidneys shrink as the abnormality progresses (Fig. 13–14; see Fig 13–25). Kidney contour remains smooth except in some advanced cases in which a "wavy" appearance develops owing to the prominence of septal cortex surrounding atrophic areas of centrilobar cortex (Fig. 13–15). Small kidneys have not been reported in S hemoglobinopathy or in uncomplicated diabetes. The fulminant form of renal papillary necrosis (see Fig. 14–20) with smooth renal enlargement and decreased function is very uncommon and is associated with urinary tract obstruction and infection, diabetes mellitus and severe acute pyelonephritis, renal vein thrombosis, homozygous-S hemoglobinopathy, and, only rarely, analgesic nephropathy. In some of these disorders, the papillary necrosis may be limited to one kidney. In most instances, the kidney size is normal and the outline is smooth.

In an early stage of the disease, papillary swelling may be the only radiologic abnormality present. This may be difficult to distinguish from the normal kidney. Necrosis of the papilla and disruption of its uroepithelial lining takes several radiologic forms. Figure 13–16 presents examples of tract formation, which is an early manifestation of necrosis. These appear as faint streaks of density oriented parallel to the long axis of the papilla, usually extending from the fornix. This pattern is commonly seen in heterozygous-S hemoglobinopathies. Tract formation can be easily overlooked unless careful attention is given to technical details such as proper

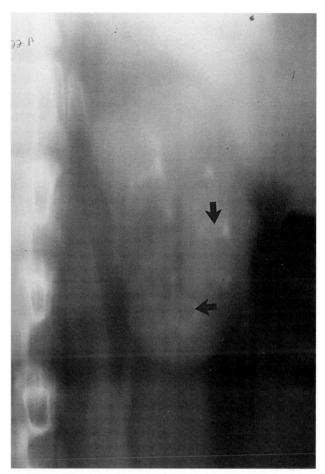

FIGURE 13–15. Renal papillary necrosis with "wavy" contour superimposed on global wasting of the kidney. Analgesic nephropathy in a 44-year-old man. All papillae are involved, and there are nonopaque filling defects representing sloughed papillae in two calyces *(arrows).* Tomogram. Same patient is illustrated in Fig. 13–23.

collimation, oblique views, and adequate calyceal distention. Conclusive evidence of tract formation requires identification on more than one film and the absence of excessive calyceal distention, either from obstruction or abdominal compression.

Papillary necrosis is readily detectable when there is cavitation of the central portion of the papilla or complete sloughing of the papillary tip. The cavitating form has been called *medullary* or *partial papillary slough,* while detachment of the whole papilla has been labeled *papillary* or *total papillary sloughing.* Medullary cavitation is often central but may also be eccentric. The long axis of the cavity parallels the long axis of the papilla. The shape of the cavity varies from long and thin to short and bulbous. Some cavities have sharp margins; others are irregular (Figs. 13–17 through 13–19). A total papillary slough can be identified by a band of density across the base of the papilla. As the papillary tip separates farther from its medullary base, the band of density widens. With complete separation, the sloughed tissue is seen as a triangular radiolucent filling defect in the opacified calyx (Fig. 13–20;

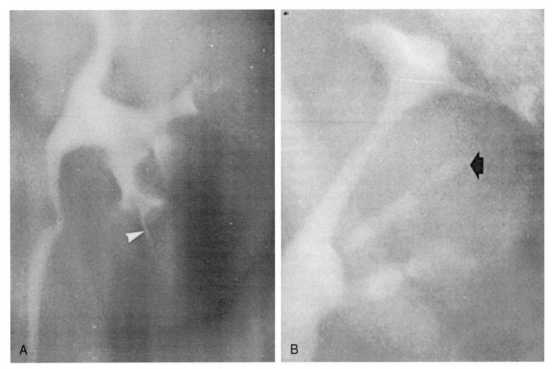

FIGURE 13–16. Renal papillary necrosis represented by tracts of contrast material extending from the fornix into the lateral aspects of medulla *(arrows)*.
  A, A 51-year-old woman with mild diabetes mellitus and normal-sized kidneys. Same patient is illustrated in Fig. 13–26.
  B, Similar finding in a patient with SA hemoglobinopathy.
  (From Eckert, D.E., et al.: Radiology *113*:59, 1974. Reproduced with kind permission of the authors and *Radiology.*)

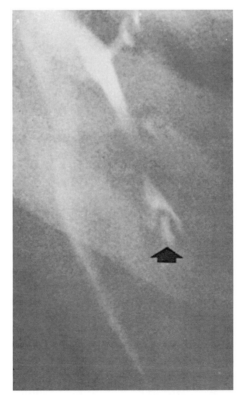

FIGURE 13–17. Renal papillary necrosis. Sharply defined elongated cavity *(arrow)* in center of papilla in a patient with SA hemoglobinopathy represents the *medullary* form of papillary necrosis. (From Eckert, D.E., et al.: Radiology *113*:59, 1974. Reproduced with kind permission of the authors and *Radiology.*)

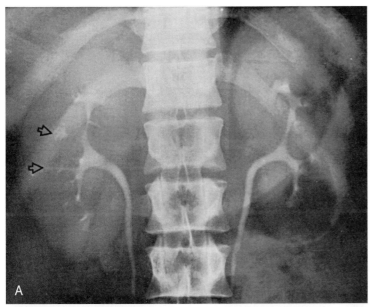

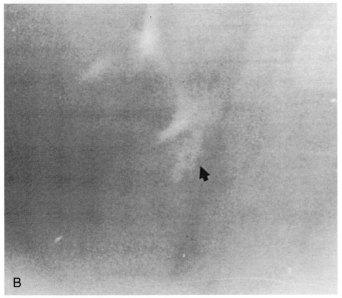

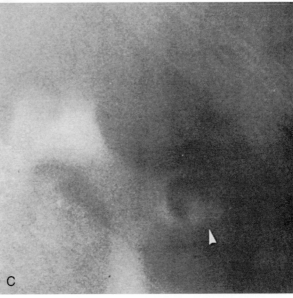

FIGURE 13–18. Renal papillary necrosis with various forms of cavitation in a 33-year-old man with SC hemoglobinopathy and hematuria.

A, Kidneys are of normal size and smooth in contour. Central cavitation is present in many papillae, particularly in right interpolar areas *(arrows).* Right lower and left upper poles are magnified in parts *B* and *C.*

B, Ill-defined smudge *(arrow)* represents early cavitation. Lucent oblique line is psoas margin, not medial border of kidney.

C, Eccentric, irregular cavity near forniceal angle *(arrow).*

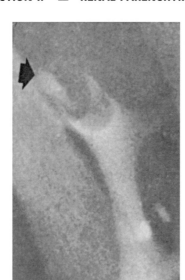

FIGURE 13–19. Renal papillary necrosis. Elongated cavity *(arrow)* situated eccentrically in the papilla of a patient with SA hemoglobinopathy. (From Eckert, D.E., et al.: Radiology *113*:59, 1974. Reproduced with kind permission of the authors and *Radiology.*)

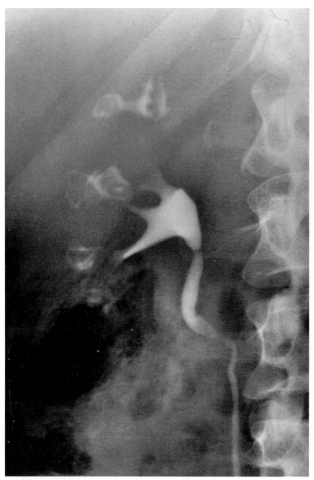

FIGURE 13–20. Renal papillary necrosis in a patient with analgesic nephropathy. Each of the papillae has separated and forms nonopaque calyceal filling defects, many of which have triangular shapes. This represents the *papillary* form of papillary necrosis.

see also Fig. 13–15). Margins at the point of separation are initially rough but later become smooth. Necrotic tissue may pass into the renal pelvis and beyond, causing obstruction. The remaining calyx has a round or saccular shape and smooth margins (Fig. 13–21).

There is a form of papillary necrosis that is difficult to diagnose because the necrotic tissue does not slough and the silhouette of the papilla is preserved. This form has been termed *necrosis in situ*. These papillae may shrink slightly over time, and some calcify or ossify. A confident radiologic diagnosis of papillary necrosis in this form requires supportive clinical evidence or other specific coexisting radiologic abnormalities, such as cavities or sloughing.

Calcification in papillary tissue (nephrocalcinosis) is common in analgesic nephropathy but has not been reported in papillary necrosis due to heterozygous-S hemoglobinopathy. Presumably, this difference reflects greater tissue damage from analgesic drugs. Nephrocalcinosis may be seen either in papillae that have no other radiologic abnormality or in those that have cavitated. In most instances, foci of calcification are round, homogeneous, and arranged in a semilunar arc that corresponds to the positions of the papillary tips (Figs. 13–22 and 13–23). This appearance is indistinguishable from that of nephrocalcinosis from causes other than papillary necrosis. On the other hand, a ring-shaped, triangular pattern of calcification is unique to papillary necrosis (Fig. 13–24). Here, calcium outlines the periphery of a necrotic papilla, which may be sloughed and moving down the urinary tract. Calci-

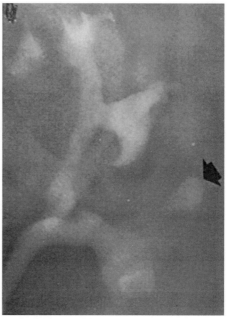

FIGURE 13–21. Renal papillary necrosis. Loss of papillary tip, either by sloughing or atrophy, leaves smooth-margined saccular calyx *(arrow)* without overlying focal contour scar in a patient with SA hemoglobinopathy. (From Eckert, D.E., et al.: Radiology *113*:59, 1974. Reproduced with kind permission of the authors and *Radiology.*)

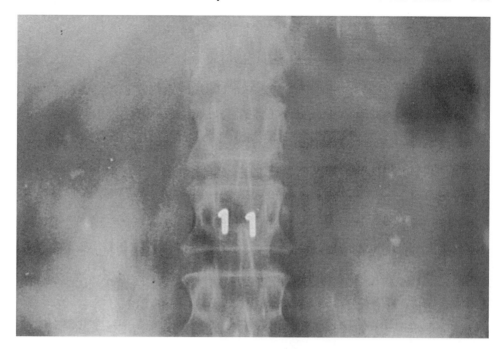

FIGURE 13–22. Papillary calcification at multiple sites in renal papillary necrosis. Preliminary tomogram. Same patient is illustrated in Fig. 13–14.

fication or ossification may be the only radiologic abnormality in the necrosis in situ form of papillary necrosis.

Enlargement of the septum of Bertin may centrally displace an adjacent calyx or infundibulum. This can create the impression of a mass (Fig. 13–25). A radionuclide scan may be necessary to identify this deformity as a pseudotumor.

Abnormal and persistent dense areas on a nephrogram have been reported in papillary necrosis in experimental animals, in infants with shock-like states, and, rarely, in adults. Although rare, such a finding on a nephrogram should alert the radiologist to the possibility of papillary necrosis.

Presumably, this finding is due to tubule obstruction by necrosis of papillary tips.

Necrotic tissue passing down the pelvocalyceal system and the ureter produces the radiologic picture of obstruction. The obstructing material is often non-opaque (Fig. 13–26). When recovered in the urine, its tissue origin can usually be established by pathologic examination. Blood clots may act similarly.

Even though histologic damage may be present in all papillae, radiologically detectable lesions may be spotty or unilateral. Usually, multiple sites of involvement are present bilaterally, although the pattern of lesions may be mixed.

PAPILLARY NECROSIS TYPICAL FINDINGS

Primary Uroradiologic Elements

Size: normal to small
Contour: smooth
Lesion distribution: bilateral (analgesic nephropathy, diabetes, S hemoglobinopathy); unilateral (obstructive uropathy, renal vein thrombosis, severe acute pyelonephritis, tuberculosis)

Secondary Uroradiologic Elements

Papillae
   Enlarged (early)
   Disrupted (cavity, tracts, or slough)
   Retracted
Collecting system
   Dilated (focal, calyx)
   Intraluminal filling defects (opaque or nonopaque)
Parenchymal thickness
   Wasted (analgesic nephropathy)
Calcification
   Papillary
   Curvilinear: ring-shaped and triangular in sloughed papilla

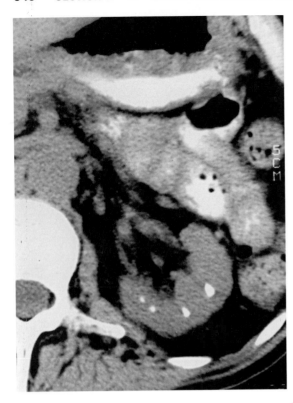

FIGURE 13–23. A semilunar arc of calcification in the tips of multiple papillae is illustrated in a patient with renal papillary necrosis. Computed tomogram, unenhanced. Same patient is illustrated in Fig. 13–15.

FIGURE 13–24. Calcification in a triangular ring pattern is unique to renal papillary necrosis. In this example, several sloughed papillae are located in the proximal ureter *(arrows)* in addition to the calyces.

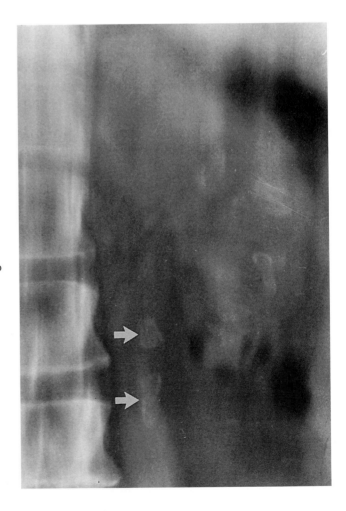

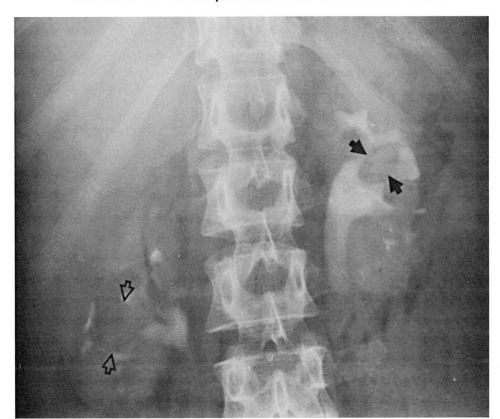

FIGURE 13–25. Focal masslike displacement *(arrows)* of pelvocalyceal systems bilaterally. This type of deformity is sometimes seen in advanced analgesic nephropathy due to hypertrophy of the septal cortex.

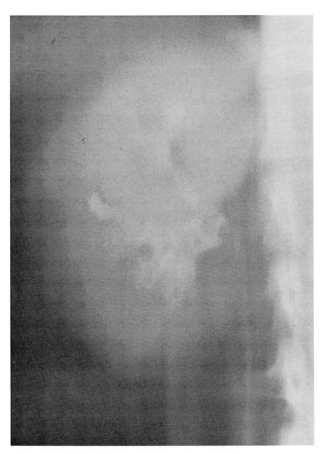

FIGURE 13–26. Multiple radiolucent filling defects in the pelvis of the right kidney, which caused intermittent obstruction. These represent blood clots, sloughed papillary tissue, or a combination of both. Obstruction and hematuria are common complications of renal papillary necrosis. Same patient is illustrated in Fig. 13–16*A*.

Diminished excretion of contrast material, reflecting renal failure, occurs in advanced stages of analgesic nephropathy but is not seen with other causes of *chronic* papillary necrosis. This usually occurs in patients with small kidneys and a long history of analgesic abuse. Impaired contrast material density is also seen with large kidneys in *acute* analgesic nephropathy, in papillary necrosis caused by overwhelming urinary tract infection in the obstructed or diabetic patient, and in sickle cell nephropathy with impaired concentration of urine.

Only a few studies of ultrasonography in papillary necrosis have been reported. Increased medullary echogenicity in the absence of calcification has been described. Sloughed papillae might be imaged as material within the collecting system lumen. These may have the sound-reflecting characteristics of stones, if calcified, or exhibit an echo pattern similar to that of renal parenchyma, if uncalcified. Calyces may be dilated at the site of a disgorged papilla, or the entire collecting system may be dilated when obstruction supervenes. Overall, the poor spatial resolution of ultrasonography limits its usefulness in the assessment of papillary necrosis.

Computed tomography is a sensitive modality for the detection of nephrocalcinosis (see Fig. 13–23). In advanced analgesic nephropathy, unenhanced computed tomography documents bilaterality of involvement, wasting of the renal parenchyma, and the "wavy" contour that is sometimes present in this condition.

TUBERCULOSIS

Definition

Tuberculosis shows a wider variety of pathologic features than any other disease of the renal parenchyma. The kidney may become focally scarred or globally enlarged or may develop single or multiple masses. It may appear grossly normal or completely destroyed. Early in the disease, however, renal size and contour are normal, and the lesion first becomes radiologically detectable as minor irregularities on the surface of a papilla and its calyx. It is for this reason that renal tuberculosis is included in this chapter.

Tuberculosis of the kidney occurs as a result of metastatic seeding of *Mycobacterium tuberculosis* in the glomerular and peritubular capillary bed from a primary infection elsewhere. The organism is usually of the human, rather than bovine, type. The organisms are disseminated through the bloodstream and therefore always involve both kidneys diffusely. The subsequent course of the infection, however, is determined by the dose and virulence of the inoculum as well as by host resistance factors. Characteristically, most of the initial lesions heal, and only one or a few progress to clinically or radiologically apparent abnormalities. This happens when the bacilli erode out of their initial vascular location and spill into the tubule lumina. As a result

of this migration, granulomas form along the nephron. Those occurring in the loop of Henle produce ulceration of the papillary tip. Granuloma formation, caseous necrosis, and cavitation are stages of progressive infection that cause single or multiple masses, which can ultimately destroy the entire kidney. Occasionally, these may cavitate and communicate with the collecting structure. Fibrosis and calcium deposition represent healing. The pattern of progression and healing is highly variable and produces asymmetric histologic, macroscopic, and radiologic abnormalities unique to each patient. In some cases the entire pathologic picture is limited to one or only a few papillae. As described in Chapter 15, pelvocalyceal and ureteral involvement appear as mucosal ulceration, focal or generalized dilatation, or cicatrix formation. Generalized or focal hydronephrosis follows localized scar formation in the pelvis or an infundibulum. Eventually the bladder and genital structures may become involved.

Brucellosis and primary fungal infection of the kidney may produce a pathologic picture identical to that of tuberculosis.

Clinical Setting

Renal tuberculosis affects adult men more commonly than women in the general population. Reflecting on the many different pathologic manifestations, it is not surprising that the clinical picture, too, is highly variable. Most, but not all, patients have a history of tuberculosis in a site other than the kidney, usually in bone or the lungs. Infection in the primary organ may be inactive by the time renal tuberculosis becomes apparent. Therefore, a normal chest radiograph is found in about 50 per cent of patients with urinary tract tuberculosis. Only 10 to 15 per cent of patients with active genitourinary tuberculosis have active pulmonary disease at the same time. In addition to affecting the general population, tuberculosis is prevalent in immunocompromised patients, notably those with acquired immunodeficiency syndrome.

Fever, anorexia, fatigue, weakness, night sweats, and weight loss are uncommon in renal tuberculosis. Frequency is the most common urinary tract symptom. Suprapubic, groin, or flank pain; hematuria; dysuria; and complaints referable to epididymitis may be symptoms of patients with urinary tract tuberculosis. On the other hand, 10 per cent of patients are asymptomatic. Pus cells in urine that is "sterile" when cultured on standard media are the classic laboratory findings. The diagnosis is established by the demonstration of acid-fast bacilli on microscopic examination of the urine with special stains, by culture on appropriate media, or by growth of tubercle bacilli in inoculated guinea pigs.

Radiologic Findings

The single most distinctive feature of renal tuberculosis is a parenchymal cavity communicating with

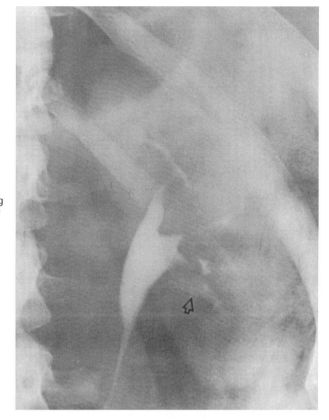

FIGURE 13–27. Tuberculosis. "Smudging" of contrast material along the medial side of the lower pole calyceal system *(arrow)* is a very early sign of tuberculosis. Excretory urogram.

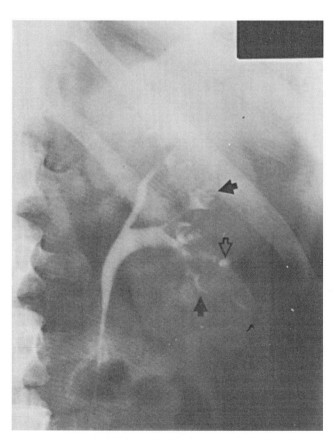

FIGURE 13–28. Tuberculosis. Involvement of several papillae is manifested by collections of contrast material in a smooth cavity at one site *(open arrow)* and in irregular linear extensions in papillae at other sites *(solid arrows)*. Excretory urogram. (Courtesy of Professor Thomas Sherwood, M.B., University of Cambridge, Cambridge, England.)

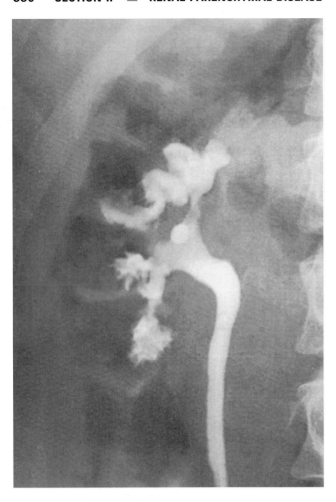

FIGURE 13–29. Tuberculosis causing extensive generalized papillary necrosis. Retrograde pyelogram.

the collecting system. Notable also are the multiplicity of genitourinary abnormalities. Tuberculous involvement of the lumbar spine, paraspinous and psoas abscess, and calcifications in the liver, spleen, adrenal glands, and lymph nodes may coexist.

The entire genitourinary system may be radiologically normal in symptomatic renal tuberculosis. The earliest urographic abnormality is irregularity of the surface of one or more papillae or calyces at a time when renal size and contour are normal. The papilla may appear "smudged" (Fig. 13–27; see Fig. 13–33), or tracts of contrast material may extend into the medulla along the side of the papilla (Fig. 13–28). Papillary necrosis can become quite extensive (Figs. 13–29 and 13–30). Despite generalized hematogenous dissemination of the tuberculosis organism, radiologic abnormalities are confined to a single kidney in over 70 per cent of cases.

Progressive involvement of renal parenchyma occurs in three forms, which may occur singly or in combination. First is the effect of granulomas that grow and coalesce, leading to unifocal or multifocal mass lesions. These may enlarge overall renal length, expand the thickness of the renal substance, and cause displacement of adjacent portions of the collecting system (see Fig. 13–30). Focal calcification, either circumscribed or amorphous, occurs at these sites, particularly as caseation occurs. These

masses may rupture into the collecting system, leaving irregular parenchymal cavities that opacify during urography, computed tomography, or retrograde pyelography (Fig. 13–31). The second form seen in advanced renal tuberculosis is caused by tissue loss and scarring, leading to surface scars over retracted papillae and dilated calyces (Fig. 13–32). Impaired excretion of contrast material may be noted in either of these two forms. A third form of renal tuberculosis is the calcified non-functioning kidney representing autonephrectomy, the so-called *putty kidney* (Fig. 13–33). Calcium deposition in this stage is usually extensive, and the overall size of the destroyed tuberculous organ is often surprisingly close to normal.

In some cases, the collecting system may be the only abnormal part of the kidney. The most common deformity is dilatation with an obstructing stricture. Dilatation may be limited to a single calyx whose draining infundibulum is narrowed by a scar, or it may involve the entire pelvocalyceal system (Figs. 13–34 and 13–35; see also Fig. 13–30). Occasionally, obstruction can be of such a high grade and so prolonged that severe hydronephrosis of all or part of the kidney develops (Fig. 13–36).

Detection of abnormalities in other portions of the genitourinary system is helpful in establishing the diagnosis of tuberculosis. The ureter may be

Text continued on page 356

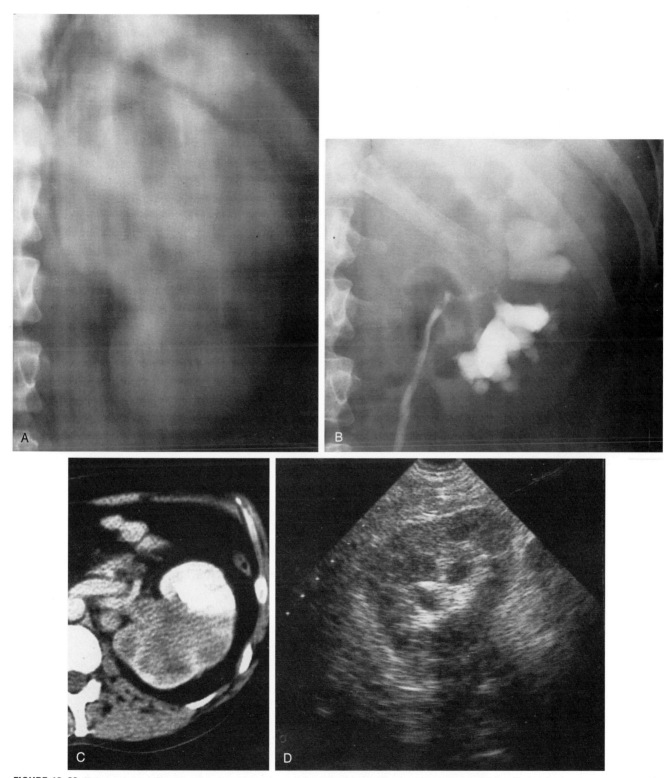

FIGURE 13–30. Tuberculosis affecting the dorsal portion of the left kidney. The involved area exhibits diminished enhancement and is generally enlarged with overall preservation of reniform shape. The calyces subserving the functioning ventral part of the kidney opacify but are dilated as a result of ureteral and pelvic involvement. Papillary necrosis is evident in the medullae of the ventral portion of the kidney.

    A, Excretory urogram, nephrographic phase. Tomogram.

    B, Excretory urogram, delayed film.

    C, Computed tomogram, contrast material–enhanced.

    D, Ultrasonogram, transverse section. The calyces within the central sinus complex are dilated.

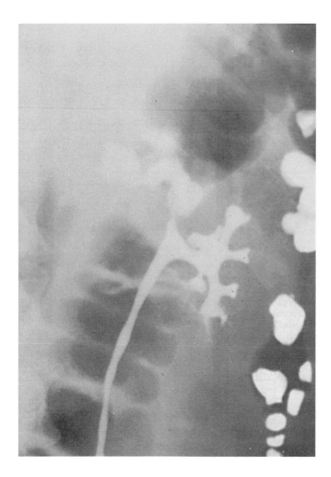

FIGURE 13–31. Tuberculosis. Cavitation of granulomatous masses in the upper pole has left irregular parenchymal cavities, which opacify during retrograde pyelography. Densities lateral to the kidney represent residual barium in the descending colon. Same patient is illustrated in Fig. 15–29.

FIGURE 13–32. Tuberculosis causing extensive tissue loss of the right kidney. The upper pole is severely scarred and contains calcium. Papillae are not visualized, and the calyces are dilated. Mild dilatation of the interpolar and lower polar calyces of the left kidney reflect bilateral involvement. Excretory urogram.

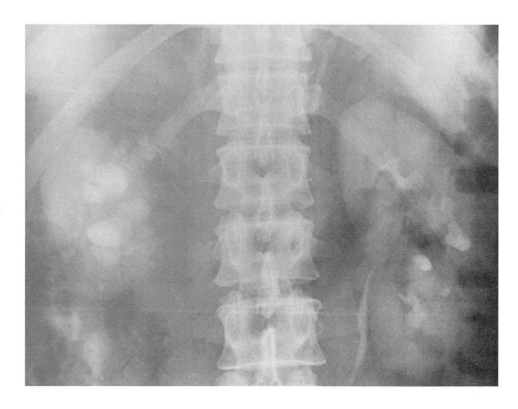

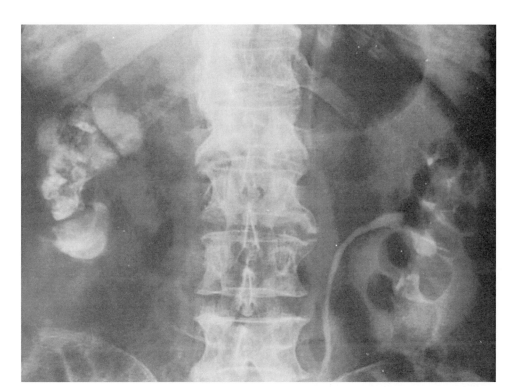

FIGURE 13–33. Tuberculosis resulting in right auto-nephrectomy. The kidney has become calcified and does not excrete contrast material. The papillae of the left kidney are disrupted, representing tuberculous involvement at an earlier stage than that seen on the right side. Excretory urogram.

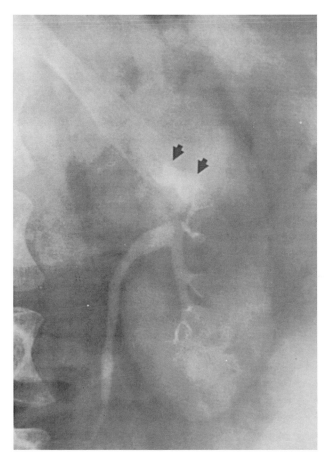

FIGURE 13–34. Tuberculosis causing focal caliectasis *(arrows)* due to scarring of the infundibulum draining the upper pole system. Excretory urogram.

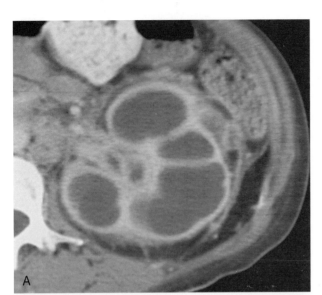

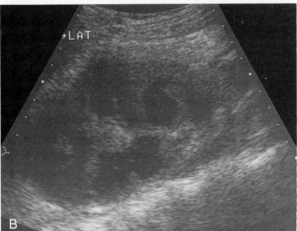

FIGURE 13–35. Tuberculosis causing chronic hydronephrosis secondary to pelvic scar formation. There is marked caliectasis and parenchymal atrophy without pelvic dilatation.
    A, Computed tomogram, contrast material–enchanced.
    B, Ultrasonogram, sagittal plane.

RENAL TUBERCULOSIS TYPICAL FINDINGS

Primary Uroradiologic Elements

Size: variable
Contour: variable; may have focal expansion or scar
Lesion distribution: unilateral (20 to 30 per cent bilateral)

Secondary Uroradiologic Elements

Papillae: irregular margin (earliest sign); retracted (late); calcified (late)
Collecting system: irregular margin; multifocal dilatation; strictured; disrupted
   (communicating with parenchymal cavities)
Parenchymal thickness: variable
Calcification: generalized, dense (autonephrectomy); focal (circumscribed, amorphous)
Nephrogram: replaced (focal or multifocal)
Echogenicity: disrupted parenchymal architecture; caliectasis; pelviectasis
Additional features: ureter (short, straight, calcified, with reflux and multiple strictures);
   bladder (thick wall, decreased capacity); seminal vesicles and epididymides (calcified)

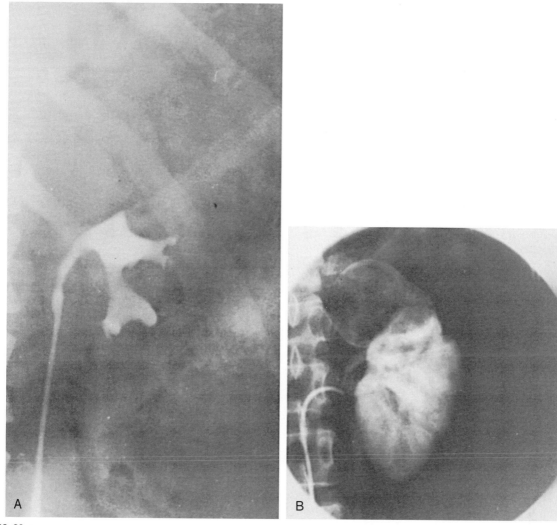

FIGURE 13–36. Tuberculosis. Scar formation in the infundibulum draining the left upper pole is so severe that advanced hydronephrosis of the upper pole has ensued.
A, Retrograde pyelogram. There is complete occlusion of the infundibulum to the upper pole.
B, Late phase of a selective angiogram. The thick-walled, hydronephrotic upper pole is well visualized.
(Courtesy of M. Korobkin, M.D., University of Michigan, Ann Arbor, Michigan.)

FIGURE 13–37. Tuberculosis. Cavitating tuberculoma of the right kidney produces an ultrasonographic image of a fluid-filled mass with low-level internal echoes. Longitudinal scan. (Courtesy of Gerald W. Friedland, M.D., Stanford University, Stanford, California.)

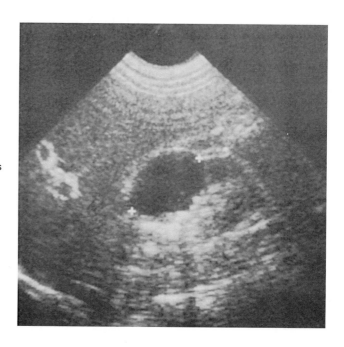

shortened, dilated, and unusually straight, or it may contain multiple strictures. Extensive calcification and thickening of the ureter has been termed *pipe-stem ureter.* The bladder becomes thick-walled and has a diminished capacity for urine storage as a result of tuberculous cystitis. Vesicoureteral reflux may occur. The epididymis or seminal vesicle may calcify. See Chapters 15 and 19 for further discussion of uroepithelial tuberculosis.

The varied features of tuberculosis can be determined by computed tomography and ultrasonography, as well as by excretory urography (see Figs. 13–30 and 13–35B). The latter method, however, is more likely to detect early abnormalities of the papillae. Granulomas appear as masses that have soft tissue density on computed tomography or are echogenic on ultrasonography. Computed tomographic attenuation values decrease with caseation and liquefaction. A tuberculoma that cavitates into the pelvocalyceal system is transformed into a hypoechoic, well-defined mass (Fig. 13–37).

DIFFERENTIAL DIAGNOSIS

The various causes of nephrocalcinosis produce a similar pattern of calcium deposition and cannot be distinguished from each other by radiologic criteria alone. The one exception to this generalization is the pattern of very dense calcium deposition throughout the medullary portions of the renal lobe seen in many, but not all, cases of **renal tubular acidosis**.

Differentiation between **medullary sponge kidney, renal papillary necrosis**, and **tuberculosis** is occasionally difficult. Unlike renal papillary necrosis and tuberculosis, destruction and sloughing of the papillae do not occur in medullary sponge kidney. Also, medullary sponge kidney calcification is rounded and clustered in cystic dilatations of collecting tubules. As contrast material flows into these cystic dilatations during urography, these baseline calcific densities are obscured while the cystic dilatations become apparent. Contrariwise, calcium deposition in both renal papillary necrosis and tuberculosis is more amorphous, involves the whole papilla, and is less uniformly patterned than in sponge kidney. Further, the baseline densities in these two entities are likely to remain discrete and identifiable after contrast material enhancement. Ring-shaped papillary calcification, however, is unique for renal papillary necrosis.

Fine linear striations of contrast material in the papillae and medulla, similar to the pattern of medullary sponge kidney, may also be seen in **Caroli's disease**, in the **juvenile form of autosomal recessive polycystic kidney disease** that is characterized by severe hepatic fibrosis, portal vein hypertension, and minimal renal failure, and as a **normal** finding, especially when excretory urography is performed with low osmolality contrast material.

Papillary and calyceal abnormalities of **reflux nephropathy** may be identical to those of renal papillary necrosis. However, reflux nephropathy can be distinguished by a focal contour scar overlying the papillary deformity, whereas wasting, when it does occur in papillary necrosis, is global. Also, papillary calcification is rare in reflux nephropathy and common in papillary necrosis.

Postobstructive atrophy affecting both kidneys has a number of features in common with papillary necrosis. Papillae disappear, and the kidney undergoes global shrinkage. Both the distribution and the severity of papillary abnormalities are more uniform in postobstructive atrophy than in papillary necrosis. In addition, a mixture of cavitation and atrophy is seen in papillary necrosis, whereas atrophy alone follows relief of obstruction.

Advanced analgesic nephropathy with chronic renal failure can be differentiated from other causes of end-stage renal failure, such as **chronic glomerulonephritis** and **malignant nephrosclerosis**, by the demonstration of papillary calcifications, a wavy contour superimposed on small, smooth kidneys or, if necessary, by the retrograde pyelographic demonstration of papillary abnormalities.

Papillary necrosis presenting as acute renal failure with enlarged, smooth kidneys may be impossible to distinguish from the many other causes of bilaterally enlarged, failed kidneys (discussed in Chapter 8), based on radiologic data alone. To make matters more difficult, evolution of papillary abnormalities may be delayed in these conditions, and serial retrograde pyelograms may be required to demonstrate characteristic papillary deformities.

Early papillary abnormalities due to **tuberculosis** may be similar in appearance to the other causes of renal papillary necrosis. Tuberculosis, however, tends to give a smudged, ill-defined, "moth-eaten" pattern to the papillary-calyceal area, whereas abnormal collections of contrast material in renal papillary necrosis due to other causes are somewhat better defined, either as linear tracts from the fornix into the medulla or as umbilicated cavities extending into the papilla. In addition, abnormalities of other forms of papillary necrosis are limited to the papillary area, while the tuberculous lesion may extend more deeply into the medulla. As these two entities progress in severity, their features diverge and differentiation becomes quite easy.

Some cases of healed tuberculosis produce a surface scar with retraction of the underlying papilla and focal calyceal dilatation. This picture, at either a single or multiple sites, is indistinguishable from **reflux nephropathy (chronic pyelonephritis)**. The diagnosis of tuberculosis can be favored only if other features, such as parenchymal calcification in the scar or stricture of the collecting system or ureter, are also present.

BIBLIOGRAPHY

Nephrocalcinosis and Medullary Sponge Kidney

Afonso, D. N., and Oliveira, A. G.: Medullary sponge kidney and congenital hemihypertrophy. Br. J. Urol. *62*:187, 1988.

Al-Murrani, B., Cosgrove, D. O., Svensson, W. E., and Blaszczyk, M.: Echogenic rings: An ultrasound sign of early nephrocalcinosis. Clin. Radiol. *44*:49, 1991.

Banner, M. P.: Nephrocalcinosis. In Pollack, H. M. (ed.): Clinical Urography. Philadelphia, W.B. Saunders Co., 1990, Chap. 57.

Brennan, R. P., Pearlstein, A. E., and Miller, S. A.: Computed tomography of the kidneys in a patient with methoxyflurane abuse. J. Comput. Assist. Tomogr. *12*:155, 1988.

Brenner, R. J., Spring, D. B., Sebastian, A., McSherry, E. M., Genant, H. K., Palubinskas, A. J., and Morris, R. C.: Incidence of radiographically evident bone disease, nephrocalcinosis and nephrolithiasis in various types of renal tubular acidosis. N. Engl. J. Med. *307*:217, 1982.

Choong, M., and Phillips, G. W. L.: Renal transitional cell carcinoma mimicking medullary sponge kidney. Br. J. Radiol. *64*:275, 1991.

Cumming, W. A., and Ohlsson, A.: Nephrocalcinosis in Bartter's syndrome: Demonstration by ultrasonography. Pediatr. Radiol. *14*:125, 1984.

Day, D. L., Scheinman, J. L., and Mahon, J.: Radiological aspects of primary hyperoxaluria. AJR *146*:395, 1986.

Duncan, P. A., Sagel, I., and Farnsworth, P. B.: Medullary sponge kidney and partial Beckwith-Wiedemann syndrome: Association with congenital asymmetry. N.Y. State J. Med. *79*:1222, 1979.

Estroff, J. A., Mandell, J., and Benacerraf, B. R.: Increased renal parenchymal echogenicity in the fetus: Importance and clinical outcome. Radiology *181*:135, 1991.

Falkoff, G. E., Rigsby, C. M., and Rosenfield, A. T.: Partial, combined cortical and medullary nephrocalcinosis: US and CT patterns in AIDS-associated MAI infection. Radiology *162*:343, 1987.

Garel, L., Filiatrault, D., and Robitaille, P.: Nephrocalcinosis in Bartter's syndrome. Pediatr. Nephrol. *2*:315, 1988.

Gedroyc, W. M., and Saxton, H. M.: More medullary sponge variants. Clin. Radiol. *39*:423, 1988.

Gilsanz, V., Fernal, W., Reid, B. S., Stanley, P., and Ramos, A.: Nephrolithiasis in premature infants. Radiology *154*:107, 1985.

Ginalski, J. M., Portmann, L., and Jaeger, P.: Does medullary sponge kidney cause nephrolithiasis? AJR *155*:299, 1990.

Ginalski, J. M., Schnyder, P., Portmann, L., and Jaeger, P.: Medullary sponge kidney on axial computed tomography: Comparison with excretory urography. Eur. J. Radiol. *12*:104, 1991.

Ginalski, J. M., Spiegel, T., and Jaeger, P.: Use of low-osmolality contrast medium does not increase prevalence of medullary sponge kidney. Radiology *182*:311, 1992.

Harrison, A. R., and Rose, G. A.: Medullary sponge kidney. Urol. Res. *7*:197, 1979.

Hermany-Schulman, M.: Hyperechoic renal medullary pyramids in infants and children. Radiology *181*:9, 1991.

Hill, G. S.: Calcium and the kidney, nephrolithiasis, and hydronephrosis. In Heptinstall, R. H. (ed.): Pathology of the Kidney, 4th ed. Boston, Little, Brown & Co., 1992, pp. 1563–1630.

Hill, S. C., Hoeg, J. M., and Avila, N. A.: Nephrocalcinosis in homozygous familial hypercholesterolemia: Ultrasound and CT findings. J. Comput. Assist. Tomogr. *15*:101, 1991.

Houseal, L. M., and Sabatini, S.: Isolated renal tubular disorders. In Schrier, R. W., and Gottschalk, C. W. (eds.): Diseases of the Kidney, 6th ed. Boston, Little, Brown & Co., 1997, pp. 591–613.

Kaver, I., Flanders, E. L., Kay, S., and Koontz, W. W., Jr.: Segmental medullary sponge kidney mimicking a renal mass. J. Urol. *141*:1181, 1989.

Kenney, I. J., Aiken, C. G., and Lenney, W.: Furosemide-induced nephrocalcinosis in very low birth weight infants. Pediatr. Radiol. *18*:323, 1988.

Maschio, G., Tessitore, N., D'Angelo, A., Fabris, A., Corgnati, A., Oldrizzi, L., Loschiavo, C., Lupo, A., Valvo, E., Gammaro, L., and Rugio, C.: Medullary sponge kidney and hyperparathyroidism: A puzzling association. Am. J. Nephrol. *2*:77, 1982.

Muther, R. S., McCarron, O. A., and Bennett, W. M.: Renal manifestations of sarcoidosis. Arch. Intern Med. *141*:643, 1981.

Ohlsson, L.: Normal collecting duct: Visualization at urography. Radiology *170*:33, 1989.

Parks, J. H., Coe, F. L., and Strauss, A. L.: Calcium nephrolithiasis and medullary sponge kidney in women. N. Engl. J. Med. *306*:1088, 1982.

Patriquin, H. B., and O'Regan, S.: Medullary sponge kidney in childhood. AJR *145*:315, 1985.

Sage, M. R., Lawson, A. D., Marshall, V. R., and Ryall, R. L.: Medullary sponge kidney and urolithiasis. Clin. Radiol. *33*:435, 1982.

Saxton, H. M.: Opacification of collecting ducts at urography. Radiology *170*:16, 1989.

Shultz, P. K., Strife, J. L., Strife, C. F., and McDaniel, J. D.: Hyperechoic renal medullary pyramids in infants and children. Radiology *181*:163, 1991.

Torres, V. E., Young, W. F., Jr., Afford, K. P., and Hattery, R. R.: Association of hypokalemia and aldosteronism and renal cysts. N. Engl. J. Med. *322*:345, 1990.

Toyoda, K., Miyamoto, Y., Ida, M., Tada, S., and Utsunomiya, M.: Hyperechoic medulla of the kidneys. Radiology *173*:431, 1989.

Whitehouse, R. W.: High- and low-osmolar contrast agents in urography: A comparison of the appearances with respect to pyelotubular opacification and renal length. Clin. Radiol. *37*:395, 1986.

Wood, B. P.: Renal cystic disease in infants and children. Urol. Radiol. *14*:284, 1992.

Yendt, E. R.: Medullary sponge kidney and nephrolithiasis. N. Engl. J. Med. *306*:1106, 1982.

Renal Papillary Necrosis

Appel, R.G., Bleyer, A.J., and Mccabe, J.C.: Analgesic nephropathy: A soda and a powder. Am. J. Med. Sci. *310*:161, 1995.

Barrett, B.J.: Acetaminophen and adverse chronic renal outcomes: An appraisal of the epidemiologic evidence. Am. J. Kidney Dis. *28*:S14, 1996.

Bennett, W.M., Henrich, W.L., and Stoff, J.S.: The renal effects of nonsteroidal anti-inflammatory drugs: Summary and recommendations. Am. J. Kidney Dis. *28*:S56, 1996.

Bengtsson, U., Angervall, L., Ekman, H., and Lehmann, L.: Transitional cell tumors of the renal pelvis in analgesic abusers. Scand. J. Urol. Nephrol. *2*:145, 1968.

Braden, G. L., Kozinn, D. R., Hampf, F. E., Parker, T. H., and Germain, M. J.: Ultrasound diagnosis of early renal papillary necrosis. J. Ultrasound Med. *10*:401, 1991.

Brezis, M., and Rosen, S.: Hypoxia of the renal medulla: Its implication for disease. N. Engl. J. Med. *332*:647, 1995.

Buckalew, V. M.: Habitual use of acetaminophen as a risk factor for chronic renal failure: A comparison with phenacetin. Am. J. Kidney Dis. *28*:S7, 1996.

Eckert, D. E., Jonutis, A. J., and Davidson, A. J.: The incidence and manifestations of urographic papillary abnormalities in patients with S-hemoglobinopathies. Radiology *113*:59, 1974.

Elseviers, M.M., Deschepper, A., Corthouts, R., Bosmans, J.L., Cosyn, L., Lins, R.L., Lornoy, W., Matthys, E., Roose, R., Van Caesbroeck, D., et al.: High diagnostic performance of CT scan for analgesic nephropathy in patients with incipient to severe renal failure. Kidney Int. *48*:1316, 1995.

Handa, S. P., and Tewari, H. D.: Urinary tract carcinoma in patients with analgesic nephropathy. Nephron *28*:62, 1981.

Hartman, G. W., Torres, V. E., Leago, G. F., Williamson, B., Jr., and Hattery, R. R.: Analgesic-associated nephropathy: Pathophysiological and radiological correlation. JAMA *251*:1734, 1984.

Heptinstall, R. H. (ed.): Pathology of the Kidney, 4th ed. Boston, Little, Brown & Co., 1992.

Hoffman, J. C., Schnur, M. J., and Koenigsberg, M.: Demonstration of renal papillary necrosis by sonography. Radiology *145*:785, 1982.

Johansson, S., Angervall, L., Bengtsson, U., and Wahlqvist, L.: Uroepithelial tumors of the renal pelvis associated with abuse of phenacetin-containing analgesics. Cancer *33*:743, 1974.

Lindvall, N.: Radiological changes of renal papillary necrosis. Kidney Int. *13*:93, 1978.

Longacre, A. M., and Popky, G. L.: Papillary necrosis in patients with cirrhosis: A study of 102 patients. J. Urol. *99*:391, 1968.

McCall, I. W., Moule, N., Desai, P., and Serjeant, G. R.: Urographic findings in homozygous sickle cell disease. Radiology *126*:99, 1978.

McCredie, M., Coates, M. S., Ford, J. M., Disney, A. P. S., Auld, J. J., and Stewart, J. H.: Geographic distribution of cancers of the kidney and urinary tract and analgesic nephropathy in Australia and New Zealand. Aust. N. Z. J. Med. *20*:684, 1990.

Palmer, B.F., and Henrich, W.L.: Clinical acute renal failure with nonsteroidal anti-inflammatory drugs. Semin. Nephrol. *15*:214, 1995.

Palmer, B. F., and Henrich, W. L.: Nephrotoxicity of nonsteroidal anti-inflammatory agents, analgesics, and angiotensin-converting enzyme inhibitors. In Schrier, R. W., and Gottschalk, C. W. (eds.): Diseases of the Kidney, 6th ed. Boston, Little, Brown, and Co., 1997, pp. 1167–1188.

Pandya, K. K., Koshy, M., Brown, N., and Presman, D.: Renal papillary necrosis in sickle cell hemoglobinopathies. J. Urol. *115*:497, 1976.

Perneger, T.V., Whelton, P.K., and Klag, M.J.: Risk of kidney failure associated with the use of acetaminophen, aspirin, and nonsteroidal antiinflammatory drugs. N. Engl. J. Med. *331*:1675, 1994.

Poynter, J. D., and Hare, W. S. C.: Necrosis *in situ*: A form of renal papillary necrosis seen in analgesic nephropathy. Radiology *111*:69, 1974.

Puvaneswary, M., and Segasothy, M.: Analgesic nephropathy: Ultrasonic features. Aust. Radiol. *32*:247, 1988.

Roberts, G. M., Evans, K. T., Bloom, A. L., and Al-Gailani, F.: Renal papillary necrosis in haemophilia and Christmas disease. Clin. Radiol. *34*:201, 1983.

Ronco, P.M., and Flahault, A.E.: Drug-induced end stage renal disease. N. Engl. J. Med. *331*:1711, 1994.

Sabatini, S.: Pathophysiologic mechanisms in analgesic-induced papillary necrosis. Am. J. Kidney Dis. *28*:S34, 1996.

Sandler, D. P., Burr, R., and Weinberg, C.R.: Nonsteroidal anti-inflammatory drugs and the risk for chronic renal disease. Ann. Intern. Med. *115*:165, 1991.

Talner, L. B., Webb, J. A. W., and Dail, D. H.: Lacunae: A urographic finding in chronic obstructive uropathy. AJR *156*:985, 1991.

Ulreich, S.: Ultrasound in the evaluation of renal papillary necrosis. Radiology *148*:864, 1983.

Wagner, E. H.: Nonsteroidal anti-inflammatory drugs and renal disease: Still unsettled (editorial). Ann. Intern. Med. *115*:227, 1991.

Walker, T.M., and Serjeant, G.R.: Increased renal reflectivity in sickle cell disease: Prevalence and characteristics. Clinical Radiol. *50*:566, 1995.

Weber, M., Braun, B., and Kohler, H.: Ultrasonic findings in analgesic nephropathy. Nephron *39*:216, 1985.

Whelton, A., and Hamilton, C. W.: Nonsteroidal anti-inflammatory drugs: Effects on kidney function. J. Clin. Pharmacol. *31*:588, 1991.

Zwergel, U. E., Zwergel, T. B. H., Neisius, D. A., and Ziegler, M.: Effects of prostaglandin synthetase inhibitors on the upper urinary tract. Urol. Res. *18*:429, 1990.

Tuberculosis

Bloom, S., Wechsler, H., and Lattimer, J. K.: Results of long term study of non-functioning tuberculous kidneys. J. Urol. *104*:654, 1970.

Cremin, B. J.: Radiological imaging of urogenital tuberculosis in children with emphasis on ultrasound. Pediatr. Radiol. *17*:34, 1987.

Goldman, S. M., Fishman, E. K., Hartman, D. S., Kim, Y. C., and Siegelman, S. S.: Computed tomography of renal tuberculosis and its pathological correlates. J. Comput. Assist. Tomogr. *9*:771, 1985.

Kollins, S. A., Hartman, G. W., Carr, D. T., Segura, J. W., and Hattery, R. R.: Roentgenographic findings in urinary tract tuberculosis: A 10-year review. AJR *121*:487, 1974.

Lattimer, J. K.: Renal tuberculosis. N. Engl. J. Med. *273*:208, 1965.

Michigan, S.: Genitourinary fungal infection. J. Urol. *116*:390, 1976.

Pasternack, M. S., and Rubin, R. H.: Urinary tract tuberculosis. *In* Schrier, R. W., and Gottschalk, C. W. (eds.): Diseases of the Kidney, 6th ed. Boston, Little, Brown & Co., 1997, pp. 989–1011.

Petereit, M. F.: Chronic renal brucellosis: A simulator of tuberculosis. Radiology *96*:85, 1970.

THE PELVOCALYCEAL SYSTEM AND URETER

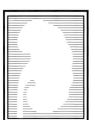

14

Intraluminal Abnormalities

UROLITHIASIS
BLOOD CLOT
TISSUE SLOUGH
   Renal Papillary Necrosis
   Cholesteatoma

FUNGUS BALL
FOREIGN MATERIAL
DIFFERENTIAL DIAGNOSIS

Abnormalities may develop within the pelvocalyceal and ureteral lumen without any attachment to the uroepithelial lining. Such precise localization is possible when an abnormality either is completely surrounded by contrast material or moves as the patient's position is altered (Figs. 14–1 and 14–2). Localization may be difficult or impossible when an intraluminal lesion is bulky enough to prevent opacified urine from surrounding it.

Adequate distention of the pelvocalyceal system or ureter and spatial reconstruction are essential mea-

sures in the accurate assessment of both mural and intraluminal abnormalities of the collecting system or ureter. During excretory urography or computed tomography, distention of the pelvocalyceal system and ureter is accomplished by either contrast material–induced diuresis, abdominal compression, or both. An oral or intravenous fluid load serves the same purpose for ultrasonography. Spatial reconstruction, which is inherent in computed tomography and ultrasonography, can be achieved indirectly from radiographs by obtaining more than one projection.

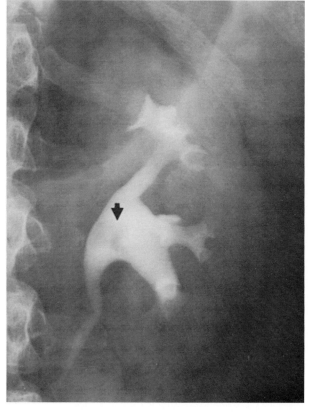

FIGURE 14–1. Uric acid stone in a 45-year-old patient undergoing treatment for non-Hodgkin's lymphoma. The stone *(arrow)* is completely surrounded by contrast material, establishing its intraluminal location. The stone was nonopaque on the preliminary film. Excretory urogram.

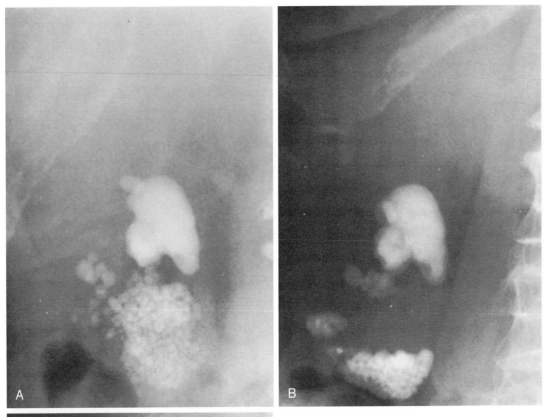

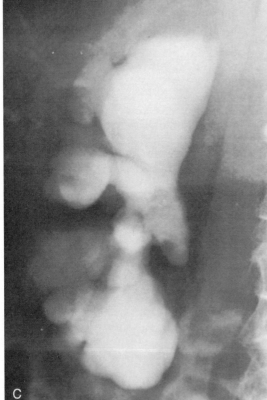

FIGURE 14–2. Multiple stones in a markedly dilated lower pole calyx. Staghorn calculus is at the ureteropelvic junction. The intraluminal location of the calyceal stones is established by their shifts as the patient's position is changed.

    A, Preliminary film, supine position.

    B, Preliminary film, upright position.

    C, Excretory urogram. Contrast material surrounds and obscures the stones.

UROLITHIASIS

Definition

Urolithiasis, or stone formation in the upper urinary tract, results from a complex series of incompletely understood events. This section covers stone formation and growth, the site of calculogenesis, and chemical composition.

Formation and Growth. Stones form in the kidney as crystalline aggregates with an ordered internal structure and growth pattern. Stone formation occurs mainly as a function of the level of saturation of a given ion or molecule in the urine. This, in turn, reflects either excessive renal excretion of the substance or reduced urine volume. When a substance can no longer remain in solution, precipitation and crystallization occur. In a biologic fluid, such as urine, this process is influenced significantly by pH, temperature, and urine volume as well as by the presence of stone "inhibitors."

The earliest step in calculogenesis is nucleation, which is the formation of the smallest crystal into a solid particle by the coming together of specific ions or molecules from a supersaturated state in the urine. This usually occurs on a nidus of noncrystalline organic and inorganic material. In some instances, a crystal of one type will be deposited on the surface of another type owing to similarities of crystalline lattice structure. This phenomenon, known as *epitaxy*, is of particular importance in the deposition of calcium oxalate crystals on a uric acid nucleus.

The physicochemical roles of supersaturation and pH are predominant in the formation of stones that are composed of uric acid, magnesium ammonium phosphate, and cystine. Urinary pH determines the concentration levels at which crystallization occurs. Uric acid and cystine stones form in acid urine and may be dissolved if the urine is alkalinized for a period of time. Alkaline conditions favor formation of magnesium ammonium phosphate and some mixed calcium phosphate stones.

Calcium calculogenesis is influenced significantly by stone inhibition factors and epitaxy as well as by supersaturation and pH. Normal urine contains substances that inhibit calculogenesis. Magnesium citrate and pyrophosphate are thought to inhibit growth of calcium phosphate crystals. Organic macromolecules resembling acid mucopolysaccharide probably exert a similar effect on calcium oxalate stone formation. Although the role of crystal inhibitors in stone formation has not been fully established, these substances may be deficient in patients in whom calcium stones form.

Two additional circumstances that favor stone formation and growth are urinary stasis and foreign material in the collecting system.

Site of Calculogenesis. In addition to an environment of maximal ionic or molecular concentration, stone formation requires a special sequestered site. The embryonic microcrystal must be protected against the normal flushing of the pelvocalyceal system by flowing urine. Several stone growth centers have been proposed: small, crystal-laden calyceal submucosal plaques (Randall's plaques), derived from tissue damaged by prior infection, toxic agents, or ischemia; the ostia of collecting tubules where minute crystals are impacted; forniceal lymphatics (Carr's pouches); and various sites in the nephron and the collecting duct. The concept of a protected stone growth center is supported by the deformity consistently found on the external surface of many calcium oxalate stones. This suggests attachment to a surface, perhaps the papillary tip, during nucleation and growth. After reaching a critical size, the stone is shed into the pelvocalyceal system.

Chemical Composition. Calculi are polycrystalline conglomerates that are composed of minerals (approximately 95 per cent) and organic matrix. Matrix, predominantly mucoprotein with lesser amounts of mucopolysaccharide, appears as concentric laminations, radial striations, or spherules in all stones. The role of matrix in calculogenesis is uncertain. It is possible that it is a template (nidus) for crystal growth, an inert coprecipitate of mineral crystals, or a marker of the site on the pyramid or calyx where nucleation and growth first occurred.

Approximately 90 per cent of stones found in the North American population contain calcium. Of these, about two-thirds are calcium oxalate monohydrate (crystal name, whewellite), calcium oxalate dihydrate (crystal name, wedellite), or mixed calcium phosphate. Pure calcium phosphate (crystal name, apatite) and pure or mixed calcium hydrogen phosphate (crystal name, brushite) account for less than 6 per cent of stones. The remaining calcium-containing stones are composed of magnesium ammonium phosphate (crystal name, struvite), and in most of these stones there is also either calcium phosphate or calcium oxalate.

Approximately 10 per cent of stones are calcium free—most of them are uric acid or cystine. Pure stones of magnesium ammonium phosphate or xanthine and matrix stones are rare, as are stones of silicates, dihydroxyadenine, and drug metabolites. A summary of the mineral composition of stones is contained in Table 14–1.

Clinical Setting

Most patients with calcium oxalate or calcium phosphate stones in industrialized countries have no identifiable underlying metabolic abnormality. The patient with *idiopathic urolithiasis* is usually male and has normal serum phosphate levels. Urinary calcium excretion is normal in up to 50 per cent of these patients. Possible factors responsible for stone formation in this group include deficiency of urine inhibitors, induction of uric acid nucleation by dietary hyperuricuria, idiopathic hyperoxaluria, or inability to acidify urine normally. The remainder of patients with idiopathic urolithiasis are hypercalciuric. Speculation on the cause of hypercalciuria has

TABLE 14–1. Mineral Composition of Renal Calculi

CRYSTAL NAME	CHEMICAL NAME	APPROXIMATE FREQUENCY (%)	ASSOCIATED WITH INFECTION	RADIOGRAPHIC OPACITY
Whewellite	Calcium oxalate monohydrate	34	No	+ + +
Wedellite	Calcium oxalate dihydrate			
	Calcium oxalate plus apatite	34	Occasionally	+ + +
Apatite, brushite, whitlockite	Calcium phosphate	6	Occasionally	+ + +
Struvite	Magnesium ammonium phosphate	1	Yes	− *
	Magnesium ammonium phosphate plus calcium phosphate	14	Yes	+ +
Uric acid, urate	Uric acid, urate	7	No	− *
Cystine	Cystine	3	No	+
(None)	Mucoprotein/mucopolysaccharide (matrix)	Rare	Yes	− *
Xanthine	Xanthine	Very rare	No	− *

*Calculi become radiographically opaque when mixed with calcium oxalate or calcium phosphate. All calculi that are nonopaque by film radiography are opaque when imaged by computed tomography.

focused on increased intestinal calcium absorption ("absorptive hypercalciuria") and increased immunoreactive parathyroid hormone secretion due to a primary renal "leakage" of calcium. In the last analysis, the diagnosis of idiopathic urolithiasis rests on the exclusion of one of the known metabolic causes, which are discussed subsequently.

Stones that form in patients with *hypercalcemia* are most often calcium phosphate and only occasionally calcium oxalate. Primary hyperparathyroidism, prolonged immobilization, milk-alkali syndrome, sarcoidosis, hypervitaminosis D, neoplastic disorders, Cushing's syndrome or disease, and hyperthyroidism may all lead to hypercalcemia and stone formation. Primary hyperparathyroidism is most frequently associated with urolithiasis.

Hyperoxaluria, either primary or secondary, also causes urolithiasis. Primary hyperoxalosis is a rare autosomal recessive inherited enzyme disorder of glyoxalate metabolism. Two forms exist. Type I, the more common of the two, causes glycolic aciduria; Type II is characterized by L-glyceric aciduria. Both cause hyperoxaluria, calcium oxalate urolithiasis, and nephrocalcinosis through increased production of endogenous oxalate. Death from renal failure usually occurs before the age of 60 years in the absence of renal dialysis.

Secondary, or acquired, hyperoxaluria occurs with conditions that cause malabsorption, rapid transit of enteric contents, and steatorrhea. These conditions include jejunoileal bypass surgery, ileal resection, and blind loop syndrome. Here, excessive intestinal fat binds intraluminal calcium ions that would normally combine with oxalate to form insoluble calcium oxalate and be eliminated in the feces. Instead, oxalate remains soluble and is absorbed in excessive amounts on reaching the colon. Hyperoxaluria and urinary tract calcium oxalate stone formation follow. These events require an intact colon.

In a nonspecific way, other chronic gastrointestinal disorders are also associated with urolithiasis, especially mixed uric acid stones. Diarrhea and op-

erations such as ileostomy induce intestinal urate and bicarbonate loss, leading to low volumes of acidic urine. Adrenocortical steroids, prolonged bedrest, and infection also predispose the patient to mixed uric acid and calcium oxalate stones. Pure uric acid stones are uncommon in these patients.

Uric acid urolithiasis is usually found in men older than 50 years without gout or any recognizable disorder of purine metabolism. Serum and urinary uric acid levels are normal. Only 25 per cent of patients with gout develop uric acid stones. Myeloproliferative disorders are associated with uric acid stones due to hyperuricemia and hyperuricuria from increased purine metabolism. Cell breakdown following chemotherapy or radiation therapy further increases the likelihood of uric acid stone formation and acute urate nephropathy.

Cystinuria is an inherited autosomal disorder of amino acid transport in the renal tubule, causing impaired reabsorption of cystine, ornithine, lysine, and arginine. The only recognized clinical consequence is cystine urolithiasis, which typically begins in the second decade of life.

Xanthinuria is a very rare autosomal recessive inherited deficiency of xanthine oxidase resulting in increased urinary excretion of xanthine and hypoxanthine. Calculi form in approximately one-third of affected patients.

Urinary tract infection may lead to magnesium ammonium phosphate (struvite) stones. *Proteus mirabilis* is the most common organism associated with urolithiasis, but some forms of *Pseudomonas aeruginosa, Klebsiella* species, *Escherichia coli,* and *Staphylococcus aureus* create conditions favorable to stone formation. These bacteria produce urease, which catalyzes the formation of ammonia from urea. Hydrolysis of ammonia produces hydroxyl (OH^-) and ammonium (NH_4^+) ions, rendering the infected urine alkaline and, in turn, increasing the concentration of trivalent phosphate ion (PO_4^{3-}). A supersaturated solution of magnesium ammonium phosphate results. High urinary pH also promotes crystallization of hydroxyapatite, which is commonly incorporated in the struvite stone. Pure matrix stones have also been described with infection, but these are very rare.

Partial urinary stasis favors stone formation by causing retention of crystal aggregates and other potential niduses. Urolithiasis does not occur with complete obstruction in the absence of infection, since no precipitating solute is excreted. Stones formed as a result of partial obstruction are usually calcium phosphate, although any of the crystal systems may participate.

Any of the metabolic conditions responsible for nephrocalcinosis also favor *de novo* formation of pelvocalyceal stones. Sometimes, the stone is simply an extrusion of a concretion originally formed in the renal parenchyma as, for example, in medullary sponge kidney. Parenchymal calcification in distal renal tubular acidosis is particularly exuberant and also frequently leads to free stones in the collecting system.

Stones may cause acute clinical symptoms. The most dramatic is renal colic, a crescendo-decrescendo pattern of pain in the flank and lateral abdomen that often radiates into the groin, scrotum, or labia. Hematuria is usually present. Occasionally, stone disease presents as symptoms of acute or chronic urinary tract infection.

Radiologic Findings

Radiography. Detection of small opaque stones is critically dependent on proper radiographic technique. The lowest feasible kilovoltage must be used to enhance density discrimination. Careful coning of the x-ray beam enhances sharpness by reducing scattered radiation. The use of clean intensifying screens eliminates artifacts resembling stones.

Proving that a density is truly within the kidney requires either a tomogram or a constant spatial relationship between the kidney and the apparent stone in two radiographic projections. In addition to the standard frontal projection, the patient should be examined in a 30-degree posterior oblique position toward the side of suspected stone, to distinguish a kidney stone from calcification in arteries, lymph nodes, rib cartilage, and gallbladder or from opaque ingested material in the bowel (Fig. 14–3).

Tomography is an important adjunct in the evaluation of kidney stones. It can be used instead of an oblique view to clarify a suspicious shadow that is seen on an initial radiograph (see Fig. 14–3). In the quest for a small stone in a patient with a strongly suggestive history, standard radiographs may be negative or suboptimal because of intestinal contents. Here, too, tomography may be of value. A range of 60 to 75 kV with a variable milliampere-second, careful coning of the x-ray beam, and the selection of an adequate number of levels to ensure proper sampling of the kidney determine whether the use of tomography will be successful.

The radiographic appearance of a stone depends on its composition. Some stones are very dense in their entirety. Others are mixed, with a central radiodense nidus; have a homogeneous intermediate radiodensity; or are nonopaque.

The radiologic search for an opaque kidney stone must be conducted before the injection of contrast material, since radiodense calcium stones will be invisible in the midst of opaque urine (Fig. 14–4; see also Fig. 14–6). Standard radiographic technique can detect opaque stones as small as 1 mm, although, in reality, obscuring bowel contents decrease the sensitivity of this modality. Mixed composition stones with a central deposit of dense calcium appear as a radiolucency that is much larger than expected on the basis of the size of the calcium density alone (Fig. 14–5). Cystine stones or struvite or uric acid calculi with small amounts of calcium have an intermediate, homogeneous density. These are slightly radiodense on preliminary films but appear radiolucent once the urine is opacified. Radiopaque ureteral stones, like kidney stones, can be detected by radiographic techniques. However, once a stone enters the ureter from the pelvocalyceal system, confirmation of its location requires opacification of the ureter, since there is no longer a closely related structure such as the kidney to serve as a spatial reference (Fig. 14–6). Nonopaque stones are revealed as radiolucent filling defects only after opacification of the pelvocalyceal system or ureter and are not detectable on preliminary films (see Fig. 14–1).

A stone that is free within the collecting system is surrounded by contrast material in all projections. A small stone may be round, smooth, or jagged. Rapidly growing stones tend to branch and may fill the entire pelvocalyceal system, forming a so-called branched or staghorn calculus (Fig. 14–7). Stones may be solitary or multiple and are found anywhere in the collecting system. Stones obstruct when they impact at points of narrowing, such as an infundibulum, the ureteropelvic junction, the point where the ureter crosses the iliac vessels, or, most commonly, the insertion of the distal ureter into the bladder, causing distention proximally (see Figs. 14–2 and 14–7). When stones move, intermittent obstruction may result.

Calcium oxalate and *calcium phosphate* stones are the most opaque and typically are uniformly dense (see Fig. 14–3). These stones vary in size but only rarely reach staghorn proportions. In some metabolic disorders, pelvocalyceal calculi coexist with nephrocalcinosis (Fig. 14–8).

Uric acid stone is nonopaque on standard radiography when pure (see Fig. 14–1). When uric acid stones are enlarged beyond 2 cm, they tend to become faintly dense, owing to impurities that have been incorporated into the lattice of the stone. Tomography is sometimes needed to demonstrate this low level of opacity. With rapid growth, a uric acid stone may form a cast of the pelvocalyceal system.

Cystine stones, when pure, are homogeneous and appear as a "frosted" or "ground-glass" radiodensity

Text continued on page 371

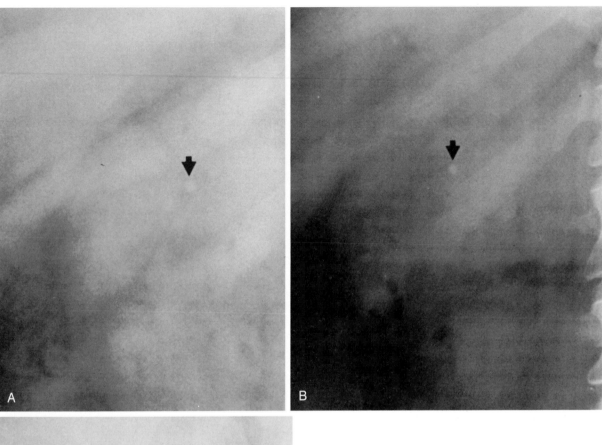

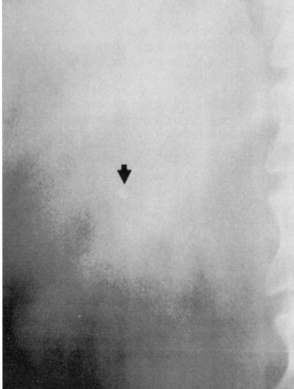

FIGURE 14–3. The position of this calcium oxalate stone *(arrow)* remains constant relative to the kidney on both frontal and oblique films, establishing its intrarenal location.

A, Preliminary film, anteroposterior projection.

B, Preliminary film, right posterior oblique projection.

C, Preliminary film, tomogram. Kidney localization can be established by demonstrating that both the stone *(arrow)* and the kidney are in focus at the same level.

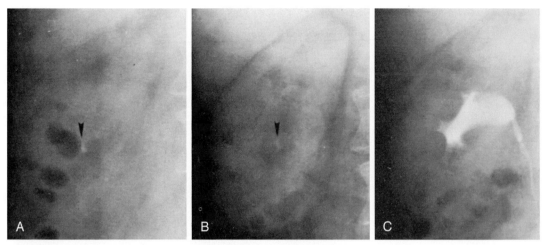

FIGURE 14–4. Radiopaque calculus obscured following injection of contrast material.
A, Preliminary film. The stone *(arrow)* overlies the region of the renal pelvis.
B, Excretory urogram, 1-minute film. The nephrogram does not affect the appearance of the stone *(arrow).*
C, Excretory urogram, 10-minute film. The stone is obscured by contrast material in the renal pelvis.

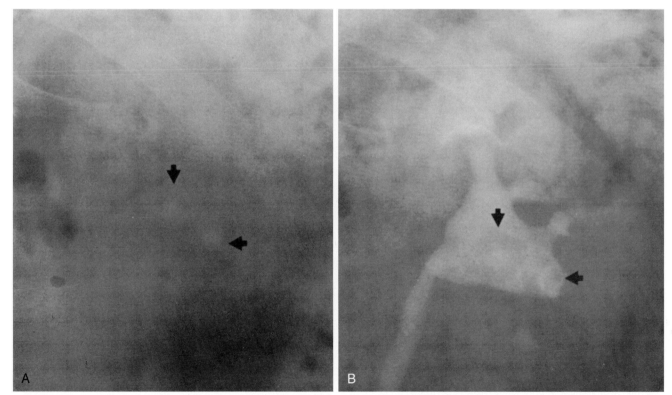

FIGURE 14–5. The size of a calculus of mixed composition is often larger than that suggested by the focal, central deposit of calcium.
A, Preliminary film. Two calculi *(arrows)* are present over the renal pelvic area. A faint band of surrounding density is suggested.
B, Excretory urogram. Opacified urine surrounding the stones reveals a thick mantle of stone material that is radiolucent relative to opacified urine *(arrows).*

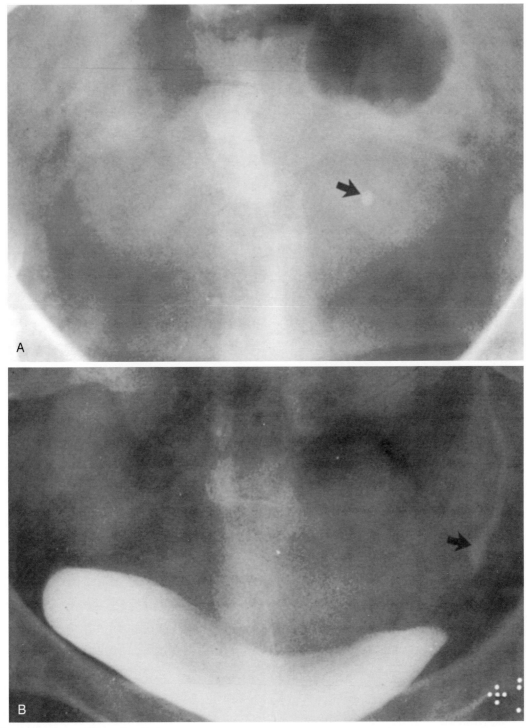

FIGURE 14–6. Radiopaque calculus, distal left ureter.
   A, Preliminary radiograph. The stone *(arrow)* is identified by its density, but its position relative to the urinary tract cannot be determined.
   B, Excretory urogram. Contrast material in the ureter surrounds and obscures the stone *(arrow),* which does not obstruct the ureter.

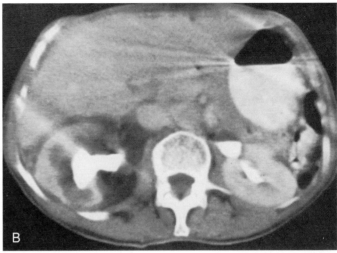

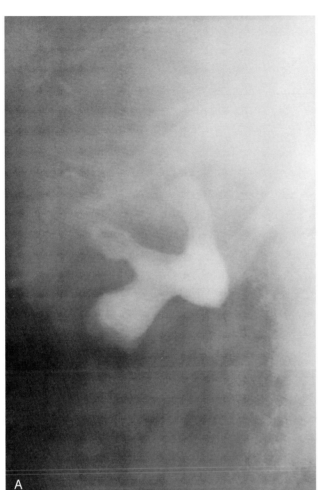

FIGURE 14–7. Staghorn struvite calculus with laminated pattern. Rapid growth of a stone leads to a branched shape that may fill the pelvocalyceal system.

A, Preliminary film.

B, Computed tomogram, contrast material–enhanced. The staghorn calculus causes chronic obstructive uropathy with diminished excretion of contrast material by the right kidney. Dilated calyces are represented by low-density areas surrounding the calculus. Low density in the parapelvic area probably represents a urinoma.

(Courtesy of Joy Price, M.D., Alta Bates Medical Center, Berkeley, California.)

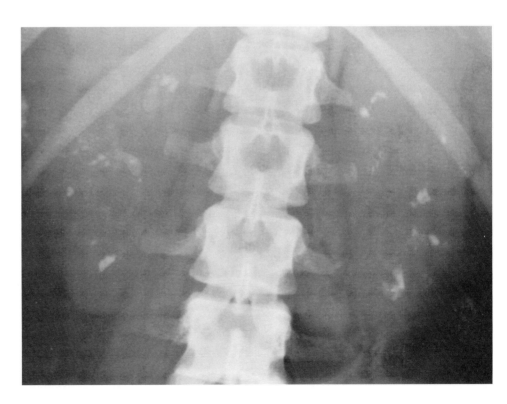

FIGURE 14–8. Urolithiasis in a 25-year-old woman with nephrocalcinosis due to renal tubular acidosis. Extensive deposits of calcium are present in the collecting system and renal parenchyma. Preliminary film. Same patient is illustrated in Figure 13–4. (Courtesy of Department of Diagnostic Radiology, Hammersmith Hospital, Royal Postgraduate Medical School, London, England.)

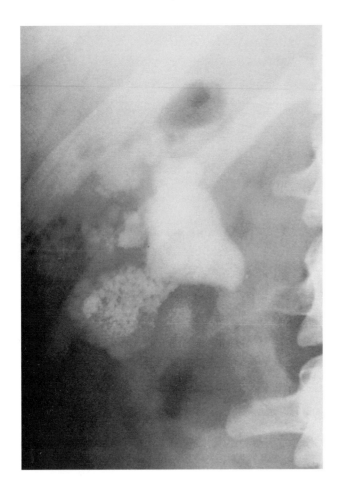

FIGURE 14–9. Pure cystine calculi in an 18-year-old man with elevated urinary cystine excretion and a family history of cystinuria. The radiographic density of these stones varies from faintly opaque to dense. Preliminary film. (Courtesy of Joy Price, M.D., Alta Bates Medical Center, Berkeley, California.)

FIGURE 14–10. Urolithiasis producing bright echoes and a sharply marginated acoustic shadow. Ultrasonogram, transverse section.

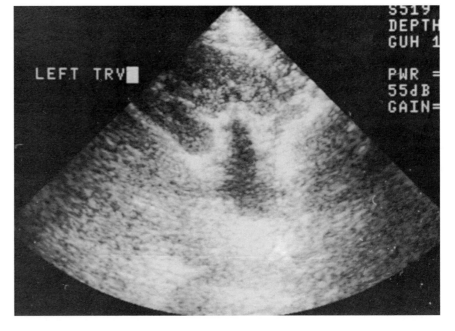

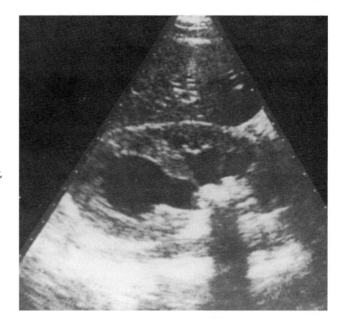

FIGURE 14–11. Calculus, ureteropelvic junction, left kidney, causing hydronephrosis. Ultrasonogram, transverse projection. The stone is highly echogenic and produces a sharply marginated acoustic shadow. (Kindly provided by Ulrike Hamper, M.D., and Sheila Sheth, M.D., The Johns Hopkins University, Baltimore, Maryland.)

intermediate between calcium and water on plain radiographs. Radiodensity, which is caused by the sulfur content of cystine, increases with size (Fig. 14–9) and laminations are absent. When small, a cystine stone is difficult to detect by radiography.

Xanthine calculus, a rare occurrence, is nonopaque, although as with uric acid stones, incorporation of impurities can result in faint, uniform opacity.

Struvite or *infection* stones have a radiographic density that is determined by the amount of calcium incorporated in the magnesium ammonium phosphate. Calcium phosphate often precipitates in layers, producing a characteristic laminated pattern of alternating bands of radiodensity and relative

radiolucency. A staghorn configuration is common (see Fig. 14–7).

Pure matrix stone is another very rare form of nonopaque calculus, but impurities may give it a stippled appearance. Typically, matrix stones are large, branched structures, but uncommonly they are small and multiple.

Ultrasonography. Stones, except for those composed of matrix as commented upon subsequently, attenuate and reflect sound. Strong echoes and a sharply marginated acoustic shadow are the ultrasonographic features that distinguish stones from other filling defects in the pelvocalyceal system and ureter (Figs. 14–10 through 14–12). Unfortunately,

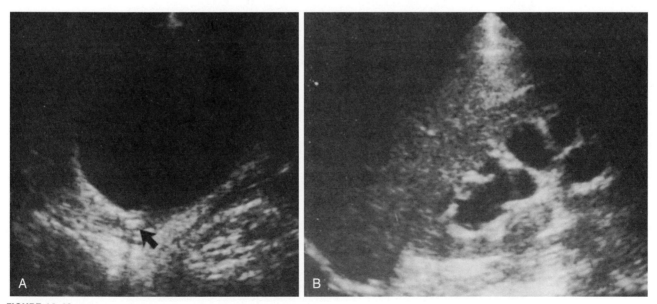

FIGURE 14–12. Calculus, distal right ureter, causing hydronephrosis. Ultrasonogram, longitudinal sections.
   A, Distal ureter. The small stone *(arrow)* is echogenic and produces some acoustic shadow. Because of the small size of the stone, however, the margins of the acoustic shadow are not sharp.
   B, Kidney. There is marked dilatation of the pelvocalyceal system.
   (Kindly provided by Ulrike Hamper, M.D., and Sheila Sheth, M.D., The Johns Hopkins University, Baltimore, Maryland.)

however, several factors may mask these features and make diagnosis by ultrasonography difficult. First, the strong echo of a stone lying centrally in a nondilated pelvis may not be discriminated from the echoes generated by the normal renal sinus. Second, stones produce a characteristic sharply marginated acoustic shadow with few, if any, low-level echoes only when the calculus is within the focal zone of the transducer and is comparable in size to the width of the incident ultrasound beam. A final potential source of error is in the ultrasonographic diagnosis of matrix stones. Limited experience suggests that a matrix stone produces low-level echoes and no acoustic shadow, regardless of size. In general, however, it is clear that although stones as small as 2 mm have been detected by ultrasonography under optimal conditions, the likelihood of error varies inversely with the size of the calculus. In females, transvaginal ultrasonography may be of value in detecting a distal ureteral stone.

Gas within the pelvocalyceal system or ureter can be confused with stone, since both conditions cause bright echoes and an acoustic shadow. However, the acoustic shadow from gas is less sharply marginated than that from stone and contains high-level reverberation echoes.

Computed Tomography. Computed tomography, like ultrasonography, detects urinary tract calculi and plays a major role in the differential diagnosis of nonopaque filling defects, especially in the pelvocalyceal system. Greater density discrimination accounts for the advantage of computed tomog-

raphy over standard radiography. Stones that are nonopaque (uric acid) or faintly opaque (cystine) by the latter technique are visually as dense as calcium-containing stones when imaged by computed tomography using standard windows (Figs. 14–13 and 14–14). However, their actual attenuation values are in a lower range than those of stone composed of calcium. Limited experience suggests that matrix stone does not have increased attenuation compared with soft tissue on computed tomography, the only apparent exception to the usual appearance of nonopaque stones on computed tomography. Calcium-containing stones are readily recognized on computed tomography by their high attenuation value (Fig. 14–15).

Stones smaller than the thickness of the computed tomographic section can be misregistered owing to partial volume effect, obscuring the true nature of the density. A thin collimator and contiguous sections minimize this source of error.

As discussed in Chapter 9, helical (spiral) computed tomography is of particular value in detecting acute obstruction caused by a ureteral stone (see Fig. 9–30). Unenhanced, contiguous helical 5-mm sections rapidly attained from kidney to bladder permit identification of the ureter as well as an obstructing calculus. This technique is superior to both ultrasonography and excretory urography in identifying a ureteral calculus and distinguishing a calculus from calcification that is not in the urinary tract, such as phleboliths or granulomatous lymph nodes.

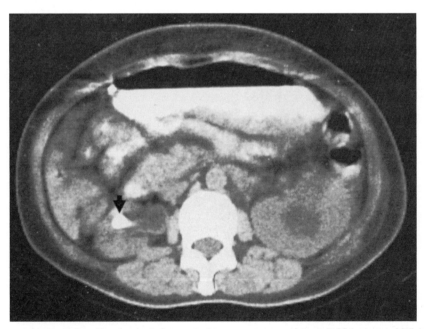

FIGURE 14–13. Cystine stone in the right calyx *(arrow).* Computed tomogram, unenhanced. (Courtesy of Michael Federle, M.D., University of Pittsburgh, Pittsburgh, Pennsylvania.)

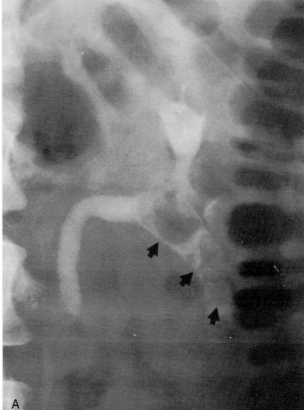

FIGURE 14–14. Multiple pure uric acid stones in the left pelvocalyceal system. The stones were not seen on the preliminary film and appear as nonopaque intraluminal filling defects during excretory urography. High attenuation values are noted by computed tomography.

A, Excretory urogram. Numerous nonopaque stones fill the pelvocalyceal system *(arrows).*

B, Computed tomogram without contrast material enhancement.

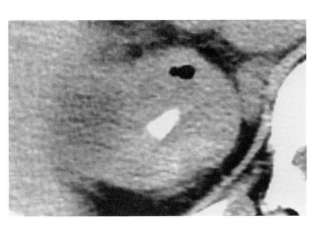

FIGURE 14–15. Cystine staghorn calculus in a patient with xanthogranulomatous pyelonephritis. Computed tomogram, unenhanced. The calcium content of the calculus yields a high attenuation value.

BLOOD CLOT

Definition

Blood clots form in the pelvocalyceal system when the volume of blood lost is large enough to cause stasis and activation of the clotting mechanism. The result is a nonopaque intraluminal mass that can obstruct the ureteropelvic junction or the ureter. Lysis occurs within 2 weeks, but, rarely, a fibrin mass remains, and this may eventually calcify.

Clots in the collecting system may develop simultaneously with bleeding into the renal parenchyma, the subcapsular space, the pelvocalyceal wall, or the retroperitoneal spaces.

Clinical Setting

The causes of urinary tract bleeding include trauma (blunt, penetrating, or iatrogenic); tumors of the kidney parenchyma, pelvocalyceal system, or ureter; nephritis and vasculitis; arteriovenous malformation or hemangioma; rupture of an arterial aneurysm; renal venous congestion; bleeding disorders; and anticoagulant therapy. Occasionally, hematuria with clot formation is idiopathic.

The radiologist should be on guard for patients who bleed after mild trauma or during the course of anticoagulant therapy when bleeding and coagulation times are within the therapeutic range. A renal tumor, congenital anomaly, or other abnormality is sometimes discovered in this way.

Clots in the pelvocalyceal system are asymptomatic unless they obstruct the pelvocalyceal system or ureter. Other signs and symptoms reflect the event that initiated the bleeding.

Radiologic Findings

In the absence of additional bleeding, blood clots become significantly smaller or disappear within 2 weeks of formation (Fig. 14–16). This unique feature aids in the differential diagnosis of nonopaque lesions of the upper urinary tract. Otherwise, blood clots exhibit radiographic features that are common to other nonopaque intraluminal lesions. Opaque urine outlines sharp margins and may dissect between clumps of clot (Fig. 14–17). The location of the clot varies with time or with a change in the position of the patient. In major hemorrhage, the clot may form a cast of the entire pelvocalyceal system, giving rise to a hand-in-glove appearance (see Fig. 29–7). Obstruction often accompanies blood clot in the upper urinary tract (see Fig. 14–16).

When a clot persists as a mass of fibrin, faintly opaque calcification may develop that resembles some urinary stones or calcified uroepithelial tumors (Fig. 14–18). This development has been described principally in patients with calcium oxalate stones after pelvic lithotomy and may reflect a specific metabolic disorder in these patients.

The ultrasonographic image of clot is a mass composed of low-level echoes that separate the strong echoes of the central sinus complex (see Fig. 14–

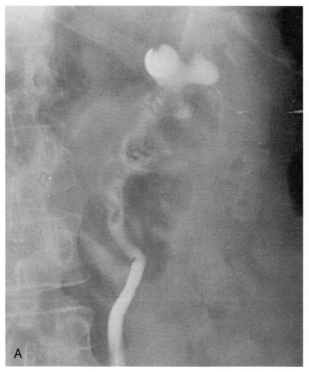
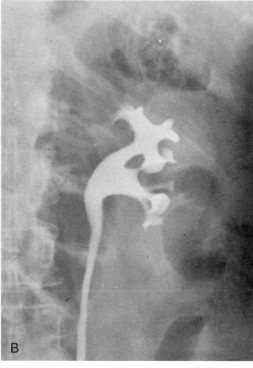

FIGURE 14–16. Blood clot, left renal pelvis and proximal ureter. Retrograde pyelograms.
A, Initial study demonstrates a worm-like filling defect in the pelvis and proximal ureter with some obstruction.
B, Examination performed 1 week later demonstrates complete disappearance of the clot.

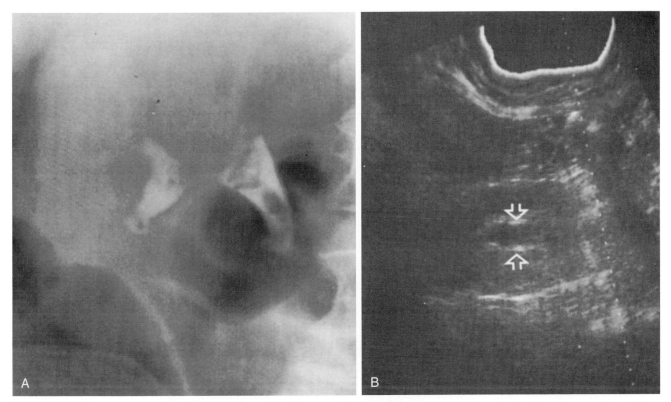

FIGURE 14–17. Blood clot in a 64-year-old woman with diabetes mellitus and severe acute pyelonephritis. Bleeding was thought to be due to renal papillary necrosis associated with the acute pyelonephritis.

A, Excretory urogram. Blood clots are of multiple size and shape. Note extension of opacified urine between the clumps of clot.

B, Ultrasonogram, longitudinal section. A mass of low-level echoes *(arrows)* separates the high-level echoes of the central sinus complex. There is no acoustic shadowing.

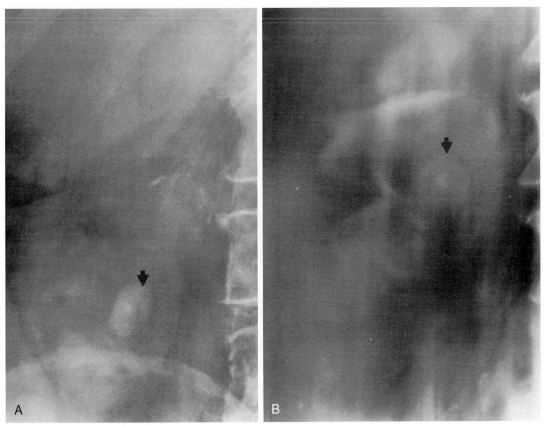

FIGURE 14–18. Calcified fibrinous mass developing as a residual complication of prior blood clot, pathologically confirmed following nephrectomy.

A, Preliminary film. *Arrow* identifies circumscribed area of calcification.

B, Excretory urogram. Tomogram. A large nonopaque mass of fibrin fills the pelvocalyceal system. Focus of calcification is centrally located *(arrow).*

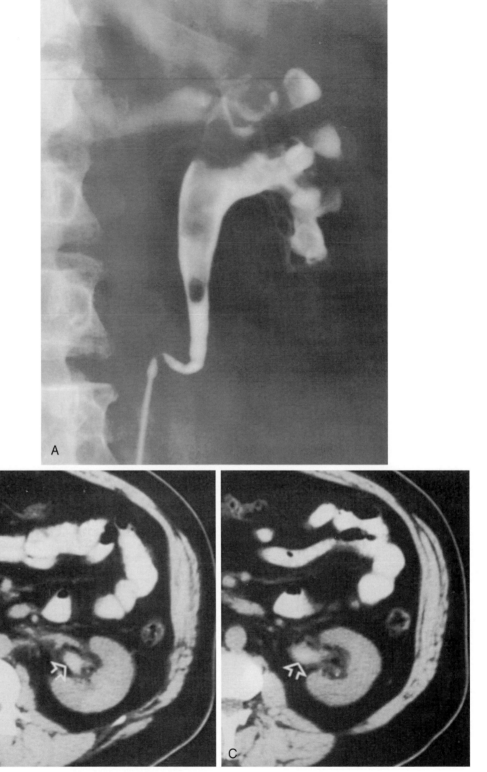

FIGURE 14–19. Blood clot recently formed in a 58-year-old man with gross hematuria due to an occult adenocarcinoma of the kidney.

A, Retrograde pyelogram. The clot forms as a nonopaque filling defect in the shape of a cast of the pelvis.

B and *C,* Computed tomograms without contrast material enhancement in two contiguous transverse planes. The clot in the pelvis *(arrows)* is identified as tissue with an attenuation value higher than that of renal parenchyma, indicating recent formation. The carcinoma is not visualized.

17B). Unlike calculus or gas, blood clot causes neither strong echoes nor acoustic shadowing. Serial ultrasonograms are an efficient way for documenting the resolution of a clot.

The computed tomographic attenuation value of clot varies with time. When the clot is fresh, its attenuation value exceeds that of soft tissue (Fig. 14–19; see Fig. 29–6). Within a week, its attenuation value decreases to a level that approximates that of nonenhanced renal parenchyma. The attenuation value of a blood clot does not increase after the administration of contrast material, as sometimes happens in transitional cell carcinoma. The intraluminal position of a blood clot is well defined by computed tomography if the pelvocalyceal system is distended enough to permit opacified urine to surround the mass. Neither ultrasonography nor computed tomography distinguishes blood clot from other soft tissue masses in the collecting system once a blood clot loses its early higher-than-normal tissue density.

TISSUE SLOUGH

Definition

Tissue sloughed from the kidney may form free, intraluminal masses. This occurs in two forms: necrosed papilla and cholesteatoma.

When *renal papillary necrosis* evolves to the stage of frank necrosis, separation may occur between the viable and dead portions of the papilla. The slough becomes a free mass that eventually moves distally from the calyx. Calcification, if it occurs, may be present at the time of separation or develop later.

Tissue slough usually develops in patients with analgesic nephropathy and less often in cases of renal papillary necrosis due to severe acute pyelonephritis or obstruction. Papillary slough does not occur in S hemoglobinopathy. A complete discussion of renal papillary necrosis is found in Chapter 13.

Cholesteatoma is an unusual form of tissue slough that results from keratinizing desquamative squamous metaplasia, or epidermization, of the transitional epithelium. In this circumstance, keratin forms into either a discrete, pearly gray–whitish mass of concentric layers or an amorphous stringy collection. Either form may obstruct. Chronic inflammation from urinary tract infection or calculus disease is generally held to be the underlying cause, although this viewpoint is not without controversy (Hertle and Androulakakis, 1982). Cholesteatoma has not been associated with malignancy of the uroepithelium. The closely related, and perhaps identical, condition of leukoplakia is discussed in Chapter 15.

Clinical Setting

A papillary slough does not produce symptoms until there is obstruction of an infundibulum, the ureteropelvic junction, or the ureter. Flank pain and colic then develop. A slough may eventually pass by the urethra. In other respects, the clinical setting is that of renal papillary necrosis in general, or of the specific causation, as discussed in Chapter 13.

Cholesteatoma develops in patients with chronic urinary tract infection or chronic stone disease. Hematuria and colic are often present. Occasionally, voided urine contains cornified squamous epithelium.

Radiologic Findings

A sloughed papilla appears as a triangle-shaped filling defect anywhere in the collecting system. One or more calyces will dilate, reflecting the loss of a papillary tip. Initially, the site of separation is irregular but later becomes smooth. When the urine is opacified, the slough that remains in its calyx appears as a nonopaque mass that fills the calyx except for a thin rim of surrounding opaque urine, the so-called *ring* sign (Fig. 14–20). (This finding may be seen in any of the nonopaque masses discussed in this chapter and is not specific for

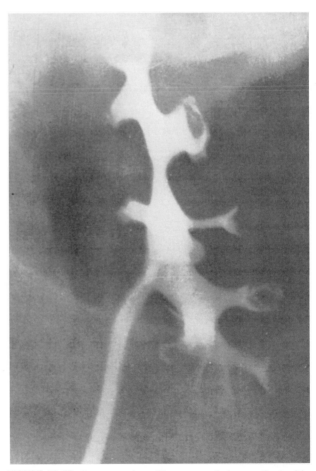

FIGURE 14–20. Acute renal papillary necrosis in a patient with diabetes mellitus and urinary tract infection. Papillary sloughs fill the calyces at multiple sites, leaving deformed medullae. Contrast material surrounds the sloughs, giving rise to the *ring* sign. Retrograde pyelogram. (Courtesy of the late A. J. Palubinskas, M.D., University of California, San Francisco.)

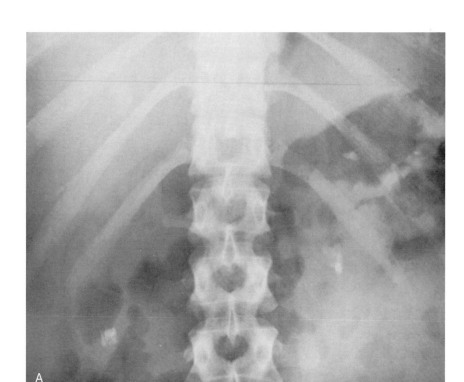

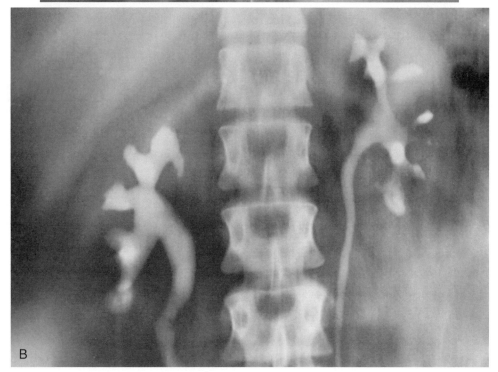

FIGURE 14–21. Renal papillary necrosis in a 27-year-old analgesic abuser. The papillary sloughs bilaterally have calcified in a ringlike pattern. These appear as nonopaque filling defects after the urine is opacified.
   A, Preliminary film.
   B, Excretory urogram. Tomogram. Note calyceal deformities characteristic of papillary necrosis.

sloughed tissue.) A slough may migrate distally, causing dilatation proximal to a point of impaction.

Calcium is sometimes deposited along the periphery of a sloughed papilla, forming a ringlike pattern (Fig. 14–21). Occasionally, the whole papilla is dense, in which case the radiographic, ultrasonographic, and computed tomographic images are indistinguishable from calculus or any other calcified mass. The use of these modalities to differentiate noncalcified slough from other causes of nonopaque filling defects is discussed at the end of this chapter.

Up to one-half of the patients with cholesteatoma have urolithiasis. A cholesteatoma is usually nonopaque. Only rarely is there faint density, presumably due to microdeposits of calcium. Cholesteatoma usually presents as a rounded, intraluminal mass in the pelvocalyceal system. Contrast material extends into the concentric laminations of a cholesteatoma to produce an "onion skin" pattern of alternating density and lucency (Fig. 14–22). In amorphous forms, the filling defects are multiple and stringy, with indistinct margins. This pattern may be indistinguishable from that produced by mural lesions of the pelvocalyceal system, as discussed in Chapter

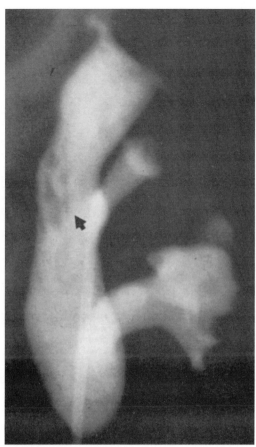

FIGURE 14–23. Cholesteatoma in a 72-year-old woman. Retrograde pyelogram. There is a cluster of multiple, linear, irregular lucencies with indistinct margins *(arrow)*. (From Wills, J. C., Pollack, H. M., and Curtis, J. A.: AJR *136*:941, 1981. Reproduced with kind permission of the authors and *American Journal of Roentgenology.*)

15 (Fig. 14–23). Cholesteatoma isolated in a single calyx has been reported. Computed tomography demonstrates a pelvocalyceal mass of relatively high attenuation value that reflects the microdeposits of calcium. Limited experience with examination of cholesteatoma by ultrasonography suggests a pattern of echogenic mass without acoustic shadowing.

FUNGUS BALL

Definition

Fungus ball, or mycetoma, is a yellow-brown mass of putty-like consistency that forms from either blood-borne or ascending infection of the urinary tract by certain species of fungus. Most mycetomas are caused by *Candida albicans. Aspergillus* species are the second most commonly found organisms. Mycetomas have also been reported in urinary tract infection with *Cryptococcus neoformans, Phycomycetes* species, and *Penicillium* species. Microscopically, the ball is usually an aggregate of the mycelia (M-form) of the fungus and necrotic debris. Occasionally, the mass is composed of clumps of yeast cells (Y-form).

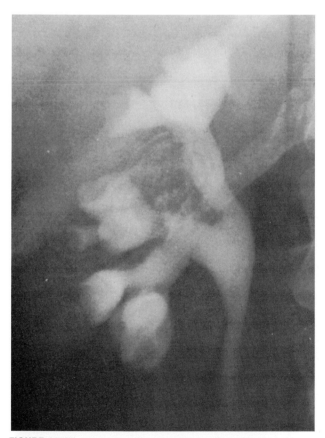

FIGURE 14–22. Cholesteatoma developing in a 46-year-old woman with a 2-year history of intermittent urinary tract infections. Excretory urogram reveals a 1.5-cm mass extending from the renal pelvis into the infundibulum of the upper pole. Contrast material outlines concentric laminations. (From Amberg, J. A., and Talner, L. B.: Urol. Radiol. *1*:192, 1980. Reproduced with kind permission of the authors and *Urologic Radiology.*)

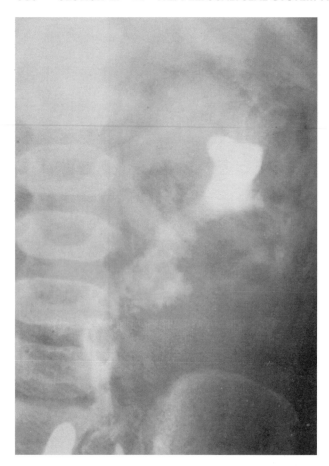

FIGURE 14–24. Candidiasis in the transplanted kidney of a young patient who had bilateral nephrectomies for Wilms' tumor. The pelvocalyceal system and proximal ureter are filled with an amorphous mass. Contrast material insinuates into the interstices to form a lacelike pattern. Retrograde pyelogram. (From Clark, R. E., Minagi, H., and Palubinskas, A. J.: Renal candidiasis. Radiology *101*:567, 1971. Reproduced with kind permission of the authors and *Radiology.*)

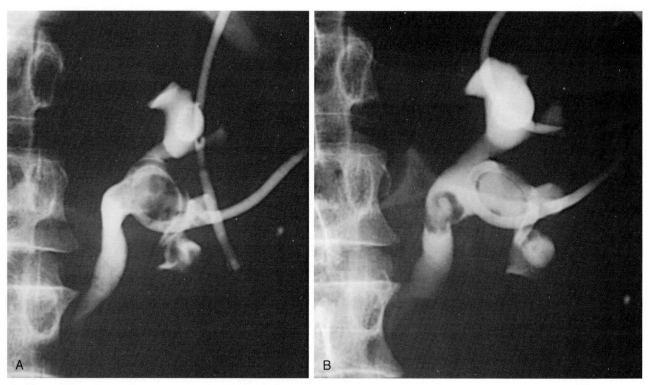

FIGURE 14–25. Candidiasis fungus ball, left kidney, causing intermittent obstruction in a 66-year-old woman with diabetes mellitus. Antegrade pyelograms.
  A, Initial study demonstrates filling defect in the renal pelvis.
  B, Two weeks later, the fungus ball has changed in shape and become smaller.

Involvement of the renal parenchyma occurs in over 90 per cent of patients with blood-borne dissemination of the *Candida* species. In these cases, the fungus ball forms from mycelia shed into the pelvis from the collecting tubules and coexists with white uroepithelial plaques of thrush.

Clinical Setting

Fungal infection of the urinary tract occurs in a setting of altered host resistance. Severe debilitating disease, acquired immunodeficiency syndrome, and administration of antibiotics, adrenal corticosteroids, immunosuppressants, and antineoplastic drugs are common factors. Diabetes mellitus, drug abuse, and prolonged use of indwelling catheters are additional clinical circumstances that favor fungal infection.

The clinical findings of fungal infection of the urinary tract vary with the route of infection, the extent of renal parenchymal involvement, and the development of obstruction by the fungus ball.

The fungus ball itself may cause colic when obstruction, usually at the ureteropelvic junction, occurs. Oliguria or anuria and azotemia result from bilateral obstructing fungus balls or obstruction in a single kidney. Other clinical findings include stranguria and funguria and passage of debris by the urethra. Pneumaturia, from fermentative gases, occurs rarely.

Radiologic Findings

A fungus ball fills the renal pelvis or the ureter with a large, nonopaque mass. Multiple masses occur. Carbon dioxide, butyric acid, and lactate are fermentative gases that sometimes create a lacy radiolucent pattern within the mass. This is best noted on a preliminary film. During enhanced studies, including pyelography, contrast material insinuates itself into the interstices, causing a similar lacelike radiodense pattern (Fig. 14–24). Over time, a mycetoma may move or change size or shape (Fig. 14–25).

Hydronephrosis and impaired pelvocalyceal opacification occur when a fungus ball causes obstruction, usually at the ureteropelvic junction. Other radiologic findings that may be present with a fungus ball are those caused by structural damage resulting from concurrent infection of the renal parenchyma (caliectasis, contour scar, papillary necrosis, and focal enlargements due to abscess) or uroepithelial thrush (mural nodules).

A fungus ball has an ultrasonographic appearance of an echogenic mass that does not cause an acoustic shadow. The computed tomographic attenuation value of a mycetoma is in the range of soft tissue (Fig. 14–26). Neither ultrasonography nor computed tomography differentiates a fungus ball from other intraluminal masses of soft tissue density, except when gas is detected.

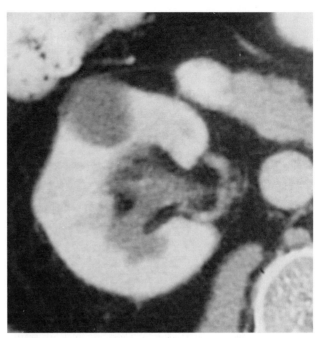

FIGURE 14–26. Mucormycosis fungus ball causing flank pain in a 55-year-old woman with diabetes mellitus. Computed tomogram, contrast material–enhanced. The fungus ball forms a cast of the pelvis and is of soft-tissue attenuation value. A simple cyst is present on the ventral aspect of the kidney.

FOREIGN MATERIAL

Definition

Foreign substances in the renal pelvis are derived from several sources and vary in density from radiolucent to radiopaque. These materials arrive in the pelvocalyceal system and ureter by migration through normal pathways, by passage through newly established channels, or, in the case of gasforming infection, by formation *in situ*.

A solid object placed in the bladder, either operatively or by self-insertion through the urethra, may migrate through the ureter into the renal pelvis. Catheters, drains, or stents inserted into the distal ureter may do likewise, presumably as a result of reverse peristalsis induced by the foreign material. Air introduced during bladder or ureteral instrumentation and gas formed by infection and fermentation also pass retrograde into the pelvocalyceal system.

Solid objects also enter the renal pelvis directly from high-velocity wounds or by penetration from adjacent sites, as with surgically placed drains, needles, or sutures. Migration of ingested objects into the renal pelvis from the alimentary tract usually occurs at the second part of the duodenum. The foreign body, often a toothpick, pin, or bone, migrates into the pelvis of the right kidney, traversing the anterior renal fascia. Much less frequently, this occurs between the fourth part of the duodenum and the left renal pelvis.

Renoalimentary fistulas unassociated with an ingested foreign body are due to trauma and are now rare. In the preantibiotic period, however, these fistulas developed from infection that complicated the traumatic wound. The most common form of renoalimentary fistula is renocolic, in which the renal parenchyma (not the renal pelvis) communicates with the ascending or descending colon. Rare fistulas between the kidney and the stomach, small intestine, appendix, rectum (in the case of a pelvic kidney), or lung have been recorded. Kidney cancer infrequently leads to alimentary fistulas. Even rarer is renocolic fistula due to primary carcinoma of the colon invading the kidney.

Air in the upper urinary tract is often seen with cutaneous nephrostomy, ureteroileostomy, and ureterosigmoidostomy.

Clinical Setting

The clinical features of a foreign body in the kidney vary with the initiating circumstances. A solid object within the renal pelvis, regardless of origin, is usually asymptomatic for a long period of time. Signs and symptoms, when they do arise, are those of infection or colic. Frequency, urgency, and pain are common complaints, and hematuria and pyuria are often present.

Urinary tract gas per se does not produce symptoms. The clinical findings of infection, either primary in the urinary tract or secondary to the fistula, usually dominate.

Radiologic Findings

Gas in the pelvocalyceal system or ureter appears as numerous, sharply defined, round radiolucencies that change with time or with alteration of the patient's position or as complete filling of the lumen (Fig. 14–27). When a large amount of gas is present, the entire lumen is radiolucent, and its wall is sharply defined as a dense, thin line. When the patient is in an upright position, gas rises to the most cephalic portion of the collecting system (Fig. 14–28).

Solid foreign bodies have the shape and radiodensity of the material of which they are composed. Nonopaque objects may become radiopaque by encrustation with calcium crystals.

Caliectasis and pyelectasis occur if the foreign body obstructs urine flow. The radiographic signs of infection may also be associated with a foreign body.

The ultrasonographic and computed tomographic findings of foreign bodies depend on the nature of the material. Strong echoes and acoustic shadows are produced by sound reflectors such as gas or solid objects. Gas causes an acoustic shadow with poorly defined margins and high-level reverberation echoes within the shadow. Foreign material is easily

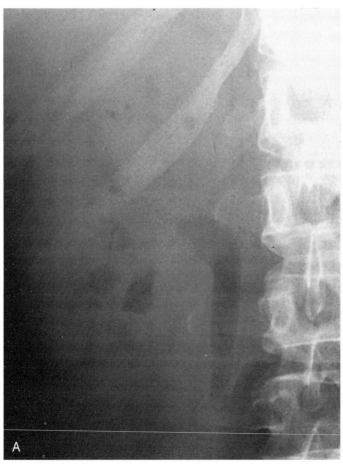

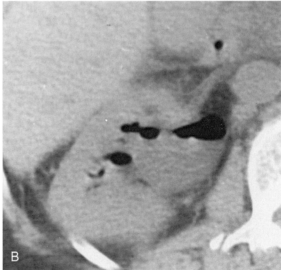

FIGURE 14–27. Pelvocalyceal and ureteral gas associated with pyelonephrosis in a 57-year-old woman with diabetes mellitus.

A, Preliminary film. The radiolucent gas outlines the proximal ureter and many calyces.

B, Computed tomogram, unenhanced. Gas is present in the renal pelvis and calyces.

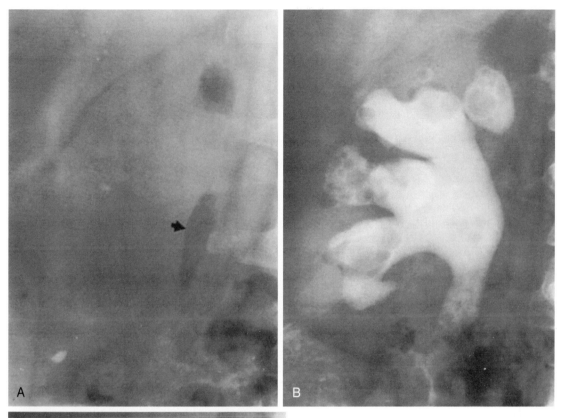

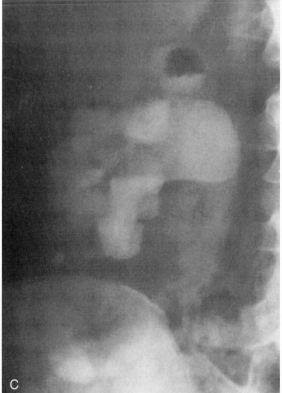

FIGURE 14–28. Air in the pelvocalyceal system and proximal ureter of a 60-year-old patient with cutaneous ureterostomy and urinary tract infection.

A, Preliminary film, supine position. Air fills a portion of the renal pelvis *(arrow).*

B, Excretory urogram, supine position. There are numerous sharply defined lucencies within the pelvocalyceal system.

C, Excretory urogram, upright position. Gas rises to form air-fluid level.

detected by computed tomography, which also demonstrates abnormalities of the perirenal and pararenal spaces in cases of renoalimentary fistulas.

DIFFERENTIAL DIAGNOSIS

The abnormalities discussed in this chapter fall into two major groups: those that are radiopaque, and those that are not. The radiolucent nature of **gas** is a unique diagnostic feature.

The major challenge lies in distinguishing nonopaque calculus from blood clot, tissue slough, or fungus ball. Mural lesions, particularly transitional cell carcinoma, must also be considered when the location of the lesion cannot be confidently established as intraluminal by the criteria set down in the beginning of this chapter.

Ultrasonography is valuable in establishing that a nonopaque filling defect is a **stone.** High-level echoes and a sharply defined acoustic shadow distinguish a calculus from noncalcified tissue slough, fungus ball, blood clot, and transitional cell tumor. Acoustic shadowing due to gas must be taken into account in this assessment. Gas, of course, is easily identified by its radiographic or computed tomographic lucency.

Computed tomography also aids in the assessment of a nonopaque intraluminal lesion. When a radiographically nonopaque filling defect is very dense by computed tomography, the diagnosis of stone is firmly established. Cholesteatoma and fresh blood clot are slightly denser than renal parenchyma, whereas most transitional cell tumors and mature blood clots will be no denser than kidney tissue. Barely detectable calcium deposits, rarely seen in some uroepithelial tumors, should be cautiously kept in mind, but these tumors are usually stippled rather than homogeneous.

Time-related changes in size, shape, and attenuation value are distinctive features of **blood clot.** Documentation requires a minimum of a few days' interval between examinations, however. In the absence of further bleeding, a clot disappears within 14 days, during which time it diminishes in computed tomographic density. Other renal abnormalities that may represent the primary cause of bleeding—papillary necrosis or tumor, for example—offer a hint as to the nature of the filling defect.

Tissue slough due to renal papillary necrosis can be recognized by the characteristic triangular shape of the shed portion of the papilla or by its location within a calyx deformed by the amputation of the papillary tip. The ring sign produced when the slough is surrounded by opacified urine may be mimicked by a mass of any origin that is located within the lumen of the calyx. The laminated appearance of cholesteatoma during contrast material–enhanced studies suggests this diagnosis. On the other hand, when a **cholesteatoma** has a stringy rather than rounded mass appearance, a specific radiologic diagnosis is not possible.

A pelvic or ureteral mass with mixed soft tissue and gas densities is characteristic of a **fungus ball.** In the absence of gas, however, there are no radiologic features that distinguish this form of nonopaque intraluminal mass from the others discussed in this chapter.

The vast majority of radiopaque intraluminal abnormalities of the pelvocalyceal system and ureter are **calculi.** These are usually diagnosed accurately by their radiopaque nature, size, location, and shape. A calcified sloughed papilla is easily distinguished from stone when the calcification is deposited on the periphery of the slough. A homogeneously calcified slough, on the other hand, cannot be distinguished from a stone, except perhaps for its triangular shape or the presence of a deformed calyx. The rare, faintly calcified old blood clot is indistinguishable from a faintly calcified calculus or tumor.

Foreign bodies should be recognized by familiarity of shape, as is the case with bullets, needles, sutures, or catheters. These characteristics may become obscured by calcific encrustations, which can mask the true nature of the lesion.

BIBLIOGRAPHY

General

Fein, A. B., and McClennan, B.: Solitary filling defects of the ureter. Semin. Roentgenol. *21*:201, 1986.

Malek, R. S., Aguilo, J. J., and Hattery, R. R.: Radiolucent filling defects of the renal pelvis: Classification and report of unusual cases. J. Urol. *114*:508, 1975.

Parienty, R. A., Ducellier, R., Pradel, J., Lubrano, J.-M., Coquille, F., and Richard, F.: Diagnostic value of CT numbers in pelvocalyceal filling defects. Radiology *145*:743, 1982.

Pollack, H. M., Arger, P. H., Banner, M. P., Mulhern, C. B., Jr., and Coleman, B. G.: Computed tomography of renal pelvic defects. Radiology *138*:645, 1981.

Williams, B., Jr., Hartman, G. W., and Hattery, R. R.: Multiple and diffuse ureteral filling defects. Semin. Roentgenol. *21*:214, 1986.

Urolithiasis

Asplin, J. R.: Uric acid stones. Semin. Nephrol. *16*:412, 1996.

Banner, M. P.: Calculous disease of the urinary tract. In Pollack, H. M. (ed.): Clinical Urography. Philadelphia, W. B. Saunders, 1990, pp. 1752–1925.

Boridy, I. C., Maklad, N., and Sandler, C. M.: Suspected urolithiasis in pregnant women: Imaging algorithm and literature review. Am. J. Roentgenol. *167*:869, 1996.

Brown, R. C., Loening, S. A., Ehrhardt, J. C., and Hawtrey, C. E.: Cystine calculi are radiopaque. AJR *135*:565, 1980.

Bruwer, A.: Primary renal calculi: Anderson-Carr-Randall progression? AJR *132*:751, 1979.

Carr, R. J.: A new theory on the formation of renal calculi. Br. J. Urol. *26*:105, 1954.

Clayman, R. V., and Williams, R. D.: Oxalate urolithiasis following jejuno-ileal bypass-mechanism and management. Surg. Clin. North Am. *59*:1071, 1979.

Coe, F. L., Parks, J. H., and Asplin, J. R.: Medical progress: The pathogenesis and treatment of kidney stones. N. Engl. J. Med. *327*:1141, 1992.

Cohen, T. D., and Preminger, G. M.: Struvite calculi. Semin. Nephrol. *16*:425, 1996.

Cooke, S. A. R.: The site of calcification in the human renal papilla. Br. J. Surg. *57*:890, 1970.

Dalrymple, N. C., Verga, M., Anderson, K. R., Bove, P., Covey, A.

M., Rosenfield, A. T., and Smith, R. C.: The value of unenhanced helical computerized tomography in the management of acute flank pain. J. Urol. 159:735, 1998.

Federle, M. P., McAninch, J. W., Kaiser, J. A., Goodman, P. C., Roberts, J., and Mall, J. C.: Computed tomography of urine calculi. AJR 136:255, 1981.

Fielding, J. R., Steele, G., Fox, L. A., Heller, H., and Loughlin, K. R.: Spiral computerized tomography in the evaluation of acute flank pain: A replacement for excretory urography. J. Urol. 157:2071, 1997.

Gearhart, J. P., Herzberg, G. Z., and Jeffs, R. D.: Childhood urolithiasis: Experiences and advances. Pediatrics 87:445, 1991.

Graves, F. T.: An experimental study of the anatomy of the tubules of the human kidney and its relation to calculus formation. Br. J. Urol. 54:569, 1982.

Hillman, B. J., Drach, G. W., Tracey, P., and Gaines, J. A.: Computed tomographic analysis of renal calculi. AJR 142:549, 1984.

Kawashima, A., Sandler, C. M., Boridy, I. C., Takahashi, N., Benson, G. S., and Goldman, S. M.: Unenhanced helical CT of ureterolithiasis: Value of the tissue rim sign. AJR 168:997, 1997.

Leroy, A. J.: Diagnosis and treatment of nephrolithiasis: Current perspectives. AJR 163:1309, 1994.

Levine, J. A., Neitlich, J., Verga, M., Dalrymple, N., and Smith, R. C.: Ureteral calculi in patients with flank pain: Correlation of plain radiography with unenhanced helical CT. Radiology 204:27, 1997.

Mall, J. C., Collins, P. A., and Lyon, E. S.: Matrix calculi. Br. J. Radiol. 48:807, 1975.

Mandel, N.: Mechanism of stone formation. Semin. Nephrol. 16:364, 1996.

Margolin, E. G., and Cohen, L. H.: Genitourinary calcification: An overview. Semin. Roentgenol. 17:95, 1982.

Menon, M., Parulkar, B. G., and Drach, G. W.: Urinary lithiasis: Etiology, diagnosis, and medical management. In Walsh, P. C., Retik, A. B., Vaughan, E. D., Jr., and Wein, A. J. (eds.): Campbell's Urology, 7th ed. Philadelphia, W. B. Saunders, 1998, pp. 2661–2734.

Olcott, E. W., Sommer, F. G., and Napel, S.: Accuracy of detection and measurement of renal calculi: In vitro comparison of three-dimensional spiral CT, radiography, and nephrotomography. Radiology 204:19, 1997.

Pak, C. Y. C.: Etiology and treatment of urolithiasis. Am. J. Kidney Dis. 18:624, 1991.

Parks, J. H., and Coe, F. L.: Pathogenesis and treatment of calcium stones. Semin. Nephrol. 16:398, 1996.

Patriquin, H., and Robitaille, P.: Renal calcium deposition in children: Sonographic demonstration of the Anderson-Carr progression. AJR 146:1253, 1986.

Prien, E. L., Sr.: The analysis of urinary calculi. Urol. Clin. North Am. 1:229, 1974.

Prien, E. L., Sr.: The riddle of Randall's plaques. J. Urol. 114:500, 1975.

Randall, A.: Papillary pathology as a precursor of primary calculus. J. Urol. 44:580, 1940.

Resnick, M. I., Kirsh, E. D., and Cohen, A. M.: Use of computerized tomography in the delineation of uric acid calculi. J. Urol. 131:9, 1984.

Sheppard, P. W., and White, F. E.: Demonstration of a matrix calculus using computed tomography. Br. J. Radiol. 60:1028, 1987.

Smith, L. H.: The pathophysiology and medical treatment of urolithiasis. Semin. Nephrol. 10:31, 1990.

Smith, L. H., and Segura, J. W.: Urolithiasis. In Kelalis, P. P., Kind, L. R., and Belman, A. B. (eds.): Clinical Pediatric Urology. Philadelphia, W. B. Saunders, 1992, pp. 1327–1352.

Sommer, F. G., and Taylor, K. J. W.: Differentiation of acoustic shadowing due to calculi and gas collections. Radiology 135:399, 1980.

Takahashi, N., Kawashima, A., Ernst R. P., Boridy, I. C., Goldman, S. M., Benson, G. S., and Sandler, C. M.: Ureterolithiasis: Can clinical outcome be predicted with unenhanced helical CT? Radiology 208:97, 1998.

Van Arsdalen, K. N.: Pathogenesis of renal calculi. Urol. Radiol. 6:65, 1984.

Vermeulen, C. W., and Lyon, E. S.: Mechanisms of genesis and growth of calculi. Am. J. Med. 45:684, 1968.

Vermeulen, C. W., Lyon, E. S., and Ellis, J. E.: The renal papilla and calculogenesis. J. Urol. 97:573, 1967.

Yilmaz, S., Sindel, T., Arslan, G., Ozkaynak, C., Karaali, K., Kabaalioglu, A., and Luleci, E.: Renal colic: Comparison of spiral CT, US and IVU in the detection of ureteral calculi. Eur. Radiol. 8:212, 1998.

Zwirewich, C. V., Buckley, A. R., Kidney, M. R., Sullivan, L. D., and Rowley, V. A.: Renal matrix calculus: Sonographic appearance. J. Ultrasound Med. 9:61, 1990.

Blood Clot

Beck, P., and Evans, K. T.: Renal abnormalities in patient with haemophilia and Christmas disease. Clin. Radiol. 23:349, 1972.

Navani, S., Bosniak, M. A., and Shapiro, J. H.: Varied radiographic manifestations of urinary tract bleeding. J. Urol. 100:339, 1968.

Schaner, E. G., Balow, J. E., and Doppman, J. L.: Computed tomography in the diagnosis of subcapsular and perirenal hematoma. AJR 129:83, 1977.

Thomas, J., Stey, A., and Aboulker, P.: Calculi on blood clots. J. Urol. (Paris) 82:496, 1976.

Wright, F. W., Matthews, J. M., and Brock, L. G.: Complication of hemophilic disorders affecting the renal tract. Radiology 98:571, 1971.

Tissue Slough

Amberg, J. A., and Talner, L. B.: Clinical Pathologic Conference: Cholesteatoma in a 46-year-old woman. Urol. Radiol. 1:192, 1980.

Carsky, E. W., Prior, J. T., Moore, R., and Hamel, J.: Cholesteatoma of the kidney: Radiographic findings. Radiology 78:796, 1962.

Eugan, J. W., Jr.: Urothelial neoplasms: Pathologic anatomy. In Hill, G. S. (ed.): Uropathology. New York, Churchill Livingstone, 1989, pp. 719–793.

Hare, W. S. C., and Poynter, J. D.: The radiology of renal papillary necrosis as seen in analgesic nephropathy. Clin. Radiol. 25:423, 1974.

Hertle, L., and Androulakakis, P.: Keratinizing desquamative metaplasia of the upper urinary tract: Leukoplakia-cholesteatoma. J. Urol. 127:631, 1982.

Osius, T. G., Harrod, C. S., and Smith, D. R.: Cholesteatoma of the renal pelvis. J. Urol. 87:774, 1962.

Sarlis, J. N., Malakates, S. K., and Papadimitriou, D.: Cholesteatoma of renal pelvis. J. Urol. 118:468, 1967.

Weitzner, S.: Cholesteatoma of the calix. J. Urol. 108:365, 1972.

Fungus Ball

Biggers, R., and Edwards, J.: Anuria secondary to bilateral ureteropelvic fungus balls. Urology 15:161, 1980.

Boldus, R. A., Brown, R. C., and Culp, D. A.: Fungus balls in renal pelvis. Radiology 102:555, 1972.

Clark, R. E., Minagi, H., and Palubinskas, A. J.: Renal candidiasis. Radiology 101:567, 1971.

Cohen, G. H.: Obstructive uropathy caused by ureteral candidiasis. J. Urol. 110:285, 1973.

Davies, S. F., and Sarosi, G. A.: Fungal urinary tract infections. In Schrier, R. W., and Gottschalk, C. W. (eds.): Diseases of the Kidney, 6th ed. Boston, Little, Brown & Co., 1997, pp. 973–988.

Fisher, J., Mayhall, G., Duma, R., Shadomy, S., Shadomy, J., and Wathington, C.: Fungus balls of the urinary tract. South. Med. J. 72:1281, 1979.

Gerle, R. D.: Roentgenographic features of primary renal candidiasis. AJR 119:731, 1973.

Irby, P. B., Stoller, M. L., and McAninch, J. W.: Fungal bezoars of the upper urinary tract. J. Urol. 143:447, 1990.

Margolin, H. N.: Fungus infection of urinary tract. Semin. Roentgenol. 6:323, 1971.

Melchior, J., Mebust, W. K., and Valk, W. L.: Ureteral colic from a fungus ball: Unusual presentation of systemic aspergillosis. J. Urol. *108*:698, 1972.

Stuck, K. J., Silver, T. M., Jaffe, M. H., and Bowerman, R. A.: Sonographic demonstration of renal fungus balls. Radiology *142*:473, 1981.

Warshowsky, A. B., Keiller, D., and Gittes, R. F.: Bilateral renal aspergillosis. J. Urol. *113*:8, 1975.

Wise, G. J.: Fungal infections of the urinary tract. In Walsh, P. C., Retik, A. B., Vaughan, E. D., Jr., and Wein, A. J. (eds.): Campbell's Urology, 7th ed. Philadelphia, W. B. Saunders, 1998, pp. 779–806.

Foreign Material

Arthur, G. W., and Morris, D. G.: Reno-alimentary fistulae. Br. J. Surg. *53*:396, 1966.

Baird, J. M., and Spence, H. M.: Ingested foreign bodies migrating to the kidney from the gastrointestinal tract. J. Urol. *99*:675, 1968.

Bissada, N. K., Cole, A. T., and Fried, F. A.: Renoalimentary fistula: An unusual urological problem. J. Urol. *110*:273, 1973.

Brust, R. W., Jr., and Morgan, A. L.: Renocolic fistula secondary to carcinoma of the colon. J. Urol. *111*:439, 1974.

Eickenberg, H.-U., Amin, M., and Lich, R., Jr.: Travelling bullets in genitourinary tract. Urology *6*:224, 1975.

Frang, D.: A swallowed needle found in the kidney pelvis. J. Urol. (Paris) *71*:647, 1978.

Osmond, J. D.: Foreign bodies in the kidney. Radiology *60*:375, 1953.

Rittenberg, G. M., and Warren, E.: Air in the pelvocalyceal system: A normal finding in patients with ureteroileostomies. AJR *128*:311, 1977.

Shukri, A. M.: Reno-alimentary fistulae. Br. J. Surg. *55*:551, 1968.

Wiscott, J. W.: Hydronephrosis from shell fragment in renal pelvis. Milit. Med. *134*:1334, 1969.

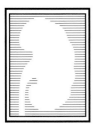

CHAPTER **15**

Mural Abnormalities

Each of the dissimilar abnormalities discussed in this chapter shares the same distinguishing characteristic—a primary involvement of the pelvocalyceal or ureteral wall. Except for pyelocalyceal diverticula and ureteroceles, these lesions, which are variably focal, multifocal, or diffuse, transform the normally smooth mucosa into a surface that is irregular, nodular, or sharply narrowed. In some situations, a free intraluminal component is also present, but only secondary to the initiating mural event.

A mural lesion maintains a constant relationship with the pelvocalyceal wall. Opacified urine surrounds only that part of the abnormality that projects into the lumen, never completely surrounding it. Focal or multifocal mural lesions are usually sharply marginated and may form an acute angle at their site of attachment to the wall. Diffuse lesions, on the other hand, are irregular.

The radiologic criteria for mural lesions are apparent only when the pelvocalyceal system and ureter are well opacified and fully distended. This requires an adequate dose of contrast material and, in some cases, carefully applied abdominal compression to distend the pelvocalyceal system. Useful adjuncts to standard radiographic techniques are multiple projections, changes in patient position, and later re-examination. Direct opacification of the collecting system by retrograde or antegrade pyelography is occasionally required. Computed tomography may be of particular value in characterizing the mural origin of a uroepithelial lesion.

Tumors of the uroepithelium, usually transitional cell carcinoma, are the most frequently encountered mural lesions in the adult's upper urinary tract and are discussed first in this chapter. Next, congenital ureteropelvic junction obstruction is discussed. Following these two sections, a variety of conditions are discussed, including uncommon infections, unusual responses to infection or inflammation, mural hemorrhage, longitudinal mucosal folds, and pseudodiverticulosis. Calyceal diverticulum is an abnormality of the collecting system wall and, therefore, is discussed in this chapter even though its radiologic appearance is that of a communicating cyst rather than a mural mass. Likewise, ureterocele is included as a prolapse of the ureter into the bladder at the ureterovesical junction.

TUMORS

Definition

Approximately 8 per cent of all malignant kidney tumors have a uroepithelial origin. Transitional cell carcinoma accounts for 85 to 95 per cent of these. The remainder, for the most part, are squamous cell carcinoma. Only a very few cases of uroepithelial mucinous adenocarcinoma have been recorded. Also rare are primary benign and malignant tumors of the nonepithelial components of the pelvocalyceal wall and direct mural metastases.

Upper tract tumors of the uroepithelium are not evenly distributed. Transitional cell carcinoma occurs two to three times more commonly in the renal pelvis than in the ureter. Of the ureteral tumors, most occur in the distal third of that structure. There is also a well-established tendency toward multicentricity and bilaterality of transitional cell carcinomas. Bilateral upper tract metachronous or synchronous, or both, transitional cell carcinoma has been reported in up to 10 per cent of patients. Metachronous transitional cell carcinoma of the bladder develops in up to 40 per cent of patients with transitional cell carcinoma of the renal pelvis and in up to 55 per cent of patients with transitional cell carcinoma of the ureter.

The histologic spectrum of *transitional cell carcinoma* extends from papilloma, a thin fibrovascular core covered by normal transitional cell mucosa, to advanced cytologic and architectural features of malignancy. The gross appearance of transitional cell carcinoma varies from papillary and bulky to sessile. Some tumors are unifocal, whereas others are multiple or diffusely spread over confluent areas of the pelvocalyceal or ureteral mucosal surface.

Squamous cell carcinoma is generally thought to arise from transitional cell epithelium that has undergone squamous metaplasia in response to chronic irritation with or without infection. Many pathologists believe that these tumors are associated with leukoplakia, but others deny the idea that such association exists. Intercellular bridges and keratin pearls are specific histologic characteristics of squamous cell carcinoma. Lesions are usually single and highly invasive.

Mucinous adenocarcinoma is the rarest form of primary uroepithelial malignancy. This tumor, like squamous cell carcinoma, develops from metaplastic transformation of transitional cells in response to chronic inflammation. It is characterized by papillary structures with gland formation, vacuolated goblet cells, and mucin. Mucinous adenocarcinoma tends to involve broad areas of the pelvic and calyceal surface, which makes recognition more difficult than if there had been an exophytic pattern of growth.

Benign mesodermal tumors of the upper urinary tract, known as *fibroepithelial polyps,* are uncommon. Most arise in the ureter and may extend retrograde into the renal pelvis. A few originate proximal to the ureteropelvic junction. The core of these polypoid masses consists of fibrous tissue, smooth muscle, blood or lymphatic vessels, or nerve cells. The fibrous component is most often predominant. A thin layer of normal urothelium covers these polyps, which are usually elongated, thin, and occasionally divided at their tip into several fingerlike branches. The bulk of the polyp lies free in the lumen of the collecting system or ureter and may be mobile.

Malignant nonepithelial sarcoma arising from the wall of the pelvis or calyces is extremely rare. This tumor may be derived from any of the mesenchymal components and is classified according to the predominant tissue type.

Most *metastatic tumors* involve the pelvocalyceal system or ureter by invasion from surrounding blood vessels, lymphatic channels, or lymph nodes; direct metastases occur rarely. Carcinoma of the stomach, prostate, breast, lung, cervix, and colon and melanoma account for most metastatic tumors.

Clinical Setting

Transitional cell carcinoma occurs most frequently in men and has a peak incidence in the seventh decade. The entire uroepithelium is at risk, although the ureter is less frequently affected than the pelvocalyceal system, while the upper tract as a whole is less frequently involved than the bladder.

Historically, certain epidemiologic factors have been associated with an increased risk for the development of transitional cell carcinoma. These include exposure to chemicals in the dye, petroleum, rubber, and cable industries as well as in occupations such as hair-dresser, leather finisher, spray painter, and textile weaver. Tobacco, coffee, artificial sweetener, tryptophan metabolites, and chronic inflammation or infection are additional risk factors. Increased prevalence of transitional cell carcinoma in patients with analgesic and Balkan nephropathy is well established. A history of transitional cell carcinoma of the bladder increases the likelihood of tumor appearing in the renal pelvis, suggesting that transitional cell carcinoma originates in unstable uroepithelium at multiple sites.

There is an 8-fold increase in the risk for transitional cell carcinoma of the renal pelvis in patients with analgesic nephropathy. One or more metabolites of phenacetin are thought to be the causal agent. Unlike the population at large, among analgesic abusers, women are more frequently affected than men; a younger age group is involved; and the renal pelvis, rather than the urinary bladder, is the predominant site of tumor. The long induction time, estimated at 22 years on average, emphasizes the need for long-term surveillance of patients with analgesic nephropathy.

Squamous cell carcinoma occurs in an older age group than does transitional cell carcinoma and is generally believed to be closely associated with chronic infection and leukoplakia of the urinary tract. Calculi are present in more than half of the patients with this tumor. The prevalence in men is approximately equal to that in women. These patients follow a rapidly lethal clinical course that reflects the highly invasive behavior of squamous cell carcinoma.

Mucinous adenocarcinoma of the renal pelvis occurs only in patients with severe infection and stone disease. Branched (staghorn) calculi and hydronephrosis are frequently noted.

Malignant tumor, including the rare mural metastasis, commonly causes painless hematuria. Clots may cause intermittent obstruction and colic. Dull, persistent flank pain may also be a prominent feature. Palpable tumor is uncommon, although a hydronephrotic kidney may be felt when the tumor causes chronic obstruction.

Benign mesenchymal tumor (fibroepithelial polyp) causes hematuria and flank pain in over 50 per cent of cases. Obstruction, however, is infrequent even though the bulk of the polyp is intraluminal. These tumors occur mainly in children.

Malignant Uroepithelial Tumors

Radiologic Findings

Excretory Urography. Most malignant tumors of the collecting system and ureter fulfill the criteria for a mural location, as outlined in the beginning of this chapter. However, these lesions may vary greatly in appearance. Some are single polypoid masses with a smooth, irregular, or lobular surface (Figs. 15–1 through 15–3). The same pattern may occur at multiple sites. Other lesions, particularly squamous cell carcinoma, are broad based and flat and are single or multiple (Fig. 15–4). Occasionally, there is a superficial spread over large areas, with

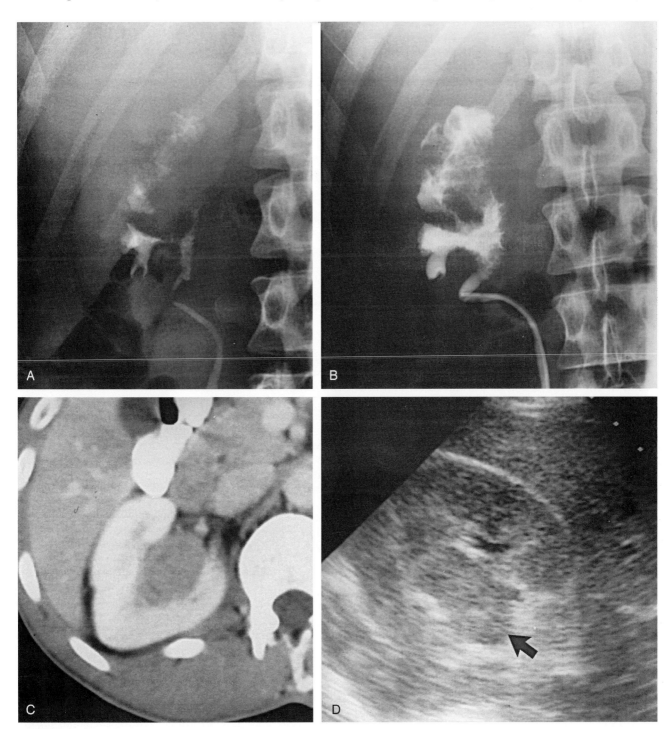

FIGURE 15–1. Transitional cell carcinoma, right renal pelvis, in a 34-year-old male. A large, lobulated, broad-based mass fills much of the pelvis of the left kidney. Contrast material filling the interstices of the tumor gives rise to a lacy appearance.

 A, Excretory urogram.

 B, Retrograde pyelogram.

 C, Computed tomogram, contrast material–enhanced. The tumor appears as a homogeneous soft tissue mass filling the pelvis.

 D, Ultrasonogram, transverse section. The tumor *(arrow)* is uniformly echogenic.

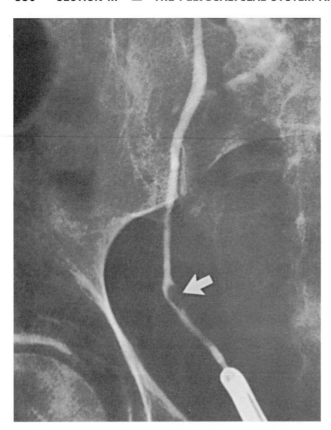

FIGURE 15–2. Transitional cell carcinoma, right distal ureter. Retrograde ureterogram. The tumor appears as a single, small, smooth, polypoid mass *(arrow)*.

an irregular mucosal pattern (Fig. 15–5). In some tumors that arise in the pelvocalyceal system, infiltration of the renal sinus or parenchyma, or both, is so advanced that the kidney loses function. In this circumstance, the involved portion of the kidney is enlarged, its reniform shape is preserved, and the density of the nephrogram is diminished as a reflection of diminished perfusion, which can be angiographically demonstrated as narrowing and irregularity of intrarenal arterial branches (Fig. 15–6).

Contrast material trapped within the interstices of a polypoid growth causes a stippled appearance when viewed *en face* or in cross section (Fig. 15–7; see also Figs. 15–1B, 15–9B). This pattern may suggest a malignant uroepithelial tumor in some cases but is generally not helpful in differentiating neoplastic from non-neoplastic filling defects of the pelvis. Transitional cell carcinoma may develop punctate calcific deposits that are detected infrequently by standard radiography (Fig. 15–8) but are readily seen by computed tomography. These deposits explain why the attenuation value of uroepithelial tumors is sometimes higher than that of renal parenchyma.

A tumor located in the pelvocalyceal system is visualized directly by excretory urography in only 60 to 70 per cent of patients owing either to high-grade hydronephrosis or loss of function from renal parenchymal infiltration by a primary lesion in the pelvocalyceal system (Figs. 15–9 and 15–10; see Fig.

15–8). In these circumstances, diagnostic accuracy can be increased by pyelography, using either a retrograde or antegrade technique (see Figs. 15–6, 15–8, and 15–9). Either of these approaches opacifies the pelvocalyceal system better than excretory urography when renal function is compromised. Antegrade pyelography is particularly valuable when the tumor is obstructive and causes hydronephrosis. Brushing of the lesion for cytologic study can be combined with either direct approach.

A tumor located in the ureter appears as a nonopaque, irregular filling defect, usually with dilatation of the ureter proximal to the mass (Fig. 15–11; see Figs. 15–2 and 15–3). The ureter just distal to the tumor is also often slightly dilated. The combination of the distal margin of a nonopaque soft tissue mass invaginating into a distended segment of an opacified ureter constitutes the *chalice* or *Bergman's* sign, which can be seen with either excretory urography or pyelography (Fig. 15–12; see Fig. 15–11B). This sign is valuable in distinguishing a nonopaque tumor from a nonopaque stone in that the latter causes spasm, rather than distention, of the segment of the ureter distal to it.

Transitional cell carcinoma located in the pelvocalyceal system sometimes invades the renal parenchyma, producing an infiltrating focal parenchymal mass, obliteration of the adjacent collecting system, and reduced nephrographic density in the involved region (see Fig. 15–10). These features must be distinguished from those of adenocarcinoma arising

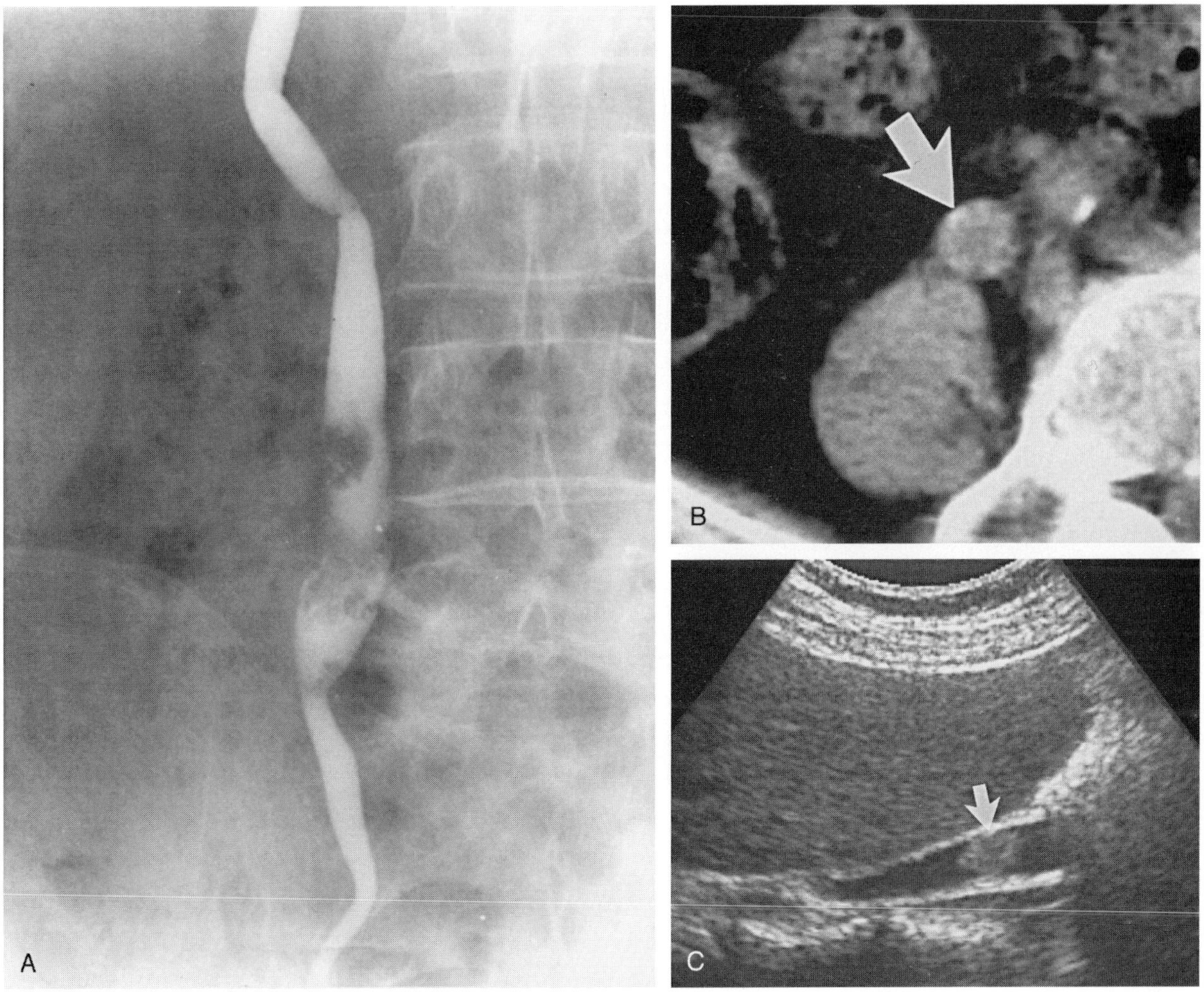

FIGURE 15–3. Transitional cell carcinoma, right mid-ureter.

A, Excretory urogram. The ureter is dilated both proximal and distal to the multilobulated mass.

B, Computed tomogram, contrast material–enhanced. The tumor is of homogeneous density and surrounded by a faint ring of opacified urine *(arrow)*. *C,* Ultrasonogram, longitudinal projection. The soft tissue echoes of the tumor *(arrow)* are sharply defined from the urine-filled, slightly dilated ureter.

in the renal parenchyma. This can be accomplished by recognizing the preservation of the reniform shape of the enlarged kidney that is characteristic of neoplasms that infiltrate the kidney in contradistinction to the ball-shaped geometry produced by tumors that expand in all directions from an epicenter originating in the renal parenchyma. This concept is amplified in Chapter 12.

A stone that coexists with a mural lesion raises the possibility of epidermoid or mucinous adenocarcinoma. When epidermoid carcinoma develops in the presence of leukoplakia, the latter may dominate the radiologic findings, and the neoplasm cannot be separately identified.

Computed Tomography. Computed tomography defines the contour and mural attachment of a uroepithelial tumor following pelvocalyceal or ureteral opacification. The soft tissue attenuation value of the tumor may increase as much as 2-fold after rapid intravenous injection of contrast material. The tumor appears as a mural mass projecting into

the uroepithelial-lined lumen, as circumferential or eccentric thickening of the pelvic or ureteric wall, or as soft tissue infiltrating the renal sinus or periureteric fat (see Figs. 15–1C, 15–3B, and 15–7B). Computed tomography offers no special advantage over excretory urography or pyelography in assessing the tumor itself. Instead, its special value is in evaluating the nature of a nonopaque filling defect in general and in staging documented uroepithelial tumors. Here, peripelvic fat obliteration, nephrographic defects, direct extension into the peripelvic or periureteric space, and lymph node enlargement provide evidence of tumor spread that may be useful in formulating therapeutic plans.

Ultrasonography. Large pelvocalyceal tumors separate the compact, dense central sinus echoes of the normal kidney and generate echoes similar in intensity to those of the renal parenchyma (see Fig. 15–1D). Tumors that are too small to separate the central sinus echoes may not be detectable by ultrasonography. Tumors of the ureter are seen as a soft

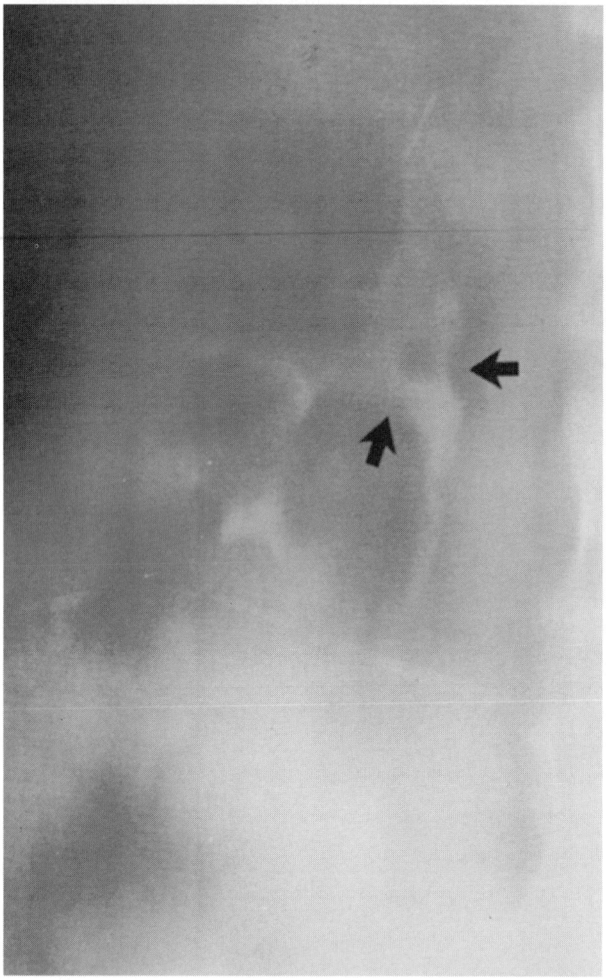

FIGURE 15–4. Transitional cell carcinoma. Multiple, broad-based, flat lesions *(arrows)* are present in the right renal pelvis of a 72-year-old man with gross, total hematuria. Excretory urogram.

tissue mass that is often situated at the distal end of a slightly dilated ureter (see Fig. 15–3C). Ultrasonographic examination does not reliably distinguish between urothelial tumor and blood clot unless the central low-level echo pattern changes with time, which is characteristic of clot.

Ultrasonography detects infiltration of the kidney parenchyma by a tumor originating in the pelvocalyceal system. Here, the kidney size is enlarged owing to regional growth, the contour remains reniform, and the echo texture of the involved portion of the kidney is altered from that of the normal parenchyma.

Magnetic Resonance Imaging. Magnetic resonance imaging in the evaluation of malignant epithelial tumors is secondary to computed tomography except in patients who have a history of prior adverse reaction to iodinated contrast material or who have renal failure. Nevertheless, magnetic resonance can provide useful information regarding parenchymal and venous invasion (Fig. 15–13).

Angiography. The angiographic features of malignant uroepithelial tumors include fine neovascularity, a homogeneous tumor blush, vascular encasement, and absence of arteriovenous shunts (see Fig. 15–5B). Central pelvic tumors are supplied by the pelviureteric artery, which may be enlarged or

displaced, or both. Tumors located in the periphery of the collecting system are supplied by branches of the main renal artery. Encasement, spreading, or straightening of interlobar or arcuate arteries and a nephrographic deficit indicate parenchymal invasion (see Figs. 15–5B and 15–10B). Angiography is no longer used in the diagnostic evaluation of uroepithelial tumors.

Miscellaneous Tumors

The radiologic features of malignant, nonepithelial (mesenchymal), and metastatic tumors of the collecting system and ureter are similar to those of epithelial malignancies described in the foregoing section. Multifocal, blood-borne mural metastases, an uncommon event, may simulate benign conditions, such as pyelitis cystica (Fig. 15–14). Computed tomography differentiates metastases that are isolated to the wall from those that invade from the peripelvic or periureteric space (Fig. 15–15).

Benign mesodermal tumors (fibroepithelial polyps) of the pelvis are smooth, long, nonopaque filling defects that move freely in both antegrade and retrograde directions. These tumors are single, bifid, or multibranched (Figs. 15–16 and 15–17). Demonstration of the point of attachment to the pelvic

Text continued on page 399

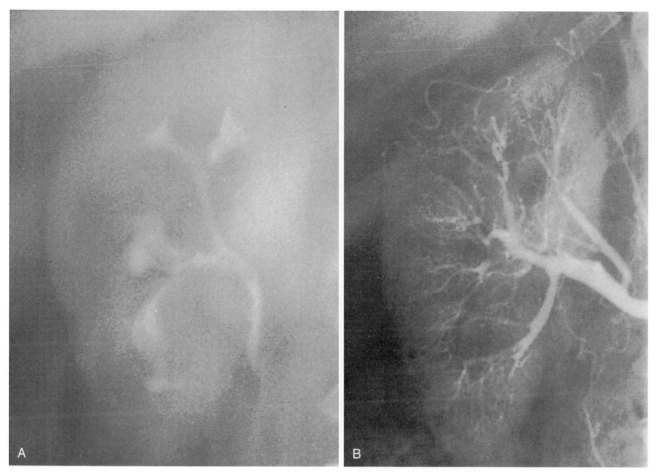

FIGURE 15–5. Transitional cell carcinoma, right kidney.

A, Excretory urogram. Superficial spread extends over a large area of the pelvocalyceal system. Caliectasis in the middle and lower poles is present. A mass effect on the inferior margin of the pelvis indicates spread of the tumor into the renal sinus fat.

B, Selective renal arteriogram, arterial phase. Encasement of the distal main renal artery and displacement of the artery to the lower pole also indicate spread of tumor into the renal sinus.

FIGURE 15–6. Transitional cell carcinoma, right kidney. Retrograde pyelogram. The collecting system is obliterated by infiltrating tumor.

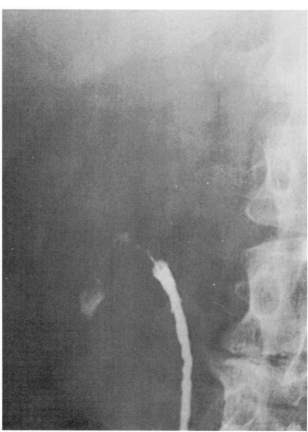

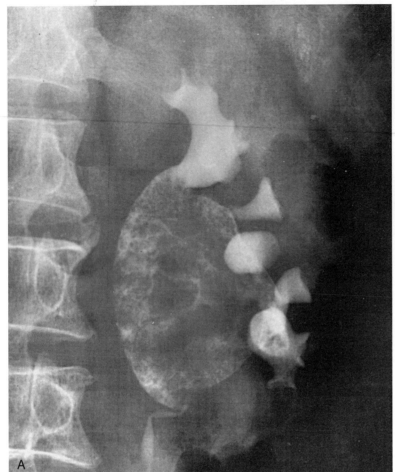

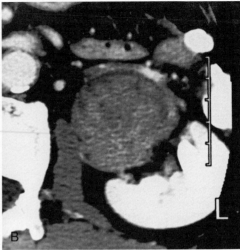

FIGURE 15–7. Transitional cell carcinoma, left renal pelvis. A lacy appearance is derived from contrast material that is trapped within the interstices of this polypoid growth.

   A, Excretory urogram.

   B, Computed tomography, contrast material–enhanced.

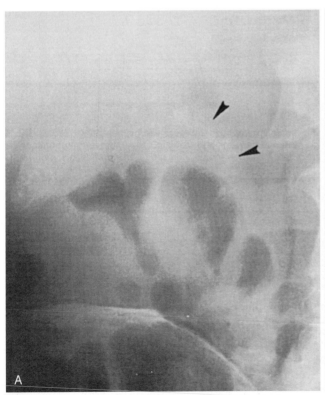

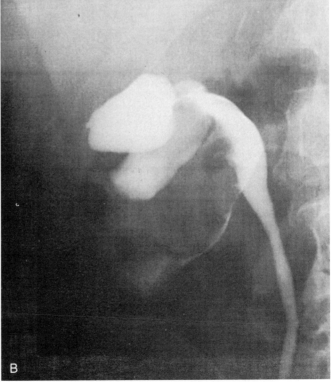

FIGURE 15–8. Transitional cell carcinoma. Stippled calcification in a bulky tumor mass, which causes obstructive uropathy.

   A, Preliminary film. Fine calcific deposits *(arrows)* are present along the upper margin of the tumor.

   B, Retrograde pyelogram. The tumor distorts and obstructs the pelvocalyceal system.

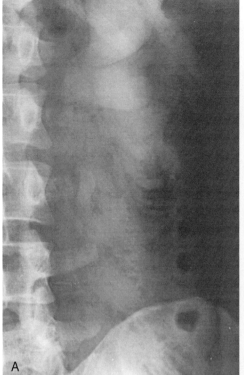

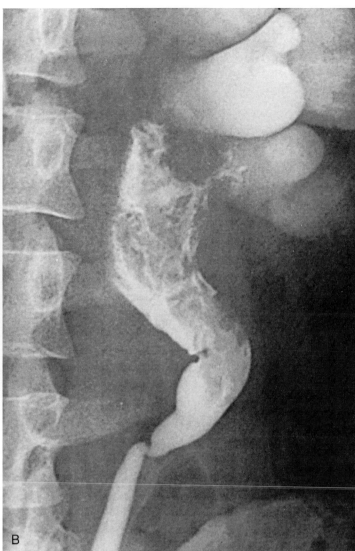

FIGURE 15–9. Transitional cell carcinoma, left pelvis, causing advanced obstructive uropathy.

A, Excretory urogram. There is only faint opacification of markedly dilated calyces.

B, Retrograde pyelogram. The tumor fills the pelvis and proximal ureter and has a lacy pattern of contrast material within its interstices.

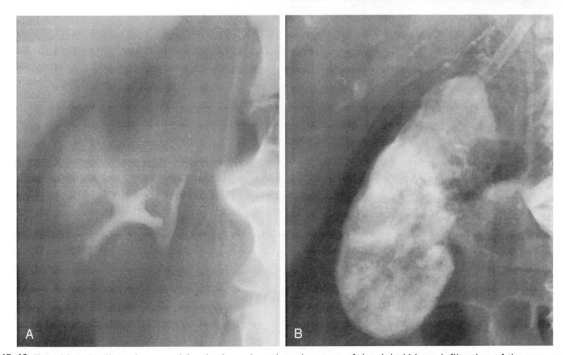

FIGURE 15–10. Transitional cell carcinoma arising in the pelvocalyceal system of the right kidney. Infiltration of the upper pole obliterates the vasculature and nephrons in this region, thereby diminishing the urographic and angiographic nephrograms. Note preservation of the reniform shape of the kidney despite the increase in size of the upper pole.

A, Excretory urogram. Tomogram. Tumor also projects into the pelvis.

B, Angiogram, nephrographic phase. There is loss of corticomedullary differentiation in addition to the decrease in the density of the upper pole nephrogram.

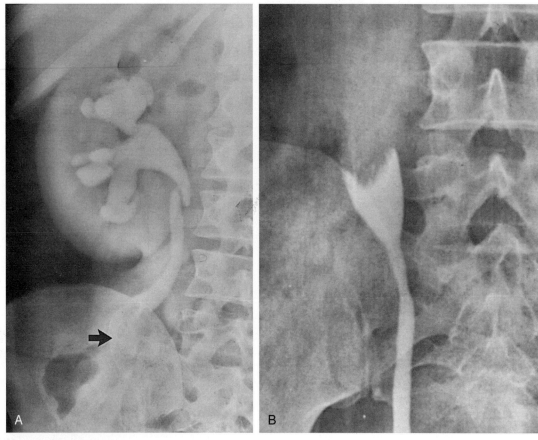

FIGURE 15–11. Transitional cell carcinoma, right ureter.
  A, Excretory urogram. The ureter is dilated proximal to the tumor, which is seen as a filling defect partially surrounded by contrast material *(arrow)*.
  B, Retrograde ureterogram. The tumor appears as a nonopaque filling defect projecting into and obstructing the ureter. The tumor invaginating into the dilated ureter constitutes the *chalice* or *Bergman's* sign.

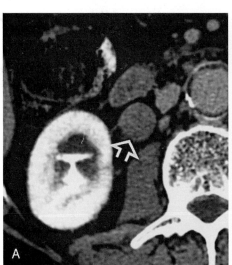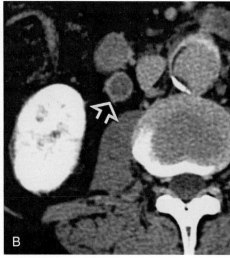

FIGURE 15–12. Transitional cell carcinoma, right ureter. Computed tomogram, contrast material–enhanced.
  A, Section proximal to the tumor demonstrates a dilated ureter *(arrow)*.
  B, Section at the level of the tumor, which is surrounded by a thin rim of opacified urine where it invaginates into the dilated ureter *(arrow)*.

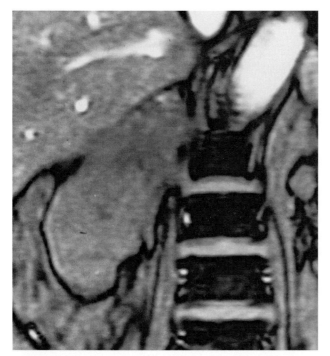

FIGURE 15–13. Transitional cell carcinoma invading the right kidney and inferior vena cava. Magnetic resonance image, coronal projection. The invasive tumor has enlarged the kidney, but the reniform shape is preserved, as is typical of tumors that grow by infiltration.

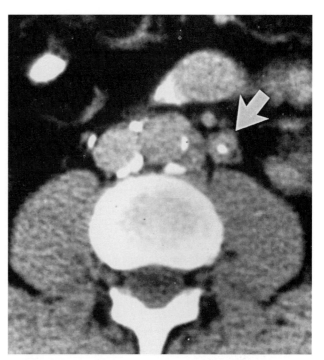

FIGURE 15–15. Non-Hodgkin's lymphoma with periureteral spread. The wall of the ureter is markedly thickened *(arrow)*. Residual lymphangiographic contrast material is present in retroperitoneal lymph nodes. Same patient is illustrated in Figure 10–20.

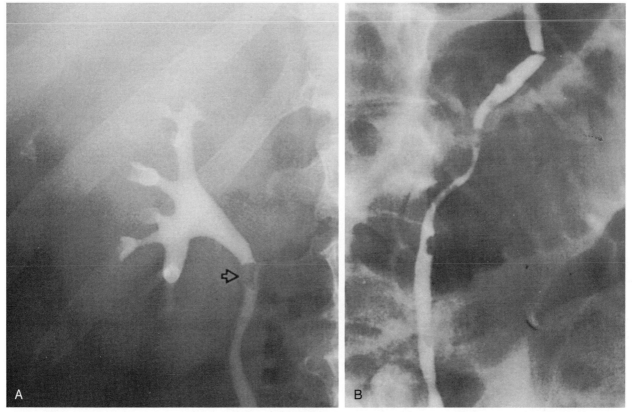

FIGURE 15–14. Mural metastases in a 59-year-old man with melanoma. There are sharply defined, oval filling defects at the right ureteropelvic junction *(arrow)* and at multiple sites in the left ureter. Some appear to be intraluminal, but all are mural. There were also blood-borne metastases to the bladder.

A, Right kidney.

B, Left mid-ureter.

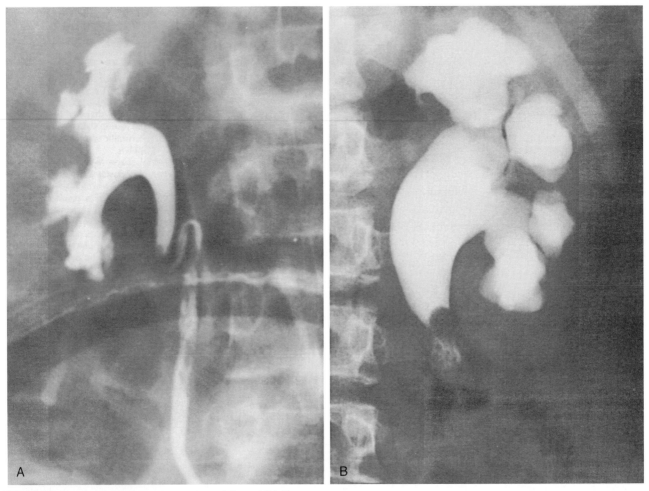

A   B

FIGURE 15–16. Fibroepithelial polyps, bilateral, in a child. Excretory urogram.
  A, Right kidney and proximal ureter. The polyp in the proximal ureter is a smooth, multibranched nonopaque filling defect that does not obstruct.
  B, Left kidney and proximal ureter. The polyp obstructs the ureteropelvic junction.

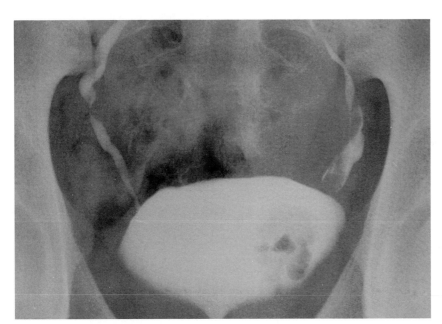

FIGURE 15–17. Fibroepithelial polyp, distal left ureter, with prolapse into the bladder. The polyp appears as a long, smooth, multibranched filling defect.

wall may require multiple projections. These lesions inconstantly cause obstruction and are best identified by excretory urography or by retrograde pyelography.

CONGENITAL URETEROPELVIC JUNCTION OBSTRUCTION

Definition

The area where the funnel-shaped renal pelvis merges into the tubule-shaped ureter is the *ureteropelvic junction*, a term embodying a general anatomic concept rather than a specific embryologic or histologic site. Congenital obstruction of this junction has been investigated extensively, but no single cause has been conclusively established. Derangement of circular and longitudinal muscle, inadequate distensibility of the ureteropelvic junctional segment due to excess inelastic collagen, and deficiency of transmitter substance at nerve endings are major theories of etiology. None of these has been validated, however. It is generally agreed that kinks, angulations, and "high insertions" of the ureter are a result, rather than a cause, of pelvic distention. Rare causes of ureteropelvic junction obstruction include crossing blood vessels, fibrous bands, ischemia, mucosal folds, aortic aneurysm, renal cyst, and eosinophilic ureteritis.

Most patients with ureteropelvic junction obstruction have no demonstrable anatomic abnormality. To explain this, Whitaker (1975) proposed a functional definition of the ureteropelvic junction as the point at which a downward moving contraction, initiated somewhere in the pelvocalyceal system, causes apposition of the ureteropelvic wall and formation of a bolus of urine. Under normal conditions, including high-flow states, efficient emptying of the pelvis follows forward propulsion of each succeeding bolus (Fig. 15–18). Whitaker theorized that congenital ureteropelvic junction obstruction occurs when the walls of the pelvis do not appose at the ureteral junction because the pelvis is not funnel-shaped. The resultant failure to create a bolus impedes urine flow across the junction (Fig. 15–19). The progressive pelvic dilatation that follows incomplete drainage leads to further inefficiency of pelvic emptying. Ultimately, there is decreased glomerular filtration and progressive hypertrophy of the pelvic musculature. In extreme circumstances, hydronephrosis results.

The radiologic findings of chronic hydronephrosis are discussed in Chapter 9. Additional discussion on the forces that propel urine forward and the various causes of the dilated pelvocalyceal system are presented in Chapter 17.

Clinical Setting

Congenital ureteropelvic junction obstruction is either discovered *in utero* during obstetrical ultrasonography or becomes apparent in an infant or child as an abdominal mass, flank or abdominal pain, failure to thrive, or nonspecific gastrointestinal complaints. The left kidney in males is more commonly involved than the right one and the frequency of congenital ureteropelvic juction obstruction is increased in association with multicystic dysplastic kidney, as discussed in Chapter 11. Infection, hypertension, hematuria, and stone formation are

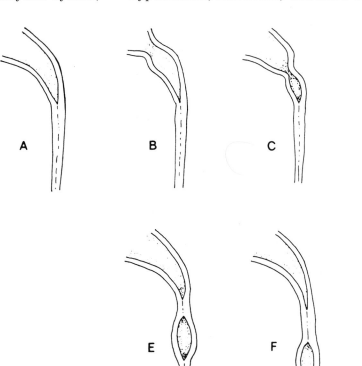

FIGURE 15–18. Schematic illustration of the sequence of peristalsis at the normal ureteropelvic junction.

A, Normal funnel shape of ureteropelvic junction in the resting state.

B and *C,* Peristaltic wave passes prograde through the pelvis.

D, Funnel shape of the pelvis leads to apposition of opposite walls as the peristaltic wave progresses toward the ureter.

E, A bolus forms as a result of circular contraction of muscles proximally and relaxation of muscles distally.

F, Progression of bolus occurs as longitudinally oriented force of the muscle contraction "pulls" the ureter over the bolus.

(Courtesy of R. H. Whitaker, Addenbrooke's Hospital, Cambridge, England, and Br. J. Urol. 47:377, 1975.)

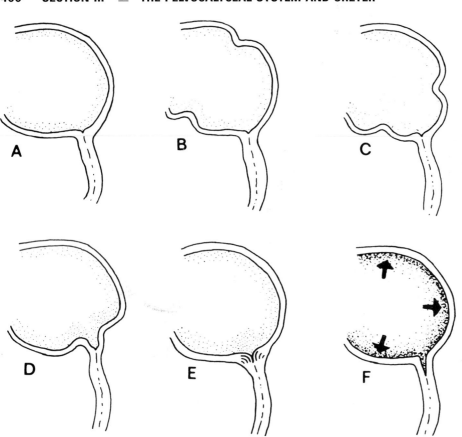

FIGURE 15–19. Schematic illustration of the sequence of peristalsis with congenital ureteropelvic junction obstruction.

A, The normal funnel shape of the distal pelvis either is absent in the resting state or is lost with rapid diuresis.

B, C, and *D,* A wave of contraction passes along the pelvic wall. The rounded shape precludes apposition of the walls and bolus formation.

E, Without a bolus on which to grip, the circular and longitudinal forces of muscular contraction are wasted. The junction is closed, and urine is prevented from passing through.

F, Some fluid drains through the orifice leading to the ureter because this is the weakest point in the high-pressure system. (Courtesy of R. H. Whitaker, Addenbrooke's Hospital, Cambridge, England, and Br. J. Urol. 47:377, 1975.)

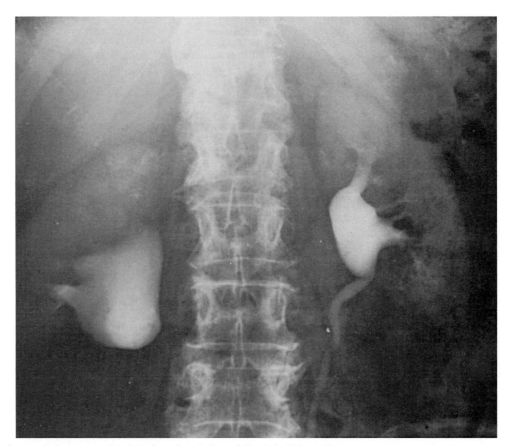

FIGURE 15–20. Congenital ureteropelvic junction obstruction of the right kidney. Excretory urogram, 20-minute prone film. The pelvocalyceal system is dilated and rounded. The ureter is unopacified despite the patient's prone position. (See Fig. 15–24 for the effect of a diuretic on this obstructed system.)

less commonly associated clinical problems. When children with congenital ureteropelvic junction obstruction sustain mild abdominal trauma, serious complications, such as hemorrhage and shock, may follow.

In adults who have congenital ureteropelvic junction obstruction, pain, hematuria, and urinary tract infection predominate. Pain is often episodic and frequently precipitated by high urine flow rates such as those produced by beer drinking.

Radiologic Findings

The classic excretory urographic findings of congenital ureteropelvic junction obstruction are a sharply defined narrowing at the junction and dilatation of the pelvocalyceal system that persists even when the patient is placed in a position that favors gravity drainage of the pelvis (Fig. 15–20). Unilateral renal enlargement, diminished parenchymal and pelvocalyceal opacification, the rim sign, and wasting of the kidney substance are late findings that reflect the long-term consequences of the inability of the collecting system to handle normal urine volume. These changes become most severe when the pelvis is surrounded by the renal parenchyma (intrarenal pelvis). An extrarenal pelvis more readily dilates in response to obstruction, thereby having less effect on parenchymal structure and function. In its most advanced form, congenital ureteropelvic junction obstruction transforms the kidney into a hydronephrotic sac.

Narrowing of the ureteropelvic junction is usually concentric (see Fig. 15–20). A sharp angulation or kink of the pelvis in relation to the proximal ureter may develop as the pelvis rotates anteriorly while it dilates (Fig. 15–21). A vessel crossing the ureteropelvic junction, usually an artery to the lower pole of the kidney, may cause a broad, tangential, sharply defined extrinsic radiolucent depression on the dilated pelvis at the junction (see Fig. 15–21). Intra-ureteral ultrasonography or magnetic resonance angiography can be used to identify a crossing vessel prior to a pyelotomy. A crossing vessel rarely, however, is the primary cause of obstruction. In severe cases, there is no opacification of the ureter beyond the obstruction.

Antegrade and retrograde pyelography clearly demonstrate the junctional narrowing and are employed when impaired function prevents adequate opacification by excretory urography (Fig. 15–22). The ability to perform urodynamic studies during antegrade pyelography makes this approach particularly advantageous.

The angiographic, ultrasonographic, and computed tomographic abnormalities of congenital ureteropelvic junction obstruction are the same as those of chronic obstructive uropathy of any etiology. These abnormalities are discussed in Chapter 9.

The collecting system is not always dilated in congenital ureteropelvic junction obstruction. Dila-

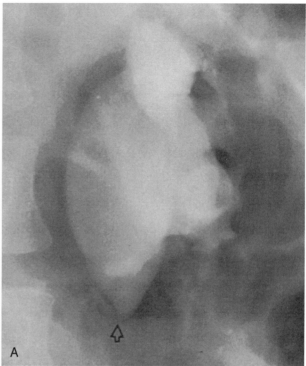

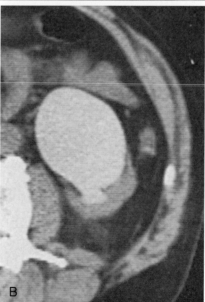

FIGURE 15–21. Congenital ureteropelvic junction obstruction.

A, Excretory urogram. A sharp angulation has developed as the pelvis dilates and rotates anteriorly *(arrow).* An artery running to the lower pole of the kidney and crossing this site tangentially was demonstrated by angiography.

B, Computed tomogram, contrast material–enhanced. The anterior rotation of the pelvis in congenital ureteropelvic junction obstruction is well illustrated in a different patient.

tation varies with both the degree of ureteropelvic dysfunction and the urine flow rate. When patients with low-grade obstruction are examined in a dehydrated state, the pelvocalyceal system may be normal or "flabby" or contain longitudinal striae representing the redundant mucosa of a usually dilated system. Long-standing obstruction leads to im-

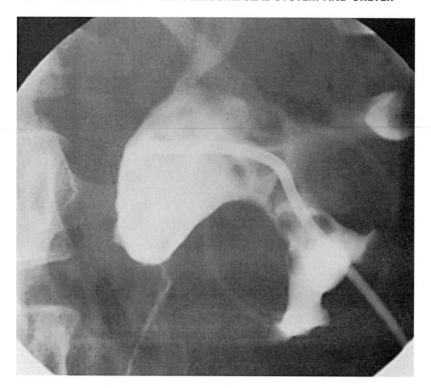

FIGURE 15–22. Congenital ureteropelvic junction obstruction complicated by urolithiasis, pyonephrosis, and loss of function of the left kidney. An antegrade pyelogram through the percutaneous nephrostomy opacifies the pelvocalyceal system and ureter.

paired renal function and a decrease in the amount of urine formed by the kidney. This, too, may obscure the urographic findings of obstruction (Fig. 15–23). On the other hand, a dilated pelvocalyceal system is not to be invariably equated with obstruction, an important concept that is discussed in Chapter 17.

All of the foregoing considerations underscore the need to search for congenital ureteropelvic junction obstruction under conditions of high urine flow rates. This can be accomplished easily by oral hydration or by combining a diuretic drug with either excretory urography or radionuclide renography (Whitfield, 1977) (Fig. 15–24).

Diuresis renography is performed in patients who are well hydrated in the manner described in Chapter 2. The pattern of radionuclide elimination by the kidneys is measured before and after intravenous furosemide, given at a dose of 0.5 mg/kg. Prolonged retention of the tracer after diuresis denotes obstruction. Various patterns are schematized in Figure 15–25. Specificity of diuresis renography has been reported at 88 per cent and sensitivity at 91 percent. False-positive results occur in some dilated but nonobstructed kidneys, in azotemia, and in patients who are inadequately hydrated.

There is a small group of patients with congenital ureteropelvic junction obstruction who will not be confidently diagnosed by any of the preceding tests, including those using drug-induced diuresis. The reason for this may be the minimal nature of the functional abnormality, nondistensibility from peripelvic fibrosis caused by previous surgery, or renal functional impairment that prevents adequate excretion of either contrast material or radionuclide

tracer. Here, the pressure-flow urodynamic study, originally described by Whitaker and modified by others, provides a direct measurement of pelvocalyceal pressures under controlled flow states (see discussion in Chapter 17). This test measures bladder pressure through a urethra-bladder catheter and renal pelvis pressure through a catheter placed percutaneously directly into the pelvis. Proximal (pelvic) and distal (bladder) pressures are recorded at variable rates of perfusion through the percutaneous catheter. Technical details and diagnostic criteria vary from one laboratory to another (Pfister and Newhouse, 1979; Whitaker, 1979, 1980). Pressure is measured at flow rates of up to 20 mL/min. Obstruction is generally held to exist if the pressure gradient rises above 15 cm of water under any of the conditions of the study. During the course of the Whitaker test, an antegrade pyelogram is performed. This must be correlated with pressure measurements.

Other causes of dilatation of the collecting structures in which urodynamic pressure-flow studies may be applied are discussed in Chapter 17.

INFECTION

Definition

Tuberculosis and candidiasis involve the pelvocalyceal and ureteral wall, whereas schistosomiasis is found in the distal ureter. Tuberculosis of the renal parenchyma is discussed in Chapter 13 and that of the bladder is presented in Chapter 19. Chapter 14 discusses fungus ball as one of the intraluminal pelvocalyceal abnormalities. A discussion of schistosomiasis of the bladder is included in Chapter 19.

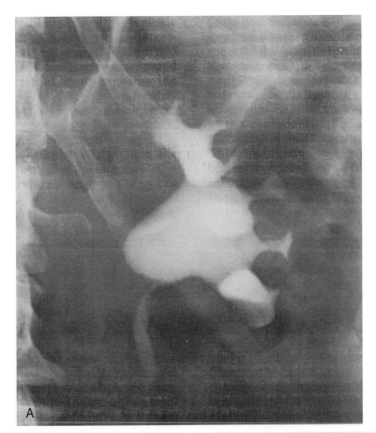

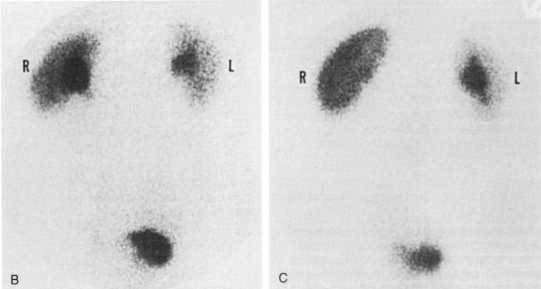

FIGURE 15–23. Congenital ureteropelvic obstruction causing decreased renal function. The diminished urine volume formed by the left kidney has led to normal pressure in the renal pelvis.

A, Retrograde pyelogram, 5-minute drainage film. Although the renal pelvis is dilated, the forniceal angles are minimally blunted.

B, 99mTc-glucoheptonate static scan, 16 minutes. Renal function on the left is 20 per cent of that on the right, but some urine is being formed, as evidenced by pelvic activity.

C, 99mTc-glucoheptonate static scan, 3 hours. Activity in the left renal pelvis persists, while there has been loss of activity in the right renal pelvis caused by normal urine flow.

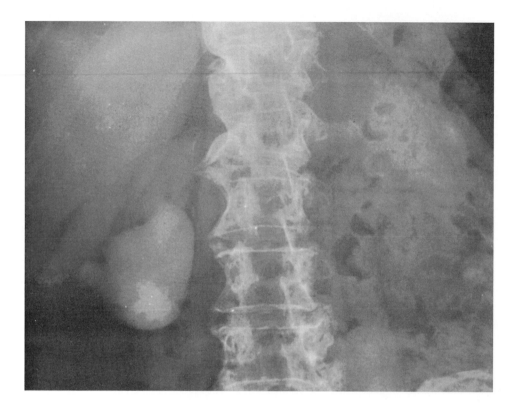

FIGURE 15–24. Congenital ureteropelvic obstruction of the right kidney. Excretory urogram. Film exposed 15 minutes after intravenous injection of furosemide (40 mg). The volume of the pelvis had increased, and the forniceal angles have dilated compared with the prediuretic state illustrated in Figure 15–20. The ureter remains unopacified. Note the washout of contrast material from the left kidney.

FIGURE 15–25. Diuresis renography. Schematized graphs of renogram activity over time in the normal, obstructed, and dilated but nonobstructed kidney. The initial slope is similar in both obstruction and nonobstructed dilatation. With injection of a diuretic drug, however, radionuclide activity decreases rapidly in nonobstructive dilatation, whereas prolonged activity is seen in obstruction.

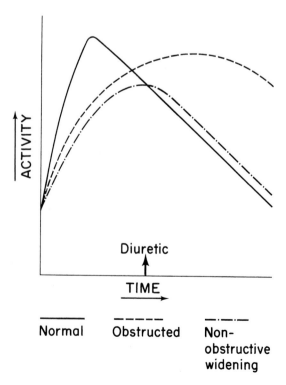

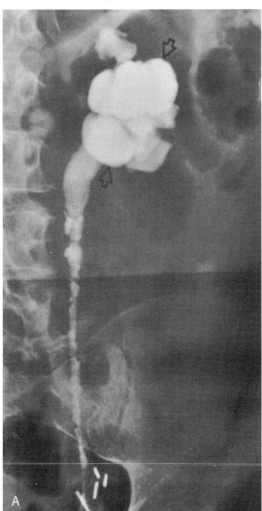

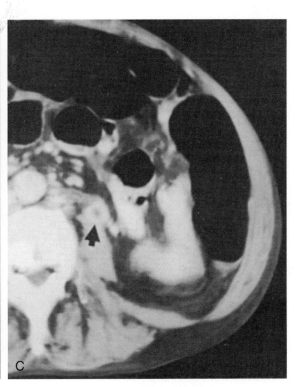

FIGURE 15–26. Renal and uroepithelial tuberculosis, active phase, in a 40-year-old man. There is extensive irregularity and ulceration of the entire ureter and pelvis. A large, cavitated granuloma in the kidney communicates with the collecting system.

A, Retrograde pyelogram. The opacified, cavitated granuloma *(arrows)* is superimposed on the pelvocalyceal system.

B, Computed tomogram with contrast material enhancement at the level of the kidney demonstrates the large cavity in the parenchyma.

C, Computed tomogram with contrast material enhancement at the level of the proximal ureter. The ureter *(arrow)* is thickened and enhances as a result of acute inflammation.

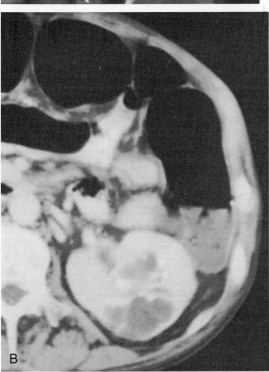

Tuberculosis. The pelvocalyceal and ureteral walls are infected by bacilli that have been shed into the urine from cavitating tuberculous granulomas in the nephrons. Thickening by granulation tissue is the earliest response of the uroepithelium to *Mycobacterium tuberculosis*. In advanced cases, the muscularis and adventitia are also involved. Mucosal ulceration develops as the granulomas enlarge and coalesce, at which time the pelvic surface is diffusely irregular.

With healing, collagen and fibrous tissue replace the granulomas. As fibrosis progresses, submucosal collagen fibers are reoriented in the submucosa and cause sharply defined scars. The collecting system and ureter proximal to the cicatrix dilate as a result of increased resistance to urine flow. When healing narrows an infundibulum to the point of obliteration, the proximal calyx dilates and becomes a fluid-filled mass that is distinguishable from a cavitated parenchymal granuloma or nephrogenic cyst only by microscopic identification of the uroepithelium. As is true of all aspects of urinary tract tuberculosis, the pattern of scarring and dilatation is variable. Involvement may be at one or several sites, from an infundibulum to the distal ureter. It is rare, however, to have involvement of the distal ureter with no proximal abnormality. Destruction and retraction of the surrounding renal parenchyma cause nonobstructive dilatation of the adjacent portion of the pelvocalyceal system without distal stenoses.

Candidiasis. The upper urinary tract is infected by *Candida albicans* by either an ascending or a hematogenous route. Uroepithelial involvement, which is uncommon, is manifested by a white membrane typical of thrush, representing infiltration of the mucosa and submucosa by fungi and inflammatory cells.

Schistosomiasis (Bilharziasis). *Schistosoma haematobium* cercariae migrate to the venules of the lamina propria of the bladder and distal ureters from the portal circulation by way of hemorrhoidal and pudendal veins. Eventually, they penetrate the muscularis and submucosa of the bladder and distal ureteral wall, where ova are deposited. The cystitis and ureteritis that subsequently develop are characterized by granulomas, superficial mucosal ulcerations, and the formation of polypoid masses of granulation tissue. Eventually, fibrosis causes strictures with obstructive dilatation and calcium deposits in the dead ova.

Clinical Setting

The clinical findings of tuberculous and fungal infections of the kidney, including the uroepithelium, are discussed in Chapters 13 and 14.

Radiologic Findings

Tuberculosis. The active phase of uroepithelial tuberculosis causes marked irregularity of part or all of the collecting system or ureter, or both, be-

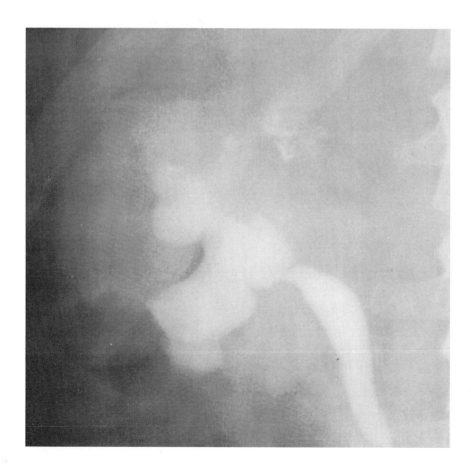

FIGURE 15–27. Uroepithelial tuberculosis, healed phase. There is a sharply defined circumferential narrowing, with proximal caliectasis due to obstruction. Excretory urogram.

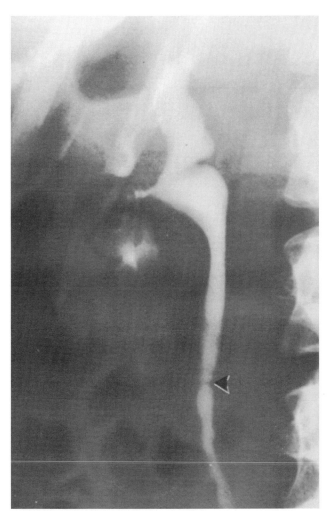

FIGURE 15–28. Uroepithelial tuberculosis, healed phase. Excretory urogram. A sharply circumscribed narrowing in the proximal ureter *(arrow)* does not cause obstruction. Eccentric narrowing at several sites is present distally.

cause of both submucosal granulomas and mucosal ulceration (Fig. 15–26). Irregularity is rarely isolated, since tuberculosis usually involves a multiplicity of sites in the kidney, pelvis, and ureter.

Fibrous scars of healed tuberculosis produce sharply defined circumferential narrowings at one or several sites in the collecting system or ureter. These are of variable thickness and often have slightly irregular margins. The portion proximal to an obstructive narrowing dilates (Figs. 15–27 and 15–28). Fibrosis may progress during the treatment of active tuberculosis, necessitating careful serial studies during this period.

Dilatation of one or more calyces, of the entire pelvocalyceal system or of long segments of the ureter may develop without obstruction as a result of either mural fibrosis or scarring of the surrounding renal parenchyma (Figs. 15–29 and 15–30). Some patients with healed urinary tract tuberculosis develop dense calcification of the pelvocalyceal wall and ureter. The latter has been termed *pipe-stem ureter* (Fig. 15–31).

Candidiasis. Uroepithelial thrush causes diffuse irregularity of the pelvocalyceal wall. This may occur as an isolated event or coexist with fungus ball, parenchymal damage, or both.

Schistosomiasis. Schistosomiasis usually involves the distal third of the ureters, although sometimes a more proximal infestation occurs. Asymmetry is common. Ureteral abnormalities are found in up to one-half of patients with bladder schistosomiasis. Very uncommonly, the radiologic findings of schistosomiasis are found only in the ureters.

Early manifestations are minimal dilatation, slight mucosal irregularity, and diminished peristalsis, leading to a failure to empty. With time, calcification, mural thickening and straightening, beading, and multiple segments of narrowing and dilatation develop (Figs. 15–32 and 15–33). In some patients, there are masses of granulation tissue, known as bilharzial polyps. These are seen as solitary or multiple filling defects. Strictures may lead to hydroureter and hydronephrosis; however, hy-

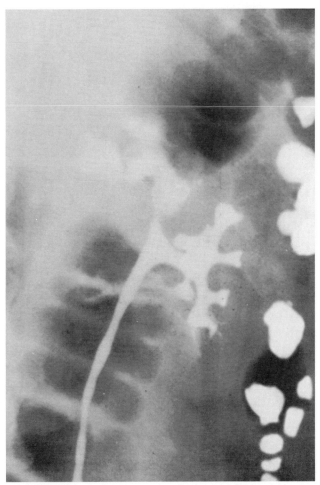

FIGURE 15–29. Uroepithelial tuberculosis, healed phase. Generalized dilatation of the renal pelvis and proximal ureter without obstruction is present. Also note the focal narrowing of the upper pole drainage system with a granulomatous mass in the upper pole. Retrograde pyelogram. Same patient is illustrated in Figure 13–31.

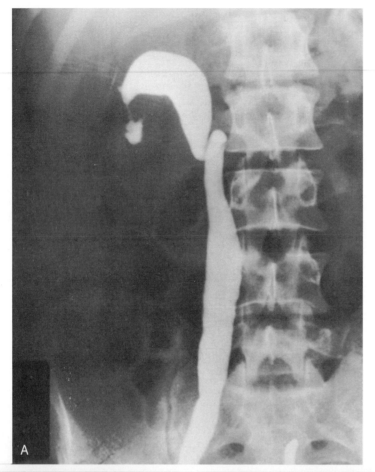

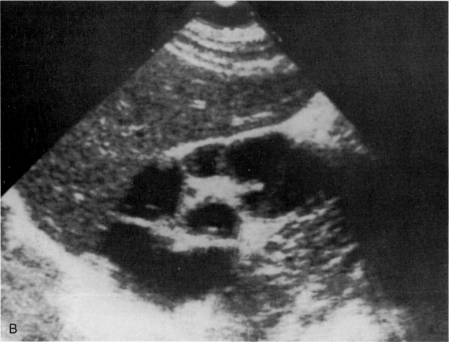

FIGURE 15–30. Uroepithelial tuberculosis, healed phase.

A, Retrograde pyelogram. Almost the entire ureter and pelvis are dilated. The proximal pelvis is tightly scarred.

B, Ultrasonogram, longitudinal section. There is marked caliectasis resulting from both the pelvic scar and the surrounding destroyed and retracted parenchyma.

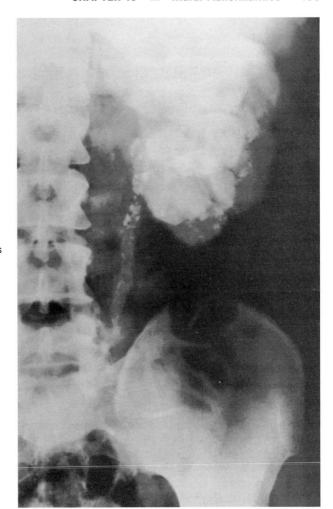

FIGURE 15–31. Healed tuberculosis with autonephrectomy. There is extensive calcification of the renal parenchyma, pelvis, and ureter. The latter is referred to as a *pipe-stem ureter*. Abdominal radiograph.

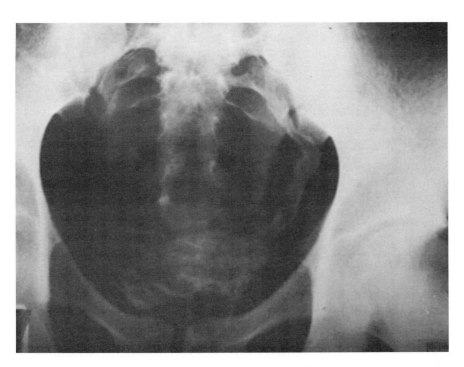

FIGURE 15–32. Schistosomiasis, left ureter and bladder. There is extensive, linear mural calcification. Abdominal radiograph.

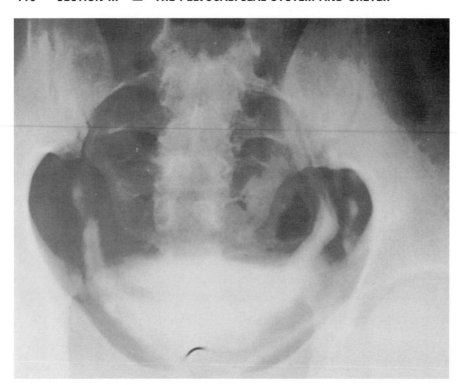

FIGURE 15–33. Schistosomiasis, both ureters and bladder. There is marked thickening and calcification of the ureteral and bladder walls. Vesicoureteral reflux is present. Cystogram.

droureter can develop from a generalized mural fibrosis and aperistalsis alone. Calcification in the wall of the ureter varies from a fine, stippled pattern to a continuous linear density. Although transitional cell carcinoma of the bladder uroepithelium develops more commonly in patients with schistosomiasis than in the general population, the same relationship does not hold for the ureter.

Excretory urography and voiding cystourethrography best demonstrate the abnormalities of ureteral schistosomiasis, including vesicoureteral reflux, if present. Computed tomography best demonstrates the marked thickening and calcification of the ureteral wall that is often present.

RESPONSES TO INFECTION OR INFLAMMATION

Pyelitis and Ureteritis Cystica

Definition

Multiple small cysts in the pelvic wall are known as *pyelitis cystica* and those in the ureteral wall are referred to as *ureteritis cystica*. These form from solid buds of uroepithelium that migrate inward from the mucosal surface, become isolated in the tunica propria, and then, through metaplasia, are transformed into glandular structures that eventually fill with clear, proteinaceous fluid. Each cyst is a discrete, small mass that elevates the uroepithelium. Some grow as large as 2 cm in diameter. Spontaneous rupture sometimes occurs.

Clinical Setting

Pyelitis and ureteritis cystica develop in older patients, particularly women. The traditional view-

point has been that the cysts form as a response to chronic infection of the urinary tract with *Escherichia coli*. However, the fact that pyelitis cystica is found in some asymptomatic patients without a history of infection casts doubt on the validity of this premise. Clinical findings, when present, include hematuria, possibly from rupture of a cyst, and signs and symptoms of urinary tract infection.

Radiologic Findings

Pyelitis and ureteritis cystica cause persistent, unchanging filling defects in the wall of the pelvocalyceal system and the proximal ureter. These are usually discrete and widely spaced and vary in size up to 2 cm in diameter (Figs. 15–34 and 15–35). The same radiologic findings, representing mural fluid-filled blebs, may be seen as part of the Stevens-Johnson syndrome. Cysts that are small and closely grouped, an uncommon occurrence, produce a ragged appearance.

Leukoplakia

Definition

Squamous metaplasia of transitional cells with keratinization, known as *epidermidalization of the uroepithelium,* is common to both leukoplakia and cholesteatoma. There is a controversy over the additional features that may characterize these two entities. The generally held view is that leukoplakia is epidermidalization plus proliferation and atypia of the basal squamous epithelial layer and that this condition is premalignant. Cholesteatoma, on the other hand, is traditionally thought of as a desquamative form of keratinizing metaplasia without malignant potential. An opposing point of view, however, proposes that leukoplakia and cholesteatoma are identical entities, characterized by metaplasia, keratinization, *and* desquamation. Proponents of this concept advocate the term *keratinizing desquamative squamous metaplasia* for both leukoplakia and cholesteatoma (Hertle and Androulakasis, 1982). Atypia and premalignant predisposition are not part of this concept. (Cholesteatoma is discussed in Chapter 14 as a rare cause of an intraluminal abnormality.)

Leukoplakia develops in the pelvocalyceal system and proximal ureter either as isolated patches or as a large confluent lesion. Renal calculus coexists in approximately 50 per cent of patients. Squamous carcinoma is said to be present in as many as 20 per cent of patients at the time that leukoplakia is diagnosed.

Clinical Setting

Leukoplakia of the upper urinary tract affects men and women equally and is most prevalent in the third to fifth decades. A history of chronic infection, often for as long as 20 years, is common. Colic and recurrent fever are frequent complaints. Passage of cornified squamous epithelium through the urethra is pathognomonic of squamous metaplasia but does not distinguish leukoplakia from cholesteatoma, if such a distinction does in fact exist.

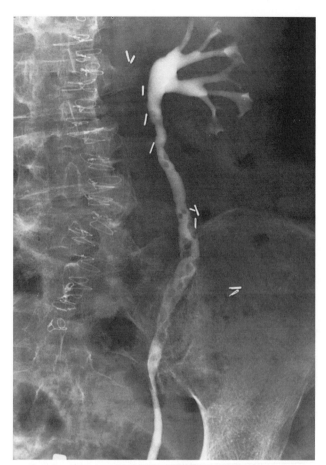

FIGURE 15–35. Ureteritis cystica. Multiple cysts appear as sharply marginated mural filling defects. Retrograde pyelogram. (Kindly provided by Wendelin S. Hayes, D.O., Georgetown University, Washington, D.C.)

Radiologic Findings

Leukoplakia causes marked irregularities of the pelvocalyceal wall that are either localized (Fig. 15–36) or generalized (Fig. 15–37). The pelvocalyceal system and proximal ureter are the usual sites of involvement. Keratin that is shed into the lumen creates an irregular intraluminal mass that has a lacy pattern of contrast material within it (see Fig. 15–36). Such a mass may obstruct at the ureteropelvic junction or more distally in the ureter. As noted earlier, stone disease coexists with leukoplakia in approximately 50 per cent of affected patients.

Malakoplakia

Definition

Malakoplakia is an uncommon response to an infection of the urinary tract with *Escherichia coli*. An intracellular abnormality of macrophages, probably at the lysosomal level, is thought to prevent complete digestion of phagocytosed bacteria. Submucosal granulomas dominated by large mononuclear cells with abundant cytoplasm develop. These cells contain intracytoplasmic inclusion bodies that are composed of calcium and iron-laden lysosomal ma-

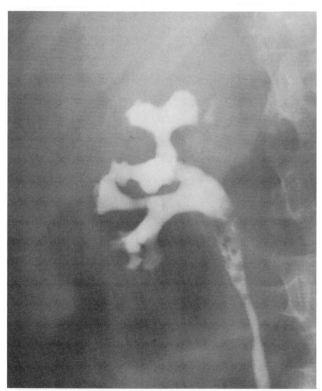

FIGURE 15–34. Pyelitis cystica. Multiple cysts of varying size appear as persistent, sharply marginated filling defects attached to the wall of the pelvocalyceal system in an elderly woman with chronic *Escherichia coli* urinary tract infection. Retrograde pyelogram.

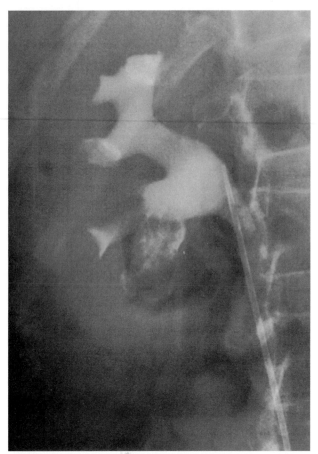

FIGURE 15–36. Leukoplakia. The filling defect in the collecting system of the lower pole contains a lacy pattern of contrast material, representing desquamated keratin. This presentation is indistinguishable from cholesteatoma and other intraluminal masses discussed in Chapter 14. Retrograde pyelogram.

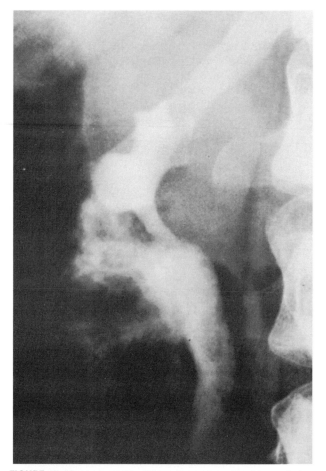

FIGURE 15–37. Leukoplakia. There is a generalized irregularity of the pelvocalyceal wall. Excretory urogram.

terial. These inclusions, known as Michaelis-Gutmann bodies, are probably bacilli in various stages of defective digestion. Michaelis-Gutmann bodies may also be found in extracellular locations. The granulomas produce multiple yellow-gray or brown elevations of the mucosa.

Malakoplakia affects the bladder most frequently, but any part of the genitourinary tract, including the testes and prostate, may be involved. Renal parenchymal malakoplakia is discussed in Chapter 11 and bladder malakoplakia is discussed in Chapter 19.

Clinical Setting

Malakoplakia develops most often in women in the fifth to sixth decade in whom altered immunity is often present. Urinary tract infection with *E. coli* is always present and accounts for the usual clinical findings of flank pain, dysuria, fever, hematuria, proteinuria, pyuria, bacilliuria, and leukocytosis. The occurrence of obstruction and renal failure depends on the site and extent of involvement.

Radiologic Findings

Malakoplakia of the collecting system and ureter causes multiple, irregular mural filling defects and

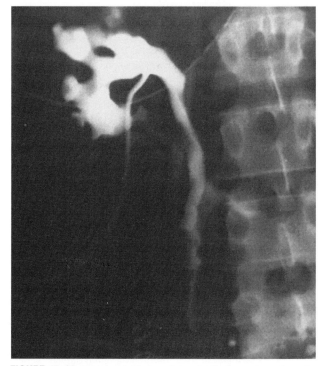

FIGURE 15–38. Malakoplakia involving both the pelvocalyceal system and the ureter. Multiple, irregular, mural filling defects are present throughout the ureter. Retrograde pyelogram.

dilatation with or without obstruction (Fig. 15–38). Abnormalities of renal parenchymal and bladder malacoplakia usually coexist (see Chapters 11 and 19.)

Xanthogranulomatous Pyelonephritis

The renal pelvis is scarred and contracted, and the calyces are dilated in xanthogranulomatous pyelonephritis. Pelvocalyceal system involvement invariably occurs as part of a process in which parenchymal abnormalities predominate. Xantho-granulomatous pyelonephritis is discussed in Chapter 9.

AMYLOIDOSIS

Definition

Amyloidosis of the upper urinary tract is rare and occurs as an isolated event except in children with familial Mediterranean fever. Amyloid deposits in the extrarenal part of the urinary tract are usually perivascular and limited to the submucosa. These are often calcified. The bladder is more frequently involved than the renal pelvis, the ureter, or the urethra. Most lesions of the upper urinary tract are unilateral. Isolated amyloidosis, unrelated to an underlying disease, usually appears as a stricture with proximal dilatation. This may be found in an infundibulum of the pelvocalyceal system, at the ureteropelvic junction, or in the ureter. In systemic amyloidosis, generalized involvement causes diffuse narrowing and irregularity of the upper urinary tract, usually in association with renal amyloidosis. Amyloidosis of the kidney parenchyma is discussed in Chapter 8, and the findings of amyloidosis of the bladder are presented in Chapter 19.

Clinical Setting

Isolated amyloidosis of the upper urinary tract is either asymptomatic or associated with hematuria. Flank pain or urinary tract infection may develop in association with stricture and obstruction. In secondary amyloidosis, renal failure and the clinical manifestations of the underlying disease are likely to dominate the clinical picture.

Radiologic Findings

A linear deposit of calcium in the submucosa is sometimes seen on standard radiographs of the pelvocalyceal system. The calcium may be dense enough to create the appearance of a pelvic cast. In this situation, a thin band of relatively radiolucent mucosa separating the opacified urine from the calcified mucosa becomes apparent during excretory urography. Hydrocalyx may also result from an isolated amyloid deposit narrowing an infundibulum.

Ureteral involvement is usually limited to a single segment in which there is an elongated, irregu-

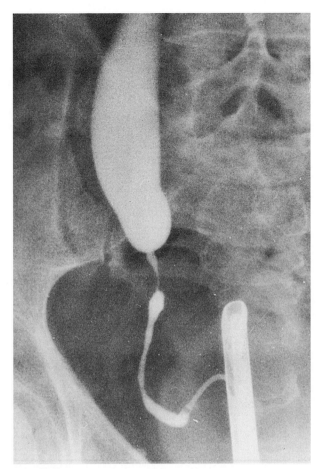

FIGURE 15–39. Amyloidosis, distal left ureter. Retrograde ureterogram. There is a smooth, concentric narrowing of a long segment of ureter with proximal dilatation.

lar stricture in the distal portion of the ureter with proximal distention (Fig. 15–39). Ureteral involvement in systemic amyloidosis, most commonly seen in patients with familial Mediterranean fever, is seen as extensive narrowing and rigidity.

POLYARTERITIS NODOSA

Upper urinary tract obstruction due to ureteral stricture has been reported as a rare event in patients with polyarteritis nodosa. The underlying pathogenesis has not been elucidated.

EOSINOPHILIC URETERITIS

Ureteral stricture due to ureteral and periureteral fibrosis and eosinophilic infiltrate is another rare cause of upper urinary tract obstruction. This has been described in patients with and without a history of allergy or parasite infestation. The pathologic appearance resembles that of eosinophilic cystitis. The radiologic appearance of the ureteral stricture is nonspecific.

MURAL HEMORRHAGE

Definition

There are clinical circumstances in which multiple, discrete mural pelvocalyceal or ureteral masses appear and disappear within a short time. The transient nature of these lesions strongly suggests that they are mural hematomas. However, an accurate pathologic description of this process is not available, since the conditions under which the lesions occur rarely yield tissue specimens. The clinical and radiologic features of these masses suggest multifocal sites of limited bleeding in the wall of the pelvis or ureter.

Clinical Setting

Mural hemorrhage may occur during anticoagulant therapy, as a result of blunt or penetrating abdominal trauma, in spontaneously acquired circulating

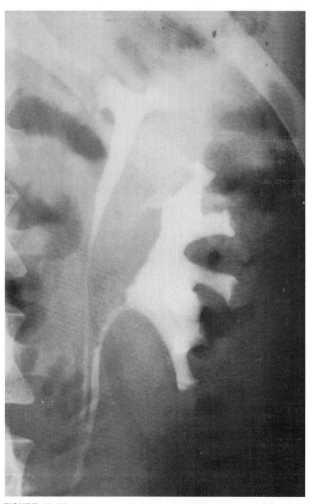

FIGURE 15–40. Mural hemorrhage. Multiple mural nodules are present in the pelvis of the left kidney of a 22-year-old man with penetrating trauma to the left retroperitoneum. Excretory urogram. (Courtesy of Jay A. Kaiser, M.D., and Hideyo Minagi, M.D., San Francisco General Hospital, San Francisco, California, and AJR *125*:311, 1975.)

anticoagulants, or as a complication of crystalluria or microurolithiasis.

Transient hematuria and flank pain are the primary clinical findings. Free blood clots, when present, are a potential cause of obstruction and renal colic.

Bleeding that develops during anticoagulant therapy, particularly when coagulation indices are within therapeutic range, may herald an underlying kidney disease, such as tumor. Radiologic studies should be carefully interpreted with this in mind.

Radiologic Findings

Mural hemorrhage produces multiple, discrete masses that project from the mucosal wall of the pelvocalyceal system or ureter (Fig. 15–40). The masses may be round or oval and discrete or irregular. Coexistent intraluminal clot can cause obstruction at the ureteropelvic junction. Computed tomography without contrast material enhancement may demonstrate thickening of the uroepithelial wall and, if performed in close proximity to the acute episode of bleeding, an attenuation value of fresh blood clot. Spontaneous clearing within 2 weeks is the usual pattern.

LONGITUDINAL MUCOSAL FOLDS

Definition

The mucosa of a normal pelvocalyceal system and proximal ureter may form multiple longitudinal ridges when collapsed or minimally distended. These folds may extend into the calyceal infundibula, as well. This normal phenomenon might be accentuated if the collecting system has been subject to prior dilatation as a result of previous or concurrent moderate to severe vesicoureteral reflux or a prior episode of obstruction.

Linear radiolucent striae identical in appearance with longitudinal mucosal folds are rarely seen in renal vein thrombosis. The basis for this mural abnormality has not been established clearly, but it may be due to either edema or dilated collateral or submucosal veins.

Clinical Setting

Longitudinal mucosal folds, when present, are usually a normal finding. This is particularly so in patients in whom low osmolality contrast material is used to opacify the urinary tract. This class of contrast material produces less of an osmotic diuresis than does high osmolality contrast material, making it likely that the upper urinary tract is visualized in a less than normal state of distention. In some individuals, however, the same finding may represent a collecting system that has become abnormally capacious as a result of moderate to severe vesicoureteral reflux or by a previously corrected severe obstructive uropathy.

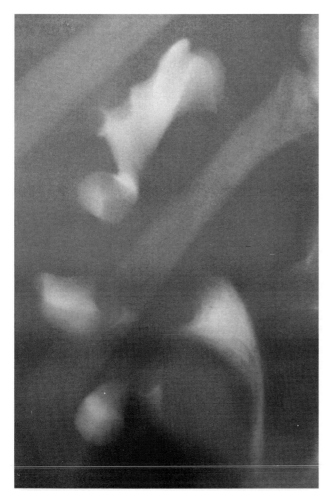

FIGURE 15–41. Longitudinal mucosal folds. Fine, regular lines of lucency are present in the right pelvis of a young woman with no history of infection, obstruction, or vesicoureteral reflux. Excretory urogram.

Radiologic Findings

Redundant mucosal folds form fine, regular, and more or less parallel longitudinal lines of lucency within an incompletely distended pelvocalyceal system that is opacified during excretory urography, pyelography, or voiding cystourethrography with reflux (Fig. 15–41). The folds disappear when the system is distended and reappear after drainage.

URETERAL PSEUDODIVERTICULOSIS

Definition

Ureteral pseudodiverticulosis is an uncommon, acquired abnormality characterized by invagination of hyperplastic transitional epithelium into the lamina propria of the ureter. The underlying muscularis is sometimes effaced but remains intact. Continuity is maintained between this outpouching and the ureteral lumen, thereby giving rise to the appearance of a diverticulum. Ureteritis cystica and ureteritis glandularis sometimes coexist with the pseudodiverticula.

Clinical Setting

Patients with ureteral pseudodiverticulosis are typically middle-aged and older. There is frequently a history of urinary tract infection, obstruction, urolithiasis, or a combination of these. However, many are asymptomatic at the time the pseudodiverticula is discovered. Studies of small populations of patients with this abnormality suggest the possibility of an increased prevalence of transitional cell carcinoma of the ureter or bladder and atypical urine cytology. These relationships, however, are not firmly established because of the small number of patients that have been investigated.

Radiologic Findings

Ureteral pseudodiverticulosis typically appears in the proximal and middle portions of both ureters as tiny (1 to 4 mm) outpouchings that are in continuity with the opacified ureter (Fig. 15–42). There are usually three to eight in each segment of involved ureter. Unilateral lesions are infrequent, and a solitary diverticulum is rare. The abnormality is best demonstrated by retrograde or antegrade ureteropyelography. Pseudodiverticulosis usually remains stable over time.

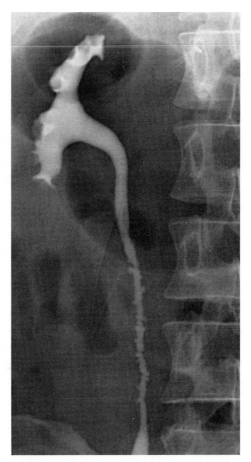

FIGURE 15–42. Pseudodiverticulosis, right mid-ureter. Retrograde ureterogram. There are multiple, small outpouchings on both sides of the ureteral wall.

PYELOCALYCEAL DIVERTICULUM

Definition

Pyelocalyceal diverticula are uroepithelium-lined pouches that extend from a peripheral point of the collecting system into the adjacent renal parenchyma. Two forms have been identified on the basis of anatomic features. Type I diverticula, the more common of the two, are connected to the calyceal cup, usually at a fornix. These lesions often have a bulbous shape with a narrow connecting infundibulum of varying length. Type I diverticula occur in the polar regions, especially in the upper pole. Most measure a few millimeters in diameter. Type II diverticula develop in the interpolar region, communicate directly into the pelvis, and are usually larger and rounder than the Type I diverticula. The neck of a Type II diverticulum is short and not easily identified.

Pyelocalyceal diverticula probably have a developmental origin. The generally held opinion is that they are ureteral bud remnants that either failed to divide into fully formed calyces or were not assimilated during the process of calyceal-lobar fusion. Support for a theory of developmental origin is derived from the equal prevalence in all age groups and the frequent, although not invariable, presence of smooth muscle below the uroepithelial lining. Explanations for the genesis of pyelocalyceal diverticula as acquired abnormalities include reflux and infection, rupture of a simple renal cyst or abscess, infundibular achalasia or spasm, and hydrocalyx secondary to inflammatory fibrosis of an infundibulum. None of these concepts is widely supported.

Stones form in as many as 50 per cent of patients with pyelocalyceal diverticulum. These stones are either single or multiple or occur in the form of milk of calcium. The latter is a colloidal suspension of precipitated calcium salts occurring either as pure calcium phosphate, calcium carbonate, or calcium oxalate, or as a mixture of any of these.

Synonyms for pyelocalyceal diverticulum are pyelogenic cyst, pericalyceal cyst, calyceal diverticulum, calyceal cyst, pyelorenal cyst, and congenital hydrocalycosis.

Clinical Setting

Pyelocalyceal diverticula are found with equal frequency at all ages and in both sexes. Most diverticula are asymptomatic and are found incidentally during excretory urography or pyelography.

Symptoms that do develop are those of infection, stone, or hemorrhage and include fever and colic. Pyuria, bacteriuria, and hematuria may develop. Some cases have been reported in which an uncomplicated diverticulum was thought to cause flank pain. Transitional cell carcinoma may arise in the uroepithelial cells that line the cavity of a pyelocalyceal diverticulum.

Radiologic Findings

Pyelocalyceal diverticula communicate with the collecting system and usually opacify during excretory urography or pyelography. However, opacification may be delayed because of a slow exchange of urine between the two structures. For similar reasons, a diverticulum can remain opacified for a longer period of time than the freely drained portions of the pelvocalyceal system.

Type I diverticula range from 1 mm to several centimeters in diameter and are mostly found extending from a point on an upper polar calyceal cup. A narrow isthmus is frequently identified connecting the opening into the calyx with the fundus of the diverticulum. Diverticular shapes are tubular, flasklike, oval, and round (Figs. 15–43 and 15–44).

Type II diverticula occur in the interpolar region and open directly into the renal pelvis rather than into a calyx. The point of connection is often obscure (Fig. 15–45). This form of diverticula may become large enough to produce a mass effect on adjacent portions of the pelvocalyceal system and cause a defect in the nephrogram (Fig. 15–46).

Both types of diverticula appear as uncomplicated fluid-filled spaces on unenhanced computed tomo-

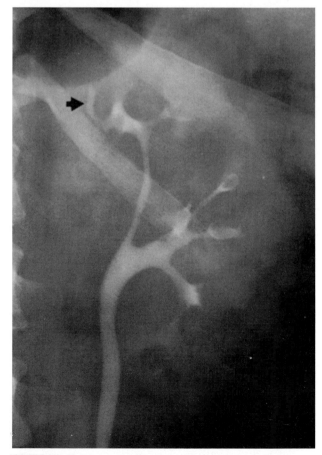

FIGURE 15–43. Pyelocalyceal diverticulum Type I. A single diverticulum *(arrow)* extends from a fornix of the upper pole calyx. A narrow isthmus is identifiable. Excretory urogram.

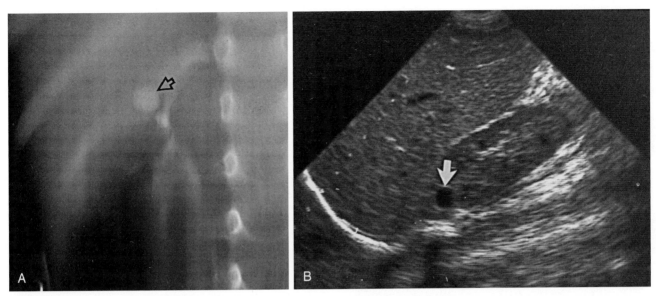

FIGURE 15–44. Pyelocalyceal diverticulum Type I.
A, Excretory urogram. The diverticulum *(arrow)* is round, extends from the upper pole calyx, and opacifies during contrast material enhancement, indicating communication with the collecting system.
B, Ultrasonogram, longitudinal section. The diverticulum *(arrow)* appears as a fluid-filled mass that is indistinguishable from a simple nephrogenic cyst.

FIGURE 15–45. Pyelocalyceal diverticulum Type II. A large communicating fluid-filled space arises from the interpolar portion of the collecting system. Retrograde pyelogram.

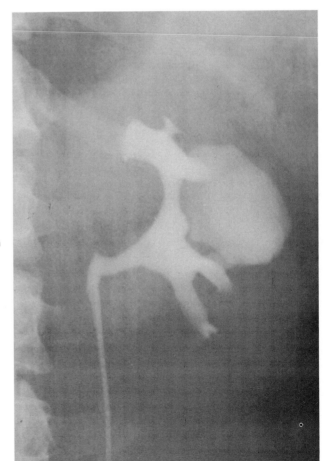

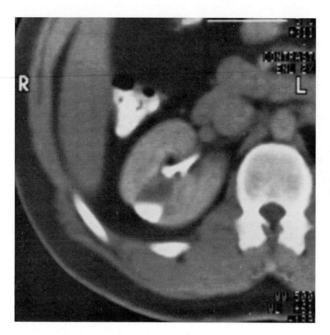

FIGURE 15–46. Pyelocalyceal diverticulum Type II. A large communicating fluid-filled space in the interpolar region extends from the collecting system to the surface of the kidney. Computed tomogram, contrast material–enhanced.

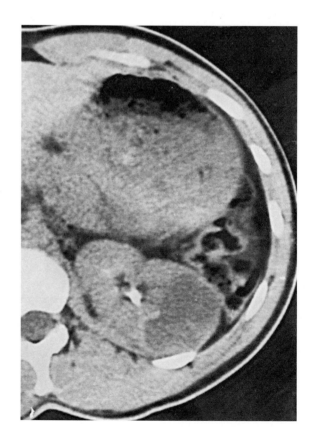

FIGURE 15–47. Pyelocalyceal diverticulum Type II appearing as a complicated cystic mass in a 27-year-old man. Computed tomogram, contrast material–enhanced. The diverticulum does not communicate, and its wall is apparently thickened as a result of expansion into the surrounding renal parenchyma.

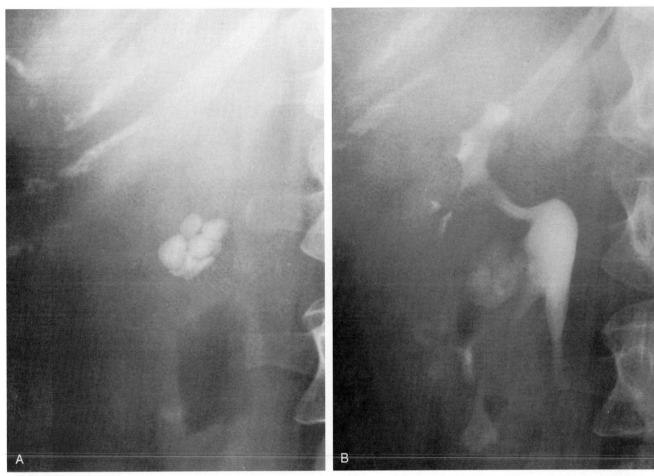

FIGURE 15–48. Pyelocalyceal diverticulum Type II with multiple stones.
A, Preliminary film.
B, Excretory urogram. Note the delayed opacification of the diverticulum.

graphic and ultrasonographic images (see Fig. 15–44). With contrast material enhancement, computed tomography demonstrates layering of contrast material in the dependent portion of the diverticulum (see Fig. 15–46).

For no apparent reason or because of occlusion of the neck from infection, edema, or scar, a diverticulum may fail to opacify during a contrast material–enhanced imaging study. In this situation, the radiologic findings, including ultrasonographic and computed tomographic, are either of a simple cyst or of a complicated cystic mass (Fig. 15–47).

A single calculus or a circumscribed collection of many small stones in the periphery of the kidney suggests a pyelocalyceal diverticulum (Fig. 15–48). These stones may change position slightly when more than one preliminary film is available for comparison. With the patient in a prone or supine position, milk of calcium forms a round, homogeneous density that may change shape slightly with varied degrees of inspiration or alteration of the patient's position. On films exposed with a horizontal x-ray beam or on computed tomograms, the dependent portion of the milk of calcium is semilunar and

there is a calcium-fluid level at the upper margin (Figs. 15–49 and 15–50). Milk of calcium is hyperechoic in the dependent portion of the diverticulum, separated from the anechoic supernatant urine by a sharp linear interface (see Fig. 15–50).

Pyelocalyceal diverticulum may be complicated by infection, hemorrhage, or transitional cell carcinoma arising from the uroepithelial lining of the diverticulum (Figs. 15–51 and 15–52). Under these circumstances, the complicating factor obscures the radiologic findings of the diverticulum.

The radiologic appearance of other fluid-filled lesions that communicate with the pelvocalyceal system may be identical to that of pyelocalyceal diverticula. These other lesions include a ruptured simple renal (nephrogenic) cyst and an evacuated abscess or hematoma. Mild forms of renal papillary necrosis and medullary sponge kidney can simulate a small diverticulum. These disorders are usually multiple, whereas a diverticulum almost always occurs singly. Focal caliectasis (hydrocalyx) due to infundibular narrowing from tuberculous cicatrix, crossing vessel, infiltrating carcinoma, or stone may also simulate a pyelocalyceal diverticulum.

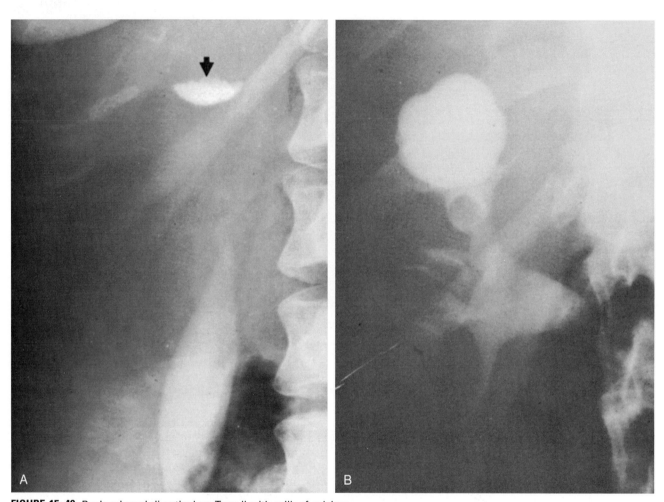

FIGURE 15–49. Pyelocalyceal diverticulum Type II with milk of calcium.
 A, Preliminary film, upright projection obtained during oral cholecystogram. The milk of calcium forms a semilunar density with a calcium-fluid level *(arrow).*
 B, Excretory urogram. Supine projection. The milk of calcium is now viewed *en face.*

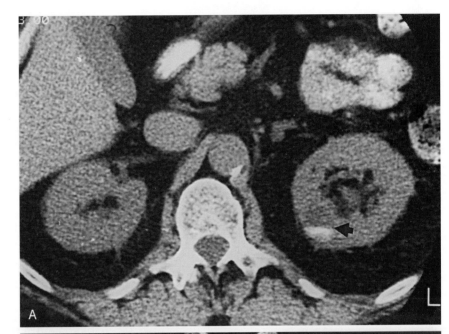

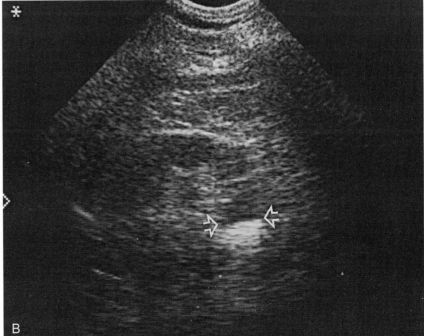

FIGURE 15–50. Pyelocalyceal diverticulum with milk of calcium, left kidney.

A, Computed tomogram, unenhanced. The diverticulum *(arrow)* appears as a round, low-density mass with high attenuation milk of calcium layered in its dependent portion.

B, Ultrasonogram, longitudinal projection. The supernatant fluid in the diverticulum *(arrows)* is echogenic, but much less so than the dependent milk of calcium.

(Kindly provided by Wendelin S. Hayes, D.O., Georgetown University, Washington, D.C.)

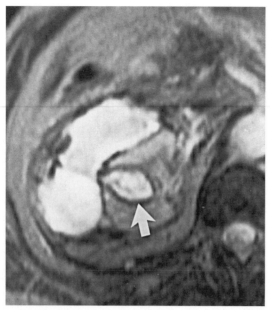

FIGURE 15–51. Pyelocalyceal diverticulum complicated by hemorrhage into the perirenal space, right kidney. Magnetic resonance image. The diverticulum *(arrow)* is filled with high signal intensity blood that extends into the perirenal space.

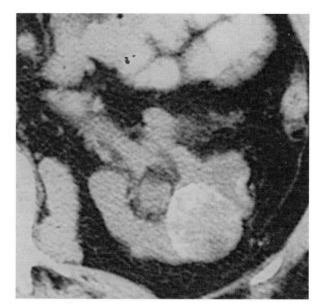

FIGURE 15–52. Pyelocalyceal diverticulum complicated by transitional cell carcinoma, left kidney. The tumor appears as an irregular filling defect within the opacified diverticulum. Computed tomogram, contrast material–enhanced.

URETEROCELE

Definition

Prolapse into the bladder of the intravesicular portion of the distal ureter with an associated dilatation of the distal ureter is known as a ureterocele, a deformity that is congenital in origin. The wall of a ureterocele is composed of a thin layer of muscle and collagen interposed between the outer surface of bladder uroepithelium and the inner surface of ureteral uroepithelium.

There are several systems for classifying ureteroceles. An appropriate classification from a radiologic point of view is one that defines an *orthotopic ureterocele* as one that forms in a ureter with a normal insertion into the trigone and an *ectopic ureterocele* as one in a ureter whose insertion is ectopic. Orthotopic ureteroceles usually occur in single systems, whereas ectopic ureteroceles usually occur in duplicated collecting systems.

A ureterocele may be complicated by partial or complete obstruction at its orifice or by the formation of a stone within its lumen. A ureterocele may also obstruct the other ureteral orifices leading into the bladder or the bladder outlet itself. Additionally, an ectopic ureterocele may deform the ureterovesical junction of a normally inserted ureter and thereby cause vesicoureteral reflux.

Ureterocele is discussed in this chapter as an abnormality of the wall of the ureter. Other topics that relate to ureterocele include the embryology and anomalies of the upper urinary tract (see Chapter 3), vesicoureteral reflux (see Chapter 5), the kidney with a duplicated pelvocalyceal system (see Chapter 9), hydronephrosis and hydroureter (see Chapters 9 and 17), renal dysplasia (see Chapter 11), and focal hydrocalyx (see Chapter 12).

Clinical Setting

Orthotopic ureteroceles are usually small, unilateral, and asymptomatic. These are most often incidental findings in an adult undergoing urinary tract evaluation for an unrelated problem. A calculus may form in the ureterocele, and in some patients there may be some obstruction to urine flow with the associated risk of infection.

Ectopic ureteroceles, on the other hand, are usually large enough to cause complications that lead to their discovery in infancy or childhood. Ectopic ureteroceles that are part of a completely duplicated upper urinary tract are usually found in females and are predominantly left-sided. These are very rare in individuals of African descent. A ureterocele that forms in a single ureter that is ectopically inserted usually occurs in males. Clinical problems that arise from the complications of an ectopic ureterocele include urinary tract infection, urine retention due to bladder neck obstruction, flank pain, stone formation, or an abdominal mass. Incontinence is present in females when the site of ectopic insertion is distal to the urogenital diaphragm. Prolapse of an ectopic ureterocele into the vagina may occur.

Radiologic Findings

Orthotopic ureteroceles are best defined radiologically during excretory urography. The distal ureter is minimally dilated and projects slightly into the lumen of the bladder. Opacified bladder urine surrounds the ureterocele and is separated from the dilated ureteral lumen by a uniformly thin line of relative radiolucency (Fig. 15–53). This represents the components of the wall of the ureterocele: the bladder and ureteral uroepithelium and the intervening muscle and collagen. This radiologic appearance, called the *cobrahead deformity,* may be simulated by conditions other than ureterocele, as described in Differential Diagnosis at the end of this chapter. A calculus in the ureterocele, which may or may not obstruct, is sometimes noted (Fig. 15–54).

An ectopic ureterocele is seen on cystography as a smooth, nonopaque, intravesicular mass that is often quite large and centered toward the base of the bladder (Fig. 15–55). When defined by excretory urography or contrast material–enhanced computed tomography, the degree of enhancement of the urine within the ureterocele and its draining ureter depends on the degree of function in the related upper pole moiety. Often, opacification is absent or diminished because of hydronephrosis or dysplasia, both caused by obstruction. In this circumstance, contrast material excreted by the functioning renal units opacifies the bladder and the ureterocele appears only as a nonopaque intravesicular mass. Ultrasonography demonstrates a ureterocele as a thin, echogenic membrane in the bladder lumen in close proximity to its associated draining ureter, which is slightly to markedly dilated (Fig. 15–56). Uncomplicated fluid (urine in the bladder and distal ureter) surrounds both sides of the membrane. Dilatation of the ureter obstructed by an ectopic ureterocele is usually moderate. However, in some patients, the ureter is so dilated and tortuous that it crosses the midline and displaces both intra-abdominal and retroperitoneal organs. This can be identified by ultrasonography, computed tomography, or percutaneous ureteropyelography as a fluid-filled, elongated mass, with multiple bends in the ureter giving the appearance of septations. The dilated ureter can be traced cephalad to its associated renal unit, which is often hydronephrotic or dysplastic or both (see Fig. 15–56). Uncommonly, the draining ureter obstructed by an ectopic ureterocele is collapsed or diminutive owing to the absence of urine produced by its renal unit.

The size and shape of a ureterocele can change with the dynamics of voiding or alterations in bladder pressure. A ureterocele may also evert and assume the appearance of a bladder diverticulum.

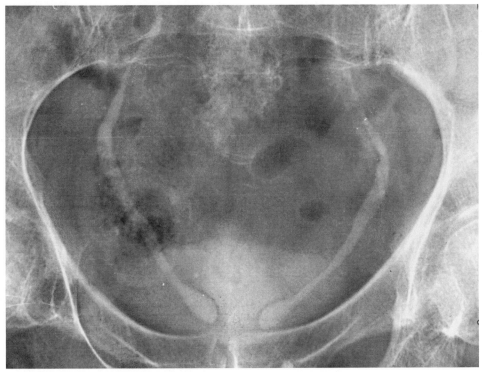

FIGURE 15–53. Ureteroceles, orthotopic, bilateral. Excretory urogram. Each ureterocele is seen as a fusiform dilatation of the distal ureter, slight prolapse of the ureter into the bladder lumen, and a thin line of relative lucency representing the wall of the ureterocele surrounded by contrast material in the ureter and bladder.

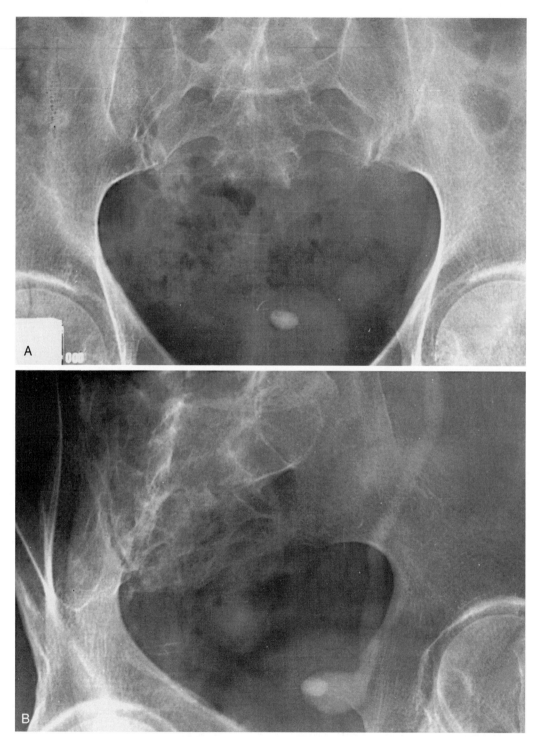

FIGURE 15–54. Ureterocele, orthotopic, complicated by stone and obstruction.
   A, Preliminary radiograph.
   B, Excretory urogram, left posterior oblique projection.

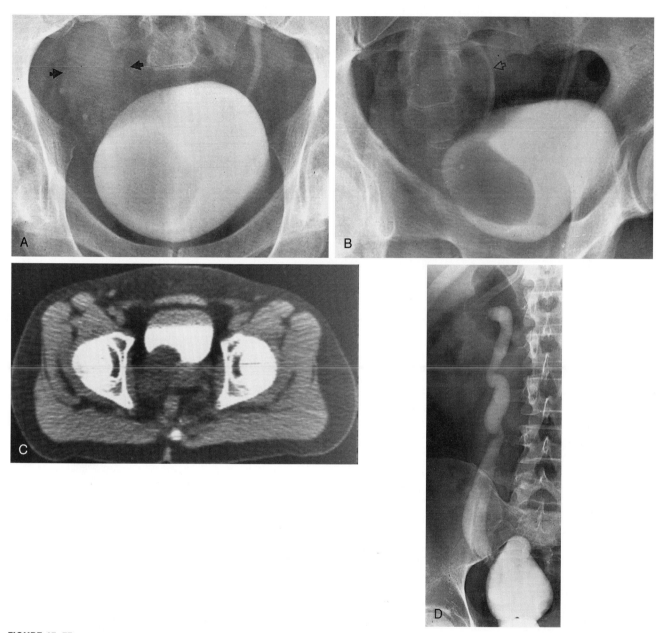

FIGURE 15–55. Ureterocele, ectopic, upper pole moiety of a completely duplicated right ureter and collecting system. The ureter to the upper pole is obstructed, dilated, and displaces the adjacent, nonobstructed ureter draining the lower pole moiety.

A, Excretory urogram. The large ectopic ureterocele projects into the lumen of the bladder as a smooth-walled filling defect. The dilated distal ureter is seen as a soft tissue mass *(arrows).*

B, Excretory urogram, left posterior oblique projection. The ureterocele projects into the bladder base. The ureter draining the lower pole moiety *(arrow)* is displaced by the obstructed, ectopically inserted ureter. There is complete duplication of the left ureter.

C, Computed tomogram, contrast material–enhanced. The ureterocele projects into the bladder base.

D, Antegrade pyelogram. The obstructed, dilated ureter draining the dystrophic upper pole moiety is opacified.

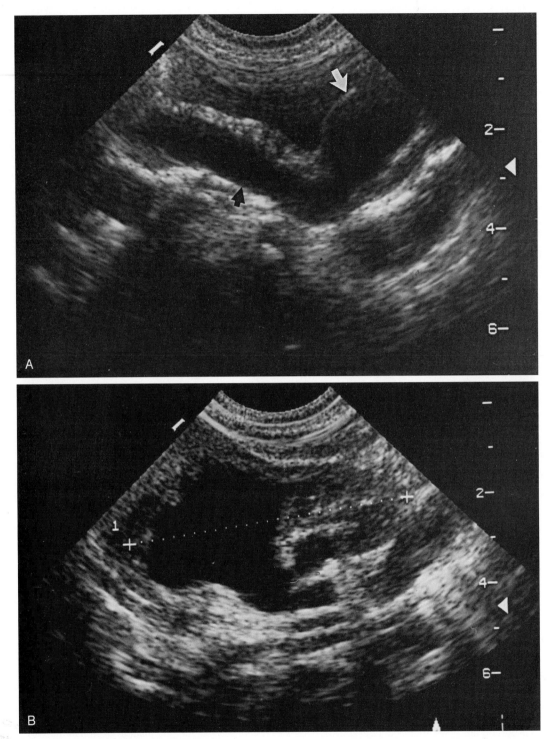

FIGURE 15–56. Ureterocele, ectopic, upper pole moiety of a completely duplicated left collecting system and ureter. Ultrasonograms, longitudinal projection.

A, Bladder. The dilated distal ectopic ureter *(black arrow)* enters the bladder. A thin, round, echogenic membrane *(white arrow)* represents the urine-filled ureterocele.

B, Kidney. The upper pole moiety is dilated as a result of obstruction by the ectopic ureterocele.

(Kindly provided by Steve Horii, M.D., Georgetown University, Washington, D.C.)

DIFFERENTIAL DIAGNOSIS

The first task in evaluating an apparent mural lesion is to verify its location. Usually, a small or medium-sized mass in the pelvocalyceal system readily satisfies criteria for a mural origin and is likely to be a **transitional cell carcinoma.** A bulky, immovable, nonopaque mass that fills the collecting system or ureter, however, may be impossible to differentiate in terms of luminal or mural location. In this circumstance, differential diagnosis must be broadly based and include intraluminal abnormalities, such as **nonopaque stone, blood clot,** and **fungus ball** as well as abnormalities of mural origin. Sorting these out depends on the unique ultrasonographic or computed tomographic features of stone, the transient nature of blood clots, and the correlation of clinical and laboratory data. This is discussed in the concluding section of Chapter 14.

Malignancy of the uroepithelium is the most common cause of an isolated focal mural mass. Uroepithelial tumors that develop in a pelvocalyceal system and invade renal tissue can be differentiated from tumors of renal parenchymal origin, such as adenocarcinoma, by an analysis of the geometry of the kidney enlargement. Tumors of uroepithelial origin preserve the reniform shape of the enlarged kidney. Most tumors of renal origin, on the other hand, grow from an epicenter and create a ball-shaped mass. This subject is discussed fully in Chapter 12. Ultimate diagnosis, of course, depends on histologic study.

Herniation of cysts from a **multilocular cystic nephroma** may also simulate a primary mural mass. These can be identified by their smooth surface and the coexistence of an expansile, large, multiloculated, cystic tumor in adjacent renal parenchyma. Extramural abnormalities that might be confused with a lesion of mural origin include **aberrant papilla,** discussed in Chapter 3, and several other entities that are discussed in Chapter 16. These include **tortuous blood vessels, focal fat deposits** projecting from the renal sinus, **endometriosis,** and **retroperitoneal metastases** invading the ureter.

Mural masses that are multifocal, discrete, and separated from each other are caused by **multifocal transitional cell carcinoma, metastases, pyelitis** or **ureteritis cystica,** or **mural hemorrhage.** The last diagnosis is favored when there is an associated intraluminal blood clot, increased attenuation value of the lesion by computed tomography, or resolution on a repeat study performed within 2 weeks. Differentiation otherwise depends on the different clinical settings in which these entities occur.

The nature of extensive, irregular mural lesions cannot be precisely established by radiologic studies. Mural tumors of any tissue type, **tuberculosis, schistosomiasis, thrush, leukoplakia, malakoplakia, xanthogranulomatous pyelonephritis,** and **amyloidosis** may have identical appearances. Tuberculosis, however, almost always has associated renal parenchymal abnormalities, and schistosomiasis is usually limited to the distal ureter and bladder. The appearance of **pseudodiverticulosis** is distinctive. Otherwise, diagnosis depends on clinical and pathologic data.

Conditions that thicken the bladder mucosa and distend the distal ureter may simulate an orthotopic ureterocele. These include carcinoma of the bladder or cervix invading the ureterovesical orifice, radiation cystitis, distal ureteral calculus, or edema of the ureterovesical junction from recent passage of stone. These **pseudoureteroceles** are identified by asymmetry of the distal lumen, thickening and irregularity of the wall, the absence of intravesicular protrusion, or the coexistence of other features of the underlying abnormality.

BIBLIOGRAPHY

General

Bechtold, R. B., Chen, M. Y. M., Dyer, R. B., and Zagoria, R. J.: CT of the ureteral wall. AJR *170*:1283, 1998.
Fein, A. B., and McClennan, B. L.: Solitary filling defects of the ureter. Semin. Roentgenol. *21*:201, 1986.
Hill, G. S.: Intrinsic and extrinsic obstruction of the urinary tract. In Hill, G. S. (ed.): Uropathology. New York, Churchill Livingstone, 1989, pp. 517–574.
Kaiser, J. A., Jacobs, R. P., and Korobkin, M.: Submucosal hemorrhage of the renal collecting system. AJR *125*:311, 1975.
Malek, R. S., Aguilo, J. J., and Hattery, R. R.: Radiolucent filling defects of the renal pelvis: Classification and report of unusual cases. J. Urol. *114*:508, 1975.
Pollack, H. M., Arger, P. H., Banner, M. P., Mulhern, C. B., Jr., and Coleman, B. G.: Computed tomography of renal pelvic defects. Radiology *138*:645, 1981.
Smith, W. L., Weinstein, A. S., and West, J. F.: Defects of renal collecting systems in patients receiving anticoagulants. Radiology *112*:649, 1974.
Williamson, B., Jr., Hartman, G. W., and Hattery, R. R.: Multiple and diffuse ureteral filling defects. Semin. Roentgenol. *21*:214, 1986.

Tumors

Ambos, M. A., Bosniak, M. A., Megibow, A. J., and Raghavendra, B.: Ureteral involvement by metastatic disease. Urol. Radiol. *1*:105, 1979.
Aufderheide, A. C., and Streitz, J. M.: Mucinous adenocarcinoma of the renal pelvis: Report of two cases. Cancer *33*:167, 1974.
Banner, M. P., and Pollack, H. M.: Fibrous ureteral polyps. Radiology *130*:73, 1979.
Bergman, H., Friedenberg, R. M., and Sayegh, V.: New roentgenologic signs of carcinoma of the ureter. AJR *86*:707, 1961.
Booth, C. M., Cameron, K. M., and Pugh, R. C. B.: Urothelial carcinoma of the kidney and ureter. Br. J. Urol *52*:430, 1980.
Brandes, D., and Katz, R. S.: Nonepithelial tumors of the ureter and bladder. In Hill, G. S. (ed.): Uropathology. New York, Churchill Livingstone, 1989, pp. 861–872.
Burnett, K. R., Miller, J. B., and Greenbaum, E. I.: Transitional cell carcinoma: Rapid development in phenacetin abuse. AJR *134*:1259, 1980.
Colgan, J. R., III, Skaist, L., and Morrow, J. W.: Benign ureteral tumors in childhood: A case report and a plea for conservative management. J. Urol. *109*:308, 1973.
Eagan, J. W.: Urothelial neoplasms: Pathologic anatomy. In Hill, G. S. (ed.): Uropathology. New York, Churchill Livingstone, 1989, pp. 719–792.
Eagan, J. W.: Urothelial neoplasms: Renal pelvis and ureter. In

Hill, G. S. (ed.): Uropathology. New York, Churchill Living-stone, 1989, pp. 843–860.

Gaakeer, H. A., and DeRuiter, H. J.: Carcinoma of the renal pelvis following the abuse of phenacetin-containing analgesic drugs. Br. J. Urol. *51*:188, 1979.

Geerdsen, J.: Tumours of the renal pelvis and ureter: Symptom-atology, diagnosis, treatment and prognosis. Scand. J. Urol. Nephrol. *13*:287, 1979.

Gonwa, T. A., Corbett, W. T., Schey, H. M., and Buckalew, V. M., Jr.: Analgesic-associated nephropathy and transitional cell carcinoma of the urinary tract. Ann. Intern. Med. *93*:249, 1980.

Gup, A.: Benign mesodermal polyp in childhood. J. Urol. *114*:619, 1975.

Hartman, D. S., Pyatt, R. S., and Dailey, E.: Transitional cell carcinoma of the kidney with invasion into the renal vein. Urol. Radiol. *5*:83, 1983.

Hughes, F. A., III, and Davis, C. S., Jr.: Multiple benign ureteral polyps. AJR *126*:723, 1976.

Joshi, K., Jain, K., Mathur, S., and Mehrota, G. C.: Mucinous adenocarcinoma of the renal pelvis. Postgrad. Med. J. *56*:442, 1980.

Kenney, P. J., and Stanley, R. J.: Computed tomography of ure-teral tumors. J. Comput. Assist. Tomogr. *11*:102, 1987.

Kinn, A. C.: Squamous cell carcinoma of the renal pelvis. Scand. J. Urol. Nephrol. *14*:77, 1980.

Leder, R. A., and Dunnick, N. R.: Transitional cell carcinoma of the pelvicalices and ureter. AJR *155*:713, 1990.

Liwnicz, B. H., Lepow, H., Schutte, H., Fernandez, R., and Ca-berwal, D.: Mucinous adenocarcinoma of the renal pelvis: Dis-cussion of possible pathogenesis. J. Urol. *114*:306, 1975.

McLean, G. K., Pollack, H. M., and Banner, M. P.: The "stipple sign"—urographic harbinger of transitional cell neoplasm. Urol. Radiol. *1*:77, 1979.

Messing, E. M., and Catalona, W.: Urothelial tumors of the urinary tract. In Walsh, P. C., Retik, A. B., Vaughan, E. D., Jr., and Wein, A. J. (eds.): Campbell's Urology, 7th ed. Philadel-phia, W. B. Saunders, 1998, pp. 2383–2410.

Murphy, D. M., Zincke, H., and Furlow, W. L.: Primary grade I transitional cell carcinoma of the renal pelvis ureter. J. Urol. *123*:629, 1980.

Narumi, Y., Sato, T., Hori, S., Kuriyama, K., Fujita, M., Kado-waki, K., Inoue, E., Maeshima, S., Fujino, Y., Saiki, S., Kuroda, M., and Kotake, T.: Squamous cell carcinoma of the uroepithe-lium: CT evaluation. Radiology *173*:853, 1989.

Nogales, F. F., Andujar, M., Beltran, A. L., Martinez, J. L., and Zuluaga, A.: Adenocarcinoma of the renal pelvis. Urol. Int. *52*:172, 1994.

Nyman, V., Oldbring, J., and Aspelin, P.: CT of carcinoma of the renal pelvis. Acta Radiol. *33*:31, 1992.

Parienty, R. A., Ducellier, R., Pradel, J., Lubrano, J.-M., Coquille, F., and Richard, F.: Diagnostic value of CT numbers in pelvo-calyceal filling defects. Radiology *145*:743, 1982.

Pollack, H. M.: Long-term follow-up of the upper urinary tract for transitional cell carcinoma: How much is enough? Radiology *167*:871, 1988.

Pollen, J. J., Levine, E., and van Blerk, P. J. P.: The angiographic evaluation of renal pelvic carcinoma. Br. J. Urol. *47*:363, 1975.

Rubinstein, M. A., Walz, B. J., and Bucy, J. G.: Transitional cell carcinoma of the kidney: 25 year experience. J. Urol. *119*:595, 1978.

Sherwood, T.: Upper urinary tract tumours following on bladder carcinoma: Natural history of uroepithelial neoplastic disease. Br. J. Radiol. *44*:137, 1971.

Subramanyam, B. R., Raghavendra, B. N., and Madamba, M. R.: Renal transitional cell carcinoma: Sonographic and pathologic correlation. J. Clin. Ultrasound *10*:203, 1982.

Tolia, B. M., Hajdu, S. I., and Whitmore, W. F., Jr.: Leiomyosar-coma of the renal pelvis. J. Urol. *109*:974, 1973.

Toppercer, A.: Fibroepithelial tumour of the renal pelvis. Can. J. Surg. *23*:269, 1980.

Urban, B. A., Buckley, J., Soyer, P., Scherrer, A., and Fishman, E. K.: CT appearance of transitional cell carcinoma of the renal pelvis. 1. Early-stage disease. AJR *169*:157, 1997.

Urban, B. A., Buckley, J., Soyer, P., Scherrer, A., and Fishman, E. K.: CT appearance of transitional cell carcinoma of the renal pelvis. 2. Advanced-stage disease. AJR *169*:163, 1997.

Wagle, D. C., Moore, R. H., and Murphy, G. P.: Squamous cell carcinoma of the renal pelvis. J. Urol. *111*:453, 1974.

Weiss, L. M., Gelb, A. B., and Medeiros, L. J.: Adult renal epithelial neoplasms. Am. J. Clin. Pathol. *103*:624, 1995.

Winalski, C. S., Lipman, J. C., and Tumeh, S. S.: Ureteral neo-plasms. Radiographics *10*:271, 1990.

Wong-You-Cheong, J. J., Wagner, B. J., and Davis, C. J., Jr.: Transitional cell carcinoma of the urinary tract: Radiologic-pathologic correlation. RadioGraphics *18*:123, 1998.

Youssem, D. M., Gatewood, O. M. B., Goldman, S. M., and Mar-shall, F. F.: Synchronous and metachronous transitional cell carcinoma of the urinary tract: Prevalence, incidence and ra-diographic detection. Radiology *167*:613, 1988.

Congenital Ureteropelvic Junction Obstruction

Bauer, S. B.: Anomalies of the kidney and ureteropelvic junction. In Walsh, P. C., Retik, A. B., Vaughan, E. D., Jr., and Wein, A. J. (eds.): Campbell's Urology, 7th ed. Philadelphia, W. B. Saunders, 1998, pp. 1708–1756.

Bernstein, G. T., Mandell, J., Lebowitz, R. L., Bauer, S. B., Colodny, A. H., and Retik, A. B.: Ureteropelvic junction ob-struction in the neonate. J. Urol. *140*:1216, 1988.

Chahlaoui, J., and Herba, M. J.: Ureteropelvic junction obstruc-tion in the adult. J. Can. Assoc. Radiol. *28*:40, 1977.

Ekelund, L., Lindstedt, E., Thiesen, V., and Jönsson, M.-B.: Di-uresis urography in equivocal pelvic-ureteric obstruction. Urol. Radiol. *1*:147, 1980.

English, P. J., Testa, H. J., Gosling, J. A., and Cohen, S. J.: Idiopathic hydronephrosis in childhood—a comparison be-tween diuresis renography and upper urinary tract morphol-ogy. Br. J. Urol. *54*:603, 1982.

Farres, M. T., Pedron, P., Gattegno, B., Haab, F., Tligui, M., Carette, M. F., and Bigot, J. M.: Helical CT and 3D reconstruc-tion of ureteropelvic junction obstruction: Accuracy in detec-tion of crossing vessels. J. Comput. Assist. Tomogr. *22*:300, 1998.

Gosling, J. A., and Dixon, J. S.: Functional obstruction of the ureter and renal pelvis: A histological and electron microscopic study. Br. J. Urol. *50*:145, 1978.

Hanna, M. K., Jeffs, R. D., Sturgess, J. M., and Barkin, M.: Ureteral structure ultrastructure: II. Congenital ureteropelvic obstruction and primary obstructive megaureter. J. Urol. *116*:725, 1976.

Hill, G. S.: Ureteropelvic junction obstruction. In Hill, G. S. (ed.): Uropathology. New York, Churchill Livingstone, 1989, pp. 575–598.

Husmann, D. A., Kramer, S. A., Malek, R. S., and Allen, T. D.: Infundibulopelvic stenosis: A long term followup. J. Urol. *152*:837, 1994.

Jaffee, R. B., and Middleton, A. W.: Whitaker test—differen-tiation of obstructive from nonobstructive uropathy. AJR *134*:9, 1980.

Johnston, J. H., Evans, J. P., Glassberg, K. I., and Shapiro, S. R.: Pelvic hydronephrosis in children: A review of 219 personal cases. J. Urol. *117*:97, 1977.

Kendall, A. R., and Karafin, L.: Intermittent hydronephrosis: Hydration pyelography. J. Urol. *98*:653, 1967.

Malek, R. S.: Intermittent hydronephrosis: The occult ureteropel-vic obstruction. J. Urol. *130*:863, 1983.

Murnaghan, G. F.: The dynamics of the renal pelvis and ureter with reference to congenital hydronephrosis. Br. J. Urol. *30*:321, 1958.

Nixon, H. H.: Hydronephrosis in children: A clinical study of seventy-eight cases with special reference to the role of aber-rant renal vessels and the results of conservative operations. Br. J. Surg. *40*:601, 1953.

Notley, R. G.: Electron microscopy of the upper ureter and pelvi-ureteric junction. Br. J. Urol. *40*:37, 1968.

Pfister, R. C., and Newhouse, J. H.: Interventional percutaneous pyeloureteral techniques: I. Antegrade pyelography and ure-teral perfusion. Radiol. Clin. North Am. *17*:341, 1979.

Powers, T. A., Grove, R. B., Bauriedel, J. K., Orr, S. C., Melton, R. E., and Bowden, R. D.: Detection of obstructed uropathy using ^{99m}technetium diethylenetriaminepentaacetic acid. J. Urol. *124*:588, 1980.

Stage, K. H., and Lewis, S.: Use of the radionuclide washout test in evaluation of suspected upper urinary obstruction. J. Urol. *125*:379, 1981.

Testa, H. J.: Nuclear medicine in diagnostic techniques. In O'Reilly, P. H., George, N. J. R., and Weiss, R. M. (eds.): Urology. Philadelphia, W. B. Saunders, 1990, pp. 99–117.

Wadsworth, D. E., and McClennan, B. L.: Benign causes of acquired ureteropelvic junction obstruction: A uroradiologic spectrum. Urol. Radiol. *5*:77, 1983.

Whitaker, R. H.: Some observations and theories on the wide ureter and hydronephrosis. Br. J. Urol. *47*:377, 1975.

Whitaker, R. H.: The Whitaker test. Urol. Clin. North Am *6*:529, 1979.

Whitaker, R. H.: Investigation of the dilated upper urinary tract. J. R. Soc. Med. *73*:377, 1980.

Whitfield, H. N., Britton, K. E., Fry, I. K., Hendry, W. F., Nimmon, C. C., Travers, P., and Wickham, J. E. A.: The obstructed kidney: Correlation between renal function and urodynamic assessment. Br. J. Urol. *49*:615, 1977.

Tuberculosis

Barrie, H. J., Kerr, W. K., and Gale, G. L.: The incidence and pathogenesis of tuberculous strictures of the renal pyelus. J. Urol. *98*:584, 1967.

Friedenberg, R. M.: Tuberculosis of the genitourinary system. Semin. Roentgenol. *6*:310, 1971.

Gow, J. G.: Genitourinary tuberculosis: A 7 year review. Br. J. Urol. *51*:239, 1979.

Kollins, S. A., Hartman, G. W., Carr, D. T., Segura, J. W., and Hattery, R. R.: Roentgenographic findings in urinary tract tuberculosis: A 10 year review. AJR *121*:487, 1974.

Pasternack, M. S., and Rubin, R. H.: Urinary tract tuberculosis. In Schrier, R. W., and Gottschalk, C. W. (eds.): Diseases of the Kidney, 6th ed. Boston, Little, Brown & Co., 1997, pp. 989–1011.

Roylance, J., Penry, J. B., Davies, E. R., and Roberts, M.: The radiology of tuberculosis of the urinary tract. Clin. Radiol. *21*:163, 1970.

Candidiasis

Margolin, H. N.: Fungus infection tract. Semin. Roentgenol. *6*:323, 1971.

McDonald, D. F., and Fagan, C. J.: Fungus balls in the urinary tract: Case report. AJR *114*:753, 1972.

Michigan, S.: Genitourinary fungal infection. J. Urol. *116*:390, 1976.

Wise, G. J., and Silver, D. A.: Fungal infections of the genitourinary system. J. Urol. *149*:1377, 1993.

Schistosomiasis

Al-Ghorab, M. M.: Radiological manifestations of genitourinary bilharziasis. Clin. Radiol. *19*:100, 1968.

Dittrich, M., and Doehring, E.: Ultrasonographical aspects of urinary schistosomiasis: Assessment of morphologic lesions in the upper and lower urinary tract. Pediatr. Radiol. *16*:225, 1986.

Hugosson, C., and Olsen, P.: Early ureteric changes in *Schistosoma haematobium* infection. Clin. Radiol. *37*:501, 1986.

Jorulf, H., and Lindstedt, E.: Urogenital schistosomiasis: CT evaluation. Radiology *157*:745, 1985.

Mahmoud, A. A.: Schistosomiasis. N. Engl. J. Med. *297*:1329, 1974.

Palmer, P. E. S., and Reeder, M. M.: Parasitic disease of the urinary tract. In Pollack, H. M. (ed.): Clinical Urography. Philadelphia, W. B. Saunders, 1990, pp. 999–1019.

Smith, J. H., and von Lichtenberg, F.: Parasitic diseases of the genitourinary system. In Walsh, P. C., Retik, A. B., Vaughan, E. D., Jr., and Wein, A. J. (eds.): Campbell's Urology, 7th ed. Philadelphia, W. B. Saunders, 1998, pp. 733–778.

Umerah, B. C.: The less familiar manifestations of schistosomiasis of the urinary tract. Br. J. Radiol. *50*:105, 1977.

Young, S. W., Khalid, K. H., Fariz, Z., and Mahmoud, A. H.: Urinary tract lesions of *Schistosoma haematobium* with detailed radiographic considerations of the bladder. Radiology *111*:81, 1974.

Pyelitis Cystica

Köhler, R.: Pyelo-ureteritis cystica. Acta Radiol. (Diagn.) *4*:123, 1966.

Limburg, D., and Zuidema, B. J.: Pyeloureteritis cystica. Diagn. Imaging *49*:141, 1980.

Loitman, B. S., and Chiat, H.: Ureteritis cystica and pyelitis cystica. Radiology *68*:345, 1957.

McNulty, M.: Pyelo-ureteritis cystica. Br. J. Radiol. *30*:648, 1957.

Leukoplakia

Besmann, E. F.: Renal leukoplakia. Radiology *88*:872, 1967.

Hertle, L., and Androulakasis, P.: Keratinizing desquamative squamous metaplasia of the upper urinary tract: Leukoplakia—cholesteatoma. J. Urol. *127*:631, 1982.

Noyes, W. E., and Palubinskas, A. J.: Squamous metaplasia of renal pelvis. Radiology. *89*:292, 1967.

Reece, R. W., and Koontz, W. W., Jr.: Leukoplakia of the urinary tract: A review. J. Urol. *114*:165, 1975.

Smith, B. A., Jr., Webb, E. A., and Price, W. E.: Renal leukoplakia: Observations of behavior. J. Urol. *87*:279, 1969.

Weitzner, S.: Cholesteatoma of the calix. J. Urol. *108*:365, 1972.

Malakoplakia

Abdou, N. I., NaPombejara, C., Sagawa, A., Ragland, C., Stechschulte, D. J., Nilsson, U., Gourley, W., Watanabe, I., Lindsey, N. J., and Ellen, M. S.: Malakoplakia: Evidence for monocytic lysosomal abnormality correctable by cholinergic agonist *in vitro* and *in vivo*. N. Engl. J. Med. *297*:1413, 1977.

Bennett, W. H.: Malacoplakia of the urinary tract: Report of three cases. J. Urol. *70*:84, 1953.

Cadnaphornchai, P., Rosenberg, B. F., Taher, S., Prosnitz, E. H., and McDonald, F. D.: Renal parenchymal malakoplakia: An unusual cause of renal failure. N. Engl. J. Med. *299*:1110, 1978.

Hartman, D. S., Davis, C. J., Jr., Lichtenstein, J. E., and Goldman, S. M.: Renal parenchymal malacoplakia. Radiology *136*:33, 1980.

O'Dea, M. J., Malek, R. S., and Farrow, G. M.: Malacoplakia of the urinary tract: Challenges and frustrations with 10 cases. J. Urol. *118*:739, 1977.

Soberon, L. M., Zawada, E. T., Jr., Cohen, A. H., and Kaloyanides, G. J.: Renal parenchymal malacoplakia presenting as acute oliguric renal failure. Nephron *26*:200, 1980.

Stanton, M. J., and Maxted, W.: Malacoplakia: A study of the literature and current concepts of pathogenesis, diagnosis and treatment. J. Urol. *125*:139, 1981.

Amyloidosis

Amendola, M. A.: Amyloidosis of the urinary tract. In Pollack, H. M. (ed.): Clinical Urography. Philadelphia, W. B. Saunders, 1990, pp. 2493–2500.

Callaghan, P., and Asklin, B.: Ureteral obstruction due to primary localized amyloidosis. Scand. J. Urol. Nephrol. *27*:535, 1993.

David, P. S., Babaria, A., March, D. E., and Goldberg, R. D. S.: Primary amyloidosis of the ureter and renal pelvis. Urol. Radiol. *9*:158, 1987.

Ferch, R., Haskell, R., and Farebrother, T.: Primary amyloidosis of the urinary bladder and ureters. Br. J. Urol. *80*:953, 1997.

Gardner, K. D., Jr., Castellino, R. A., Kempson, R., Young, B. W., and Stamey, T. A.: Primary amyloidosis of the renal pelvis. N. Engl. J. Med. *284*:1196, 1971.

German, K. A., and Morgan, R. J.: Primary amyloidosis of the renal pelvis and upper ureter. Br. J. Urol. *73*:99, 1994.

Lee, K. T., and Deeths, T. M.: Localized amyloidosis of the ureter. Radiology *120*:60, 1976.

Moul, J. M., and McLeod, D. C.: Bilateral organ-limited amyloidosis of the distal ureter associated with osseous metaplasia and radiographic calcifications. J. Urol. *139*:807, 1988.

Pirnar, T., and Coruh, M.: Radiologic findings in renal amyloidosis of children. Pediatr. Radiol. *1*:72, 1973.

Thomas, S. D., Sanders, P. W., III, and Pollack, H. M.: Primary amyloidosis of the urinary bladder and ureter: Cause of mural calcification. Urology 9:586, 1977.

Willen, R., Willen, H., Lindstedt, E., and Ekelund, L.: Localized primary amyloidosis of the ureter. Scand. J. Urol. Nephrol. 17:385, 1983.

Polyarteritis Nodosa

Hefty, T. R., Bonafede, P., and Stenzel, P.: Bilateral ureteral stricture from polyarteritis nodosa. J. Urol. 141:600, 1989.

Eosinophilic Ureteritis

Hellstrom, H. R., Davis, B. K., Shonnard, J. W., and MacPherson, T. A.: Eosinophilic pyeloureteritis: Report of a case. J. Urol. 122:833, 1979.

Uyama, T., Moriwaki, S., Aga, Y., and Yamamoto, A.: Eosinophilic ureteritis? Regional ureteritis with marked infiltration of eosinophils. Urology 18:615, 1981.

Mural Hemorrhage

Antolak, S. J., Jr., and Mellinger, C. T.: Urologic evaluation of hematuria during anticoagulant therapy. J. Urol. 101:111, 1969.

Brannen, G. E., Wettlaufer, J. N., Stables, D. P., and Weil, R.: Intramural bleeding into a renal allograft pelvis during heparin anticoagulation. Br. J. Radiol. 52:838, 1979.

Buntley, D. W., and McDuffie, R.: Pyeloureteral filling defects associated with anticoagulation: A case report. J. Urol. 115:335, 1976.

Eisenberg, R. L., and Clark, R. E.: Filling defects in the renal pelvis and ureter owing to bleeding secondary to acquired circulating anticoagulants. J. Urol. 116:662, 1976.

Higenbottam, T., Ogg, C. S., and Saxton, H. M.: Acute renal failure from the use of acetazolamide (Diamox). Postgrad. Med. J. 54:127, 1978.

Kaiser, J. A., Jacobs, R. P., and Korobkin, M.: Submucosal hemorrhage of the renal collecting system. AJR 125:311, 1975.

Kossol, J. M., and Patel, S. K.: Suburoepithelial hemorrhage: The value of preinfusion computed tomography. J. Comput. Assist. Tomogr. 10:157, 1986.

Miller, V., Witten, D. M., and Shin, M. S.: Computed tomographic findings in suburothelial hemorrhage. Urol. Radiol. 4:11, 1982.

Smith, W. L., Weinstein, A. S., and Wiot, J. F.: Defects of the renal collecting system in patients receiving anticoagulants. Radiology 113:649, 1974.

Viamonte, M., Roen, S. A., Viamonte, M., Jr., Casal, G. L., and Rywlin, A. M.: Subepithelial hemorrhage of renal pelvis simulating neoplasm (Antopol-Goldman lesion). Urology 16:647, 1980.

Longitudinal Mucosal Folds

Astley, R.: Striation (longitudinal mucosal folds) in the upper urinary tract: III. Urinary tract striation in children: Some experimental observations. Br. J. Radiol. 44:452, 1971.

Cremin, B. J., and Stables, D. P.: Striation (longitudinal mucosal folds) in the upper urinary tract: II. A comparison in children and adults. Br. J. Radiol. 44:449, 1971.

Daughtridge, T. G.: Mucosal folds in the upper urinary tract. AJR 107:743, 1969.

Friedland, G. W., and Forsberg, L.: Striation of the renal pelvis in children. Clin. Radiol. 23:58, 1972.

Hyde, I., and Wastie, M. L.: Striation (longitudinal mucosal folds) in the upper urinary tract: I. Striated renal pelvis and ureter in children. Br. J. Radiol. 44:445, 1971.

Parker, M. D., and Clark, R. L.: Urothelial striations revisited. Radiology 198:89, 1996.

Silber, I., and McAllister, W. H.: Longitudinal folds as an indirect sign of vesicoureteral reflux. J. Urol. 103:89, 1970.

Ureteral Pseudodiverticulosis

Cochran, S. T., Waisman, J., and Barbaric, Z. L.: Radiographic and microscopic findings in multiple ureteral diverticula. Radiology 137:631, 1980.

Wasserman, N. F., LaPointe, S., and Posalaky, I. P.: Ureteral pseudodiverticulosis. Radiology 155:561, 1985.

Wasserman, N. F., Posalaky, I. P., and Dykoski, R.: The pathology of ureteral pseudodiverticulosis. Invest. Radiol. 23:592, 1988.

Pyelocalyceal Diverticulum

Healey, T., and Grundy, W. R.: Milk of calcium in calycine diverticula. Br. J. Radiol. 53:845, 1980.

Middleton, A. W., Jr., and Pfister, R. C.: Stone-containing pyelocaliceal diverticulum: Embryonic, anatomic, radiologic and clinical characteristics. J. Urol. 111:2, 1974.

Pomerantz, R. M., Kirschner, L. P., and Twigg, H. L.: Renal milk of calcium collection: Review of literature and report of case. J. Urol. 103:18, 1970.

Rosenberg, M. A.: Milk of calcium in a renal calyceal diverticulum: Case report and review of literature. AJR 101:714, 1967.

Siegel, M. J., and McAlister, W. H.: Calyceal diverticula in children: Unusual features and complications. Radiology 131:79, 1979.

Spence, H. M., and Singleton, R.: Cysts and cystic disorders of the kidney: Types, diagnosis, treatment. Urol. Surv. 22:131, 1972.

Timmons, J. W., Jr., Malek, R. S., Hattery, R. R., and de Weerd, J. H.: Caliceal diverticulum. J. Urol. 114:6, 1975.

Williams, G., Blandy, J. P., and Tressider, G. C.: Communicating cysts and diverticula of the renal pelvis. Br. J. Urol. 41:163, 1969.

Wulfsohn, M. A.: Pyelocaliceal diverticula. J. Urol. 123:1, 1980.

Ureteroceles

Bauer, S. B., and Retik, A. B.: The non-obstructive ectopic ureterocele. J. Urol. 119:804, 1978.

Conlin, M. J., Skoog, S. J., and Tank, E. S.: Current management of ureteroceles. Urology 45:357, 1995.

Mandell, J., Colodny, A. H., Lebowitz, R., Bauer, S. B., and Retik, A. B.: Ureteroceles in infants and children. J. Urol. 123:921, 1980.

Mitty, H. A., and Schapira, H. E.: Ureterocele and pseudoureterocele: Cobra vs cancer. J. Urol. 117:557, 1977.

Morse, F. P., III, Sears, B., and Brown, H. P.: Carcinoma of the bladder presenting as simple adult ureterocele. J. Urol. 111:36, 1974.

Nussbaum, A. R., Dorst, J. P., Jeffs, R. D., Gearhart, J. P., and Sanders, R. C.: Ectopic ureter and ureterocele: Their varied sonographic manifestations. Radiology 159:227, 1986.

Prewitt, L. H., Jr., and Lebowitz, R. L.: The single ectopic ureter. AJR 127:941, 1976.

Schlussel, R. N., and Retik, A. B.: Anomalies of the ureter. In Walsh, P. C., Retik, A. B., Vaughan, E. D., Jr., and Wein, A. J. (eds.): Campbell's Urology, 7th ed. Philadelphia, W. B. Saunders, 1998, pp. 1814–1858.

Share, J. C., and Lebowitz, R. L.: Ectopic ureterocele without ureteral and calyceal dilatation (ureterocele disproportion): Findings on urography and sonography. AJR 152:567, 1989.

Sherwood, T., and Stevenson, J. J.: Ureteroceles in disguise. Br. J. Radiol. 42:899, 1969.

Tanagho, E. A.: Anatomy and management of ureteroceles. J. Urol. 107:729, 1972.

Thompson, G. J., and Kelalis, P. P.: Ureterocele: A clinical appraisal of 176 cases. J. Urol. 91:488, 1964.

Thornbury, J. R., Silver, T. M., and Vinson, R. K.: Ureteroceles vs pseudoureteroceles in adults. Radiology 122:81, 1977.

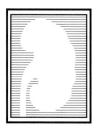

Renal Sinus and Periureteral Abnormalities

PARAPELVIC CYST
RENAL SINUS LIPOMATOSIS
VASCULAR ABNORMALITIES
SOLID TUMORS OF THE RENAL SINUS

ENDOMETRIOSIS
NEOPLASTIC AND INFLAMMATORY INFILTRATION
URETERAL DEVIATION
DIFFERENTIAL DIAGNOSIS

The abnormalities discussed in this chapter originate either in the renal sinus or in the tissue that surrounds the ureter. The renal sinus is the extension of the perinephric space into the deep recess situated on the medial border of the kidney. Contained within this space are the pelvocalyceal system, fat, and lymph nodes. Arteries, veins, lymphatic channels, and nerves of the autonomic nervous system traverse the sinus and enter or exit the kidney by penetrating the extension of the renal capsule that is invaginated into the inner recess of the sinus. The fat that fills this space surrounds the tips of the septa of Bertin and the calyces at their point of attachment to the papillae. Medially, the sinus fat is continuous with the fat of the perinephric space through which the proximal two-thirds of the ureter passes to where it pierces the caudal fusion of the anterior and posterior renal fascia at the level of the iliac crest. From this point to the ureterovesical junction, the ureter is in the pelvic extraperitoneal space.

Most abnormalities of the renal sinus are focal and are best described as parapelvic, using the prefix *para* to mean "alongside" or "beside." These abnormalities cause focal displacement and smooth effacement of the pelvocalyceal system as seen with excretory urography or pyelography and a circumscribed mass as seen with cross-sectional tomographic techniques such as ultrasonography, computed tomography, and magnetic resonance imaging. Disorders that surround the pelvocalyceal system are described as peripelvic, using the prefix *peri* to mean "around." This distribution, which occurs mainly with renal sinus lipomatosis, causes generalized attenuation of the pelvocalyceal system.

Parapelvic cyst, renal sinus lipomatosis, vascular abnormalities, and solid tumors of the renal sinus are each discussed in the initial sections of this chapter. Some of these entities, such as pelvocalyceal impressions caused by normal blood vessels

and some forms of peripelvic fat deposition, produce radiologic abnormalities but are of no clinical significance in themselves. Others cause only subtle abnormalities on excretory urography or pyelography but are readily identified by cross-sectional imaging techniques. The final sections of this chapter describe abnormalities that arise outside the ureter but, nevertheless, are in close enough proximity to deform or displace that structure. These include endometriosis, neoplastic and inflammatory infiltration, and certain causes of deviation in the course of the ureter. Other aspects of normal and abnormal ureteral course are discussed in Chapter 3 (anatomy of the ureter), Chapter 10 (lymphoma of the renal sinus), Chapter 19 (the bladder), and Chapter 21 (the retroperitoneum).

PARAPELVIC CYST

Definition

Parapelvic cysts are spherical or ovoid, blue-gray masses that intimately attach to the renal pelvis or calyx and are filled with clear yellow fluid containing albumin, lipids, and cholesterol. Previously, these cysts, which do not communicate with the pelvocalyceal system, were thought to be mostly solitary and unilocular. Experience with computed tomography and ultrasonography, however, has shown that parapelvic cysts are often multiple or multilocular. They may fill the sinus and surround the entire collecting system, causing a pattern of effacement and stretching that is usually associated with peripelvic abnormalities such as sinus lipomatosis. Rarely, a solitary cyst will insinuate itself deeply into the sinus and deform only a single calyx or infundibulum.

Parapelvic cysts are extraparenchymal lesions that probably arise from ectatic lymphatic channels. There is no consensus on the terminology for parapelvic cysts, which have also been called *pyelolym-*

phatic, peripelvic, or, simply, *renal sinus* or *hilar cysts.* Regardless of terminology, these cysts are uncommonly of clinical importance and are rarely subject to pathologic study.

A large parapelvic cyst may extrude from the renal sinus and cause stretching of the vascular pedicle of the kidney. Compression and displacement of a part of the pelvocalyceal system to the point of obstruction is another complication of a large cyst. Rarely, a parapelvic cyst disappears, presumably following spontaneous rupture.

Clinical Setting

Parapelvic cysts occur in all age groups. Most cysts are asymptomatic. Dull flank pain, hematuria, and the signs and symptoms of urinary tract infection, presumably secondary to obstruction, are ascribed to these lesions. If the vascular pedicle is severely stretched by a large parapelvic cyst, hyperreninemic hypertension may develop. This can be reversed by evacuation of the cyst.

Radiologic Findings

Excretory Urography. A soft tissue density in the renal sinus that causes focal displacement and smooth effacement of the adjacent portion of the pelvocalyceal system make up the findings on excretory urography of a single parapelvic cyst (Fig. 16–1). Rarely, a halo of lucency around the mass is detected on tomograms, owing to the displacement of sinus fat. Multiple or multiloculated parapelvic cysts fill the renal sinus and cause generalized, rather than focal, effacement and stretching of the collecting system (Fig. 16–2). This pattern closely resembles that of sinus lipomatosis, except the tissue surrounding the distorted pelvocalyceal system has the radiodensity of water rather than of fat. Obstructive caliectasis occasionally may occur with either the focal or the generalized form of parapelvic cyst (see Figs. 16–1 and 16–2). The urographic nephrogram shows normal findings, however, as would be expected of a cyst that has a sinus rather than parenchymal origin. Curvilinear calcification of the cyst wall occurs rarely.

Ultrasonography. An anechoic mass with a well-defined far wall and acoustic enhancement are the findings on ultrasonographic examination of parapelvic cyst (Fig. 16–3). These cysts are located within the normally echogenic central sinus complex, which may be either focally displaced or separated. Distinction between parapelvic cyst and hydronephrosis is dependent on the demonstration of continuity between a dilated pelvis and its branching calyces in the case of hydronephrosis (Fig. 16–4; see Fig. 17–11) and the absence of branching in the case of a parapelvic cyst. Distinction on ultrasonography between a parapelvic cyst and other fluid-containing structures of the renal sinus, such as a renal artery aneurysm, a nephrogenic cyst protruding into the sinus, or a Type II

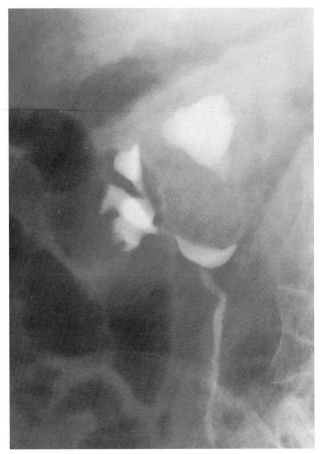

FIGURE 16–1. Solitary parapelvic cyst. An oval mass with the density of water focally displaces the collecting system. Effacement of the infundibula has caused caliectasis. Excretory urogram.

pyelocalyceal diverticulum, may be impossible without the use of other diagnostic modalities, including Doppler ultrasonographic evaluation.

Computed Tomography. The location of a parapelvic cyst within the renal sinus is best demonstrated by computed tomography (see Figs. 16–2 and 16–4). These lesions have a homogeneous appearance with an attenuation value close to that of water. Rarely, the attenuation value of a cyst may be greater than water owing to either an elevated protein content or prior bleeding. Some cysts are single and have a smooth outline; others are multiple, bilateral, and lobulated. Individual cysts separated by vessels and the collecting system can be identified occasionally. Contrast material enhancement is required to visualize the effaced pelvocalyceal system and ensure that the fluid-filled structure in the renal sinus, seen on unenhanced computed tomograms, is not a dilated pelvis (see Fig. 16–4). The attenuation value of parapelvic cysts is not changed by intravenous contrast material.

Magnetic Resonance Imaging. The magnetic resonance image of a parapelvic cyst shows a mass of water signal intensity surrounded by high signal renal sinus fat on T1-weighted scans. As with most

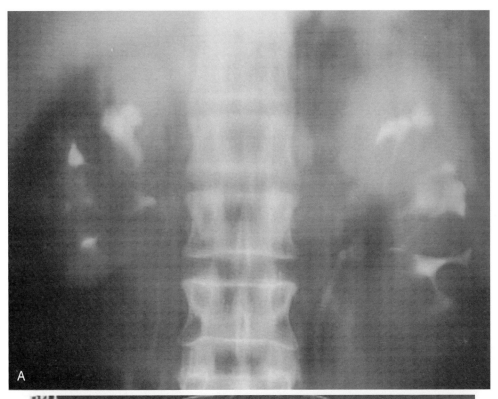

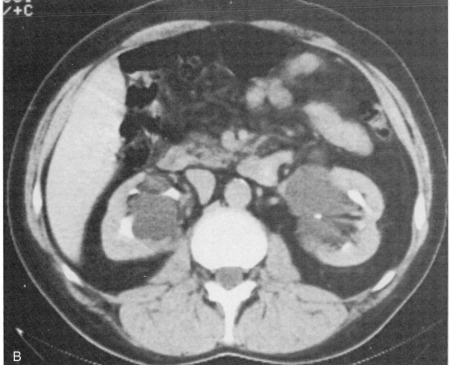

FIGURE 16–2. Multiple, bilateral parapelvic cysts in a 58-year-old hypertensive man. There is generalized effacement and stretching of the pelvis and infundibula of both kidneys. The tissue filling the sinuses is the density of water. Caliectasis is generalized.

A, Excretory urogram. Tomogram.

B, Computed tomogram, contrast material–enhanced. Note the smoothly marginated, homogeneous cysts.

(Courtesy of Carol Weinstein, M.D., Good Samaritan Hospital, Portland, Oregon.)

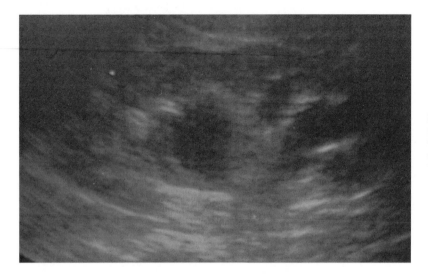

FIGURE 16–3. Parapelvic cysts. Ultrasonogram. Multiple fluid-filled structures with well-defined walls are seen. These do not communicate, in contradistinction to the findings in obstructive uropathy.

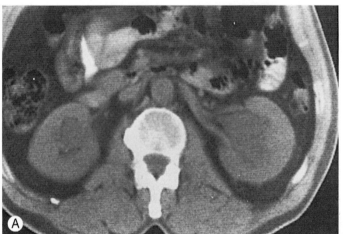

FIGURE 16–4. Parapelvic cysts, bilateral and multiple.
A, Computed tomogram, unenhanced. A mass of water attenuation values fills both renal sinuses. This could represent either parapelvic cysts or hydronephrosis.
B, Computed tomogram, contrast material–enhanced. Opacification of an attenuated collecting system surrounded by the cystic masses indicates the diagnosis of parapelvic cysts.
C, Ultrasonogram, left kidney. Coronal projection. Multiple septated cystic masses fill the renal sinus.
(Kindly provided by Giovanna Casola, M.D., University of California, San Diego.)

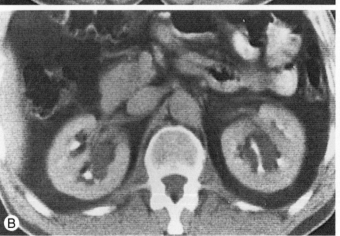

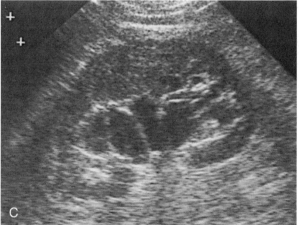

cysts, signal increases within parapelvic cysts on T2-weighted scans.

RENAL SINUS LIPOMATOSIS

Definition

A thin layer of loose fatty tissue in continuity with fat of the perirenal space normally envelops the other structures in the renal sinus. The amount of fat is minimal in young and lean individuals. Conversely, there is a normal increase in sinus fat with aging and obesity.

Proliferation of sinus fat also occurs abnormally in association with processes causing destruction or atrophy of renal tissue (see Fig. 16–9). In this situation, increased fat deposits preserve some of the overall kidney mass that would otherwise be reduced as renal parenchyma is lost. In rare cases, renal bulk is larger than normal and virtually the entire kidney is accounted for by greatly expanded

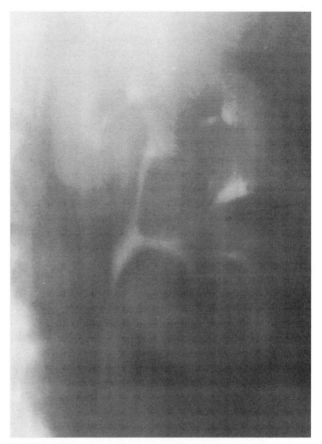

FIGURE 16–6. Sinus lipomatosis of the left kidney. There is diffuse elongation and attenuation of the pelvis and infundibula, mild caliectasis, and thinning of the renal parenchyma. Excretory urogram. Tomogram.

sinus fat capped only by a very thin mantle of renal parenchyma. This extreme, which may have inflammatory cells infiltrating the proliferative sinus fat, has been referred to as *replacement lipomatosis* of the kidney.

Normal sinus fat does not affect the distensibility of the pelvocalyceal system. When fat proliferates, however, the entire collecting system becomes attenuated and loses its distensibility. Occasionally, fat collects in a single focus that deforms the adjacent pelvocalyceal system. Rarely, this projects into the wall of the pelvis and simulates a mural mass.

Synonyms for renal sinus lipomatosis are *peripelvic lipomatosis, renal fibrolipomatosis* (a misnomer), and, simply, *peripelvic fat proliferation.*

Clinical Setting

Renal sinus lipomatosis is normal in aged and obese individuals and is sometimes found in patients without known current or previous disease. By itself, fatty proliferation is asymptomatic. Clinical abnormalities that might be present reflect the primary process causing wasting, such as reflux nephropathy, atherosclerosis, or recurrent urinary tract infection.

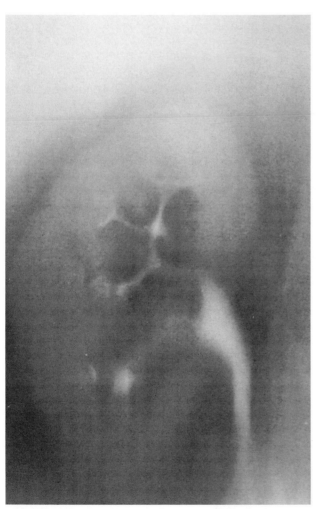

FIGURE 16–5. Normal renal sinus fat. The lucency in the central part of the kidney has an irregular fan shape and attenuates the pelvocalyceal system. Excretory urogram. Tomogram.

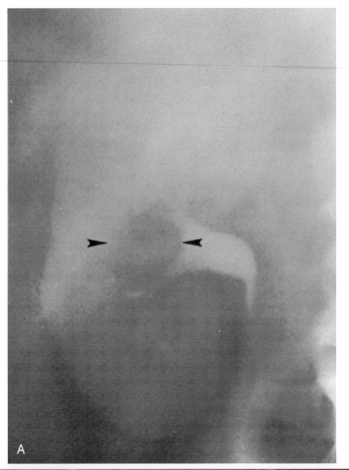

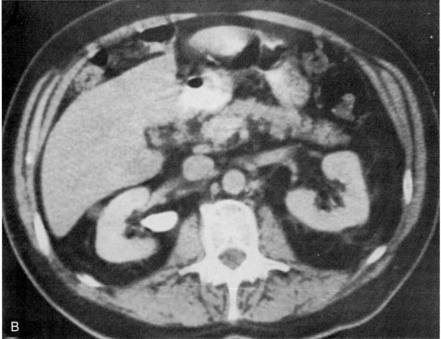

FIGURE 16–7. Focal sinus lipomatosis of the right kidney. The midportion of the pelvis is displaced around a radiolucent mass *(arrows)*.

A, Excretory urogram. Tomogram.

B, Computed tomogram, contrast material–enhanced. The tissue at the site of pelvic distortion has the same attenuation value as perirenal fat.

(Courtesy of Joy Price, M.D., Alta Bates Medical Center, Berkeley, California.)

Radiologic Findings

Normal sinus fat causes a fan-shaped, irregular radiolucency in the central part of the kidney (Fig. 16–5). Tomography is a useful adjunct when overlying gas obscures the renal sinus. A serrated interface between deep sinus fat and adjacent renal parenchyma is accentuated during the nephrographic phase of excretory urography.

Once opacified, the pelvocalyceal system appears diffusely elongated or "spider-like" when the sinus fat has proliferated. The infundibula radiate from the hilus toward the parenchyma in a pattern that has been likened to the spokes of a wheel. The calyces reflect the state of the renal parenchyma and are typically normal. Renal parenchymal thickness is diminished when there is a primary underlying parenchymal disease (Fig. 16–6).

Lipomatosis is usually diffusely distributed in the renal sinus. Occasionally, fat deposits in a single focus, causing a localized deformity of the pelvis, infundibulum, or calyx. This deformity is similar in radiologic appearance to that of any other parapelvic mass except for its radiolucency (Fig. 16–7). Rarely, the focal fat deposit is small and deeply invaginates the adjacent pelvic wall, simulating a mural mass. Defining the parapelvic nature of this lesion requires a well-distended and opacified pelvocalyceal system, exposures in steep oblique projections, and, ultimately, identification of the fatty nature of the lesion by ultrasonography, computed tomography, or magnetic resonance imaging.

Sinus lipomatosis leads to hyperechoic enlargement of the renal sinus (Fig. 16–8). Usually, the central sinus complex is more extensive than normal, although this finding may be obscured unless the plane of the image passes through the central axis of the sinus.

Computed tomography or magnetic resonance im-

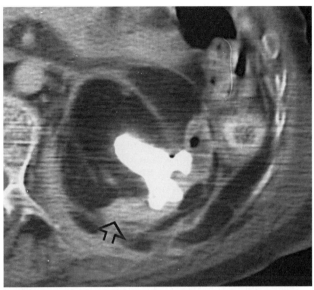

FIGURE 16–9. Renal sinus lipomatosis, left kidney, in a 76-year-old woman with severe chronic urinary tract infection and staghorn calculus. Computed tomogram, contrast material–enhanced. A tumor-like mass of fat fills the left perirenal space medially and surrounds the staghorn calculus. The loss of renal parenchyma *(arrow)* is so advanced that the renal sinus is no longer a discrete region. Gas is present in a ventral calyx. Same patient is illustrated in Figure 21–19.

aging unequivocally defines the fatty nature of sinus lipomatosis (Fig. 16–9; see Fig. 16–7). Computed tomography is especially useful in examining patients with focal fat deposits that mimic other focal masses of the renal sinus.

VASCULAR ABNORMALITIES

Definition

Both arteries and veins impress on the pelvocalyceal system and ureter, either as closely opposed normal vessels or as aneurysms, collateral vessels, or varices.

Pelvocalyceal impressions by normal dorsal and ventral branches of the renal artery are common in patients with an intrarenal pelvis. Most branches cross the infundibulum to the upper pole. Other frequent sites of normal arterial impressions are the pelvis itself and the ureteropelvic junction. Normal veins passing anterior to the pelvocalyceal system produce impression in similar locations and patterns. The gonadal vein may cause a normal impression on the ureter as it follows a parallel course or, on the right side, where it crosses the ureter at approximately the level of the third lumbar vertebra.

Renal artery aneurysms are classified morphologically as either saccular or fusiform and histologically by the number of components of the arterial wall that are preserved. A "true" aneurysm is one in which intima, muscularis, and serosa are intact. The designation "false" aneurysm is used when one or more of these components are absent. An arterial

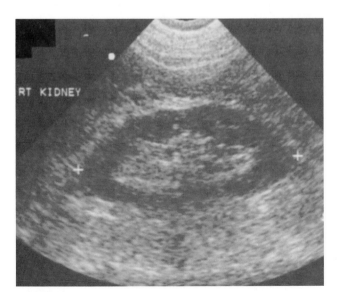

FIGURE 16–8. Sinus lipomatosis associated with end-stage renal failure. Ultrasonogram, longitudinal projection. There is increased prominence of the central sinus echo complex.

aneurysm that communicates directly with dilated renal veins is described as an *arteriovenous aneurysm* or *fistula*.

Another useful classification of aneurysms is etiologic and includes the terms *atherosclerotic, dysplastic, post-stenotic, post-traumatic* or *spontaneous arteriovenous,* and *mycotic*. Atherosclerosis causes true, saccular aneurysms within the most proximal 2 cm of the main renal artery and at its major bifurcations. Atherosclerotic aneurysm of the aorta and common iliac artery also affect the course of the ureter, as discussed later. The aneurysm of arterial dysplasia is a false aneurysm, or pseudoaneurysm, that forms as a result of dissection. These may be large and saccular but, unlike atherosclerotic aneurysms, occur along the nonbifurcating portions of the artery. Post-stenotic aneurysms are fusiform as a result of hemodynamic forces distal to a stenosis. Arteriovenous aneurysms or fistulas are false aneurysms that follow penetrating trauma or spontaneous rupture of an atherosclerotic or mycotic aneurysm into an adjacent vein. Congenital arteriovenous malformation (hemangioma) is discussed in Chapter 12.

Extrinsic impressions on the pelvocalyceal system and ureter are also caused by collateral arteries and veins and by varices. Collateral arterial circulation develops in response to main vessel occlusion and provides channels for renal arterial flow around a major arterial stenosis or occlusion or for venous drainage when the main renal vein or inferior vena cava is occluded. Collateral arteries also form in response to increased blood flow as occurs in vascular tumor or arteriovenous aneurysm (fistula). Collateral pathways develop from existing vascular systems, such as the pelvic, ureteral, gonadal, adrenal, capsular, or lumbar arteries or veins as well as the ascending lumbar veins. Vascular dilatation in response to increased blood flow causes multiple impressions on the pelvocalyceal system and proximal ureter. Varices do not necessarily indicate renal vein obstruction. Any condition that increases renal blood flow, such as arteriovenous aneurysm (fistula) and vascular adenocarcinoma, may cause varices, just as they may cause arterial collaterals to form. Varices are also associated with congenital extrarenal venous malformations (left-sided or double inferior vena cava and circumaortic or retroaortic left renal vein), occlusion of the inferior vena cava, or portal vein hypertension with splenorenal shunt. Compression of the left renal vein between the aorta and the superior mesenteric artery, known as the *nutcracker syndrome,* is another cause of a renal varix that is invariably left-sided. Chapters 6 and 21 contain additional discussions of aneurysms and collateral circulation.

Clinical Setting

Normal arteries or veins impinging on the pelvocalyceal system or ureter rarely cause symptoms. Nephralgia due to the partial obstruction, by cross-

ing vessels, of the infundibulum that drains upper pole calyces, the so-called *Fraley's syndrome,* occurs rarely.

Atherosclerotic aneurysms are usually discovered in older patients, frequently those beyond the sixth decade. Clinical abnormalities ascribed to renal artery aneurysms include flank pain, palpable mass, bruit, and hematuria. Spontaneous rupture, hyperreninemic hypertension, and distal embolization are major complications. Aneurysms in women of childbearing age are predisposed to spontaneous rupture during pregnancy.

Arterial dysplasia develops most frequently in women before the fifth decade. Renovascular hypertension dominates the clinical findings in these patients. Spontaneous dissection may lead to renal infarction with flank pain and hematuria. Dysplastic aneurysm per se does not cause symptoms.

The signs and symptoms of arteriovenous aneurysm (fistula) are caused by high-volume shunts. A continuous bruit in the flank or abdomen associated with a thrill is frequently present. Wide pulse pressure and diastolic hypertension may be noted. The latter is caused by the renal ischemia that follows

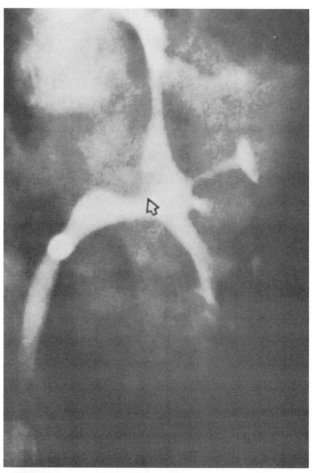

FIGURE 16–10. Arterial impression on the renal pelvis *(arrow).* A normal artery was identified by angiography. Excretory urogram.

(Courtesy of Thomas A. Freed, M.D., Marin General Hospital, Greenbrae, California.)

Radiologic Findings

Normal Artery and Vein

Normal arteries produce extrinsic impressions on the pelvocalyceal system in several locations and patterns that are seen during excretory urography. The most common one is a thin linear radiolucency that crosses the superior pole infundibulum, the ureteropelvic junction, or the pelvis itself. Proximal dilatation and delayed emptying may be noted. Caliectasis due to narrowing of an infundibulum by a crossing vessel is a rare cause of nephralgia, a condition known as Fraley's syndrome. Another pattern caused by a normal artery is a concave impression on an infundibulum or the pelvis, which viewed *en face* may simulate a mural or intraluminal lesion. Steep oblique projections establish the parapelvic origin of the "filling defect" (Fig. 16–10).

Normal renal veins cause smooth linear radiolucencies that are oriented in a horizontal or slightly oblique direction across the renal pelvis or infundibula—especially the one draining the upper pole (Figs. 16–11 and 16–12). Venous impressions are wider than those caused by arteries and change in size during the Valsalva maneuver or as the patient's position is changed. Distention of the pelvis or ureter usually effaces a venous impression but will not completely obliterate an arterial one. Steep oblique projections help to establish the parapelvic location of normal renal veins. The normal

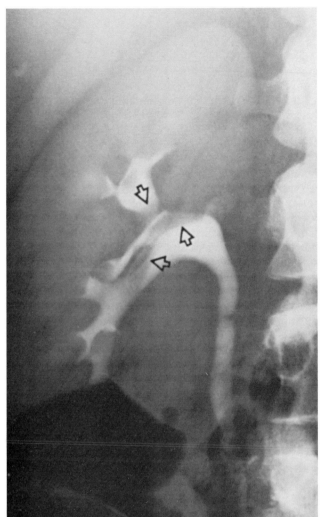

FIGURE 16–11. Venous impression on the renal pelvis *(arrows)*. Normal veins were identified by venography. Excretory urogram. (Courtesy of Jonathan Fish, M.D., and Daniel Kaplan, M.D., John Muir Hospital, Walnut Creek, California.)

shunting of arterial blood away from functional renal tissue. Patients with large-volume shunts are at risk for high-output congestive failure.

Renal arterial collateral circulation develops in patients with renovascular hypertension and causes no direct clinical abnormalities. Renal varices, on the other hand, cause both flank pain and hematuria, presumably from congestion of submucosal venous channels. The nutcracker syndrome may cause hematuria or proteinuria, or both, that originates in the left kidney.

Right flank pain and urinary tract infection in young, parous women with dilatation of the proximal ureter has been called the *ovarian vein syndrome*. These findings have been ascribed to varix or thrombosis of the right ovarian vein, which crosses the right ureter at approximately the level of the third lumbar vertebra. This syndrome, however, has not been established as a definite clinical entity.

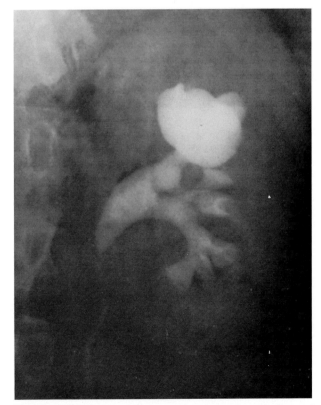

FIGURE 16–12. Caliectasis caused by a renal vein crossing and compressing the infundibulum of the upper pole calyx. Excretory urogram.

right gonadal vein may produce an impression on the right ureter at approximately the level of the third lumbar vertebra.

Aneurysm

Excretory Urography. Annular calcification, which occurs in more than 50 per cent of atherosclerotic renal artery aneurysms may be confused with curvilinear calcification in kidney or gallbladder stones; lymph nodes; splenic artery aneurysms; or adrenal, parapelvic, or nephrogenic cysts (Fig. 16–13; see also Fig. 6–1). Distinction between a

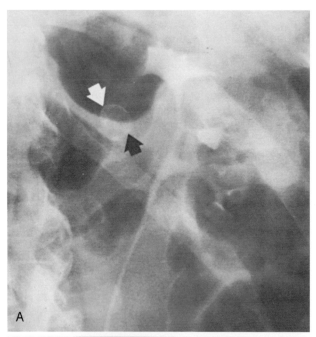

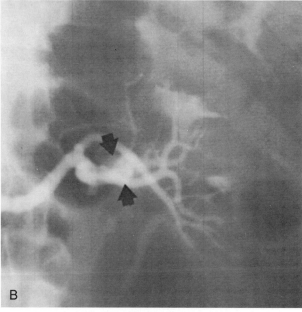

FIGURE 16–13. Saccular, atherosclerotic renal artery aneurysm with annular calcification *(arrows)*.
A, Excretory urogram.
B, Renal arteriogram, arterial phase. Arrows define opacification of the aneurysmal sac.

calculus and a calcified renal artery aneurysm is especially important before undertaking extracorporeal shock wave lithotripsy. Occasionally, an aneurysm is detected as a soft tissue mass that is accentuated by surrounding sinus fat. A large renal artery aneurysm produces a concave extrinsic deformity on the adjacent portion of the pelvocalyceal system (Fig. 16–14). If viewed *en face*, this may simulate a mural mass. An aneurysm that causes renovascular ischemia may also produce notching of the pelvis by collateral arteries and other urographic features of renovascular ischemia, which are described in Chapter 6. Dysplastic or arteriovenous aneurysms of the renal artery cause urographic abnormalities that are similar to those of atherosclerosis (Fig. 16–15). Renal vein varices caused by arteriovenous aneurysm (fistula) may form a parapelvic mass as well as peripelvic and periureteral notches.

Atherosclerotic aneurysm of the aorta may cause lateral displacement of the left ureter in a manner similar to the various retroperitoneal masses that are discussed in Chapter 21. An aneurysm of the common iliac artery causes an abrupt deviation of the ureter, which passes anterior to the artery.

Angiography. Angiography is the definitive method for studying aneurysms. Atherosclerotic aneurysms are located in the proximal portion of the main renal artery or distally at bifurcations. Most are saccular (see Figs. 16–13 and 16–14). The lumen is sometimes partially filled with thrombus that obscures the true size of the aneurysm. Washout of injected contrast material from the aneurysmal sac is often delayed (Fig. 16–16). Fusiform aneurysms usually form just distal to an arterial stenosis (Fig. 16–17). Occasionally, atherosclerotic narrowing or occlusion is found in the arterial segment just distal to the aneurysm. An aortogram as well as a selective renal arteriogram is necessary to demonstrate the collateral circulation completely.

The appearance of renal arterial dysplasia varies with the histologic type. Fusiform dilatation just distal to a narrow annular radiolucent band characterizes intimal fibroplasia (Fig. 16–18). These occur in major segmental branches as well as in the main renal artery. The occurrence of multiple, small, repetitive circumarterial dilatations that protrude beyond the circumference of the normal proximal artery, the so-called "string of beads," is the angiographic pattern of medial fibroplasia (Fig. 16–19). The other form of renal artery dysplasia, subadventitial fibroplasia, is associated with deformities that are not, strictly, aneurysmal in that true dilatation is absent (Fig. 16–20).

Angiography of arteriovenous aneurysms (fistulas) requires large volumes of rapidly injected contrast material because of the rapid blood flow through these lesions. Nearly immediate venous opacification is the hallmark of arteriovenous aneurysm (see Fig. 16–15). Frequently, multiple serpentine arteriovenous channels are opacified. Large shunts cause decreased nephrographic density.

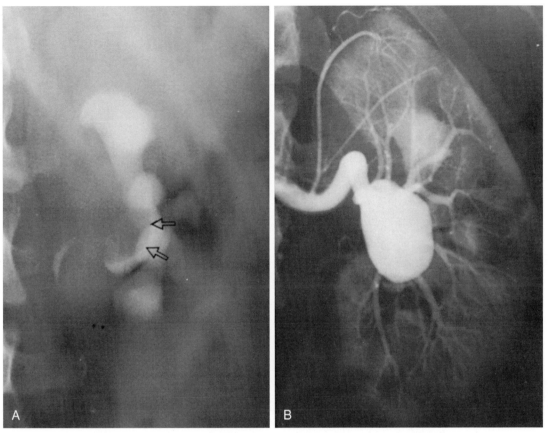

FIGURE 16–14. Saccular, atherosclerotic aneurysm at bifurcation of the main renal artery, causing an extrinsic deformity of the adjacent portion of the pelvis *(arrows)*.
  A, Excretory urogram.
  B, Renal arteriogram, arterial phase.

These angiographic findings can be duplicated occasionally by a highly vascular adenocarcinoma.

Ultrasonography. On ultrasonography, any saccular aneurysm produces findings of a fluid-filled mass. Flow patterns are accurately established by both spectral and color Doppler techniques.

Computed Tomography and Magnetic Resonance Imaging. Computed tomography and magnetic resonance angiography are useful adjuncts in the evaluation of renal artery aneurysm and dysplasia (Fig. 16–21). On unenhanced images, a saccular aneurysm appears as a renal sinus mass with attenuation values between those of water and soft tissue. The vascular nature of the mass is established by the demonstration of flow characteristics on magnetic resonance imaging and by its rapid enhancement immediately following intravenous injection of a bolus of contrast material with either computed tomography or magnetic resonance images. Magnetic resonance angiography with gadolinium enhancement may replace conventional angiography in the future.

Collateral Circulation and Varices

Excretory Urography. Collateral arterial channels cause multiple, small, extrinsic indentations on the distended pelvocalyceal system and proximal ureter. The number and location of these indenta-

tions are determined by the site of renal artery narrowing or occlusion (Figs. 16–22 and 16–23). Notching may be limited to a single calyx or infundibulum when a segmental artery is occluded. Varices produce similar impressions on the collecting system and ureter but are usually broader or "scalloped" in comparison with the "notched" appearance of arterial collaterals (Figs. 16–24 and 16–25). Additionally, varices may change in size as the patient moves from the prone to supine position or performs the Valsalva maneuver. Arterial collaterals are not subject to such variation.

Computed Tomography. Collateral arterial channels and varices are visualized as small soft tissue structures in the renal sinus or periureteral tissue. These may be confused with lymph nodes. Enhancement with contrast material, however, establishes the vascular nature of these structures (see Fig. 16–25).

Angiography. Arterial collaterals opacify during aortography and selective renal arteriography. Feeding vessels are enlarged and the collaterals are serpiginous; opacification is delayed (see Fig. 16–22 and 16–23). Branches of the renal artery distal to the occlusion also opacify late. Renal varices are gently undulating channels with broad lumina that opacify during the venous phase of an arteriogram or a dynamic computed tomogram (see Figs. 16–24

Text continued on page 450

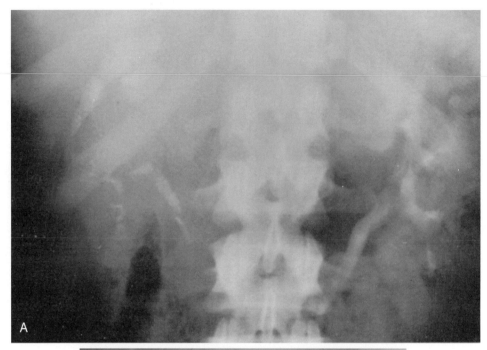

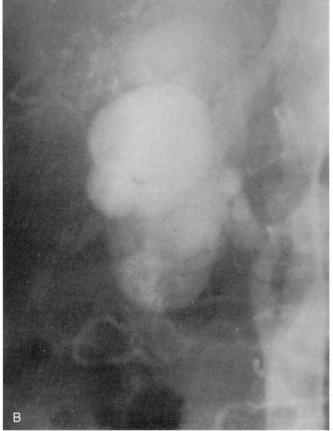

FIGURE 16–15. Post-traumatic arteriovenous aneurysm (fistula) following a penetrating wound of the right flank. The patient developed hypertension and a right abdominal bruit.
   A, Excretory urogram. The upper pole and interpolar collecting systems are displaced and obstructed by the aneurysm.
   B, Aortogram. A large arterial and venous chamber is opacified.

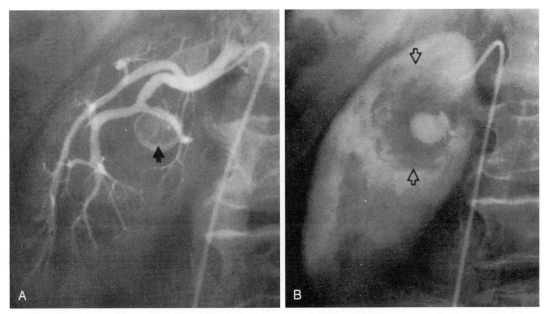

FIGURE 16–16. Saccular, atherosclerotic aneurysm with a thrombus partially filling the lumen *(solid arrow)*. The aneurysm had bled spontaneously and was surrounded by hematoma *(open arrows)*.
  A, Renal arteriogram, arterial phase.
  B, Renal arteriogram, nephrographic phase. There is delayed washout of contrast material from the aneurysmal sac.
  (Courtesy of Joy Price, M.D., Alta Bates Medical Center, Berkeley, California.)

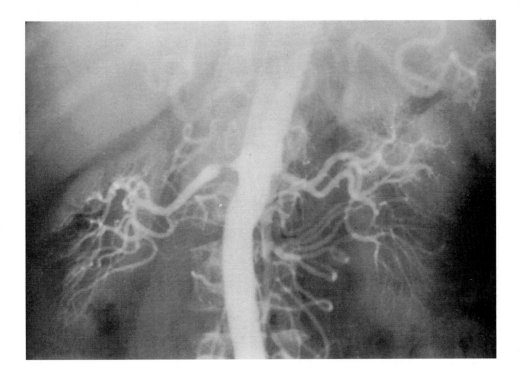

FIGURE 16–17. Fusiform atherosclerotic aneurysm in the right renal artery. Dilatation develops as a result of hemodynamic alterations, caused by an atherosclerotic stenosis immediately proximal to the aneurysm. Aortogram.

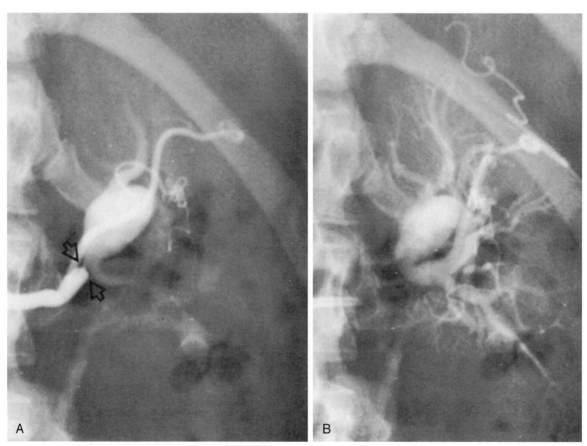

FIGURE 16–18. Intimal fibroplasia with post-stenotic fusiform aneurysm. This form of arterial dysplasia is characterized by a narrow annular band *(arrow)*. Same patient is illustrated in Figures 6–4 and 16–22.
  A, Renal arteriogram, early phase.
  B, Renal arteriogram, late phase.
  (Courtesy of Janet Dacie, M.B., St. Bartholomew's Hospital, London, England.)

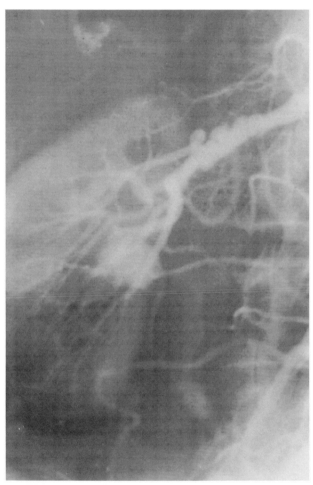

FIGURE 16–19. Medial fibroplasia. In this form of renal artery dysplasia, there are repetitive circumarterial dilatations that protrude beyond the margin of the normal artery. Aortogram. Same patient is illustrated in Figure 6–7.

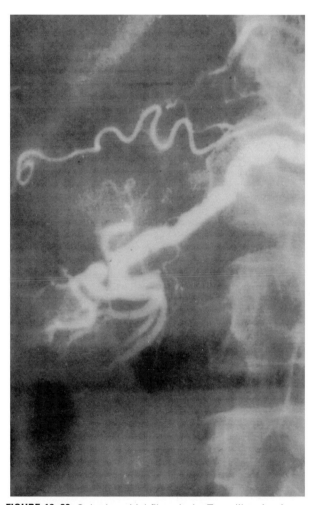

FIGURE 16–20. Subadventitial fibroplasia. True dilatation is absent in this type of renal artery dysplasia. Aortogram.

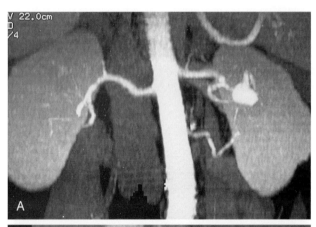

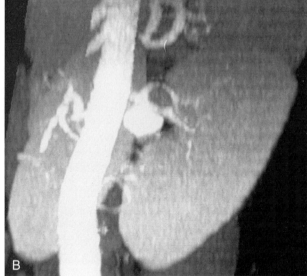

FIGURE 16–21. Renal artery aneurysm. Computed tomographic arteriogram. Same patient is illustrated in Figures 1–9 and 6–8.
 A, Coronal reconstruction, frontal projection. An aneurysm is present at the bifurcation of the main renal artery.
 B, Coronal reconstruction, oblique projection.

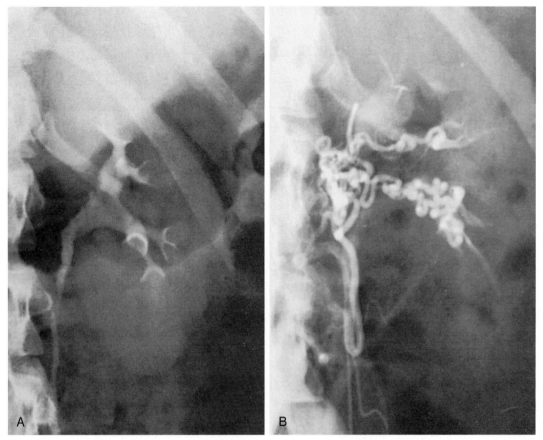

FIGURE 16–22. Renal arterial collaterals have caused multiple, small extrinsic indentations on the pelvis and proximal ureter of a 16-year-old girl with intimal fibroplasia of the left renal artery. Same patient is illustrated in Figures 6–4 and 16–18.

A, Excretory urogram.

B, Renal arteriogram, delayed film. There are dilated, tortuous periureteric and peripelvic collaterals that correspond to the abnormalities depicted in part *A*.

(Courtesy of Janet Dacie, M.B., St. Bartholomew's Hospital, London, England.)

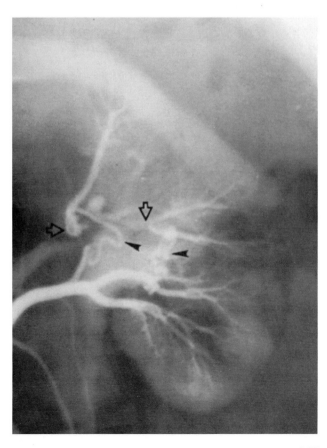

FIGURE 16–23. Intrarenal arterial collateral vessels *(solid arrows)* providing circulation to arcuate arteries distal to a major segmental artery occlusion *(open arrow)*. This collateral pattern is of the type that causes notching limited to an infundibulum. Renal arteriogram. (Courtesy of Helen C. Redman, M.D., University of Texas at Dallas, Dallas, Texas.)

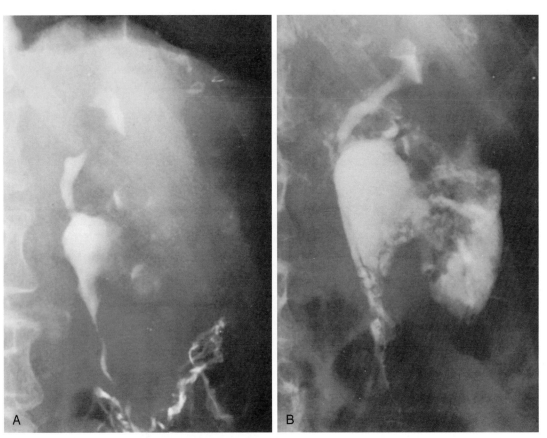

FIGURE 16–24. Venous collaterals. There are broad scalloped deformities of the pelvocalyceal system that correspond to dilated pelviureteric and peripelvic venous channels.
    A, Excretory urogram.
    B, Renal arteriogram, venous phase. Only a few of several renal veins have become opacified.

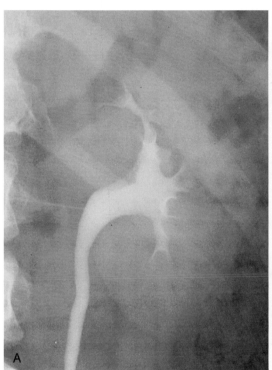

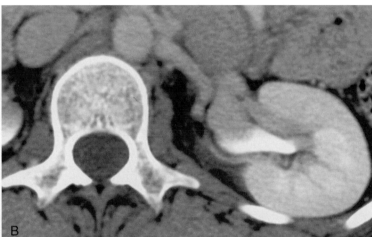

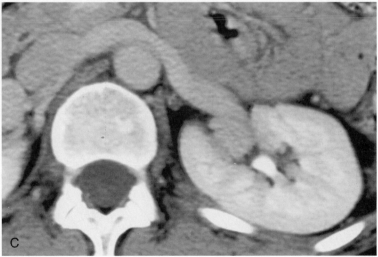

FIGURE 16–25. Renal vein varix, left kidney.
 A, Excretory urogram. There is a broad-based impression on the superior aspect of the pelvis.
 B and *C,* Computed tomograms, contrast material–enhanced, obtained sequentially from cranial to caudal. The renal vein is enhanced and includes a varix deforming the pelvis.

and 16–25). Venographic demonstration often requires selective catheterization augmented by contrast material injection during the Valsalva maneuver, a balloon-occluding selective venous catheter, and venous injection immediately following selective renal artery injection of 6 to 8 mg of epinephrine to reduce renal blood flow and prolong venous washout time.

SOLID TUMORS OF THE RENAL SINUS

Definition

Primary tumors of the renal sinus develop from any tissue within the renal sinus space. The various forms of lymphoma commonly involve sinus nodes, as discussed in Chapter 10. Fibroma, plasmacytoma, and myeloid metaplasia have also been reported in these structures. Metastases to sinus lymph nodes occur either as part of a generalized retroperitoneal process or as an isolated involvement, as with primary gonadal tumors.

Urine that leaks from the fornices of an obstructed pelvocalyceal system usually collects within the cone of the renal fascia that defines the outer limits of the perirenal space and forms a urinoma or uriniferous perirenal pseudocyst, which is discussed in Chapter 21. Uncommonly, leaked urine causes a granulomatous reaction in the renal sinus fat. A parapelvic urine granuloma containing loculated fluid is the result. These granulomas usually resolve spontaneously.

Clinical Setting

Primary renal sinus tumors may cause flank pain owing to obstructive uropathy or urinary tract infection. Symptoms of the primary underlying disease predominate in the case of renal sinus metastases.

Radiologic Findings

Soft tissue mass and focal deformity of the adjacent portion of the pelvocalyceal system are the major radiologic findings of renal sinus tumors and parapelvic urine granuloma (Fig. 16–26). A very large tumor displaces the kidney laterally and may cause anterior rotation. When renal sinus tumor is part of a diffuse infiltrating process, loss of perirenal fat, straightening, and displacement of the ureter and obliteration of the renal outline are noted.

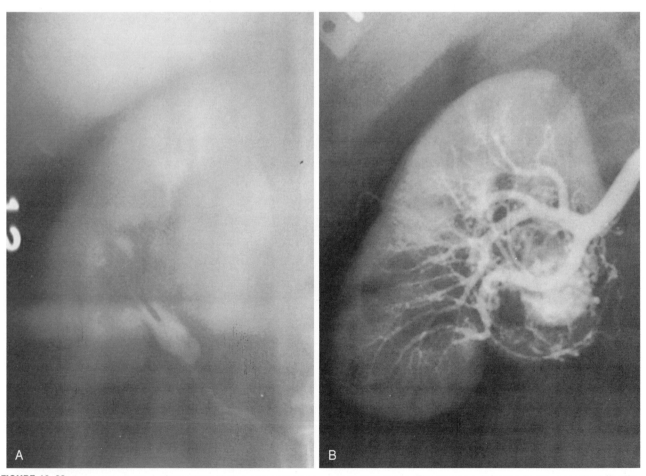

FIGURE 16–26. Adenocarcinoma of the right kidney presenting as a parapelvic mass. The tumor originates in the superior hilar lip and displaces the pelvocalyceal system downward.

A, Excretory urogram. Tomogram.

B, Renal arteriogram, arterial phase.

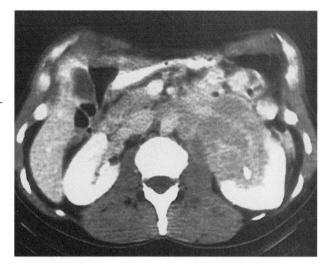

FIGURE 16–27. Lymphoma invading the left renal sinus in a 54-year-old man. Computed tomogram, contrast material–enhanced. The kidney is displaced laterally. The tumor fills the renal sinus, causing obstructive uropathy without dilatation of the pelvis. A dilated calyx is present. The combination of caliectasis without pelviectasis is characteristic of large, infiltrating masses in the renal sinus.

Ultrasonography and computed tomography are particularly useful in identifying renal sinus masses (Fig. 16–27). Solid lesions cause echoes of varying intensity. Lymphoma, in particular, is associated with low-intensity echoes. Attenuation values on computed tomography are those of soft tissue. Following administration of intravenous contrast material, sinus masses enhance variably, if at

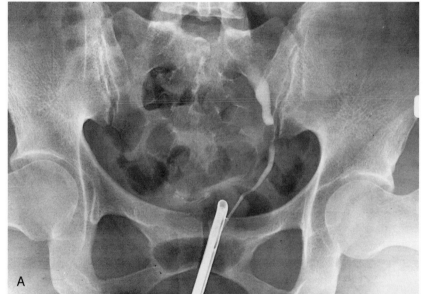

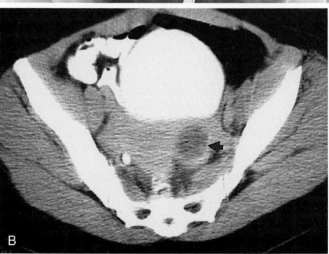

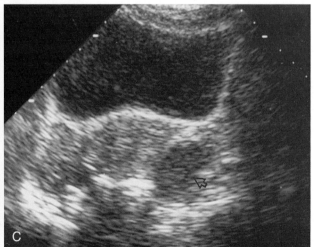

FIGURE 16–28. Endometriosis, left ureter.
A, Retrograde ureterogram. There is a sharply defined, smooth, concentric narrowing of a short segment of the ureter at the inferior margin of the sacroiliac joint. The proximal ureter is dilated.
B, Computed tomogram, contrast material–enhanced. The endometrioma *(arrow)* is of low attenuation, representing cystic degeneration.
C, Ultrasonogram, transverse projection. The cystic endometrioma *(arrow)* is hypoechoic and contains low-level echoes.
(Courtesy of Wendelin S. Hayes, D.O., Georgetown University, Washington, D.C.)

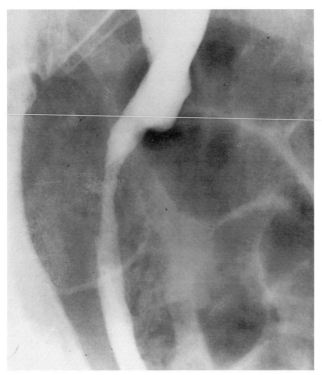

FIGURE 16–29. Endometriosis, distal right ureter. Retrograde ureterogram. A long segment of ureter is smoothly narrowed. There is proximal dilatation.

all, depending on their tissue type. Usually, retroperitoneal tumors are hypovascular. However, some, such as leiomyosarcoma, may be very vascular.

A tumor that infiltrates the sinus often causes obstructive uropathy at the level of the renal pelvis. This is seen with contrast-enhanced studies or ultrasonography as caliectasis without pelviectasis, the pelvis being prevented from distention by the surrounding infiltrative mass (see Fig. 16–27). The correct diagnosis of obstructive uropathy may be missed in this circumstance because of the absence of a dilated pelvis.

Studies of parapelvic urine granuloma with ultrasonography or computed tomography demonstrate an anechoic central component to these inflammatory soft tissue masses, which also have a corresponding area in which the attenuation value is that of water.

ENDOMETRIOSIS

Definition

Urinary tract involvement is very uncommon and usually occurs in patients with endometriosis involving other parts of the pelvis. The bladder is far more often involved than is the ureter, as discussed in Chapter 19. The ectopic endometrium is usually extrinsic to the ureter and located in the adventitia and periureteral tissue. The endometrial tissue itself may cause distortion of the ureter, or fibrosis may develop as a result of bleeding. As described

subsequently, ureteral involvement is most often located at the level of the posterior attachment of the uterosacral ligament, a structure that is frequently involved in cases of pelvic endometriosis.

Clinical Setting

Ureteral endometriosis may be asymptomatic or cause flank pain, frequency, dysuria, or hematuria. Uncommonly, these clinical findings are related to the menstrual cycle.

Radiologic Findings

A smooth, tapered narrowing of a short segment of the distal one-third of the ureter is the radiologic appearance of endometriosis of the ureter (Fig. 16–28). The ureter distal to the stricture is normal. In some patients, a long segment of distal ureter is smoothly narrowed by surrounding endometrial implants (Fig. 16–29). The portion of the ureter that is involved is usually within 3 cm of the inferior margin of the sacroiliac joint, a level that corresponds to the attachment of the uterosacral ligament. Because the obstruction is often severe enough to cause hydronephrosis, visualization of the narrowed ureter may require direct retrograde or antegrade ureterography. Computed tomography or ultrasonography demonstrates the endometrial implant as a soft tissue mass (see Fig. 16–28).

NEOPLASTIC AND INFLAMMATORY INFILTRATION

The ureter may be displaced or obstructed at any level by adjacent lymph nodes that become enlarged by metastatic deposits from a distant primary neoplasm. The most common primary sites are breast, gastrointestinal tract, lung, or lymphoma. These are presented in Chapter 21 as part of a broader discussion of tumors in the retroperitoneum.

Neoplasms that originate in pelvic organs may obstruct the distal ureter by direct extension to and invasion of the periureteral tissue. This complication is most often associated with carcinoma arising in the cervix, prostate, bladder, or rectosigmoid colon. A primary origin in the uterus or ovary may also grow in a similar pattern.

Ureteral deformity and obstruction may also be caused by Crohn's disease, appendicitis, diverticulitis, and pelvic inflammatory disease. Usually, the ureter is involved by direct extension of a phlegmon, abscess, or fistula. However, in some cases, periureteral fibrosis is the dominant response, and this may be remote from the primary site of inflammation. Crohn's disease of the terminal ileum and right colon and appendicitis affect the right ureter, whereas Crohn's disease of the jejunum or left colon and diverticulitis involve the left ureter. Ureteral involvement in these cases usually affects several centimeters of the ureter at the level of the pelvic brim.

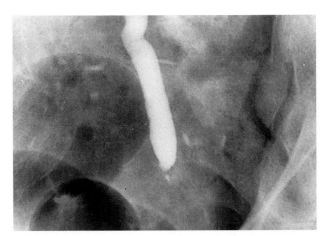

FIGURE 16–30. Local invasion of distal left ureter by metastatic carcinoma of the prostate. Antegrade pyelogram. There is irregular narrowing of the ureter with proximal dilatation.

Involvement of the ureter by neoplastic or inflammatory processes variably produces ureteral displacement, smooth or irregular narrowing, obstruction and hydronephrosis, or any combination of these (Fig. 16–30). Depending on the particular form and severity, these can be visualized by excretory urography or by antegrade or retrograde pyeloureterography. Computed tomography best demonstrates the periureteral component, which may be a mass that is isolated or one that is contiguous with a primary tumor or inflammatory process. Fibrosis alone causes thickening of the periureteral tissue.

URETERAL DEVIATION

The normal course of the ureter and the anomaly of retrocaval ureter are described in Chapter 3. There are numerous abnormalities extrinsic to the ureter that deviate its course. Aortic and iliac artery aneurysms are discussed earlier in this chapter. Others are described in Chapters 10 (lymphoma of the kidney), 19 (the bladder), and 21 (the retroperitoneum).

DIFFERENTIAL DIAGNOSIS

A mass in the renal sinus is usually manifested by focal displacement and effacement of the pelvocalyceal system. Unequivocal radiolucency, either on standard or tomographic films, strongly suggests the diagnosis of the **focal form of renal sinus lipomatosis.** Most often, the abnormality is of radiographic soft tissue density. Here, the diagnostic possibilities include **parapelvic cyst, saccular aneurysm,** and **primary** or **metastatic tumor.**

Ultrasonography, including Doppler evaluation, is valuable in the investigation of a parapelvic mass to establish the fluid content of a parapelvic cyst or the vascular nature of a saccular aneurysm. In addition to flow characteristics, aneurysm is suggested when mural echoes generated by a thrombus are present. Solid tumor is the leading diagnostic

possibility when a mass without evidence of fluid is noted.

A negative computed tomographic attenuation value equal to that of perirenal fat conclusively identifies a tumorous fatty deposit. A diagnosis of saccular aneurysm is confidently established by rapid and marked enhancement of the "mass" after a bolus of intravenous contrast material is given. Angiography may still be necessary to characterize an aneurysm. Computed tomography provides unequivocal evidence of the solid nature of primary and metastatic masses. Its application to the search for tumor in other parts of the retroperitoneum is basic. Finally, computed tomography may be useful in the assessment of parapelvic cyst or urine granuloma when these lesions yield equivocal findings on ultrasonographic evaluation.

Occasionally, a smooth extrinsic deformity of the collecting system develops from a process that originates in the renal parenchyma rather than in the renal sinus (see Fig. 16–26). This occurs either with normal variants, such as **lobar dysmorphism** or a **prominent hilar lip** (see Chapter 3), or with true parenchymal masses, such as **abscess, simple cyst,** and **adenocarcinoma** (see Chapter 12). Normal variants usually deform infundibula or calyces, while abscess, tumor, or cyst alters the renal pelvis in addition to the peripheral collecting system. Invasion of the collecting system by malignant parenchymal tumor causes irregular pelvocalyceal deformities that simulate primary mural lesions, which are discussed in Chapter 15.

The key to differentiating extraparenchymal from parenchymal lesions that deform the pelvocalyceal system is the evaluation of the nephrogram of the area adjacent to the mass. Finding of an intact nephrogram favors a diagnosis of a disorder that arises in the renal sinus. A disrupted nephrogram indicates a renal parenchymal process that extends into a portion of the renal sinus. This holds true except when a malignant process of the renal sinus invades the adjacent parenchyma, a very uncommon event. The technique used to evaluate the integrity of the renal parenchyma varies with individual circumstances and might include excretory urography with tomography, radionuclide scan, computed tomography, or renal angiography (see discussion in Chapter 27).

Generalized attenuation of the pelvocalyceal system due to **diffuse renal sinus lipomatosis** can be reliably determined when the fatty nature of the excessive peripelvic tissue is established by characteristic findings on radiographs, tomograms, computed tomograms, ultrasonograms, or magnetic resonance imaging. These findings are absent when the collapse of the pelvocalyceal system is due to other causes, such as those discussed in Chapter 18. **Generalized parapelvic cysts** may deform the pelvocalyceal system in the same manner as renal sinus lipomatosis. In this situation, the fluid nature of the masses in the sinus is established by ultrasonography or computed tomography and their differentiation from hydronephrosis is established by enhancement of the attenuated pelvocalyceal system by contrast material.

Impressions on the pelvis or ureter by **normal** or **abnormal blood vessels** can be differentiated from other causes by demonstration of contrast material enhancement of the arteries or veins during computed tomography, by documenting flow with color Doppler ultrasound or magnetic resonance imaging, or by direct visualization of the responsible vessels during angiography.

Ureteral narrowing or deformity due to the extrinsic causes discussed in this chapter are often identical in appearance to those produced by many of the mural abnormalities presented in Chapter 15. Differentiation is usually dependent on a distinctive clinical history or the demonstration of coexistent pathology such as **endometriosis, Crohn's disease, diverticulitis,** or the other entities that are discussed.

BIBLIOGRAPHY

General

Fein, A. B., and McClennan, B. L.: Solitary filling defects of the ureter. Semin. Roentgenol. *21*:201, 1986.
Malek, R. S., Aguilo, J. J., and Hattery, R. R.: Radiolucent filling defects of the renal pelvis: Classification and report of unusual cases. J. Urol. *114*:508, 1975.
Williamson, B., Jr., Hartman, G. W., and Hattery, R. R.: Multiple and diffuse ureteral filling defects. Semin. Roentgenol. *21*:214, 1986.

Parapelvic Cyst

Amis, E. S., Jr., and Cronan, J. J.: The renal sinus: An imaging review and proposed nomenclature for sinus cysts. J. Urol. *139*:1151, 1988.
Amis, E. S., Jr., Cronan, J. J., and Pfister, R. C.: Pseudohydronephrosis on noncontrast computed tomography. J. Comput. Assist. Tomogr. *6*:511, 1982.
Amis, E. S., Jr., Cronan, J. J., and Pfister, R. C.: The spectrum of peripelvic cysts. Br. J. Urol. *55*:150, 1983.
Androvlakakis, P. A., Kirayiannis, B., and Deliveliotis, A.: The parapelvic renal cyst: A report of 8 cases with particular emphasis on diagnosis and management. Br. J. Urol. *52*:342, 1980.
Bernstein, J.: The classification of renal cysts. Nephron *11*:91, 1973.
Chan, J. C. M., and Kodroff, M. B.: Hypertension and hematuria secondary to parapelvic cyst. Pediatrics *65*:821, 1980.
Cronan, J. J., Amis, E. S., Jr., Yoder, I. C., Kopans, D. B., Simeone, J. F., and Pfister R. C.: Peripelvic cysts: An impostor of sonographic hydronephrosis. J. Ultrasound Med. *1*:229, 1982.
Crummy, A. B., and Madsen, P. O.: Parapelvic renal cyst: The peripheral fat sign. J. Urol. *96*:436, 1966.
Dana, A., Musset, D., Ody, B., Rethers, C., Lepage, T., Moreau, J.-F., and Michel, J.-R.: Abnormal renal sinus: Sonography patterns of multilocular parapelvic cysts. Urol. Radiol. *5*:227, 1983.
Hidalgo, H., Dunnick, N. R., Rosenberg, E. R., Ram, P. C., and Korobkin, M.: Parapelvic cysts: Appearance on CT and sonography. AJR *138*:667, 1982.
Morag, B., Rubinstein, Z. J., and Solomon, A.: Computed tomography in the diagnosis of renal parapelvic cysts. J. Comput. Assist. Tomogr. *7*:833, 1983.
Ralls, P. W., Esensten, M. L., Boger, D., and Halls, J. M.: Severe hydronephrosis and severe renal cystic disease: Ultrasonic differentiation. AJR *134*:473, 1980.

Steel, J. F., Howe, G. E., Feeney, M. J., and Blum, J. A.: Spontaneous remission of peripelvic renal cysts. J. Urol. *114*:10, 1975.

Renal Sinus Lipomatosis

Ambos, M. A., Bosniak, M. A., Gordon, R., and Madayag, M. A.: Replacement lipomatosis of the kidney. AJR *130*:1087, 1978.
Case records of the Massachusetts General Hospital. Case 14-1974. N. Engl. J. Med. *290*:845, 1974.
Honda, H., McGuire, C. W., Barloon, T. J., and Hashimoto, K.: Replacement lipomatosis of the kidney: CT features. J. Comput. Assist. Tomogr. *14*:229, 1990.
Hurwitz, R. S., Benjamin, J. A., and Cooper, J. F.: Excessive proliferation of peripelvic fat of the kidney. Urology *11*:448, 1978.
Scheinman, L. J., and Reibman, S. J.: Peripelvic fat simulating renal pelvic tumor. J. Urol. *123*:564, 1980.
Subramanyam, B. R., Bosniak, M. A., Horii, S. C., Megibow, A. J., and Balthazar, E. J.: Replacement lipomatosis of the kidney: Diagnosis by computed tomography and sonography. Radiology *148*:791, 1983.

Vascular

Abrams, H. L., and Cornell, S. H.: Patterns of collateral flow in renal ischemia. Radiology *84*:1001, 1965.
Altebarmakian, V. K., Caldamone, A. A., Dachelet, R. J., and May, A. G.: Renal artery aneurysm. Urology *13*:257, 1979.
Angel, J. L., and Knuppel, R. A.: Computed tomography in diagnosis of puerperal ovarian vein thrombosis. Obstet. Gynecol. *63*:61, 1984.
Baum, S., and Gillenwater, J. Y.: Renal artery impressions on the renal pelvis. J. Urol. *95*:139, 1966.
Beckman, C. F., and Abrams, H. L.: Idiopathic renal vein varices: Incidence and significance. Radiology *143*:649, 1982.
Beinart, C., Sniderman, K. W., Saddekni, S., Weiner, M., Vaughn, E. D., Jr., and Sos, T. A.: Left renal vein hypertension: A cause of occult hematuria. Radiology *145*:647, 1982.
Boijsen, E., and Köhler, R.: Renal artery aneurysm. Acta Radiol. (Diagn.) *1*:1077, 1963.
Castaneda-Zuniga, W., Zollikofer, C., Valdez-Davila, O., Nath, P. H., and Amplatz, K.: Giant aneurysms of the renal arteries: An unusual manifestation of fibromuscular dysplasia. Radiology *133*:327, 1979.
Cerny, J. C., Chang, C.-Y., and Fry, W. J.: Renal artery aneurysms. Arch. Surg. *96*:653, 1968.
Chait, A., Matasar, K. W., Fabian, C. E., and Mellins, H. Z.: Vascular impressions on the ureters. AJR *111*:729, 1971.
Cleveland, R. H., Fellows, K. E., and Lebowitz, R. L.: Notching of the ureter and renal pelvis in children. AJR *129*:837, 1977.
Derrick, F. C., Rosenblum, R. R., and Lynch, K. M., Jr.: Pathological association of the right ureter and right ovarian vein. J. Urol. *97*:633, 1967.
Dykhuizen, R. F., and Roberts, J. A.: The ovarian vein syndrome. Surg. Gynecol. Obstet. *130*:443, 1970.
Ekelund, L., Boijsen, E., and Lindstedt, E.: Pseudotumor of the renal pelvis caused by renal artery aneurysm. Acta Radiol. (Diagn.) *20*:753, 1979.
Fishman, M. C., Pollack, H. M., Arger, P. H., and Banner, M. P.: Radiographic manifestations of spontaneous renal sinus hemorrhage. AJR *142*:161, 1984.
Fraley, E. E.: Vascular obstruction of superior infundibulum causing nephralgia. N. Engl. J. Med. *275*:1403, 1966.
Hayashi, M., Kume, T., and Nihira, H.: Abnormalities of renal venous system and unexplained renal hematuria. J. Urol. *124*:12, 1980.
Kreel, L., and Pyle, R.: Arterial impressions on the renal pelvis. Br. J. Radiol. *35*:609, 1962.
Lefleur, R. S., Ambos, M. A., and Rotheberg, M.: An unusual vascular impression on the renal pelvis. Urol. Radiol. *1*:117, 1979.
Lien, H. H., and vonKrogh, J.: Varicosity of the left renal ascending lumbar communicant vein: A pitfall in CT diagnosis. Radiology *152*:484, 1984.
Meng, C.-H., and Elkin, M.: Venous impression on the calyceal system. Radiology *87*:878, 1966.

Mintz, M. C., Levy, D. W., Axel, L., Kressel, H. Y., et al.: Puerperal ovarian vein thrombosis: MR diagnosis. AJR *149*:1273, 1987.

Painter, W. E., Di Donato, R. R., and White, R.: Renal arteriovenous aneurysm causing hydronephrosis and renal atrophy. AJR *104*:306, 1968.

Pearson, J. C., Tanagho, E. A., and Palubinskas, A. J.: Nonoperative diagnosis of pyelocalyceal deformity due to venous impressions. Urology *13*:207, 1979.

Poutasse, E. F.: Renal artery aneurysms. J. Urol. *113*:443, 1975.

Rosenthal, J. T., Costello, P., and Roth, R. A.: Varicosities of renal venous system. Urology *15*:427, 1980.

Slominski-Laws, M. D., Kiefer, J. H., and Vermeulen, C. W.: Arteriovenous aneurysm of the kidney. J. Urol. *75*:586, 1956.

Smith, J. N., and Hinman, F., Jr.: Intrarenal arterial aneurysms. J. Urol. *97*:990, 1967.

Stewart, B. H., Dustan, H. P., Kiser, W. S., Meaney, T. F., Straffon, R. A., and McCormack, L. J.: Correlation of angiography and natural history in evaluation of patients with renovascular hypertension. J. Urol. *104*:231, 1970.

Wendel, R. G., Crawford, E. D., and Hehman, K. N.: "Nutcracker" phenomenon: Unusual cause for renal varicosities with hematuria. J. Urol. *123*:761, 1980.

Tumor of the Renal Sinus

Ambos, M. A., Bosniak, M. A., Megibow, A. J., and Raghavendra, B.: Ureteral involvement by metastatic disease. Urol. Radiol. *1*:105, 1979.

Barbaric, Z. L., and Frank, I. N.: Peripelvic renal pseudocyst due to obstruction. AJR *129*:1097, 1977.

Friedman, A. C., Hartman, D. S., Sherman, J., Lautin, E. M., and Goldman, M.: Computed tomography of abdominal fatty masses. Radiology *139*:415, 1981.

Grossman, I. W., and Kopilnick, M. D.: Peripelvic renal fibroma: Radiographical, pathological and ultrastructural study of a unique lesion. J. Urol. *105*:174, 1971.

Olivares, R. L., Jr., McDaniel, E. C., McCallum, D. C., and Mackenzie, J. R.: Peripelvic urine granuloma simulating a renal neoplasm. J. Urol. *107*:693, 1972.

Redlin, L., Francis, R. S., and Orlando, M. M.: Renal abnormalities in agnogenic myeloid metaplasia. Radiology *12*:605, 1976.

Rubin, B. E.: Computed tomography in the evaluation of renal lymphoma. J. Comput. Assist. Tomogr. *3*:759, 1979.

Silver, T. M., Thornbury, J. R., and Teears, R. J.: Renal peripelvic plasmacytoma: Unusual radiographic findings. AJR *128*:313, 1977.

Endometriosis

Bennington, J. L., and Beckwith, J. B.: Tumors of the kidney, Renal Pelvis, and Ureter. AFIP Atlas of Tumor Pathology, second series, fascicle 12. Washington, D.C., Armed Forces Institute of Pathology, 1975.

Hill, G. S.: Uropathology. New York, Churchill Livingstone, 1989.

Kane, C., and Drovin, P.: Obstructive uropathy associated with endometriosis. Am. J. Obstet. Gynecol. *151*:207, 1985.

Langmade, C. F.: Pelvic endometriosis and ureteral obstruction. Am. J. Obstet. Gynecol. *122*:463, 1975.

Laube, D. W., Calderwood, G. S., and Benda, J. A.: Endometriosis causing ureteral obstruction. Obstet. Gynecol. *65*:695, 1985.

Lucero, S. P., Wise, H. A., Kirsh, G., Devoe, K., Hess, M. L., Kandawalla, N. C., and Drago, J. R.: Ureteric obstruction secondary to endometriosis. Br. J. Urol. *61*:201, 1988.

Older, R. A.: Endometriosis of the genitourinary tract. In Pollack, H. M. (ed.): Clinical Urography. Philadelphia, W.B. Saunders, 1990, pp. 2485–2492.

Olive, D. L., and Schwartz, L. B.: Endometriosis. N. Engl. J. Med. *328*:1759, 1993.

Pollack, H. M., and Wills, J. J.: Radiographic features of ureteral endometriosis. AJR *131*:627, 1978.

Reddy, A. N., and Evans, A. T.: Endometriosis of the ureters. J. Urol. *111*:474, 1974.

Shook, T. E., and Nyberg, L. M.: Endometriosis of the urinary tract. Urology *31*:1, 1988.

Stiehm, W. D., Becker, J. A., and Weiss, R. M.: Ureteral endometriosis. Radiology *102*:563, 1972.

Neoplastic and Inflammatory Infiltration

Abrams, H. L., Spiro, R., and Goldstein, N.: Metastases in carcinoma: Analysis of 1000 autopsied cases. Cancer *3*:74, 1950.

Cohen, W. M., Freed, S. Z., and Hasson, J.: Metastatic cancer of the ureter: A review of the literature and case presentations. J. Urol. *112*:188, 1974.

Demos, T. C., and Moncada, R.: Inflammatory gastrointestinal disease presenting as genitourinary disease. Urology *13*:115, 1979.

Gelister, J. S. K., Falzon, M., Crawford, R., Chapple, C. R., and Hendry, W. F.: Urinary tract metastasis from renal carcinoma. Br. J. Urol. *69*:250, 1992.

Geller, S. A., Lin, C.-S.: Ureteral obstruction from metastatic breast carcinoma. Arch Pathol *99*:476, 1975.

Miller, W. A., and Spear, J. L.: Periureteral and ureteral metastases from carcinoma of the cervix. Radiology *107*:533, 1973.

Recloux, P., Weiser, M., Piccart, M., and Sculier, J. P.: Ureteral obstruction in patients with breast cancer. Cancer *61*:1904, 1988.

Richie, J. P., Withers, G., and Ehrlich, R. M.: Ureteral obstruction secondary to metastatic tumors. Surg. Gynecol. Obstet. *148*:355, 1979.

Shield, D. E., Lytton, B., Weiss, R. M., Schiff, M., Jr.: Urologic complications of inflammatory bowel disease. J. Urol. *115*:701, 1976.

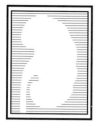

17

The Dilated Pelvocalyceal System and Ureter

The uroradiologic tradition that equated dilatation of the urinary tract with obstruction has been in question ever since voiding cystourethrography first demonstrated that dilatation of nonobstructed upper tracts occurred solely as a consequence of vesicoureteral reflux. Now the concept of nonobstructive dilatation of the renal collecting system and ureter is firmly established and multiple causes have been identified. Thus, proper analysis of a dilated upper urinary tract requires consideration of both obstructive and nonobstructive factors.

In the first section of this chapter, the discussion is of the forces that propel urine from the calyces to the bladder. These forces are fundamental to an understanding of dilatation of the upper urinary tract, regardless of cause. Next, the variable pathophysiologic expressions of urinary tract obstruction and their radiologic analogues are described as a function of a continuum of time extending from acute to chronic. This discussion also takes into account those cases in which obstruction is intermediate, intermittent, or equivocal. The numerous specific causes of obstruction (e.g., congenital, neoplastic, inflammatory), presented in other chapters, are not enumerated. The concluding section of this chapter is a discussion of nonobstructive dilatation, particularly the specific conditions that are associated with this finding.

DYNAMICS OF URINE PROPULSION

The upper urinary tract is normally a low pressure system that contains a small volume of urine. *Peristalsis* is the principal force that propels urine forward. *Nephronic pressure* and *gravity* also contribute to the transport of urine through this system. It is useful to consider each of these factors when trying to understand the various circumstances of pelvocalyceal and ureteral dilatation.

Nephronic Pressure

Nephronic pressure is the hydrodynamic force imparted to tubule fluid by glomerular filtration and by the secretion and reabsorption of water and solutes by tubule cells. Each of these factors influences upper tract dilatation by their effect on the pressure and the volume of formed urine. For example, urine formation in acute extrarenal obstruction persists because the balance between continued perfusion of the glomerular capillaries and uninterrupted reabsorption of water by the distal tubules favors ongoing glomerular filtration, although at a reduced rate. The continued formation of urine in the presence of outflow obstruction, however, leads to slight dilatation of the upper tract to the point of the obstruction and invariable blunting with occasional rupture of the calyceal fornices, reflecting both volume and pressure increases. In diabetes insipidus, on the other hand, dilatation occurs without an obstructing lesion because nephrons produce a larger than normal volume of urine as a result of their inability to reabsorb water at the distal tubule and collecting duct level.

Peristalsis

Peristalsis originates in the proximal portion of the pelvocalyceal system, presumably at a pacemaker site in specially adapted calyceal muscle. The stimulus for contraction is thought to be passive stretching of the calyceal wall by urine. The electrical excitation that stimulates the contractile wave spreads from one smooth muscle cell to another through very close anatomic contacts called nexuses. Nerves play no role in the propagation of peristalsis. Muscle contraction first becomes visible in the renal pelvis and continues distally as a coordinated wave. The frequency of peristaltic contractions increases as the volume of urine increases. At very high urine flow rates, peristalsis ceases, and urine flows in a continuous column into the bladder, propelled by nephronic pressure and, when the patient is upright, by gravity.

The concepts of Whitaker (1975) provide a comprehensive basis for understanding normal and abnormal peristalsis. The contraction wave that moves down the renal pelvis does not propel urine forward until it reaches a point at which the pelvis becomes funnel-shaped, a configuration that permits apposition of its walls. The ureteropelvic junction is the site at which apposition first occurs. It is Whitaker's contention that apposition of the walls is essential for bolus formation, and that bolus formation, in turn, is a prerequisite for peristalsis. Propulsion of urine from the ureteropelvic junction forward is the result of the resolution of the forces of contraction of the spirally arranged ureteric mus-

cle into circular and longitudinal vectors in relation to the bolus. Effective peristalsis requires obliteration of the lumen of the ureter at the top of the bolus by a strong circular contraction, by relaxation ahead of the bolus, and by a longitudinally directed muscle contraction that has the effect of pulling the ureter over the bolus. This sequence is illustrated in Figures 17–1 and 17–2.

A variety of disorders of peristalsis cause dilatation of the renal pelvis and ureter. These include abnormality in the shape of the ureteropelvic junction (discussed in Chapter 15), congenital or acquired deficiencies of the wall of the pelvis and ureter, and functional incoordination between the longitudinal and circular forces of muscular contraction, discussed in the concluding section of this chapter.

Gravity

The upright position favors forward flow of urine by adding the effect of gravity to that of nephron pressure and peristalsis. Under low to moderate flow conditions, peristalsis is very effective, and the relative contribution of gravity is minimal. This is not the case, however, when a high urine flow rate converts the pelvis and ureter into a wide column of continuously moving urine. Here, the contribution of peristalsis is negligible compared with that of nephronic pressure and gravity.

The role of gravity in emptying the collecting system is assessed by radiologic examination of the patient in the upright or prone position. This is an

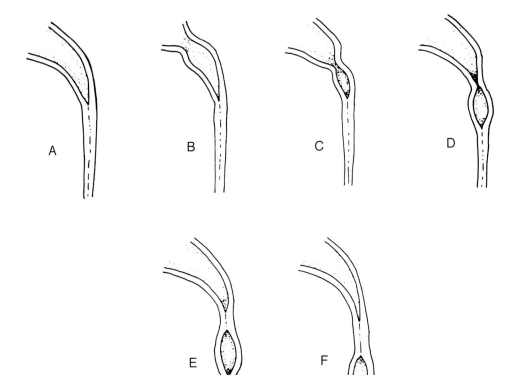

FIGURE 17–1. Schematic illustration of sequence of peristalsis at the normal ureteropelvic junction.

A, Normal funnel shape of the ureteropelvic junction at rest.

B and *C,* Peristaltic wave passes prograde through the pelvis.

D, Funnel shape of the pelvis leads to apposition of opposite walls as peristaltic wave progresses toward the ureter.

E, A bolus forms as a result of circular contraction of muscles proximally and relaxation of muscles distally.

F, Progression of bolus occurs as the longitudinally oriented force of muscle contraction "pulls" the ureter over the bolus.

(Courtesy of R. H. Whitaker, Addenbrooke's Hospital, Cambridge, England, and Br. J. Urol. 47:377, 1975.)

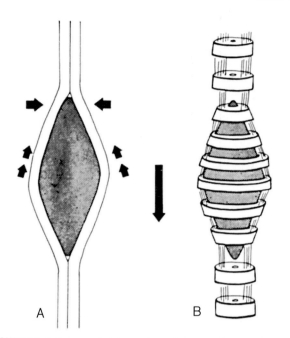

FIGURE 17–2. Schematic illustration of the resolution of forces and the ureteral muscle action in normal ureteral peristalsis.

A, Resolution of forces into circular and longitudinal sectors in relation to the bolus.

B, Representation of muscle contraction and relaxation in relation to the bolus.

(Courtesy of R. H. Whitaker, Addenbrooke's Hospital, Cambridge, England, and Br. J. Urol. 47:377, 1975.)

important step in evaluating the dilated pelvis and ureter. Emptying of a dilated system by placing a patient upright for a few minutes is evidence against obstruction. However, caution is required in interpretation of findings because in some cases of partial obstruction, gravity contributes the extra force needed to empty the contents of a proximally dilated system across a narrowed segment. On the other hand, dilatation proximal to a narrowing that persists in the upright position is evidence for obstruction.

OBSTRUCTIVE UROPATHY

Whitaker defines urinary tract obstruction as a "narrowing such that the proximal pressure must be raised to transmit the usual flow through it" (1975). This implies that neither *dilatation nor increased pelvic pressure is invariably present in obstruction,* although some degree of dilatation is usually present. According to this definition, the diagnosis of obstruction requires the measurement of hydrostatic pressure proximal and distal to a demonstrable narrowing at known urine flow rates. The pressure-flow technique of Whitaker, described in Chapter 15, is the invasive method by which these parameters can be studied directly. However, the goal for assessing the dilated upper urinary tract is to use the various imaging modalities that indirectly measure these elements, allowing the radiologist to avoid, in almost all instances, the need for invasive techniques.

In obstruction, the degree of collecting system dilatation and of damage to the structure and function of the kidney is determined by both the chronicity and the severity of the offending lesion. Acute obstruction creates a constellation of abnormalities quite distinct from those created by chronic obstruction (Fig. 17–3). Radiologic patterns in intermittent obstruction differ from those seen with unrelenting lesions. Each of these is considered in the following sections.

Acute Obstruction

Driven by hemodynamic pressure from perfusion of glomerular capillaries, urine production continues in acute obstruction, although at a greatly reduced rate. Hydrostatic pressure proximal to the obstruction rises as newly formed urine moves into the obstructed system. Urine formation eventually would cease if it were not for factors that partially compensate for the increasing pressure. These include continued water reabsorption by the distal tubules and collecting ducts and leakage of urine into veins, lymphatics, and the renal sinus through ruptured calyceal fornices. Some urine may also pass between tubule cells and into the interstitial space of the kidney. The passage of urine around the obstructing lesion is yet another compensating factor. The net effect is a balanced state in which urine formation continues, although at a reduced rate.

The foregoing considerations indicate that the major impact of acute obstruction on the kidney is functional, rather than structural. Blunting of the forniceal angles is the most reliable and consistent anatomic representation of increased hydrostatic pressure in the pelvocalyceal system, and forniceal rupture is the extreme consequence of elevated urine pressure. Dilatation of the upper urinary tract to the point of obstruction is always minimal to moderate (Fig. 17–4). Other anatomic alterations caused by acute obstruction include increased renal

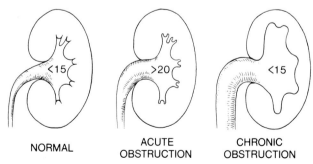

NORMAL   ACUTE OBSTRUCTION   CHRONIC OBSTRUCTION

FIGURE 17–3. Schematic illustration of the differences in pelvocalyceal dilatation, renal function (pelvic pressure), and structural kidney damage between acute and chronic obstruction. In acute obstruction, there is minimal dilatation, marked increase in pelvic pressure, and no structural damage. Chronic obstruction is characterized by marked dilatation and normal pelvic pressures as nephron damage permanently slows the rate of urine formation. Numbers refer to intrapelvic pressure in centimeters of water.

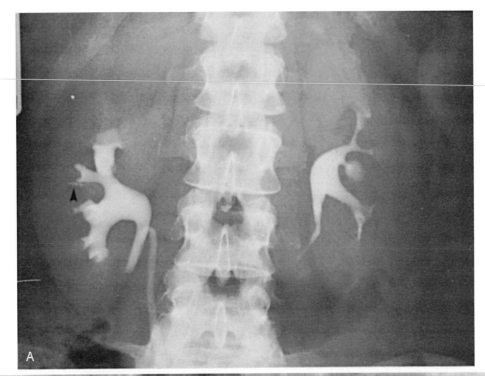

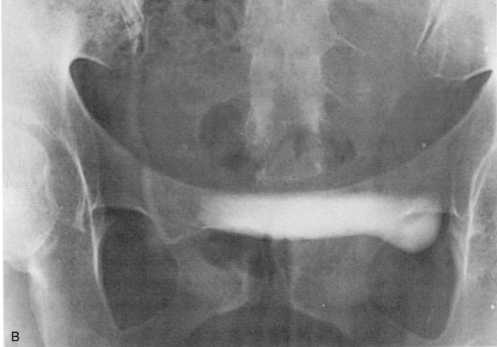

FIGURE 17–4. Acute obstructive uropathy due to stone in the distal right ureter. There is minimal enlargement of the pelvocalyceal system. Dilatation of the forniceal angles and leakage of contrast material into the sinus *(arrowhead)* through a ruptured fornix reflect elevated hydrostatic pressure in the pelvis of the kidney. Despite the added force of gravity when the patient is upright, the system does not drain. Same patient is illustrated in Figure 9–21.

    A, Excretory urogram, 20-minute film.
    B, Upright, postvoid film of the bladder.

parenchymal thickness, linear strands of edema coursing through the perinephric space, and edematous thickening of the ureter at the site of an impacted calculus, the *tissue-rim sign* (see Fig. 9–30). Delayed appearance of either contrast material during contrast material–enhanced imaging studies or of radioactivity during radionuclide studies with a filtered agent reflects a decrease in glomerular filtration rate caused by elevated tubule pressure. Nevertheless, glomerular filtration does continue, and a gradual increase over time in nephrographic radiodensity or radioactivity occurs in these respective studies. As contrast material or tracer slowly passes antegrade through the tubule lumina and collecting ducts, the minimally dilated collecting system and ureter proximal to the obstruction are visualized. Leakage of urine through ruptured fornices is shown by contrast material in renal sinus tissue or, more rarely, in the medullary interstitium, renal veins, or lymphatics. This is classified, respectively, as *pyelosinus, pyelointerstitial, pyelovenous,* or *pyelolymphatic backflow.* The dense nephrographic appearance and dilated collecting structures persist over time and are not influenced by gravity when the patient is examined in the upright position. The upright position, however, is useful in moving contrast material distally to visualize the point of obstruction. The functional defects of acute obstruction are most pronounced in patients whose pelvocalyceal systems are "intrarenal"

and thus not readily distensible (Fig. 17–5). In comparison, "extrarenal" systems dilate more and have a less severe functional defect.

Of all the features of acute obstruction noted on contrast material–enhanced studies, blunting of the calyceal fornices, forniceal rupture, and failure of a dilated system to drain under the influence of gravity are most specific. In patients with acute colic, however, unenhanced spiral computed tomography usually establishes the diagnosis of acute urinary tract obstruction and precludes the need for contrast material–enhanced studies when increased parenchymal thickness, perinephric edema, and the tissue-rim sign are demonstrated. Of course, computed tomographic demonstration of an obstructing ureteral calculus is diagnostic.

Ultrasonography is highly sensitive in detecting moderate to marked dilatation of the collecting system. This degree of dilatation, however, is not a usual feature of acute obstruction. Therefore, there is always a significant possibility of a false-negative result when ultrasonography, even when combined with an abdominal radiograph to detect opaque calculus, is used to diagnose acute obstruction in patients with acute colic and hematuria. Likewise, it is impossible to distinguish by ultrasonography mild dilatation due to obstruction from a normal extrarenal pelvis. As discussed in Chapter 9, the potential value of Doppler ultrasonography has not been realized in the diagnosis of obstructive uropathy.

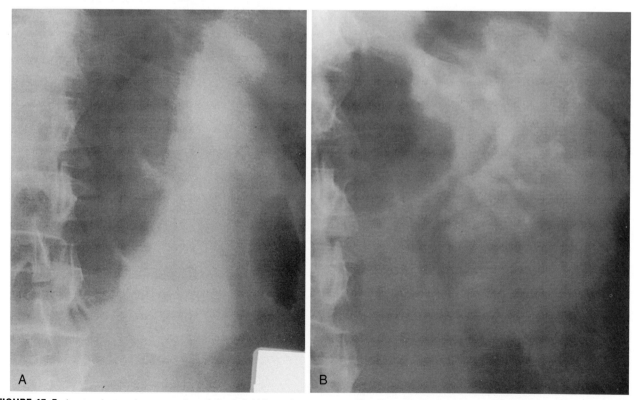

FIGURE 17–5. Acute obstructive uropathy of the left kidney due to stone. The "intrarenal" location of the pelvis causes pronounced transitory functional effects, seen as an increasingly dense nephrogram and a marked delay in pelvocalyceal opacification.
A, Excretory urogram, 10-minute film.
B, Excretory urogram, 1-hour film. There has been spontaneous passage of a stone into the bladder.

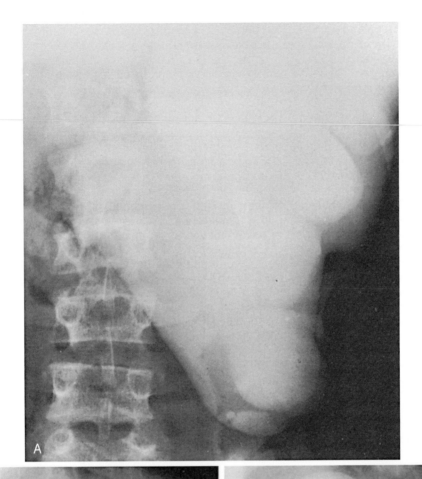

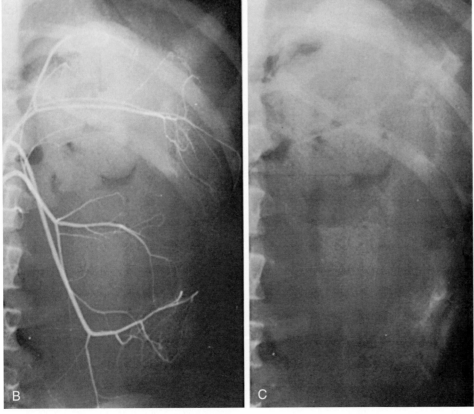

FIGURE 17–6. Chronic obstructive uropathy due to ureteropelvic junction obstruction in a 16-year-old boy with congenital unilateral kidney and renal failure. In this extreme example, the kidney has become a large, urine-filled sac with minimal perfusion by stretched, branchless arteries.

A, Antegrade pyelogram.

B, Renal arteriogram, arterial phase.

C, Renal arteriogram, late phase. Thin bands of compressed renal tissue, the *rim sign,* are opacified.

Chronic Obstruction

The elevated hydrostatic pressure of acute unrelieved obstruction eventually causes moderate to marked dilatation of the collecting system and ureter to the level of obstruction, wasting of the renal parenchyma, and reduction in renal blood flow. These features of chronic obstruction evolve over time and represent both structural and functional changes. As nephrons atrophy and renal blood flow diminishes, the amount of urine formed progressively diminishes to equal the amount that can leave the system. Thus, the pelvocalyceal system eventually converts from an initial high-pressure, minimally dilated, acutely obstructed structure to a passively dilated, low-pressure, chronically obstructed sac, with a slow exchange of urine (see Fig. 17–3).

Chronic obstruction is usually associated with mild and nonspecific symptoms or is asymptomatic. Causes of chronic obstruction include ureteropelvic junction obstruction; urolithiasis; ureteral stricture; periureteral fibrosis; primary or metastatic retroperitoneal tumors; congenital anomalies; and a wide variety of bladder and bladder outlet abnormalities, as discussed in other chapters.

The extent of renal damage caused by a chronic obstructive lesion is determined by both duration and degree of obstruction. In extreme cases, the kidney is transformed into a functionless, fluid-filled flank mass composed of a thin rim of severely atrophied parenchyma and is minimally perfused by stretched, branchless arteries (Fig. 17–6). In this instance, a flank mass is detectable by abdominal radiography alone and by excretory urography. The fluid-filled nature of the mass is established by either ultrasonography or computed tomography. Pyelography can demonstrate the site of obstruction. When performed by the antegrade route, pressure in the hydronephrotic kidney, usually less than 10 cm of water, can be measured.

Abnormalities less severe than the preceding extreme example are more common. Even with moderate to marked dilatation, the pelvis can usually be distinguished from the calyces. The renal parenchyma is variably thinned. The density of the nephrogram is diminished because of the decreased clearance of contrast material by compromised nephrons. An increasingly dense nephrogram is not seen in chronic obstruction, reflecting the normal hydrostatic pressure of urine in the collecting system. Early in the course of the excretory urogram, thin bands of slightly radiodense parenchyma, the *rim sign,* surround the dilated, not yet opacified calyces, producing a *negative pyelogram* (Figs. 17–7 and 17–8). In some patients with chronic obstruction, a thin curvilinear area of enhancement develops during the course of urography at the interface between the inner medulla and the adjacent dilated calyces. This *calyceal crescent sign* represents concentrated contrast material in distal collecting ducts whose orientation has been distorted by caly-

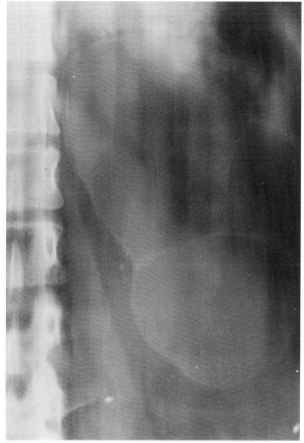

FIGURE 17–7. Chronic obstructive uropathy causing a *rim sign.* Excretory urogram. There is nephrographic enhancement of strikingly thin renal parenchyma representing residua of atrophied cortex and medulla.

ceal dilatation (Fig. 17–9). Collecting system opacification is delayed. In less severe circumstances, only moderate dilatation of the collecting system and wasting of the renal parenchyma are noted (Fig. 17–10). In some patients, obstruction is partial and nonprogressive. In these cases, dilatation of the collecting system may disappear and the radiologic findings of obstruction can be evoked only when the patient is in a diuretic state.

Slow uptake and prolonged activity in the radioisotope renogram are the hallmarks of moderate chronic obstructive uropathy, but these can also be seen in dilated nonobstructed systems. Renography, including diuresis renography, is discussed subsequently and in Chapter 2.

Screening for chronic obstructive uropathy is most efficaciously performed with ultrasonography, using the criteria described in Chapter 9 (Fig. 17–11). When combined with a radiograph of the abdomen to exclude a false-negative result caused by staghorn calculus, the sensitivity of ultrasonography in detecting a dilated collecting system approaches 100 per cent. Other, very uncommon sources of false-negative results are acute renal failure superimposed on chronic obstruction and neoplastic, inflammatory, or desmoplastic processes in

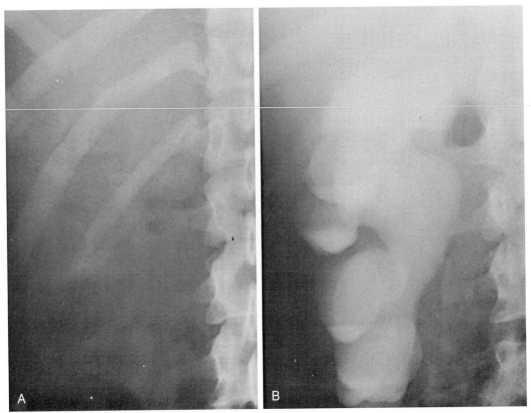

FIGURE 17–8. Chronic obstructive uropathy in a 27-year-old woman with long-standing ureteropelvic junction obstruction. Same patient is illustrated in Figure 9–27.
A, Excretory urogram. Early film demonstrates the nephrogram of compressed parenchyma surrounding the nonopacified calyces, the *negative pyelogram.*
B, Excretory urogram. The previously radiolucent dilated calyces are opacified on a delayed upright film.

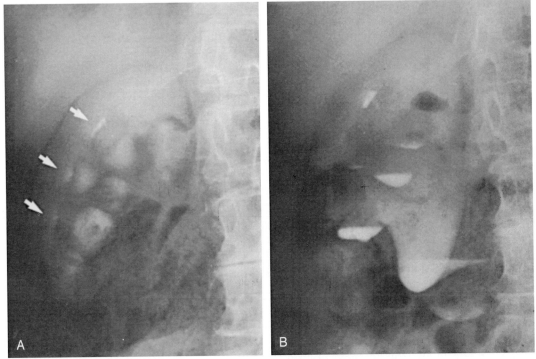

FIGURE 17–9. Chronic obstructive uropathy. Early demonstration of a dilated collecting system on an upright film.
A, Excretory urogram, supine film. Narrow, semilunar bands of contrast material *(arrows)* called *calyceal crescents* are present at the interface between renal parenchyma and the faintly opacified dilated calyces.
B, Excretory urogram, upright film. Layering of contrast material facilitates visualization of the dilated calyces.

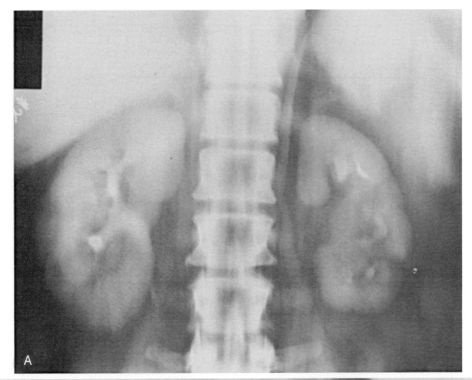

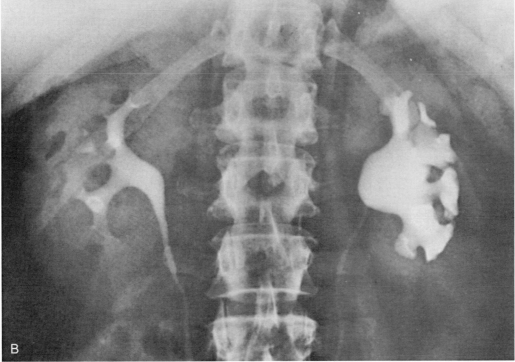

FIGURE 17–10. Chronic obstructive uropathy of the left kidney, intermediate grade. There is moderate parenchymal thinning and collecting system dilatation, but the time-density pattern of the nephrogram is normal, indicating a stable state.
  A, Excretory urogram, 3-minute tomogram.
  B, Excretory urogram, 10-minute film.

the renal sinus and periureteral tissue that prevent dilatation of the obstructed collecting system and ureter. Not all dilated systems are caused by obstruction, however. Therefore, false-positive tests occur and account for a specificity of approximately 75 per cent. These results, however, are to be ex-

pected in a screening test and do not detract from the value of ultrasonography as the primary technique for the diagnosis of chronic obstruction. The causes of nonobstructive dilatation of the collecting system that account for false-positive results are discussed in the last section of this chapter.

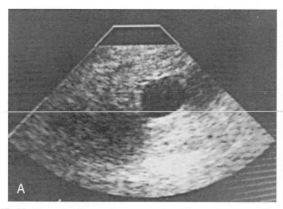
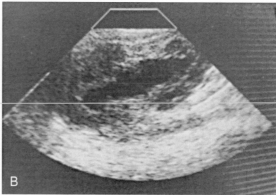

FIGURE 17–11. Chronic obstructive uropathy. Ultrasonogram. The dilated oval pelvis, seen on a medial longitudinal section *(A)*, communicates with the intrarenal portion of the pelvocalyceal system, seen on a more lateral longitudinal section *(B)*.

Computed tomography is also a very accurate technique for the detection of dilatation of the collecting system (Fig. 17–12). Contrast material–enhancement is sometimes needed to establish that the dilated fluid-filled structure is in fact the pelvocalyceal system rather than a noncommunicating parapelvic cyst (see Fig. 16–4). Additionally, computed tomography is more likely than ultrasonography to image the obstructing lesion. Often, however, computed tomography will only identify dilatation and not provide the information needed to separate obstructive from nonobstructive causes. The ultimate identification of a lesion responsible for the obstruction often requires retrograde or antegrade pyelography (see Fig. 17–6). Additional features of chronic obstructive uropathy are discussed in Chapter 9.

Intermediate, Intermittent, and Equivocal Forms of Obstruction

Diagnosis of acute and chronic obstruction is straightforward in most patients when excretory urography and ultrasonography are used, with occasional assistance from radionuclide renography,

computed tomography, or pyelography. There is a group of patients in whom these standard studies produce normal or equivocal results, yet in whom there is convincing clinical evidence for obstruction. Most of these patients have functional obstructions at the ureteropelvic junction, as discussed in Chapter 15. In patients who experience obstruction intermittently, correct diagnosis requires examination during symptomatic periods, so-called acute urography. Other patients have obstructive lesions of intermediate severity that are occult except when studied during a condition of diuresis that challenges the ability of the collecting system and the ureter to accommodate large urine flow rates. Equivocal findings of obstruction may also be encountered in patients whose dilatation is due to nonobstructive causes or in patients whose collecting systems are not distensible because of prior surgery and peripelvic fibrosis.

To evaluate any of these possibilities, standard tests must be modified to evoke evidence of obstruction. *Diuresis renography* assesses the ability of the upper tract to transport urine under conditions of high flow rates. This technique evaluates the shape of the renographic curve before and after a diuresis provoked by intravenous furosemide. This test helps to separate patients whose obstruction is mild or intermittent from those whose dilated pelvis is not caused by obstruction at all. When diuresis renography fails to resolve the question of obstruction, a pressure-flow urodynamic study permits direct measurement of pressure in the renal pelvis and bladder under conditions of controlled flow, as discussed in Chapter 15.

In patients with obstruction, the goal is to select for surgery those patients who have periods of continuous or intermittent high pelvic pressure under conditions of usual urine flow rates, since this is the circumstance that eventually causes deterioration of renal function.

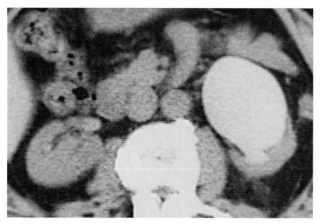

FIGURE 17–12. Chronic obstructive uropathy of the left kidney. Computed tomogram, contrast material–enhanced. There is marked dilatation of the collecting system and thinning of the renal parenchyma. The nephrogram no longer demonstrates the increasingly dense pattern of acute obstruction. Same patient is illustrated in Figure 9–24.

NONOBSTRUCTIVE DILATATION
Vesicoureteral Reflux

Persistent reflux of large volumes of urine through the vesicoureteral junction may dilate the ureter and pelvocalyceal system (Fig. 17–13). Reflux is often found in infants or children and most commonly results from an abnormally short segment of terminal ureter traversing the bladder wall, commonly with a more obtuse angle of insertion than is normally present in nonrefluxing ureters. Usually, this mural segment of the distal ureter lengthens and its angle of insertion becomes more acute as the child grows. Reflux then disappears spontaneously and without consequence. There are some children, however, in whom this does not occur. In them, reflux may be massive and persistent, causing the collecting system and the ureter to dilate and the kidney to suffer global atrophy as a result of a "water-hammer" effect on the parenchyma (Fig. 17–14). This is termed *reflux atrophy* and is discussed in Chapter 6 as one cause of the unilateral, small, smooth kidney. Reflux atrophy is distinct from another complication of major vesicoureteral reflux, the focal scarring of reflux nephropathy (chronic atrophic pyelonephritis) (see discussion in Chapter 5). Either of these reflux-induced structural alterations of the kidney persist into adulthood as permanent damage, although both originate in infancy or early childhood.

Vesicoureteral reflux is not always caused by a short, obtusely angled, mural segment of distal ureter. A bladder diverticulum located adjacent to the ureteral orifice may become large enough to transform a nonrefluxing orifice into one that allows vesicoureteral reflux. This sometimes occurs in infants and children as a result of a congenital deficiency of muscle in the posterolateral wall of the bladder where the ureter inserts. Known as a *Hutch* or *congenital bladder diverticulum,* this deformity may actually incorporate the ureteral orifice into the diverticulum itself. Reflux may also occur in patients with bladder outlet obstruction, such as posterior urethral valves in male children, or in dysmorphic conditions, such as prune-belly syndrome. At any age, reflux can develop *de novo* as a consequence of neurologic disorders of the bladder.

One potentially misleading appearance associated with massive vesicoureteral reflux in children is the coexistence of a large capacity, thin-walled bladder and marked upper urinary tract dilatation. This combination has been termed *megacystis-megaureter syndrome* but is actually nothing more than the effect of large volumes of refluxed urine refilling the bladder after voiding and maintaining its distended state.

Pelvocalyceal dilatation due to recurrent overdistention by refluxed urine is usually persistent. The appearance on excretory urography or ultrasonography is indistinguishable from that of pelvocalyceal dilatation due to other causes discussed in this chapter. In some patients, the dilatation of the collecting system may not be apparent when the patient is examined in an antidiuretic state. Instead, the collecting system appears redundant or flaccid or longitudinal folds are noted, as discussed in Chapter 15 (see Fig. 15–41). The dilated nature of the collecting system in these cases becomes apparent only when the examination is repeated with diuresis. It should be kept in mind, however, that longitudinal folds may be a normal finding, especially when low osmolality contrast material is used to enhance the urinary tract.

Although reflux as a cause of dilatation of the pelvocalyceal system and ureter is sometimes demonstrable by voiding cystourethrography in the adult, dilatation may be the residual effect of prior, spontaneously corrected reflux, in which case voiding cystourethrography fails to identify the etiology (Fig. 17–15). In this circumstance, vesicoureteral reflux cannot be distinguished from other nonobstructive causes of dilatation.

Infection

Dilatation of the pelvocalyceal system and ureter sometimes occurs with acute pyelonephritis (Fig. 17–16). Presumably, this results from inhibition of the muscular activity of the ureter and the pelvis by pathogens, possibly through release of endotoxin. Appropriate antibiotic therapy quickly reverses this effect. Other imaging abnormalities seen during the early phase of acute pyelonephritis are described in Chapter 9.

High Flow States

Diabetes insipidus, osmotic diuresis, and unilateral kidney are all examples of high flow states. *Diabetes insipidus* occurs when the kidney is unable to maximally concentrate urine. Normally, vasopressin pro-

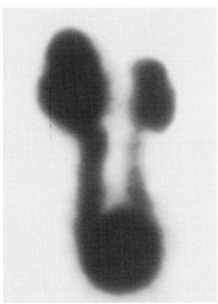

FIGURE 17–13. Vesicoureteral reflux, grade V, bilateral. ^{99m}Tc-pertechnetate voiding cystogram. Refluxed urine fills the markedly dilated ureters and pelvocalyceal systems. Same patient is illustrated in Figure 5–2. (Courtesy of Massoud Majd, M.D., Children's National Medical Center, Washington, D.C.)

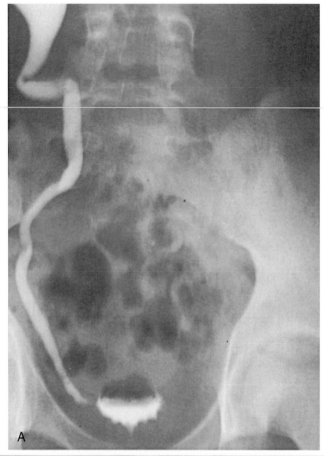

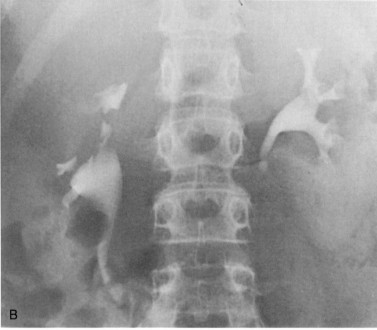

FIGURE 17–14. Vesicoureteral reflux into the right pelvocalyceal system of an 11-year-old girl with recurrent urinary tract infection. This reflux has led to dilatation of the pelvocalyceal system and global parenchymal atrophy. Same patient is illustrated in Figure 5–7.

A, Voiding cystourethrogram.

B, Excretory urogram. Note the longitudinal mucosal folds in the right pelvis due to incomplete distention of the collecting system.

duced by the hypothalamus-hypophysis acts on distal tubules and collecting ducts to increase water reabsorption and thereby concentrate the urine. Either deficient hypothalamic-hypophyseal production of vasopressin or insensitivity of the renal tubules to normal amounts of endogenous vasopressin causes diabetes insipidus.

Hypothalamic diabetes insipidus develops when vasopressin production is reduced by more than 90 per cent. This usually occurs following pituitary destruction by tumor (usually craniopharyngioma), by surgery, or as a complication of meningitis or head trauma. Rarely, hypothalamic diabetes insipidus is present on a hereditary basis. Hypothalamic

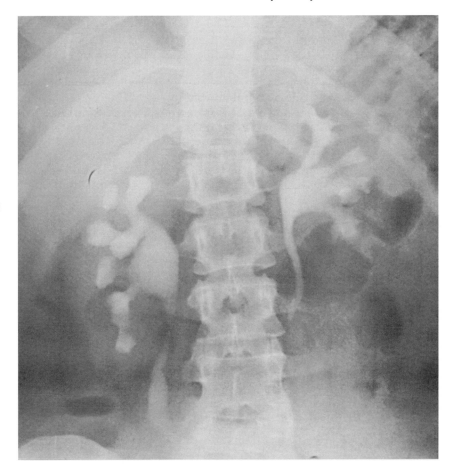

FIGURE 17–15. Pelvocalyceal dilatation and global parenchymal wasting in the right kidney of a 26-year-old woman without prior urologic history. In the absence of concurrent reflux and a pertinent history, it is impossible to determine a responsible cause. Excretory urogram.

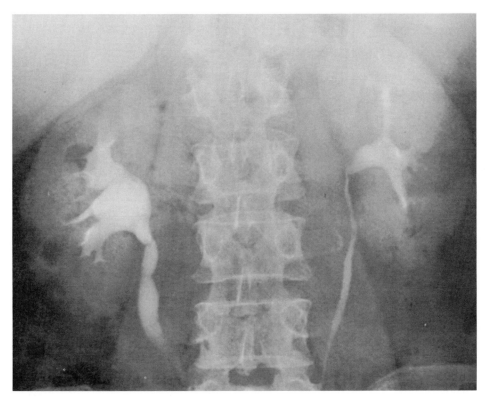

FIGURE 17–16. Dilatation of the pelvocalyceal system of the right kidney during an episode of acute pyelonephritis. Excretory urogram.

diabetes insipidus is characterized by the ability of the kidney to concentrate urine in response to exogenous vasopressin and its inability to do so with water deprivation alone.

Another form of diabetes insipidus is caused by compulsive intake of large amounts of water, a condition known as *psychogenic water intoxication*. In this condition, excessive fluid intake inhibits normal hypothalamic-hypophyseal production of vasopressin. Increased concentration of urine following water deprivation characterizes this form of diabetes insipidus.

Primary nephrogenic diabetes insipidus occurs when distal tubules and collecting ducts are unable to respond to either endogenous or exogenous vasopressin. This is a rare sex-linked recessive genetic disorder found mainly in infants and young males.

As part of a major renal disorder, the kidney may become incapable of maximally concentrating urine. *Secondary nephrogenic diabetes insipidus* develops in association with drug toxicity, analgesic nephropathy, sickle cell anemia, hypokalemia or hypercalcemia from any cause, chronic uremic nephropathy, postobstructive nephropathy, reflux nephropathy (chronic atrophic pyelonephritis), amyloidosis, and sarcoidosis. No specific tubule lesion that accounts for polyuria in these conditions has been identified.

Patients with diabetes insipidus complain of poly-uria, polydipsia, and constipation, and they excrete hypotonic urine. Excessive water excretion may cause severe dehydration, which in infants or children can lead to convulsions and death.

The pelvocalyceal systems, ureters, and bladder are dilated in all forms of diabetes insipidus as the volume of urine formed overwhelms the peristaltic capacity of the ureter (Fig. 17–17). Overdistention eventually leads to loss of ureteral muscle tone. The ureter then becomes a passive conduit between the kidney and the bladder, and urine is propelled only by nephronic pressure and gravity. Marked distention of the bladder may contribute further to upper tract distention of obstructing the ureterovesical junction. Global wasting of the kidney, including effacement of the papillae, occurs as increased hydrostatic pressure causes renal parenchymal atrophy. Collecting system dilatation and renal wasting are readily visualized by excretory urography, ultrasonography, and computed tomography.

Moderate dilatation of the calyces, pelvis, and ureter is also seen during osmotic diuresis from any cause and in the single kidney that has undergone compensatory hypertrophy (Fig. 17–18).

Congenital Megacalyces

Uniform dilatation of the calyces due to underdevelopment of the papillae constitutes congenital mega-

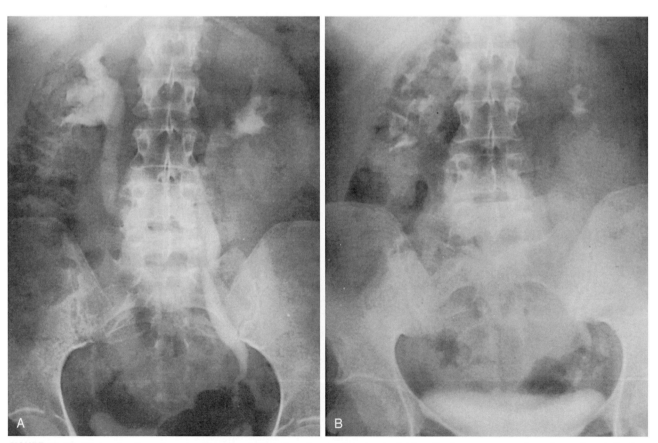

FIGURE 17–17. Bilateral pelvocalyceal and ureteral dilatation due to diabetes insipidus. Drainage occurs when the patient is in the upright position.
  A, Excretory urogram. Patient is supine.
  B, Excretory urogram. Patient is upright.

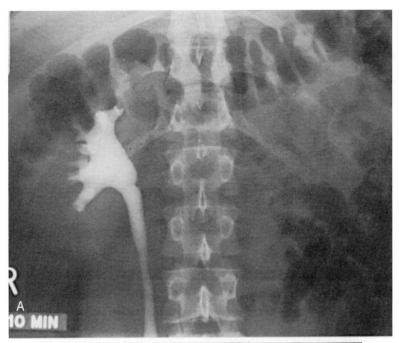

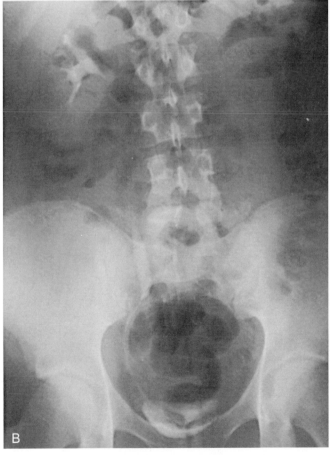

FIGURE 17–18. Pelvocalyceal and ureteral dilatation due to a high flow state in a patient with congenital absence of one kidney. Drainage occurs when the patient is in the upright position.
   A, Excretory urogram. Patient is supine.
   B, Excretory urogram. Patient is upright.

calyces. The medullary tip is of a semilunar shape that caps, rather than projects as a cone into the calyx. The calyces are polygonal and have a mosaic or faceted appearance.

The pathogenesis of congenital megacalyces has not been established. Suggested possibilities are faulty ureteral bud division, primary hypoplasia of

glomeruli in the juxtamedullary cortex, functional infundibular achalasia due to maldevelopment of smooth muscle fibers of the pelvocalyceal junction, and transient collecting system obstruction *in utero,* caused by involuting folds in the proximal portion of the fetal ureter.

The diagnosis of congenital megacalyces should

be considered only in patients whose characteristic calyceal deformities exist without prior or concurrent obstruction. Vesicoureteral reflux must also be excluded. Stasis of urine in the enlarged calyces predisposes the patient to infection and stone formation, which are the major clinical abnormalities in these patients.

Renal function, as measured by creatinine clearance or serum creatinine, is normal in patients with congenital megacalyces. This is an important feature in differentiating this abnormality from postobstructive atrophy. Some data suggest a moderate defect in concentrating ability of kidneys with congenital megacalyces (Talner and Gittes, 1974).

Congenital megacalyces are usually unilateral. Contrast material appears at the same time in the affected and the normal kidney during excretory urography, but maximum opacification of the pelvocalyceal system is delayed in the abnormal kidney because of the dilution effect of the large volume of urine in its collecting system. The renal pelvis and infundibula are often capacious but otherwise normal (Fig. 17–19). Other features of congenital megacalyces on excretory urography are normal to increased number of calyces, normal to increased length of kidney, and decreased thickness of renal parenchyma due to both expanded calyceal volume and thinning of the medulla. The papillary tips are either absent or very shallow. Congenital megacalyces are not progressive. The occasional finding of a dilated ureter has been cited as evidence for obstruction as a pathogenetic factor.

Stones and infection complicate the urographic appearance of congenital megacalyces and preclude confident distinction from other entities, especially postobstructive atrophy.

Ultrasonography and computed tomography demonstrate dilatation of the calyces and reduction in thickness of the renal parenchyma. Neither of these techniques, however, is useful in distinguishing congenital megacalyces from other nonobstructive causes of a dilated collecting system.

Quantitative renal radionuclide studies with either ^{99m}Tc-DTPA or ^{99m}Tc-DMSA demonstrate normal glomerular function in the kidney with congenital megacalyces and distinguish these kidneys from those whose similar structural deformity is accompanied by a permanent loss of nephrons. Examples of the latter include postobstructive atrophy or pressure atrophy from vesicoureteral reflux. Radionuclide renograms with tracers that measure excretion show marked prolongation of the excretory phase in the congenital megacalyces kidney. This result, simulating obstruction, is due to the gradual mixing of isotope with the large volume of urine in the dilated calyces (see Fig. 17–19). The diuresis renogram will exclude obstruction in this situation. These aspects of radionuclide imaging are discussed further in Chapter 2.

Postobstructive Atrophy

The renal changes following relief of urinary tract obstruction include generalized papillary atrophy, global thinning of the parenchyma, and generalized dilatation of the pelvocalyceal system. Some of the dilatation, particularly that involving the calyces, is due to atrophy of surrounding tissue. Altered smooth muscle morphology may also contribute to postobstructive pelvocalyceal dilatation.

Persistent collecting system dilatation after surgical correction of obstruction raises the possibility of ineffective surgery. Diuresis renography or pressure-flow measurement usually resolves this question.

Pelvocalyceal dilatation in postobstructive atrophy produces abnormalities on urography, ultrasonography, and computed tomography that are identical to the findings of nonobstructive dilatation caused by other forms of parenchymal atrophy or maldevelopment (see Fig. 17–15). Impaired function of the postobstructive kidney is detectable by radionuclide techniques and is a basis for distinction from congenital megacalyces. (A discussion of other aspects of postobstructive atrophy appears in Chapter 6.)

Pregnancy

As a result of pregnancy, the collecting systems and ureters dilate, and peristaltic activity diminishes.

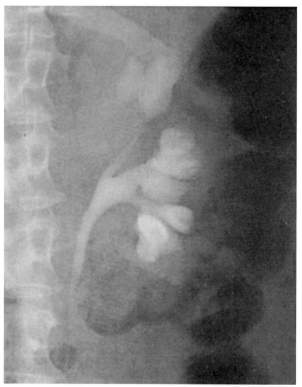

FIGURE 17–19. Congenital bilateral megacalyces (presumed diagnosis) in a 57-year-old woman with a normal urologic history and normal renal function. The excretory urogram was performed because a radionuclide bone scan suggested bilateral obstruction. Dilatation of calyces, polycalycosis, and flattened papillae are present.

Microscopically, there is hypertrophy of ureteropelvic smooth muscle and hyperplasia of connective tissue. These changes affect about 90 per cent of women during the course of pregnancy, appearing as early as the end of the first trimester and becoming maximal in the third trimester. Dilatation of the ureter extends only to the level of the pelvic brim; distal to this point the caliber is normal. Dilatation during pregnancy far more often involves the right collecting system and ureter than the left. Only one-third of patients demonstrate any left-sided changes at all, and even less often does left-sided dilatation predominate. Most changes arising from pregnancy resolve within a few weeks after delivery. Persistent dilatation after parturition is usually caused by urinary tract infection acquired during pregnancy.

The cause of upper tract dilatation during pregnancy has been debated extensively but never precisely defined. The muscle-relaxing effects of progesterone-like hormones and partial mechanical obstruction are two likely contributing factors. Suggested causes of obstruction include thickening of muscle and connective tissue in the distal segment of the ureter, compression by a dilated ovarian vein, compression by iliac vessels, and pressure from the gravid uterus, which rotates to the right as it enlarges. Hypertrophy of Waldeyer's sheath, a connective tissue envelope around the distal ureter, might cause dilatation either by direct compression or by preventing hormonally induced relaxation of the distal ureter. None of these considerations alone explains the predominant involvement of the right side, the absence of distal ureteral dilatation, and the appearance of these changes early in pregnancy before the uterus is large enough to produce pressure on the ureter. It is likely that the cause is multifactorial.

The dilated collecting system and ureter associated with sluggish peristalsis predisposes the patient to urinary tract infection. Otherwise, this condition is without consequence.

Ultrasonography detects the dilatation of pregnancy and, of course, establishes the presence of pregnancy as the cause.

Prune-Belly Syndrome

Congenital absence or deficiency of abdominal musculature, cryptorchidism, and dystrophic urinary tract abnormalities constitute the major findings of the prune-belly syndrome. This condition, which occurs predominantly in males, is also known as the *Eagle-Barrett* or *triad syndrome*.

Urinary tract abnormalities in prune-belly syndrome are dominated by marked dilatation, elongation, and tortuosity of the ureters. Obstruction of the ureter or of the lower urinary tract is only rarely present. Ureteral dilatation is most marked distally, and vesicoureteral reflux is usually present. Diminished to absent peristalsis reflects a patchy absence of ureteral muscle interspersed with abnormal amounts of fibrous and collagenous tissue. Similar histologic findings are present in the bladder, which is usually dilated, but not trabeculated. A urachal cyst or diverticulum often coexists. The prostatic urethra is dilated and elongated, the prostate is hypoplastic, and the verumontanum is absent to small. (See Chapter 19 for further discussion of the bladder in prune-belly syndrome.) The kidneys variably demonstrate pelvocalyceal dilatation, parenchymal dysplasia, small size, and diminished function. In some cases, the kidneys are normal.

The clinical consequences of prune-belly syndrome vary from death *in utero* or in the neonatal period with Potter's syndrome to minimal symptoms and an extended life span. Renal failure and urosepsis are the principal complications of those who survive with moderate to severe expression of this disorder.

Excretory urography, ultrasonography, and voiding cystourethrography demonstrate the previously described abnormalities of the urinary tract in patients with prune-belly syndrome (Fig. 17–20). In some cases, the question of a coexistent obstructing lesion must be resolved with the pressure-flow study of Whitaker.

Primary Megaureter

The term *primary megaureter* is used here to describe a ureter that has a normally tapered distal segment but is otherwise dilated over a varying length, from a few centimeters immediately proximal to the distal tapered end to and including the

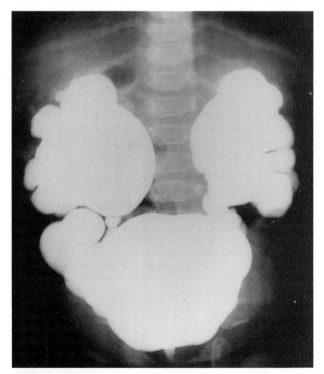

FIGURE 17–20. Prune-belly syndrome in a newborn with renal failure. Cystogram. There is marked dilatation of the bladder and the upper urinary tracts with renal parenchymal wasting.

pelvocalyceal system. In extreme examples, renal atrophy accompanies hydronephrosis and hydroureter. Excluded from this definition are dilatation of the ureter due to vesicoureteral reflux and the other causes of nonobstructed dilatation discussed in the preceding sections as well as ureters obstructed by demonstrable mechanical obstruction.

The nature of primary megaureter has not been fully elaborated. The tapered distal segment is normal in caliber, freely allows passage of a retrograde catheter, but is aperistaltic. This is the segment that is thought to be abnormal. The more proximal dilated segment, on the other hand, exhibits normal or increased peristalsis and the bolus of urine within this segment is often incompletely propelled into the bladder. These abnormalities are generally considered secondary to the defect of the distal aperistaltic segment. Despite these observations, no consistent, specific histologic abnormality has been identified either in the tapered distal or the more proximal dilated segments. These findings, however, point to a functional impairment of peristalsis in the distal ureter, perhaps because of disordered arrangement of muscle.

Inclusion of primary megaureter in this section on nonobstructed dilatation of the ureter is arbitrary and based on the absence of a mechanical obstructing lesion. A valid argument could be made to classify this entity as a functional obstruction in the same manner as most cases of ureteropelvic junction obstruction. Indeed, moderate to severe primary megaureter meets Whitaker's criteria for obstruction, as discussed earlier in this chapter.

As a congenital abnormality, primary megaureter is found in all ages, although severe instances usually come to medical attention in infancy and childhood. A tendency toward predominance in males and left-sided involvement has been reported. Bilaterality has been noted in up to 50 per cent of patients and other anomalies in up to 40 per cent of cases. These include ipsilateral ureteropelvic junction obstruction, contralateral agenesis, contralateral or ipsilateral vesicoureteral reflux, contralateral ureteral ectopia or duplication, and ipsilateral megacalyces, among others.

Severity of primary megaureter varies from the commonly encountered minimal and inconsequential to the rare, severe functional obstruction with

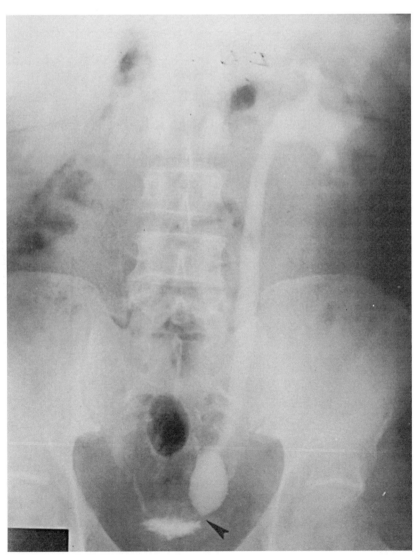

FIGURE 17–21. Primary megaureter with dilatation that includes the pelvocalyceal system as well as the ureter. Note fusiform narrowing of the most distal portion of the left ureter *(arrow)*. Excretory urogram, postvoid film.

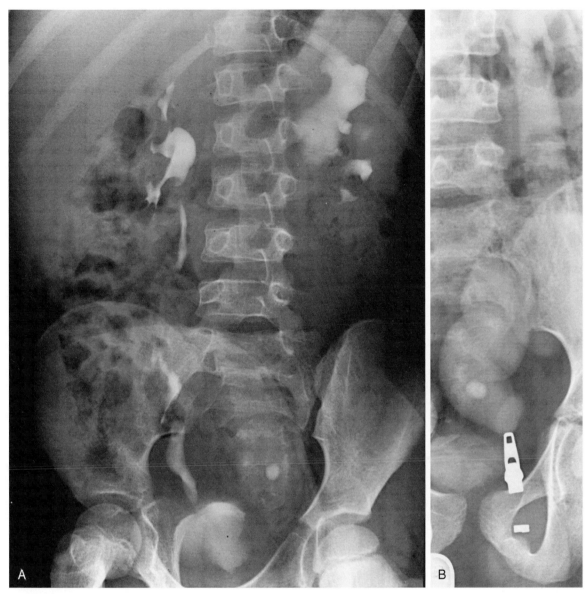

FIGURE 17–22. Primary megaureter causing marked dilatation of the left ureter and pelvis as well as wasting of the renal parenchyma. A nonobstructing stone is present in the pelvic portion of the ureter.

A, Excretory urogram, right posterior oblique projection. The left pelvis is dilated and the renal parenchyma wasted. A stone is seen overlying the coccyx. The bladder is deformed and effaced by the adjacent dilated, but unopacified, distal ureter.

B, Delayed film. The markedly dilated ureter with a dense stone is well visualized.

(Courtesy of Wendelin S. Hayes, D.O., Georgetown University, Washington, D.C.)

hydroureter, hydronephrosis, and impaired kidney function. Clinical findings, when present, include pain, hematuria, abdominal mass, or the signs and symptoms of urinary tract infection.

Primary megaureter is best studied by excretory urography. In mild cases, there is a 2 to 3 cm fusiform dilatation of the distal ureter just proximal to a tapered extravesical distal segment of up to 4 cm in length. With increased severity, the ureter dilates more proximally to include the pelvocalyceal system (Fig. 17–21). In extreme cases, there is wasting of the renal parenchyma and evidence of impaired excretion of contrast material (Fig. 17–22). Characteristically, the ureters lack tortuosity despite considerable dilatation. Fluoroscopy during excretory

urography or real-time ultrasonography permit visualization of peristalsis, which, depending on severity, may be normal, increased, or diminished. Ineffective emptying and a to and fro movement of the urine in the dilated portion of the ureter is a frequent finding. Patients with advanced degrees of primary megaureter demonstrate obstructive patterns in diuresis urography or renography and in pressure-flow urodynamic studies.

DIFFERENTIAL DIAGNOSIS

Separating intermediate, intermittent, and equivocal forms of obstruction from the various nonobstructive causes of dilatation is the first challenge in evaluating patients whose radiologic findings do not clearly point to obstruction. Diuresis renography meets this challenge in most instances by demonstrating prolonged retention of radioactivity in those who are obstructed or the rapid washout of radionuclide in those who are not. The use of urodynamic pressure-flow studies is required only when a diuresis study yields inconclusive results.

Once **obstruction** is eliminated as a cause of upper tract dilatation, **vesicoureteral reflux** must be considered. Voiding cystourethrography, using either radiographic or radionuclide techniques, accomplishes this with a high degree of accuracy but only when reflux is concurrent. Unfortunately, this is not the rule in adults whose renal damage occurred during infancy or childhood from reflux that has long since been resolved. Unless identified by relevant historical data, often not available in this frequently asymptomatic condition, these patients will be indistinguishable from those with other causes of nonobstructive collecting system dilatation.

Nonobstructive and nonreflux dilatation of the pelvocalyceal system and ureter is sometimes accompanied by wasting of the renal parenchyma in patients with prior reflux, in the various forms of **high flow states**, in **postobstructive atrophy**, in **prune-belly syndrome**, and in **primary megaureter**. In each of these, atrophy is accompanied by impaired function of the affected kidney, as measured by radionuclide techniques. Dilatation of the collecting system and decreased parenchymal thickness are also features of congenital megacalyces, but in this circumstance radionuclide studies of the affected kidney demonstrate normal function.

If nonobstructive dilatation occurs unaccompanied by thinning of the renal parenchyma, identification of a specific cause will be solely dependent on correlation with clinical data, if available. Radiologic criteria alone are insufficient.

Finally, in the evaluation of patients with a dilated upper urinary tract, awareness should be maintained of the occasional coexistence of two independent abnormalities, the radiologic findings of which may overlap. **Combinations of ureteropelvic and ureterovesical junction obstruction, congenital megacalyces and primary megaureter,** and **primary megaureter and vesicoureteral reflux** have been documented in a few instances. Also, it is important to exclude the effect of **elevated bladder pressure** as a cause of a dilated ureter. This may be seen not only in patients with bladder outflow obstruction but also in patients with voluntary infrequent voiding or, simply, filled bladders.

BIBLIOGRAPHY

Techniques

Choyke, P. L.: The urogram: Are rumors of its death premature? Radiology *184*:33, 1992.

Coley, B. D., Arellano, R. S., Talner, L. B., Baker, K. B., Peterson, T., and Mattrey, R. F.: Renal Resistive Index in experimental partial and complete ureteral obstruction. Acad. Radiol. *2*:373, 1995.

Cronan, J. J., and Tublin, M. E.: Role of the resistive index in the evaluation of acute renal obstruction. AJR *164*:377, 1995.

Ekelund, L., Lindstedt, E., Thiesen, V., and Jönsson, M.-B.: Diuresis urography in equivocal pelvic-ureteric obstruction. Urol. Radiol. *1*:147, 1980.

Fielding, J. R., Steele, G., Fox, L. A., Heller, H., and Loughlin, K. R.: Spiral computerized tomography in the evaluation of acute flank pain: A replacement for excretory urography. J. Urol. *157*:2071, 1997.

Haddad, M. C., Sharif, H. S., Shahed, M. S., Mutaiery, M. A., Samihan, A. M., Sammak, B. M., Southcombe, L. A., and Crawford, A. D.: Renal colic: Diagnosis and outcome. Radiology *184*:83, 1992.

Jaffe, R. B., and Middleton, A. W.: Whitaker test: Differentiation of obstructive from nonobstructive uropathy. AJR *134*:9, 1980.

Keogan, M. T., Kliewer, M. A., Hertzberg, B. S., Delong, D. M., Tupler, R. H., and Carroll, B. A.: Renal resistive indexes: Variability in Doppler US measurement in a healthy population. Radiology *199*:165, 1996.

Koff, S. A., Thrall, J. H., and Keyes, J. W., Jr.: Diuretic radionuclide urography: Non-invasive method for evaluating nephroureteral dilatation. J. Urol. *122*:451, 1979.

Lupton, E. W., O'Reilly, P. H., Testa, H. J., Gosling, J. A., and Dixon, J. S.: Diuresis renography in idiopathic hydronephrosis. Ann. R. Coll. Surg. Engl. *62*:216, 1980.

Mallek, R., Bankier, A. A., Etele-Hainz, A., Kletter, K., and Mostbeck, G. H.: Distinction between obstructive and nonobstructive hydronephrosis: Value of diuresis duplex Doppler sonography. AJR *166*:113, 1996.

Nilson, A. E., Avrell, M., Bratt, C. G., and Nilsson, S.: Diuretic urography in the assessment of obstruction of the pelviureteric junction. Acta Radiol. (Diagn.) *21*:499, 1980.

O'Reilly, P. H.: Investigation of obstructive uropathy. In O'Reilly, P. H., George, N. J. R., Weiss, R. M. (eds.): Diagnostic Techniques in Urology. Philadelphia, W. B. Saunders, 1990, pp. 401–425.

O'Reilly, P., Aurell, M., Britton, K., Kletter, K., Rosenthal, L., and Testa, T.: Consensus on diuresis renography for investigating the dilated upper urinary tract. J. Nucl. Med. *37*:1872, 1996.

Sanders, R. C., and Hartman, D. S.: The sonographic distinction between multicystic kidney and hydronephrosis. Radiology *151*:621, 1984.

Scola, F. H., Cronan, J. J., and Schepps, B.: Grade I hydronephrosis: Pulsed Doppler US evaluation. Radiology *171*:519, 1989.

Smith, R. C., Verga, M., McCarthy, S., and Rosenfield, A. T.: Diagnosis of acute flank pain: Value of unenhanced helical CT. AJR *166*:97, 1996.

Tublin, M. E., Dodd, G. D., III, and Verdile, V. P.: Acute renal colic: Diagnosis with duplex Doppler US. Radiology *193*:697, 1994.

Whitaker, R. H.: Perfusion pressure flow studies. In O'Reilly, P. H., George, N. J. R., and Weiss, R. M. (eds.): Diagnostic Techniques in Urology. Philadelphia, W. B. Saunders, 1990, pp. 135–142.

Obstructive Uropathy

Bernstein, G. T., Mandell, J., Lebowitz, R. L., Bauer, S. B., Colodny, A. H., and Retik, A. B.: Ureteropelvic junction obstruction in the neonate. J. Urol. *140*(part 2):1216, 1988.

Brown, T., Mandell, J., and Lebowitz, R. L.: Neonatal hydronephrosis in the era of sonography. AJR *148*:959, 1987.

Clark, W. R., and Malek, R. S.: Ureteropelvic junction obstruction: I. Observations on the classic type in adults. J. Urol. *138*:276, 1987.

Clautice-Engel, T., Anderson, N. G., Allan, R. B., and Abbott, G. D.: Diagnosis of obstructive hydronephrosis in infants: Comparison sonograms performed 6 days and 6 weeks after birth. AJR *164*:963, 1995.

Cronan, J. J., and Tublin, M. E.: Role of the resistive index in the evaluation of acute renal obstruction. AJR *164:*377, 1995.

Curry, N. S., Gobien, R. P., and Schabel, S. I.: Minimal-dilatation obstructive nephropathy. Radiology *143:*531, 1982.

Deyoe, L. A., Cronan, J. J., Breslaw, B. H., and Ridlen M. S.: New techniques of ultrasound and color Doppler in the prospective evaluation of acute renal obstruction: Do they replace the intravenous urogram? Abdom. Imaging *20:*58, 1995.

Dixon, J. S., and Gosling, J. A.: An evaluation of idiopathic hydronephrosis using light and electron microscopy. Ann. R. Coll. Surg. Engl. *62:*216, 1980.

Editorial: The dilated upper urinary tract. Br. Med. J. *1:*1382, 1979.

Fernbach, S. K.: The dilated urinary tract in children. Urol. Radiol. *14:*34, 1992.

Friedland, G. W.: Miscellaneous congenital anomalies of the genitourinary tract. In Pollack, H. M. (ed.): Clinical Urography. Philadelphia, W. B. Saunders, 1990, pp. 771–787.

Gosling, J. A., and Dixon, J. S.: Functional obstruction of the ureter and renal pelvis: A histological and electron microscopic study. Br. J. Urol. *50:*145, 1978.

Gulmi, F. A., Felsen, D., and Vaughan, E. D.: Pathophysiology of urinary tract obstruction. In Walsh, P. C., Retik, A. B., Vaughan, E. D., Jr., and Wein, A. J. (eds.): Campbell's Urology, 7th ed. Philadelphia, W. B. Saunders, 1998, pp. 342–386.

Heneghan, J. P., Dalrymple, N. C., Verga, M., Rosenfield, A. T., and Smith, R. C.: Soft-tissue "rim" sign in the diagnosis of ureteral calculi with use of unenhanced helical CT. Radiology *202:*709, 1997.

Hill, G. S.: Basic physiology and morphology of hydronephrosis. In Hill, G. S. (ed.): Uropathology. New York, Churchill Livingstone, 1989, pp. 467–515.

Hill, G. S.: Intrinsic and extrinsic obstruction of the urinary tract. In Hill, G. S. (ed.): Uropathology. New York, Churchill Livingstone, 1989, pp. 467–515 and 517–574.

Hill, G. S.: Ureteropelvic junction obstruction. In Hill, G. S. (ed.): Uropathology. New York, Churchill Livingstone, 1989, pp. 575–598.

Hoffer, F. A., and Lebowitz, R. L.: Intermittent hydronephrosis: A unique feature of ureteropelvic junction obstruction caused by a crossing renal vessel. Radiology *156:*655, 1985.

Koff, S. A.: Problematic ureteropelvic junction obstruction. J. Urol. *138:*390, 1987.

McGrath, M. A., Estroff, J., and Lebowitz, R. L.: The coexistence of obstruction at the ureteropelvic and ureterovesical junction. AJR *149:*403, 1987.

Peters, C. A.: Urinary tract obstruction in children. J. Urol. *154:*1874, 1995.

Platt, J. F., Rubin, J. M., Ellis, J. H., and DiPietro, M. A.: Duplex Doppler US of the kidney: Differentiation of obstructive from nonobstructive dilatation. Radiology *171:*515, 1989.

Smith, R. C., Verga, M., Dalrymple, N., McCarthy, S., and Rosenfield, A. T.: Acute ureteral obstruction: Value of secondary signs on helical unenhanced CT. AJR *167:*1109, 1996.

Takahashi, N., Kawashima, A., Ernst, R. D., Boridy, I. C., Goldman, S. M., Benson, G. S., and Sandler, C. M.: Ureterolithiasis: Can clinical outcome be predicted with unenhanced helical CT? Radiology *208:*97, 1998.

Talner, L. B.: Urinary obstruction. In Pollack, H. M. (ed.): Clinical Urography. Philadelphia, W. B. Saunders, 1990, pp. 1535–1628.

Talner, L. B.: Specific causes of obstruction. In Pollack, H. M. (ed.): Clinical Urography. Philadelphia, W. B. Saunders, 1990, pp. 1629–1751.

Weiss, R. M.: Physiology and pharmacology of the renal pelvis and ureter. In Walsh, P. C., Retik, A. B., Vaughan, E. D., Jr., and Wein, A. J. (eds.): Campbell's Urology, 7th ed. Philadelphia, W. B. Saunders, 1998, pp. 839–868.

Whitaker, R. H.: Investigation of the dilated upper urinary tract. J. R. Soc. Med. *73:*377, 1980.

Whitaker, R. H.: Pathophysiology of ureteric obstruction. In Williams, D. I., and Chisholm, G. D. (eds.): Scientific Foundation of Urology, Vol. II. Urogenital Tract: Oncology and the Urologic

Armamentarium. London, William Heinemann, 1976, pp. 18–22.

Whitaker, R. H.: Some observations and theories on the wide ureter and hydronephrosis. Br. J. Urol. *47:*377, 1975.

Whitaker, R. H., and Johnson, J. H.: A simple classification of wide ureters. Br. J. Urol. *47:*781, 1976.

Nonobstructive Dilatation

Atala, A., and Keating, M. A.: Vesicoureteral reflux and megaureter. In Walsh, P. C., Retik, A. B., Vaughan, E. D., Jr., and Wein, A. J. (eds.): Campbell's Urology, 7th ed. Philadelphia, W. B. Saunders, 1998, pp. 1859–1915.

Bailey, R. R., and Rolleston, G. L.: Kidney length and ureteric dilatation in the puerperium. J. Obstet. Gynaecol. Br. Common. *78:*55, 1971.

Blickman, J. G., and Lebowitz, R. L.: The coexistence of primary megaureter and reflux. AJR *143:*1053, 1984.

Burbige, K. A., Amodio, J., Berdon, W. E., Hensle, T. W., Blanc, W., and Lattimer, J. K.: Prune-belly syndrome. J. Urol. *137:*86, 1987.

Burbige, K. A., Lebowitz, R. L., Colodny, A. H., Bauer, S. B., and Retik, A. B.: The megacystic-megaureter syndrome. J. Urol. *131:*113, 1984.

Connolly, L. P., Treves, S. T., Connolly, S. A., Zurakowski, D., Share, J. C., BarSever, Z., Mitchell, K. D., and Bauer, S. B.: Vesicoureteral reflux in children: Incidence and severity in siblings. J. Urol. *157:*2287, 1997.

Garcia, C. J., Taylor, K. J. W., and Weiss, R. M.: Congenital megacalyces: Ultrasound appearance. J. Ultrasound Med. *6:*163, 1987.

Greskovich, F. J., III, and Nyberg, L. M.: The prune-belly syndrome: A review of its etiology, defects, treatment and prognosis. J. Urol. *140:*707, 1988.

Hamilton, S., and Fitzpatrick, J. M.: Primary non-obstructive megaureter in adults. Clin. Radiol. *38:*181, 1987.

Hanna, M. K., and Wyatt, J. K.: Primary obstructive megaureter in adults. J. Urol. *113:*328, 1975.

Harrison, R. B., Ramchandani, P., and Allen, J. T.: Psychogenic polydipsia: unusual cause for hydronephrosis. AJR *133:*327, 1979.

Hellström, M., Jodal, V., Märild, S., and Wettergren, B.: Ureteral dilatation in children with febrile urinary tract infection or bacteruria. AJR *148:*483, 1987.

Johnston, J. H.: Megacalicosis: A burnt-out obstruction? J. Urol. *110:*344, 1973.

Kass, E. J., Silver, T. M., Konnak, J. W., Thornbury, J. R., and Wolfman, M. G.: The urographic findings in acute pyelonephritis: Non-obstructive hydronephrosis. J. Urol. *116:*544, 1976.

King, L. R.: Megaloureter: Definition, diagnosis and management. J. Urol. *123:*222, 1980.

Manson, A. D., Yalowitz, P. A., Randall, R. V., and Greene, L. F.: Dilatation of the urinary tract associated with pituitary and nephrogenic diabetes insipidus. J. Urol. *103:*327, 1970.

Marchant, D. J.: Effects of pregnancy and progestational agents on the urinary tract. Am. J. Obstet. Gynecol. *112:*487, 1972.

Mark, L. K., and Möel, M.: Primary megaloureter. Radiology *93:*345, 1969.

McLoughlin, A. P., III, Pfister, R. C., Leadbetter, W. F., Salzstein, S. L., and Kessler, W. D.: The pathophysiology of primary megaloureter. J. Urol. *109:*805, 1973.

O'Reilly, P. H., Lawson, R. S., Shields, R. A., Testa, H. J., Carroll, R. N. P., and Charlton-Edwards, E.: The dilated, nonobstructed renal pelvis. Br. J. Urol. *53:*205, 1981.

Paltiel, H. J., and Lebowitz, R. L.: Neonatal hydronephrosis due to primary vesicoureter reflux: Trends in diagnosis and treatment. Radiology *170:*787, 1989.

Parker, M., and Clark, R. L.: Urothelial striations revisited. Radiology *198:*89, 1996.

Pfister, R. C., and Hendren, W. H.: Primary megaureter in children and adults: Clinical and pathophysiologic features of 150 ureters. Urology *12:*160, 1978.

Pfister, R. C., McLaughlin, A. P., III, and Leadbetter, W. F.: Radiological evaluation of primary megaureter. Radiology *99:*503, 1971.

Schulman, A., and Herlinger, H.: Urinary tract dilatation in pregnancy. Br. J. Radiol. *48:*638, 1975.

Shapiro, S. R., Woerner, S., Adelman, R. D., and Palmer, J. M.: Diabetes insipidus and hydronephrosis. J. Urol. *119:*715, 1979.

Spiro, F. I., and Fry, I. K.: Ureteric dilatation in non-pregnant women. Proc. Royal Soc. Med. *63:*462, 1970.

Talner, L. B., and Gittes, R. F.: Megacalyces: Further observations and differentiation from obstructive renal disease. AJR *121:*473, 1974.

Vargas, B., and Lebowitz, R. L.: The coexistence of congenital megacalyces and primary megaureter. AJR *147:*313, 1986.

Waltzer, W. C.: The urinary tract in pregnancy. J. Urol. *125:*271, 1981.

Weber, A. L., Pfister, R. C., James, A. E., Jr., and Hendren, W. H.: Megaureter in infants and children: Roentgenologic, clinical and surgical aspects. AJR *112:*170, 1971.

Whitaker, R. H., and Flower, C. D. R.: Megacalices—how broad a spectrum? Br. J. Urol. *53:*1, 1981.

Willi, U. V., and Lebowitz, R. L.: The so-called megaureter-megacystis syndrome. AJR *133:*409, 1979.

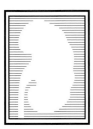

CHAPTER

18

The Effaced Pelvocalyceal System and Ureter

EXTRINSIC COMPRESSION
   Global Enlargement of Renal Parenchyma
   Masses or Masslike Abnormalities of the Renal
   Sinus and Perirenal Space

SPASM AND/OR INFLAMMATION
INFILTRATION
OLIGURIA

The abnormalities discussed in this chapter have in common the feature of a collapsed pelvocalyceal system or ureter or both. Four broad categories account for this appearance: *extrinsic compression* by diseases of the renal parenchyma, renal sinus, or perirenal space, *spasm* and/or *inflammation, infiltration* of the upper urinary tract, and *oliguric states,* in which the volume of urine formed is insufficient to distend the collecting system.

Specific entities in these categories are discussed in other chapters. In this chapter they are brought together only in summary form because generalized effacement of the collecting system is sometimes the predominant finding and the point of departure in radiologic diagnosis. Table 18–1 is a list of the various causes of effacement.

EXTRINSIC COMPRESSION
Global Enlargement of Renal Parenchyma

Generalized enlargement of the renal parenchyma often causes indistensibility of the collecting system. Excessive renal bulk occurs with cellular infiltration or proliferation, with deposition of abnormal proteins, or with the accumulation of interstitial edema or blood. These processes often reduce urine volume, which also contributes to the collapse of the pelvocalyceal system and ureter.

Bilateral renal enlargement by cellular infiltration or proliferation occurs with proliferative or necrotizing disorders of glomeruli. Neoplastic infiltrations are associated with leukemia and lymphoma, while inflammatory cell infiltration causes bilateral

---

TABLE 18–1. Causes of Effacement of the Pelvocalyceal System and Ureter

Extrinsic Compression
  Global enlargement of renal parenchyma—bilateral
    Proliferative or necrotizing disorders of glomeruli
    Amyloidosis
    Multiple myeloma
    Neoplastic infiltrates (leukemia, lymphoma)
    Acute tubular necrosis
    Acute cortical necrosis
    Acute interstitial nephritis
    Acute urate nephropathy
  Global enlargement of renal parenchyma—unilateral
    Renal vein thrombosis
    Acute arterial infarction
    Acute pyelonephritis
    Neoplastic infiltrates (e.g., mesoblastic nephroma, medullary carcinoma)
  Masses or masslike abnormalities of the renal sinus and perirenal space
    Renal sinus lipomatosis
    Parapelvic cyst
    Hemorrhage

Extrinsic Compression *continued*
    Renal sinus or perirenal neoplasm (e.g., lymphoma, metastatic lymphadenopathy, primary perirenal neoplasm)
    Retroperitoneal fibrosis
    Abdominal aortic aneurysm

Spasm and/or Inflammation
  Infection
    Acute pyelonephritis
    Acute tuberculosis and candidiasis
    Xanthogranulomatous pyelonephritis
  Hematuria

Infiltration
  Malignant uroepithelial tumors

Oliguria
  Antidiuretic state
  Renal ischemia
  Oliguric renal failure

nephromegaly in acute interstitial nephritis. Amyloidosis and multiple myeloma are examples of renal enlargement due to deposition of abnormal proteins. Acute tubular necrosis and acute cortical necrosis have a similar effect as a result of abnormal fluid accumulation within the renal parenchyma. Intratubular and interstitial depositions of uric acid crystals cause large smooth kidneys in acute urate nephropathy. Each of these processes affects both kidneys uniformly, and both are discussed in Chapter 8.

Unilateral renal enlargement with effacement of the collecting system may follow renal vein thrombosis or acute arterial infarction with swelling of the interstices of the kidney by blood and congested intrarenal capillaries and veins. Engorgement may be so severe and urine production so limited that retrograde pyelography is needed to opacify the collapsed collecting system. Generalized effacement of the pelvocalyceal system is also found in cases of severe acute pyelonephritis. Effacement in this circumstance is caused by acute inflammatory cell infiltrate, reduced urine flow, and spasm of the collecting system. In addition, renal neoplasms that grow by infiltration, such as mesoblastic nephroma or medullary carcinoma, may be associated with collapse of the collecting system. Chapters 9 and 12 discuss in detail causes of unilateral renal enlargement that might be associated with an effaced collecting system.

Masses or Masslike Abnormalities of the Renal Sinus and Perirenal Space

Renal sinus lipomatosis characteristically elongates and attenuates the pelvis and infundibula. This condition, which is usually bilateral, is associated with aging and obesity or occurs as a response to pathologic loss of renal parenchyma. The surrounding renal parenchyma is sometimes wasted. Excessive fat deposition in the renal sinus is most readily detected by computed tomography or ultrasonography.

Some parapelvic cysts insinuate themselves around the pelvis and infundibula and cause a urographic appearance similar to that of renal sinus lipomatosis. Distinction between these two disorders is rarely of clinical importance but can be made reliably by ultrasonography, computed tomography, or magnetic resonance imaging. Renal sinus lipomatosis and parapelvic cyst are discussed in Chapter 16.

Spontaneous hemorrhage into the renal sinus has been described in patients on anticoagulant therapy. This self-limiting process causes attenuation of the pelvocalyceal system, impaired excretion of contrast material, and, occasionally, caliectasis. Blood in the sinus produces an initially high-density mass that disappears within a few weeks.

A neoplasm in the renal sinus, either primary or metastatic, may surround the pelvocalyceal system and proximal ureter. As a result, the predominant radiologic finding may be a lack of distensibility of these structures. Lymphoma invading the kidney by a trans-sinus route, as described in Chapter 10, characteristically causes such an abnormality. Other entities that produce similar findings in the ureter are discussed in Chapter 16.

Neoplastic and non-neoplastic processes that develop in the perirenal space may surround or severely displace and stretch all or part of the ureter. Retroperitoneal fibrosis, abdominal aortic aneurysm, metastatic periaortic lymphadenopathy, and primary tumors of the retroperitoneum are examples. These are discussed in Chapter 21.

SPASM AND/OR INFLAMMATION

One manifestation of acute pyelonephritis is generalized effacement of the pelvocalyceal system. The precise mechanism for this is unclear. Spasm of the smooth muscles of the collecting system wall is the likely explanation, although swelling of the kidney may play a role as well. Paradoxically, some patients with acute pyelonephritis have a dilated pelvocalyceal system and ureter as a result of paralysis of the smooth muscle by bacterial endotoxins. In severe forms of acute pyelonephritis, effacement of the pelvis and calyces is always present due to oliguria, parenchymal swelling, and spasm. Acute infection is discussed in Chapter 9.

Uroepithelial tuberculosis and candidiasis cause submucosal granulomas, mucosal ulcerations, and, eventually, fibrosis and mural thickening. These conditions render the collecting system and ureter nondistensible. They are discussed in Chapter 15.

Upper urinary tract bleeding, whether from the kidney or directly from uroepithelial structures, can cause effacement of the collecting system, presumably as a result of irritation of pelvocalyceal smooth muscle. This reverts to normal as bleeding ceases.

INFILTRATION

Malignant uroepithelial tumors, most commonly transitional cell carcinoma, may either grow superficially or infiltrate deeply over a large area of the pelvocalyceal system or ureter. Either of these patterns may cause generalized effacement of the upper tract in association with a nodular mucosal pattern, which is discussed in Chapter 15.

OLIGURIA

The pelvocalyceal system and ureter are collapsed in the oliguric kidney, just as they are distended by a large volume of urine in high flow states, such as diabetes insipidus. Collapse is readily reversed by a fluid load when oliguria is due to the antidiuretic effect of water deprivation. However, no such easy reversal occurs when oliguria reflects primary renal vascular or parenchymal disease. In these situations, effacement of the pelvocalyceal system is one radiologic abnormality among many that reflect the underlying disorder. For example, a collapsed upper urinary tract due to oliguria caused by severe renal artery stenosis will be a unilateral phenomenon, accompanied by those other radiologic signs of ischemia that are discussed in Chapter 6. On the other hand, oliguria caused by acute renal failure will be associated with bilaterally enlarged smooth kidneys, which are discussed in Chapter 8.

BIBLIOGRAPHY

Global Enlargement: Bilateral

See Bibliography for Chapter 8.

Global Enlargement: Unilateral

See Bibliography for Chapter 9.

Masses or Masslike Abnormalities of the Renal Sinus and Perirenal Space

See Bibliography for Chapters 16 and 21.

Spasm and/or Inflammation

See Bibliographies for Chapter 9 (Acute Pyelonephritis and Xanthogranulomatous Pyelonephritis); Chapter 15 (Acute Tuberculosis, Candidiasis, and Xanthogranulomatous Pyelonephritis).

Infiltration

See Bibliography for Chapter 15.

Oliguria

See Bibliographies for Chapter 6 (Renal Ischemia) and Chapter 8 (Acute Renal Failure).

SECTION IV

THE LOWER URINARY TRACT

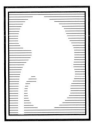
The Urinary Bladder

The pathologic processes that involve the urinary bladder mostly arise from the urothelium and are similar to those involving the renal pelvis and ureter. Additionally, the bladder is susceptible to involvement by abnormalities that originate in surrounding structures, which include both the extravesical portions of the pelvic retroperitoneum and the intraperitoneal space.

The entities discussed in this chapter are presented in the context of their most commonly encountered cross-sectional or cystographic imaging patterns. This approach, while valuable, nevertheless carries certain inconsistencies that the reader should keep in mind. First, disparate pathologic processes may share identical or similar radiologic patterns. Thus, radiologic interpretation of bladder abnormalities is often limited to a differential diagnosis. Second, several of the diseases that affect the bladder may become manifest by more than one pattern. These are cross-referenced in the text.

Trauma of the bladder is presented in Chapter 29.

ANATOMY

The urinary bladder is a distensible, muscular pouch that changes in size as it distends with urine.

As the bladder enlarges, its contour changes from oval to ellipsoid. The bladder is predominantly a pelvic organ, lying behind the pubic symphysis when empty and rising above the symphysis when full. The bladder is located anterior to the vagina, uterus, and cervix in the female, while in the male it is superior to the prostate and anterosuperior to the seminal vesicles. Fat and connective tissue surround the lateral aspects of the bladder and allow expansion as filling occurs. Anteroinferiorly, the bladder is supported by the symphysis pubis. The space between the anterior bladder wall and the posterior aspect of the symphysis pubis is known as the *anterior perivesical space* or *space of Retzius*. The *dome* of the bladder is its superior surface, which is covered by peritoneum. The superoanterior portion of the bladder, the *apex*, is attached to the anterior abdominal wall by the *median umbilical ligament*, a remnant of the urachus. The posteroinferior wall is also referred to as the *base* and is contiguous with the bladder neck.

The anterior reflection of peritoneum that passes over the superior surface of the bladder is lifted away from the anterior abdominal wall as the bladder fills. In males, the peritoneum extends over the posterior aspect of the bladder and is reflected over the anterior aspect of the rectum to form the *rectovesical pouch*. In females, the peritoneum extends inferiorly along the posterior bladder surface and is

Portions of this chapter, authored by Wendelin S. Hayes, were published in Chapter 19 of the previous edition of *Radiology of the Kidney and Urinary Tract.*

reflected back over the anterior aspect of the uterus, forming the *cul-de-sac,* or *pouch of Douglas.*

The mucosa of the bladder is the same multilayered transitional epithelium that lines the ureter and pelvocalyceal system. The triangular area between the two ureteral orifices and the urethra, the *trigone,* is composed of smooth urothelium over muscle that supports and stabilizes the distal ureters and bladder neck. A ridge of muscle, the *interureteric ridge,* extends between the ureteral orifices and forms the posterior aspect of the trigone. The pubovesical ligament in women and the puboprostatic ligament in men also provide support for the bladder neck. The muscular component of the bladder wall is composed of longitudinal and circular smooth muscle bundles that form distinct layers near the bladder neck.

The dominant arterial blood supply to the bladder is from the superior, middle, and inferior vesical arteries, which are branches of the hypogastric artery. Lymphatic drainage of the bladder is primarily to the external iliac chain of lymph nodes.

ANOMALIES

Exstrophy and Epispadias

Exstrophy of the bladder and epispadias occur as a spectrum of defects in the formation of the anterior abdominal wall caused by varying degrees of failure of midline fusion of the mesodermal tissue below the umbilicus. Exstrophy is the most common anomaly of the bladder. Males are affected more often than females by a ratio of 2:1. In its most severe manifestation, the rectus abdominus muscle is widely separated and the bladder lies open and everted on the anterior abdominal wall. The bladder mucosa is continuous with the skin. The exposed transitional cell mucosa often undergoes metaplasia, creating an increased risk for adenocarcinoma of the bladder. With an associated epispadias, the urethral mucosa covers the dorsum of a short penis and the urethra opens on the dorsal surface of the penis. In the female, the urethra is short, the labia are widely separated, and the clitoris is cleaved. The upper urinary tract is usually normal.

A radiograph of the pelvis in the exstrophy/epispadias anomaly demonstrates diastasis of the pubic symphysis (Fig. 19–1). On excretory urography, there is a wide lateral curve of the pelvic portion of the distal ureters, which then turn medially and slightly upward and pass through the bladder wall in a perpendicular direction. The most distal portion of the ureters is slightly dilated. The remainder of the upper tracts is usually normal.

Congenital Bladder Diverticulum

A congenital bladder diverticulum is uncommon and develops as a result of herniation of bladder mucosa through the detrusor muscle of the bladder, usually at a location slightly above and lateral to a ureteral orifice. This so-called *Hutch diverticulum* may vary from small to quite large and cause either obstruction of or vesicoureteral reflux into the ipsilateral ureter. In male infants, bladder diverticula must be distinguished from protrusions of the urinary bladder bilaterally into the inguinal rings anteriorly. These outpouchings, known as "bladder ears," are transient and usually disappear with aging.

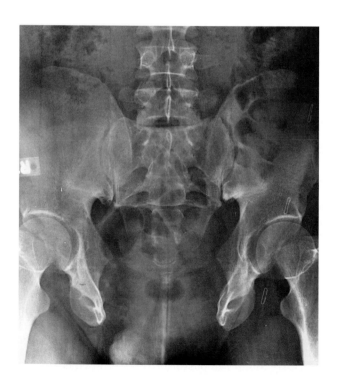

FIGURE 19–1. Bladder exstrophy. The radiograph of the pelvis reveals diastasis of the symphysis pubis.

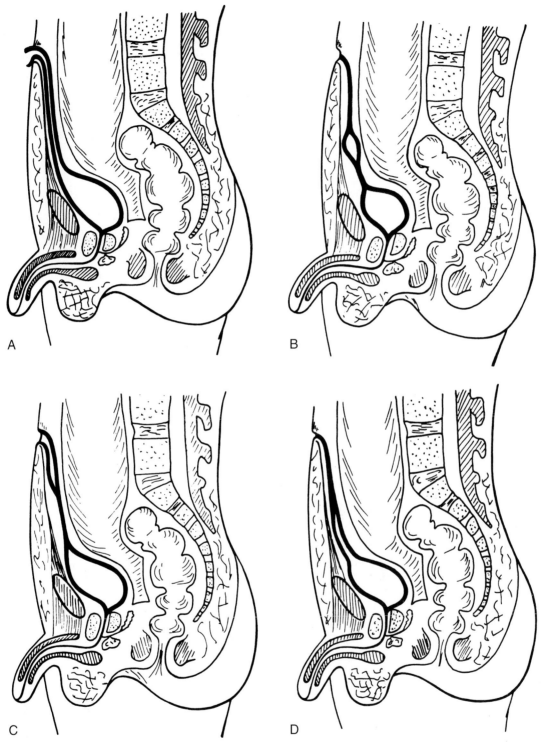

FIGURE 19–2. Congenital urachal anomalies.
A, Patent urachus.
B, Urachal cyst.
C, Urachal sinus.
D, Urachal diverticulum.
(From Schnyder, A., and Candardjis, G.: Vesicourachal diverticulum: CT diagnosis in two adults. AJR *137:*1063, 1981. Reproduced with kind permission of the authors and *American Journal of Roentgenology.)*

Prune-Belly Syndrome

Prune-belly syndrome *(Eagle-Barrett syndrome, triad syndrome)* is a congenital deficiency of the abdominal wall musculature associated with abnormal testicular descent, dilated ureters, and an enlarged abnormally positioned bladder. Of unknown etiology, the condition affects males exclusively. A variety of skeletal, gastrointestinal, cardiac, and pulmonary anomalies occasionally are associated with prune-belly syndrome. The syndrome is named for the wrinkled appearance of the distended and lax abdominal wall that results from absent musculature.

The bladder is often enlarged and elongated, but lacks trabeculation. A urachal anomaly may be present. The wall of the bladder is thickened by connective tissue replacement of normal smooth muscle. A similar process involves the ureters, although ureteral dilatation may also be secondary to vesicoureteral reflux, which is present in approximately 85 per cent of cases. Reflux may also contribute to the frequent urinary tract infections, hydronephrosis, and renal dysplasia that occur in these patients. Dilatation of the prostatic urethra (megalourethra) is an additional characteristic radiologic feature that can mimic posterior urethral valve on voiding cystourethrography. Prune-belly syndrome may be indistinguishable from posterior urethral valve *in utero.*

The appearance of the ureter in prune-belly syndrome is discussed in Chapter 17.

Urachal Anomalies

The urachus develops from the superior portion of the urogenital sinus and connects the dome of the bladder to the allantoic duct during fetal life. The urachus is located behind the abdominal wall and anterior to the peritoneum in the space of Retzius. Before birth, the urachus obliterates and becomes a vestigial structure known as the *medial umbilical ligament.* In the absence of complete obliteration, the urachus persists in one of four types: *patent urachus, urachal cyst, urachal sinus,* or *urachal diverticulum* (Fig. 19–2).

Patent urachus represents the failure of the entire course of the urachus to close, resulting in an open channel between the bladder and the umbilicus. A patent urachus is usually diagnosed in the newborn when urine is noted leaking from the umbilicus. Patent urachus is directly demonstrated by retrograde injection of contrast material into its orifice at the umbilicus. This anomaly may also be identified during a voiding cystourethrogram in the lateral projection or by ultrasonography as a fluid-filled tubular structure extending from the bladder to the umbilicus (Fig. 19–3). Urethral atresia or posterior urethral valve with bladder outlet obstruction coexists with patent urachus in up to 30 per cent of cases. Here, voiding cystourethrography demonstrates these additional, complicating features.

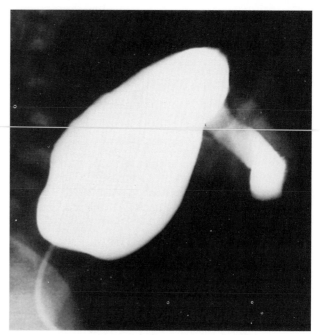

FIGURE 19–3. Patent urachus. A voiding cystourethrogram demonstrates contrast material in a patent urachus, which extends through the umbilicus into the umbilical stump, ending in a blind pouch.

A *urachal cyst* forms when both the umbilical and the vesical ends of the urachal lumen close, but an intervening portion remains patent and fluid-filled. This generally occurs in that part of the urachus that is closest to the bladder. Urachal cysts usually remain obscure until complicated by infection, or, more rarely, tumor. The clinical findings that result, such as midabdominal or suprapubic pain, fever, dysuria, or a palpable mass with associated urinary tract symptoms often mimic a variety of acute abdominal or pelvic inflammatory processes. Rarely, spontaneous drainage of a urachal cyst through the umbilicus occurs. Radiologically, an uncomplicated urachal cyst or sinus appears as a collection of simple fluid localized in the midline of the anterior abdominal wall between the umbilicus and the pubis and often contiguous with the bladder dome. A urachal cyst complicated by infection or neoplasm demonstrates features of mixed echogenicity, attenuation values and signal characteristics that deviate upward from those of water, or soft tissue components and thickening of the urachal wall (Figs. 19–4 and 19–5).

Urachal sinus is a blind-ending dilatation of the urachus at the umbilical end, whereas *urachal diverticulum* is a similar deformity that communicates with the anterosuperior aspect of the bladder as a result of failure of closure of the urachus at the bladder. A urachal diverticulum sometimes occurs in boys with urethral obstruction and may also be associated with prune-belly syndrome without outlet obstruction. A urachal diverticulum is identified as a urine-filled anterosuperior extension from the bladder dome demonstrated by cystography,

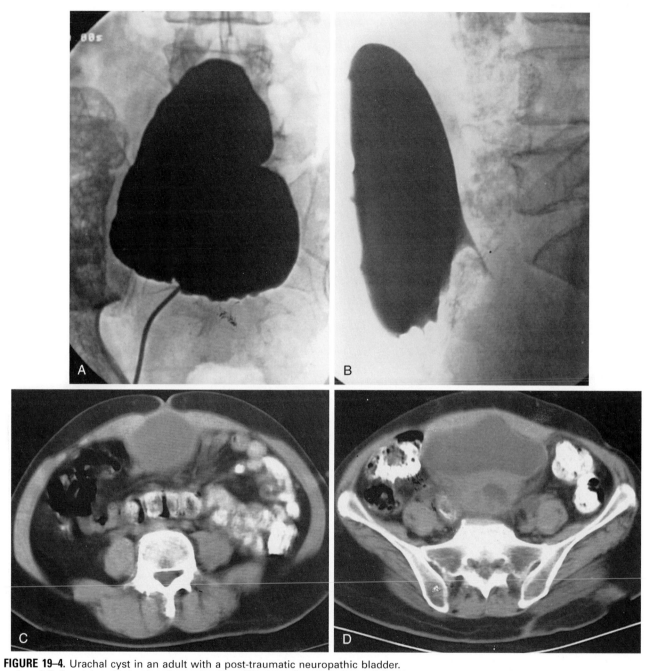

FIGURE 19–4. Urachal cyst in an adult with a post-traumatic neuropathic bladder.

A and *B,* Frontal and lateral radiographs. Opacification of a urachal cyst following percutaneous puncture reveals a predominantly smooth wall cyst. There is no communication to the bladder.

C and *D,* Computed tomograms without contrast material enhancement at the level of the umbilicus and pelvis demonstrate the extent of the cyst.

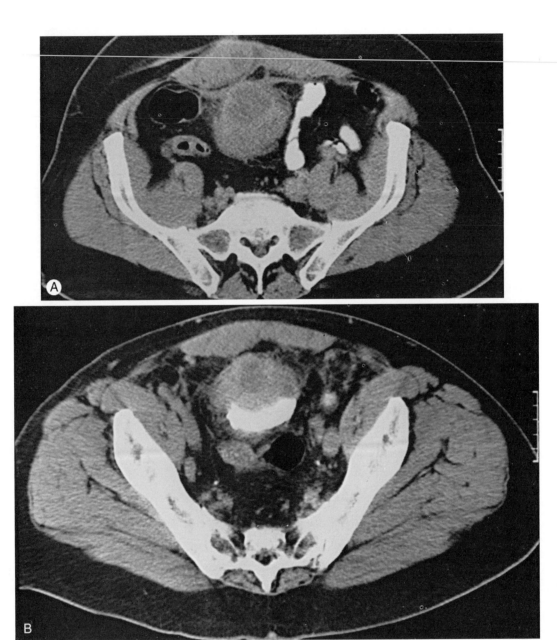

FIGURE 19–5. Infected urachal cyst in an adult with persistent lower abdominal pain. Computed tomograms with contrast material enhancement demonstrate an irregular mass of variable attenuation values that extend from the level of the umbilicus to the dome of the bladder.

A, Upper section demonstrates involvement of the rectus abdominis muscle.

B, Section at the level of dome of the opacified bladder shows surrounding inflammation as stranding density extending into adjacent fat.

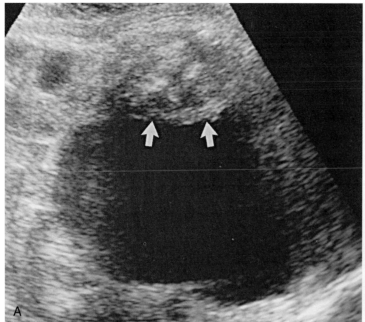

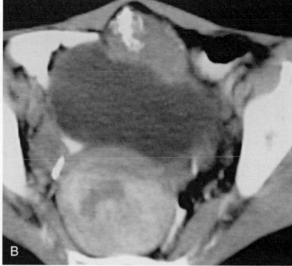

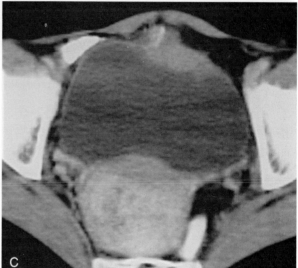

FIGURE 19–6. Urachal adenocarcinoma in a 46-year-old woman with recurrent cystitis and hematuria.

A, Ultrasonogram. There is a heterogeneous mass projecting into the lumen of the bladder *(arrows).* Echogenic foci are present, but there is no definite shadowing.

B and *C,* Contrast material–enhanced computed tomograms. Large calcifications within the mass are noted. Although the mass is predominantly exophytic, a portion projects into the bladder lumen.

voiding cystourethrography, ultrasonography, computed tomography, or magnetic resonance imaging.

Urachal anomalies retain a mucosal lining of transitional cell urothelium from which a malignancy, often adenocarcinoma, may arise (Fig. 19–6). This is discussed in a section that follows.

INTRALUMINAL FILLING DEFECTS

In a manner similar to that described in Chapter 14 for the renal pelvis and ureter, certain abnormalities are located within the bladder lumen. Unattached to the bladder mucosa, these lesions are completely surrounded by contrast material, move as the position of the patient changes, or change their appearance over time.

Calculus

Calculus is the most commonly encountered intraluminal filling defect of the bladder. Most calculi originate in the kidney and descend into the bladder where they form a nidus for progressive enlargement. Stone formation and growth is promoted by urine stasis, as is found in bladder outlet obstruction, neuropathic bladder, or diverticulum. Long-term instrumentation, other foreign bodies, and infection also favor calculogenesis. *Proteus mirabilis* is the organism most commonly associated with bladder infection and stone formation. Because of the relationship to bladder outlet obstruction, bladder stones are seen far more frequently in males than females. Calculi are associated with an increased risk of bladder carcinoma.

Almost all bladder stones are sufficiently calcified to be opaque on radiographs. Calculi tend to be smooth and round or oval in shape (Fig. 19–7). A laminated appearance of alternating high and medium opacity may be seen, presumably as a reflection of a prolonged asymptomatic period before detection. Once surrounded by contrast material, a bladder calculus may be perceived as relatively lucent, opaque, or obscured depending on the relative baseline opacity and the size of the calculus as well

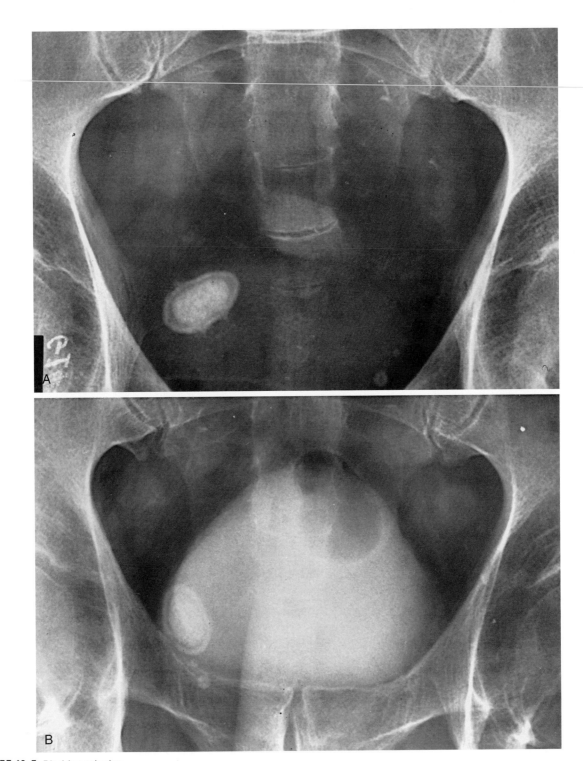

FIGURE 19–7. Bladder calculus.
  A, Radiograph of the pelvis demonstrates a laminated bladder calculus.
  B, Excretory urogram, right lateral decubitus view. The calculus has moved with the change in position of the patient.

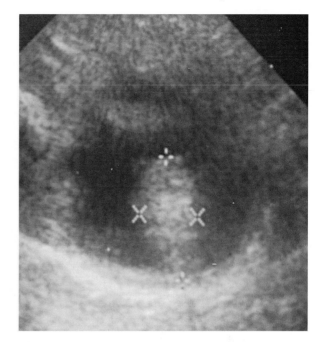

FIGURE 19–8. Intraluminal blood clot in a premature infant with hematuria secondary to renal vein thrombosis. Ultrasonogram, transverse decubitus view. The echogenic intraluminal mass *(cursors)* moved with change of the patient's position.

as the iodine concentration of the contrast material used to opacify the bladder.

Blood Clot

Blood clot within the bladder requires substantial hemorrhage from a source either in the bladder itself or from the upper urinary tract. Often a patient's clinical history points to a specific cause. Gross hematuria is usually present unless obstruction has occurred.

Standard radiography is normal unless there is pre-existing stone disease or bladder distention due to obstructing clot. The identification of a filling defect implies active or recent hemorrhage, because lysis is usually rapid owing to endogenous urinary anticoagulants. Thus, a decrease in the size of an intraluminal clot would be expected soon after the cessation of active bleeding. The clot, which is either smooth or irregular in contour, is mobile, unless

quite large (Fig. 19–8). Large clots tend to conform to the surrounding bladder, but this feature depends on the degree of bladder filling (Fig. 19–9).

Fungus Ball

Fungus ball is an uncommon cause of an intraluminal bladder filling defect. However, in immunocompromised patients, including diabetic patients, hyphae may become so numerous within the bladder as to form a mass, which may become sufficiently large as to cause outlet obstruction. A fungus ball may be associated with an irregular laminated appearance of alternating lucency and opacity owing to gas formation (Fig. 19–10). More often, however, no gas is present, and the process is seen as a mobile filling defect during excretory urography or cystography. One should remember to look carefully for upper tract disease in these patients, although

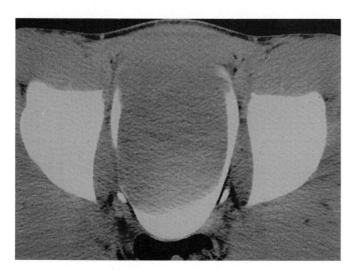

FIGURE 19–9. Intraluminal blood clot in a 22-year-old man who had a kidney biopsy 8 hours earlier. Computed tomogram, contrast material–enhanced. The clot forms a large, smooth filling defect within the bladder.

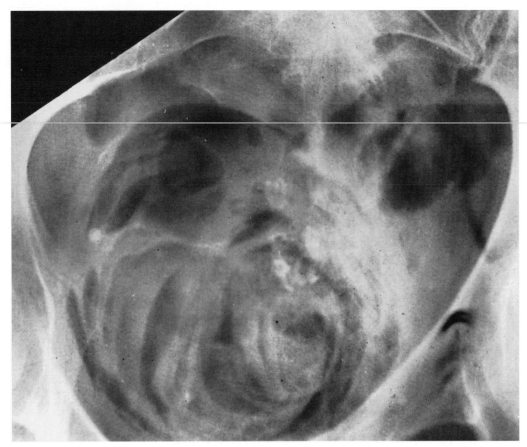

FIGURE 19–10. Fungus ball in bladder due to candidiasis. Radiograph of the pelvis demonstrates a laminated, gas-containing filling defect within the bladder.

only a minority of patients will have imaging evidence for upper tract abnormality.

Tissue Slough

Tissue slough is an uncommon cause of an intraluminal filling defect and may be either calcified or nonopaque. Renal papillary necrosis is discussed in detail in Chapter 13.

MURAL-BASED FILLING DEFECTS

The disorders that characteristically assume the radiologic appearance of a mural-based filling defect have in common the imaging features of contiguity with the bladder wall and projection into the bladder lumen. Mural-based lesions fall into three groups: (1) a group that is nearly always solitary; (2) a group that creates the appearance of a solitary mural lesion, but in reality results from a process that extends through the bladder wall from a dominant site of origin in the extravesical space; and (3) a group of abnormalities that forms multiple small filling defects that involve the entire mucosal surface but do not cause generalized thickening of the bladder wall. The abnormalities in this third group must be distinguished from lesions that cause a diffuse mucosal irregularity in conjunction with marked mural thickening, as discussed in detail in the section Mural Thickening, later in this chapter.

Imaging criteria for mural-based abnormalities are straightforward. Cystography, or late-phase excretory urography or computed tomography, reveals a fixed, relative lucency within the contrast material–filled bladder. Ultrasonography demonstrates a protrusion of tissue with medium level echoes into the fluid-filled bladder. Focal echogenicity with shadowing may be seen in those disorders that are sometimes associated with calcification, such as urachal carcinoma or hemangioma. Computed tomographic criteria for a mural abnormality include a lesion that is variably hyperdense to unopacified urine. On delayed contrast material–enhanced scans, the mural mass is seen as hypodense relative to opacified urine. A mural lesion is slightly hyperintense to urine on T1-weighted and slightly hypointense on T2-weighted magnetic resonance images. The lesion may enhance to a variable degree following injection of contrast material during dynamic scanning. On delayed images, as the concentration of contrast material within the bladder lumen increases, the signal intensity of the urine on T1-weighted images forms a trilevel pattern of darker signal intensity in the urine above and below a midzone of bright signal intensity.

Epithelial Neoplasms

Nephrogenic Adenoma. Nephrogenic adenoma has been classified as a benign neoplasm by some, while others view this lesion as a metaplastic uro-epithelial response to chronic inflammation associated with bladder calculi, chronic indwelling catheter, prior surgery, or trauma. Histologically, a nephrogenic adenoma is composed of papillary fronds and tubules that are usually covered by transitional epithelium. These produce a polypoid or papillary lesion that in gross appearance may be mistaken for carcinoma.

Nephrogenic adenoma is encountered most frequently in young adults, and males are affected more commonly than females. Unlike most benign tumors, the clinical setting for nephrogenic adenoma includes signs and symptoms of chronic irritation or infection, including dysuria, urgency, frequency, and microscopic hematuria.

On radiologic investigation, nephrogenic adenoma appears as a single tumor or as multiple mural masses that have no distinguishing features from other benign or malignant tumors.

Transitional Cell Papilloma. Most pathologists consider transitional cell papilloma to be a very low-grade transitional cell carcinoma. This emphasizes the potential for both recurrence and evolution into a higher-grade tumor. Others contend that the expected life span of an individual is not significantly altered by a papilloma, although it is acknowledged that such a patient may be at risk for recurrence. The radiologic features of a papilloma are indistinguishable from those of a small transitional cell carcinoma.

Transitional Cell Carcinoma. Transitional cell carcinoma accounts for more than 90 per cent of all malignant tumors of the bladder and reaches a peak prevalence in the seventh decade of life. Males have a risk that is threefold greater than that of females. Transitional cell carcinoma appears in the bladder approximately 10 times more often than in other urothelial-lined structures, presumably due to the relatively large mucosal surface area of the renal pelvis and ureter. Multiple transitional cell carcinomas occur in 34 per cent of cases. These additional lesions may occur anywhere along the urinary tract. Thorough preoperative and postoperative imaging, therefore, is essential.

Numerous risk factors have been described for transitional cell carcinoma, including a wide variety of chemical toxins that presumably become carcinogenic when excreted and concentrated in the urinary tract. Inhaled tobacco smoke, which leads to the excretion of multiple carcinogens, represents the chemical exposure most frequently associated with transitional cell carcinoma. Occupational exposure to aniline dyes, chemicals used in plastic and rubber manufacturing, and some industrial solvents have also been implicated as risk factors. Iatrogenic causes include the use of cyclophosphamide and therapeutic radiation. Bladder calculus

and recurrent urinary tract infection may also lead to a slight increase risk of transitional cell carcinoma.

Hematuria, either gross or microscopic, occurs in 90 per cent of patients with bladder transitional cell carcinoma. Some patients present with signs or symptoms of obstruction, depending on the size and location of the tumor. Less commonly, initial symptoms arise from a metastasis rather than from the primary tumor in the bladder.

An irregular mass projecting into the bladder lumen from a fixed mural site is the imaging hallmark of a transitional cell carcinoma (Fig. 19–11). The lesion is typically branched or frondlike, as is characteristic of tumors that grow in a papillary pattern. Contrast material outlines the branches of the lesion and fills the interstices in an irregular fashion. The attachment to the bladder wall may be either sessile or stalklike (Fig. 19–12). Ultrasonography depicts a transitional cell carcinoma as a soft tissue structure of low to intermediate echo texture projecting into the urine-filled bladder lumen (see Fig. 19–12B). Many transitional cell carcinomas are so small that they escape radiologic detection despite careful cystographic, ultrasonographic, or computed tomographic technique. Cystoscopy, too, may fail to visualize these very small tumors, the detection of which requires random biopsy. At the other extreme, some transitional cell carcinomas fill the entire bladder lumen and extend through the muscular wall at the time of diagnosis. Calcification is detected in transitional cell carcinoma in less than 2 per cent of cases.

Transitional cell carcinoma enhances rapidly after contrast material administration, whether imaged by computed tomography or by magnetic resonance imaging (see Fig. 19–12C and D). Images generally should be obtained in the first minute after the administration of a bolus of contrast mate-

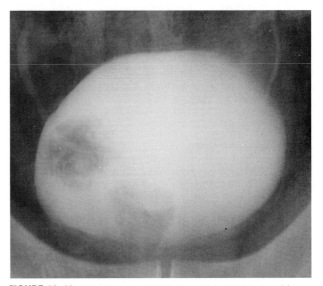

FIGURE 19–11. Transitional cell carcinoma in a 52-year-old man. Excretory urogram. An irregular filling defect arises from the lateral wall of the bladder.

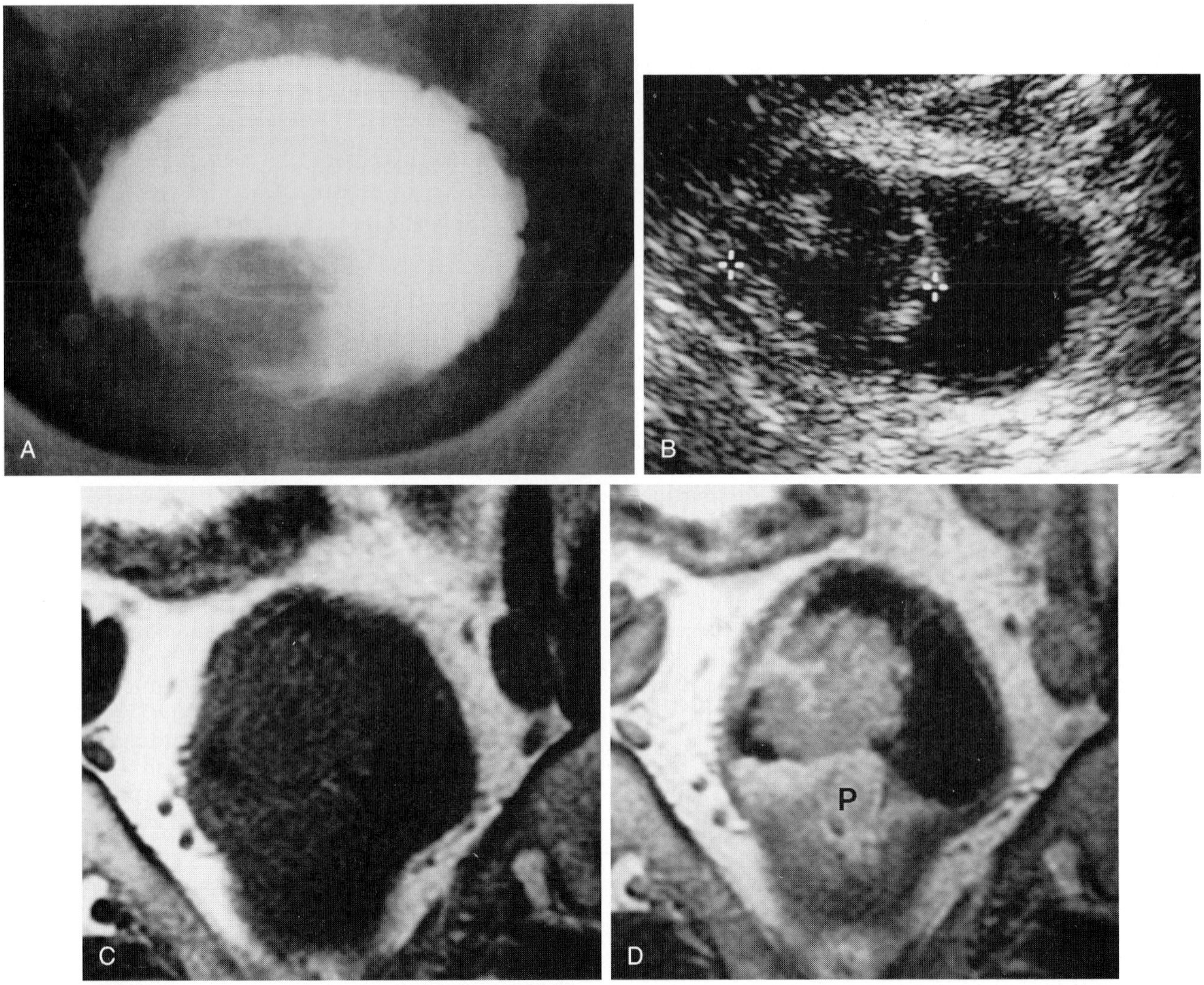

FIGURE 19–12. Transitional cell carcinoma in a 52-year-old man.

A, Cystogram demonstrates mild trabeculation of the bladder due to outlet obstruction caused by benign prostatic hyperplasia. The tumor forms an irregular filling defect of the right lateral wall.

B, Ultrasonogram, transverse plane. The tumor *(cursors)* is hypoechoic.

C, T1-weighted magnetic resonance image in a coronal plane shows that the mass is of only slightly greater signal intensity than urine.

D, T1-weighted magnetic resonance image after gadolinium administration. The mass enhances and its point of attachment to the right lateral bladder wall is delineated. The scan was obtained immediately after administration of the contrast material and therefore the signal intensity of surrounding urine has not yet been altered. There is no evidence of extension of the tumor into the perivesical fat. The depth of muscular invasion cannot be confidently assessed. *P,* prostate.

rial. Delayed images, obtained several minutes later, depict increasing enhancement of the surrounding urine and rapid loss of tumor tissue enhancement (Fig. 19–13).

An important prognostic determinant in transitional cell carcinoma is the microscopic assessment of the tumor relative to the muscularis propria. Those lesions that do not invade the muscularis propria are termed *superficial,* whereas those that have grown into the muscularis propria or beyond are characterized as *invasive.* A high level of accuracy in differentiating superficial tumors from those with deep muscle invasion using either computed tomography or magnetic resonance imaging has not been clearly established. Three-dimensional magnetic resonance imaging techniques may eventually contribute to accurate local staging of the depth of tumor invasion. Contrast material–enhanced computed tomography or magnetic resonance imaging may be used to determine the presence or absence of transmural extension into the perivesical fat and lymph node enlargement. Lymph nodes larger than 10 mm in their short axis or 13 mm in their long axis are considered abnormal. However, using these criteria, a node may be enlarged without metastatic disease (false-positive), just as one of normal size may contain metastatic tumor (false-negative).

Squamous Cell Carcinoma. Squamous cell carcinoma accounts for between 5 and 10 per cent of bladder neoplasms and is associated with mechanical irritation of the bladder mucosa by calculi, chronic indwelling catheter, chronic or recurrent infection, and schistosomiasis.

Squamous cell carcinoma appears as an irregular mural-based mass projecting into the bladder lumen. In this respect it is radiologically similar to some transitional cell carcinomas. However, transitional cell carcinoma is more likely to exhibit a branching morphology and attachment to the bladder wall by a narrow stalk and is also more likely to be associated with synchronous or metachronous lesions elsewhere within the urinary tract.

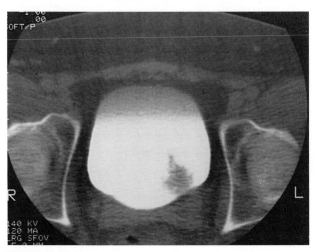

FIGURE 19–13. Transitional cell carcinoma. Computed tomogram, contrast material–enhanced. An irregular mural-based mass protrudes into the bladder lumen.

Adenocarcinoma. Adenocarcinoma of the bladder itself is very uncommon. On the other hand, approximately 85 per cent of malignant neoplasms that arise in anomalous remnants of the urachus are adenocarcinomas, the result of metaplasia of the transitional cell mucosal lining of these structures. Similarly, adenocarcinoma is the most frequent malignancy that arises in patients with extrophy of the bladder. Most urachal malignancies are clinically silent until they invade through the bladder wall and disrupt the mucosa, producing hematuria or the passage of mucin in the case of adenocarcinoma. Thus, when a cystoscopic biopsy of a midline anterior tumor of the bladder mucosa is interpreted as adenocarcinoma, a urachal origin with bladder invasion is the usual explanation.

In contrast to transitional cell carcinoma, urachal adenocarcinoma frequently contains calcification, often has an extravesical component, and is invariably found in the superoanterior midline (see Fig. 19–6). Calcification is typically coarse and may be curvilinear. The extraluminal component of the mass can be traced toward the umbilicus on cross-sectional imaging. The tumor may be of heterogeneous or low attenuation computed tomographic values due to the presence of mucin.

Miscellaneous Nonepithelial Neoplasms

Leiomyoma. Leiomyoma is the most common mesenchymal tumor of the bladder. This benign lesion virtually never undergoes malignant transformation to a leiomyosarcoma. Nevertheless, surgical removal is required for definitive diagnosis, as well as for treatment.

A leiomyoma is composed of benign smooth muscle cells and fibrous stroma. Characteristically, a smooth, well-defined mass projects into both the bladder lumen and the extravesical space in equal portions (Fig. 19–14). The smoothness of the surface of a leiomyoma results from the tumor originating in the wall rather than the mucosa of the bladder, in contradistinction to the mucosal neoplasms discussed in the preceding section. Because they are generally slow-growing, necrosis and hemorrhage are rare. Disruption of the overlying mucosa is also very uncommon.

Leiomyosarcoma. Leiomyosarcoma is a rare bladder neoplasm that grows rapidly into a large, invasive mass that projects into the bladder lumen as well as extending into the extravesical space (Fig. 19–15). However, this appearance is the same as that which would be noted in the case of a large, invasive transitional cell carcinoma that had extended into the extravesical space. Indeed, in the presence of this morphologic finding, the frequency of transitional cell carcinoma compared with the rarity of a leiomyoma would favor the former diagnosis.

Rhabdomyosarcoma. Rhabdomyosarcoma is the most common pelvic malignancy in children. In males, the tumor typically arises from the prostate

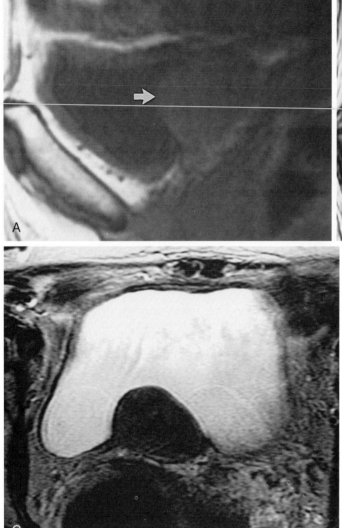

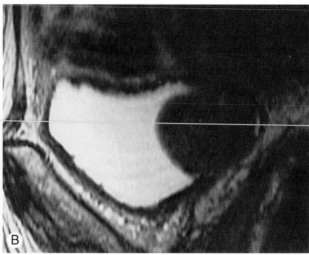

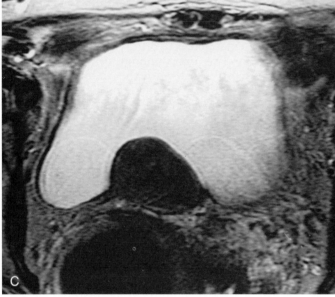

FIGURE 19–14. Leiomyoma. Magnetic resonance images.
A, Sagittal T1-weighted image shows a posterior, well-circumscribed mass *(arrow)* that is nearly isointense to urine.
B, Sagittal T2-weighted image demonstrates a low signal, homogeneous, well-marginated mass.
C, Axial T2-weighted image shows both an intraluminal and a smaller extraluminal component.

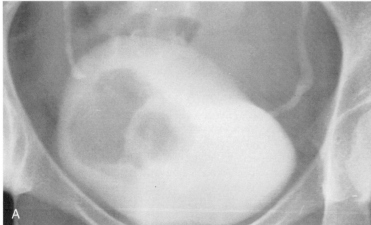

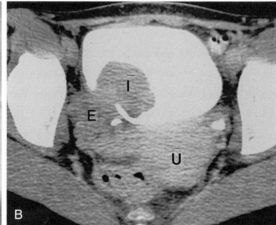

FIGURE 19–15. Leiomyosarcoma in a 22-year-old woman.
A, Excretory urogram. A large, lobulated filling defect is present in the right side of the bladder.
B, Contrast material–enhanced computed tomography confirms both intraluminal *(I)* and extraluminal *(E)* portions of the tumor. *U,* uterus.

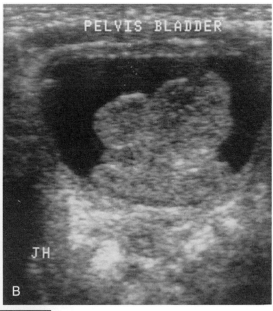

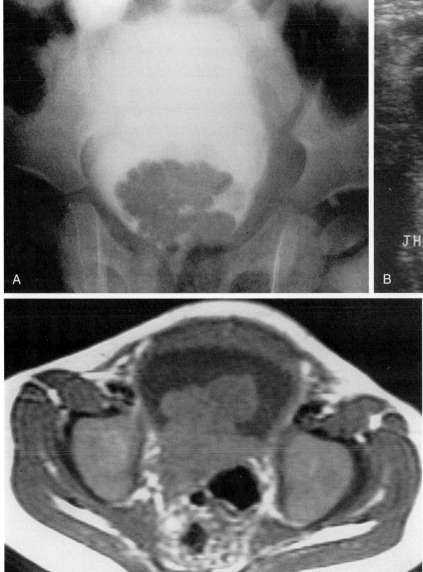

FIGURE 19–16. Rhabdomyosarcoma, bladder, in a 15-month-old female infant.
A, Excretory urogram. The mass is composed of multiple, grapelike lobules.
B, Ultrasonogram demonstrates a lobulated soft tissue mass within the bladder.
C, Magnetic resonance image, T1-weighted, axial projection. Posterior extension of the tumor is demonstrated.

or bladder wall, whereas in females, it most commonly arises from the vagina. Testicle, pelvic floor, perineum, and retroperitoneum are other potential tissues of origin. Because they are usually quite large at the time of diagnosis and invasion into the bladder base is common, the exact site of origin of these tumors is often difficult to establish.

Rhabdomyosarcoma that grows in a hollow viscus such as the bladder or vagina may assume a grapelike, polypoid appearance, referred to as *sarcoma botryoides.* Symptoms of bladder outlet obstruction, palpable lower abdominal mass, and hematuria are the usual clinical findings.

Radiologic findings of rhabdomyosarcoma include a lobulated, soft tissue mass in the base of the bladder detected either on cystography, delayed contrast material–enhanced imaging studies or as echogenic soft tissue projecting into the urine-filled bladder by ultrasonography (Fig. 19–16).

Hemangioma. Hemangioma is a rare, benign mural tumor of the bladder that projects into the bladder lumen from a mural base. Phleboliths are often seen within this tumor as rounded calcifications (Fig. 19–17). The radiologic appearance of a hemangioma overlaps that of many of the other entities discussed in this section. Diagnosis therefore requires surgical excision.

Paraganglioma. Paraganglioma is a rare bladder tumor of neurogenic origin that accounts for less than 1 per cent of all extra-adrenal paragangliomas. Paraganglioma in the bladder produces a mural soft tissue mass of similar gross morphology to other forms of benign and malignant tumors. The trigone is the most common location, followed by the dome and the lateral walls of the bladder. A bladder paraganglioma that is metabolically active creates the setting for a unique clinical presentation in which hypertension, palpitation, headache, blurred vision,

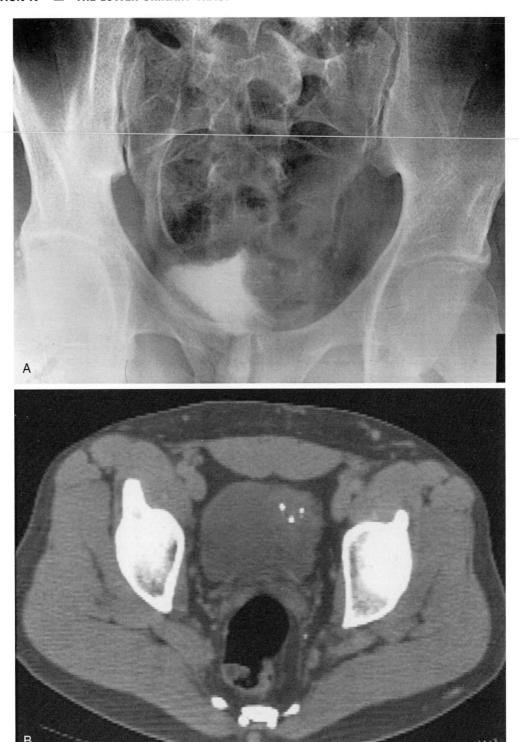

FIGURE 19–17. Hemangioma.
A, Excretory urogram. There is a large mass attached to the wall of the bladder. Faint, punctate densities within the mass represent phleboliths.
B, Computed tomogram without contrast material–enhancement demonstrates the mural mass and phleboliths protruding into the urine-filled bladder lumen.

diaphoresis, anxiety, and syncope are variably exacerbated during urination. Hematuria is frequently present.

Paraganglioma of the bladder appears on radiologic studies as an intramural mass that is indistinguishable from other tumor types (Fig. 19–18). Distinctive features that are often present are a high signal intensity on T2-weighted magnetic resonance images, tumor uptake using the radionuclide meta-iodobenzylguanidine, and, less distinctively, neovas-

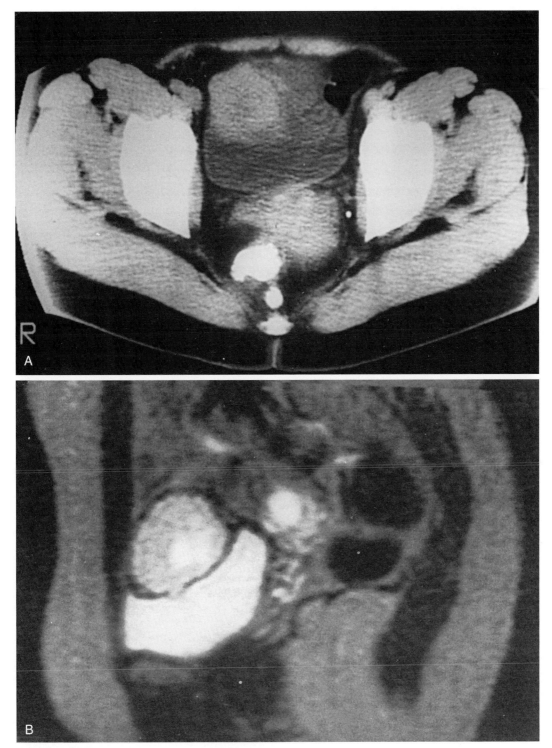

FIGURE 19–18. Paraganglioma.
  A, Computed tomogram, unenhanced. There is a round mass in the dome of the bladder.
  B, Magnetic resonance image, T2-weighted, sagittal plane. The mass in the dome of the bladder has a high signal intensity.

cularity and tumor stain demonstrated by angiography. With magnetic resonance imaging, moderately T2-weighted sequences delineate the lesion from urine. These and other aspects of adrenal and extra-adrenal paraganglioma are discussed in Chapters 21 and 22.

Secondary Neoplasms

Extravesical Primary Neoplasm and Pelvic Lymph Node Metastasis. Direct extension of a malignant neoplasm from tissues and organs adjacent to the bladder is not uncommon. Cervical carci-

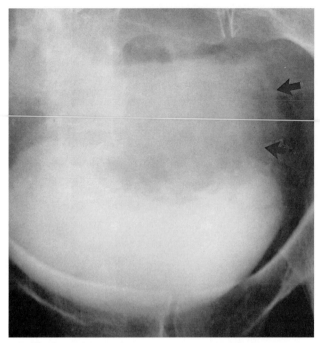

FIGURE 19–19. Recurrent carcinoma of the colon with involvement of the bladder wall in a 51-year-old woman. Late phase excretory urogram shows focal mucosal irregularity and the extrinsic component of the mass *(arrows).*

noma in women and prostate carcinoma in men are common examples of tumors that may form a focal mural mass as a consequence of bladder invasion. Imaging findings vary with the extent and location of the primary tumor and include focal wall thickening as an early manifestation of transmural extension into the bladder lumen in large tumors (Fig. 19–19). Fistula formation may occur, as well.

Lymphoma. Lymphoma usually affects the bladder by enlargement of iliac lymph nodes, as discussed in the section Abnormal Contour, at the end of this chapter. Lymphoma may involve the bladder wall directly and produce either multiple focal mural-based masses projecting into the bladder lumen or focal thickening of the bladder wall (see Fig. 19–33). This manifestation of lymphoma, however, is very uncommon.

Hematogenous Metastasis. Blood-borne metastases to the bladder, as might be seen in melanoma, are very uncommon. When present, these appear as multiple, sharply defined, mural-based projections into the bladder lumen.

Cystitis Glandularis and Cystitis Cystica. Cystitis glandularis is composed of glands in the lamina propria that are lined by cuboidal to columnar cells surrounded by urothelial cells. There are two histologic types, *typical,* or *nonmucinous,* which is common, and *intestinal,* or *mucinous,* an uncommon form. The intestinal type usually occurs in chronically irritated bladders, such as those with long-term catheters or stones, and may be diffuse and extensive. This uncommon form is associated with a slightly increased risk of bladder carcinoma. The common typical type of cystitis glandularis, on

the other hand, occurs for the most part as microscopic foci in as many as 70 per cent of otherwise normal bladders, most notably in the trigone, and is not associated with an increased risk of carcinoma.

Cystitis cystica consists of Brunn's nests whose central cells have degenerated to form small cystic cavities. Like cystitis glandularis, microscopic evidence of cystitis cystica is widespread in the bladders of both adults and children without other evidence of disease. Cystitis cystica frequently coexists with cystitis glandularis.

In view of the high prevalence of microscopic cystitis glandularis and cystitis cystica, only a small number of patients have related clinical or radiologic findings. Dysuria, hematuria, or other nonspecific symptoms may prompt radiologic evaluation. Furthermore, bladder biopsy may be positive for either or both of these lesions in patients with no imaging abnormalities.

Radiologic findings of both cystitis glandularis and cystica depict multiple irregular rounded or nodular elevations of the mucosa. This appearance may mimic advanced or multicentric carcinoma (Fig. 19–20).

Ureteritis cystica and pyelitis cystica are similar conditions occurring in the upper urinary tract. These are discussed in Chapter 15.

Inflammation

Schistosomiasis. Schistosomiasis may sometimes produce one or more mural lesions that project into the bladder lumen. More commonly, how-

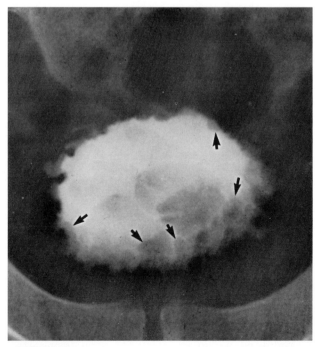

FIGURE 19–20. Cystitis cystica and cystitis glandularis. There are multiple filling defects *(arrows)* throughout the bladder wall, giving rise to a cobblestone appearance. Excretory urogram.

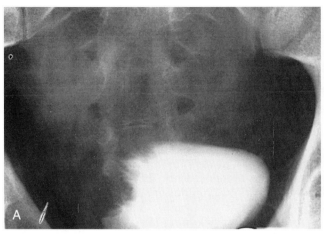

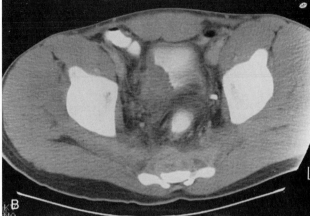

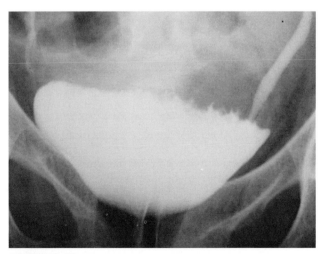

FIGURE 19–21. Crohn's disease in a young male patient with dysuria.

A, Excretory urogram. The right side of the bladder has a tethered or spiculated appearance.

B, Computed tomogram with contrast material enhancement at the level of the bladder base. There is thickening of the right lateral wall of the bladder, strands of soft tissue density in the perivesical fat, and increased presacral soft tissue.

C, Computed tomogram with contrast material enhancement at the level of the bladder dome. The thickened terminal ileum deforms the right side of the bladder.

ever, this parasitic infection causes marked, generalized mural thickening and is, therefore, discussed in the relevant section that follows. It must be kept in mind that the detection of a focal, mural-based lesion in a patient with schistosomiasis may represent a complicating carcinoma.

Extravesical Processes. *Diverticulitis, Crohn's disease, appendicitis, urachal abscess,* and *pelvic inflammatory disease* are diseases that may lead to a focal irregularity or thickening of the mucosa when the inflammatory process extends through the bladder wall.

Clinical parameters may differ among these entities. Appendicitis, for example, generally has a more acute clinical course than the other abnormalities. Other clinical and imaging features can be used to differentiate diverticulitis from Crohn's disease. For example, patients with Crohn's disease are generally younger and the bladder abnormality is more likely to affect the right surface of the bladder (Fig. 19–21). By comparison, diverticulitis is more likely to occur in the sigmoid and, as a result, the posterior left surface of the bladder is affected, although exceptions to this pattern may, of course, occur (Fig. 19–22). Using similar analysis, an infected urachal cyst is a likely diagnosis when a bladder lesion is anterosuperior and midline in location.

Conventional cystography or late phase excretory urography is usually of limited value in that these

techniques identify only the mural and urothelial portion of a process that, by definition, has a large extravesical component. Therefore, computed tomography, usually with intravenous and enteric contrast material, is the best test for demonstration of the bladder, perivesical fat, adnexae, and adjacent bowel.

FIGURE 19–22. Focal cystitis secondary to adjacent bowel inflammation in a 65-year-old patient with diverticulitis. Excretory urogram. There is an irregular mucosal thickening across the dome of the bladder. The remainder of the bladder mucosa is smooth.

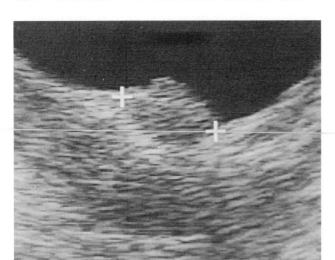

FIGURE 19–23. Endometriosis. Oblique longitudinal ultrasonogram shows an irregular mass *(cursors)* arising from the posterior wall of the bladder and projecting into the lumen. On this image, the intraluminal and extraluminal portions are approximately evenly distributed.

Endometriosis

The bladder is the most common site of urinary tract involvement by endometriosis. Such involvement is not common, however, occurring in less than 3 per cent of women with pelvic endometriosis. Endometriosis that affects the bladder wall appears as blue-black nodules that protrude into the bladder lumen. Implants may also be present on the serosal surface of the bladder.

Patients with endometriosis are generally younger than those who develop bladder neoplasia, although older women on postmenopausal hormone replacement therapy may develop the complication of endometriosis. Symptoms, such as dysuria, frequency, and hematuria, may be cyclic in relation to menstruation.

Endometrial deposits in the wall of the bladder are seen radiologically as mural filling defects that are indistinguishable from many of the other abnormalities that are discussed in this section, including carcinoma. These are best detected radiologically by cystography or ultrasonography as an irregular mass of medium echogenicity surrounded by urine within the bladder (Fig. 19–23). Computed tomography, while nonspecific, may allow localization and assessment of extent of involvement, including extravesical disease. Magnetic resonance imaging is often used in the evaluation of patients with suspected endometriosis, but this modality has not been studied with specific regard to the assessment of genitourinary tract involvement.

Endometriosis of the ureter is discussed in Chapter 16.

MURAL THICKENING

The bladder wall may be either uniformly thickened or have an irregular thickening, known as *trabecu-*

lation, in response to a variety of pathologic processes. Cystography or late phase excretory urography permits identification of mural thickening as increased soft tissue density between the contrast material–filled bladder lumen and the surrounding perivesical fat when the bladder is fully distended. This same pattern can be identified on cross-sectional imaging studies, which has the added advantage of direct visualization of the thickness of the bladder wall. The degree of bladder filling must always be taken into account when assessing bladder wall thickness. Generally, the wall of a well-distended bladder that exceeds 3 mm is considered abnormal. Fortunately, conditions that result in thickening also typically cause irregularity of the mucosa, and it may be the combination of these findings that allows classification of the abnormality.

It is useful to characterize bladder wall thickening as to whether involvement is *diffuse* or *focal* in extent. Diffuse thickening is more likely to represent a disease that is intrinsic to the bladder. Examples of this form include acute cystitis, schistosomiasis, malakoplakia, or chronic bladder outlet obstruction. Focal wall thickening, on the other hand, usually represents either invasion by an extravesical process, such as endometriosis, inflammatory bowel disorders, or extrinsic neoplasm, mural invasion of a mucosal neoplasm, such as transitional cell carcinoma, or focal lymphoma of the bladder (see Fig. 19–33). These causes of focal thickening are described in the foregoing section of this chapter.

Diffuse Wall Thickening

Acute Cystitis. Acute cystitis due to bacterial infection is most commonly the result of transurethral invasion of the bladder by coliform bacteria that have colonized the perineum. The short length of the female urethra contributes to the striking preponderance of acute cystitis in females compared with males. *Escherichia coli* is the most common organism causing acute cystitis. Immunosuppressed patients are at increased risk for acute cystitis. Most patients with the diagnosis do not have a defined risk factor, however.

Dysuria, urinary frequency and urgency, and gross hematuria are the most common clinical features of acute cystitis. However, patients may be asymptomatic. Pyuria and bacteriuria are the dominant laboratory findings.

The acutely infected bladder often appears normal on radiologic studies. Cystography is usually not performed in patients with acute symptoms because of the risk of inducing bacteremia. Mucosal inflammation and edema may cause thickened bladder mucosa with a cobblestone appearance. Bladder irritability may lead to reduced bladder capacity.

Acute bacterial cystitis in patients with diabetes mellitus may sometimes be associated with the formation of both intraluminal and intramural bladder gas, a condition known as *emphysematous cystitis.* *E. coli* is the most common pathogen. The gas in emphysematous cystitis is carbon dioxide, which is produced by bacterial fermentation of urine glucose within the bladder wall.

Most patients with emphysematous cystitis are elderly and have a history of long-standing or poorly controlled diabetes mellitus. In addition to the symptoms of cystitis described in the previous section, pneumaturia may be present. Unlike emphysematous pyelonephritis, which is described in Chapter 9, emphysematous cystitis is not life threatening and usually responds to appropriate antimicrobial therapy and control of the patient's diabetes mellitus.

Standard radiographs of the lower abdomen or computed tomograms demonstrate gas within the bladder wall as a mottled or streaky radiolucency (Fig. 19–24). Gas is also often present in the bladder lumen. A contrast material–enhanced imaging study confirms the location of the mural gas. The bladder wall may appear thickened and irregular, reflecting inflammation and edema.

Occasionally, gas extends into the ureters or perivesical soft tissue. Intraluminal gas due to infection must be differentiated from that due to vesicovaginal or vesicoenteric fistula or recent surgical or diagnostic instrumentation (Fig. 19–25).

Schistosomiasis. Schistosomiasis, or bilharziasis, of the urinary tract is the result of infection with *Schistosoma haematobium,* a parasite found throughout southwest Asia, eastern Africa, and the Middle East. Individuals become infected when exposed to water inhabited by snails harboring the organism. The cercariae penetrate the skin, gain access to the bloodstream, and migrate to the venules of the lamina propria of the bladder and distal ureters. Through these venous channels, eggs are

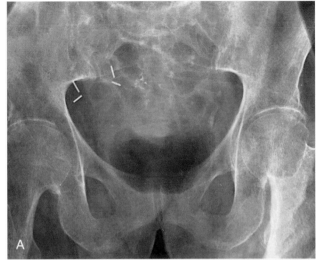
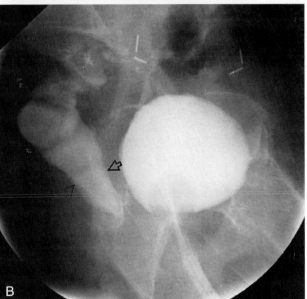

FIGURE 19–25. Intraluminal bladder gas secondary to a vesicoenteric fistula.
A, Radiograph of the pelvis demonstrates gas lucency within the bladder.
B, Cystogram. The rectosigmoid colon *(arrows)* opacifies with contrast material introduced into the bladder.

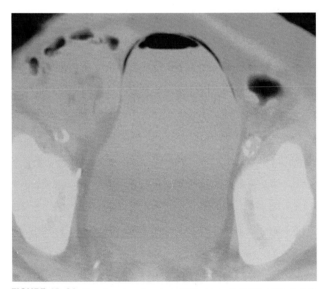

FIGURE 19–24. Emphysematous cystitis in a patient with renal transplant and severe urinary tract infection. Computed tomogram, unenhanced. Gas is present in the wall of the bladder as well as within the lumen.

deposited within the bladder submucosa and give rise to a granulomatous inflammatory response that includes superficial mucosal ulcerations and polypoid masses of granulation tissue. Ultimately, fibrosis and calcium deposition in dead ova develop.

Dysuria, hematuria, frequency, and ureteral obstruction are commonly present. Obstructive uropathy may be of insidious development and eventually cause renal insufficiency.

The radiologic features of bladder schistosomiasis vary with the duration of infestation. Initially, the bladder mucosa demonstrates a prominent and irregular pattern representing nonspecific acute inflammation, edema, and granulomas in the submucosa. As a late manifestation, calcification forms in a pattern that varies from focal to curvilinear, the

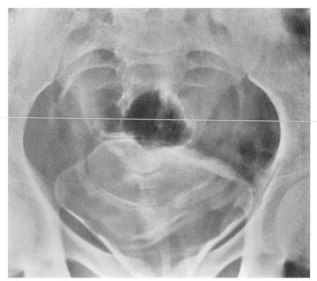

FIGURE 19–26. Schistosomiasis. There is dense calcification of the bladder wall and distal ureters. Radiograph.

latter being a very suggestive radiologic sign of urinary schistosomiasis (Fig. 19–26). Ultimately, the bladder becomes contracted. Focal filling defects may represent either an inflammatory polypoid component of schistosomiasis or a uroepithelial carcinoma. Such carcinomas occur with increased frequency in these patients.

Schistosomiasis of the ureter is discussed in Chapter 15.

Tuberculosis. In contrast to acute bacterial cystitis, which arises in a retrograde manner, tuberculosis of the bladder results from organisms that have descended antegrade from the kidneys. Therefore, bladder involvement usually coexists with evidence of ureteral and renal tuberculosis. Initially, the ureteral orifice becomes edematous and ulcerated. Ureteral obstruction may follow. The inflammatory process may progress to involve any portion of the bladder, resulting in multiple mural irregularities. Eventually, fibrosis of the bladder wall causes asymmetry and contraction of the bladder. If fibrosis involves the ureteral orifice, either stricture or a rigid, dilated ureteral orifice with vesicoureteral reflux develops. The reader is referred to Chapter 13 for a discussion of tuberculosis of the kidney and to Chapter 15 for a discussion of tuberculosis of the pelvocalyceal system and ureter.

Radiation Cystitis. Cystitis sometimes develops as a result of external or intracavitary radiation therapy for primary urothelial neoplasms or other pelvic malignancies. This is usually mild. In some patients, however, a severe cystitis occurs either in an *acute* or a *delayed* form.

In acute radiation cystitis, edema, hyperemia, petechiae, and ulceration of the bladder wall develop. Clinically, symptoms of bladder inflammation, such as frequency and dysuria as well as hematuria, become manifest. Radiologic studies, if abnormal, demonstrate prominence and irregularity of bladder

mucosa, bladder irritability, and increased contractility. These findings, however, are not specific for radiation.

Delayed radiation cystitis develops up to 4 years following therapy, depending on dose and host susceptibility. Here, the pathologic findings are interstitial fibrosis, obliterative endarteritis, and telangiectasia of the bladder mucosa. Severe hematuria may be a complicating factor. The radiologic findings in delayed radiation cystitis are dominated by extensive fibrosis causing reduced bladder capacity, a thickened bladder wall, and, in some cases, upper tract obstruction (Fig. 19–27). Calcification is rare. An increased attenuation value of the perivesical fat and the presence of surgical clips suggesting prior lymph node dissection may be clues to the diagnosis in the absence of available history. In addition, atrophy and fatty replacement of the pyriformis muscles or other muscles about the pelvis may be seen (Fig. 19–28).

Cyclophosphamide Cystitis. Cyclophosphamide, used as an antineoplastic or immunosuppressive agent, produces metabolites that are cytotoxic to uroepithelium. The bladder is especially susceptible, presumably reflecting more prolonged exposure than in the upper urinary tract. Cystitis occurs in as many as 40 per cent of patients receiving cyclophosphamide. Patients with significant cyclophosphamide exposure should be screened with urine cytology because of the higher risk of bladder cancer.

In acute cyclophosphamide cystitis, the bladder mucosa becomes edematous and hyperemic. Ulceration and hemorrhage may ensue. Radiologic findings at this stage include bladder wall thickening and irregularity with intraluminal filling defects due to blood clots (Fig. 19–29). Acute cyclophosphamide cystitis may evolve into a chronic form charac-

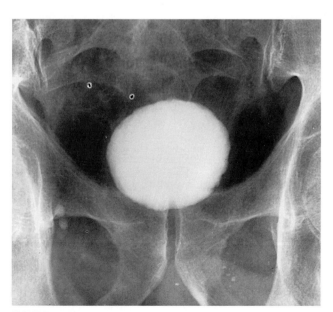

FIGURE 19–27. Radiation cystitis. The bladder wall is slightly irregular and contracted. Excretory urogram.

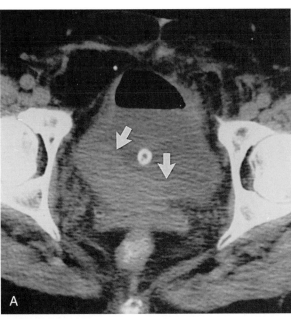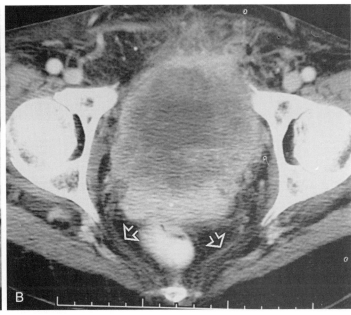

FIGURE 19–28. Radiation cystitis in an 84-year-old woman with hematuria.

A, Computed tomography, unenhanced. There is a large soft tissue mass of the bladder base *(arrows)* which extends to the bladder outlet and causes obstruction. The mass is nearly isodense with urine. A urethral catheter is in place, but was clamped prior to scan.

B, Three months later, after therapeutic radiation, the mass is no longer seen. The bladder wall is now thickened and irregular. Additionally, there is an ill-defined increase in the density of the fat anterior to the bladder. Fatty replacement of the pyriformis muscles *(arrows)* has occurred.

terized by bladder fibrosis, and, in some patients, persistent bladder hemorrhage. Radiologically, this stage is seen as a contracted, low-capacity bladder, sometimes with upper urinary tract dilatation (Fig. 19–30). Mural calcification may be similar to that seen in schistosomiasis.

Malakoplakia. Malakoplakia is an uncommon granulomatous response to an infection of the urinary tract, predominantly with *E. coli.* An intracellular abnormality of macrophages, probably at the lysosomal level, is thought to prevent complete digestion of phagocytosed bacteria. Submucosal granulomas dominated by large mononuclear cells with abundant cytoplasm develop. Intracellular and extracellular inclusion bodies composed of calcium and iron-laden lysosomal material are present. These inclusions, known as Michaelis-Gutmann bodies, are probably bacilli in various stages of defective digestion. The granulomas produce multiple yellow-gray or brown elevations of the mucosa.

Malakoplakia affects any part of the genitourinary tract, including the testes and prostate, but the bladder is involved most frequently. Malakoplakia of the kidney is discussed in Chapter 11 and that of the pelvis and ureter in Chapter 15.

Malakoplakia affects females most often, predominantly in the fifth to sixth decades of life. Symptoms are generally those of urinary tract infection and bladder irritability. Hematuria is commonly present.

In addition to diffuse bladder thickening, the radiologic appearance of malakoplakia of the bladder includes single or multiple mural filling defects, especially in the trigone or bladder base (Fig. 19–31). Radiologic differentiation from neoplasm is not possible.

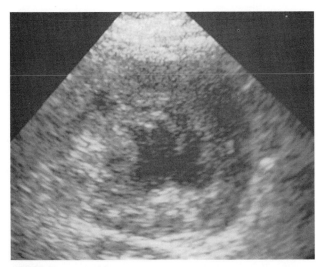

FIGURE 19–29. Hemorrhagic cystitis secondary to cyclophosphamide. Transverse ultrasonogram of the bladder shows pronounced irregular wall thickening. (Kindly provided by Jade J. Wong-You-Cheong, M.D., University of Maryland, Baltimore, Maryland.)

Focal Wall Thickening

See discussion on page 494 under Mural-Based Filling Defects.

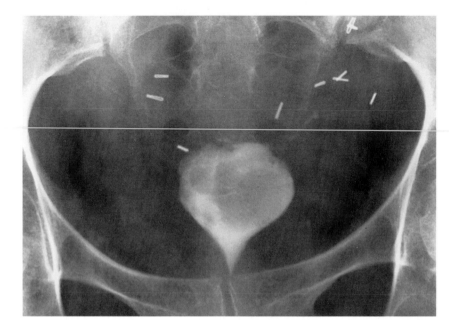

FIGURE 19–30. Cyclophosphamide cystitis. The bladder is contracted and deformed by fibrosis. Filling defects within the bladder represent blood clots. Excretory urogram.

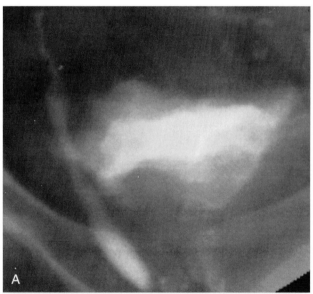

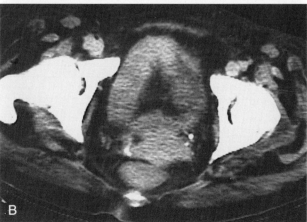

FIGURE 19–31. Malakoplakia, bladder.
  A, Excretory urogram. Extensive, irregular filling defects are seen throughout the bladder wall.
  B, Computed tomogram demonstrates diffuse thickening of the bladder.

ABNORMAL CONTOUR

Symmetric Narrowing

There is a group of disorders of the extravesical space that cause symmetric compression of the lateral aspects of the bladder, an appearance that has been referred to as "teardrop" bladder. Characteristically, the bladder base appears rounded and the dome tapered. The bladder mucosa is generally spared in the wide variety of disorders that produce this abnormal bladder contour.

Pelvic Lipomatosis. Proliferation of mature fat in the extraperitoneal space of the pelvis occurs as an idiopathic process and is the most common cause of symmetric bladder narrowing. Limited demographic studies of this poorly understood abnormality suggest a predominance in black males of all ages, although this association has been questioned. Symptoms are usually absent. When present, however, they reflect bladder inflammation, obstruction of the bladder outlet or rectum, diminished bladder capacity, venous compression, or ureteral obstruction.

Symmetric, circumferential external compression, elongation and elevation of the bladder and the rectosigmoid, and medial deviation of the distal ureters can be observed in pelvic lipomatosis. The iliac veins and the caudal portion of the inferior vena cava may be similarly narrowed. In the inflammatory form of pelvic lipomatosis, cystitis, including cystitis glandularis and cystica, may also be noted. In severe cases, this may be associated with ureteral obstruction and obstructive uropathy.

Fat proliferation is recognizable on standard radiographs as increased lucency in the perivesical soft tissue and as an increased amount of fat density tissue with computed tomography or magnetic resonance imaging. The deformities of the bladder, rectosigmoid, and ureters described previously are best demonstrated radiologically by cystography, excretory urography, barium enema, or computed tomography (Fig. 19–32). Ultrasonography demonstrates the abnormal bladder contour as well as the surrounding echogenic fat without evidence of a definite mass.

Pelvic Hematoma. The symmetric deformity of

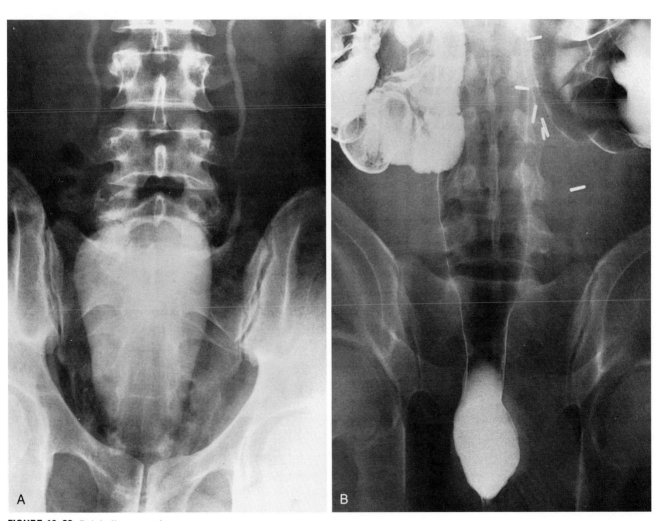

FIGURE 19–32. Pelvic lipomatosis.
A, Excretory urogram demonstrates symmetric compression of the bladder.
B, Barium enema. There is extrinsic compression and straightening of the rectum and rectosigmoid.

the bladder caused by pelvic hematoma is the same as that caused by pelvic lipomatosis. However, the tissue density of blood rather than fat in the extravesical space, as well as different clinical circumstances readily differentiate the two. Recent blunt trauma, penetrating trauma, including transfemoral arteriography and anticoagulation therapy, are common causes of pelvic hematoma. Patients who have sustained blunt trauma sufficient to cause pelvic hematoma often have radiographically apparent fractures.

Computed tomography or magnetic resonance imaging confirm the presence of hematoma, the exact characteristics of which vary with time. The same modalities permit differentiation of hematoma from other masses, such as lymphadenopathy or primary pelvic tumor, based on the relatively well-defined margins of the latter two entities. A symmetric deformity of the bladder as seen on cystography may also be caused by a urinoma that forms in association with blunt trauma. Again, computed tomography or magnetic resonance imaging serves to distinguish urinoma from the other abnormalities discussed in this section. Bladder trauma is discussed in detail in Chapter 29.

Lymphoma. Lymphoma of the bladder can have a variety of appearances, including multifocal mural masses and focal wall thickening, as discussed in a preceding section of this chapter (Fig. 19–33). However, lymphoma is more likely to cause symmetric narrowing of the bladder contour as a result of lymphadenopathy (Fig. 19–34). Indeed, lymphoma is the most common neoplastic cause of symmetric bladder narrowing. Nonlymphomatous malignancies of the pelvis also may occasionally produce substantial lymphadenopathy and similar radiologic findings. In either case, computed tomography or magnetic resonance imaging will confirm the soft tissue masses, which will seldom be limited

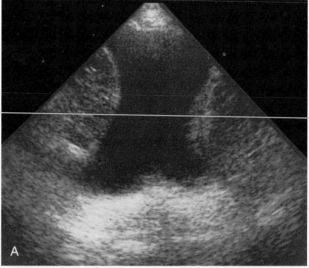

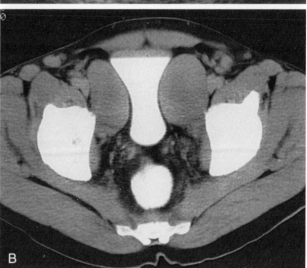

FIGURE 19–34. Lymphoma, retroperitoneal lymph nodes, causing bilateral and symmetric extrinsic compression of the bladder.
A, Ultrasonogram, transverse projection.
B, Computed tomogram, contrast material–enhanced.

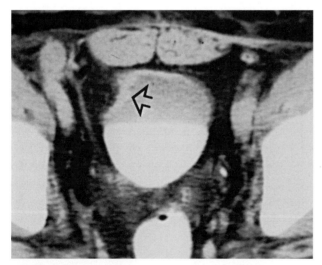

FIGURE 19–33. Non-Hodgkin's lymphoma in a 63-year-old man. Contrast material–enhanced computed tomogram. There is focal thickening of the bladder wall *(arrow)* with minimal mucosal component.

to the pelvis, and allow easy differentiation from pelvic lipomatosis.

Iliopsoas Hypertrophy. In young athletic individuals, iliopsoas hypertrophy may occasionally produce symmetric narrowing of the bladder as well as deviation of the mid- and distal ureter. The deviation of the mid-ureter distinguishes this condition from pelvic lipomatosis, which does not usually affect the proximal two-thirds of the ureter. Generalized adenopathy, on the other hand, can be identical to iliopsoas hypertrophy in terms of its impact on the course of the ureter. Computed tomography or magnetic resonance imaging are definitive in documenting the prominence of the iliopsoas muscles, as well as the absence of either fatty proliferation or lymphadenopathy.

Miscellaneous. Extrinsic compression of the bladder and medial deviation of the distal ureter are also caused by a *narrow bony pelvis, nonlympho-*

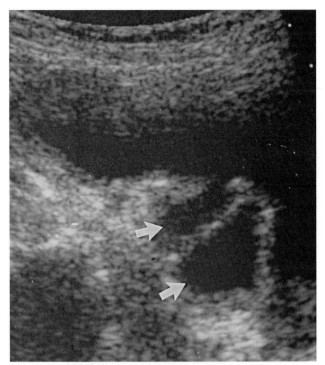

FIGURE 19–35. Diverticula in an 80-year-old man with benign prostatic hyperplasia, difficulty voiding, and recurrent urinary tract infection. The ultrasonogram shows the diverticula as multiple fluid-filled outpouchings *(arrows)*.

matous lymphadenopathy, lymphocele, lymphangioma, iliac artery aneurysm, and *iliac vein varices* associated with occlusion of the inferior vena cava. While usually symmetric and bilateral, these may sometimes be eccentric and focal. *Seminal vesicle cyst* also may cause extrinsic bladder compression, as discussed in Chapter 25. Many of these conditions have a distinctive clinical setting with associated characteristic radiologic findings that permit an accurate diagnosis.

Asymmetric Contour

Diverticulum. Most bladder diverticula are acquired in association with long-standing bladder outlet obstruction, including those due to neuropathic disorders of the bladder. Most commonly, diverticula are encountered in older men with benign prostatic enlargement, prostatitis, or carcinoma of the prostate. Other causes include urethral stricture and, in infants, congenital urethral valve or stricture. In females, bladder diverticula may develop in outlet obstruction owing to neuropathic disorders, urethral carcinoma, or diverticulum. *Congenital* bladder diverticulum is discussed in the section Anomalies, earlier in this chapter.

An *acquired* bladder diverticulum begins as a small outpouching of mucosa that evaginates between hypertrophied detrusor muscle bundles but does not extend beyond the outer margin of the bladder wall. This structure is called a *cellule*. Only when the cellule protrudes beyond the outer margin of the bladder wall is it referred to as a diverticulum. Most acquired diverticula develop in the base of the bladder, often just anterolateral to a ureteral orifice. Diverticula can vary in size and become much larger than the bladder. They may be single or multiple (Fig. 19–35). Large diverticula may cause ureteral deviation or obstruction, vesicoureteral reflux, urinary tract infection, or calculi (Fig. 19–36). Some diverticula grow large enough to deform the bladder and cause urinary retention. Diverticula are lined by uroepithelium and, therefore, may be the site of carcinoma of the bladder (Fig. 19–37). Because a diverticulum lacks a layer of muscle, invasive carcinoma arising in a diverticulum is likely to spread faster than one that arises in the bladder lumen.

The imaging appearance of bladder diverticula varies with location, size, effect on adjacent structures, and the presence of complicating stone or

FIGURE 19–36. Bladder diverticula. A cystogram demonstrates a large right-sided diverticulum and a small left-sided diverticulum. The narrow neck leading through the bladder wall is visualized in both. Reflux of contrast material into the right ureter is present.

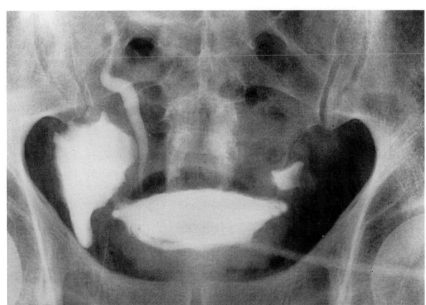

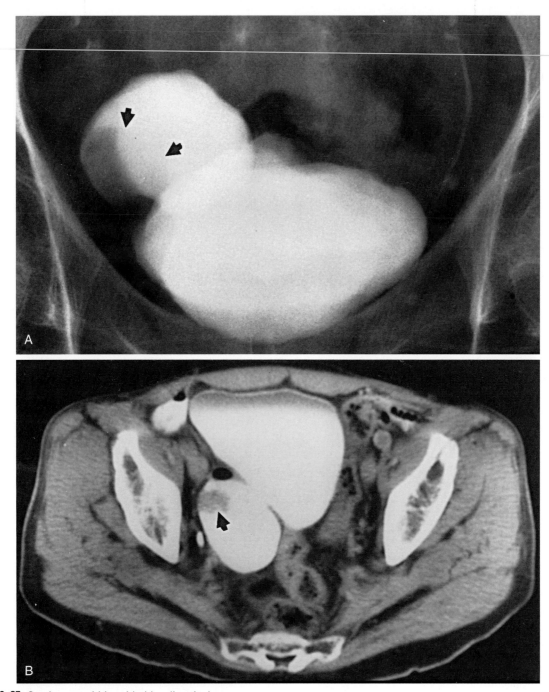

FIGURE 19–37. Carcinoma within a bladder diverticulum.
   A, Excretory urogram demonstrates an intraluminal filling defect *(arrows)* within a right-sided bladder diverticulum.
   B, Computed tomogram with contrast material enhancement reveals an irregular mural-based mass *(arrow)* protruding into the lumen of the bladder diverticulum.

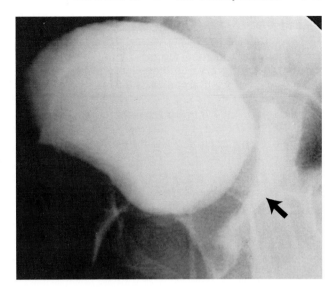

FIGURE 19–38. Vesicovaginal fistula following hysterectomy. Cystogram. The oblique lateral view demonstrates contrast material in the vagina *(arrow)*. (Kindly provided by Jade J. Wong-You-Cheong, M.D., University of Maryland, Baltimore, Maryland.)

tumor. A wide-neck diverticulum fills and empties readily with the bladder, whereas one with a narrow neck leads to urine stasis, chronic infection, and stone formation. Radiographs obtained after voiding are valuable in this regard.

Fistula. Fistula formation is included in this section on asymmetric abnormal contour because the most common imaging finding is extension of contrast material outside the normal confines of the bladder. Fistulae vary greatly in etiology, location, and severity. Not surprisingly, then, imaging techniques may have to be adapted to a given individual's unique circumstance.

Inflammatory causes of fistulae to the lower urinary tract include diverticulitis, most commonly, and Crohn's disease. Advanced malignancy, chronic appendicitis, therapeutic radiation, and pelvic surgery are also associated with fistula formation. Fistulae are often "unidirectional" during imaging studies. For example, a rectovesical communication may only be seen during cystography and not during a positive contrast enema. A clinically signifi-

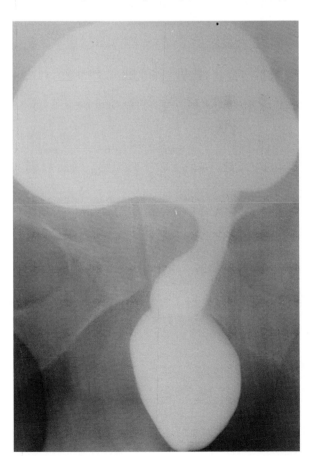

FIGURE 19–39. Inguinal hernia. Cystogram. The bladder extends into left hemiscrotum. (Kindly provided by Jade J. Wong-You-Cheong, M.D., University of Maryland, Baltimore, Maryland.)

cant fistula is, at times, undetectable by either imaging route. Generally, however, administration of water-soluble contrast material demonstrates the fistulous communication between one viscus and the other in at least one direction (Fig. 19–38).

Hernia. Rarely, a portion of the bladder herniates through the inguinal ring into the scrotum (Fig. 19–39). Sometimes the distal ureter also extends into the hernia. This may mimic hydrocele formation by physical examination or ultrasonography.

BIBLIOGRAPHY

Anatomy and Anomalies

Brooks, J. D.: Anatomy of the lower urinary tract and male genitalia. In Walsh, P. C., Retik, A. B., Vaughan, E. D., Jr., and Wein, A. J. (eds.): Campbell's Urology, 7th ed. Philadelphia, W. B. Saunders, 1998, pp. 89–128.
Gearhart, J. P., and Jeffs, R. D.: Exstrophy-epispadias complex and bladder anomalies. In Walsh, P. C., Retik, A. B., Vaughan, E. D., Jr., and Wein, A. J. (eds.): Campbell's Urology, 7th ed. Philadelphia, W. B. Saunders, 1998, pp. 1939–1990.
Goldman, I. L., Caldamone, A. A., Gauderer, M., Hampel, N., Wesselhoeft, C. W., and Elder, J. S.: Infected urachal cysts: A review of 10 cases. J. Urol. 140:375, 1988.
Spataro, R. F., Davis, R. S., McLachlan, M. S. F., Linke, C. A., and Barbaric, Z. L.: Urachal abnormalities in the adult. Radiology 149:659, 1983.

Intraluminal Filling Defects

Amendola, M. A., Sonda, L. P., Diokno, A. C., and Vidyasagar, M.: Bladder calculi complicating intermittent clean catheterization. AJR 141:751, 1983.
Lebowitz, R. L., and Vargas, B.: Stones in the urinary bladder in children and young adults. AJR 148:491, 1987.

Neoplasms

Amendola, M. A., Glazer, G. M., Grossman, H. B., Aisen, A. M., and Francis, I. R.: Staging of bladder carcinoma: MRI-CT-Surgical correlation. AJR 146:1179, 1986.
Baker, M. E., Silverman, P. M., and Korobkin, M.: Computed tomography of prostatic and bladder rhabdomyosarcomas. J. Comput. Assist. Tomogr. 9:780, 1985.
Barentsz, J. O., Ruijs, S. H. J., and Strijk, S. P.: The role of MR imaging in carcinoma of the urinary bladder. AJR 160:937, 1993.
Barentsz, J. O., Jager, G., Mugler, J. P. III, Oosterhof, G., Peters, H., Erning, L. T. J. O., and Ruijs, S. H. J.: Staging urinary bladder cancer: Value of T1-weighted three-dimensional magnetization-prepared-rapid gradient echo and two-dimensional spin-echo sequences. AJR 164:109, 1995.
Belis, J. A., Post, G. J., Rochman, S. C., and Milam, D. F.: Genitourinary leiomyomas. Urology 13:424, 1979.
Bornstein, I., Charboneau, J. W., and Hartman, G. W.: Leiomyoma of the bladder: Sonographic and urographic findings. J. Ultrasound Med. 5:407, 1986.
Brenner, D. W., and Schellhammer, P. F.: Upper tract urothelial malignancy after cyclophosphamide therapy: A case report and literature review. J. Urol. 137:1226, 1987.
Brick, S. H., Friedman, A. C., Pollack, H. M., Fishman, E. K., Radecki, P. D., Siegelbaum, M. H., Mitchell, D. G., Lev-Toaff, A. S., Caroline, D. F.: Urachal carcinoma: CT findings. Radiology 169:377, 1988.
Bryan, P. J., Butler, H. E., LiPuma, J. P., Resnick, M. I., and Kursh, E. D.: CT and MR imaging in staging bladder neoplasms. J. Comput. Assist. Tomogr. 11:96, 1987.
Buy, J. N., Moss, A. A., Guinet, C., Ghossain, M. A., Malbec, L., Arrive, L., and Vadrot, D.: MR staging of bladder carcinoma: Correlation with pathologic findings. Radiology 169:695, 1988.

Caceres, J., Mata, J. M., Lucaya, J., Palmer, J., and Donoso, L.: Hemangioma of the bladder. Radiographics 11:161, 1991.
Charnsangavej, C.: Lymphoma of the genitourinary tract. Radiol. Clin. North Am. 28:865, 1990.
Cheng, D., and Tempany, C. M. C.: MR imaging of the prostate and bladder. Semin. Ultrasound CT MR 19:67, 1998.
Ellis, J. H., McCullough, N. B., Francis, I. R., Grossman, H. B., and Platt, J. F.: Transitional cell carcinoma of the bladder: Patterns of recurrence after cystectomy as determined by CT. AJR 157:999, 1991.
Husband, J. E. S., Olliff, J. F. C., Williams, M. P., Heron, C. W., and Cherryman, G. R.: Bladder cancer: Staging with CT and MR imaging. Radiology 173:435, 1989.
Jacobs, M. A., Bavendam, T., and Leach, G. E.: Bladder leiomyoma. Urology 34:56, 1989.
McCulloch, C. J.: A comparison of clinical and MR staging of bladder carcinoma. Clin. Radiol. 50:878, 1995.
Messing, E. M., and Catalona, W. L.: Urothelial tumors of the urinary tract: Bladder cancer. In Walsh, P. C., Retik, A. B., Vaughan, E. D., Jr., and Wein, A. J. (eds.): Campbell's Urology, 7th ed. Philadelphia, W. B. Saunders, 1998, pp. 2329–2382.
Montague, D. K., and Boltuch, R. L.: Primary neoplasms in vesical diverticula: Report of 10 cases. J. Urol. 116:41, 1976.
Narumi, Y., Sato, T., Kuriyama, K., Fujita, M., Saiki, S., Kuroda, M., Miki, T., and Kotake, T.: Vesical dome tumors: Significance of extravesical extension on CT. Radiology 169:383, 1988.
Nesbitt, J. A., and Walther, P. J.: Computed tomographic imaging of microscopic dystrophic calcification in urachal adenocarcinoma. Urology 27:184, 1986.
Neuerburg, J. M., Bohndorf, K., Sohn, M., Teufl, F., Guenther, R. W., and Daus, H. J.: Urinary bladder neoplasms: Evaluation with contrast-enhanced MR imaging. Radiology 172:739, 1989.
Rholl, K. S., Lee, J. K. T., Heiken, J. P., Ling, D., and Glazer, H. S.: Primary bladder carcinoma: Evaluation with MR imaging. Radiology 163:117, 1987.
Tanimoto, A., Yuasa, Y., Imai, Y., Izutsa, M., Hiramatsu, K., Tachibana, M., and Tazaki, H.: Bladder tumor staging: Comparison of conventional and gadolinium-enhanced dynamic MR imaging and CT. Radiology 185:741, 1992.
Whitmore, W. F., Jr.: Bladder cancer: An overview. CA 38:213, 1988.
Yousem, D. M., Gatewood, O. M. B., Goldman, S. M., and Marshall, F. F.: Synchronous and metachronous transitional cell carcinoma of the urinary tract: Prevalence, incidence, and radiographic detection. Radiology 167:613, 1988.

Cystitis Glandularis and Cystitis Cystica

Davies, G., and Castro, J. E.: Cystitis glandularis. Urology 10:128, 1977.
Edwards, P. D., Hurm, R. A., and Jaeschke, W. H.: Conversion of cystitis glandularis to adenocarcinoma. J. Urol. 108:568, 1972.
Young, R. H., and Eble, J. N.: Non-neoplastic disorders of the urinary bladder. In Bostwick, D. G., and Eble, J. N. (eds.): Urologic Surgical Pathology. St. Louis, Mosby, 1997, pp. 174–175.

Infection and Inflammation

Aron, B. S., and Schlesinger, A.: Complications of radiation therapy: The genitourinary tract. Semin. Roentgenol. 9:65, 1974.
Gow, J. E.: Genitourinary tuberculosis. In Walsh, P. C., Retik, A. B., Vaughan, E. D., Jr., and Wein, A. J. (eds.): Campbell's Urology, 7th ed. Philadelphia, W. B. Saunders, 1998, pp. 807–836.
Hanno, P.: Interstitial cystitis and related diseases. In Walsh, P. C., Retik, A. B., Vaughan, E. D., Jr., and Wein, A. J. (eds.): Campbell's Urology, 7th ed. Philadelphia, W. B. Saunders, 1998, pp. 631–662.
Harold, D. L., Koff, S. A., and Kass, E. J.: Candida albicans "fungus ball" in bladder. Urology 9:662, 1977.
Jorulf, H., and Lindstedt, E.: Urogenital schistosomiasis: CT evaluation. Radiology 157:745, 1985.
Klein, F. A., and Smith, M. J. V.: Urinary complications of cyclophosphamide therapy: Etiology, prevention, and management. South. Med. J. 76:1413, 1983.

Maatman, T. J., Novick, A. C., Montague, D. K., and Levin, H. S.: Radiation-induced cystitis following intracavitary irradiation for superficial bladder cancer. J. Urol. *130:*338, 1983.

Olmo, J. M. C., Carcamo, P., Deiriarte, E. G., Jimenez, F., Martinezpineiro, L., and Martinezpineiro, J. A.: Genitourinary malakoplakia. Br. J. Urol. *72:*6, 1993.

Pollack, H. M., Bauner, M. P., Martinez, L. O., and Hodson, C. J.: Diagnostic considerations in urinary bladder wall calcification. AJR *136:*791, 1981.

Quint, H. J., Drach, G. W., Rappaport, W. D., and Hoffman, C. J.: Emphysematous cystitis: A review of the spectrum of disease. J. Urol. *147:*134, 1992.

Schaeffer, A. J.: Infections of the urinary tract. In Walsh, P. C., Retik, A. B., Vaughan, E. D., Jr., and Wein, A. J. (eds.): Campbell's Urology, 7th ed. Philadelphia, W. B. Saunders, 1998, pp. 587–595.

Shook, T. E., and Nyberg, L. M.: Endometriosis of the urinary tract. Urology *31:*1, 1988.

Sircus, S. I., Sant, G. R., and Ucci, A. A.: Bladder detrusor endometriosis mimicking interstitial cystitis. Urology *32:*339, 1988.

Smith, J. H., and von Lichtenberg, F.: Parasitic diseases of the genitourinary system. In Walsh, P. C., Retik, A. B., Vaughan, E. D., Jr., and Wein, A. J. (eds.): Campbell's Urology, 7th ed. Philadelphia, W. B. Saunders, 1998, pp. 733–778.

Stanton, M. J., and Maxted, W.: Malacoplakia: A study of the literature and current concepts of pathogenesis, diagnosis and treatment. J. Urol. *125:*139, 1981.

Tomaszewski, J. E.: Cystitis. In Hill, G. S. (ed.): Uropathology. New York, Churchill Livingstone, 1989, pp. 431–454.

Extravesical Lesions

Banner, M. P.: Genitourinary complications of inflammatory bowel disease. Radiol. Clin. North Am. *25:*199, 1987.

Carpenter, A. A.: Pelvic lipomatosis: Successful surgical treatment. J. Urol. *110:*397, 1973.

Chang, S. F.: Pear-shaped bladder caused by large iliopsoas muscles. Radiology *128:*349, 1978.

Enzinger, F. M., and Weiss, S. W.: Rhabdomyosarcoma. In Enzinger, F. M., and Weiss, S. W. (eds.): Soft Tissue Tumors. St. Louis, C. V. Mosby Co., 1995, pp. 539–578.

Heyns, C. F.: Pelvic lipomatosis: A review of its diagnosis and management. J. Urol. *146:*267, 1991.

Hill, G. S.: Intrinsic and extrinsic obstruction of the urinary tract. In Hill, G. S. (ed.): Uropathology. New York, Churchill Livingstone, 1989, pp. 235–278 and 517–574.

Merine, D., Fishman, E. K., Kuhlman, J. E., Jones, B., Bayless, T. M., and Siegelman, S.: Bladder involvement in Crohn disease: Role of CT in detection and evaluation. J. Comput. Assist. Tomogr. *13:*90, 1989.

Resnick, M. I., and Kursh, E. D.: Extrinsic obstruction of the ureter. In Walsh, P. C., Retik, A. B., Vaughan, E. D., Jr., and Wein, A. J. (eds.): Campbell's Urology, 7th ed. Philadelphia, W. B. Saunders, 1998, pp. 387–422.

Diverticulum

Hill, G. S.: Lower urinary tract obstruction. In Hill, G. S. (ed.): Uropathology. New York, Churchill Livingstone, 1989, pp. 599–622.

Jarow, J. P., and Brendler, C. B.: Urinary retention caused by a large bladder diverticulum: A simple method of diverticectomy. J. Urol. *139:*1260, 1988.

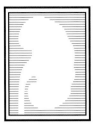

CHAPTER **20**

The Urethra

This chapter describes the normal anatomy, anomalies, and acquired diseases of the urethra. Trauma of the urethra is discussed in Chapter 29.

ANATOMY

The Male Urethra

The most commonly used approach to male urethral anatomy divides the urethra into two parts: *posterior* and *anterior.* The posterior urethra is made up of the *prostatic* and *membranous* portions, and the anterior is composed of the *bulbous* or *bulbar* and *penile* or *pendulous* urethra (Figs. 20–1 and 20–2).

The prostatic urethra extends from the bladder neck to the proximal margin of the urogenital diaphragm and is surrounded by the prostate gland. The *prostatic ducts* drain directly into the prostatic urethra. A mound of smooth muscle along its posterior wall forms a prominent landmark, the *verumontanum.* On either side of the verumontanum are the openings of the ejaculatory ducts. The orifice of the prostatic *utricle,* a vestige of the müllerian duct, is located in the midline of the proximal verumontanum.

The membranous urethra is that portion of the posterior urethra that traverses the *urogenital dia-phragm,* which is also known as the *external sphincter.* The membranous urethra is between 1 and 2 cm in length.

The bulbous urethra, which is immediately distal to the membranous urethra, is the intrascrotal portion of the anterior urethra. The proximal one-half of the bulbous urethra is dilated and has a symmetric cone shape at its proximal end when distended.

The penile urethra, which extends from the penoscrotal junction to the external meatus distally, lies ventral to the corpora cavernosa and is surrounded by the corpus spongiosum. The *fossa navicularis* is the slightly dilated, 1- to 1.5-cm segment of the penile urethra that narrows just proximal to the meatus.

Mucus-producing glands, known as the *paraurethral glands of Littré,* are located along the anterior urethra. These glands are most numerous in the bulbous urethra. The *bulbourethral glands,* which are also called *Cowper's glands,* are situated within the urogenital diaphragm. The ducts that drain these glands, however, insert into the bulbous urethra.

The Female Urethra

The female urethra is much shorter than the male urethra, measuring only about 4 cm in total length (Fig. 20–3). Although there is a continuation of the muscle layers from the bladder base to surround

Portions of this chapter, authored by Wendelin S. Hayes, were published in Chapter 20 of the previous edition of *Radiology of the Kidney and Urinary Tract.*

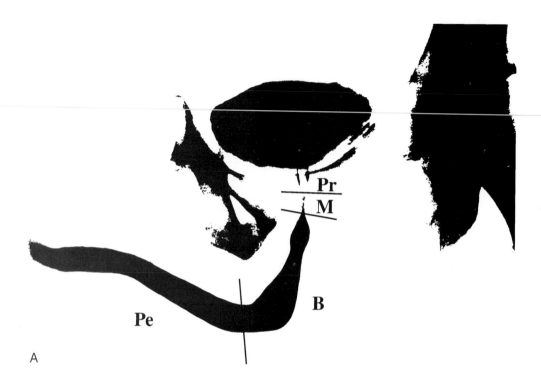

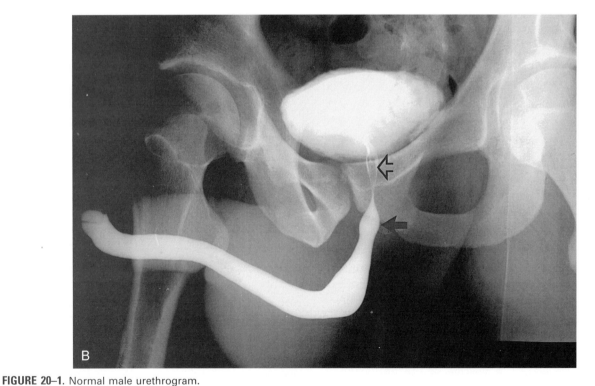

FIGURE 20–1. Normal male urethrogram.
A and *B,* Retrograde urethrogram demonstrating prostatic *(Pr),* membranous *(M),* bulbar *(B),* and penile *(Pe)* portions of the urethra. The verumontanum *(open arrow)* and the normal urethrographic cone shape of the proximal bulbar urethra *(closed arrow)* are also noted.

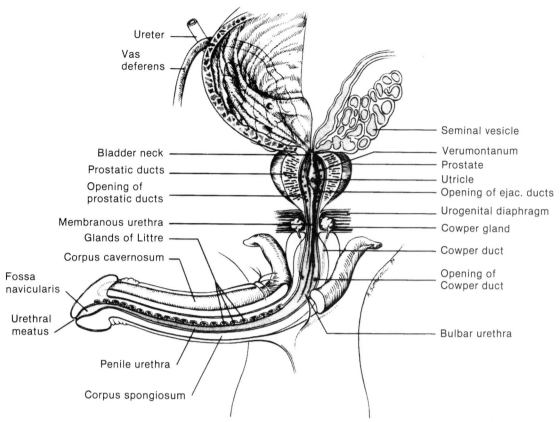

Ureter

Vas deferens

Seminal vesicle

Verumontanum

Bladder neck

Prostatic ducts

Opening of prostatic ducts

Prostate

Utricle

Opening of ejac. ducts

Membranous urethra

Glands of Littre

Corpus cavernosum

Urogenital diaphragm

Cowper gland

Cowper duct

Fossa navicularis

Urethral meatus

Opening of Cowper duct

Bulbar urethra

Penile urethra

Corpus spongiosum

FIGURE 20–2. Schematic drawing of male urethral anatomy. (From Amis, E. S., Newhouse, J. H., and Cronan, J. J.: Radiology of male periurethral structures. AJR *151*:321–324, 1988. Reproduced with kind permission of the authors and *American Journal of Roentgenology.*)

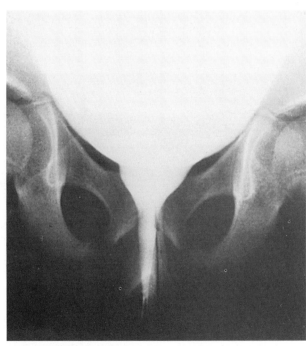

FIGURE 20–3. Normal female urethra. Voiding cystourethrogram. (Courtesy of William H. Bush, Jr., M.D., University of Washington, Seattle.)

the urethra, there is no inner circular layer functioning as an external sphincter as there is in men. Although most conditions of the urethra are more common in men than in women, important exceptions include primary urethral carcinoma and diverticulum.

ANOMALIES

Posterior Urethral Valve

There are two types of posterior urethral valve anomalies that lead to obstruction of the proximal male urethra. *Type I* morphology, which accounts for 95 per cent of posterior urethral valves, results from the formation of a thick, valvelike membrane from tissue of wolffian duct origin. This courses obliquely from the verumontanum to the most distal portion of the prostatic urethra. A variable-sized opening in the posterior central aspect of this membrane produces a foldlike appearance.

A Type II urethral valve was originally described as a mucosal fold that extended from the verumontanum to the bladder neck. It is now generally acknowledged that this type does not exist. Thus, the anomalous designation of a second variety of urethral valve is *Type III*. A Type III valve consists of a disklike membrane that is oriented across the urethral lumen at the level of the membranous urethra. An orifice of variable size is typically located centrally.

Clinical features of Type I and Type III posterior urethral valves are similar and vary with the severity of the obstruction that they cause. Not surprisingly, the higher the degree of obstruction, the younger the age at presentation. A posterior urethral valve is a common cause of bilateral hydronephrosis in a male fetus (Fig. 20–4). Severe cases are detected by ultrasonography *in utero* as oligohydramnios and growth retardation. Urinary ascites

may also be present, the result of bladder rupture. In the neonatal period, Potter's syndrome, including pulmonary hypoplasia, is apparent and associated with a high mortality rate. Additionally, bladder distention, bladder wall thickening, bilateral hydronephrosis, and renal dysplasia are noted both in obstetric ultrasonograms and in the neonate (see Fig. 20–4). Mild degrees of obstruction may not be detected until early adulthood when they become apparent as renal insufficiency or recurrent urinary tract infections. Because of compensatory bladder hypertrophy, an abnormality of urinary stream may not be present in these patients.

Voiding cystourethrography is the study of choice for the evaluation of suspected posterior urethral valve. In Type I posterior urethral valve, a catheter can often be passed retrograde without unusual difficulty, despite the presence of significant obstruction of voided urine. In contrast, Type III posterior urethral valve often impedes the passage of a catheter past the web. Radiologic findings include dilatation and elongation of the posterior urethra and, occasionally, a linear radiolucent band representing the valve (Figs. 20–5 through 20–7). The verumontanum is often enlarged. The bladder neck commonly hypertrophies and, thus, appears narrow in relationship to the dilated posterior urethra. Unilateral or bilateral vesicoureteral reflux is present in as many as 50 per cent of patients whose posterior urethral valve is discovered within the first year of life. Bladder hypertrophy, trabeculation, sacculation, and diverticula are also demonstrated by cystography.

Pelvic ultrasonography can be of value in the diagnosis of posterior urethral valve. Because the pubis is not ossified in the neonate, a clear view of the dilated posterior urethra is possible. On sagittal projections, the bladder and dilated posterior urethra create the appearance of a "keyhole," a finding that is highly suggestive of posterior urethral valve.

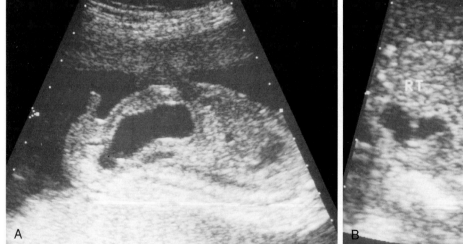
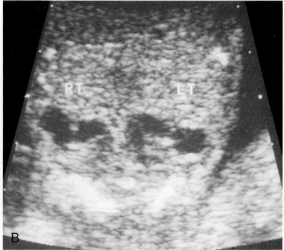

FIGURE 20–4. Posterior urethral valve demonstrated by ultrasonography *in utero*.
A, Longitudinal projection demonstrates dilatation of the bladder and posterior urethra. The degree of obstruction is not severe enough to cause oligohydramnios.
B, Transverse scan at the level of the kidneys. There is moderate bilateral hydronephrosis.

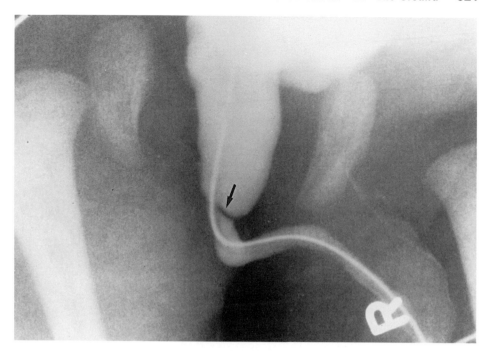

FIGURE 20–5. Posterior urethral valve in a newborn. Voiding cystourethrogram. The posterior urethra is dilated proximal to the sharply defined valve *(arrow)*. The eccentric orifice through which the catheter passes and the anterior bulge are characteristic of a Type I valve.

Diverticulum of the Anterior Urethra and Anterior Urethral Valve

What has been called anterior urethral valve is, in reality, nearly always a congenital diverticulum of the anterior urethra. A diverticulum of the anterior urethra develops on the ventral surface of the penile urethra, either as a result of incomplete development of the corpus spongiosum focally or incomplete fusion of a segment of the urethral plate. The diverticulum is usually oval, and its distal lip is thin and valvelike. It is this thin, anterior lip that has been called an anterior urethral valve.

The diverticulum fills during voiding, thereby narrowing and obstructing the true urethra. Incomplete bladder emptying and bladder infections are complications. Dribbling at the end of urination may also be present.

During voiding cystourethrography, the typical saccular diverticulum of the anterior urethra fills with contrast material and appears as an oval structure on the ventral aspect of the anterior urethra (Fig. 20–8). With distention of the diverticulum, partial or complete outflow obstruction occurs.

Congenital Meatal Stenosis

A pinpoint narrowing of the meatus on a congenital basis is a rare condition that is sometimes present in conjunction with hypospadias. More commonly, meatal stenosis is due to meatitis complicating circumcision. Diagnosis of meatal stenosis is usually by physical examination rather than by urethrography, which documents dilatation of the anterior and posterior urethra.

Megalourethra

Megalourethra is a rare anomaly that results from abnormal development of the corpus spongiosum and, less frequently, the corpus cavernosum. Nonobstructive congenital dilatation of the penile urethra is the result. This anomaly may coexist with other urinary tract anomalies, including prune-belly syndrome, renal dysplasia, megaureter, megacystis, and bladder diverticulum, as well as vesicoureteral reflux. Both the phallus and the urethra are enlarged in megalourethra. Because sepsis may follow instrumentation of the urethra, radiologic investigation of this disorder is best conducted by antegrade voiding techniques rather than retrograde urethrography.

Hypospadias/Epispadias

Hypospadias is a condition in which the urethral meatus opens onto the ventral surface of the penis at a point proximal to the tip of the glans. In epispadias, in contradistinction, the urethral orifice is located on the dorsal aspect of the penis. Epispadias is usually seen in association with the various forms of exstrophy, which are discussed in Chapter 19. Epispadias in the female is associated with a short, patulous urethra, widely separated labia, and a bifid clitoris.

In either hypospadias or epispadias, voiding cystourethrography demonstrates a foreshortened urethra.

Urethral Duplication

Urethral duplication can be either complete or incomplete. *Complete* duplication takes several forms: two separate urethras originate from the bladder and persist with separate external drainage; a common urethra originates from the bladder and duplicates distally; or a duplicated origin unites distally into a single external orifice. In *incomplete* duplica-

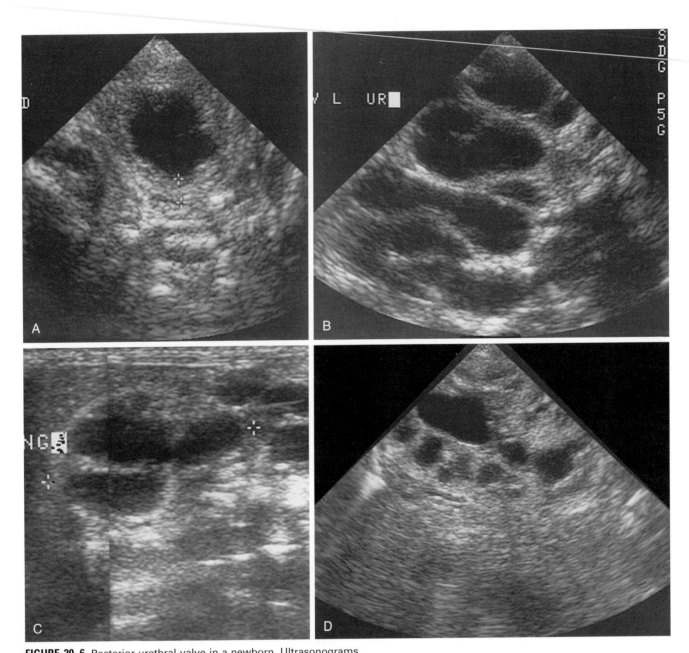

FIGURE 20–6. Posterior urethral valve in a newborn. Ultrasonograms.
  A, Bladder, transverse section. The bladder wall *(cursors)* is thickened.
  B, Left ureter, transverse section. The ureter is dilated and tortuous.
  C, Right kidney and *D,* left kidney, longitudinal sections. Bilateral hydronephrosis and renal dysplasia are present.

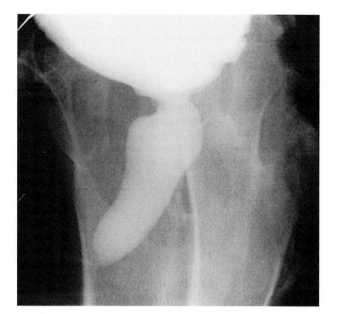

FIGURE 20–7. Posterior urethral valve in a newborn. Voiding cystourethrogram. There is dilatation and elongation of the posterior urethra with an abrupt change in caliber at the site of the valve as well as a prominent indentation on the posterior aspect of the bladder neck.

tion, an accessory urethra that does not communicate with either the bladder or the main urethra opens on the dorsal or ventral surface of the penis. Uncommonly, an accessory urethra arises from the main urethra and ends blindly in the periurethral tissue. In most cases, both the primary urethra and the accessory urethra are in the midline. The ventrally positioned urethra is usually the more functional one and also the urethra that is more easily catheterized regardless of its meatal position. Urethral duplication also occurs as a component of partial or complete caudal duplication anomalies, which include bladder duplication.

Specific clinical symptoms vary with the type of duplication. Patients with patent urethral duplication are either asymptomatic or exhibit a double urinary stream. Incontinence, infection, and dysuria are present occasionally.

A voiding cystourethrogram and a retrograde urethrogram, which may require two catheters in some patients, demonstrate the two urethral channels.

Congenital Urethral Stricture

A true congenital urethral stricture is one that is limited to a localized narrowing at the junction of the posterior and anterior urethra. Segmental urethral stenosis or complete atresia is rarely seen, often in association with severe cases of prune-belly syndrome.

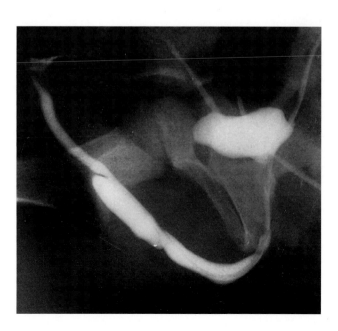

FIGURE 20–8. Congenital diverticulum of the urethra. Voiding cystourethrogram. The saccular diverticulum is an elongated, oval structure on the ventral aspect of the anterior urethra. (Courtesy of Stanford M. Goldman, M.D., University of Texas, Houston, Texas.)

NEOPLASMS

Urethral neoplasms are among the least common malignancies of the urinary tract. The histology of these lesions varies with their site of origin in the urethra. The proximal half of the female urethra is lined by transitional epithelium, whereas the mucosa of the distal half is composed of stratified squamous epithelium. The epithelium of the male urethra is more variable. Transitional epithelium lines the prostatic urethra whereas the membranous and most of the anterior urethra is lined by pseudostratified columnar epithelium. The mucosa of the distal urethra, near the meatus, is characterized by stratified squamous epithelium.

Benign Tumors

Fibrous Polyp

This benign lesion arises in the region of the verumontanum and is a rare cause of bladder obstruction in boys. The polyp is pedunculated and composed of a loose, fibrous, connective tissue core covered by transitional cell epithelium.

Both retrograde and voiding cystourethrography demonstrate the mobility of a fibrous polyp, which appears as an oval filling defect, often on a stalk, in the posterior urethra. Prolapse either into the bladder or into the membranous or bulbous urethra occurs during voiding (Fig. 20–9). Ultrasonographically, a fibrous polyp appears as an echogenic polypoid mass in the bladder base.

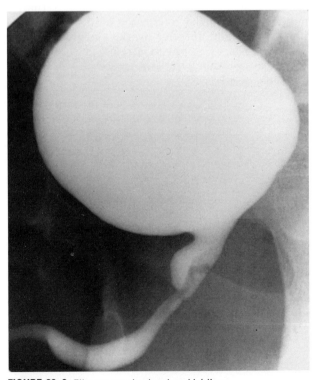

FIGURE 20–9. Fibrous urethral polyp. Voiding cystourethrogram. The polyp appears as an elongated structure in the posterior urethra. (Courtesy of Stanford M. Goldman, M.D., University of Texas, Houston, Texas.)

Papilloma

Urothelial papilloma is an uncommon mucosal lesion with a frondlike morphology and no invasion or significant cellular atypia. Still, it is considered by some to represent a Grade I papillary urothelial carcinoma in view of its risk, albeit low, of recurrence, sometimes as a higher-grade lesion. On urethrography, a small solitary filling defect is seen in a patient with dysuria or hematuria. This lesion should not be confused with squamous papilloma, which is commonly referred to as condylomata acuminata and is discussed later.

Other benign tumors that rarely occur in the urethra or periurethral tissue include *leiomyoma, hemangioma,* and *benign prostatic epithelial polyp.*

Malignant Tumors

Transitional Cell Carcinoma Extending from Bladder

Most cases of transitional cell carcinoma of the urethra represent extension from bladder carcinoma. Therefore, most occur in males, and the prostatic urethra is the most common site involved. Among patients with bladder carcinoma who are to be treated with cystectomy, the incidence of urethral involvement is approximately 10 per cent. In those patients who undergo cystectomy but not urethrectomy for a bladder transitional cell carcinoma, urethral surveillance is required, owing to the risk of subsequent development of malignancy. This typically is not an issue in women in whom cystectomy generally includes urethrectomy.

Primary Urethral Carcinoma

Primary urethral carcinoma is rare, especially in males. Histology parallels the epithelium characteristic of the site of origin. Most urethral carcinomas are of squamous cell origin and arise in the bulbomembranous region of the urethra. The proximal urethra gives rise to transitional cell carcinoma. Adenocarcinoma of the urethra is the least common of all urethral carcinomas and originates in either Cowper's glands or the glands of Littré. In males, the prognosis for transitional cell carcinoma is worse than that for squamous cell carcinoma, possibly because of its location in the proximal urethra where invasion into adjacent pelvic viscera is more likely to occur compared with a tumor of more distal location. Predisposing factors for squamous cell carcinoma of the urethra include chronic irritation, gonoccocal urethritis, urethral trauma, and stricture.

Urethrography demonstrates a long segment of irregular narrowing (Figs. 20–10 and 20–11). With advanced disease, a diffusely infiltrating mass is identified by computed tomography or magnetic resonance imaging (Figs. 20–12 and 20–13). A change in the appearance of a pre-existing stricture or recurrent stricture after urethroplasty raises the suspicion of urethral carcinoma.

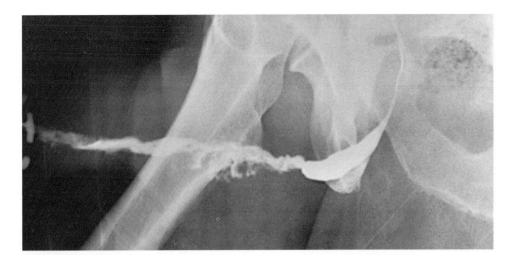

FIGURE 20–10. Squamous cell carcinoma, anterior urethra. Retrograde urethrogram. The tumor produces an irregular narrowing of a long segment of the anterior urethra.

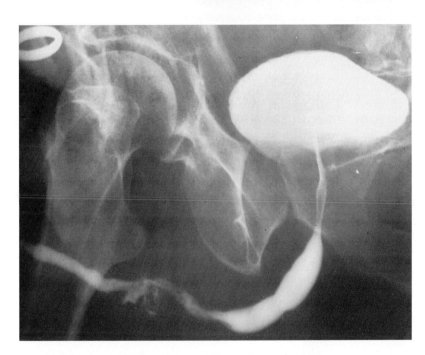

FIGURE 20–11. Squamous cell carcinoma, anterior urethra. Retrograde urethrogram. There is a mass in the distal urethra associated with a long, irregular stricture.

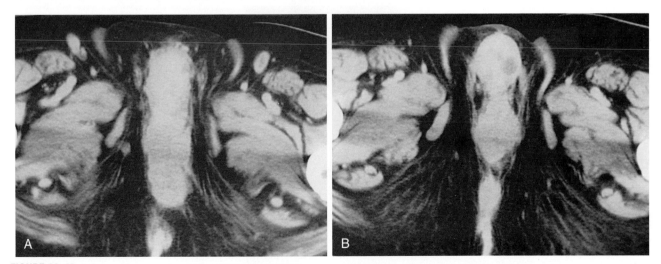

FIGURE 20–12. Advanced squamous cell carcinoma, urethra.
A and *B,* Contrast material–enhanced computed tomogram, transverse sections. The penis is enlarged, irregular and enhances in a heterogeneous pattern. There is extension of tumor into the perineum. (Courtesy of Jade J. Wong-You-Cheong, M.D., University of Maryland, Baltimore, Maryland.)

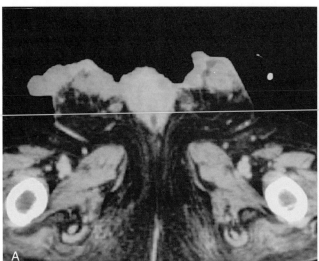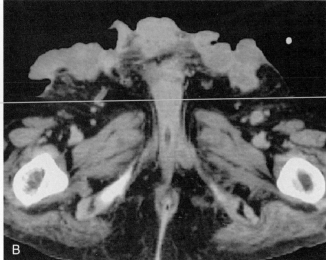

FIGURE 20–13. Advanced squamous cell carcinoma, urethra.
A and *B,* Contrast material–enhanced computed tomogram, transverse sections. A large ulcerated mass involving the base of the penis and surrounding soft tissue is present. (Courtesy of Jade J. Wong-You-Cheong, M.D., University of Maryland, Baltimore, Maryland.)

In women, approximately three-fourths of urethral carcinomas are squamous cell. The distal third of the urethra is the most frequent site for squamous cell carcinoma, whereas transitional cell carcinoma and adenocarcinoma usually involve the proximal urethra. Females with malignant urethral tumors usually develop a bleeding mass. Although urethrography may be useful in some patients, it is often quite limited, owing to difficulty in depicting the female urethra. Cross-sectional techniques, such as magnetic resonance imaging or computed tomography, generally show an invasive mass in the region of the urethra.

Sarcoma

Sarcoma of the urethra is extremely rare. Histologic types include *rhabdomyosarcoma, myxosarcoma,*

malignant fibrous histiocytoma, and *leiomyosarcoma.* These aggressive tumors may infiltrate the soft tissues of the perineum both above and below the urogenital diaphragm and invade adjacent midline viscera.

INFECTION

Gonorrhea

Infection of the urethra by *Neisseria gonorrhoeae* most commonly involves the glands of Littré in the bulbous urethra and frequently leads to stricture formation in this part of the urethra. However, any portion of the urethra may be involved. The bacteria provoke an inflammatory response in the urethral submucosa that is characterized by cell necrosis

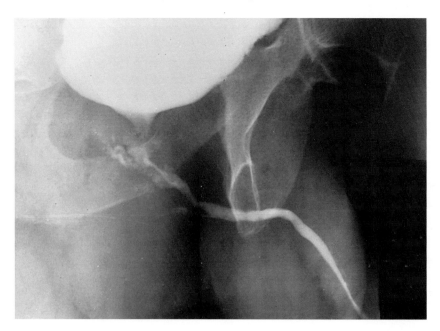

FIGURE 20–14. Gonorrheal urethritis complicated by fistulas and sinuses. Retrograde urethrogram. There is irregular narrowing of the bulbar urethra with multiple sinuses.

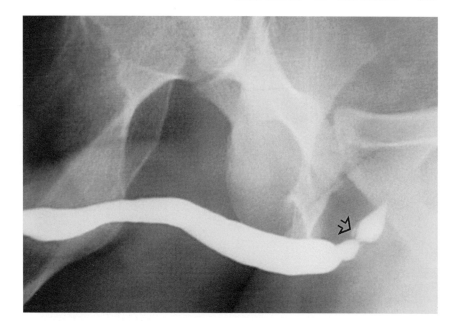

FIGURE 20–15. Gonorrheal urethritis with late stricture. Retrograde urethrogram. There is focal urethral narrowing of the bulbar urethra. Cowper's ducts are faintly seen *(arrow)*.

and granulation tissue. A periurethral abscess that sometimes follows may eventually drain into the urethra and appear as a communicating diverticulum during urethrography. Periurethral abscesses may also evolve into multiple fistulas between the urethra and the perineum, forming the so-called "watering pot" perineum.

The clinical hallmarks of acute gonococcal urethritis are a purulent urethral discharge and dysuria. Acute symptoms may resolve without antibiotic therapy. In the absence of effective therapy for the acute infection, the organism may persist in the glands of Littré, causing a thin urethral discharge and favoring the development of fibrosis and stricture. Obstructive voiding symptoms may occur

months to years after the initial gonococcal infection.

Radiologic evaluation by retrograde urethrography in gonococcal urethritis is usually limited to circumstances in which there are complications of the acute infection. A periurethral abscess that has drained into the urethra is seen as a diverticulum-like collection of contrast material that communicates with the urethra. Fistulas between the urethra and the skin, the "watering pot" perineum, are also opacified during retrograde urethrography (Fig. 20–14). Postgonoccocal strictures are often irregular in appearance, are several centimeters in length, and most often involve the bulbous urethra (Figs. 20–15 and 20–16). There is often associated

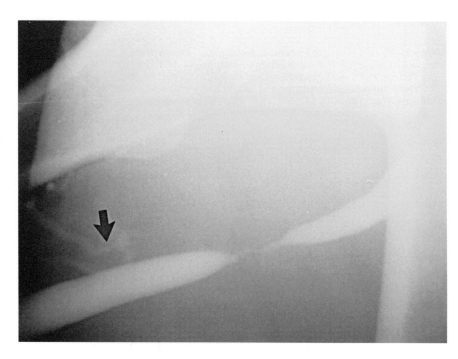

FIGURE 20–16. Gonorrheal urethritis with late stricture. Retrograde urethrogram. There is a long stricture in the bulbous urethra. A small amount of venous intravasation is present *(arrow)*, a result of the pressure required to visualize the stricture. (Courtesy of Jade J. Wong-You-Cheong, M.D., University of Maryland, Baltimore, Maryland.)

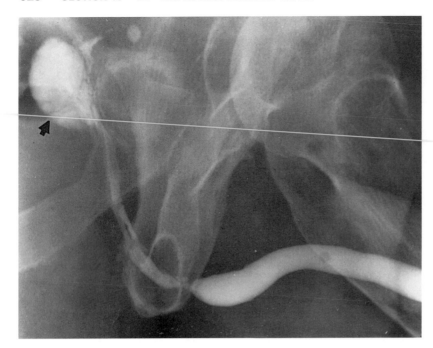

FIGURE 20–17. Gonorrheal urethritis and stricture. Retrograde urethrogram. There is a long stricture of the proximal portion of the bulbous urethra and reflux of contrast material into the prostate *(arrow)*.

FIGURE 20–18. Condylomata acuminata. Retrograde urethrogram. There are multiple filling defects throughout the entire urethra. (From Pollack, H. M., DeBenedictis, T. J., Marmar, J. L., and Praiss, D. E.: Urethrographic manifestations of venereal warts (condylomata acuminata). Radiology *126*:643–646, 1978. Reproduced with kind permission of the authors and *Radiology*.)

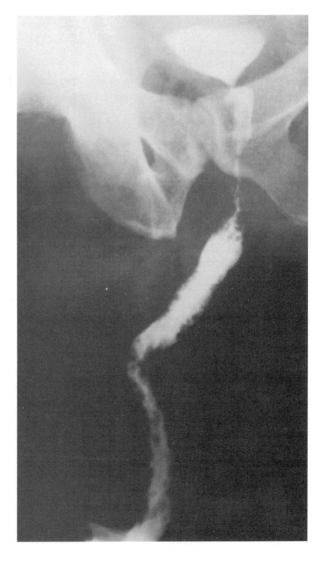

filling of the glands of Littré as well as Cowper's duct and gland. In some patients the stricture may be quite localized. Stricture formation in the most proximal part of the bulbous urethra leads to a loss of the normal cone shape of this segment. When the urethra is examined by voiding cystourethrography, reflux of contrast material into dilated prostatic ducts may be noted (Fig. 20–17). This represents increased hydrostatic pressure proximal to a stricture.

Condylomata Acuminata

Condylomata acuminata, often referred to as *genital warts*, are the result of infection with human papillomavirus. This sexually transmitted disease usually becomes apparent as verrucae on the skin of the penis, perineum, or perianal region. Mucosal lesions occur only in a minority of patients and virtually never in patients without detectable external condylomata. Urethral discharge and irritative voiding symptoms are the usual clinical indicators of urethral mucosal lesions. Involvement of the bladder may also occur.

Urethrography demonstrates multiple filling defects, which may line the entire urethra (Fig. 20–18). The appearance of urethral condylomata may mimic urethral carcinoma. However, a history of sexually transmitted disease and the presence of external condylomata typically point to the correct diagnosis.

Tuberculosis

Tuberculosis of the urethra results from a descending infection from the upper urinary tract or is secondary to tuberculosis of the prostate. Although the prostate is involved in up to 70 per cent of cases of genital tuberculosis, the urethra is rarely affected. When the urethra is involved, the bulbous and membranous segments are the most common sites. Periurethral and prostatic caseating granulomas as well as fistulas between the urethra and the perineum are frequently present. The latter complication causes the same "watering pot" appearance as that described in gonorrhea.

Tuberculosis of the kidney is discussed in Chapter 13, that of the pelvis and ureter in Chapter 15, and that of the bladder in Chapter 19.

Schistosomiasis

Urethritis secondary to *Schistosomiasis haematobium* occurs in association with bladder involvement. Fistulas that develop involve the bulbar urethra, the scrotum, and the perineum. Long strictures of the penile urethra also occur. Schistosomiasis of the prostate often coexists.

Schistosomiasis of the ureter is discussed in Chapter 15 and that of the bladder in Chapter 19.

MISCELLANEOUS
Diverticulum of the Female Urethra

A diverticulum of the female urethra, unlike a congenital diverticulum of the male urethra, is an acquired abnormality that arises from dilatation of periurethral mucous glands. Maternal birth trauma has also been considered as a possible cause. Urinary stasis within the diverticulum leads to stone formation in some patients (Fig. 20–19).

An uncomplicated diverticulum may cause dribbling after completion of voiding. If the diverticulum becomes infected, the clinical findings are those of purulent discharge, dyspareunia, and a palpable mass.

Conventional voiding cystourethrography may demonstrate a diverticulum but is often normal (Fig. 20–20). A calculus may make the diverticulum more conspicuous. Double-balloon urethrography is a consistently successful technique for detecting a diverticulum in the female urethra (Fig. 20–21). This method is often gainfully employed in a patient with strong clinical suspicion for urethral diverticulum and a normal conventional voiding cysto-

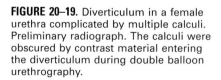

FIGURE 20–19. Diverticulum in a female urethra complicated by multiple calculi. Preliminary radiograph. The calculi were obscured by contrast material entering the diverticulum during double balloon urethrography.

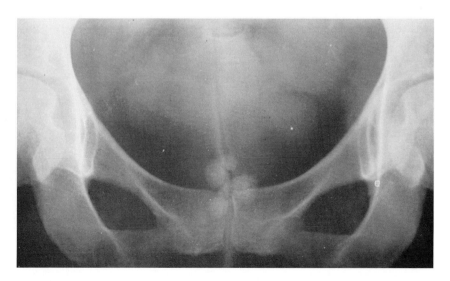

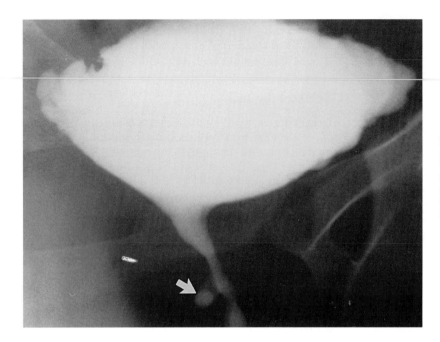

FIGURE 20–20. Small diverticulum of the urethra in a 31-year-old woman with dysuria. Voiding cystourethrogram, oblique view. The diverticulum *(arrow)* is seen posterior to the urethra. (Courtesy of Jade J. Wong-You-Cheong, M.D., University of Maryland, Baltimore, Maryland.)

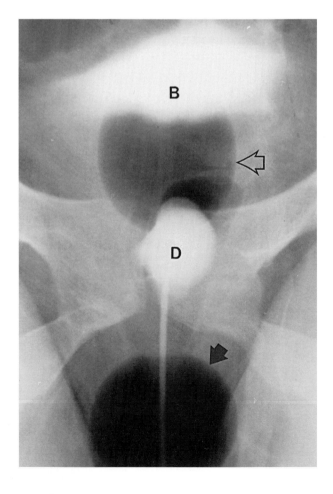

FIGURE 20–21. Diverticulum, female urethra. Double balloon urethrogram. The internal balloon *(open arrow)* of the catheter is at the bladder neck and the external balloon *(closed arrow)* at the urethral orifice. The diverticulum *(D)* is distended with contrast material. A small amount of contrast material is in the bladder *(B)*.

urethrogram. The two balloons are used to increase intraluminal pressure within the urethra by occluding both the internal and external orifices. The goal of this approach is to enlarge the diverticulum and thereby increase the likelihood of detection.

The success of visualizing the diverticulum with transperineal, transvaginal, or transrectal ultrasonography, computed tomography, or magnetic resonance imaging varies with the size and location of the lesion (Fig. 20–22). A diverticulum appears as a structure of bright signal intensity on T2-weighted magnetic resonance images.

Cowper's Duct Cyst

Cowper's glands are paired structures located on either side of the membranous urethra within the urogenital diaphragm. Their ducts enter the proximal bulbar urethra. Cowper's glands function as accessory male sex organs that contribute to semen coagulation and urethral lubrication.

Abnormalities of Cowper's duct are uncommon. Cowper's duct cyst, also called a *syringocele,* occurs most commonly in infants and young children secondary to narrowing of the duct orifice. Clinical findings include recurrent urinary tract infection or irritative and obstructive voiding symptoms. Rarely, Cowper's duct cyst appears as a perineal mass.

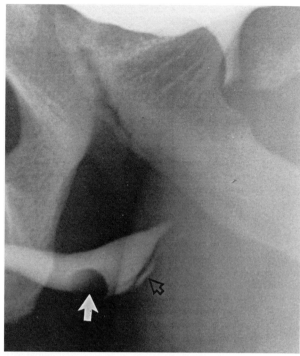

FIGURE 20–23. Cowper's duct cyst. Retrograde urethrogram. The smooth filling defect in the bulbous urethra *(solid arrow)* results from dilatation of the terminal portion of one of Cowper's ducts. The cyst, itself, does not fill with contrast material. There is faint visualization of the contralateral Cowper's duct *(open arrow).* Only a portion of the prostatic urethra is visualized on this study.

The dilated duct is seen radiologically most often as a negative filling defect on the ventral surface of the opacified bulbar urethra (Fig. 20–23). Reflux of contrast material into a patulous or perforated syringocele opacifies the dilated duct.

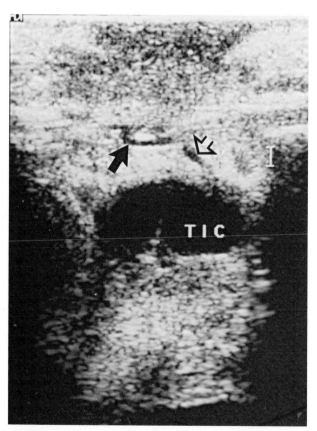

FIGURE 20–22. Diverticulum, female urethra. Ultrasonogram, transverse projection. The diverticulum *(tic)* is connected to the urethra *(closed arrow)* by a thin channel *(open arrow).* (Courtesy of Jade J. Wong-You-Cheong, M.D., University of Maryland, Baltimore, Maryland.)

BIBLIOGRAPHY

Anatomy

Amis, E. S., Jr., Newhouse, J. H., and Cronan, J. J.: Radiology of male periurethral structures. AJR *151*:321, 1988.

Brooks, J. D.: Anatomy of the lower urinary tract and male genitalia. In Walsh, P. C., Retik, A. B., Vaughan, E. D., Jr., and Wein, A. J. (eds.): Campbell's Urology, 7th ed. Philadelphia, W. B. Saunders, 1998, pp. 89–128.

McCallum, R. W.: The adult male urethra: Normal anatomy, pathology and method of urethrography. Radiol. Clin. North Am. *17*:227, 1979.

Siegel, C. L., Middleton, W. O., Teefey, S. A., Weinstein, M. A., McDougall, E. M., and Klutke, C. G.: Sonography of the female urethra. AJR *170*:1269, 1998.

Strohbehn, K., Quint, L. E., Prince, M. R., Wojno, K. J., and Delancey, J. O.: Magnetic resonance imaging anatomy of the female urethra: A direct histologic comparison. Obstet. Gynecol. *88*:750, 1996.

Tan, I. L., Stoker, J., Zwanborn, A. W., Entius, K. A. C., Calame, J. J., and Lameris, J. S.: Female pelvic floor: Endovaginal MR imaging of normal anatomy. Radiology *206*:777, 1998.

Anomalies

Appel, R. A., Kaplan, G. W., Brock, W. A., and Streit, D.: Megalourethra. J. Urol. *135*:747, 1986.

Cremin, B. J.: A review of the ultrasonic appearances of posterior urethral valve and ureteroceles. Pediatr. Radiol. 16:357, 1986.

Das, S., and Brosman, S. A.: Duplication of the male urethra. J. Urol. 117:452, 1977.

Duckett, J. W.: Hypospadias. In Walsh, P. C., Retik, A. B., Vaughan, E. D., Jr., and Wein, A. J. (eds.): Campbell's Urology, 7th ed. Philadelphia, W. B. Saunders, 1998, pp. 2093–2119.

Effmann, E. L., Lebowitz, R. L., and Colodny, A. H.: Duplication of the urethra. Radiology 119:179, 1976.

Gonzales, E. T.: Posterior urethral valves and other urethral anomalies. In Walsh, P. C., Retik, A. B., Vaughan, E. D., Jr., and Wein, A. J. (eds.): Campbell's Urology, 7th ed. Philadelphia, W. B. Saunders, 1998, pp. 2069–2091.

Hill, G. S.: Anomalies of the bladder and urethra. In Hill, G. S. (ed.): Uropathology. New York, Churchill Livingstone, 1989, pp. 235–277.

Hulbert, W. C., and Duckett, J.: Current views on posterior urethral valves. Pediatr. Ann. 17:31, 1988.

Hutton, K. A. R., Thomas D. F. M., and Davies, B. W.: Prenatally detected posterior urethral valves: Qualitative assessment of second trimester scans and prediction of outcome. J. Urol. 158:1022, 1997.

Kirks, D. R., and Grossman, H.: Congenital saccular anterior urethral diverticulum. Radiology 140:367, 1981.

Macpherson, R. I., Leithiser, R. E., Gordon, L., and Turner, W. R.: Posterior urethral valves: An update and review. Radiographics 6:753, 1986.

Mahony, B. S., Callen, P. W., and Filly, R. A.: Fetal urethral obstruction: US evaluation. Radiology 157:221, 1985.

Nurenberg, P., and Zimmern, P. E.: Role of MR imaging with transrectal coil in the evaluation of complex urethral abnormalities. AJR 169:1335, 1997.

Psihramis, K. E., Colodny, A. H., Lebowitz, R. L., Retik, A. B., and Bauer, S. B.: Complete patent duplication of the urethra. J. Urol. 136:63, 1986.

Rosenfeld, B., Greenfield, S. P., Springate, J. E., and Feld, L. G.: Type III posterior urethral valves: Presentation and management. J. Pediatr. Surg. 29:81, 1994.

Scherz, H. C., Kaplan, G. W., and Packer, M. G.: Anterior urethral valves in the fossa navicularis in children. J. Urol. 138:1211, 1987.

Shrom, S. H., Cromie, W. J., and Duckett, J. W.: Megalourethra. Urology 17:152, 1981.

Neoplasms

Bagley, F. H., and Davidson, A. I.: Congenital urethral polyp in a child. Br. J. Urol. 48:278, 1976.

Bolduan, J. P., and Farah, R. N.: Primary urethral neoplasms: Review of 30 cases. J. Urol. 125:198, 1981.

Caro, P. A., Rosenberg, H. K., and Snyder, H. M., III: Congenital urethral polyp. AJR 147:1041, 1986.

Cornella, J. L., Larson, T. R., Lee, R. A., Magrina, J. F., and Kammerer-Doak, D.: Leiomyoma of the female urethra and bladder: Report of twenty-three patients and review of the literature. Am. J. Obstet. Gynecol. 176:1278, 1997.

Craig, J. R., and Hart, W. R.: Benign polyps with prostatic-type epithelium of the urethra. Am. J. Clin. Pathol. 63:343, 1975.

Grabstald, H.: Tumors of the urethra in men and women. Cancer 32:1236, 1973.

Hopkins, S. C., Nag, S. K., and Soloway, M. S.: Primary carcinoma of male urethra. Urology 23:128, 1984.

Kaplan, G. W., Bulkley, G. J., and Grayhack, J. T.: Carcinoma of the male urethra. J. Urol. 98:365, 1967.

Katz, R. S.: Tumors and tumorlike conditions of the male urethra. In Hill, G. S. (ed.): Uropathology. New York, Churchill Livingstone, 1989, pp. 1369–1380.

Kimche, D., and Lask, D.: Congenital polyp of the prostatic urethra. J. Urol. 127:134, 1982.

Levine, R. L.: Urethral cancer. Cancer 45:1965, 1980.

Morikawa, K., Togashi, K., Minami, S., Dodo, Y., Imura, T., Matsumoto, M., and Konishi, J.: MR and CT appearance of urethral clear cell adenocarcinoma in women. J. Comput. Assist. Tomogr. 19:1001, 1995.

Reuter, V. E.: Urethra. In Bostwick, D. G., and Eble, J. N. (eds.): Urologic Surgical Pathology. St. Louis, Mosby–Year Book, 1997, p. 435.

Infection

Berger, R. E.: Sexually transmitted diseases: The classic diseases. In Walsh, P. C., Retik, A. B., Vaughan, E. D., Jr., and Wein, A. J. (eds.): Campbell's Urology, 7th ed. Philadelphia, W. B. Saunders, 1998, pp. 663–684.

Bissada, N. K., Cole, A. T., and Fried, F. A.: Extensive condylomas acuminata of the entire male urethra and the bladder. J. Urol. 112:201, 1974.

McCallum, R. W.: The adult male urethra: Normal anatomy, pathology and method of urethrography. Radiol. Clin. North Am. 17:227, 1979.

Osegbe, D. N., and Amaku, E. O.: Gonococcal strictures in young patients. Urology 18:37, 1981.

Osoba, A. O., and Alausa, O.: Gonococcal urethral stricture and watering-can perineum. Br. J. Vener. Dis. 52:387, 1976.

Pollack, H. M., DeBenedictis, T. J., Marmar, J. L., and Praiss, D. E.: Urethrographic manifestations of venereal warts (condyloma acuminata). Radiology 126:643, 1978.

Sawczuk, I., Badillo, F., and Olsson, C. A.: Condylomata acuminata: Diagnosis and follow-up by retrograde urethrography. Urol. Radiol. 5:273, 1983.

Singh, M., and Blandy, J. P.: The pathology of urethral stricture. J. Urol. 115:673, 1976.

Symes, J. M., and Blandy, J. P.: Tuberculosis of the male urethra. Br. J. Urol. 45:432, 1973.

Tomaszewski, J. E.: Urethritis. In Hill, G. S. (ed.): Uropathology. New York, Churchill Livingstone, 1989, pp. 455–466.

Miscellaneous

Kim, B., Hricak, H., and Tanagho, E. A.: Diagnosis of urethral diverticula in women: Value of MR imaging. AJR 161:809, 1993.

Maizels, M., Stephens, F. D., King, L. R., and Firlit, C. F.: Cowper's syringocele: A classification of dilatations of Cowper's gland duct based upon clinical characteristics of 8 boys. J. Urol. 129:111, 1983.

Neitlich, J. D., Foster, H. E., Glickman, M. G., and Smith, R. C.: Detection of urethral diverticula in women: Comparison of a high resolution fast spin echo technique with double balloon urethrography. J. Urol. 159:408, 1998.

Redman, J. F., and Rountree, G. A.: Pronounced dilatation of Cowper's gland duct manifest as a perineal mass: A recommendation for management. J. Urol. 139:87, 1988.

Sant, G. R., and Kaleli, A.: Cowper's syringocele causing incontinence in an adult. J. Urol. 133:279, 1985.

Siegelman, E. S., Banner, M. P., Ramchandani, P., and Schnall, M. D.: Multicoil MR imaging of symptomatic female urethral and periurethral disease. RadioGraphics 17:349, 1997.

Vargas-Serrano, B., Cortina-Moreno, B., Rodriguez-Romero, R., and Ferreiro-Arguelles, I.: Transrectal ultrasonography in the diagnosis of urethral diverticula in women. J. Clin. Ultrasound 25:21, 1997.

Yaffe, D., and Zissin, R.: Cowper's gland duct: Radiographic findings. Urol. Radiol. 13:123, 1991.

THE RETROPERITONEUM AND ADRENAL

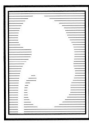

The Retroperitoneum

The advent of computed tomography, ultrasonography, and magnetic resonance imaging has opened a new era for the anatomic study of the retroperitoneum. The spatial and density resolution and cross-sectional anatomic display of computed tomography, augmented by the intrinsic contrast provided by abundant fat usually found in the retroperitoneum, combine to yield images of exquisite accuracy and clinical usefulness. The same attributes apply to images generated by magnetic resonance. Ultrasonography, although effective in defining fluid collections and solid tumors whose echo pattern is distinctive from the normally echogenic retroperitoneal fat, is not as efficacious in evaluating retroperitoneal disorders.

This chapter first presents the anatomy of the retroperitoneum and then describes the various pathologic processes that affect each of the three compartments that constitute the retroperitoneum. This is followed by a discussion of primary retroperitoneal neoplasms, retroperitoneal lymphadenopathy, retroperitoneal fibrosis, and pseudotumors of the retroperitoneum. Excluded from consideration are the solid organs other than the kidney that are contained within the retroperitoneum.

ANATOMY

The retroperitoneum is a large space bounded anteriorly by the posterior parietal peritoneum and posteriorly by the transversalis fascia (Figs. 21–1 through 21–5). The diaphragm marks the cephalic limits, and the level of the pelvic brim marks the approximate caudal extent of this area.

Each side of the retroperitoneum is divided into three compartments by two separate layers of medium to dense collagenous connective tissue fascia, mainly oriented in a coronal plane, one anterior and the other posterior to the kidney and adrenal gland. The *anterior renal fascia* (Gerota's fascia) is a thin layer of connective tissue that is sometimes difficult to distinguish, whereas the *posterior renal fascia* (Zuckerkandl's fascia) is slightly thicker and consistently identifiable. A normal fascial thickness of up to 3 mm has been reported, although most fasciae measure approximately 1 mm (Fig. 21–6). These two sheaths, which together constitute the *renal fascia,* blend together laterally to form a single membrane, the *lateroconal fascia.* This structure extends posterolateral to the ascending or descending colon, where it fuses with the parietal peritoneum. Superiorly, both layers of renal fasciae blend with the diaphragmatic fascia to form the cephalic limit of the retroperitoneum. Inferiorly, the caudal extent is marked by the fusion of anterior and posterior leaves with the iliac fascia and the periureteric connective tissue at the level of the iliac crest. The medial extent of the anterior renal fascia blends into the connective tissue and fat that surrounds the great vessels behind the pancreas and duodenum. The posterior renal fascia fuses along its medial margin with the fascia of the psoas and the quadratus lumborum muscles. These medial relationships effectively close one perirenal space from direct communication with the other side in most instances.

The *renal capsule* is a firm, smooth sheet of fibrous tissue with a thin layer of smooth muscle

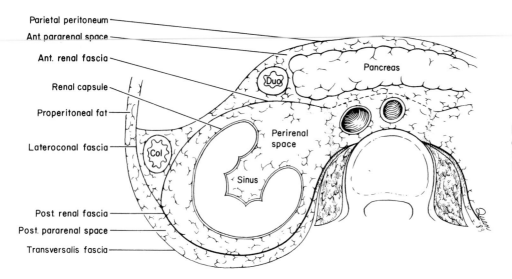

Parietal peritoneum
Ant. pararenal space
Ant. renal fascia
Renal capsule
Properitoneal fat
Lateroconal fascia
Post. renal fascia
Post. pararenal space
Transversalis fascia

Pancreas
Duo
Perirenal space
Col
Sinus

FIGURE 21–1. Diagram of the cross-sectional anatomy of the right retroperitoneum at the level of the renal sinus.

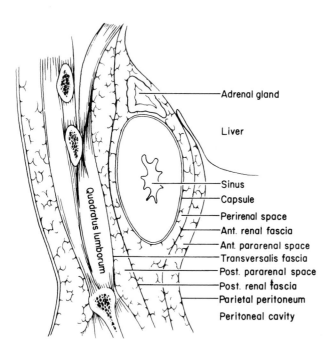

Adrenal gland
Liver
Sinus
Capsule
Perirenal space
Ant. renal fascia
Ant. pararenal space
Transversalis fascia
Post. pararenal space
Post. renal fascia
Parietal peritoneum
Peritoneal cavity
Quadratus lumborum

FIGURE 21–2. Diagram of the parasagittal anatomy of the right retroperitoneum at the level of the renal sinus.

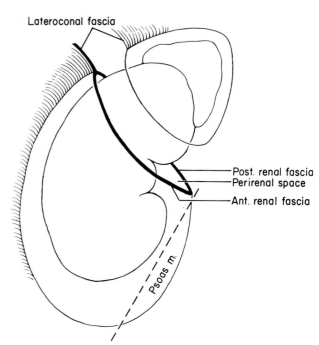

Lateroconal fascia
Post. renal fascia
Perirenal space
Ant. renal fascia
Psoas m.

FIGURE 21–3. Diagram of the right renal fascia in a frontal projection.

FIGURE 21–4. Anatomy of the retroperitoneum. Helical computed tomograms, contrast material–enhanced.

A, Section at the level of the renal sinus. A portion of the left renal vein *(closed arrow)* passes anterior to the renal artery *(open arrow)* and crosses the midline between the aorta and the superior mesenteric artery before entering the inferior vena cava *(c).* Note the relationship of the descending duodenum *(d)* to the right kidney.

B, Section at the level of the lower poles. Note the relationship of the ascending and descending colon *(arrows)* and the descending duodenum *(d)* to the kidneys and perirenal spaces. The various compartments and structures can be identified using Figure 21–1.

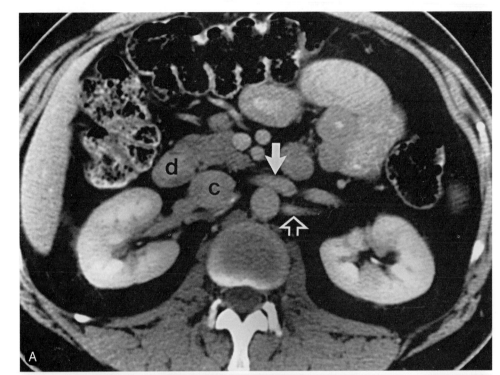

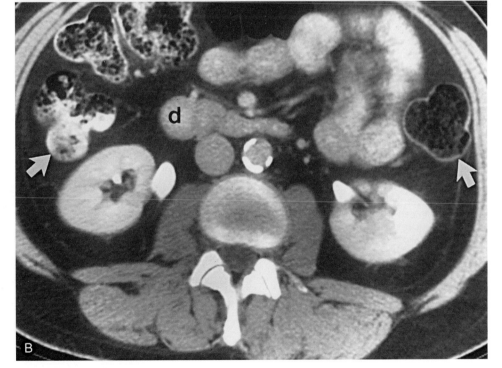

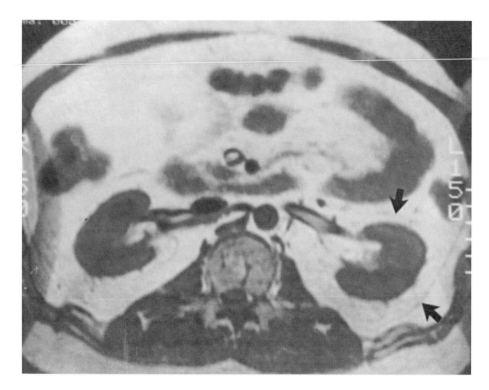

FIGURE 21–5. Anatomy of the retroperitoneum. Magnetic resonance, T1-weighted image. Fat in the perirenal and pararenal space and the renal sinuses is represented by high intensity signal. The fascia around the left kidney is well visualized *(arrows)*.

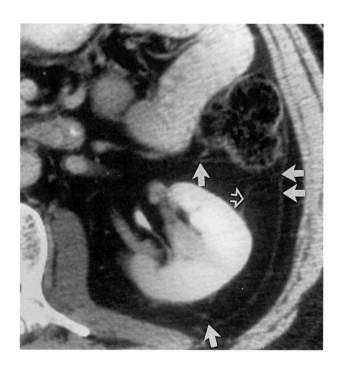

FIGURE 21–6. Normal renal fascia. Computed tomogram, contrast material–enhanced. Anterior and posterior renal fascia *(closed arrows)*; lateroconal fascia *(double solid arrow)*; bridging septum in perirenal space *(open arrow)*.

that invests the kidney. The capsule adheres to the underlying parenchyma through fine connective tissue processes and bridging blood vessels that allow easy stripping of the capsule away from the normal kidney. With disease, the capsule thickens and becomes more adherent. The subcapsular area is a potential space where fluid can collect.

The *perirenal space,* encompassed by the anterior and posterior renal fasciae, contains the kidney and adrenal gland. Abundant fat fills this space, particularly posterior and inferior to the lower pole of the kidney. This fat acts as natural contrast material and accounts for the visualization of the renal outline and the upper one-half of the psoas muscle on standard radiographs (Fig. 21–7). The superior and inferior capsular arteries that originate variably from the main renal artery, its proximal major branches, and the inferior adrenal artery course through the perirenal fat in proximity to the kidney and supply blood to both the capsule and the perirenal fat. The middle capsular artery is a recurrent artery extending from the superior or inferior artery or arising directly from an arcuate branch of the renal artery that perforates the cortex and extends into the perirenal fat. Capsular veins parallel the arteries but have an extensive potential collateral network. The renal sinus is a continuation of the perirenal space where it invaginates into the hilum

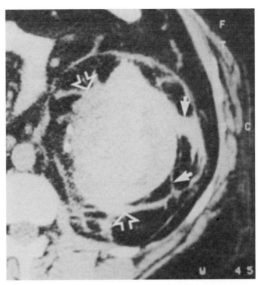

FIGURE 21–8. Prominent bridging septa. Computed tomogram, unenhanced. Extracorporeal shock wave lithotripsy was complicated by perirenal hemorrhage. Blood surrounds the kidney *(open arrows)* and is contained by bridging septa *(solid arrows)* that are parallel to the renal capsule. Perpendicular septa extending to the renal fascia are thickened.

of the kidney. The contents of the sinus (pelvocalyceal system, proximal ureter, and neurovascular and lymphatic structures) are thus contents of the perirenal space. (These are discussed separately in Chapter 16.) The perinephric fat is traversed by fibrils, called *bridging septa* (see Fig. 21–6). These extend from the renal capsule to the renal fascia and are easily visualized when they become thickened by fluid or other disease processes (Fig. 21–8). In addition to connecting the renal capsule and fascia, some of these septations connect the anterior and posterior leaves of the renal fascia, whereas others arise from the capsule and are more or less parallel to the surface of the kidney. The posterior renorenal septum is an important structure that runs from the anterolateral to the posteromedial aspect of the renal capsule.

The *anterior pararenal space* is limited anteriorly by the posterior parietal peritoneum and posteriorly by the anterior renal fascia. The pancreas; the descending, transverse, and ascending duodenum; the ascending and descending colon; and the splenic, hepatic, and proximal superior mesenteric arteries are contained within this space. Unlike the two perirenal spaces, the anterior pararenal space communicates across the midline. Fat deposition in this space is usually sparse. The anterior and posterior pararenal spaces potentially communicate along their inferior margin.

The *posterior pararenal space* is bounded by the transversalis fascia. The medial extent of this space is limited by the fusion of the posterior renal fascia with the fasciae of the psoas and quadratus lumborum muscles. Nevertheless, there is a potential communication with the prevertebral retrocrural

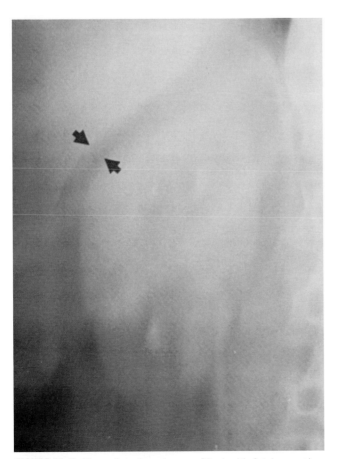

FIGURE 21–7. Normal perirenal space filled with fat *(arrows).* Excretory urogram, tomogram.

space, which, in turn, leads to the mediastinum. Laterally, the fat of the posterior pararenal space continues as the properitoneal "flank stripe." The fat of this space outlines the lower one-half of the psoas muscle. The posterior pararenal space contains no organs.

ABNORMALITIES OF THE RETROPERITONEAL SPACES

Renal Fasciae

The renal fasciae, even when abnormal, are visualized infrequently during excretory urography and then almost always with tomography. During computed tomography, on the other hand, the fasciae are seen in most normal individuals. Edema, hyperemia, or fibrosis thicken the fasciae in a variety of conditions, including nephrolithiasis, upper urinary tract infection, carcinoma, lymphoma, subcapsular hematoma, renal infarction, and prior renal surgery (Figs. 21–9, 21–10). Nonrenal causes of fascial thickening include leaking abdominal aneurysm, infection of the perinephric space, acute or chronic pancreatitis, retroperitoneal tumor, pancreatic carcinoma, peritonitis, ascites due to cirrhosis, retroperitoneal fibrosis, and radiation therapy.

Perirenal Space

Fluid. Abnormalities that arise either within the kidney or within structures of the adjacent retroperitoneal spaces may cause fluid to accumulate in the perirenal space. The most common fluid accumulations are blood, pus, and urine.

Fluid that collects slowly and in small to moderate amounts usually localizes in the posterior and inferior aspects of the perirenal space, behind and below the lower pole of the kidney (Figs. 21–11, 21–12). Acute distention of the perirenal space by a large amount of fluid transforms the normal inferomedial orientation of this space into a vertical axis, obliterates the outline of the kidney and upper one-half of the psoas muscle, and displaces the kidney in an anterior, medial, and superior direction. When the volume of fluid is extensive, anterior displacement of the descending duodenum or lateral displacement of the retroperitoneal part of the ascending or descending colon, or both, may occur depending on the location of the fluid. Occasionally a large perirenal collection of fluid causes a concave deformity of the renal contour similar to that seen with a subcapsular fluid collection (Fig. 21–13).

A *perirenal hematoma* may result from trauma; leaking aneurysm; renal, adrenal, or other retroper-

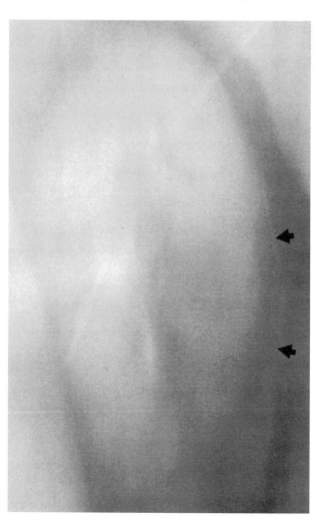

FIGURE 21–9. Thickened renal fascia *(arrows)* in a 70-year-old man with chronic urinary tract infection. Excretory urogram.

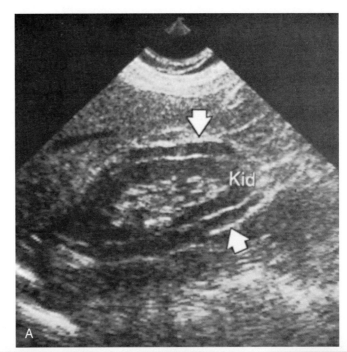

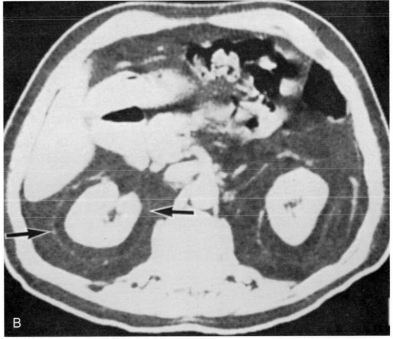

FIGURE 21–10. Thickened renal fascia.
A, Ultrasonogram, longitudinal section, supine. Right kidney *(Kid).* The renal fascia is identified by arrows.
B, Computed tomogram. Arrows identify thickened fasciae.
(Courtesy of Department of Radiology, Vancouver General Hospital, Vancouver, British Columbia, Canada.)

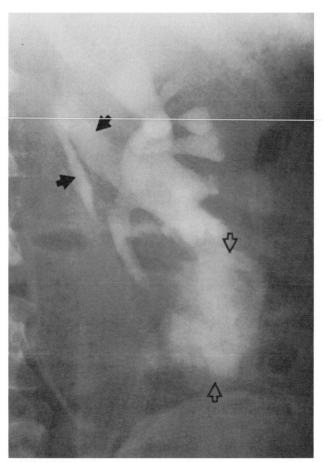

FIGURE 21–11. Perirenal leakage of urine due to subacute obstruction 7 days after pyelolithotomy. Opacified urine has collected medial to the kidney *(solid arrows)* and posterior and inferior to the lower pole of the kidney *(open arrows)*. Excretory urogram.

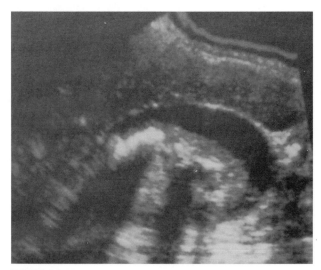

FIGURE 21–12. Large perirenal fluid collection of urine in a patient with chronic obstruction of the right kidney due to urolithiasis. The localization of the urine is atypical in being mainly anterior. Note the acoustic shadows caused by urolithiasis and the thickened renal fascia. Ultrasonogram, longitudinal axis, supine. (Courtesy of Hedvig Hricak, M.D., University of California, San Francisco.)

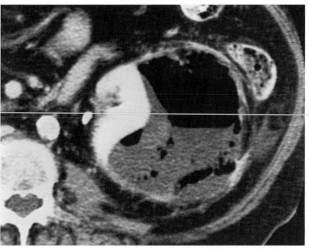

FIGURE 21–13. Perinephric abscess. The kidney is compressed by fluid and gas in the perinephric space. The renal fascia is thickened. Computed tomogram, contrast material–enhanced.

itoneal tumors; vasculitis; bleeding diathesis; renal infarct; or renal cyst. Fresh blood typically has a homogeneous attenuation value of 50 to 80 Hounsfield units. Five to 15 days after hemorrhage, clumps of high attenuation material are usually intermingled with surrounding water-density fluid (Fig. 21–14). Nontraumatic perirenal hemorrhage is often termed *spontaneous* (Fig. 21–15). Carcinoma and angiomyolipoma of the kidney are each the cause of approximately 30 per cent of cases of spontaneous perirenal hematoma. For patients with a spontaneous perirenal hematoma in whom a mass is not detected on initial computed tomography, serial repeat examinations should be performed until the hematoma has completely resolved.

Pus from suppurative processes, either in the kidney or in the pararenal spaces, may extend into the perirenal space (see Fig. 21–13). In pancreatitis, this is facilitated by the release of digestive enzymes, which, at a minimum, increase the density of perirenal fat owing to edema.

Urine may leak into the perirenal space as a result of an acute or subacute outflow obstruction, as occurs with ureteral obstruction or penetrating or blunt trauma (Fig. 21–16). In the case of acute obstruction due to stone, urine enters the perirenal space through rupture of a calyceal fornix that is distended by increased hydrostatic pressure in the pelvocalyceal system. When patients are studied with excretory urography, the contrast material–induced osmotic diuresis adds to the already elevated pressure of urine in the renal pelvis. Thus, the likelihood of forniceal rupture and urine leakage increases with the amount of contrast material given. Rupture may also occur from a previously dilated calyx and progress directly through the renal parenchyma and into the subcapsular and perirenal spaces. This situation is likely to occur when pre-existing disease has thinned the parenchyma. Acute leakage of urine into the perirenal space due

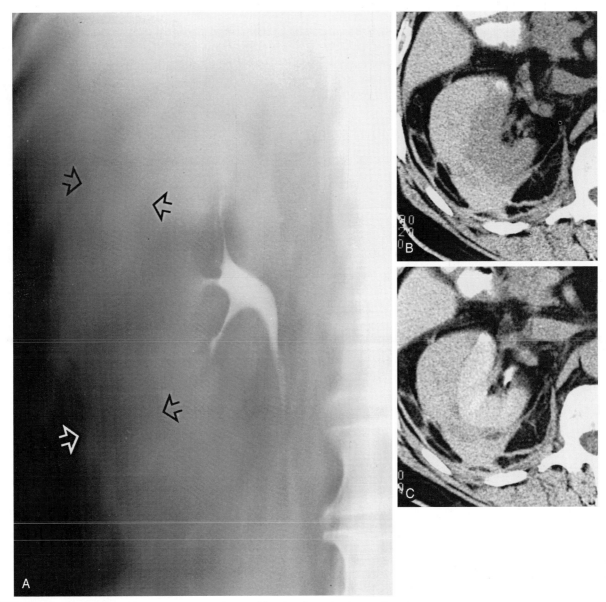

FIGURE 21–14. Acute perirenal hematoma secondary to bleeding in a simple renal cyst.

A, Excretory urogram. Blood in the perirenal space replaces perirenal fat and creates a soft tissue mantle *(open arrows)* surrounding the enhanced kidney.

B, Computed tomogram, unenhanced. The fresh blood that fills the perirenal space is of higher density than the unenhanced renal parenchyma.

C, Computed tomogram, contrast material–enhanced. With enhancement, the perirenal blood becomes less dense relative to the renal parenchyma.

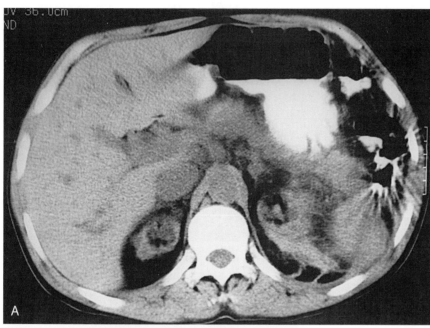

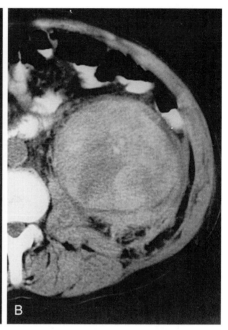

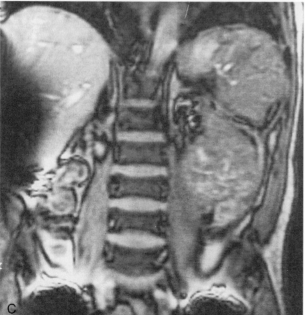

FIGURE 21–15. Large left retroperitoneal hematoma secondary to hemorrhage from left kidney. End-stage renal disease complicated by acquired cystic kidney disease in a 42-year-old man. Same patient is illustrated in Figure 7–16.

A, Computed tomogram, unenhanced at level of kidneys, which are bilaterally small with multiple cysts. Fresh blood of a density slightly higher than that of the kidney is present in the posterior aspect of the left kidney.

B, Computed tomogram, unenhanced, lower abdomen. There is a large hematoma expanding the caudal aspect of the perirenal space.

C, T1-weighted gradient echo sequence magnetic resonance image. The hematoma exhibits mixed signal intensity.

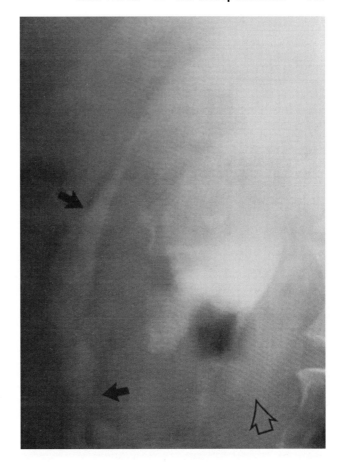

FIGURE 21–16. Perirenal urine collection following subacute obstruction of the right proximal ureter by a metastasis from a colon tumor in a 71-year-old man. Opacified urine can be detected in the perirenal space *(closed arrows)* and the renal sinus *(open arrow)*. Excretory urogram.

to trauma occurs at any point where the pelvocalyceal system or proximal ureter is disrupted.

Urine that slowly leaks into the perirenal space over a long period of time creates a unique condition known as *urinoma*. This urine collection has also been termed a *uriniferous perirenal pseudocyst, pseudohydronephrosis, hydrocele renalis, perirenal cyst, perinephric cyst,* and *pararenal pseudocyst.* Here, an encapsulated extrapelvocalyceal collection of urine forms from urine leakage through a rent in the collecting system or the proximal ureter when chronic ureteral obstruction is present. Accidental or surgical trauma, congenital obstruction in children, ureteral tumor, stone, blood clot, and periureteric fibrosis are among the usual causes of the obstruction. As urine leaks into the perirenal space, normal fat is transformed into a dense, reddish fibrous mass that is covered by distended veins. The wall of this pseudocyst contains fatty or fibrous debris, blood clot, and crystals of urine salts. The mature pseudocyst is the end result of this process of lipolysis and fibroblastic round cell stimulation. A false capsule forms within 2 weeks and matures in approximately 6 weeks.

Clinical manifestations of urinoma are a palpable flank mass and vague abdominal distress or tenderness. There is little, if any, fever. The mass appears slowly after the initiating event, often with a latent period of 4 or more months.

Urinoma has a radiologic appearance of a soft tissue mass whose axis usually, but not always, approximates the cone of renal fascia (see Fig. 21–3). Large lesions displace the kidney superiorly and deviate the lower pole laterally. The proximal ureter is sometimes displaced medially, occasionally to an extreme degree. Perirenal fat remote from the urinoma remains uninvolved so that both the upper psoas margin and the contour of the superior half of the kidney are preserved. Additionally, radiologic and ultrasonographic findings of chronic obstruction are present. Active extravasation is sometimes seen following injection of contrast material (Fig. 21–17). The fluid nature of the urinoma can be accurately defined by ultrasonography, computed tomography, or magnetic resonance imaging. Debris or blood may produce low-level echoes or raise the computed tomographic attenuation values.

Tumor. Tumor involvement of the perirenal space usually occurs by direct extension from the kidney or the pararenal spaces, although rarely primary tumors arise directly from perirenal fat (see Figs. 21–25 and 21–26). Primary tumors arising in the perirenal space are discussed in the following section. Whereas fluid in the perirenal space usually has a homogeneous density and is smoothly marginated, as seen by cross-sectional imaging methods, malignant tumors are often inhomogeneous and have irregular margins and attenuation values that are greater than the patient's normal fat. Contrast material enhancement often occurs in

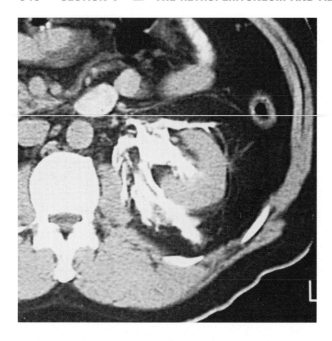

FIGURE 21–17. Urinoma complicating acute obstruction. Computed tomogram, contrast material–enhanced. Contrast material fills the renal sinus and perirenal space.

solid perirenal tumors. Tumors in the perirenal space may obstruct lymphathic channels, leading to linear strands of density in the fat of the perinephric space. This is particularly true with lymphoma and other malignancies with lymphatic involvement.

Caution should be exercised in assessing invasiveness of a tumor by computed tomography or magnetic resonance imaging. A bulky tumor may intimately contact an adjacent space or organ without actual invasion. Contiguity of structures, therefore, should not by itself be used as evidence for invasion in the staging of tumors.

Gas. Gas may extend into the perirenal space from a gas-forming renal infection, from penetrat-

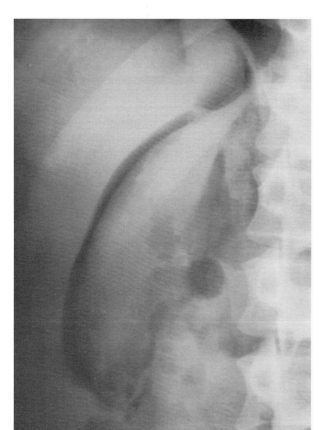

FIGURE 21–18. Gas in the right perirenal space due to perforation of descending duodenum. (Courtesy of Hedvig Hricak, M.D., University of California, San Francisco.)

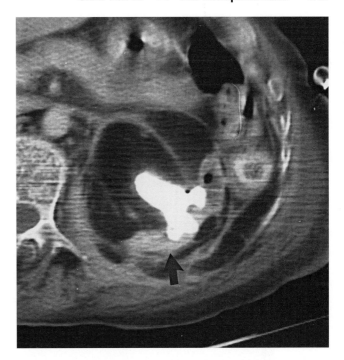

FIGURE 21–19. Replacement lipomatosis, left kidney, in a patient with chronic urinary tract infection and staghorn calculus. Computed tomogram, contrast material–enhanced. The left kidney *(arrow)* is wasted and a large staghorn calculus is present. There is marked proliferation of renal sinus and perirenal fat. Same patient is illustrated in Figure 16–9.

ing trauma, by extension from the pararenal space, or by spread from the extraperitoneal portion of the true pelvis (see Fig. 21–13). Pancreatic inflammation, perforated duodenum, and diverticulitis are the usual causes of perirenal gas that originates in the anterior pararenal space (Fig. 21–18).

Fat. Peripelvic fat, including that of the renal sinus, as well as pararenal fat, may become diffusely increased in obesity, in pelvic lipomatosis, in Cushing's syndrome, and in association with aging. Severe renal parenchymal atrophy may be associated with massive fat deposition in the renal sinus and perinephric space. This phenomenon is known as *replacement lipomatosis* and is usually associated with long-standing renal inflammatory disease (Fig. 21–19).

Abnormal Vessels. Renal venous collaterals enlarge in renal vein thrombosis and are seen by computed tomography as a network of fine, linear densities in the perirenal fat that may be difficult to distinguish from fibrous septa (Fig. 21–20). A multitude of pathways exist and include the following veins: renoazygous, gastrorenal, adrenolumbar, inferior phrenic, adrenorenal, splenorenal, reno-

FIGURE 21–20. Renal venous collaterals in a patient with occlusion of the left renal vein secondary to metastatic deposits in the left renal sinus and around the aorta and inferior vena cava. Fine linear densities in the perirenal fat represent venous collaterals. These may be difficult to distinguish from fibrous septa. Computed tomogram, contrast material–enhanced.

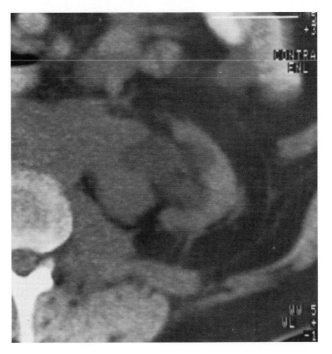

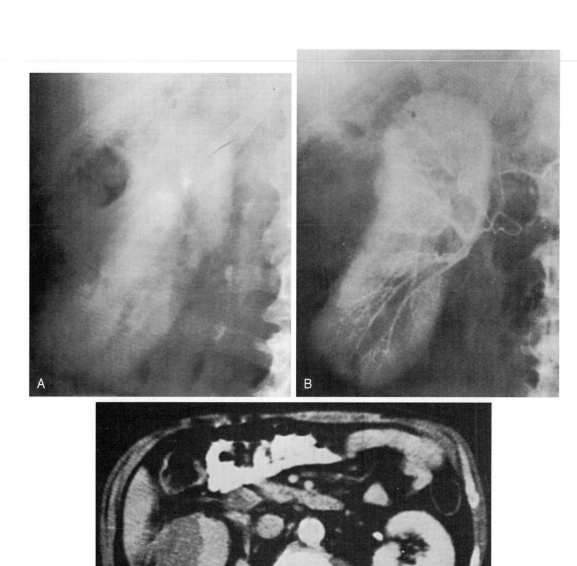

FIGURE 21–21. Subcapsular hematoma forming in the right kidney as a result of an acute lobar infarction. The fluid is confined by the capsule and causes a broad concave deformity of the underlying renal parenchyma. Note absence of a beak sign indicating the extrarenal location of the hematoma.

A, Excretory urogram.

B, Selective arteriogram, late arterial phase.

C, Computed tomogram, contrast material–enhanced.

(Courtesy of Stuart London, M.D., Oakland, California.)

lumbar, gonadal, and ureteral. These veins pass through perirenal fat and provide systemic or portal drainage from the kidney by way of subcapsular and perforating renal veins.

Subcapsular Space

Fluid is considered subcapsular, or potentially within a renorenal septum, when it is immediately contiguous with a portion of the renal parenchyma and flattens its normal convex border. Typically, fat is present between the fluid collection and Gerota's fascia, which is preserved. In contrast, a fluid collection is diagnosed as perinephric when it surrounds a major portion of the kidney, is contiguous with and obliterates the renal fascia, replaces the normal perinephric fat, and typically does not flatten or distort the renal contour.

The most common subcapsular or localized perinephric fluid collection is blood. Although there are many non-neoplastic causes such as trauma, vasculitis, bleeding diathesis, renal infarction, and intrinsic renal disease (Fig. 21–21), carcinoma or angiomyolipoma of the kidney must always be considered as the cause, especially in a nontraumatic or spontaneous setting. Pus is less likely to accumulate in the subcapsular space or localized perinephric space, as the proteolytic enzymes often enable direct extension through the capsule, septa, and even the renal fascia into the paranephric spaces. Occasionally, a subcapsular or localized perinephric hematoma becomes secondarily infected, resulting in a thick-walled localized inflammatory mass. Most frequently, subcapsular or localized perinephric fluid collections are identified following trauma. Management is usually conservative, and most cases resolve spontaneously. Less commonly, however, the hematoma does not resolve and becomes chronic. Renovascular (ischemic) hypertension may follow, a phenomenon known as *Page kidney*. Biconvex, lentiform calcification is characteristic of chronic subcapsular or loculated perinephric hemorrhage (Fig. 21–22).

Anterior Pararenal Space

Pancreatitis is the most common cause of a fluid collection in the anterior pararenal space. Large fluid collections in the anterior pararenal space extend toward the peritoneal cavity, displacing the small intestine ventrally and the ascending or descending colon laterally (Fig. 21–23). The properitoneal "flank stripe," renal outline, perirenal fat, and psoas margins are maintained. Proteolytic enzymes disrupt the small septal fibers that connect the lateral conal fascia to the anterior renal fascia. Fluid dissects between the two major layers of the posterior renal fascia, producing a characteristic wedge-shaped appearance of the retrorenal fluid. Typically the fat within the posterior pararenal space is compressed but preserved.

Posterior Pararenal Space

Abnormalities of the posterior pararenal space develop through the spread of disease from the anterior pararenal space, the retrocrural space, extraperitoneal pelvic structures, the perirenal space, or adjacent organs. Spontaneous hemorrhage, extension of osteomyelitis of the spine, and lymphatic extension of tumor from the pelvis or lower extremities are several examples. Primary tumors of posterior pararenal fat and connective tissue occur as well.

Abnormalities that extend into the posterior pararenal space obliterate the lower one-half of the

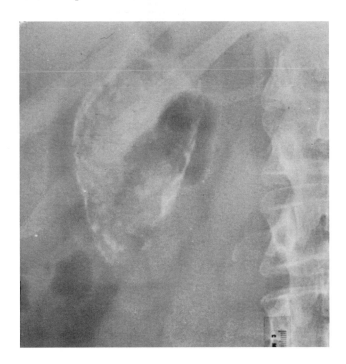

FIGURE 21–22. Chronic, calcified subcapsular or localized perinephric hemorrhage. Plain abdominal film. There is a biconvex, lentiform calcification overlying the lateral margin of the right kidney.

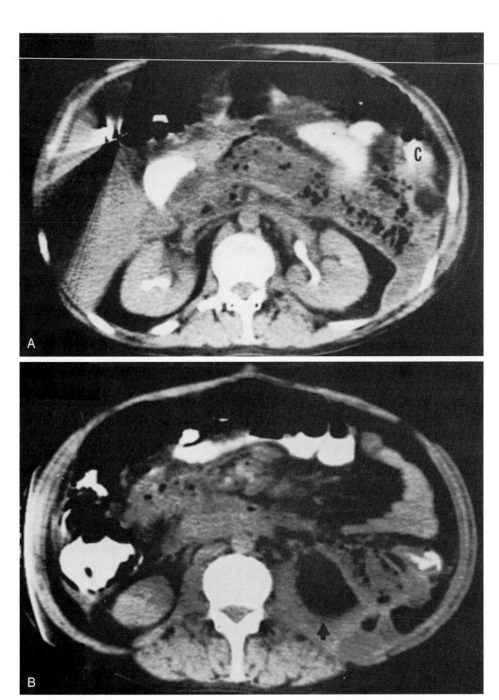

FIGURE 21–23. Abscess in the anterior pararenal space due to acute pancreatitis. The abscess, which also contains gas, points toward the peritoneal cavity and displaces the descending colon *(C)* anteriorly and laterally. Note preservation of the integrity of the renal fascia and the perirenal space.

    A, Computed tomogram with contrast material enhancement at the level of the renal sinus.

    B, Computed tomogram at the level of the inferior cone of the renal fascia. Note the extension of the abscess into the posterior pararenal space *(arrow)* and preservation of the perirenal space within the cone of the renal fascia.

    (Courtesy of Philip M. Weinerman, M.D., Ohio State University, Columbus, Ohio.)

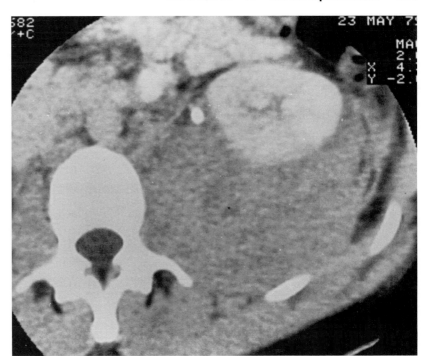

FIGURE 21–24. Posterior paranephric and perinephric hemorrhage following renal biopsy. Computed tomogram, contrast material–enhanced. The hematoma, which is less dense than the enhanced kidney, displaces the kidney anteriorly and obliterates both the psoas muscles and the posterior renal fascia.

psoas muscle and the properitoneal flank stripe. The kidney may be displaced in an anterior and superior direction (Fig. 21–24). Fluid collections have an inferomedial axis similar to that of the inferior cone of the perirenal fascia.

PRIMARY RETROPERITONEAL TUMORS

The term *primary retroperitoneal tumor* is reserved for a neoplasm that originates within the soft tissue between the parietal peritoneum and transversalis fascia but does not arise from a retroperitoneal organ such as the kidney or adrenal gland. Most primary retroperitoneal neoplasms arise from mesenchyme, neurogenic tissue, or embryonic rests, as summarized in Table 21–1. Using this definition, and by including lymph nodes as a retroperitoneal organ, lymphoma is not considered a primary retroperitoneal tumor. Lymphangioma, although best considered a developmental malformation and not a true neoplasm, is an important retroperitoneal mass that can be confused with primary retroperitoneal tumors.

To establish the diagnosis of a primary retroperitoneal tumor radiologically and pathologically, it is necessary to demonstrate that the mass is truly retroperitoneal in location, yet one that does not originate from a retroperitoneal organ. This can be quite difficult or impossible when the tumor is very large or there has been invasion into adjacent viscera. Of principal importance for surgical planning, however, is establishing the extent of involvement and the relationship of the tumor to normal structures.

Because of the obscure nature of symptoms produced by retroperitoneal tumors, they tend to be large at the time of diagnosis. Initial radiologic investigation often includes abdominal radiography and contrast material studies of the gastrointestinal tract or urinary tract. These typically demonstrate a soft tissue mass and displacement of organs without intrinsic involvement. Calcification may be present, but is rarely specific enough to be useful in refining diagnostic choices. Formed bone suggests teratoma or, very rarely, mesenchymoma. Fat, seen as a radiolucency on radiographs, occurs in liposarcoma, lipoma, teratoma, or extra-adrenal myelolipoma. However, fat-containing renal angiomyolipoma or adrenal myelolipoma may sometimes simulate the same findings as a fatty primary retroperitoneal tumor.

Once a retroperitoneal tumor is suspected, computed tomography or magnetic resonance imaging should be used (Fig. 21–25). These imaging modalities can determine the likely site of origin and describe the gross morphology. In some cases a specific histologic diagnosis can be confidently predicted on the basis of radiologic features, as in liposarcoma or teratoma. In most cases, however, a differential diagnosis is all that is possible.

Unlike computed tomography, magnetic resonance imaging provides images in the coronal and sagittal planes that are sometimes advantageous in defining the relationship of a retroperitoneal tumor to the kidney, the adrenal gland, or other organs and in assessing the patency of the large vessels of the abdomen (Fig. 21–26). Regarding staging, however, it is important to realize that demonstration of contiguity between a tumor and an adjacent organ, such as the liver, kidney, or bowel, does not necessarily signify invasion. Invasion is most reliably demonstrated by the angiographic demonstration of neovascularity derived from the principal arterial supply to the organ in question. This phe-

TABLE 21–1. Differential Features of the Most Common Primary Retroperitoneal Tumors

TUMOR	FEATURES
Mesenchymal Neoplasms	
Liposarcoma	Fatty component on computed tomography or magnetic resonance imaging (inconstant)
Leiomyosarcoma	Nonfatty; conspicuous necrosis; intravascular component
Malignant fibrous histiocytoma	Nonfatty; less necrotic than leiomyosarcoma; no vascular invasion
Neurogenic Neoplasms	
Nerve sheath tumors	History of neurofibromatosis; dumbbell growth through neural foramen; bone erosion
Neuroblastoma	Occurs in children; paraspinal; elevated vanillylmandelic acid levels; 80% calcify
Ganglioneuroma	Young adults; paraspinal location; bone erosion
Paraganglioma	Hypertension; elevated vanillylmandelic acid levels; paraspinal; very bright on T2-weighted magnetic resonance imaging; positive MIBG scan
Neoplasms Derived from Embryonic Remnants	
Teratoma	Children and young adults; calcification (clumps or shards); cystic component; fat (sebum or adipose tissue); dermoid (Rokitansky) plug
Germ cell malignancies (e.g., yolk sac tumor)	Children or young adults; elevated tumor tissue markers
Extrarenal Wilms' tumor	Children; very rare; arise along urogenital ridge between kidney and gonad
Developmental Malformation	
Lymphangioma	Elongated shape; uniloculated or multiloculated cystic mass, crosses multiple spaces

nomenon is known as *parasitization* of blood vessels by the invading tumor. Radionuclide techniques are of limited use in the evaluation of most retroperitoneal tumors except for specific situations such as the metaiodobenzylguanidine (MIBG) radionuclide scan for suspected paraganglioma. This is discussed in Chapters 2 and 22.

Mesenchymal

Liposarcoma is the most common primary retroperitoneal malignancy of mesenchymal origin. Most lipoposarcomas occur between the fourth and sixth decades of life. Women are slightly more commonly affected than are men. Liposarcoma is a malignancy of undifferentiated mesenchymal cells from its in-

ception rather than a malignant transformation of previously normal retroperitoneal fat. Like other retroperitoneal tumors, symptoms caused by liposarcoma are insidious and the tumor is usually quite large before it is detected. Computed tomographic and magnetic resonance images correlate closely with the histologic findings. Well-differentiated tumors contain fat that has imaging characteristics indistinguishable from those of normal retroperitoneal or subcutaneous fat (Fig. 21–27). Poorly differentiated pleomorphic, round cell, or myxoid liposarcomas often have little to no radiologically detectable fat and therefore are impossible to differentiate from other forms of retroperitoneal tumors that are not fat bearing (Fig. 21–28; see also Fig. 21–26). Eighty to 90 per cent of retroperitoneal liposarcomas have sufficient fat for detection by radiologic techniques. In well-differentiated liposarcoma, the margins of the tumor may be difficult to determine, as tumor fat blends imperceptibly with normal retroperitoneal fat. Complete surgical removal of retroperitoneal liposarcoma is often difficult owing to its infiltrating margins. Recurrence or distant metastases, or both, are common.

Leiomyosarcoma is the second most common primary retroperitoneal tumor derived from mesenchyme. It is thought to arise from smooth muscle within the retroperitoneum, including the wall of the inferior vena cava. Two-thirds to three-fourths of these tumors occur in women, usually in the fifth or sixth decade of life. Three dominant growth patterns for leiomyosarcoma have been identified: completely extravascular (62 per cent), completely intravascular within the lumen of the inferior vena cava (5 per cent), and a pattern of combined extraluminal and intraluminal growth (33 per cent) (Hartman et al., 1992). Extravascular tumors usually present as mass, pain, and weight loss. Tumors with an intraluminal vena caval component may present with Budd-Chiari syndrome, nephrotic syndrome, or lower extremity edema, depending on the extent and location of the tumor thrombus. Necrosis is a conspicuous, pathologic feature of retroperitoneal leiomyosarcoma and is seen radiologically as attenuation values and signal intensities intermediate between soft tissue and uncomplicated fluid. A leiomyosarcoma that does not have a vascular component is seen radiologically as a usually necrotic mass that displaces retroperitoneal organs (Fig. 21–29). This appearance is similar to that of many other primary, non–fat-containing tumors of the retroperitoneum. Radiologic studies are suggestive of leiomyosarcoma when a solid tumor has both extravascular and intravascular components or is completely intravascular and expands the lumen of the inferior vena cava (Fig. 21–30).

Malignant fibrous histiocytoma is the third most common mesenchymal primary retroperitoneal malignancy. These are most commonly detected during the sixth decade of life. Males are slightly more frequently affected than are females. Presenting complaints and physical findings are nonspecific

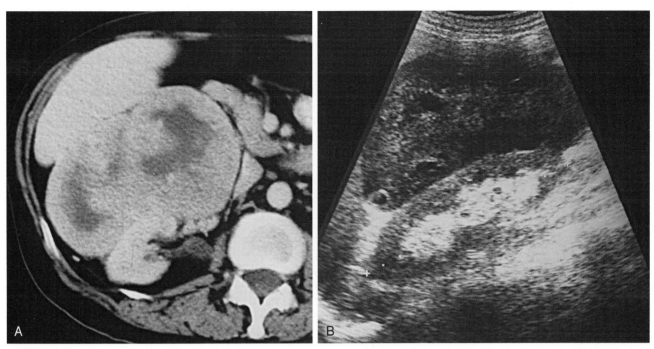

FIGURE 21–25. Large retroperitoneal malignant fibrous histiocytoma in a 61-year-old woman.
   A, Computed tomogram, contrast material–enhanced. The tumor is of heterogeneous density, indicating areas of necrosis, and does not appear to involve the kidney.
   B, Ultrasonogram, longitudinal section. The tumor is of mixed echogenicity and is sharply delineated from the kidney.

and include pain, fever, mass, and weight loss. Radiologic studies usually demonstrate a noncalcified mass displacing adjacent retroperitoneal organs. On computed tomography and magnetic resonance images, malignant fibrous histiocytoma does not contain fat and tends to demonstrate less evidence of necrosis than does the typical leiomyosarcoma (see Fig. 21–25). Most malignant fibrous histiocytomas are moderately vascular or hypervascular. Unlike retroperitoneal leiomyosarcoma, malignant fi-

brous histiocytoma does not involve the inferior vena cava.

Miscellaneous tumors of mesenchymal origin are less common than liposarcoma, leiomyosarcoma, and malignant fibrous histiocytoma. These include malignancies of cartilage, bone, mesothelial tissue,

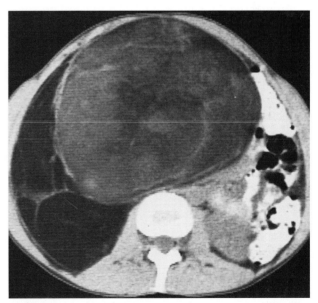

FIGURE 21–27. Liposarcoma. Computed tomogram. A large tumor displaces the aorta and bowel. The tissue in the lateral part of the tumor is well-differentiated fat and is identical in attenuation values to normal retroperitoneal or subcutaneous fat. The medial portion of the tumor is of higher density and represents areas of hemorrhage or poorly differentiated tumor.

FIGURE 21–26. Perinephric liposarcoma. T1-weighted coronal magnetic resonance image. A large mass fills the right perinephric space. The kidney is displaced but is otherwise normal. The tumor does not contain detectable fat.

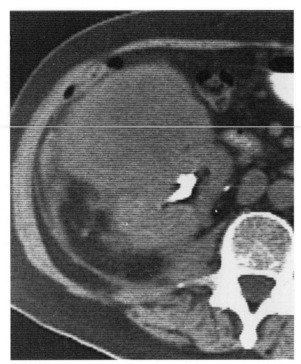

FIGURE 21–28. Liposarcoma, poorly differentiated, invading the kidney. Computed tomogram, contrast material–enhanced. The tumor contains no detectable fat and is inseparable from the kidney.

and blood vessels. There are no distinctive radiologic features associated with any of these tumors.

Neurogenic

Nerve sheath tumors, such as schwannoma or neurofibroma, may present either as a solitary retroperitoneal mass or, in the case of neurofibroma, as a complication of neurofibromatosis. These tumors are usually encountered in patients who are younger than those with mesenchymal tumors. Both males and females are equally affected. Nerve sheath tumors occur along the course of peripheral or sympathetic nerves. They may be benign or malignant. Small tumors are usually well defined and sharply circumscribed (Fig. 21–31). Large tumors often demonstrate necrosis. Although computed tomography and magnetic resonance imaging define, localize, and determine tumor extent, they do not permit differentiation between benign and malignant nerve sheath tumors. The radionuclide gallium, on the other hand, may be useful in this regard, since uptake occurs in malignant but not in benign neural neoplasms.

A diagnosis of nerve sheath tumor may be suggested by clinical or radiologic manifestations of neurofibromatosis, a bilobed dumbbell-shaped mass with one component extending into a neural foramen, or a well-defined mass associated with adjacent smooth erosion of the spine or the undersurface of a rib.

Neuroblastoma, ganglioneuroblastoma, and *ganglioneuroma* are derived from sympathetic ganglion cells. Although most originate within the adrenal medulla, these tumors may arise anywhere along the chain of sympathetic ganglia. Extra-adrenal forms of these tumors, therefore, are paraspinal or presacral-retrorectal in location. Neuroblastoma is the malignant tumor of sympathetic ganglion cells, while ganglioneuroma is the benign form. Ganglioneuroblastoma contains both differentiated and undifferentiated elements, and its biologic behavior is variable. In the newborn, neuroblastoma may rarely differentiate into a less aggressive ganglioneuroblastoma or benign ganglioneuroma, which may persist into adulthood as an asymptomatic tumor (Fig. 21–32).

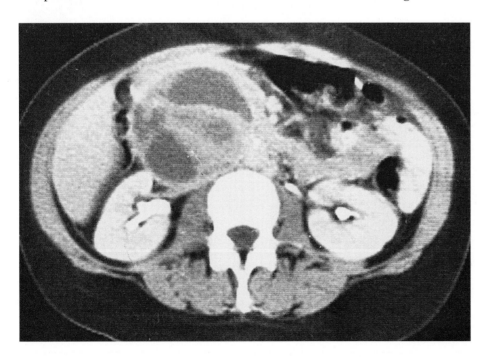

FIGURE 21–29. Extravascular leiomyosarcoma. Computed tomogram, contrast material–enhanced. There is a large mass with low density areas representing necrosis.

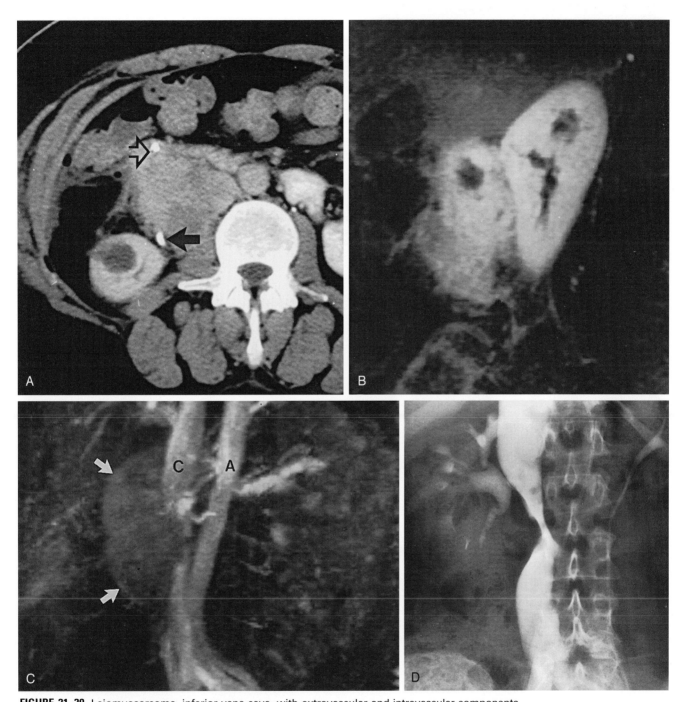

FIGURE 21–30. Leiomyosarcoma, inferior vena cava, with extravascular and intravascular components.

A, Computed tomogram, contrast material–enhanced. The tumor obscures the inferior vena cava and displaces both the duodenum *(open arrow)* and the proximal ureter *(closed arrow).*

B, T1-weighted magnetic resonance image, contrast material–enhanced, sagittal projection. The heterogeneous enhancing mass impresses on the anterior and inferior surface of the kidney.

C, Magnetic resonance angiogram. The mass *(arrows)* arises from the anterolateral wall of the inferior vena cava *(C). A,* Aorta.

D, Inferior vena cavogram. The tumor both displaces the cava and protrudes into its lumen.

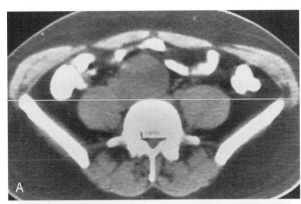

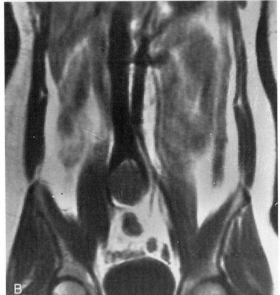

FIGURE 21–31. Nerve sheath tumor. There is a well-defined soft tissue mass near the bifurcation of the aorta and inferior vena cava.
  A, Computed tomogram.
  B, Magnetic resonance image, T1-weighted, coronal section.

FIGURE 21–32. Ganglioneuroma, extra-adrenal, in a 55-year-old asymptomatic woman. The tumor is sharply defined and homogeneous and partially surrounds the inferior vena cava. Computed tomogram, contrast material–enhanced.

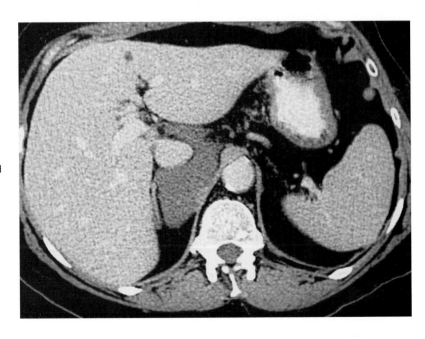

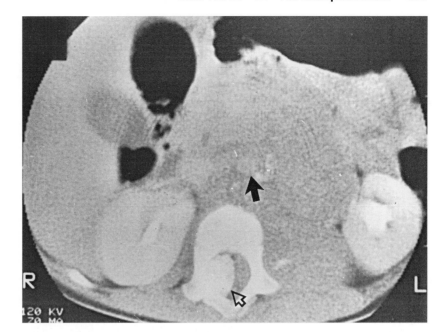

FIGURE 21–33. Neuroblastoma. Computed tomogram after intrathecal and intravenous administration of contrast material. A large calcified mass displaces and partially obstructs the left kidney. The aorta *(solid arrow)* is displaced ventrally. The tumor has invaded the spinal canal and displaces the thecal sac *(open arrow)* to the right.

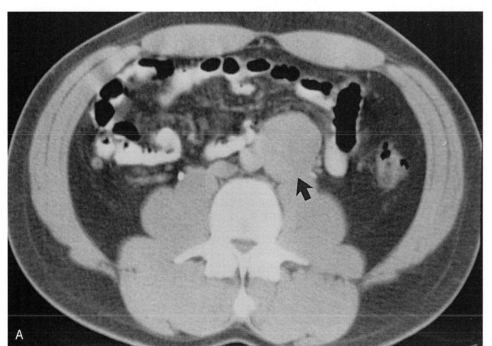

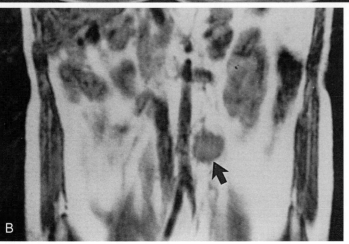

FIGURE 21–34. Paraganglioma located in the organ of Zuckerkandl. There is a well-defined mass *(arrow)* near the aortic bifurcation.
A, Computed tomogram, contrast material–enhanced.
B, Magnetic resonance image, T1-weighted, coronal section.

The clinical and radiologic features of the extra-adrenal sympathoblast-derived tumors are similar to those that arise in the adrenal gland, as discussed in Chapter 22. These include presentation in childhood for neuroblastoma and ganglioneuroblastoma and in young adults for ganglioneuroma, abnormally high levels of urinary vanillylmandelic acid (especially with neuroblastoma and ganglioneuroblastoma), origin in a paraspinal or presacral-retrorectal location, punctate tumoral calcification, and invasion of the spinal canal (Fig. 21–33).

Paraganglioma, like the neuroblastoma line of tumors, usually arises within the adrenal medulla, where it is termed *pheochromocytoma.* Paragangliomas may, however, arise from paraganglionic cells located anywhere along the chain of sympathetic ganglia. Approximately 10 per cent of all paragangliomas are extra-adrenal. Males are affected more frequently than are females. Most patients are diagnosed between the ages of 30 and 45 years. Most paragangliomas are hormonally active and cause clinical findings related to excess secretion of catecholamine. These include headache, sweating, palpitations, and hypertension. Approximately 10 per cent of paragangliomas are multiple and separate. Rarely, a continuous chain of paragangliomas occurs in a paraspinal location, a condition known as *paragangliomatosis.*

The most common location of extra-adrenal, retroperitoneal paraganglioma is between the origin of the inferior mesenteric artery and the aortic bifurcation, a region known as the *organ of Zuckerkandl* (Fig. 21–34). The second most common site of occurrence is the renal hilum (Fig. 21–35). The least frequently involved location is suprarenal and extra-adrenal. Ten to 15 per cent of extra-adrenal paragangliomas are malignant. Although malignant paragangliomas are larger than benign paragangliomas, distinction between benign and malignant cannot be achieved radiologically unless metastases are identified.

Computed tomography typically demonstrates a well-defined para-aortic mass. Tumors less than 7 cm are usually homogeneous and sharply marginated. Larger tumors frequently demonstrate irregular margins and heterogeneous density. Some paragangliomas exhibit very high signal intensity on T2-weighted magnetic resonance images in at least a portion of the tumor. Radionuclide studies with MIBG demonstrate increased activity in the tumor. This technique is especially useful for identifying multiple tumors or metastases, as described in Chapter 2. Imaging features of paraganglioma are similar to those of adrenal pheochromocytoma and are discussed in Chapter 22 (see Figs. 22–13 through 22–15).

Clinical and radiologic features that support a diagnosis of paraganglioma include abnormally high levels of serum catecholamine (75 to 90 per cent of cases), a history of a previously resected paraganglioma or of a predisposing familial syn-

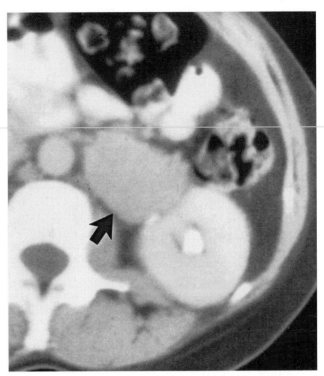

FIGURE 21–35. Paraganglioma, left renal hilum. Computed tomogram, contrast material–enhanced. There is a well-defined extrarenal mass *(arrow)* adjacent to the left renal hilum.

drome such as von Hippel-Lindau disease, neurofibromatosis, or multiple endocrine neoplasias (MEN II), a para-aortic location, high signal intensity on T2-weighted magnetic resonance images, and a positive MIBG radionuclide scan.

Embryonic Remnants

Teratoma is the most common primary retroperitoneal tumor arising from an embryonic rest. Females are more commonly involved than males by a ratio of 3:1. Age distribution is bimodal, with a peak in the first 6 months of life and a second peak in early adulthood. Most retroperitoneal teratomas are mature and displace rather than invade adjacent organs. Complete excision of a mature teratoma is curative, since they neither metastasize nor recur.

The radiologic findings of retroperitoneal teratoma are illustrated in Figure 21–36. Ninety per cent of retroperitoneal teratomas calcify, usually in a pattern of congealed clumps or linear shards. Unlike in ovarian teratomas, formed teeth are very uncommon in primary retroperitoneal teratomas. Seventy-five per cent of retroperitoneal teratomas have a cystic component. A characteristic feature of a cystic teratoma is an eccentric protrusion of either solid or solid and cystic tissue into the cyst. This protrusion, known as a *dermoid plug* or *Rokitansky's body,* is detected in less than 50 per cent of cases. Fat is detected by radiologic techniques in 60 per cent of cases, usually in the form of adipose tissue or, far less commonly, as sebum. Sebum is fat

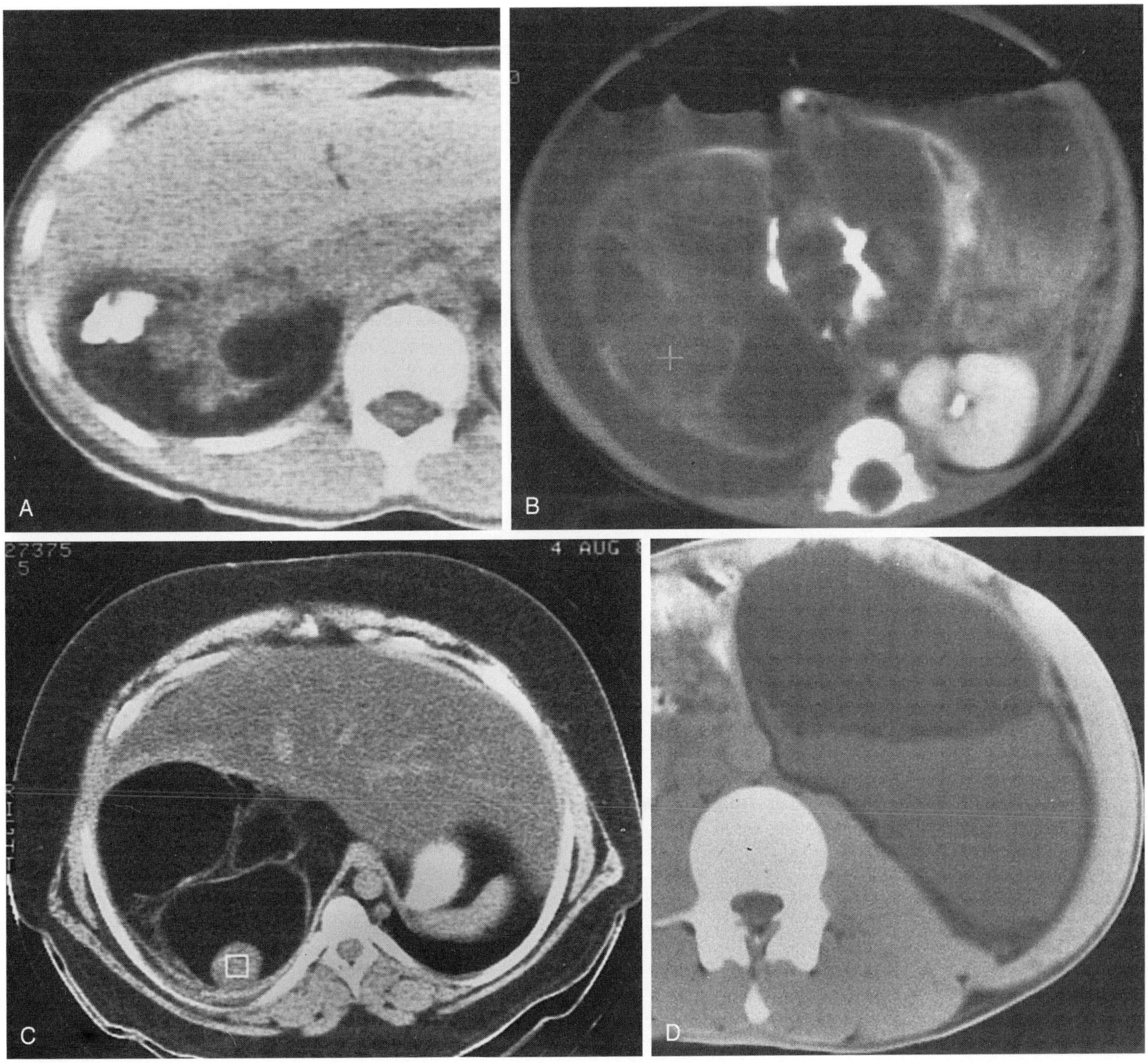

FIGURE 21–36. Teratoma, retroperitoneum. Characteristic radiologic features are illustrated in four different cases.
A, Computed tomogram, contrast material–enhanced. Congealed calcification and adipose tissue.
B, Computed tomogram, contrast material–enhanced. Linear shards of calcification and prominent cysts.
C, Computed tomogram, contrast material–enhanced. Multiple cysts with dermoid plug or Rokitansky's body (cursor).
D, Computed tomogram, unenhanced. Fat-fluid level is representative of sebum.

that is liquid at body temperature and is recognized on computed tomography as a fat-fluid level composed of a negative attenuation value supernatant material and a dependent fluid collection with an attenuation value of water. A fat-containing retroperitoneal tumor in childhood is most likely a teratoma, although a benign lipoma may produce similar features.

Primary retroperitoneal tumors other than teratoma that are derived from embryonic tissue include *germ cell tumors* (Fig. 21–37) and *extrarenal Wilms' tumor.* Primary retroperitoneal germ cell tumors are rare. Most are thought to be metastases from a primary tumor in the testicle that is either occult or has involuted into a fibrotic scar. Similar

to primary germ cell tumors of the testicle, tumor tissue markers, such as alpha-fetoprotein and human chorionic growth hormone, may be elevated in primary germ cell tumors of the retroperitoneum. Extrarenal Wilms' tumor is extremely rare and is thought to originate from the metanephric blastema of the embryonic urogenital ridge. Most, therefore, arise near the midline and between the kidney and the ovary or testicle.

Developmental Malformation

Lymphangioma is a developmental malformation in which lymphangiectasia follows the failure of developing lymphatic tissue to establish normal commu-

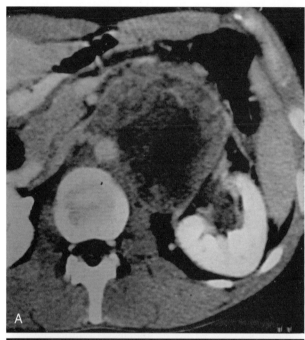

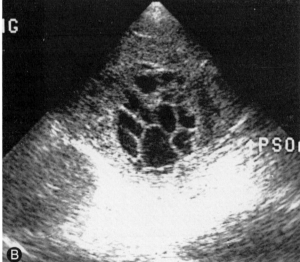

FIGURE 21–37. Endodermal sinus tumor originating in the retroperitoneum. The cystic and necrotic tumor displaces adjacent structures.
  A, Computed tomogram, contrast material–enhanced.
  B, Ultrasonogram, longitudinal section.

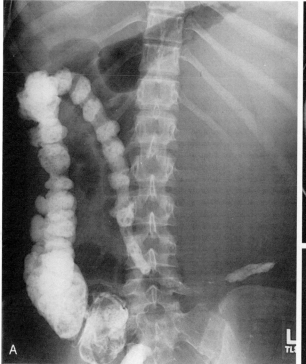

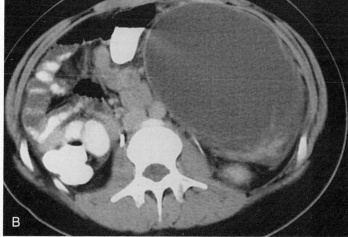

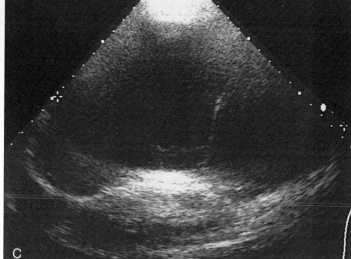

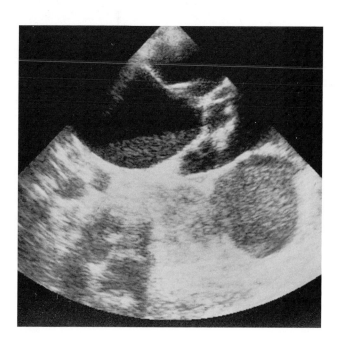

FIGURE 21–38. Lymphangioma, retroperitoneum, in a 17-year-old female. The mass is composed of multiple locules separated by thin septa and containing uncomplicated fluid.

A, Abdominal radiograph. The large left-sided mass displaces the barium-filled transverse colon and splenic flexure caudally.

B, Computed tomogram, contrast material–enhanced.

C, Ultrasonogram, longitudinal section.

FIGURE 21–39. Lymphangioma, retroperitoneum, complicated by hemorrhage or infection. Ultrasonogram, transverse section. Echogenic debris in cysts is shown, some of which is layered in dependent portions of locules.

nication with the remainder of the lymphatic system. Although not a true neoplasm, it must be considered in the diagnosis of retroperitoneal masses. In lymphangioma, abnormal lymphatic channels dilate to form a unilocular or multilocular cystic mass. Lymphangioma is usually discovered early in life, but it may occur in adulthood as well. There is no sex predilection. The most common clinical findings include pain, abdominal distention, fever, fatigue, weight loss, and hematuria.

The most characteristic radiologic features of lymphangioma include a unilocular or multilocular cystic elongated mass that crosses more than one compartment of the retroperitoneum (Fig. 21–38). The ultrasonographic and computed tomographic characteristics of the cyst contents are usually those of uncomplicated fluid. Some solid elements may be present as a result of infection or hemorrhage (Fig. 21–39). Calcification and chyle are uncommon.

RETROPERITONEAL LYMPHADENOPATHY

Retroperitoneal lymph nodes may be para-aortic, paracaval, interaortocaval, renal hilar, and suprahilar. Lymph nodes are recognized as abnormal when they are enlarged, are increased in number, or exhibit abnormal internal architecture.

Spiral computed tomography is the best technique for detecting enlarged retroperitoneal lymph nodes. Structures that must be differentiated from adenopathy include bowel loops, left-sided inferior vena cava, retroaortic or circumaortic left renal vein, dilated normal veins, the diaphragmatic crus, and

retroperitoneal hemorrhage (especially due to aneurysm), and retroperitoneal fibrosis. Accurate assessment requires complete opacification of the small bowel with dilute oral contrast material to distinguish loops of intestine. Intravenous contrast material may be required to identify vascular structures.

Normal lymph nodes are between 3 and 10 mm in diameter and are round or oval structures of soft tissue density in the para-aortic and paracaval areas. Isolated nodes that measure 10 to 15 mm in diameter are suspicious for abnormality. Lymph nodes that exceed 15 mm in cross-sectional diameter are definitely abnormal. It is useful to remember that between the aorta and the left psoas muscle there is normally no extranodal structure larger than 5 mm in diameter. Loss of the normal lateral contour of the aorta strongly suggests para-aortic adenopathy.

Abnormal lymph nodes may be solitary or multiple and may occur in clusters or conglomerate masses (Figs. 21–40, 21–41). In patients with known lymphoproliferative disease, clusters of more than the usual number of normal-sized lymph nodes are usually abnormal. The attenuation value of abnormal lymph nodes varies from low values associated with tissue necrosis through normal tissue density to high density corresponding to hemorrhage (Fig. 21–42). These may be homogeneous or heterogeneous. Very negative attenuation values are seen in *lipoplastic lymphadenopathy* or fatty replacement of lymph nodes. Attenuation values of up to approximately 120 Hounsfield units have been described in patients with Hodgkin's disease or with

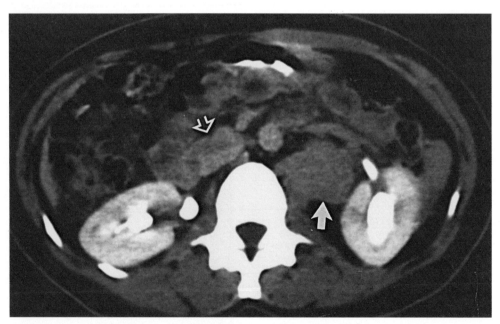

FIGURE 21–40. Retroperitoneal adenopathy due to Castleman's disease. Computed tomogram, contrast material–enhanced. A conglomeration of lymph nodes *(solid arrow)* displaces and obstructs the left kidney. Paracaval lymphadenopathy is also present *(open arrow)* but is difficult to distinguish from intestinal loops because of insufficient oral contrast material.

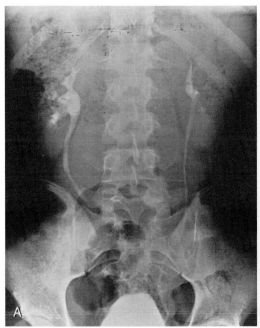

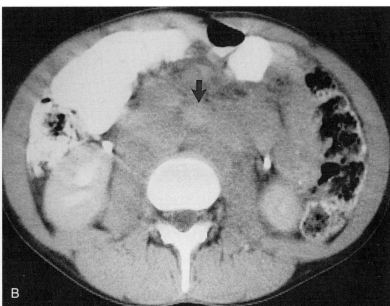

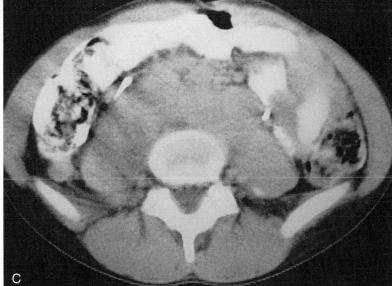

FIGURE 21–41. Lymphadenopathy presenting as a large, bilateral confluent retroperitoneal mass.

A, Excretory urogram. The proximal and mid-ureters are displaced laterally and the left kidney is rotated by the mass of enlarged lymph nodes.

B and *C,* Computed tomograms, contrast material–enhanced. Individual lymph nodes have consolidated into a single large midline and parasagittal mass that displaces the aorta ventrally *(arrow)* and the urinary tract laterally.

(Kindly provided by William R. Corse, D.O., National Naval Medical Center, Bethesda, Maryland.)

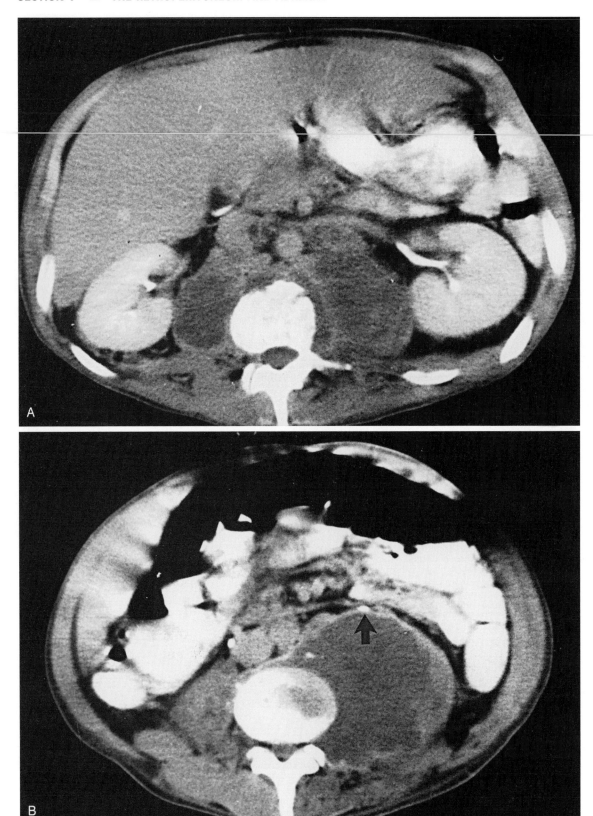

FIGURE 21–42. Lymphoma associated with necrotic lymph nodes extending into the psoas muscles.

A, Computed tomogram, contrast material–enhanced. The mass lateral to the aorta is a necrotic left para-aortic lymph node. Lymph nodes are also present behind the aorta and between the aorta and the inferior vena cava. Enlarged nodes surround and distort the inferior vena cava. Both psoas muscles are involved.

B, Computed tomogram with contrast material enhancement caudal to the area shown in part *A.* The ureter *(arrow)* is displaced anteriorly by an enlarged psoas muscle infiltrated by tumor.

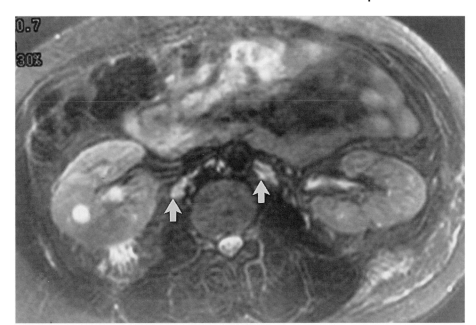

FIGURE 21–43. Lymphadenopathy due to metastatic renal adenocarcinoma detected by magnetic resonance imaging. Fat-suppressed fast spin-echo T2-weighted image demonstrates multiple small lymph nodes *(arrows)* adjacent to the inferior vena cava and aorta. A high signal intensity cyst and perinephric strands are present on the right.

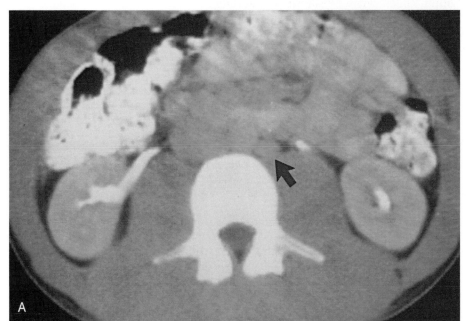

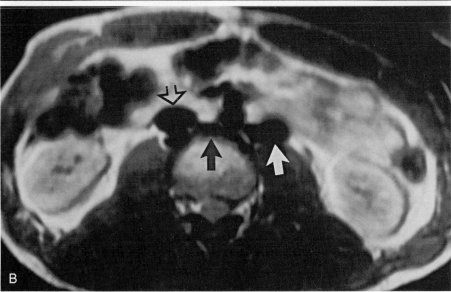

FIGURE 21–44. Retroaortic left renal vein mimicking lymphadenopathy.
A, Computed tomogram, contrast material–enhanced. A 1-cm soft tissue mass *(arrow)* has the appearance of an enlarged lymph node.
B, T2-weighted magnetic resonance scan demonstrates the "mass" *(closed white arrow)* in continuity with the retroaortic renal vein *(closed black arrow)* and inferior vena cava *(open arrow).* The low signal intensity of this structure indicates a vascular structure.

metastases from primary carcinoma of the breast or ovary. Calcification of lymph nodes may occur following chemotherapy or in patients with retroperitoneal lymph node metastases from a primary testicular tumor. It is impossible to differentiate benign and malignant causes for node enlargement by computed tomography alone. Likewise, computed tomography cannot depict focal architectural change in either normal-sized or consistently enlarged nodes. Thus, a negative examination does not exclude lymph node pathology.

Magnetic resonance imaging may provide useful complementary information when computed tomography is inconclusive. Abnormal lymph nodes usually exhibit low or intermediate signal intensity on T1-weighted or proton-density images. On T2-weighted images, abnormal lymph nodes have a high signal intensity and may resemble fat. Fat-suppressed magnetic resonance scans are also effective in detecting retroperitoneal adenopathy (Fig. 21–43). Magnetic resonance techniques can also be used to differentiate abnormal lymph nodes with high signal intensity from blood vessels in which the flow void phenomenon produces low signal intensity (Fig. 21–44). Active adenopathy typically enhances with gadolinium chelates.

RETROPERITONEAL FIBROSIS

Retroperitoneal fibrosis results from the proliferation of fibrous tissue in a midline and para-aortic distribution. Cases of retroperitoneal fibrosis that are idiopathic are known as *Ormond's disease.* A number of specific etiologies for retroperitoneal fibrosis have been established. These include *aortic hemorrhage, aortitis,* and *aortic atherosclerosis. Retroperitoneal malignancy,* especially metastases, may also produce this abnormality by provoking a desmoplastic response to tumor cells. Sclerosing Hodgkin's disease, in particular, has been associated with this occurrence. Other conditions that may be associated with retroperitoneal fibrosis are *methysergide toxicity, inflammatory bowel disease, extravasation of blood or urine* into the retroperitoneum, *prior surgery* or *radiation* to the region, and *collagen vascular disease.* The last may also occur with Riedel's thyroiditis and sclerosing mediastinitis.

Idiopathic retroperitoneal fibrosis most commonly occurs in patients between 40 and 60 years of age. Males are more commonly affected than are females by a ratio of 2:1. Pathologically, the fibrotic mass is predominantly sagittal and parasagittal, typically extending from below the level of the kidneys to the bifurcation of the great vessels. The fibrotic tissue may involve the inferior vena cava, aorta, ureters, and occasionally the iliac and renal veins in a symmetric or asymmetric distribution. Microscopically idiopathic retroperitoneal fibrosis is characterized by collagen, fibroblasts, and inflammatory cells when it is at a mature stage of development. Considerable vascularity is present initially. The presence of neoplastic cells excludes the diagnosis of idiopathic retroperitoneal fibrosis and confirms that the fibrotic process is a desmoplastic response to malignancy.

The clinical and laboratory findings of idiopathic retroperitoneal fibrosis are nonspecific and include fever, back pain, and elevated erythrocyte sedimentation rate. Less common signs and symptoms include lower extremity swelling due to venous occlusion, oliguria or anuria caused by ureteral obstruction, and constipation due to rectal involvement.

Excretory urography typically demonstrates bilateral hydronephrosis, which may be asymmetric and sometimes even unilateral. Rarely, the ureters and kidneys are uninvolved. Retrograde studies demonstrate a smooth tapering of the ureters that is most pronounced at the pelvic brim (Fig. 21–45). The ureteral narrowing may vary from focal to involvement of a long segment. Despite the ureteral narrowing and obstructive uropathy, there is little or no impediment to the retrograde passage of a ureteral catheter. Ureteral encasement by retroperitoneal fibrosis is usually not associated with medial displacement, although a slight degree of medial deviation sometimes occurs.

Computed tomography typically demonstrates a homogeneous soft tissue mass that extends from the infrarenal para-aortic region to the bifurcation of the aorta and encases the aorta, inferior vena cava, and ureters. Ureteral involvement with subsequent proximal ureteral dilatation and hydronephrosis may be asymmetric or unilateral. The aorta is usually not displaced ventrally (see Fig. 21–45). Contrast material enhancement varies with the age of the process. In its earliest stages of development, enhancement occurs as a manifestation of increased vascularity associated with active inflammation. Later, the dense organized fibrous tissue has less vascularity and, correspondingly, does not enhance.

It has been suggested that magnetic resonance imaging might permit distinction between benign or non-neoplastic retroperitoneal fibrosis and malignant retroperitoneal fibrosis (Fig. 21–46). In nonmalignant retroperitoneal fibrosis, a low or intermediate signal intensity on T1- and T2-weighted images has been reported in contrast to a higher signal intensity on T2-weighted images in most malignancies. Magnetic resonance imaging also demonstrates the effect of the fibrotic mass on the aorta and inferior vena cava.

Ultrasonography demonstrates retroperitoneal fibrosis as a poorly marginated, periaortic mass that is typically echo free or hypoechoic. Associated hydronephrosis is easily evaluated by ultrasonography as well. Body habitus, bowel gas, and adjacent bony structures may degrade the ultrasonographic imaging of retroperitoneal fibrosis.

Atypical manifestations of retroperitoneal fibrosis include ventral displacement of the aorta (Fig. 21–47), disease confined to the pelvis, involvement of the perirenal space, displacement of the retroperito-

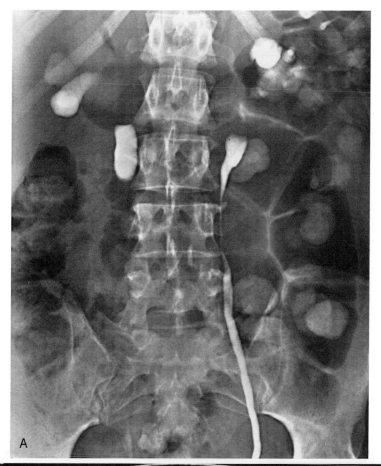

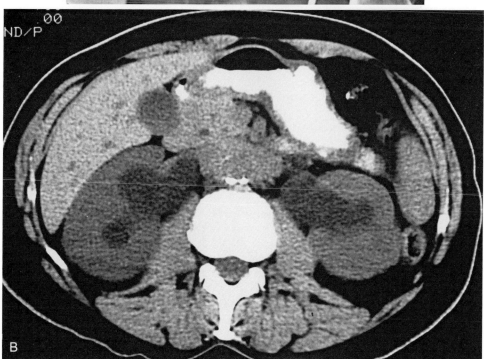

FIGURE 21–45. Retroperitoneal fibrosis.
A, Retrograde pyelogram. The fibrotic mass encases the left ureter, resulting in a long, smooth stricture and hydronephrosis. Similar findings were present involving the right ureter.
B, Computed tomogram, unenhanced. The attenuation value of the fibrotic mass is similar to that of the psoas muscles. The fibrotic mass surrounds the partially calcified aorta and the inferior vena cava. Note that the aorta maintains its normal position just ventral to the spine.

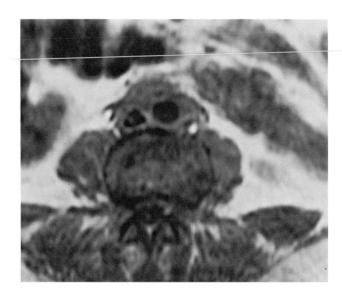

FIGURE 21–46. Retroperitoneal fibrosis. T1-weighted spin-echo magnetic resonance image. There is a mass of low to intermediate signal intensity surrounding the aorta and inferior vena cava. The vena cava is slightly compressed.

FIGURE 21–47. Retroperitoneal fibrosis. Computed tomogram, contrast material–enhanced. Unilateral hydronephrosis and the ventral displacement of the aorta from the spine are unusual manifestations of retroperitoneal fibrosis. Confident radiologic differentiation from lymphoma is impossible.

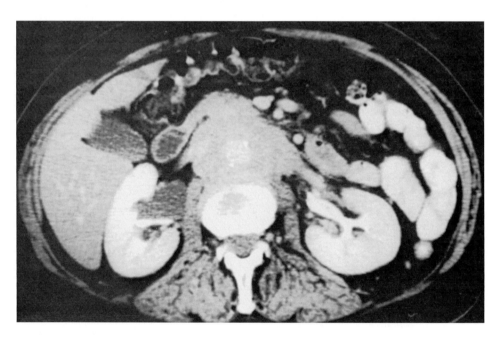

neal bowel, and vascular occlusion. Very rarely, the results of computed tomography are normal.

PSEUDOTUMORS OF THE RETROPERITONEUM

Left para-aortic pseudotumors can be a source of error in interpreting transverse cross sections of the retroperitoneum. These are caused by normal or variant vascular or intestinal structures, such as a duplicated inferior vena cava, a normal splenic artery or vein, an enlarged azygos vein from congenital or acquired processes, a circumaortic or retroaortic left renal vein, an enlarged left gonadal vein, loops of small bowel, displaced organs as a result of prior surgery, an extrarenal pelvis, and duplicated ureters (see Fig. 21–44). Oral and intravenous administration of contrast material, dynamic scans, magnetic resonance, and color Doppler ultrasonography are valuable techniques for ruling out pseudotumors that cause potential interpretative errors.

BIBLIOGRAPHY

Retroperitoneal Anatomy and Spaces

Aizenstein, R. I., Owens, C., Sabnis, S., Wilbur, A. C., Hibbein, J. F., and O'Neil, H. K.: The perinephric space and renal fascia: Review of normal anatomy, pathology and pathways of disease spread. Crit. Rev. Diagnost. Imaging 38:325, 1997.

Aizenstein, R. I., Wilbur, A. C., and O'Neil, H. K.: Interfascial and perinephric pathways in the spread of retroperitoneal disease: Refined concepts based on CT observations. Am. J. Roentgenol. 168:639, 1997.

Bechtold, R. E., Dyer, R. B., Zogoria, R. J., and Chen, M. Y. M.: The perirenal space: Relationship of pathologic processes to normal retroperitoneal anatomy. Radiographics 16:841, 1996.

Dodds, W. J., Darweesh, R. M. A., Lawson, T. L., Stewart, E. T., Foley, W. D., Kishk, S. M. A., and Hollwarth, M.: The retroperitoneal spaces revisited. AJR 157:1155, 1986.

Feuerstein, I. M., Zeman, R. K., Jaffe, M. H., Clark, L. R., and David, C. L.: Perirenal cobwebs: The expanding CT differential diagnosis. J. Comput. Assist. Tomogr. 8:1128, 1984.

Honda, H., McGuire, C. W., Barloon, T. J., and Harshimoto, K.: Replacement lipomatosis of the kidney: CT features. J. Comput. Assist. Tomogr. 14:229, 1990.

Kneeland, J. B., Auh, Y. H., Rubenstein, W. A., Zirinsky, K., Morrison, H., Whalen, J. P., and Kazam, E.: Perirenal spaces: CT evidence for communication across the midline. Radiology 164:657, 1987.

Korobkin, M., Silverman, P. M., Quint, L. E., and Francis I. R.: CT of the extraperitoneal space: Normal anatomy and fluid collections. AJR 159:933, 1992.

Kunin, M.: Bridging septa of the perinephric space: Anatomic, pathologic and diagnostic considerations. Radiology 158:361, 1986.

Mastromatteo, J. F., Mindell, H. J., Mastromatteo, M. F., Magnant, M. B., Sturtevant, N. V., and Shuman, W. P.: Communications of the pelvic extraperitoneal spaces and their relation to the abdominal extraperitoneal spaces: Helical CT cadaver study with pelvic extraperitoneal injections. Radiology 202:523, 1997.

Meyers, M. A.: Uriniferous perirenal pseudocyst: New observations. Radiology 117:539, 1975.

Mindell, H. J., Mastromatteo, J. F., Dickey, K. W., Sturtevant, N. V., Shuman, W. P., Oliver, C. L., Leister, K. L. and Barth, R. A.: Anatomic communications between the three retroperitoneal spaces: Determination of CT-guided injections of contrast material in cadavers. AJR 164:1173, 1995.

Mitchell, G. A. G.: Renal fascia. Br. J. Surg. 37:257, 1950.

Molmenti, E. P., Balfe, D. M., Kanterman, R. Y., and Bennett, H. F.: Anatomy of the retroperitoneum: Observations of the distribution of pathologic fluid collections. Radiology 200:95, 1996.

Raptopoulos, V., Kleinman, P. K., Marks, S., Jr., Snyder, M., and Silverman, P. M.: Renal fascial pathway: Posterior extension of pancreatic effusions within the anterior pararenal space. Radiology 158:367, 1986.

Raptopoulos, V., Lei, Q. F., Touliopoulos, P., Vrachliotis, T. G., and Marks, S. C.: Why perirenal disease does not extend into the pelvis: The importance of closure of the cone of the renal fasciae. AJR 164:1179, 1995.

Raptopoulos, V., Touliopoulos, P., Lei, Q. F., and Marks, S. C.: Medial border of the perirenal space: CT and anatomic correlation. Radiology 205:777, 1997.

Rubenstein, W. A., and Whalen, J. P.: Extraperitoneal spaces. AJR 157:1162, 1986.

Thornbury, J. R.: Perirenal anatomy: Normal and abnormal. Radiol. Clin. North Am. 17:321, 1979.

Winfield, A. C., Gerlock, A. J., Jr., and Shaff, M. I.: Perirenal cobwebs: A CT sign of renal vein thrombosis. J. Comput. Assist. Tomogr. 5:705, 1981.

Retroperitoneal Tumors

Brandes, S. B., Chelsky, M. J., Petersen, R. O., and Greenberg, R. E.: Leiomyosarcoma of the renal vein. J. Surg. Oncol. 63:195, 1996.

Brietta, L. K., and Watkins, D.: Giant extra-adrenal myelolipoma. Arch. Pathol. Lab. Med. 118:188, 1994.

Choyke, P. L., Hayes, W. S., and Sesterhenn, I. A.: Primary extragonadal germ cell tumors of the retroperitoneum: Differentiation of primary and secondary tumors. Radiographics 13:1365, 1993.

Davidson, A. J., and Hartman, D. S.: Imaging strategies for neoplasms of the kidney, adrenal gland and retroperitoneum. CA 37:151, 1987.

Davidson, A. J., Hartman, D. S., and Goldman, S. M.: Mature teratoma of the retroperitoneum: Radiologic, pathologic, and clinical correlation. Radiology 172:421, 1989.

Enzinger, F. M., and Weiss, S. W.: Soft Tissue Tumors, 3rd ed. St. Louis, C. V. Mosby, 1995.

Goss, P. E., Schwertfeger, L., Blackstein, M. E., Iscoe, N. A., Ginsberg, R. J., Simpson, W. J., Jones, D. P., and Shepperd, F. A.: Extragonadal germ cell tumors. Cancer 73:1971, 1994.

Hartman, D. S., Hayes, W. S., Choyke, P. L., and Tibbetts, G. P.: Leiomyosarcoma of the retroperitoneum and inferior vena cava: Radiologic-pathologic correlation. Radiographics 12:1203, 1992.

Henricks, W. H., Chu, Y. C., Goldblum, J. R., and Weiss, S. W.: Dedifferentiated liposarcoma: A clinicopathological analysis of 155 cases with a proposal for an expanded definition of dedifferentiation. Am. J. Surg. Pathol. 21:271, 1997.

Keslar, P. J., Buck, J. L., Suarez, E. S.: Germ cell tumors of the sacrococcygeal region: Radiologic pathologic correlation. Radiographics 14:607, 1994.

Kilkenny, J. W., Bland, K. I. and Copeland, E. M.: Retroperitoneal sarcoma: The University of Florida experience. J. Am. Coll. Surgeons 182:329, 1996.

Kim, T., Murakami, T., Oi, H., Matsushita, M., Tomoda, K., Fukuda, H., and Nakamura, H.: CT and MR imaging of abdominal liposarcoma. AJR 166:829, 1996.

Lee, J. K. T.: Magnetic resonance imaging of the retroperitoneum. Urol. Radiol. 10:48, 1988.

Levine, E., Huntarakoon, M., and Wetzel, L. H.: Malignant nerve-sheath neoplasms in neurofibromatosis: Distinction from benign tumors by using imaging techniques. AJR 149:1059, 1987.

Lipton, M., Sprayregen, S., Kutcher, R. and Frost, A.: Venous invasion in renal vein leiomyosarcoma: Case report and review of the literature. Abdom. Imaging 20:64, 1995.

Radin, R., David, C. L., Goldfarb, H., and Francis I. R.: Adrenal and extra-adrenal retroperitoneal ganglioneuroma: Imaging findings in 13 adults. Radiology 202:703, 1997.

Sneiders, A., Zhang, G. and Gordon, B. E.: Extra-adrenal perirenal myelolipoma. J. Urol. 150:1496, 1993.

Todd, C. S., Michael, H., and Sutton, G.: Retroperitoneal leiomyosarcoma: Eight cases and a literature review. Gynecol. Oncol. *59*:333, 1995.

Retroperitoneal Lymphadenopathy

Einstein, D. M.: Abdominal lymphadenopathy: Spectrum of CT findings. Radiographics *11*:457, 1991.

Hartman, D. S.: Retroperitoneal tumors and lymphadenopathy. Urol. Radiol. *12*:132, 1990.

Lien, H. H., et al.: Normal and anomalous structures simulating retroperitoneal lymphadenopathy at computed tomography. Acta Radiol. *29*:385, 1988.

Moul, J. W., Maggio, M. I., Hardy, M. R., and Hartman, D. S.: Retroaortic left renal vein in testicular cancer patient: Potential staging and treatment pitfall. J. Urol. *147*:454, 1992.

Sagel, S. S., and Lee, J. K. T.: Retroperitoneal lymphadenopathy. In Taveras, J. E. Ferrucci, J. T. (eds.): Radiology: Diagnosis–Imaging–Intervention. Philadelphia, J. B. Lippincott, 1988.

Retroperitoneal Fibrosis

Amis, E. S.: Retroperitoneal fibrosis. AJR *157*:321, 1991.

Gilkeson, G. S., and Allen, N. B.: Retroperitoneal fibrosis: A true connective tissue disease. Rheum. Dis. Clin. North Am. *22*:23, 1996.

Mulligan, S. A., Holley, H. C., Koehler, R. E., Koslin, D. B., Rubin, E., Berland, L. L., and Kenney, P. J.: CT and MR imaging in the evaluation of retroperitoneal fibrosis. J. Comput. Assist. Tomogr. *13*:277, 1989.

Rominger, M. G., and Kenney, P. J.: Perirenal involvement by retroperitoneal fibrosis: The usefulness of MRI to establish diagnosis. Urol. Radiol. *13*:173, 1992.

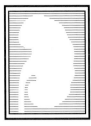

CHAPTER

22

The Adrenal

NORMAL ANATOMY
IMAGING MODALITIES
APPROACH TO ADRENAL IMAGING
ABNORMAL ADRENAL FUNCTION
    Cushing's Syndrome (Hypercortisolism)
    Hyperaldosteronism
    Virilization
    Feminization
    Mixed Endocrine Syndrome
    Neuroblastoma/Ganglioneuroblastoma
    Pheochromocytoma
    Addison's Disease

ABNORMAL ADRENAL MORPHOLOGY WITH
NORMAL FUNCTION
    Nonhyperfunctioning Adenoma
    Metastases
    Lymphoma
    Cyst
    Hemorrhage
    Myelolipoma
    Ganglioneuroma
    Granulomatous Disease
    Rare Adrenal Masses
DIAGNOSTIC SETS

NORMAL ANATOMY

The adrenal glands are located within the perinephric space and are completely surrounded by perirenal fat. Each gland weighs approximately 4 gm, 90 per cent of which is cortex and only 10 per cent medulla. The two portions of the adrenal, each of different embryologic origin, are autonomous with respect to hormone production and pathologic states.

The adrenal cortex is derived from mesoderm and is involved in the synthesis of mineralocorticoids, glucocorticoids, androgens, and estrogens. Cortical neoplasms include adenoma and carcinoma, both of which may hyperfunction. Cortical hyperplasia usually results from excessive stimulation of adrenocorticotropic hormone (ACTH) but may be autonomous.

The adrenal medulla is derived from neural crest ectoderm and is involved in the synthesis of epinephrine and norepinephrine. Medullary tumors include neuroblastoma, ganglioneuroblastoma, ganglioneuroma, and pheochromocytoma.

The right adrenal gland is suprarenal and at a more cephalic position than the left adrenal gland (Fig. 22–1). It is usually detected on axial images at the level just superior to the upper pole of the right kidney and dorsal to the inferior vena cava. Right adrenal masses are truly suprarenal, and large masses often displace the right kidney inferiorly. The medial limb of the right gland is more conspicuous than the lateral (horizontal) limb. The limbs of the normal adrenal gland are usually thinner than the adjacent diaphragmatic crura, al-

though the medial limb of the right gland normally can be as thick as 5 mm.

The normal left adrenal is slightly more caudal relative to the kidney than is the right gland (see Fig. 22–1). It is usually detected on axial sections obtained at the same level as the upper pole of the left kidney. Left adrenal masses often compress the ventral surface of the kidney, but unlike right adrenal masses they usually do not displace the kidney inferiorly. On axial sections the left adrenal has the appearance of an inverted V or Y.

The splenic vein is another useful landmark to identify the left adrenal gland and to determine the origin of retroperitoneal masses. The left adrenal gland is positioned between the left kidney and the splenic vein. Adrenal masses classically arise dorsal to the splenic vessels, whereas pancreatic masses originate ventral to the splenic vein (see Fig. 22–13). Normal adrenal glands vary in size and shape but are always straight or concave. Glands that are round or convex are abnormal and signify either enlargement or a mass.

There are several conditions that may simulate an adrenal mass. On the left side, a "pseudotumor" may be due to fluid-filled gastric fundus or gastric diverticulum, accessory spleen, tortuous splenic vein, inferior phrenic vein, exophytic upper pole renal mass, pancreatic mass, or diaphragmatic crura. On the right side, interposition of colon between liver and kidney, a fluid-filled duodenum, a caudate lobe of the liver, or an exophytic upper pole renal mass may be confused with an adrenal mass.

571

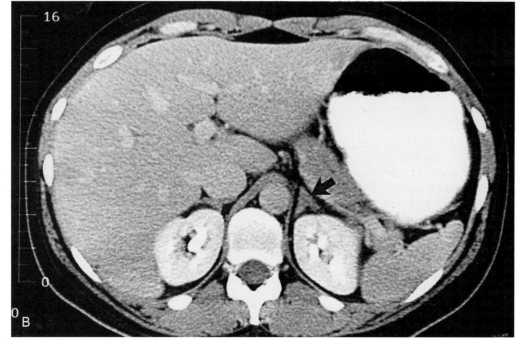

FIGURE 22–1. Normal adrenal glands. Computed tomograms, contrast material–enhanced.

A, The medial limb of the right adrenal gland *(arrow)* is dorsal to the inferior vena cava and ventral to the upper pole of the kidney.

B, The left adrenal gland *(arrow)* has an inverted V appearance.

Most of these misleading appearances can be distinguished by a carefully performed, contrast material–enhanced, dynamic computed tomogram with an adequate amount of oral contrast material or by magnetic resonance imaging in several planes.

IMAGING MODALITIES

Although there are many imaging modalities to evaluate the adrenal glands, no single technique is perfect for all clinical problems. In most cases,

multiple modalities are used. It is imperative to correlate all images with biochemical results and clinical findings.

Computed tomography allows outstanding spatial resolution of normal and abnormal adrenal glands. Spiral computed tomography avoids misregistration artifacts, thereby improving accuracy. Although it provides excellent morphologic information, computed tomography does not provide functional data.

Although the spatial resolution of magnetic resonance imaging is slightly inferior to that of computed tomography, it may be very helpful in selected cases. Coronal or sagittal images may confirm the adrenal gland origin of a mass when axial images are equivocal. The flow void phenomenon seen with magnetic resonance imaging allows excellent evaluation of vascular patency, especially when other modalities are indeterminate. Contrast resolution of magnetic resonance imaging is superior to that of computed tomography. Pheochromocytoma often has a characteristic high signal on T2-weighted images, particularly when conventional spin-echo, rather than fast spin-echo, technique is used. Likewise, magnetic resonance enables differentiation of metastases from nonhyperfunctioning adenoma in many cases.

Radionuclide imaging of the adrenal is most useful when functional information is required. There are two main pharmaceuticals that have potential for general use. Metaiodobenzylguanidine (MIBG) is an analogue of norepinephrine and is useful in detecting functioning medullary tumors. NP-59 (beta-iodomethyl-19-norcholesterol) depicts glucocorticoid, mineralocorticoid, and androgen secretion. Both are labeled with iodine 131 or iodine 123.

MIBG is especially useful in detecting extra-adrenal paraganglioma, multiple paragangliomas, metastatic or recurrent paraganglioma, and neuroblastoma. MIBG is, however, costly and time consuming, taking up to 3 days to complete a study.

NP-59 is not commonly used because of its lack of general availability. Because it accumulates in areas of cortical hormone synthesis, its primary application is in the evaluation of incidentally detected adrenal masses with normal adrenal function. The term *nonfunctioning* adenoma is a misnomer. Those greater than 2 cm in diameter usually demonstrate some accumulation of NP-59. Thus, they are better considered non*hyper*functioning adenomas. In contrast, absence of discernible NP-59 uptake in an adrenal mass greater than 2 cm in diameter indicates a hypofunctioning or nonfunctioning lesion, such as metastasis. Disadvantages of NP-59 include a 5- to 7-day interval between injection of the radiopharmaceutical and the imaging study and a relatively high radiation dose to the adrenal gland.

Preliminary investigations indicate that positron emission tomography may be helpful in differentiating benign from malignant adrenal lesions. Radionuclide evaluation of the adrenal gland is discussed further in Chapter 2.

Adrenal venous sampling, although somewhat technically difficult, provides functional information by obtaining blood samples for metabolic assay. This is especially useful when morphologic data are equivocal or contradictory with clinical or laboratory data. Venous sampling is most widely used in differentiating adenoma from hyperplasia in patients with hyperaldosteronism. In these cases the adenoma is often small and difficult to image. Bilateral samples are required, and, ideally, these should be collected simultaneously. Sampling before and after the administration of ACTH also provides useful information. With this technique, a ratio of aldosterone to cortisol should be calculated before and after ACTH stimulation to correct for varying dilution of adrenal vein blood in each sample.

Venous samples obtained with an adenoma demonstrate elevated levels of aldosterone in the ipsilateral vein with a positive response to stimulation with ACTH. The contralateral gland has suppressed or normal levels of aldosterone. Hyperplasia, on the other hand, demonstrates elevated aldosterone levels from both adrenal veins, with further increase after ACTH.

Inferior vena cavography may be required to detect the intraluminal component of an adrenal malignancy, such as carcinoma or pheochromocytoma. This technique may be especially useful in those cases in which magnetic resonance imaging, ultrasonography, or computed tomography are equivocal.

Adrenal arteriography is rarely required. It is potentially dangerous in patients with pheochromocytoma and rarely diagnostic for a specific histologic diagnosis. Computed tomography and magnetic resonance imaging almost always provide the morphologic information required for surgical planning.

APPROACH TO ADRENAL IMAGING

Adrenal imaging can be conveniently divided into two main categories: (1) the radiologic evaluation of abnormal adrenal function and (2) the evaluation of abnormal adrenal morphology with normal adrenal function (nonhyperfunctioning adrenal masses). Abnormal adrenal function can be further subdivided into hyperfunction, either cortical or medullary, or adrenal insufficiency (Addison's disease).

In patients with abnormal adrenal function, the primary task of the radiologist is to detect and characterize the adrenal pathology and pathophysiology. For example, in a patient with known hypercortisolism, it is the radiologist's objective to determine whether the cause is hyperplasia, adenoma, or carcinoma.

When confronted with abnormal adrenal morphology and apparent normal adrenal function, it is essential to confirm by laboratory studies that the adrenal glands are truly not hyperfunctioning. In many cases cortical or medullary hormones will be mildly elevated, thus allowing a specific diagnosis. These so-called nonfunctional masses are usually encountered as incidental findings while imaging other clinical problems. Although there are many causes for a nonhyperfunctioning adrenal mass, differential features are often present that will enable a specific diagnosis.

ABNORMAL ADRENAL FUNCTION

Cushing's Syndrome (Hypercortisolism)

Cushing's syndrome (hypercortisolism) is the result of excessive glucocorticoid production. Clinical features include truncal obesity, "buffalo hump," "moon" face, hirsutism, and muscle atrophy. Hypertension is common. The diagnosis of Cushing's syndrome is established by finding elevated levels of free cortisol in a 24-hour urine collection.

Once the diagnosis has been established, determination of the etiology is important, as outlined in Table 22–1. Excluding exogenous sources, 70 to 85 per cent of cases in adults are due to ACTH-producing pituitary adenoma causing bilateral hyperplasia. Ten to 20 per cent of cases result from an adrenal adenoma, and 5 to 10 per cent are caused by adrenal carcinoma. In children, Cushing's syndrome is usually caused by carcinoma.

Most cases of adrenal hyperplasia result from excessive ACTH production by a pituitary adenoma, which is known as *Cushing's disease*. In 1 to 2 per cent of cases of hyperplasia, however, excessive ACTH is produced not by a pituitary adenoma but rather by a nonpituitary tumor such as oat cell carcinoma, bronchial carcinoid, or pheochromocytoma. Rare etiologies of adrenal hyperplasia include hypothalamic tumors and primary pigmented nodular adrenocortical disease.

Patients with Cushing's syndrome should be initially evaluated with computed tomography of the adrenal glands. Adrenal imaging in these patients is facilitated by the abundant retroperitoneal fat that is usually present. Hyperplasia is suggested when one of four patterns is present: bilateral adrenal enlargement, normal glands, multiple small nodules, or a multinodular gland with a dominant nodule. Diffuse bilateral enlargement is the most common pattern, recognized as enlargement of the entire gland without a focal mass (Fig. 22–2). The limbs are thicker and sometimes longer than normal. If both adrenals are enlarged, the diagnosis of hyperplasia can be made confidently because bilateral adenomas are extremely rare.

Hyperplastic adrenal glands frequently appear normal or only slightly enlarged on computed tomography (Fig. 22–3). A normal computed tomographic study never excludes the diagnosis of adrenal hyperplasia, which can be established on the basis of biochemical studies demonstrating hypercortisolism alone.

Uncommonly, adrenal hyperplasia is multinodular. The nodules are almost always less than 3 cm in diameter and frequently less than 1 cm in diameter. In most cases there is enlargement of the gland between individual nodules.

Rarely, a multinodular gland may have a single dominant nodule that may be mistaken for an adenoma (Fig. 22–4). If ipsilateral adrenalectomy were performed in this circumstance, Cushing's syndrome would persist postoperatively owing to the occult contralateral hyperplasia. In these cases it is especially important to not overlook subtle signs of hyperplasia such as other, smaller nodules or slight adrenal enlargement. This is in contradistinction to cases of adenoma in which remaining adrenal tissue is atrophic, as discussed below.

Careful evaluation of the computed tomographic pattern of hyperplasia may be useful in determining its pathophysiology. In classic Cushing's disease caused by an ACTH-producing pituitary tumor, approximately one-half of the adrenal glands appear normal and one-half are mildly enlarged. Marked enlargement, that is, a right medial limb that is larger than 10 mm in thickness, is not seen in classic pituitary-dependent Cushing's disease and usually signifies ectopic ACTH production (Fig. 22–5).

Petrosal venous sampling is more accurate than computed tomography in determining the pathogenesis of the adrenal hyperplasia. Bilateral simultaneous sampling of the inferior petrosal sinuses is extremely sensitive, specific, and accurate for diagnosing Cushing's disease and distinguishing that entity from ectopic ACTH sources. Lack of an ACTH gradient across the pituitary gland indicates an ectopic source for ACTH production.

Ten to 20 per cent of cases of Cushing's syndrome are caused by an adrenal adenoma. A functioning adenoma that causes hypercortisolism is usually easily detected on computed tomography because it is usually larger than 2 cm in diameter and is surrounded by abundant retroperitoneal fat (Fig. 22–6). Most adenomas have a smooth, round, or oval contour that is well delineated. The contralateral adrenal gland is usually smaller than normal because of ACTH suppression by the functioning adenoma. Computed tomographic features that differentiate adenoma from carcinoma include smooth contour, sharp margination, a size less than 5 cm in diameter, and absence of hemorrhage or necrosis. Because approximately 15 per cent of adenomas calcify, this feature is not helpful in differentiating adenoma from carcinoma.

Although two-thirds of adrenal cortical carcinomas demonstrate some degree of biochemical hyperfunction, only 5 to 10 per cent of adult cases of Cushing's syndrome are caused by carcinoma. In contrast, most childhood cases of Cushing's syndrome are caused by carcinoma. Adrenal cortical carcinoma is suspected when any of the following

TABLE 22–1. Causes of Cushing's Syndrome

Exogenous adrenal steroids
Adrenal hyperplasia (70%–85%)
  Pituitary adenoma (Cushing's disease)
  Ectopic adrenocorticotropic hormone
    Oat cell carcinoma
    Bronchial carcinoid
    Pheochromocytoma
    Islet cell tumor
    Medullary thyroid carcinoma
    Thymic carcinoid
    Ovarian tumor
  Hypothalamus (rare)
  Primary pigmented nodular adrenal disease (rare)
Adrenal adenoma (10%–20%)
Adrenal carcinoma (5%–10%)

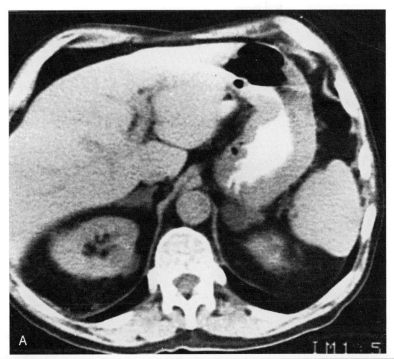

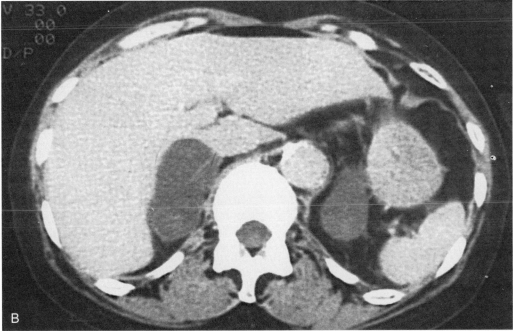

FIGURE 22–2. Hyperplasia, adrenal, in two patients.

A, Computed tomogram, contrast material–enhanced. Both adrenal glands are mildly enlarged.

B, Computed tomogram, contrast material–enhanced. There is marked enlargement of both glands, which are lobular with convex contours.

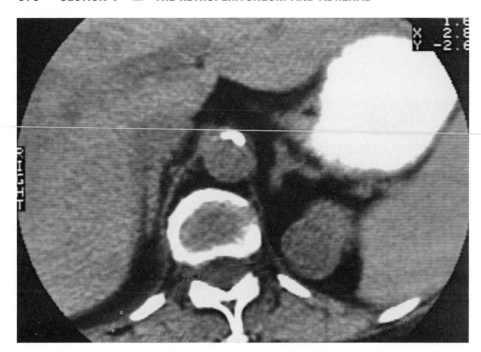

FIGURE 22–3. Hyperplasia with minimal enlargement. Computed tomogram without contrast material. Both glands maintain their normal shape, but the limbs are thicker than the adjacent diaphragmatic crura.

computed tomographic findings are present: a mass greater than 5 cm in diameter, necrosis, hemorrhage, inhomogeneous enhancement, venous extension into an adrenal or renal vein or into the inferior vena cava, distant metastases (especially lung, lymph nodes, liver), or invasion into adjacent viscera (Fig. 22–7). Thirty to 40 per cent of carcinomas calcify.

Magnetic resonance imaging is usually not necessary in most cases of Cushing's syndrome but may be useful in selected circumstances (Fig. 22–8; see Fig. 22–7B and C). Adrenal carcinoma is typically hypointense compared with liver on T1-weighted images and is hyperintense compared with liver on T2-weighted images. The coronal or sagittal images may help define adrenal from renal origin if axial computed tomography is equivocal (see Fig. 22–7B). Magnetic resonance imaging is also useful for documenting the extent of venous invasion and may be helpful in differentiating tumor thrombus from nontumor venous thrombus when gadolinium-enhanced scans are performed.

Hyperaldosteronism

Primary hyperaldosteronism is the result of elevated aldosterone production by the adrenal cortex with subsequent hypertension, hypokalemia, and suppression of plasma renin activity. Approximately 80 per cent of cases of primary hyperaldosteronism have a unilateral cortical adenoma, a condition known as *Conn's syndrome*. Most of the remaining cases have bilateral micronodular or macronodular hyperplasia. It is very rare to have an adrenal carcinoma that produces only aldosterone. Differentiation is extremely important because surgical resection of an adenoma usually results in improvement

or cure of hypertension and electrolyte disturbances, whereas surgical intervention in hyperplasia usually does not result in prolonged improvement of these abnormalities.

Computed tomography in patients with hyperaldosteronism is less often diagnostic than in patients with Cushing's syndrome because in the former the tumor is usually smaller and there is no increase in periadrenal retroperitoneal fat compared with the latter. The average aldosterone-producing adenoma measures only 1.7 cm in diameter, with a range of 0.5 to 3.5 cm (Fig. 22–9). Overlapping sections of 1.5- to 3.0-mm thickness, therefore, are recommended. Because of increased cytoplasmic lipid in aldosterone-producing adenoma, the computed tomographic attenuation values in patients with primary aldosteronism are usually lower than in patients with Cushing's syndrome. Occasionally, the attenuation value is similar to water and an adenoma mimics a small adrenal cyst.

Patients with clinical findings that support the diagnosis of an adenoma and who also have an obvious unilateral nodule and a normal contralateral gland on computed tomography do not require venous sampling. Utilizing thin-section computed tomography, two-thirds of patients with hyperplasia have small micronodules whereas one-third have normal-appearing adrenal glands. In cases with multiple bilateral nodules, computed tomography cannot reliably permit distinction between hyperplasia and adenoma. Occasionally it is difficult to decide if a nodule less than 2 cm in diameter seen on computed tomography represents an adenoma or a single nodule in hyperplastic glands (Fig. 22–10). Therefore, all patients with bilateral nodules or equivocal findings on computed tomography require venous sampling, as do patients with bilaterally normal glands.

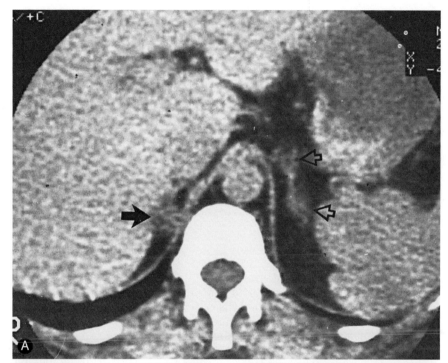

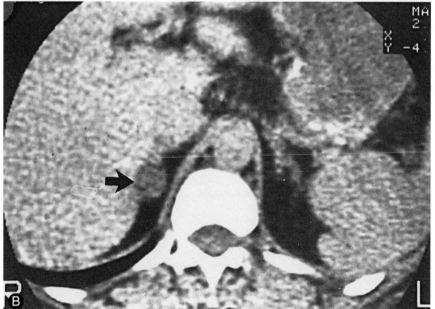

FIGURE 22–4. Macronodular hyperplasia with a dominant nodule.

A and *B,* Computed tomograms without contrast material at two contiguous levels. There is a small right adrenal mass *(solid arrows)* that could be confused with an adenoma. Careful evaluation of the left gland, however, demonstrates two additional nodules *(open arrows).* In a patient with adrenal hyperfunction, these findings are most consistent with macronodular hyperplasia.

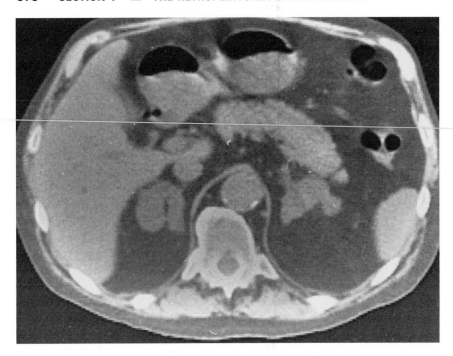

FIGURE 22-5. Hyperplasia, adrenal, due to ectopic adrenocorticotropic hormone produced by a small cell carcinoma of the lung. Computed tomogram, unenhanced. The increased amount of retroperitoneal fat facilitates evaluation of the massively enlarged adrenal glands. Enlargement to this degree usually results from an ectopic rather than a pituitary source of adrenocorticotropic hormone.

Virilization

Virilization refers to the appearance of adult masculine characteristics in prepubertal males or in females of any age. It is often called the *adrenogenital syndrome* and can be caused by congenital adrenal cortical hyperplasia or neoplasia. Most cases occur in children.

Congenital adrenal hyperplasia is caused by an enzymatic deficiency (usually 21-hydroxylase) in the biosynthetic pathway of adrenal steroids. This results in ineffective adrenal steroid production with overproduction and accumulation of cortisol precursors, some of which produce androgenic effects. Overproduction of androgens causes masculinization, owing to inhibition of differentiation of the embryonic genital tract along female lines. In 30 per cent of cases, mineralocorticoid production is also impaired, leading to hyponatremia, hyperkalemia, hypoglycemia, and hypotension. The hyperplastic adrenal glands are usually larger than normal while maintaining a normal shape.

Adrenal adenoma or carcinoma may also produce virilization. However, this occurs in the neonatal period with extreme rarity, which helps in differentiation from congenital adrenal hyperplasia. With a virilizing adrenal tumor, size is not as reliable a criterion in differentiating adenoma from carcinoma as it is in Cushing's syndrome. In children, some benign adenomas are larger than 5 cm in diameter. In adults, the majority of adrenal virilizing tumors are malignant.

Feminization

Feminization from adrenal hyperfunction is very rare. It usually occurs in adult males who present with gynecomastia, testicular atrophy, feminizing hair changes, and loss of libido. In the adult, feminization is almost always due to carcinoma, whereas in children, it is more likely caused by an adenoma.

Mixed Endocrine Syndrome

Mixed endocrine syndrome refers to any combination of hypercortisolism, hyperaldosteronism, virilization, or feminization syndromes. These are usually associated with adrenal cortical carcinoma. Cushing's syndrome caused by adrenal adenoma or hyperplasia may be associated with increased levels of sex hormones and/or their precursors, but actual clinical signs of virilization or feminization with Cushing's syndrome are usually seen only in adrenal carcinoma.

Neuroblastoma/Ganglioneuroblastoma

Neuroblastoma is a highly malignant neoplasm that arises most commonly in the adrenal medulla but may also originate in any sympathetic ganglia in an extra-adrenal location. Neuroblastoma is the most common solid, extracranial tumor in infants and children and the second most common intra-abdominal tumor in children after Wilms' tumor. Both sexes are equally affected. Ninety per cent of neuroblastomas become manifest within the first 8 years of life, whereas 50 per cent of patients are younger than 2 years of age when diagnosed. Rarely, neuroblastoma is congenital or present in the first month of life. Fetal neuroblastoma can be diagnosed by prenatal ultrasonography. In these patients, fetal hydrops is suggestive of metastatic tumor.

About one-half of patients with neuroblastoma present with a palpable mass, often with accompanying pain and fever. In 90 per cent of patients,

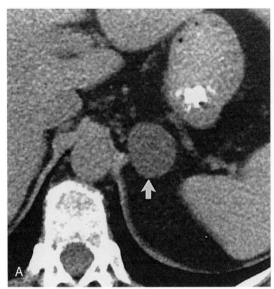

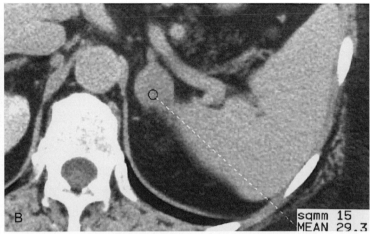

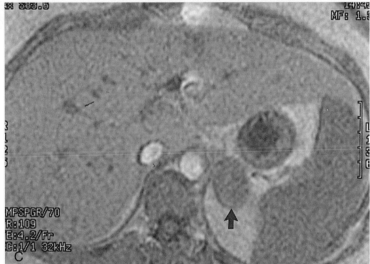

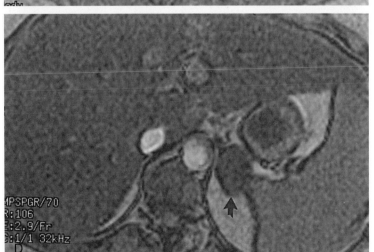

FIGURE 22–6. Adrenal adenoma in three patients.

A, Unenhanced computed tomogram. The adenoma *(arrow)* is well defined and has an attenuation value of −7.1 Hounsfield units.

B, Computed tomogram, contrast material–enhanced. The adenoma is well defined and homogeneous. The attenuation value measures 29.3 Hounsfield units 1 hour after contrast material was administered.

C and *D,* Magnetic resonance images. In-phase *(C)* and opposed-phase *(D)* gradient-echo images demonstrate the adenoma *(arrow)* to be hypointense to spleen in *D.*

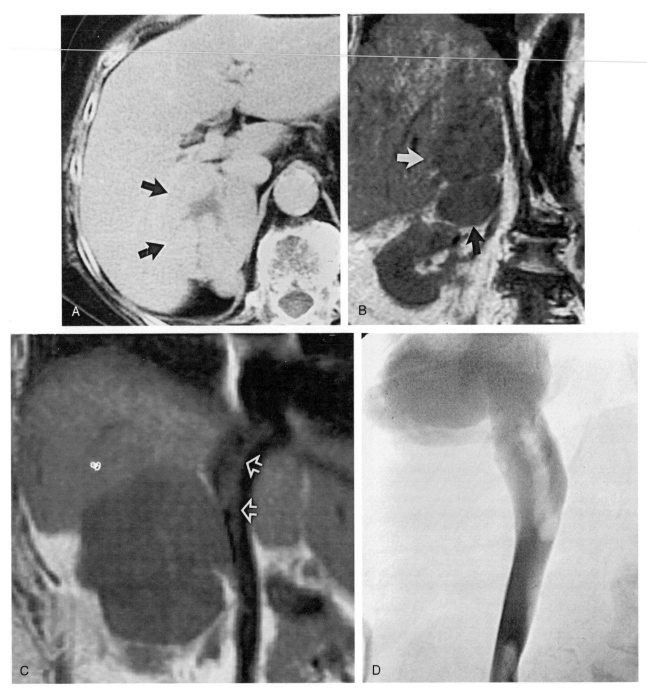

FIGURE 22–7. Adrenal carcinoma with inferior vena cava invasion.

A, Computed tomogram, contrast material–enhanced. The carcinoma *(arrows)* is large and heterogeneous.

B, Magnetic resonance image. Coronal T1-weighted image. The tumor *(arrows)* is bilobed. The extrarenal location is verified in the coronal plane.

C, Magnetic resonance image. Oblique T1-weighted image. There is a linear filling defect *(arrows)* in the inferior vena cava.

D, Inferior vena cavogram, lateral projection. The filling defect, which was tumor thrombus, is confirmed.

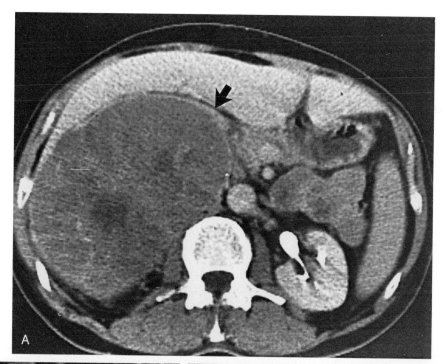

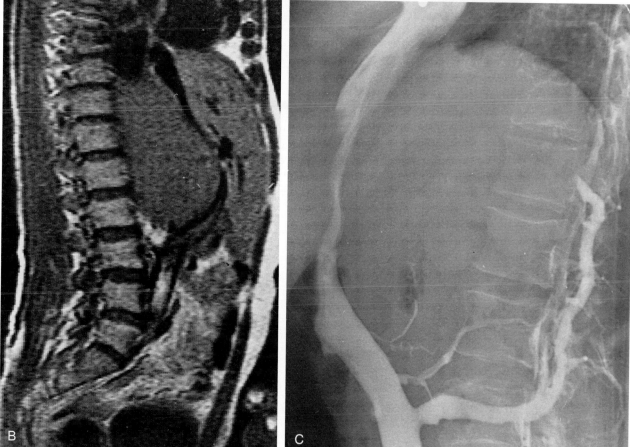

FIGURE 22–8. Adrenal carcinoma displacing the inferior vena cava.

A, Computed tomogram, contrast material–enhanced. A large inhomogeneous mass displaces the inferior vena cava ventrally *(arrow).* It is impossible to be certain whether tumor has extended into the inferior vena cava.

B, Magnetic resonance image, T1-weighted, sagittal section. The inferior vena cava is displaced but patent.

C, Cavogram. The inferior vena cava is narrowed but is free of tumor thrombus. Posterior collateral veins are prominent.

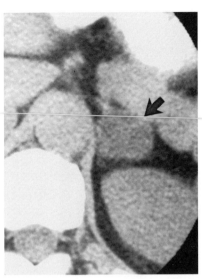

FIGURE 22–9. Adrenal adenoma causing secondary hyperaldosteronism (Conn's syndrome). Computed tomogram, unenhanced. There is a well-defined mass *(arrow)* arising in the left adrenal. Characteristically, mineralocorticoid-secreting adrenal adenomas have abundant tumor lipid with a resultant attenuation value near that of water.

there is an elevated level of vanillylmandelic acid that is the basis of the diagnosis. If there is intraspinal extension of tumor, then pain, paraplegia, limb weakness, urinary retention, constipation, or loss of bladder and bowel control become manifest. Neuroblastoma may be associated with spontaneous chaotic eye movements, particularly when voluntary eye movement is attempted, a condition known as opsoclonus-myoclonus. Watery diarrhea with hypokalemic hypochlorhydria due to a vasoactive polypeptide is present in approximately 10 per cent of patients with neuroblastoma.

Staging is extremely important in patient management and prognosis. A tumor confined to the adrenal gland is Stage I, whereas one that extends in continuity with the adrenal gland but remains on one side of the body is Stage II. Stage III is a localized tumor that crosses the midline, whereas Stage IV involves distant metastases. In Stage IV-S (special), metastases are confined to skin, bone marrow, or liver.

Pathologically, neuroblastoma is a solid, poorly defined tumor with conspicuous areas of hemorrhage and necrosis. Large tumors frequently engulf the aorta and other retroperitoneal structures. The kidneys and ureters are usually displaced laterally. Direct invasion into liver, kidney, pancreas, or the spinal canal is common. Rarely, neuroblastoma is cystic as a result of extensive hemorrhage and necrosis.

Ganglioneuroblastoma is a composite tumor that contains both mature ganglion cells and primitive neuroblastomal elements and is, in fact, a differentiating or maturing neuroblastoma. As such, a ganglioneuroblastoma has a better prognosis than a neuroblastoma. It is impossible to differentiate the two tumors radiologically.

Surgical excision remains the most successful means of therapy for neuroblastoma and ganglioneuroblastoma. The role of the radiologist is to determine extent of tumor, and, if possible, resectability. Regardless of size, tumors that invade major vessels, such as aorta, celiac plexus, or superior mesenteric artery, are not resectable. Tumors that cross the midline but do not come into contact with large vessels or are adherent to only one side of a vessel may be resectable. Intraspinal extension is treated by decompressive laminectomy and debulking of tumor.

The ultrasonographic appearance of most abdominal neuroblastomas is that of a tumor of variable echogenicity with irregular hyperechoic areas intermixed with less echogenic areas. These correspond to foci of hemorrhage, necrosis, and microcalcification. Ultrasonography is usually able to demonstrate that the mass is extrarenal, thus establishing neuroblastoma rather than Wilms' tumor as the most likely diagnosis.

Computed tomography typically demonstrates a calcified, inhomogeneous solid mass with areas of hemorrhage and necrosis. Enhancement is usually inhomogeneous. Computed tomography nicely demonstrates the relation of the tumor to adjacent organs and blood vessels. Neuroblastoma arising from the adrenal is similar in appearance to extra-adrenal neuroblastoma (see Fig. 21–33).

Magnetic resonance imaging is sometimes helpful in evaluating the extent of a tumor for planning either radiation or surgical therapy, as well as for monitoring tumor size as a follow-up (Fig. 22–11). Magnetic resonance imaging does require sedation in very young patients but eliminates the need for intrathecal injection of contrast material. On T1-weighted images, metastases in the medullary cavities of bones can also be imaged as low-signal foci relative to higher signal in bone marrow. Spinal extension is best detected by magnetic resonance imaging, which precludes the need for myelography.

On any imaging modality, a cystic neuroblastoma may be difficult to distinguish from adrenal hemorrhage, as discussed subsequently in this chapter. Differential features favoring neuroblastoma include elevated levels of vanillylmandelic acid, discovery beyond the neonatal period, and the presence of a solid component (Fig. 22–12).

Neuroblastoma that develops in infants younger than 1 year of age is less aggressive and associated with a better prognosis than neuroblastoma that arises in older children. Rarely, a neonatal neuroblastoma matures into a well-differentiated, benign neoplasm (i.e., a ganglioneuroma).

Pheochromocytoma

Pheochromocytoma is a neoplasm of the adrenal medulla composed of paraganglionic cells that produce catecholamines. The term pheochromocytoma should be restricted to tumors that arise within the adrenal gland. The same tumor arising in the

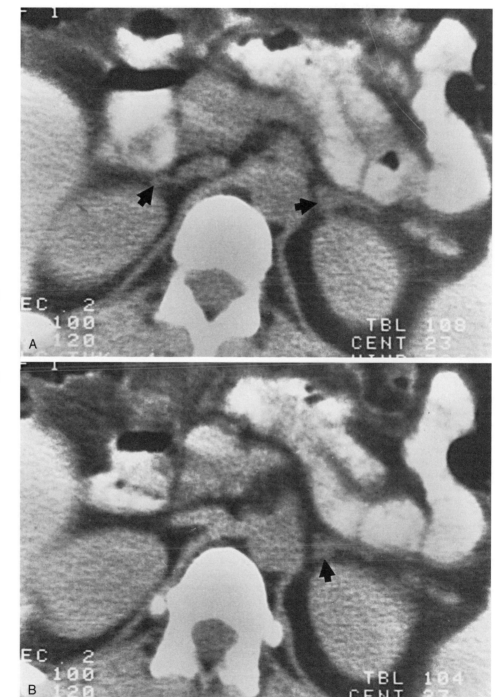

FIGURE 22–10. Adrenal hyperplasia, bilateral, causing hyperaldosteronism.

A and *B,* Computed tomograms, contrast material–enhanced, consecutive 4-mm-thick sections. There is a small nodular mass in each adrenal gland *(arrows).* Venous sampling demonstrated elevated levels of mineralocorticoids in each gland.

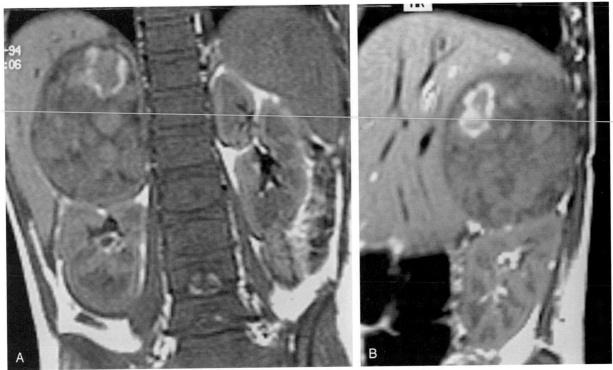

FIGURE 22–11. Neuroblastoma presenting as a large, smooth, heterogeneous right suprarenal mass in a 7-year-old boy. Magnetic resonance images.
    A, T1-weighted image. Coronal projection.
    B, T2-weighted image. Sagittal plane. The heterogeneous signal characteristics indicate areas of hemorrhage and necrosis. The extrarenal origin of the tumor is well demonstrated in both projections.

sympathetic chain outside the adrenal gland should be referred to as a paraganglioma rather than an extra-adrenal pheochromocytoma. These are discussed in Chapter 21.

Excess catecholamine production causes labile or sustained hypertension combined with episodes of perspiration, palpitations, and anxiety. The 24-hour urine vanillylmandelic acid level is elevated in more than 90 per cent of patients. The presence of free norepinephrine in a 24-hour urine specimen is the most sensitive indicator of functioning paraganglioma. Plasma catecholamine measurement is less accurate than assays of urine because secretion by a paraganglioma is often intermittent and because

intravenous sampling may cause a stress-related increase in plasma catecholamine levels.

Pheochromocytoma has been associated with *Type IIA* and *Type IIB multiple endocrine neoplasia (MEN) syndromes, von Hippel-Lindau disease, neurofibromatosis,* and *Carney's triad.* Fifty per cent of patients with multiple endocrine neoplasia syndromes and pheochromocytoma are asymptomatic.

The mean diameter of a pheochromocytoma is 6 cm, although in association with multiple endocrine neoplasia syndromes the tumor is often smaller and difficult to image. The term *medullary hyperplasia* has been applied to hyperfunctioning nodules less than 1 cm in diameter in association with multiple

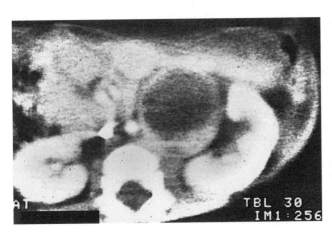

FIGURE 22–12. Neuroblastoma, cystic, in a 4-month-old infant with an abdominal mass. Computed tomogram, contrast material–enhanced. There is a thick-walled, cystic adrenal mass displacing and distorting the left kidney.

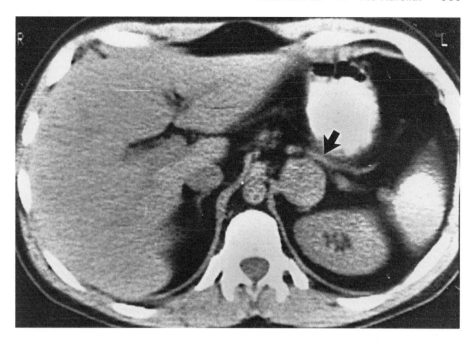

FIGURE 22–13. Pheochromocytoma, left adrenal. Computed tomogram, unenhanced. There is a small, well-defined mass dorsal to the splenic artery *(arrow)* and ventral to the left kidney.

endocrine neoplasia syndromes. Hemorrhage and necrosis are common in large pheochromocytomas. Indeed, the tumor may become cystic as a result of extensive hemorrhage. About 10 per cent of pheochromocytomas calcify and 10 per cent are associated with extra-adrenal paragangliomas or are bilateral.

Approximately 10 per cent of pheochromocytomas are malignant. However, both the radiologic and histologic diagnosis of malignancy is dependent on the presence of metastases rather than an inherent, distinctive set of features. Frequent sites of metastases include bone, lymph nodes, lung, and liver. Extension or direct invasion into the inferior vena cava is not common. Recurrence of metastases may occur 3 to 5 years after resection of a primary malignant pheochromocytoma.

The optimal strategy for the radiologic evaluation of a patient with suspected pheochromocytoma is controversial. Computed tomography has a high sensitivity (more than 90 per cent) in the detection of functioning pheochromocytoma. Contrast material is rarely required. If, however, a nonionic contrast material is used, no subsequent increase in epinephrine or norepinephrine levels has been demonstrated. Glucagon is contraindicated because it may provoke a hypertensive crisis. A small tumor is usually homogeneous, whereas a large tumor often contains areas of diminished attenuation reflecting necrosis (Fig. 22–13). Those with extensive hemorrhage may be confused radiologically with an adrenal cyst (Fig. 22–14). As stated earlier, bilateral pheochromocytomas are present in about 10 per cent of cases (Fig. 22–15).

There are, however, several important limitations of computed tomography. It is impossible to differentiate pheochromocytoma from other types of adrenal tumors by computed tomography alone. Clip artifacts often make evaluation for recurrence after surgery difficult. Computed tomography appears to be less reliable than magnetic resonance imaging studies for very small nodules (medullary hyperplasia) and less sensitive than magnetic resonance and radionuclide studies for extra-adrenal tumors and metastatic disease. Despite these limitations, computed tomography is the preferred technique for initial evaluation of a patient with clinical evidence of a catecholamine-producing tumor.

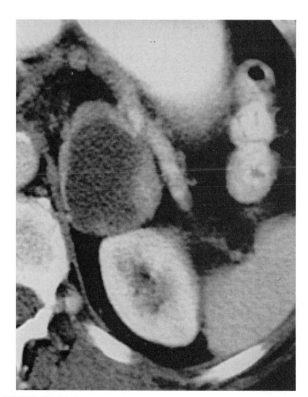

FIGURE 22–14. Pheochromocytoma, cystic, left adrenal. Computed tomogram, unenhanced. There is a 5.5-cm thick-walled cystic adrenal mass ventral to the left kidney.

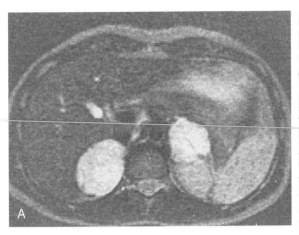

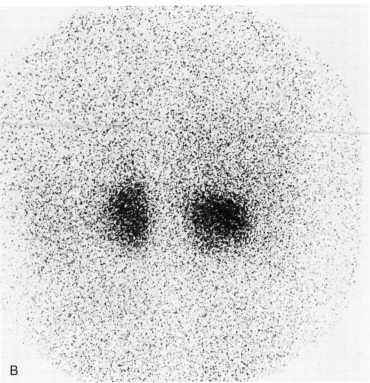

FIGURE 22–15. Pheochromocytoma, bilateral.
   A, Magnetic resonance image, T2-weighted. Both tumors have a very bright signal.
   B, MIBG scan. There is uptake of radionuclide by both tumors.

Magnetic resonance imaging is another excellent technique to evaluate a patient with suspected pheochromocytoma. Magnetic resonance imaging is particularly useful in detecting extra-adrenal paragangliomas, especially those arising in the wall of the bladder and paracardiac region, in evaluating the postoperative patient, in patients with hypertension and only mildly elevated catecholamine levels, and in patients at increased risk for developing paraganglioma (e.g., von Hippel-Lindau syndrome).

On T1-weighted images, a pheochromocytoma has a signal intensity that is lower than or equiva-lent to that of liver, kidney, or muscle. In many patients the signal intensity is high on T2-weighted images (see Fig. 22–15A). These signal characteristics readily support the diagnosis of pheochromocytoma in the appropriate clinical setting. However, a pheochromocytoma may demonstrate atypical signal characteristics, which emphasizes the importance of correlating radiologic abnormalities with clinical and laboratory findings.

MIBG is a norepinephrine analogue that may be useful as a radionuclide agent when other imaging modalities are equivocal because it accumulates at

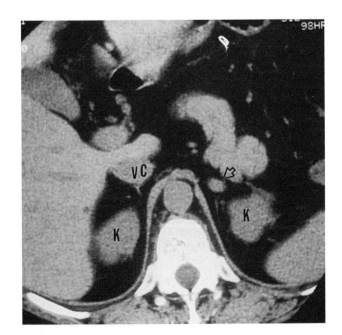

FIGURE 22–16. Addison's disease, destructive pattern. Computed tomogram, unenhanced. The adrenal glands are barely visible as thin linear densities between the right kidney *(K)* and the inferior vena cava *(VC)* and between the left kidney *(K)* and the splenic vein *(arrow)*.

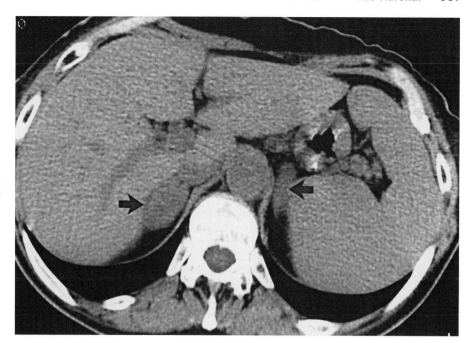

FIGURE 22–17. Addison's disease, replacement pattern, in a patient with histoplasmosis. Computed tomogram, unenhanced. Both glands *(arrows)* are enlarged with convex margins.

sites of norepinephrine synthesis. It is especially helpful in detecting medullary hyperplasia, recurrence, metastases, or extra-adrenal paragangliomas (see Fig. 22–15B). MIBG has the advantage of imaging the entire body with one dose of the radionuclide. Disadvantages of MIBG include limited availability, relatively poor spatial resolution, and the length of the procedure (1 to 3 days). The specificity of an MIBG scan is not 100 per cent. Other tumors, such as neuroblastoma, carcinoid, medullary thyroid carcinoma, choriocarcinoma, and atypical schwannoma can also accumulate the radionuclide, although in a clinical setting different from that of pheochromocytoma. This technique is also discussed in Chapter 2.

Addison's Disease

Addison's disease (adrenal insufficiency) results from reduced secretion of adrenal steroid hormones to a level below that required for endocrine homeostasis. Advanced cases are usually readily apparent clinically. Recognition of early disease, however, is often difficult. The most common symptoms of adrenal insufficiency are slowly progressive fatigability, weakness, anorexia, weight loss, cutaneous and mucosal pigmentation, hypotension, and, occasionally,

TABLE 22–2. Causes of Adrenal Insufficiency

Idiopathic atrophy (autoimmune)
Replacement diseases
  Tuberculosis
  Histoplasmosis
  Blastomycosis
  Amyloidosis
  Hemorrhage
  Metastatic disease
  Lymphoma

hypoglycemia. These features are nonspecific and easily confused with other, more common, chronic illnesses. Occasionally, sudden, massive adrenal destruction due to sepsis or adrenal hemorrhage causes acute adrenal insufficiency that presents as fulminating shock.

Although there are many causes of Addison's disease, as enumerated in Table 22–2, two radiologic patterns dominate. The most common pattern is that of adrenal atrophy with diminutive glands (Fig. 22–16). In these cases, glandular atrophy is idiopathic and presumed to be due to autoimmune destruction. These patients are often cachectic and not efficaciously examined by computed tomography because of absent retroperitoneal fat and the small size of both adrenal glands. The other major pattern seen in Addison's disease is that of bilateral adrenal enlargement with preservation of the adrenal shape (Fig. 22–17). This occurs when the adrenal gland is replaced by inflammatory or neoplastic cells, abnormal metabolites, or hemorrhage.

ABNORMAL ADRENAL MORPHOLOGY WITH NORMAL FUNCTION

The most common causes of an adrenal mass with normal adrenal function are a nonhyperfunctioning adenoma, metastatic disease, cyst, hemorrhage, myelolipoma, ganglioneuroma, and granulomatous disease. Rare causes of a nonfunctioning mass include mesenchymal tumor (e.g., leiomyosarcoma), primary melanoma, and hemangioma. Rare causes of bilateral adrenal enlargement include extramedullary hematopoiesis and Wolman's disease. Additionally, the functional adrenal masses previously discussed must also be considered because occasionally they are nonfunctional, as, for example, the one-third of adrenal cortical carcinomas that do not hyperfunction.

Nonhyperfunctioning Adenomas

Nonhyperfunctioning adenomas 3 cm in diameter or larger occur in approximately 3 per cent of autopsies. Prevalence increases slightly with age. An increased prevalence of adenoma also has been reported in patients with diabetes, hypertension, renal adenocarcinoma, and hereditary colonic adenomatosis.

Radiologic diagnosis is directed at identifying the unique morphologic or physiologic characteristics of nonhyperfunctioning adenomas. Adenomas are usually smaller than 5 cm in diameter, are non-necrotic, and often contain intracellular lipid. Cortical hormones are synthesized but not in excessive quantities, hence the term *nonhyperfunctioning* rather than *nonfunctioning* adenoma.

Computed tomographic findings that favor adenoma are a homogeneous mass, a diameter less than 5 cm, and an attenuation value between −5 and 10 Hounsfield units on an unenhanced computed tomogram (see Fig. 22–6A). Computed tomographic scans obtained 15 minutes to 1 hour after administration of contrast material are often helpful in differentiating an adenoma from a metastasis (see Fig. 22–6B). The typical adenoma demonstrates homogeneous enhancement and more rapid washout of contrast material than does the typical metastasis.

An adenoma is typically isointense or slightly hypointense to liver on T1- and T2-weighted spin-echo magnetic resonance sequences. If an opposed-phase gradient-echo scan is used, an adenoma with sufficient intracellular lipid demonstrates signal dropout relative to spleen. (see Fig. 22–6C and *D*).

Low attenuation value (<10 Hounsfield units) on unenhanced computed tomography and signal dropout on opposed-phase gradient-echo magnetic resonance scans correlate with intracellular lipid and are sensitive indicators in differentiating an adenoma from a metastasis. However, both of these techniques can yield indeterminate values. In these cases, measurement of attentuation values 15 minutes to 1 hour after contrast material–enhanced computed tomography may be useful. If none of these techniques produces definitive results and differentiation is critical for patient management, biopsy is required.

Metastases

The adrenal gland is the fourth most common site for metastatic disease, surpassed only by lung, liver, and bone. At autopsy about one-fourth of patients with epithelial malignancy have metastases to the adrenal. The most common primary neoplasms that metastasize to the adrenal are carcinoma of lung, breast, thyroid, or colon, lymphoma, and melanoma.

In most patients, metastases to the adrenal gland are not apparent clinically. A large tumor or one that is complicated by hemorrhage may cause flank pain or a palpable mass. Even with complete re-

placement of both glands, adrenal insufficiency is uncommon. Steroids used as part of a chemotherapeutic regimen may mask Addison's disease.

There are five pathologic and radiologic patterns of metastases to the adrenal gland: (1) small (less than 5 cm in diameter) mass, (2) large (more than 5 cm in diameter) mass, (3) multiple masses, (4) diffuse adrenal enlargement, and (5) normal-appearing glands.

Typically the small (less than 5 cm in diameter) mass is homogeneous but may have mixed density (Fig. 22–18). Rarely, an increased attenuation value caused by hemorrhage or calcification is present. Computed tomographic findings that favor a diagnosis of metastasis over adenoma include an attenuation value greater than 15 Hounsfield Units on an unenhanced scan and heterogeneous enhancement. Computed tomographic scans obtained 15 minutes to 1 hour after the administration of contrast material may be helpful. A metastasis tends toward greater enhancement and slower contrast material washout than does an adenoma.

Magnetic resonance imaging may be helpful in differentiating a metastasis from a benign mass. Metastases to the adrenal gland are typically isointense with liver on T1-weighted images and brighter than liver on T2-weighted images (Fig. 22–19). Using liver signal intensity as a reference, however, may be misleading when the liver is affected by pathologic processes such as iron deposition, hepatitis, or fatty infiltration. With the use of opposed-phase gradient-echo scanning, metastases (with no intracellular lipid) show no signal dropout relative to spleen (Fig. 22–20).

Positron emission tomography with ^{18}F-fluorodeoxyglucose (FDG) is another technique that may be useful in differentiating metastases from benign lesions. FDG is a D-glucose analogue preferentially taken up by tumor cells because of increased glu-

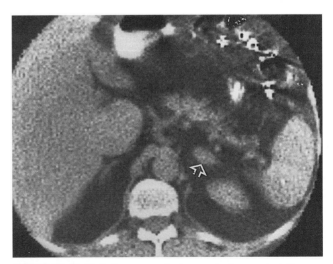

FIGURE 22–18. Metastases producing a small mass in left adrenal. Computed tomogram, contrast material–enhanced. The metastasis *(arrow)* was from a small cell carcinoma of the lung.

FIGURE 22–19. Metastases to both adrenal glands from renal cell carcinoma. There are masses in both adrenal glands *(arrowheads)*, as well as a mass in the liver *(arrows)*. On the T2-weighted image *(B)* the signal intensity of the metastases is greater than that of the uninvolved liver. Compare with the signal intensity of an adenoma illustrated in Figure 22–6*C*.

A, T1-weighted magnetic resonance image.

B, T2-weighted magnetic resonance image at the same level.

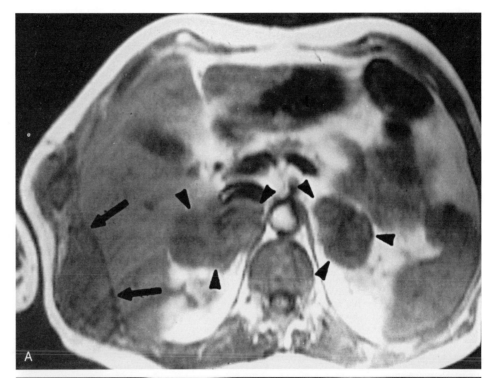

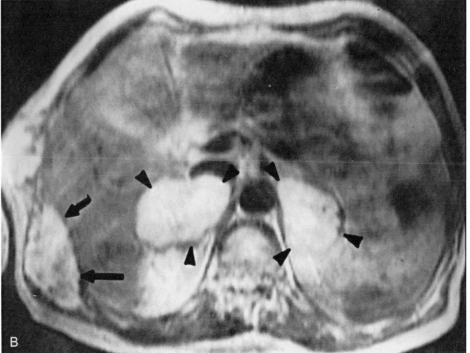

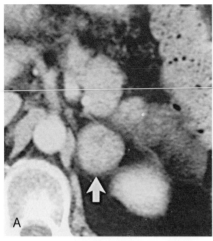

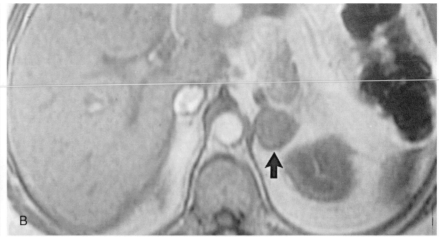

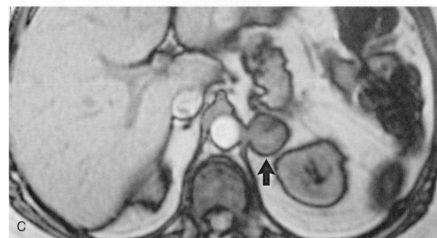

FIGURE 22–20. Metastasis, left adrenal gland, in a 42-year-old woman with primary carcinoma of the lung. The metastasis *(arrows)* measures 2.4 cm in diameter.

A, Computed tomogram, contrast material–enhanced. The tumor is smooth in outline and is heterogeneous in enhancement.

B, In-phase gradient-echo magnetic resonance image (TR = 150 msec, TE = 4.2 msec, flip angle = 60 degrees). The mass is of intermediate signal intensity.

C, Opposed-phase gradient-echo magnetic resonance image (TR = 150 msec, TE = 2.5 msec, flip angle = 60 degrees). There is no appreciable signal loss, a finding that does not support the diagnosis of adenoma.

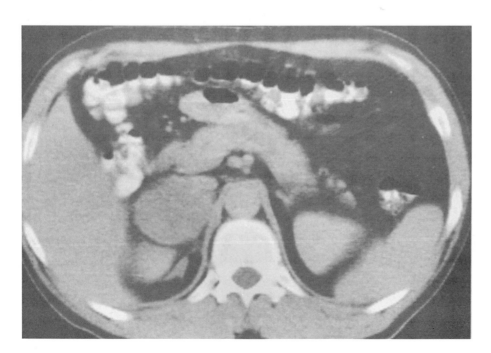

FIGURE 22–21. Metastases producing a large mass in the right adrenal. Computed tomogram, contrast material–enhanced. A melanoma had been excised several years previously.

cose metabolism. Typically, a benign adrenal lesion shows normal FDG activity.

An adrenal metastasis larger than 5 cm in diameter is less of a diagnostic problem than is a small metastatic nodule in that the former is usually associated with advanced disease and a known primary site (Fig. 22–21). Large metastases are often inhomogeneous, owing to hemorrhage or necrosis. Occasionally, hemorrhage extends into the perinephric space (Fig. 22–22).

Multiple adrenal masses or bilateral adrenal enlargement signifying diffuse infiltration are additional manifestations of metastatic disease to the adrenal gland (Figs. 22–23, 22–24). When the metastases are small, the intervening gland is of normal size. With both patterns there is frequently other evidence of abdominal metastases, such as adenopathy or liver metastases. Calcification, most likely the result of prior hemorrhage and/or necrosis, may occur in approximately 16 per cent of cases with these patterns.

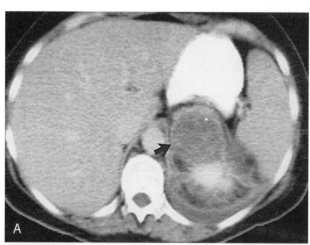

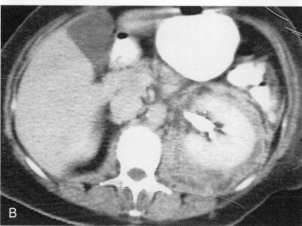

FIGURE 22–22. Metastasis to the adrenal complicated by perinephric hemorrhage.

A, Computed tomogram with contrast material enhancement through the upper pole of the left kidney. There is a large inhomogeneous adrenal mass *(arrow)* that is separate from the kidney.

B, Computed tomogram with contrast material enhancement caudal to *A.* There is blood in the perinephric space.

The radiologic identification of a normal adrenal gland does not always exclude microscopic metastatic disease. Accuracy may depend on the primary neoplasm. In one series of patients with small cell lung carcinoma, biopsy specimens from adrenal glands that appeared normal on computed tomography were found to contain malignant cells in 17 per cent of patients (Pagani, 1983). In contrast, 100 per cent of 119 adrenal glands that were normal by computed tomography in patients with ipsilateral carcinoma of the kidney were also normal histologically (Gill et al., 1994).

Lymphoma

Adrenal gland involvement is found in up to 25 per cent of patients with lymphoma at autopsy. Non-Hodgkin's lymphoma is more likely to involve the adrenal than is Hodgkin's disease. The most common pattern is diffuse enlargement with oval, round, or triangular glands (see Fig. 22–23). Bilateral involvement occurs in 50 per cent of cases and is frequently accompanied by retroperitoneal lymphadenopathy. Necrosis is uncommon in the absence of prior chemotherapy or radiation therapy. Primary lymphoma of the adrenal gland is extremely rare.

Cyst

An adrenal cyst is an uncommon, fluid-filled, non-neoplastic mass that is usually detected as an incidental finding in a patient with no other evidence of adrenal disease. Usually discovered between the third and sixth decades, adrenal cysts are more common in women than in men by a ratio of 3:1. A large cyst may cause pain, but hemorrhage and rupture are rare. Although the exact cause in many cases is uncertain, the majority are believed to be pseudocysts that have evolved from prior adrenal hemorrhage, as discussed in the section that follows. Neonates with Beckwith-Wiedemann syndrome may have benign hemorrhagic cysts within the adrenal capsule or cortex.

A typical adrenal cyst has a fluid-filled center surrounded by a thin wall that does not enhance. This radiologic appearance is similar to a renal cyst, except that up to 15 per cent of adrenal cysts develop peripheral calcification (Fig. 22–25). However, a cystic neoplasm, such as a pheochromocytoma, or rarely an adrenal abscess may produce a similar appearance (see Fig. 22–14).

Hemorrhage

Hemorrhage is the most common cause of an adrenal mass in the neonatal period. This usually occurs in association with birth trauma, hypoxia, renal vein thrombosis, sepsis, coagulopathy, or macrosomia related to maternal diabetes mellitus. The clinical triad of mass, blood loss anemia, and prolonged jaundice is characteristic for neonatal adre-

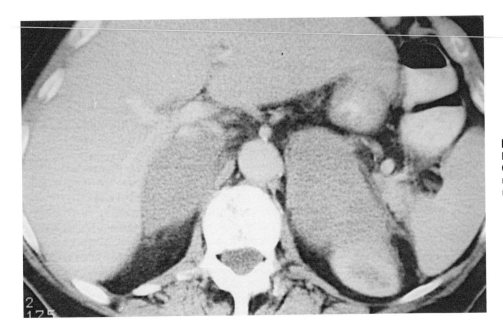

FIGURE 22–23. Metastases, bilateral, secondary to lymphoma. Computed tomogram, contrast material–enhanced. Large masses replace both adrenal glands.

FIGURE 22–24. Metastases, bilateral, secondary to thyroid carcinoma. Computed tomogram, contrast material–enhanced. Large, heterogeneous masses are in both adrenal glands.

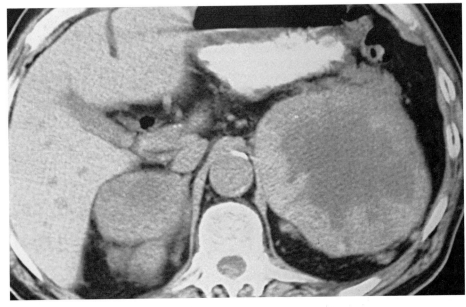
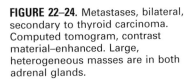

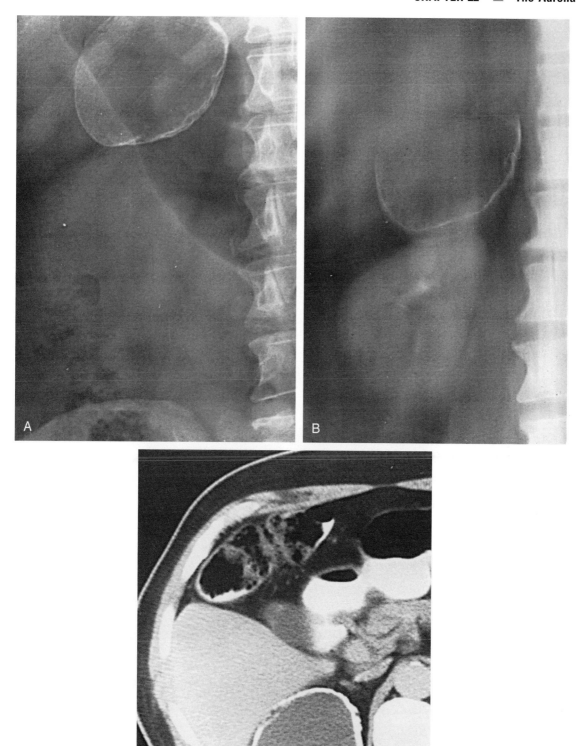

FIGURE 22–25. Cyst, calcified, right adrenal. There is a well-defined, suprarenal mass with peripheral calcification and a homogeneous water density center.
A, Abdominal radiograph.
B, Excretory urogram, tomogram.
C, Computed tomogram, contrast material–enhanced.

nal hemorrhage. In hemorrhage due to birth trauma, the right gland is more frequently involved than the left, possibly because the right adrenal gland is compressed between the spine and the liver. Although 10 per cent of cases of neonatal adrenal hemorrhage are bilateral, adrenal insufficiency is very uncommon.

Adrenal hemorrhage in the older child should raise concern for child abuse. In these cases a search for other evidence of unsuspected trauma should be undertaken.

In the adult, adrenal hemorrhage may result from severe stress, burns, sepsis, hypertension, renal vein thrombosis, liver transplantation affecting the right adrenal, underlying adrenal disease (especially tumors), anticoagulation therapy, primary antiphospholipid syndrome, and trauma. Rarely, adrenal hemorrhage is spontaneous. *Waterhouse-Friderichsen syndrome* was originally described as bilateral adrenal hemorrhage complicating meningococcal septicemia. Recently, this definition has been expanded to include bilateral adrenal hemorrhage as a complication of any cause of sepsis. Bilateral adrenal hemorrhage in the adult may cause acute adrenal insufficiency and death if not recognized and treated with adrenal corticosteroids. The

diagnosis is frequently delayed, however, because clinical findings are often nonspecific.

The ultrasonographic appearance of adrenal hemorrhage varies with the acuteness of the process. Acute hemorrhage often appears as a round or oval suprarenal mass that is slightly hyperechoic relative to liver. Occasionally the echo pattern suggests a solid mass. With time, the lesion becomes more hypoechoic and cystlike. An organizing hematoma decreases in size, becomes multiloculated, and, typically, resolves or calcifies over time (Figs. 22–26, 22–27). If a suspected hematoma does not resolve, regress, or calcify, or if the patient becomes febrile or demonstrates an elevated urinary vanillylmandelic acid value, alternative diagnoses must be considered. These would include adrenal abscess complicating adrenal hemorrhage or a rare neonatal adrenal neoplasm, such as a congenital neuroblastoma.

The computed tomographic findings of adrenal hemorrhage vary with the age of the lesion and whether it is infiltrative or masslike. Initially, a hematoma exhibits increased attenuation values in the range of 50 to 90 Hounsfield Units. The infiltrative pattern appears as an enlarged gland that is hyperdense relative to unenhanced renal paren-

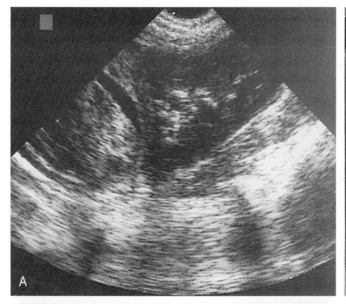

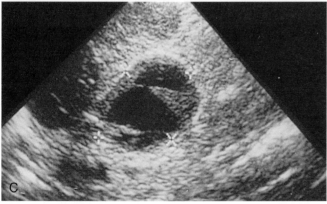

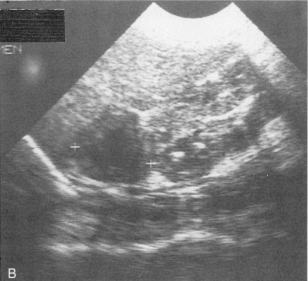

FIGURE 22–26. Hemorrhage, adrenal, in three patients with different ultrasonographic patterns.

A, Solid-appearing hemorrhage.

B, Cystic hemorrhage with a thick wall and internal echoes *(cursors)*.

C, Multiloculated, organizing hemorrhage *(cursors)*.

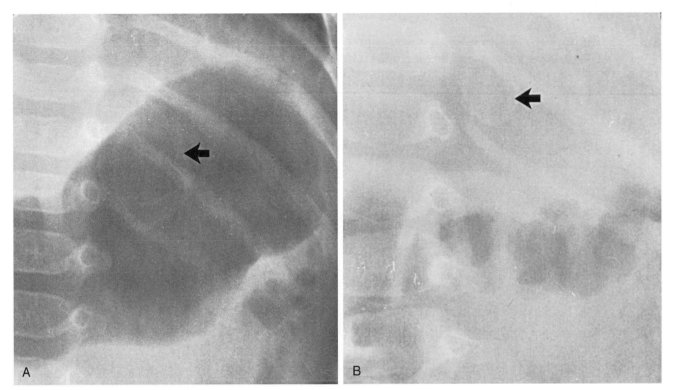

FIGURE 22–27. Hemorrhage, left adrenal, with calcification and decrease in size over time.

A, Abdominal radiograph at 1 month of age. A mass with peripheral calcification *(arrow)* overlies the 11th and 12th posterior ribs.

B, Abdominal radiograph. Ten months later the calcified mass *(arrow)* has diminished in size.

chyma. Typically, there is convex thickening of the limbs (Fig. 22–28). This appearance may simulate one of the infiltrative diseases listed in Table 22–8. However, high attenuation values are distinctive of hemorrhage. Less commonly, hemorrhage presents in the form of a mass that is usually heterogeneous. Bleeding may extend into the perinephric space (Fig. 22–29). This appearance may be identical to an adrenal tumor that has bled.

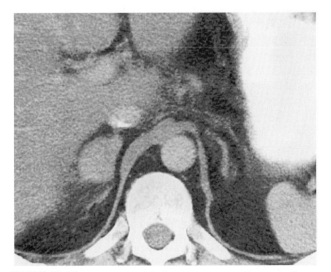

FIGURE 22–28. Hemorrhage, infiltrative pattern. Computed tomogram, contrast material–enhanced. The right adrenal gland is enlarged with a convex lateral margin. The attenuation value measured 51.7 Hounsfield units.

As the hematoma organizes, the attenuation values decrease and the lesion becomes cystic (Fig. 22–30). The wall of the cystic hematoma is initially thick and irregular but eventually becomes thin and frequently calcifies. At this stage, differentiation between an adrenal cyst and a mature cystic hematoma becomes impossible. Indeed, many apparent adrenal cysts are likely the result of an organized adrenal hemorrhage.

The appearance of adrenal hemorrhage with magnetic resonance imaging varies with the evolution of hemoglobin breakdown. Immediately after a hematoma is formed, it appears relatively hypointense on T1-weighted images and hyperintense on T2-weighted images. Over time, T1-weighted images may reveal the formation of a relatively bright ring that progresses inward toward the center of the lesion. The periphery, which may contain hemosiderin-laden macrophages, may produce a thin dark rim on both T1- and T2-weighted images in subacute or chronic hematoma (Fig. 22–31). Although fat and hemorrhage are both bright on T1-weighted images, distinction can usually be made on T2-weighted images because fat will not appear brighter than normal fat elsewhere in the body, whereas hemorrhage often does. This, in addition to the ringlike pattern, is highly suggestive of hemorrhage.

Myelolipoma

Myelolipoma is an uncommon, benign, metabolically inactive tumor composed of adipose and my-

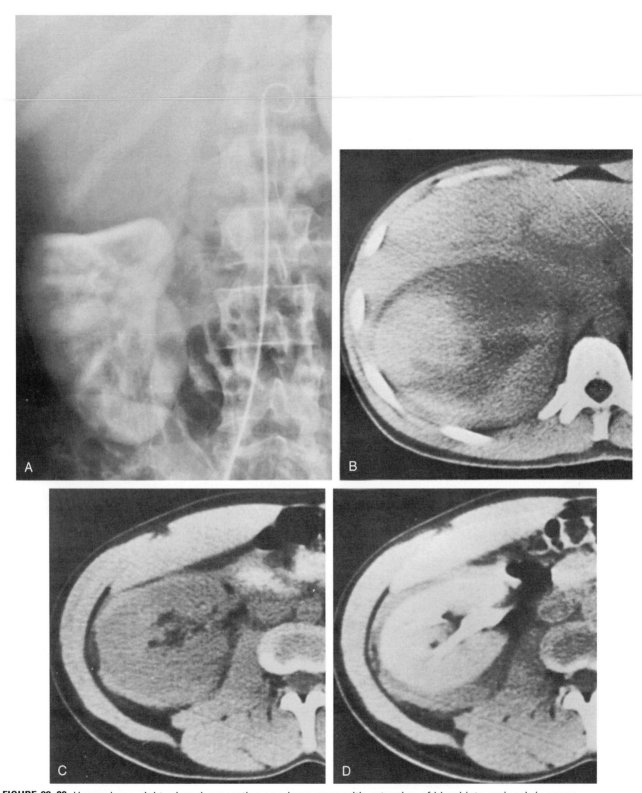

FIGURE 22–29. Hemorrhage, right adrenal, presenting as a large mass with extension of blood into perinephric space.

A, Aortogram, nephrographic phase. There is inferior displacement of the right kidney by a large, extrarenal mass.

B, Computed tomogram without contrast material enhancement through the mass demonstrates mixed densities. The high density area corresponds to fresh hemorrhage.

C, Computed tomogram without contrast material enhancement at the level of the right renal pelvis. The high density blood in the perinephric space forms a thin rim around the unenhanced kidney.

D, Computed tomogram, contrast material–enhanced at the same level as *C* confirms the nonenhancing perinephric hemorrhage.

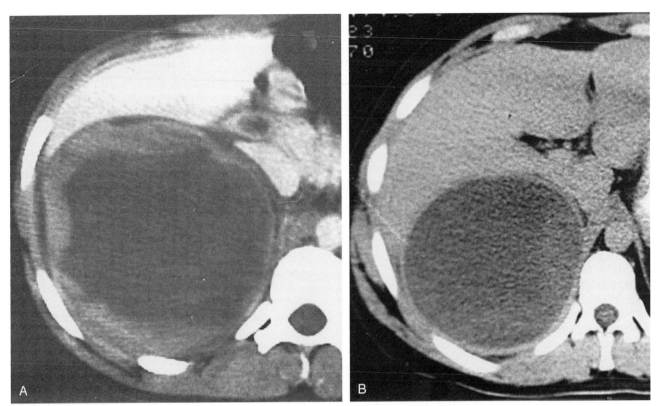

FIGURE 22–30. Hemorrhage, organizing in right adrenal in two patients. Computed tomogram, contrast material–enhanced. As hemorrhage organizes, its attenuation value approaches that of water. The wall may be thick and irregular *(A)* or thin and smooth *(B)*. In the latter case, differentiation from an adrenal cyst is extremely difficult. (Compare with Fig. 22–25.)

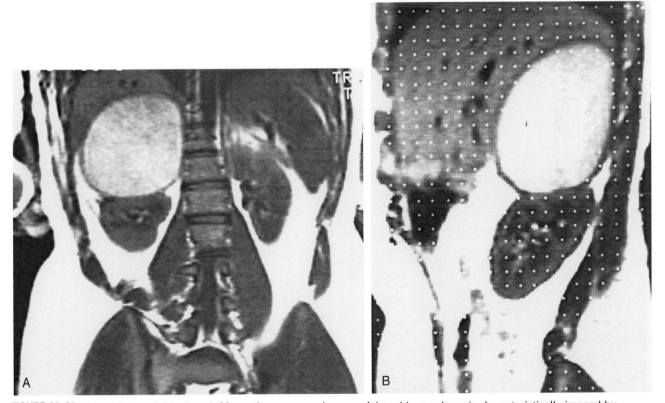

FIGURE 22–31. Hemorrhage, right adrenal. Magnetic resonance images. Adrenal hemorrhage is characteristically imaged by magnetic resonance as a well-defined, mildly heterogeneous mass with a signal that is slightly less intense than that of adjacent retroperitoneal fat. Differentiation from myelolipoma is difficult when utilizing T1-weighted images. (Compare with Fig. 22–32*B.*)
A, T1-weighted image, coronal section.
B, T1-weighted image, sagittal section.

eloid tissue that is usually detected as an incidental finding in adults undergoing a radiologic examination for unrelated clinical indications. Myelolipomas occur in four distinct clinicopathologic patterns: (1) isolated adrenal myelolipoma, (2) adrenal myelolipoma with hemorrhage, (3) extra-adrenal myelolipoma, and (4) myelolipoma with other adrenal disease.

Autopsy series have shown a prevalence of less than 0.2 per cent and an equal sex distribution. Almost all adrenal myelolipomas originate in the adrenal cortex and are often 10 cm in diameter or larger. Approximately 10 per cent of adrenal myelolipomas are bilateral. All myelolipomas contain fat as adipose tissue and myeloid elements in proportions that vary considerably. However, most have sufficient fat to permit detection by computed tomography or magnetic resonance imaging.

Although most patients have otherwise normal adrenal glands, myelolipoma can coexist with Cushing's syndrome, congenital adrenal hyperplasia, and nonhyperfunctioning adenoma. Rarely, a myelolipoma arises in an extra-adrenal site, such as the retroperitoneum, thorax, or pelvis.

Acute hemorrhage is a significant complication of myelolipoma. Spontaneous bleeding can cause acute flank pain or even hypovolemic shock. Large tumors are more likely to bleed than are small ones.

The radiologic appearance of myelolipoma de-pends on the relative amount of fat and myeloid tissue and whether there has been hemorrhage. In most lesions, the fatty component is predominant and recognizable as radiolucency on abdominal radiographs, as a hyperechoic mass on ultrasonograms, as a mass with attenuation values less than −30 Hounsfield units on computed tomograms, or as a high signal intensity on T1-weighted magnetic resonance images (Fig. 22–32).

A myelolipoma that is composed primarily of myeloid tissue may be hypoechoic on ultrasonography and have characteristics of red marrow on other imaging studies. Hemorrhage results in areas that are hypoechoic compared with fat on ultrasonography and are of high attenuation value on computed tomography. The margins of a myelolipoma that is complicated by bleeding may be irregular, owing to blood dissecting into the retroperitoneal fat. Here, the findings of hemorrhage may dominate and obliterate radiologic evidence of fat. Calcification, which is often present as a result of previous hemorrhage, is readily apparent on computed tomography and can be suggested by ultrasonography as hyperechoic areas with acoustic shadowing.

Demonstration of a fat-containing, well-marginated tumor in the region of the adrenal gland strongly suggests the diagnosis of myelolipoma. Rarely, an adenoma or an aggressive metastasis or carcinoma that engulfs normal retroperitoneal fat

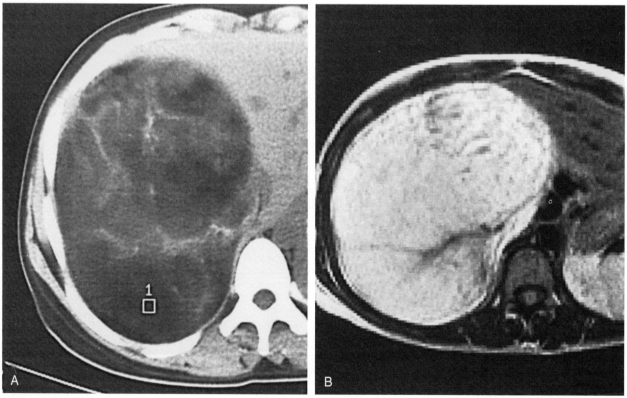

FIGURE 22–32. Myelolipoma, right adrenal. Fatty areas within the tumor are similar to normal subcutaneous fat. The higher density strands on computed tomography and the low signal areas on the magnetic resonance image correspond to areas of hemorrhage or myeloid tissue.
A, Computed tomogram, unenhanced.
B, Magnetic resonance image, T1-weighted.

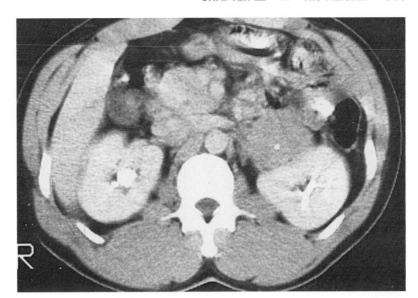

FIGURE 22–33. Ganglioneuroma, left adrenal. Computed tomogram, contrast material–enhanced. A well-defined 5-cm homogeneous adrenal mass compresses the left kidney.

as it spreads may simulate the appearance of a fat-containing tumor. If evidence of fat is absent or equivocal, a radiologic diagnosis of myelolipoma is not possible. Biopsy may be required.

Ganglioneuroma

Ganglioneuroma is a benign neoplasm that is composed of ganglion cells, Schwann cells, and collagen. Rarely, ganglioneuroma coexists with a pheochromocytoma or a peripheral nerve sheath tumor. Ganglioneuroma occurs at all ages. Most are asymptomatic. Adrenal ganglioneuroma is rarely associated with hypertension despite the fact that levels of urinary catecholamines and their metabolites are often elevated. *Verner-Morrison syndrome* consists of watery diarrhea, hypochlorhydria, and alkalosis due to secretion of a vasoactive intestinal polypeptide by a ganglioneuroma. Additional symptoms include sweating, virilization, and myasthenia gravis.

Ganglioneuromas are usually oval or spherical and sharply marginated. Calcification may be present. Large amounts of hemorrhage and necrosis are uncommon. Most tumors are uniformly solid.

Radiologic features of ganglioneuroma generally are nonspecific (Fig. 22–33). On unenhanced computed tomography, a ganglioneuroma has an attenuation value less than that of muscle. On T1-weighted magnetic resonance images, the tumor is homogeneous with relatively low signal intensity, whereas on T2-weighted images the tumor is heterogeneous with a predominantly high signal intensity.

The diagnosis of ganglioneuroma can be suggested in a nonhypertensive patient with an adrenal mass and an elevated level of catecholamine and/or catecholamine metabolites or with Verner-Morrison syndrome. In asymptomatic patients without laboratory abnormalities, a specific diagnosis requires either biopsy or surgical removal.

Granulomatous Disease

Infections that produce granulomatous reaction in the adrenal glands (usually tuberculosis or histoplasmosis) typically cause bilateral enlargement. Adrenal destruction with Addison's disease occurs in the absence of appropriate treatment. Historically, tuberculosis was the most common cause of Addison's disease.

Adrenal glands enlarged by granulomatous disease have rounded contours and resemble inflated balloons. Extension beyond the adrenal is very unusual. On computed tomography, enlarged glands usually contain lucent areas that represent necrosis. The contour may be smooth or lobular (see Fig. 22–17). With treatment, the glands often decrease in size and may become normal in appearance. Calcification may be stippled or solid when it occurs. Occasionally, a dense zone of calcification without evidence of a normal adrenal remnant is the only manifestation of healed granulomatous disease.

Uncommonly, granulomatous disease of the adrenal gland forms a mass, such as a tuberculoma. Such an appearance is impossible to differentiate from the nonfunctioning masses discussed earlier.

Rare Adrenal Masses

Rare adrenal tumors include mesenchymal tumors, such as *leiomyosarcoma, primary melanoma,* and *hemangioma.* These usually present as a large adrenal mass with normal adrenal function. Although the presence of phleboliths and contrast material pooling on angiography has been reported as characteristic for hemangioma, an accurate diagnosis is rarely made prospectively. Likewise, a specific radiologic diagnosis is rarely possible in cases of mesenchymal adrenal tumors.

Extramedullary hematopoiesis is a rare cause of adrenal enlargement. It may be seen in diseases associated with decreased red blood cell production

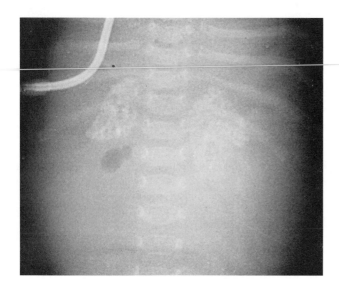

FIGURE 22–34. Wolman's disease. Abdominal radiograph. Both adrenal glands are enlarged and diffusely calcified.

TABLE 22–3. Diagnostic Set: Small (<5 cm) Solid Mass (See Fig. 22–6)

> Hyperfunction
>   Adenoma
>   Hyperplasia (dominant nodule)
>   Pheochromocytoma
>   Neuroblastoma/ganglioneuroblastoma
> Normal function
>   Metastasis
>   Adenoma
>   Myelolipoma
>   Ganglioneuroma

TABLE 22–4. Diagnostic Set: Large (>5 cm) Solid Mass (See Fig. 22–8)

> Hyperfunction
>   Carcinoma
>   Pheochromocytoma
>   Neuroblastoma/ganglioneuroblastoma
> Normal function
>   Carcinoma
>   Metastasis
>   Myelolipoma
>   Ganglioneuroma
>   Granuloma (e.g., tuberculoma)
>   Hemorrhage
>   Rare tumors (e.g., mesenchymal tumor)

TABLE 22–5. Diagnostic Set: Cystic Adrenal Mass (see Fig. 22–14)

> Hyperfunction
>   Pheochromocytoma
>   Neuroblastoma
> Normal function
>   Cyst
>   Organizing hemorrhage

TABLE 22–6. Diagnostic Set: Multiple Adrenal Masses (see Fig. 22–15)

> Hyperfunction
>   Pheochromocytoma
>   Multinodular hyperplasia
> Normal function
>   Metastasis

TABLE 22–7. Diagnostic Set: Adrenal Enlargement (see Fig. 22–2)

Hyperfunction
    Hyperplasia
    Pheochromocytoma
Normal or diminished function
    Granulomatous disease
    Metastasis
    Hemorrhage
    Extramedullary hematopoiesis
    Wolman's disease

by bone marrow. Adrenal enlargement in extramedullary hematopoiesis may, in part, result from hemorrhage that sometimes is a complicating factor.

Wolman's disease (familial xanthomatosis) is a rare metabolic disease that involves the adrenal glands. A disturbance in fat metabolism results in an abnormal accumulation of triglyceride and cholesterol esters. Characteristically, affected patients are children with hepatosplenomegaly and enlarged adrenals with punctate calcifications in areas of tissue necrosis (Fig. 22–34).

DIAGNOSTIC SETS

When confronted with an adrenal mass, it is useful to categorize the lesion in one of the following diagnostic sets:

Small Adrenal Mass (Less Than 5 cm Diameter)
Large Adrenal Mass (More Than 5 cm Diameter)
Cystic Adrenal Mass
Multiple Adrenal Masses
Adrenal Enlargement
Adrenal Calcification

Each of these diagnostic sets includes entities that can be further characterized as to whether the patient in question exhibits adrenal hyperfunction, normal function, or diminished function. Each diagnostic set is formulated in Tables 22–3 through 22–8. Other radiologic features that might enable a specific diagnosis should be sought. Usually, however, only a differential diagnosis is possible.

TABLE 22–8. Adrenal Lesions That Calcify (see Fig. 22–25)

Adenoma
Carcinoma
Neuroblastoma/ganglioneuroblastoma
Ganglioneuroma
Pheochromocytoma
Metastasis
Mesenchymal tumors
Hemangioma (phleboliths)
Cyst
Hemorrhage
Myelolipoma
Granulomatous disease
Wolman's disease

BIBLIOGRAPHY

Approach to Adrenal Imaging

Bilbey, J. H., McLoughlin, R. F., Kurkjian, P. S., Wilkins, G. E. L., Chan, N. H. L., Schmidt, N., and Singer, J.: MR imaging of adrenal masses: Value of chemical-shift imaging for distinguishing adenomas from other tumors. AJR *164*:637, 1995.

Boland, G. W., Goldberg, M. A., Lee, M. J., Mayo-Smith, W. W., Dixon, J., McNicholas, M. M., and Mueller, P. R.: Indeterminate adrenal mass in patients with cancer: Evaluation at PET with 2-[F-18]-fluoro-2-deoxy-D-glucose. Radiology *194*:131, 1995.

Boland, G. W., Hahn, P. F., Pena, C., and Mueller, P. R.: Adrenal masses: Characterization with delayed contrast-enhanced CT. Radiology *202*:693, 1997.

Choyke, P. L.: Invited commentary. RadioGraphics *14*:1029, 1994.

Choyke, P. L.: From needles to numbers: Can noninvasive imaging distinguish benign and malignant lesions? World J. Urol. *16*:29, 1998.

Cirillo, R. L., Bennett, W. F., Vitellas, K. M., Poulos, A. G., and Bova, J. G.: Pathology of the adrenal gland: Imaging features. AJR *170*:429, 1998.

Doppman, J. L.: Problems in endocrinologic imaging. Endocrinol. Metab. Clin. North Am. *26*:973, 1997.

Dunnick, N. R., Korobkin, M., and Francis, I.: Adrenal radiology: Distinguishing benign from malignant adrenal masses. AJR *167*:861, 1996.

Gilfeather, M., and Woodward, P. J.: MR imaging of the adrenal glands and kidneys. Semin. Ultrasound CT MRI *19*:53, 1998.

Korobkin, M., Brodeur, F. J., Francis, I. R., Quint, L. E., Dunnick, N. R., and Goodsitt, M.: Delayed enhanced CT for differentiation of benign from malignant adrenal masses. Radiology *200*:737, 1996.

Korobkin, M., Brodeur, F. J., Yutzy, G. G., Francis, I. R., Quint, L. E., Dunnick, N. R., and Kazerooni, E. A.: Differentiation of adrenal adenomas from nonadenomas using CT attenuation values. AJR *166*:531, 1996.

Korobkin, M., and Dunnick, N. R.: Characterization of adrenal masses. AJR *164*:643, 1995.

Korobkin, M., Giordano, T. J., Brodeur, F. J., Francis, I. R., Siegelman, E. S., Quint, L. E., Dunnick, N. R., Heiken, J. P., and Wang, H. H.: Adrenal adenomas: Relationship between histologic lipid and CT and MR findings. Radiology *200*:743, 1996.

Korobkin, M., Lombardi, T. J., Aisen, A. M., Francis, I. R., Quint, L. E., Dunnick, N. R., Londy, F., Shapiro, B., Gross, M. D., and Thompson, N. W.: Characterization of adrenal masses with chemical shift and gadolinium-enhanced MR imaging. Radiology *197*:411, 1995.

Lee, M. J., Mayo-Smith, W. W., Hahn, P. F., Goldberg, M. A., Boland, G. W., Saini, S., and Papanicolaou, N.: State-of-the-art MR imaging of the adrenal gland. RadioGraphics *14*:1015, 1994.

Mayo-Smith, W. W., Lee, M. J., McNicholas, M. M. J., Hahn, P. F., Boland, G. W., and Saini, S.: Characterization of adrenal masses (<5 cm) by use of chemical shift MR imaging: Observer performance versus quantitative measures. AJR *165*:91, 1995.

McNicholas, M. M. J., Lee, M. J., Mayo-Smith, W. W., Hahn, P. F., Boland, G. W., and Mueller, P. R.: An imaging algorithm for the differential diagnosis of adrenal adenomas and metastases. AJR *165*:1453, 1995.

Outwater, E. K., Siegelman, E. S., Huang, A. B., and Birnbaum, B. A.: Adrenal masses: Correlation between CT attenuation value and chemical shift ratio at MR imaging with in-phase and opposed-phase sequences. Radiology *200*:749, 1996.

Outwater, E. K., Siegelman, E. S., Radecki, P. D., Piccoli, C. W., and Mitchell, D. G.: Distinction between benign and malignant adrenal masses: Value of T1-weighted chemical-shift MR imaging. AJR *165*:579, 1995.

Peppercorn, P. D., and Reznek, R. H.: State-of-the-art CT and MRI of the adrenal gland. Eur. Radiol. 7:822, 1997.

Peppercorn, P. D., Grossman, A. B., and Reznek, R. H.: Imaging of incidentally discovered adrenal masses. Clin. Endocrinol. *48*:379, 1998.

Reinig, J. W., Stutley, J. E., Leonhardt, C. M., Spicer, K. M., Margolis, M., and Caldwell, C. B.: Differentiation of adrenal masses with MR imaging: Comparison of techniques. Radiology *192*:41, 1994.

Schwartz, L. H., Panicek, D. M., Doyle, M. V., Ginsberg, M. S.,

Herman, S. K., Koutcher, J. A., Brown, K. T., Getrajdman, G. I., and Burt, M.: Comparison of two algorithms and their associated charges when evaluating adrenal masses in patients with malignancies. AJR 168:1575, 1997.

Szolar, D. H., and Kammerhuber, F.: Quantitative CT evaluation of adrenal gland masses: A step forward in the differentiation between adenomas and nonadenomas? Radiology 202:517, 1997.

Welch, T. J., Sheedy, P. F., Stephens, D. H., Johnson, C. M., and Swensen, S. J.: Percutaneous adrenal biopsy: Review of a 10 year experience. Radiology 193:341, 1994.

Westra, S. J., Zaninovic, A. C., Hall, T. R., Kangarloo, H., and Boechat, M. I.: Imaging of the adrenal gland in children. RadioGraphics 14:1323, 1994.

Abnormal Adrenal Function

Abramson, S. J.: Adrenal neoplasms in children. Radiol. Clin. North Am. 35:1415, 1997.

Carney, J. A.: The triad of gastric epithelioid leiomyosarcoma, pulmonary chondroma, and functioning extra-adrenal paraganglioma: A five-year review. Medicine 62:159, 1983.

Doppman, J. L.: The dilemma of bilateral adrenocortical nodularity in Conn's and Cushing's syndromes. Radiol. Clin. North Am. 31:1039, 1993.

Doppman, J. L., and Gill, J. R.: Hyperaldosteronism: Sampling the adrenal veins. Radiology 198:309, 1996.

Doppman, J. L., Travis, W. D., Nieman, L., Miller, D. L., Chrousos, G. P., Gomez, M. T., Cutler, G. B., Loriaux, D. L., and Norton, J. A.: Cushing syndrome due to primary pigmented nodular adrenocortical disease: Findings at CT and MR imaging. Radiology 172:415, 1989.

Efremidis, S. C., Harsoulis, F., Douma, S., Zafiriadou, E., Zamboulis, C., and Kouri, A.: Adrenal insufficiency with enlarged adrenals. Abdom. Imaging 21:168, 1996.

Findling, J. W., and Doppman, J. L.: Biochemical and radiologic diagnosis of Cushing's syndrome. Endocrinol. Metab. Clin. North Am. 23:511, 1994.

Forman, H. P., Leonidas, J. C., Berdon, W. E., Slovis, T. L., Wood, B. P., and Samudrala, R.: Congenital neuroblastoma: Evaluation with multimodality imaging. Radiology 175:365, 1990.

Hattner, R. S.: Practical considerations in the scintigraphic evaluation of endocrine hypertension—the adrenal cortex and medulla. Radiol. Clin. North Am. 31:1029, 1993.

Jennings, R. W., LaQuaglia, M. P., Leong, K., Hendren, W. H., and Adzick, N. S.: Fetal neuroblastoma: Prenatal diagnosis and natural history. J. Pediatr. Surg. 28:1168, 1993.

Litchfield, W. R., and Dluhy, R. G.: Primary aldosteronism. Endocrinol. Metab. Clin. North Am. 24:593, 1995.

Marotti, M., Sucic, Z., Krolo, I., Dimanovski, J., Klaric, R., Ferencic, Z., Karapanda, N., Babic, N., and Pavlekovic, K.: Adrenal cavernous hemangioma: MRI, CT, and US appearance. Eur. Radiol. 7:691, 1997.

Melby, J. C.: Diagnosis of hyperaldosteronism. Endocrinol. Metab. Clin. North Am. 20:247, 1991.

Mukherjee, J. J., Peppercorn, P. D., Reznek, R. H., Patel, V., Kaltsas, G., Besser, M., and Grossman, A. B.: Pheochromocytoma: Effect of nonionic contrast medium in CT on circulating catecholamine levels. Radiology 202:227, 1997.

Zografos, G. C., Driscoll, D. L., Karakousis, C. P., and Huben, R. P.: Adrenal adenocarcinoma: A review of 53 cases. J. Surg. Oncol. 55:160, 1994.

Abnormal Adrenal Morphology with Normal Function

Casey, L. R., Cohen, A. J., Wile, A. G., and Dietrich, R. B.: Giant adrenal myelolipomas: CT and MRI findings. Abdom. Imaging 19:165, 1994.

Commons, R. R., and Callaway, C. P.: Adenomas of the adrenal cortex. Arch. Intern. Med. 81:37, 1948.

Cyran, K. M., Kenney, P. J., Memel, D. S., and Yacoub, I.: Adrenal myelolipoma. AJR 166:395, 1996.

Erasmus, J. J., Patz, E. F., McAdams, H. P., Murray, J. G., Herndon, J., Coleman, R. E., and Goodman, P. C.: Evaluation

of adrenal masses in patients with bronchogenic carcinoma using ^{18}F-fluorodeoxy-glucose positron emission tomography. AJR 168:1357, 1997.

Ferrozzi, F., and Bova, D.: CT and MR demonstration of fat within an adrenal cortical carcinoma. Abdom. Imaging 20:272, 1995.

Gill, I. S., McClennan, B. L., Kerbl, K., Carbone, J. M., Wick, M., and Clayman, R. V.: Adrenal involvement from renal cell carcinoma: Predictive value of computerized tomography. J. Urol. 152:1082, 1994.

Gross, M. D., and Shapiro, B.: Clinical review of 50 clinically silent adrenal masses. J. Clin. Endocrinol. Metab. 77:885, 1993.

Han, M., Burnett, A. L., Fishman, E. K., and Marshall, F. F.: The natural history and treatment of adrenal myelolipoma. J. Urol. 57:1213, 1997.

Hibbert, J., Howlett, D. C., Greenwood, K. L., MacDonald, L. M., and Saunders, A. J. S.: The ultrasound appearances of neonatal renal vein thrombosis. Br. J. Radiol. 70:1191, 1997.

Hoeffel, C., Legmann, P., Luton, J. P., Chapuis, Y., and Fayet-Bonnin P.: Spontaneous unilateral adrenal hemorrhage: Computerized tomography and magnetic resonance imaging findings in 8 cases. J. Urol. 154:1647, 1995.

Ichikawa, T., Ohtomo, K., Araki, T., Fujimoto, H., Nemoto, K., Nanbu, A., Onoue, M., and Aoki, K.: Ganglioneuroma: Computed tomography and magnetic resonance features. Br. J. Radiol. 69:114, 1996.

Johnson, G. L., Hruban, R. H., Marshall, F. F., and Fishman, E. K.: Primary adrenal ganglioneuroma: CT findings in four patients. AJR 169:169, 1997.

Kenney, P. J., Wagner, B. J., Rao, P., and Heffess, C. S.: Myelolipoma: CT and pathologic features. Radiology 208:87, 1998.

Korobkin, M., Francis, I. R., Kloos, R., and Dunnick, N. R.: The incidental adrenal mass. Radiol. Clin. North Am. 34:1037, 1996.

Korobkin, M., Brodeur, F. J., Francis, I. R., Quint, L. E., Dunnick, N. R., and Londy, F.: CT time-attenuation washout curves of adrenal adenomas and nonademonas. AJR 190:749, 1998.

McCauley, R. G. K., Beckwith, J. B., Elias, E. R., Faerber, E. N., Prewitt, L. H., and Berdon, W. E.: Benign hemorrhagic adrenocortical macrocysts in Beckwith-Wiedemann syndrome. AJR 157:549, 1991.

Miyake, H., Takaki, H., Matsumoto, S., Yoshida, S., Maeda, T., and Mori, H. Adrenal nonhyperfunctioning adenoma and nonadenoma: CT attenuation value as discriminative index. Abdom. Imaging 20:559, 1995.

Nimkin, K., Teeger, S., Wallach, M. T., DuVally, J. C., Spevak, M. R., and Kleinman, P. K.: Adrenal hemorrhage in abused children: Imaging and postmortem findings. AJR 162:661, 1994.

Provenzale, J. M., Ortel, T. L., and Nelson, R. C.: Adrenal hemorrhage in patients with primary antiphospholipid syndrome: Imaging findings. AJR 165:361, 1995.

Pagani, J. J.: Normal adrenal glands in small cell lung carcinoma: CT-guided biopsy. AJR 140:949, 1983.

Radin, R., David, C. L., Goldfarb, H., and Francis, I. R.: Adrenal and extra-adrenal retroperitoneal ganglioneuroma: Imaging findings in 13 adults. Radiology 202:703, 1997.

Rao, P., Kenney, P. J., Wagner, B. J., and Davidson, A. J.: Imaging and pathologic features of myelolipoma. RadioGraphics 17:1373, 1997.

Rozenblit, A., Morehouse, H. T., and Amis, E. S.: Cystic adrenal lesions: CT features. Radiology 201:541, 1996.

Sanders, R., Bissada, N., Curry, N., and Gordon, B.: Clinical spectrum of adrenal myelolipoma: Analysis of 8 tumors in 7 patients. J Urol 153:1791, 1995.

Sato, N., Watanabe, Y., Saga, T., Mitsudo, K., Dohke, M., and Minami, K.: Adrenocortical adenoma containing a fat component: CT and MR image evaluation. Abdom. Imaging 20:489, 1995.

Shifrin, R. Y., Bechtold, R. E., and Scharling, E. S.: Metastatic adenocarcinoma within an adrenal adenoma: Detection with chemical shift imaging. AJR 167:891, 1996.

Szolar, D. H., and Kammerhuber, F. H.: Adrenal adenomas and nonadenomas: Assessment of washout at delayed contrast-enhanced CT. Radiology 207:369, 1998.

Tung, G. A., Pfister, R. C., Papanicolaou, N., and Yoder, I. C.: Adrenal cysts: Imaging and percutaneous aspiration. Radiology 173:107, 1989.

VI

THE GENITAL TRACT

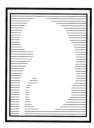

23

Ovary and Adnexa

Most women referred for pelvic imaging are evaluated by ultrasonography for the purpose of confirming or characterizing a clinically detected adnexal mass. Computed tomography and magnetic resonance imaging are usually reserved for problem-solving in selected situations. Most adnexal masses prove to be of ovarian origin, although some arise from the fallopian tube or an extragenital site, such as the appendix. This chapter discusses the imaging of normal anatomy and the common disorders of the ovaries and fallopian tubes.

ANATOMY AND PHYSIOLOGY

The ovaries are attached to the lateral aspect of the uterus by the ovarian ligament and to the pelvic side wall by a suspensory ligament. The ovary is fixed by the mesovarium to the broad ligament, which itself is a reflection of peritoneum. The arterial blood supply to the ovary is derived from branches of both the uterine artery and the aorta. Venous drainage is through paired gonadal veins. On the left side, the gonadal vein drains directly to the left renal vein, whereas on the right side drainage is to the inferior vena cava. The normal ovary is variable in volume but generally is between 8 and 14 mL. In premenarchal and postmenopausal women, the ovary is considerably smaller.

In contrast to the testicle, the gross morphology of the premenopausal ovary varies with its physiologic activity, which represents both reproductive and hormonal functions. The central stroma of the ovary is covered by a surface epithelium of modified peritoneal cells that are the site of follicle formation, rupture, and repair. The epithelial covering of the ovary is derived from the urogenital ridge in proximity to the site of müllerian duct development. This may account for the fact that the epithelial neoplasms of the ovary histologically resemble müllerian structures, such as the fallopian tube (serous), endometrium (endometrioid), and cervix (mucinous).

The histology of the ovary varies with the menstrual cycle. Granulosa cells surround individual germ cells, known as *oocytes,* and enclose a fluid-filled space, the *graafian follicle.* Under the influence of pituitary luteinizing hormone, the graafian follicle enlarges and matures during the first half of the menstrual cycle. At midcycle the follicle ruptures and expels the oocyte. The residual follicle becomes the *corpus luteum,* which is the main source of progesterone during the second half of the cycle. In the absence of pregnancy, the corpus luteum involutes. However, it is a very vascular structure and, in some instances, may enlarge and become symptomatic as a result of hemorrhage.

PHYSIOLOGIC CYSTS
Follicular Cyst

The follicular cyst is one of the most common of adnexal masses. This lesion is thought to arise either from hemorrhage into a non–dominant follicle or as a reflection of disrupted repair following follicular rupture. This benign lesion may produce pelvic pain, which is typically self-limited. A follicular cyst

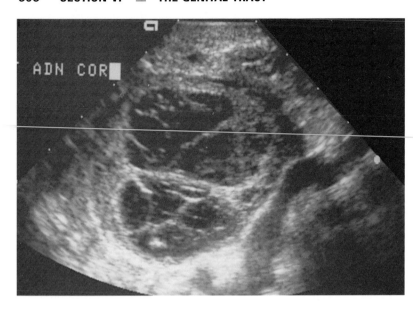

FIGURE 23–1. Hemorrhagic right ovarian cyst in a 27-year-old woman with intermittent pelvic pain of several weeks duration. Transvaginal pelvic ultrasonogram. There are two locules located centrally within the ovary with incomplete echogenic lines, the so-called "fish-net" appearance (same patient illustrated in Fig. 23–30).

almost always resolves spontaneously. Differential diagnosis includes neoplasm and endometriosis, as discussed in following sections.

The ultrasonographic appearance of a follicular cyst varies from that of a simple cyst, with an absence of internal echoes and a smooth inner wall to a heterogeneous mass with an irregular, ill-defined wall (Figs. 23–1 and 23–2). Much of this variability is related to hemorrhage within the cyst. A reticulated internal echotexture that consists of interrupted linear echogenic foci has been characterized as a "fish net" appearance (see Figs. 23–1 and 23–2B). An irregular, eccentric echogenicity may be seen due to a resolving clot. This may mimic a neoplasm (Fig. 23–3). A "ground glass" appearance of diffuse, homogeneous medium-level echogenicity with acoustic enhancement may be seen in a follicu-

lar cyst, although this appearance is more commonly associated with endometriosis.

Corpus Luteum Cyst

A corpus luteum cyst, like a follicular cyst, results from slight variations in normal ovarian physiology and is generally self-limited. The corpus luteum itself is typically unrecognized clinically and ultrasonographically in a nonpregnant patient unless complicated by hemorrhage. Although the corpus luteum cyst is more likely to have a slightly thickened irregular wall than is seen in a hemorrhagic follicular cyst, the two lesions demonstrate significant overlap in their ultrasonographic appearance and cannot be reliably differentiated (Fig. 23–4). In any event, such distinction is rarely of clinical

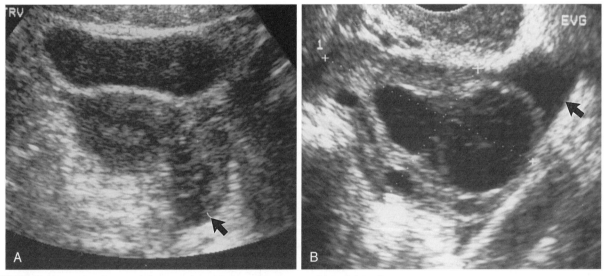

FIGURE 23–2. Hemorrhagic cyst, left ovary, in a 21-year-old woman with pelvic pain.
A, Transabdominal ultrasonogram. There is an ill-defined adnexal mass *(arrow)* posterior and lateral to the uterus.
B, Transvaginal ultrasonogram. The complex mass is composed of incomplete intersecting linear echoes, the so-called "fish-net" appearance. Free fluid is present *(arrow).*

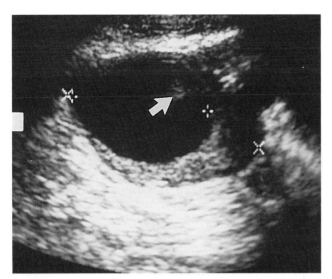

FIGURE 23–3. Hemorrhagic ovarian cyst. A small area of echogenicity *(arrow)* within an otherwise simple cyst is consistent with an eccentric clot.

importance, because follicular cysts or corpus luteum cysts, whether or not they are complicated by hemorrhage, are usually nonsurgical lesions.

Magnetic resonance imaging of a corpus luteum cyst occasionally shows homogeneous high-signal intensity on T1-weighted images as a result of hemorrhage. This finding, however, is variable, and the technique is rarely needed in the setting of any suspected physiologic cyst.

Theca Lutein Cyst

The theca lutein cyst is of importance because it is more likely to mimic a neoplasm than the two cystic masses that have been previously discussed. While physiologic, a theca lutein cyst is typically the result of *abnormal* physiology, being associated with high circulating levels of the beta subunit of human chorionic gonadotropin (beta-hCG) as occurs in patients with hydatidiform mole or other forms of gesta-

tional trophoblastic disease. Theca lutein cyst is also associated with twin gestations, fetal hydrops, and occasionally normal pregnancy. Additionally, this form of physiologic cyst occurs with hyperstimulation of the ovary associated with treatment for infertility, both with clomiphene citrate (Clomid) and, more commonly, exogenous gonadotropins (Pergonal).

A theca lutein cyst is multilocular and generally has a smooth outer surface. Septations are quite thin and smooth. The morphology of a theca lutein cyst may closely resemble that of a mucinous cystadenoma, but the clinical setting of the two generally permit differentiation. Because it occurs in a relatively specific setting, with correlative ultrasonographic or clinical findings, the theca lutein cyst does not require surgical intervention unless complicated by torsion or hemorrhage.

By ultrasonography, thin smooth septations are well seen in a theca lutein cyst. Minimal solid tissue is present, in contrast to most cystic neoplasms (Fig. 23–5). When detected, theca lutein cysts are often bilateral and may be quite large. Obviously, the causative factor in pregnancy-related theca lutein cysts will eventually resolve. Gradual resolution, sometimes over many months, also follows dilatation and curettage for a hydatidiform mole. A similar improvement follows cessation of ovarian-stimulating agents.

Serous (Epithelial) Inclusion Cyst

A serous (epithelial) inclusion cyst may be seen at any age. Nearly 10 per cent of postmenopausal patients in whom the ovaries are often thought to be inactive may have simple cysts exceeding 15 mm in diameter (Levine et al., 1992). The importance of serous (epithelial) inclusion cyst lies in the necessity that they may require follow-up in view of the

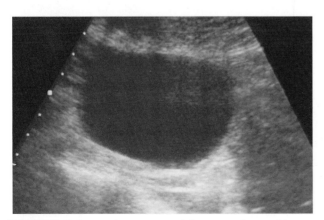

FIGURE 23–4. Corpus luteum cyst, right ovary, detected in a patient with an intrauterine pregnancy of 7 weeks duration. Transabdominal ultrasonogram. A simple cyst of 6.5 cm diameter is consistent with a corpus luteum cyst.

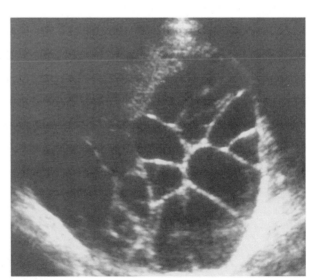

FIGURE 23–5. Theca lutein cyst in a patient with a hydatidiform mole and a high serum beta-hCG. The multiloculated cystic mass exhibits a smooth outer margin and thin smooth septations.

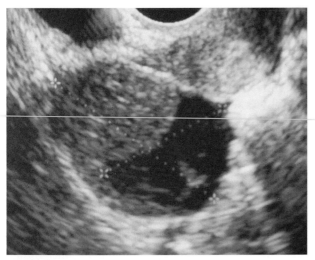

FIGURE 23–6. Tubo-ovarian abscess, right adnexa. Transvaginal ultrasonogram. There is a complex crescentic fluid collection immediately adjacent to the uniformly echogenic ovary.

overlap in the ultrasonographic appearance of small neoplasms and serous (epithelial) inclusion cysts.

POLYCYSTIC OVARIAN (STEIN-LEVENTHAL) SYNDROME

Polycystic ovarian, or Stein-Leventhal, syndrome is a nonheritable condition that consists of abnormal menses (including amenorrhea and oligomenorrhea), hirsutism, and infertility. Excessive luteinizing hormone secretion by the pituitary is the likely cause. The macroscopic features of polycystic ovarian disease range from nearly normal to bilaterally enlarged ovaries with multiple moderate-sized cysts. Imaging findings reflect this range of findings. Most commonly noted is a predominance of small peripheral follicles that are large enough to

be seen ultrasonographically. Occasionally, only ovarian enlargement without recognizable cysts is present.

INFECTION

Abscess

Pelvic inflammatory disease is often limited to the fallopian tube as *salpingitis.* Sometimes, though, infection may extend to the ovary itself and cause a *tubo-ovarian abscess.* A tubo-ovarian abscess may have an echogenic fluid collection with septations and a thickened irregular inner wall (Figs. 23–6 and 23–7). This ultrasonographic appearance is, however, nonspecific and may mimic an ovarian neoplasm. Clinical features, such as fever and leukocytosis, generally suggest the diagnosis of infection.

One of the confounding aspects of adnexal imaging is the close anatomic relationship that the ovary and fallopian tubes share with surrounding structures, especially small and large bowel. The differential diagnosis of an adnexal inflammatory mass, therefore, should include intestinal disorders. Both diverticulitis and appendicitis occasionally manifest clinical and ultrasonographic features that are indistinguishable from those of tubo-ovarian abscess. In patients in whom intestinal sources for inflammatory masses are a possibility, computed tomography with enteric contrast material may be more useful than ultrasonography in providing a comprehensive view of the pelvic anatomy.

Fallopian Tube Dilatation

Hydrosalpinx. Hydrosalpinx often follows prior pelvic inflammatory disease as a sequela of salpingitis or pyosalpinx. Clinical manifestations include pelvic pain, infertility, and a palpable pelvic mass.

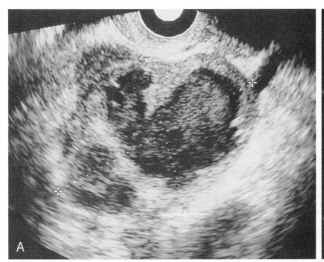
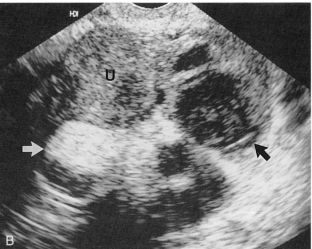

FIGURE 23–7. Tubo-ovarian abscess, left adnexa, in a 26-year-old woman with fever and pelvic pain.
A, Transvaginal ultrasonogram, longitudinal projection. A complex, thick-walled mass is present in the adnexa.
B, Transvaginal ultrasonogram, transverse projection. The complex mass *(black arrow)* is to the left of the uterus (U). The echogenic mass in the right adnexa *(white arrow)* is an incidentally discovered mature teratoma (dermoid cyst).

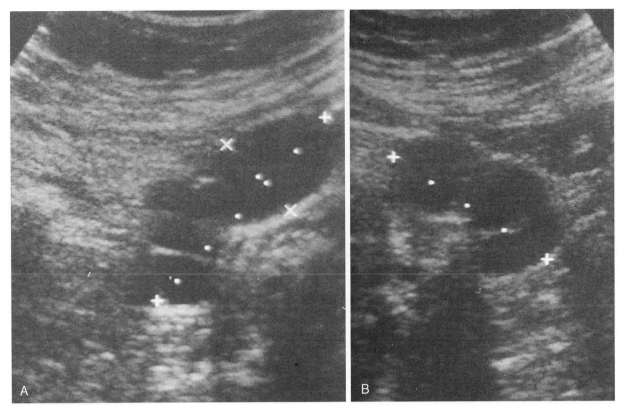

FIGURE 23–8. Hydrosalpinx, left adnexa, in a 30-year-old woman. Transabdominal ultrasonograms. *(A)* Longitudinal and *(B)* transverse projections. The cystic mass *(cursors)* has an elongated, serpentine shape with eccentric, linear echogenic folds.

Radiologic distinction from a neoplasm is often of importance in patient management. The characteristic imaging finding, which may be seen with any imaging modality but is typically seen ultrasonographically, is an elongated, predominantly cystic structure that resembles the dilated fallopian tube (Fig. 23–8). Critical features in differentiating hydrosalpinx from ovarian neoplasm include the absence of a significant soft tissue component, the lack of the spherical or ovoid shape that characterizes most ovarian neoplasms, and a history of pelvic inflammatory disease.

Pyosalpinx/Hematosalpinx. Pyosalpinx or hematosalpinx may appear identical to hydrosalpinx, but the fluid is typically more echogenic, reflecting the presence of pus or blood within the tube. The clinical setting generally facilitates the differentiation of hydrosalpinx, pyosalpinx, and hematosalpinx.

ENDOMETRIOSIS

Endometrial tissue implanted outside the endometrial cavity constitutes the condition known as endometriosis. The most common extrauterine site is the ovary and its surrounding peritoneal reflections. However, virtually any site within the peritoneal cavity may be involved. Rarely, implants involve the abdominal wall, urinary tract, or even the thorax. Endometriosis of the ureter and bladder is discussed in Chapters 16 and 19.

Endometriosis takes two forms: solid implants, which tend to be small, and cysts, which can be quite large. Both may coexist and be multiple. Symptoms, including pelvic pain, dyspareunia, and tubal dysfunction leading to infertility, are characteristic of endometriosis and may be caused by very small implants that are not radiologically demonstrable. Because the endometrial tissue responds to cyclic hormonal changes, monthly bleeding may occur. As a result, the implants enlarge over time with products of recurrent hemorrhage and surrounding fibrosis. These masses are variably referred to as *endometriomas, endometriotic cysts,* or *chocolate cysts.* The latter term refers to the thick, dark-colored nature of the cyst contents.

Despite marked variability in the frequency and chronicity of hemorrhage in endometriomas, most exhibit a characteristic ultrasonographic appearance of a moderately thick wall and diffuse homogeneous medium-level echogenicity, which has been characterized as "ground glass" in appearance. Because the content of an endometrioma is liquid, although somewhat echogenic, acoustic enhancement is usually demonstrated (Figs. 23–9 and 23–10A). Septation and soft-tissue projections into the lumen of the endometrioma are unusual, two characteristics that help differentiate an endometrioma from a neoplasm.

Endometriomas often exhibit characteristic features on magnetic resonance imaging (Fig. 23–10B, C). On T1-weighted images, the hemorrhagic degra-

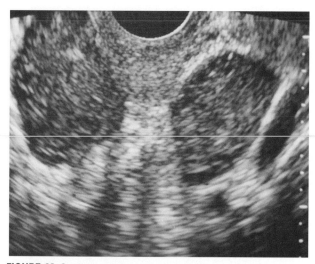

FIGURE 23–9. Endometrioma, bilateral. Transvaginal ultrasonogram. Hypoechoic, slightly heterogeneous masses represent an endometrioma in each ovary.

dation products within an endometrioma produce homogeneous high-signal intensity. A relatively lower signal intensity is seen on corresponding T2-weighted images. Occasionally, a gradation of signal intensity, consisting of lower signal in the dependent portion of the mass, is seen on T2-weighted images. This has been termed "shading." Additionally, an endometrioma exhibits considerable enhancement with gadolinium chelate contrast material.

Additional findings of endometriosis include multiplicity of lesions and ill-defined tissue planes between the pelvic viscera and surrounding bowel loops. Although these features suggest the diagnosis of endometriosis, it should be kept in mind that the same findings may be seen with hemorrhagic neoplasms. Nevertheless, the ability to suggest a benign process may support a modified surgical approach. A significant limitation in the imaging of endometriosis is the lack of sensitivity for detecting peritoneal implants, which may be the source of significant symptoms even when they are quite small. Endometriomas that are implanted on the serosal surface of the gastrointestinal tract may cause a tethered appearance to the bowel wall on imaging studies (Fig. 23–11). This is especially common along the anterior aspect of the midrectum, which is the dependent portion of the pelvis.

NEOPLASMS

Primary tumors of the ovary arise from one of three tissues: epithelial, germ cell, or gonadal stroma. Table 23–1 list the specific subtypes that occur in each of these categories, as well as secondary tumors. Only the more common of the primary tumors are discussed in this section.

Epithelial Tumors

Epithelial tumors account for slightly more than one-half of all ovarian neoplasms, but they represent 90 per cent of ovarian malignancies. Thus, when one speaks of ovarian cancer, an epithelial neoplasm is the most likely histology. These lesions arise from the surface epithelium of the ovary and include *serous, mucinous, endometrioid, clear cell,* and *Brenner* tumors. Not all epithelial tumors occur on the ovarian surface, however. Epithelial inclusion cysts, which are found within the stroma of normal ovaries, may be the source of an epithelial neoplasm that actually arises within the ovarian parenchyma.

Although epithelial tumors may occur at any age, they are more common in older women. Indeed, malignant epithelial tumors are unusual before the age of 25 years. However, women of families with more than one first-degree relative affected with ovarian carcinoma clearly have an increased risk for development of the tumor at an earlier age. Most ovarian malignancies are discovered after disease has spread beyond the ovary itself (Fig. 23–12). Thus, while ovarian cancer is less common than other gynecologic malignancies, it is a more common cause of death than either cervical or uterine carcinoma. Aside from hereditary factors, other markers for increased risk for the development of both malignant and benign epithelial tumors include nulliparity, early menses, infertility, celibacy,

TABLE 23–1. Common Neoplasms of the Ovary

HISTOLOGIC TYPE	MALIGNANT	BENIGN
Epithelial		
	Serous cystadenocarcinoma	Serous cystadenoma
	Mucinous cystadenocarcinoma	Mucinous cystadenoma (Benign form rare)
	Endometrioid carcinoma	
	Clear cell carcinoma (Malignant form rare)	(Benign form rare) Brenner tumor
Germ Cell		
	Mature teratoma, malignant transformation	Teratoma, mature (dermoid cyst)
	Teratoma, immature	
	Dysgerminoma	
	Embryonal	
	Choriocarcinoma	
	Yolk sac (endodermal sinus tumor)	
Sex Cord-Stromal[1]		
	Granulosa cell tumor	Fibroma
		Thecoma
		Fibrothecoma
		Sertoli-Leydig cell
		Steroid cell
Metastatic		
	Krukenberg	
	Other (especially colon)	

[1]Although most of these tumors generally have a benign clinical course, they are potentially malignant.

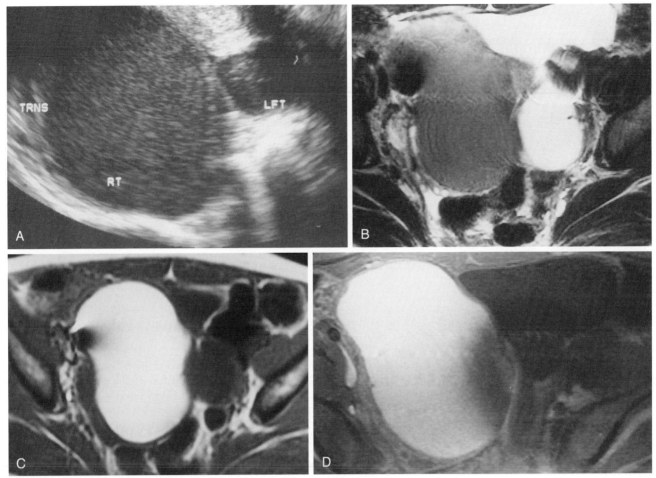

FIGURE 23–10. Endometrioma, bilateral, in a 41-year-old woman with pelvic pain.

A, Ultrasonogram, transverse projection. Both the larger right *(RT)* and the smaller left *(LFT)* endometriomas manifest diffuse, homogeneous medium level ("ground-glass") echogenicity. Posterior acoustic enhancement suggests a fluid content. Variable magnetic resonance signal intensities are illustrated in *B, C,* and *D.*

B, T2-weighted image demonstrates low-to-intermediate signal of the large, right-sided mass and homogeneous high-signal intensity of the small left-sided mass.

C, T1-weighted image at the same level shows homogeneous high-signal intensity of the larger, right-sided mass and low-signal intensity of the smaller, left-sided mass.

D, T1-weighted image with fat suppression demonstrates no significant decrease in signal intensity, suggesting hemorrhage as the most likely cause of the high-signal intensity.

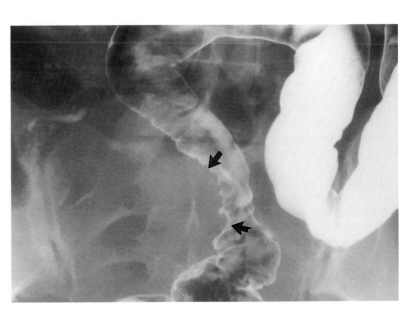

FIGURE 23–11. Endometriosis involving the serosa of the rectosigmoid. Barium enema, anteroposterior projection. The rectosigmoid colon is displaced to the left by a large endometrioma. The mucosa is intact but irregular as a result of serosal implantation *(arrows).*

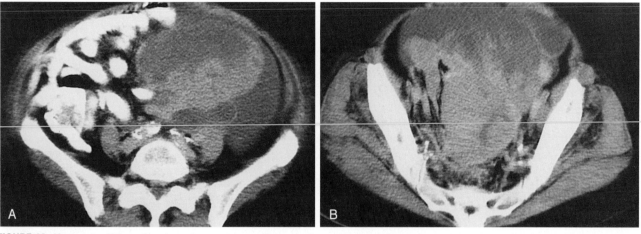

FIGURE 23–12. Poorly differentiated carcinoma, ovary. Computed tomograms, contrast material–enhanced at level of lower abdomen *(A)* and pelvis *(B)*. There is a heterogeneous soft tissue mass with extensive mesenteric and peritoneal spread.

endometrial carcinoma, and breast carcinoma. Smoking and other environmental agents, including talc and asbestos, have been implicated in some studies but are generally not thought to be causally related to the development of ovarian tumors. Oral contraceptives are associated with a decreased risk of ovarian malignancy.

Approximately 60 per cent of epithelial neoplasms are benign, 30 per cent are malignant, and 10 per cent are classified as being of "low malignant potential." This latter group, formerly called "borderline" tumors, consists of lesions that exhibit cellular atypia without stromal invasion to suggest frank malignancy. Tumors of low malignant potential have a significantly better prognosis than frank malignancies, even in the presence of implantation on the peritoneum and spread to regional lymph nodes, with a 5-year survival rate approaching 95 per cent.

Many ovarian neoplasms are discovered as incidental findings during routine pelvic examination. Symptoms, when present, include mild pain due to mass effect or acute pain associated with torsion. Ascites may be the presenting feature for patients with malignant tumors, although very uncommonly the same finding can be caused by benign lesions. Advanced malignancy may become manifest as a result of spread to other structures, such as the gastrointestinal tract. Whereas any ovarian neoplasm might present with hormonal effects, such as postmenopausal bleeding or virilization, such manifestations are less likely with epithelial tumors than with gonadal stromal tumors, as discussed in a following section.

There is a variety of potential serum tumor markers for ovarian cancer, but none is widely used for screening. One marker, CA-125, is elevated in 85 per cent of patients with ovarian cancer and, thus, can serve as a baseline for the serial evaluation of patients following surgery. Because this marker may be elevated in a variety of nonmalignant disorders, especially in premenopausal patients, it lacks specificity for use in ovarian cancer screening. Addi-

tionally, the sensitivity of CA-125 as a screening test is undermined by the fact that only one-half of patients with carcinoma limited to the ovary have an abnormal CA-125 level.

The terminology for the more common mucinous and serous epithelial tumors is often modified by the addition of the prefix *cyst-* when the tumor contains defined fluid-filled spaces. Likewise, the suffix *-fibroma* may be added when the solid portion of the tumor includes at least 50 per cent fibrous tissue. Thus, one may see a wide variety of histologic descriptions of epithelial tumors of the ovary, including, for example, *serous cystadenocarcinoma, mucinous cystadenofibroma,* or *serous cystadenoma of low malignant potential.*

Serous Tumors. Of the various epithelial ovarian neoplasms, the serous category is the most common. In some series, these account for nearly one-half of all malignant and approximately one-quarter of all benign ovarian neoplasms. However, because the majority of ovarian neoplasms overall are benign, most serous tumors are also benign.

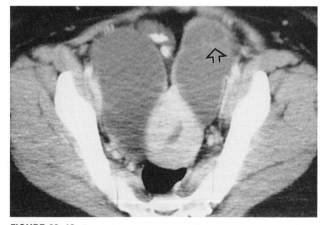

FIGURE 23–13. Serous cystadenoma of both ovaries in a 45-year-old woman. Computed tomogram with contrast material enhancement. Both ovarian tumors are homogeneous, hypodense, and predominantly cystic. A slightly thickened septum *(arrow)* is present in the anterolateral aspect of the left ovarian cystadenoma. The uterus is normal.

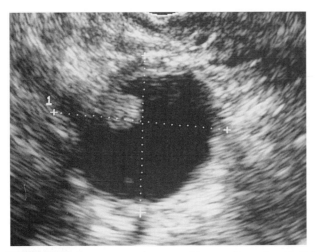

FIGURE 23–14. Serous cystadenoma of low malignant potential in a 24-year-old woman. Ultrasonogram. The tumor is a unilocular cystic mass with a papillary excrescence projecting into the lumen (same patient illustrated in Fig. 23–28).

Benign and low-malignant-potential serous tumors are typically unilocular with a predominantly smooth inner wall. However, they often include a slightly irregular focus of soft tissue that projects into the cyst lumen (Figs. 23–13 and 23–14). This papillary excrescence may be seen in other neoplasms as well, but it is clearly a more common finding in serous tumors. In contrast to benign serous neoplasms, malignant tumors are more likely to be bilateral and contain more solid tissue components, including a thickened wall and irregular septations. Enhancement following contrast material during computed tomography or magnetic resonance imaging is seen, but this feature is nonspe-

cific, as it occurs with most, if not all, ovarian neoplasms.

Mucinous Tumors. Mucinous neoplasm of the ovary is nearly as common as serous tumor but is malignant in only 10 to 15 per cent of cases. The mucin designation refers to microscopic features of the cells of the lining of the tumor. The contents of the cystic locules may contain mucin, but this is quite variable. A mucinous tumor is typically composed of multilocular cysts with thin and smooth septations separating the locules in those tumors that are benign (Figs. 23–15 and 23–16). A malignant mucinous tumor is generally indistinguishable from a serous cystadenocarcinoma. Unlike mucinous tumors of the colon or urachus, mucinous ovarian neoplasms typically do not calcify.

Mucinous tumors of low malignant potential may occasionally cause *pseudomyxoma peritonei*, a protracted condition in which affected women suffer from extensive proliferative deposition of gelatinous material within the peritoneal space. This condition often requires repeated surgical procedures in an effort to ameliorate the mass effect on the gastrointestinal tract and other abdominal viscera.

Endometrioid Tumors. Although less common than mucinous tumors, endometrioid tumors are important because they are nearly always malignant. In contrast to the cystic nature of serous and mucinous tumors, an endometroid tumor is more apt to be predominantly solid. Hemorrhage and necrosis lead to a heterogeneous architecture as imaged by ultrasonography, computed tomography, or magnetic resonance imaging.

Endometrioid tumors are more likely than other epithelial neoplasms to be associated with abnormalities of the uterine endometrium. Approxi-

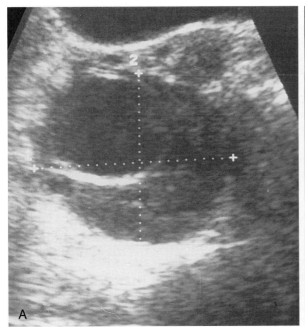
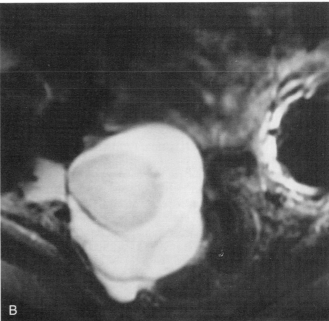

FIGURE 23–15. Mucinous cystadenocarcinoma in a 66-year-old woman. Transvaginal ultrasonogram *(A)* and T2-weighted magnetic resonance image *(B)*. There is a multiloculated, predominantly cystic mass in the right ovary.

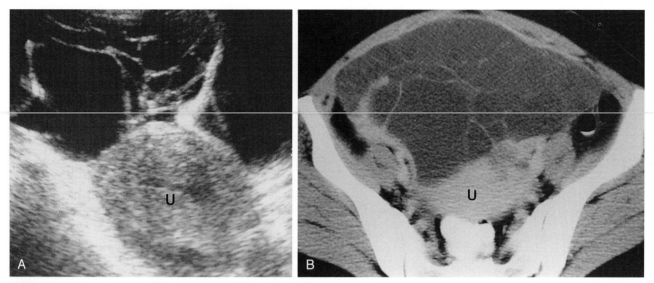

FIGURE 23–16. Mucinous cystadenocarcinoma of the ovary with low malignant potential in a 24-year-old woman.
A, Transabdominal ultrasonogram, longitudinal projection. A large, multilocular cystic mass is situated superior to the bladder and anterosuperior to the uterus.
B, Computed tomogram with contrast material enhancement. The tumor is well marginated and contains fine septations. U = uterus (same patient illustrated in Fig. 23–27).

mately one in four patients with an ovarian endometrioid neoplasm has either hyperplasia or carcinoma of the endometrium. In the latter situation, the uterine component is a separate primary tumor rather than a metastasis. In view of this association, some women with endometrioid carcinoma of the ovary present with abnormal vaginal bleeding caused by the related, but independent, uterine carcinoma.

Clear Cell Tumors. Clear cell carcinoma of the ovary is a less common epithelial cell type. Like endometrioid tumor, clear cell carcinoma is virtually always malignant. *In utero* exposure to diethylstilbestrol is not thought to be a risk factor for the development of ovarian clear cell carcinoma, as it is for the rare gynecologic malignancies of clear cell tumors of the vagina and cervix.

The gross features of clear cell carcinoma are extremely variable. These include a predominantly cystic appearance that may mimic that of malignant serous tumors, a multicystic appearance, or a predominantly solid appearance that may resemble that of endometrioid carcinoma.

Brenner Tumor. The rare Brenner tumor is the only epithelial tumor that is nearly always benign. A preoperative diagnosis is rarely made, principally because patients with a Brenner tumor often come to medical attention as a result of a coexistent mucinous cystic tumor or mature teratoma. The Brenner tumor is generally small, homogeneous, and solid and is composed of transitional cells and a dense fibrous stroma. This lesion should not be confused with the even rarer transitional cell carcinoma of the ovary, which shares some histologic similarities.

Germ Cell Tumors

Ovarian germ cell tumors are only slightly less common than epithelial tumors of the ovary. However,

because most ovarian germ cell tumors are mature teratomas, malignant germ cell tumors are quite rare. Indeed, mature teratomas account for nearly one-half of all ovarian neoplasms.

Mature Teratoma (Dermoid Cyst). A mature teratoma contains a variable mixture of ectodermal, mesodermal, and endodermal elements. When ectodermal elements, such as skin, hair follicles and sebaceous or sweat glands, predominate, the tumor is designated a dermoid cyst. Most, but not all, mature teratomas of the ovary are dermoid cysts.

These benign lesions are most commonly found in women of child-bearing years and are among the more common causes of an ovarian mass in children, as well. They often become clinically manifest as nonspecific pelvic pain but can also be detected as incidental findings during imaging or surgery for unrelated uterine or ovarian conditions. Uncommonly, ovarian torsion precipitates diagnosis. Rupture with chemical peritonitis caused by the spillage of cyst contents is rare. As many as 15 per cent of mature teratomas are bilateral. Malignant transformation of a mature teratoma occurs rarely.

A mature teratoma may be detected by standard radiography by virtue of the presence of fat, calcification, teeth, or bone within the mass (Fig. 23–17). Ultrasonographically, dermoid cysts are typically unilocular with a thin or slightly thickened wall. An eccentric echogenic mural nodule, the *Rokitansky body,* is often seen (Figs. 23–18 and 23–19). The echogenicity of these lesions represents calcification and/or the multiple tissue interfaces created by the heterogeneous mixture of tissues within the mass (see Fig. 23–7*B*). Calcification is also readily seen by computed tomography. A confident diagnosis of mature teratoma is based on the detection of lipid in the form of sebum in the cyst fluid. This is seen as negative attenuation values by computed tomog-

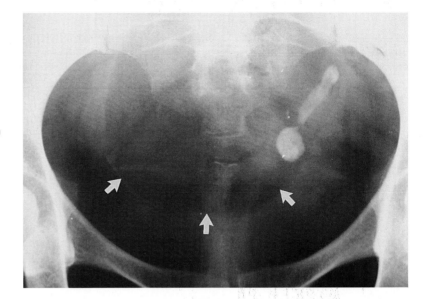

FIGURE 23–17. Mature teratoma of the ovary in a 22-year-old woman with pelvic pain. Frontal radiograph. Left-sided calcification represents bone or teeth. A large area of lucency *(arrows)* represents fat within the teratoma.

raphy or high signal intensity on T1-weighted images (see Fig. 23–19C). Fat-suppressed magnetic resonance imaging reveals a significant decrease in signal of fat-containing cyst fluid (Fig. 23–20).

Dysgerminoma. The most common of the malignant germ cell tumors is the dysgerminoma. While histologically similar to seminoma of the testicle, dysgerminoma has a less favorable prognosis, presumably because it progresses to a much larger size prior to detection than does seminoma. In common with other ovarian germ cell tumors, dysgerminoma is predominantly a solid tumor that occurs in older adolescents and young adults. Imaging techniques demonstrate a heterogeneous solid tumor. In some malignant germ cell tumors, markers such as alphafetoprotein for endodermal sinus tumors and beta-

hCG for choriocarcinoma may be positive, but negative results are not helpful.

Sex Cord–Stromal Tumors

Sex cord–stromal tumors, also called gonadal stromal tumors, occur much less commonly than epithelial or germ cell tumors. Their clinical importance lies in their occasional malignant behavior and hormonal activity. Except for the juvenile form of granulosa cell tumor, sex cord–stromal tumors are most common in women of reproductive age and older.

Fibrothecoma. Whereas fibroma and thecoma sometimes occur as separate entities, they more often coexist in a composite lesion known as a fibrothecoma. For the most part, these tumors are indistinguishable from each other by imaging criteria, with the possible exception of the magnetic resonance imaging findings in fibroma, as discussed subsequently.

The most common of the sex cord–stromal tumors is fibroma, which is a well-circumscribed, solid lesion of uniform composition. Hemorrhage or necrosis is very uncommon. Calcification, although unusual, may involve the entire tumor. Ultrasonographically, a fibroma is homogeneous and hypoechoic. Significant acoustic shadowing behind a fibroma represents attenuation of sound presumably caused by the compact cellular makeup that is characteristic of a fibroma. Computed tomographic findings of a homogeneous mass of soft tissue attenuation are nonspecific. Magnetic resonance imaging may show a relatively homogeneous low signal on T2-weighted images, presumably due to the low water content of a fibroma. This finding is distinctly different from those of other solid ovarian masses, such as endometroid carcinoma, that are likely to have a higher signal intensity on T2-weighted images. This difference may be of diagnostic value, especially in view of the similar ultrasonographic appearance of most solid ovarian masses. The clinical impact of these

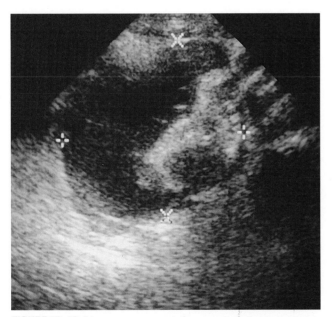

FIGURE 23–18. Mature teratoma, left ovary, in a 9-year-old girl. The highly echogenic mass, known as a *Rokitansky body,* is in a characteristic eccentric location with the unilocular cyst.

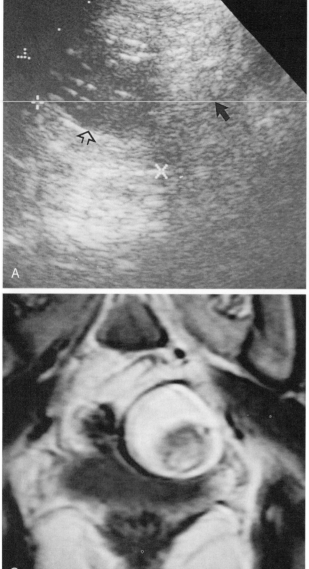

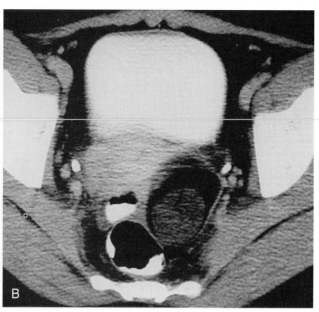

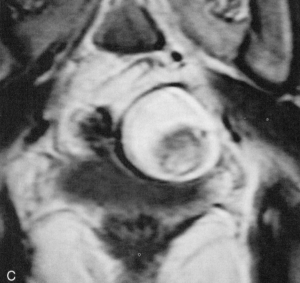

FIGURE 23–19. Mature teratoma, left ovary, in a 32-year-old woman.

A, Transvaginal ultrasonogram, transverse projection. There is a complex mass consisting of a region of increased echogenicity *(closed arrow)* and a cystic area *(open arrow).*

B, Computed tomogram with contrast material enhancement. The mass in the left adnexa contains both fat and a focus of soft tissue in the dependent portion of the teratoma.

C, T1-weighted magnetic resonance image, oblique coronal projection. The mass is predominantly isointense with fat. The area of low-signal intensity within the fat represents debris and the Rokitansky body.

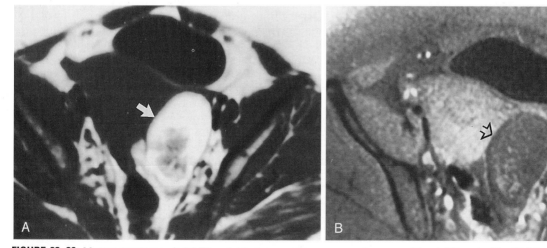

FIGURE 23–20. Mature teratoma. Axial T1-weighted magnetic resonance images without *(A)* and with *(B)* fat suppression. Lipid material within the cyst *(arrows)* results in decrease in signal intensity.

differences is limited, however, because a fibroma is generally removed either for control of symptoms or to eliminate the risk of torsion.

A thecoma often produces estrogen with clinical manifestations that vary with the age of the patient. As a result, though, endometrial hyperplasia and carcinoma are associated with thecoma or fibrothecoma. The ultrasonographic appearance of a thecoma is that of any solid ovarian mass. Magnetic resonance imaging demonstrates a higher signal intensity on T2-weighted images than does a pure fibroma. Differentiation is not of clinical importance, however, as neither fibroma nor thecoma exhibit malignant potential, and both are treated by surgical resection.

Granulosa Cell Tumor. Granulosa cell tumor takes two forms: *juvenile* and *adult*. The less common juvenile form occurs in younger adolescents, whereas the adult form affects peri- or postmenopausal women. Either form may produce estrogen and thereby lead to pseudoprecocious puberty in girls or endometrial hyperplasia or carcinoma in adults. Granulosa cell tumor is a low-grade malignancy that has a low rate of recurrence. When it does recur, it often appears many years after the initial resection.

The gross appearance and imaging findings for the two types of granulosa cell tumors are identical: well-defined, solid tumors with multiple cystic spaces, some of which may be hemorrhagic (Fig. 23–21). Ultrasonography, computed tomography, or magnetic resonance imaging depict these features with similar accuracy.

Sertoli-Leydig Cell Tumor. A pure Sertoli or pure Leydig cell tumor is a rarity. More commonly, these cell types are combined in a single malignant tumor of low grade. Sertoli-Leydig cell tumors account for less than 1 per cent of all ovarian neo-

plasms and usually occur in women younger than 30 years of age. Although this tumor is the most common virilizing tumor of the ovary, this manifestation is present in only a minority of patients. Imaging studies demonstrate the typically solid nature of these tumors. Occasionally, cystic areas are identified.

Secondary Tumors

A metastasis to the ovary is most commonly the result of a primary carcinoma of the colon. The lesion itself is nonspecific, both macroscopically and by imaging criteria. However, a pattern of bilaterality, especially in the clinical context of a known primary colonic tumor, makes the diagnosis of metastases likely.

A distinctive form of metastasis, the *Krukenberg tumor,* is almost always the result of a gastric adenocarcinoma. This tumor is recognized histologically by a characteristic signet-ring appearance of the cells comprising the ovarian tumor. A Krukenberg tumor is more likely to occur in a younger patient, presumably due to the relatively large size of and blood flow to the ovary that is normal for premenopausal women. These tumors are typically bilateral but are otherwise nonspecific in their imaging appearance. Both cystic and solid components are usually identified.

ECTOPIC PREGNANCY

In any female of reproductive age with symptoms referable to the abdomen or pelvis, the possibility of an ectopic pregnancy should be evaluated with a pregnancy test measuring the urine or serum b-hCG level. With a positive pregnancy test, a diagnosis of ectopic pregnancy first requires a careful

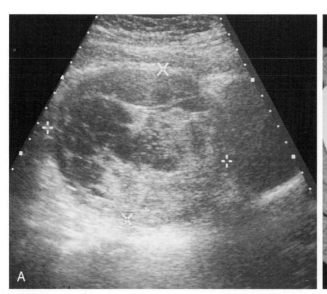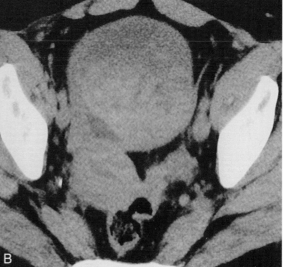

FIGURE 23–21. Granulosa cell tumor of ovary complicated by torsion in a 45-year-old woman with acute abdominal pain and a 3-week history of uterine bleeding.
A, Transabdominal ultrasonogram. The tumor is of mixed echogenicity, suggesting both fluid and solid elements.
B, Computed tomogram without enhancement. The mass is heterogeneous.

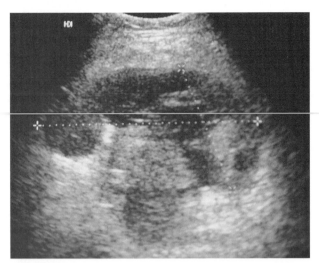

FIGURE 23–22. Ectopic pregnancy, right fallopian tube. The cursors delineate a large, complex mass in the right adnexa. Surgical findings included extensive hematoma and adhesions from previous laparoscopic tubal surgery.

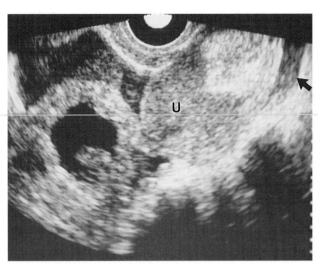

FIGURE 23–24. Ectopic pregnancy, left fallopian tube. Ultrasonogram, longitudinal projection. There is a mixed fluid-filled and solid mass near the uterine fundus (U). The echogenicity of the ascites (arrow) suggests hemoperitoneum.

clinical and ultrasonographic assessment for the presence of a normal intrauterine pregnancy. Once an intrauterine pregnancy is excluded, the adnexa must be scanned for a living embryo. Transvaginal ultrasonography reveals an embryo in as many as 25 per cent of patients with an ectopic pregnancy. Most ectopic pregnancies are located within the ampullary or isthmic portion of the fallopian tube. Any adnexal mass should be regarded as a possible ectopic pregnancy, although one must remember that a corpus luteum cyst is an expected finding in the first trimester of pregnancy (Figs. 23–22 through 23–24). Ascites, especially echogenic fluid suggesting hemoperitoneum, is additional evidence for the diagnosis of ectopic pregnancy in the proper clinical setting. It is of great importance to keep in mind that the combination of a positive pregnancy test, the absence of an intrauterine pregnancy, and a normal pelvic ultrasonogram *does not* exclude ectopic pregnancy. With this combination of findings, serial quantitative b-hCG values and follow-up pelvic ultrasonography should be performed.

ISCHEMIC TORSION

Owing, in part, to its relative mobility within the pelvis, the ovary may occasionally undergo torsion on its supporting ligaments. As a result, both venous drainage and, eventually, arterial supply may be compromised to the point of ischemia or infarction. Whereas torsion may occur at any age, it is more common in adolescence and younger adults

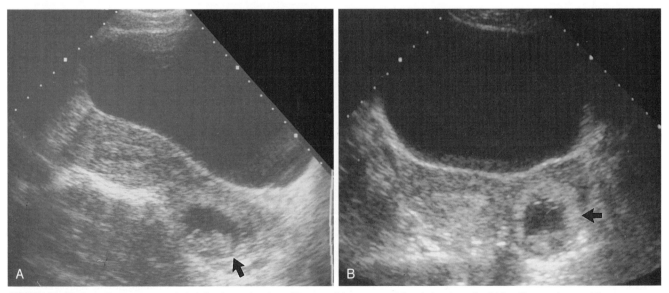

FIGURE 23–23. Ectopic pregnancy, left fallopian tube, in a 26-year-old woman with minimal vaginal bleeding and a positive pregnancy test result. Ultrasonograms in the oblique (A) and transverse (B) projections. There is a thick-walled cystic mass (arrows) adjacent to the normal uterus.

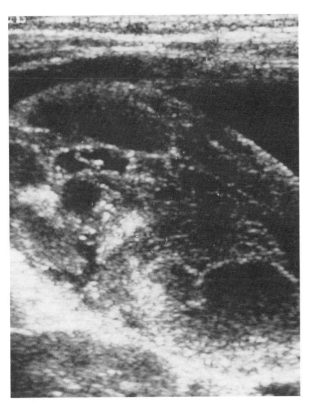

FIGURE 23–25. Torsion of the ovary in a neonate with abdominal distention. Ultrasonogram. The ovary is enlarged and manifests a prominent follicular pattern. There is surrounding ascites.

and in the presence of an ovarian neoplasm or physiologic cyst. Severe pelvic pain, often with remission and recurrence over days or weeks, is the usual clinical presentation of ovarian torsion. In contrast to other common acute conditions of ovarian origin, such as tubo-ovarian abscess and ectopic pregnancy, clinical features and laboratory test results are usually normal or nonspecific.

The most common ultrasonographic manifestation of torsion is an enlarged ovary with a prominent follicular pattern (Fig. 23–25; see Fig. 23–21). This finding is best perceived when compared with that of the contralateral ovary. It is often quite difficult to demonstrate flow in a normal ovary, especially if the patient is postmenopausal. It is important to keep in mind this possibility of a false-positive test result for torsion if color Doppler is used. Additionally, the dual blood supply to the ovary occasionally allows for blood flow even in the setting of torsion. As a result, Doppler ultrasonography to compare blood flow to both ovaries often may lead to a false-negative interpretation. This is in contrast to the established value of Doppler flow analysis in testicular torsion as discussed in Chapter 26.

PARAOVARIAN CYST

Most paraovarian cysts are of mesothelial origin, often arising from the broad ligament. These are usually incidental findings in asymptomatic patients. In this circumstance, surgery is not required for further diagnosis provided that the ovary can be identified as a separate structure. Even if surgery is to be performed, the knowledge that the lesion is separate from the ovary precludes the need for preoperative staging procedures because the identification of the mass as unrelated to the ovary is strong evidence that the mass is not only benign but also likely non-neoplastic. Symptoms due to paraovarian cyst, when present, are variable.

A paraovarian cyst is usually unilocular and simple, although it may be quite large at the time of diagnosis. The demonstration that the cystic lesion is separate from the ovary is the key to the diagnosis. This is usually accomplished by ultrasonography or by magnetic resonance imaging.

RADIOLOGIC EVALUATION OF AN ADNEXAL MASS

Prior to the advent of pelvic ultrasonography, most pelvic masses that were excised were non-neoplastic and, hence, benign. Many of these were follicular or corpus luteum cysts. With contemporary ultrasonography, the challenge now is to avoid unnecessary surgery for these self-limiting, benign processes. Further, the advent of laparascopic techniques that obviate surgical laparatomy provides additional impetus for the radiologist to identify small, likely benign lesions.

Clinical context is a fundamental consideration in formulating diagnostic possibilities in a patient with adnexal disease. A symptomatic patient with a positive pregnancy test result but no evidence of an intrauterine pregnancy is presumed to have an **ectopic pregnancy** until proved otherwise. Imaging strategies are those described in the preceding section on that subject. Fever and leukocytosis suggest the likely diagnosis of **tubo-ovarian abscess,** whereas a patient with severe acute pain and negative or moderately abnormal laboratory results should be evaluated for **torsion.** Although any ovarian lesion may produce symptoms, these three lesions are more likely to lead to dominant symptoms and, thus, are considered together.

Patients who are asymptomatic or who lack dominant symptoms can be divided into two groups based on age. Since a *postmenopausal* patient only rarely has a hemorrhagic follicular cyst, a corpus luteum cyst, or endometriosis, any lesion in this age group that is not a small simple cyst should be considered suspicious for a **neoplasm.** A small, simple cyst, less than 5 cm in diameter, may be initially presumed to be a **serous (epithelial) inclusion cyst** and monitored by serial ultrasonography. If enlargement occurs over time, laparoscopic removal for diagnosis may be required.

In a *premenopausal* patient, a small, simple cyst that is less than 3.5 cm in diameter can be assumed to be a **follicle** or **small follicular cyst** and, generally, does not require further evaluation. Lesions

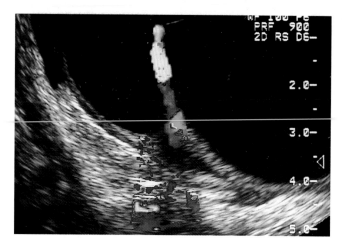

FIGURE 23–26. Mucinous cystadenoma, ovary. Color Doppler ultrasonogram. There is flow within a smooth septation.

larger than 3.5 cm in diameter but less than 6 cm in diameter, which are either simple cysts or have features of a hemorrhagic cyst, are best assessed with follow-up ultrasonography in 1 to 2 months. Here, the presumed diagnosis is **physiologic, either follicular or corpus luteum, cyst.** One must remember that physiologic processes tend not to enlarge beyond 6 cm in diameter. Thus, any mass that achieves this size, even when the ultrasonographic findings remain those of a simple cyst, should be considered as potentially neoplastic. Finally, a mass that exhibits soft tissue along the inner wall of a cyst or irregular thick septations should be presumed to be **neoplastic** and potentially malignant.

Some adnexal lesions have distinctive features. **Mature teratoma,** or **dermoid cyst,** is generally recognized by an echogenic mural nodule, the Rokitansky body described previously. Confirmation of the diagnosis using computed tomography or magnetic resonance imaging is usually possible. Identi-

fication of an adjacent but separate ovary is the basis for a diagnosis of **paraovarian cyst.** An **endometrioma** often exhibits a ground-glass appearance on ultrasonography and typically yields high signal intensity on T1-weighted images and low-to-intermediate signal intensity on T2-weighted images. A **theca lutein cyst** may resemble a neoplasm, but if present in a patient with conditions such as medication with ovarian-stimulating agents or with hydatidiform mole, the need to resect the ovarian component is eliminated unless complicated by hemorrhage or infarction.

The role of Doppler ultrasonography in the evaluation of ovarian neoplasms is controversial. The potential value of this modality was proposed by Kurjak in 1991 based on the low vascular resistance of malignant vessels within a neoplasm. The technique employs color or amplitude Doppler ultrasound to localize a vessel within the lesion (Figs. 23–26 through 23–30). Analysis of the Doppler spectrum of this vessel should identify a malignant ves-

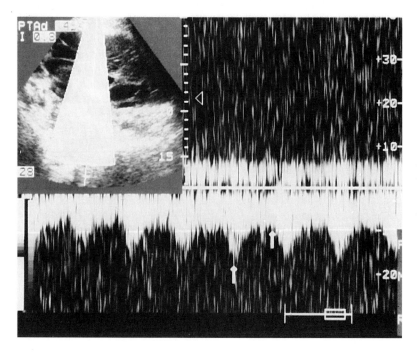

FIGURE 23–27. Mucinous cystadenoma of the ovary with low malignant potential. Doppler analysis demonstrates a low resistance waveform (resistive index = 0.44) suggesting malignant neovascularity (same patient illustrated in Fig. 23–16).

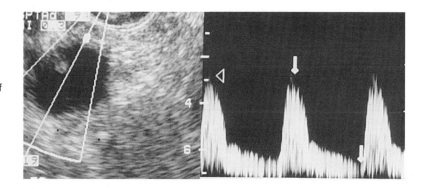

FIGURE 23-28. Serous cystadenoma of the ovary with low malignant potential. Spectral Doppler of wall of mass shows a high (normal) resistance waveform (resistive index = 0.88) (same patient illustrated in Fig. 23-14).

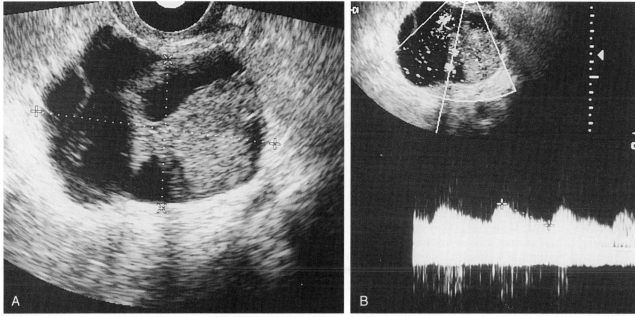

FIGURE 23-29. Endometriosis, atypical, in a 30-year-old with pelvic pain.

A, Transvaginal ultrasonogram. The complex nature of the mass with an irregular soft tissue component suggests a neoplasm.

B, Doppler evaluation demonstrates a relatively low resistance waveform (resistive index = 0.48). Although this value is in the benign range, it is very close to the threshold of 0.45 that is used to indicate malignancy.

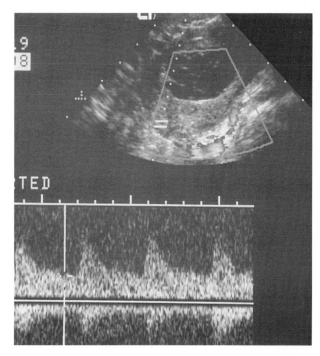

FIGURE 23-30. Ovarian cyst, hemorrhagic. Doppler shows normal pulsatility (resistive index = 0.58), which supports a benign etiology. This additional information is of limited value in this example, however, in that the internal morphology of the lesion strongly suggests the correct diagnosis (same patient illustrated in Fig. 23-1).

sel as one that lacks a normal muscular wall and demonstrates an increased diastolic flow. The low-resistance flow can be quantified as either a resistive index or pulsatility index. The normal lower thresholds are 0.50 for resistive index and 1.0 for pulsatility index. Values below these levels suggest increased diastolic flow as might be found in the vasculature of a malignancy.

Although there is considerable evidence that confirms a statistically significant difference between malignant and benign lesions based on low resistance flow, considerable overlap occurs (Salem et al., 1994). Thus, the value of the result in an individual patient is limited. Furthermore, a common premenopausal mass, the corpus luteum cyst, is highly vascular and is characterized by low-resistance flow. Endometriosis and pelvic inflammatory disease, including tubo-ovarian abscess, also have flow characteristics of malignant masses.

Doppler techniques might be applied to the evaluation of a postmenopausal patient when the ultrasonographic findings of a mass are equivocal. For example, if standard gray-scale images show a complex mass with a large amount of irregular solid tissue, Doppler ultrasonography stands to add little to the correct diagnosis as the findings overwhelmingly favor a malignant neoplasm. On the other hand, a lesion with a few septations and a minimally irregular wall may have a low or intermediate likelihood of malignancy, in which case the Doppler information may guide the surgeon in the direction of either a probably benign or probably malignant histology.

BIBLIOGRAPHY

Alcazar, J. L., Errasti, T., Jurado, M.: Blood flow in functional cysts and benign ovarian neoplasms in premenopausal women. J. Ultrasound Med. 16:819, 1997.

Andreotti, R. F., Zusmer, N. R., Sheldon, J. J., and Ames, M.: Ultrasound and magnetic resonance imaging of pelvic masses. Surg. Gynecol. Obstet. 155:327, 1988.

Arrive, L., Hricak, H., and Martin, M. C.: Pelvic endometriosis: MR imaging. Radiology 171:687, 1989.

Benacerraf, B. R., Finkler, N. J., Wojciechowski, R. N., and Knapp, R. C.: Sonographic accuracy in the diagnosis of ovarian masses. J. Reprod. Med. 35:491, 1990.

Bromley, B., and Benacerraf, B.: Adnexal masses during pregnancy: Accuracy of sonographic diagnosis and outcome. J. Ultrasound Med. 16:447, 1997.

Brown, D. L., Doubilet, P. M., Miller, F. H., Frates, M. C., Laing, F. C., DiSalvo, D. N., Benson, C. B., and Lerner, M. H.: Benign and malignant ovarian masses: Selection of the most discriminating gray-scale and Doppler sonographic features. Radiology 208:103, 1998.

Carter, J. R., Fowler, J. M., Carlson, J. W., Carson, L. F., Adcock, L. L., and Twiggs, L. B.: Prediction of malignancy using transvaginal color flow Doppler in patients with gynecologic tumors. Int. J. Gynecol. Cancer 3:279, 1993.

Clement, P. B.: Anatomy and histology of the ovary. In Kurman, R. J.: Blaustein's Pathology of the Female Genital Tract, 4th ed. New York, Springer-Verlag, 1994, pp. 563–595.

Clement, P. B.: Nonneoplastic lesions of the ovary. In Kurman, R. J.: Blaustein's Pathology of the Female Genital Tract, 4th ed. New York, Springer-Verlag, 1994, pp. 597–703.

Fleischer, A. C., Cullinan, J. A., Kepple, D. M., and Williams, L. L.: Conventional and color Doppler transvaginal sonography of pelvic masses: A comparison of relative histologic specificities. J. Ultrasound Med. 12:705, 1993.

Fleischer, A. C., Rodgers, W. H., Kepple, D. M., Williams, L. L., Jones, H. W., and Gross, P. R.: Color Doppler sonography of benign and malignant ovarian masses. Radiographics 12:879, 1992.

Goldstein, S. R., Subramanyam, B., Snyder, J. R., Beller, U., Raghavendra, B. N., and Beckman, E. M.: The postmenopausal cystic adnexal mass: The potential role of ultrasound in conservative management. Obstet. Gynecol. 73:8, 1989.

Jain, K. A., Friedman, D. L., Pettinger, T. W., Alagappan, R., Jeffrey, R. B., and Sommer, F. G.: Adnexal masses: Comparison of specificity of endovaginal US and pelvic MR imaging. Radiology 186:697, 1993.

Kier, R., Smith R. C., and McCarthy S. M.: Value of lipid- and water-suppression MR images in distinguishing between blood and lipid within ovarian masses. AJR 158:321, 1992.

Kim J. S., Lee, H. J., Woo, S. K., and Lee, T. S.: Peritoneal inclusion cysts and their relationship to the ovaries: Evaluation with sonography. Radiology 204:481, 1997.

Kimura, I., Togashi, K., Kawakami, S., Nakano, Y., Takakura, K., Mori, T., and Konishi, J.: Polycystic ovaries: Implications of diagnosis with MR imaging. Radiology 201:549, 1996.

Kinkel, K., Ariche, M., Tardivon, A. A., Spatz, A., Castaigne, D., Lhommé, C., and Vanel, D.: Differentiation between recurrent tumor and benign conditions after treatment of gynecologic pelvic carcinoma: Value of dynamic contrast-enhanced subtraction MR imaging. Radiology 204:55, 1997.

Koonings, P. P., Campbell, K., Mishell, D. R., and Grimes, D. A.: Relative frequency of primary ovarian neoplasms: A 10-year review. Obstet. Gynecol. 74:921, 1989.

Koonings, P. P., and Grimes, D. A.: Adnexal torsion in postmenopausal women. Obstet. Gynecol. 73:11, 1989.

Korbin, C. O., Brown, D. L., and Welch, W. R.: Para ovarian cystadenomas and cystadenofibromas: Sonographic characteristics in 14 cases. Radiology 208:459, 1998.

Kurjak, A., and Predanic, M.: New scoring system for prediction of ovarian malignancy based on transvaginal color Doppler sonography. J. Ultrasound Med. 11:631, 1992.

Kurjak, A., Zalud, I., and Alfirevic, Z.: Evaluation of adnexal masses with transvaginal color ultrasound. J. Ultrasound Med. 10:295, 1991.

Levine, D., Gosink, B. B., Wolf, S. I., Feldesman, M. R., and Pretorius, D. H.: Simple adnexal cysts: The natural history in postmenopausal women. Radiology 184:653, 1992.

NIH Consensus Conference: Ovarian cancer: Screening, treatment, and follow-up. JAMA 273:491, 1995.

Nishimura, K., Togashi, K., Itoh, K., Fujisawa, I., Noma, S., Kawamura, Y., Nakano, Y., Itoh, H., Torizuka, K., and Ozasa, H.: Endometrial cysts of the ovary: MR imaging. Radiology 162:315, 1987.

Outwater E., Schiebler, M. L., Owen, R. S., and Schnall, M.D.: Characterization of hemorrhagic adnexal lesions with MR imaging: Blinded reader study. Radiology 186:489, 1993.

Parker, W. H., and Berek, J. S.: Management of selected cystic adnexal masses in postmenopausal women by operative laparoscopy: A pilot study. Am. J. Obstet. Gynecol. 163:1574, 1990.

Parker, W. H., and Berek, J. S.: Laparoscopic management of the adnexal mass. Obstet. Gynecol. Clin. North Am. 21:79, 1994.

Roberts, C. L., and Weston, M. J.: Bilateral massive ovarian edema: A case report. Ultrasound Obstet. Gynecol. 11:65, 1998.

Rulin, M. C., and Preston, A. L.: Adnexal masses in postmenopausal women. Obstet. Gynecol. 70:578, 1987.

Russell, P.: Surface epithelial-stromal tumor of the ovary. In Kurman, R. J.: Blaustein's Pathology of the Female Genital Tract, 4th ed. New York, Springer-Verlag, 1994, pp. 705–782.

Salem S., White L. M., and Lai, J.: Doppler sonography of adnexal masses: The predictive value of the pulsatility index in benign and malignant disease. AJR. 163:1147, 1994.

Sassone, A. M., Timor-Tritsch, I. E., Artner, A., Westhoff, C., and Warren, W. B.: Transvaginal sonographic characterization of ovarian disease: Evaluation of a new scoring system to predict ovarian malignancy. Obstet. Gynecol. 78:70, 1991.

Silverman, P. M., Osborne, M., Dunnick, N. R., and Bandy, L. C.: CT prior to second-look operation in ovarian cancer. AJR 150:829, 1988.

Stevens, S. K., Hricak, H., and Campos, Z.: Teratomas versus cystic hemorrhagic adnexal lesions: Differentiation with proton-selective fat saturation MR imaging. Radiology 186:481, 1993.

Talerman, A.: Germ cell tumors of the ovary. In Kurman, R. J.: Blaustein's Pathology of the Female Genital Tract, 4th ed. New York, Springer-Verlag, 1994, pp. 849–914.

Timor-Tritsch, I. E., Lerner, J. P., Monteagudo, A., and Santos, R.: Transvaginal ultrasonographic characterization of ovarian masses by means of color flow-directed Doppler measurements and a morphologic scoring system. Am. J. Obstet. Gynecol. 168:909, 1993.

Troiano, R. N., Lazzarini, K. M., Scoutt, L. M., Lange, R. C., Flynn, S. D., and McCarthy, S.: Fibroma and fibrothecoma of the ovary: MR imaging findings. Radiology 204:795, 1997.

Wagner, B. J., Buck, J. L., Seidman, J. D., and McCabe, K. M.: Ovarian epithelial neoplasms: Radiologic-pathologic correlation. Radiographics 14:1351, 1994.

Wheeler, T. C., and Fleisher, A. C.: Complex adnexal mass in pregnancy: Predictive value of Doppler sonography. J. Ultrasound Med. 16:425, 1997.

Young, R. H., and Scully R. E.: Sex cord–stromal, steroid cell, and other ovarian tumors with endocrine, paraendocrine, and paraneoplastic manifestations. In Kurman, R. J.: Blaustein's Pathology of the Female Genital Tract, 4th ed. New York, Springer-Verlag, 1994, pp. 783–847.

Zaloudek, C.: The ovary. In Gompel, C., and Silverberg, S. (eds): Pathology in Gynecology and Obstetrics, 4th ed. Philadelphia, J. B. Lippincott Co., 1994, pp. 312–413.

Zawin, M., McCarthy, S., Scoutt, L., and Comite, F.: Endometriosis: Appearance and detection at MR imaging. Radiology 171:693, 1989.

Zinn, H. L., Cohen, H. L., and Zinn, D. L.: Ultrasonographic diagnosis of ectopic pregnancy: Importance of transabdominal imaging. J. Ultrasound Med. 16:603, 1997.

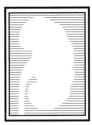

CHAPTER

24

Uterus

This chapter discusses the anatomy, physiology and common diseases of the nongravid uterus. Some of the same components of reproductive physiology that were described in Chapter 23 for the ovary also apply to the uterus. However, most clinically important uterine conditions are the result of either congenital or acquired disorders rather than slight alterations in normal physiology.

ANATOMY AND PHYSIOLOGY

The uterus is located in the midline, posterior to the bladder and anterior to the rectum. A deep reflection of peritoneum extends posterior to the uterus and forms the *cul-de-sac,* or *pouch of Douglas,* which is the most dependent portion of the pelvic cavity in both the supine and standing positions. The uterus is attached to the pelvic side wall by the paired *round ligaments.* The *broad ligament* is a peritoneal reflection over the round ligament, the fallopian tube, and the ligament of the ovary. The uterine artery, which is the principal blood supply to the uterus, arises from the internal iliac (hypogastric) artery, traverses the lateral aspect of the uterus, and forms anastamoses with the ovarian artery. There is a rich plexus of veins, especially along the lateral aspects of the inferior uterine body and cervix.

The uterus is divided into three regions, the *fundus,* the *body,* and the *cervix* and three tissue layers, the *endometrium,* the *myometrium,* and the *serosa.* The endometrium is composed of two dis-tinct tissues: *decidualis,* which is the most physiologically active layer, and *basalis.* Imaging of the individual layers is seldom important in the non-gravid patient. In a woman of childbearing years, the imaging characteristics of the endometrium vary during the normal menstrual cycle. The first day of menses is considered to be the first day of the cycle. Immediately following menses, rebuilding of the endometrium occurs as a result of estrogen stimulation. This is referred to as the *proliferative phase.* In the idealized situation, ovulation occurs on day 14 of a 28-day cycle and marks the beginning of the *secretory phase,* which occurs under the influence of both estrogen and progesterone. The endometrium is thinnest immediately following menses and thickest during the secretory phase of the cycle. The myometrium, which accounts for most of the bulk of the uterus, is composed of a complex arrangement of smooth muscle cells. A thin serosal covering of visceral peritoneum forms the outermost surface of the uterus.

Ultrasonography is the most commonly used modality for imaging the uterus, using either a trans-abdominal or a transvaginal approach. The transvaginal approach offers the advantage of better resolution and, thus, enhanced sensitivity for detection of disease. Although there is a broad variation among individuals, the ultrasonographic image of the uterus is influenced by both age and the menstrual cycle. Premenarchal and postmenopausal uteri are much smaller than in women of childbearing years. Enlargement of the uterus in children

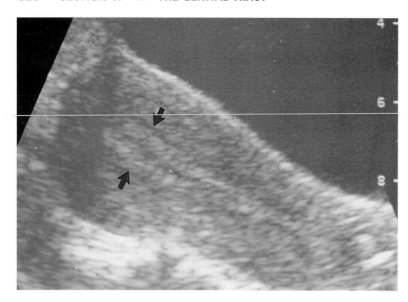

Figure 24–1. Normal uterus. Transabdominal ultrasonogram, longitudinal projection through a filled bladder. A rim of decreased echogenicity *(arrows)* representing the innermost aspect of the myometrium surrounds the endometrium. The bulk of the endometrium is homogeneously echogenic. Although somewhat variable, the layered appearance of the endometrium is typical of the proliferative phase of the menstrual cycle.

can result from precocious puberty syndrome, whereas enlargement in postmenopausal women can be due to hormone replacement, endometrial hyperplasia, or tumor and fibroids. In most women, the endometrium can be identified as a central echogenic line of varying width surrounded by the rather homogeneous medium-level echogenicity of the myometrium. A multilayered appearance to the endometrium is seen in many women (Fig. 24–1).

Magnetic resonance imaging is used far less commonly than ultrasonography for evaluation of the uterus. In some circumstances, however, the superior contrast resolution of magnetic resonance imaging is more advantageous than ultrasonography. This is especially true for characterizing some congenital disorders, evaluating adenomyosis, staging carcinoma, and, occasionally, detecting leiomyoma. Three distinct layers characterize the normal uterus on T2-weighted images (Fig. 24–2). The central *endometrium* is of high-signal intensity. The majority of the *myometrium* is of intermediate-signal intensity and comprises the outer portion of the uterus. A thin layer of low-signal intensity separates these two areas and is referred to as the *junctional zone.* Histologically, the junctional zone is the innermost layer of the myometrium. The low-signal intensity on T2-weighted images is due to the relatively low cellular water content of the junctional zone as compared with the remainder of the myometrium.

Computed tomography in patients with suspected or proven uterine malignancy is usually limited to staging of a known malignancy rather than evaluating the primary uterine abnormality. In that setting lymph node enlargement, ureteral obstruction, and liver metastases should be sought as manifestations of metastases.

ANOMALIES

During embryogenesis, the paired müllerian ducts unite in the midline to form the uterine body, the

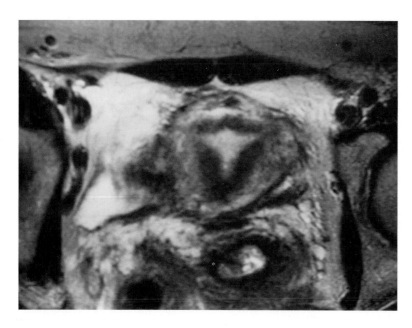

Figure 24–2. Normal uterus. Zonal anatomy as depicted by T2-weighted magnetic resonance image. The central endometrium is of high-signal intensity, the outer myometrium of intermediate-signal intensity, and the inner myometrium (or junctional zone) is of low-signal intensity.

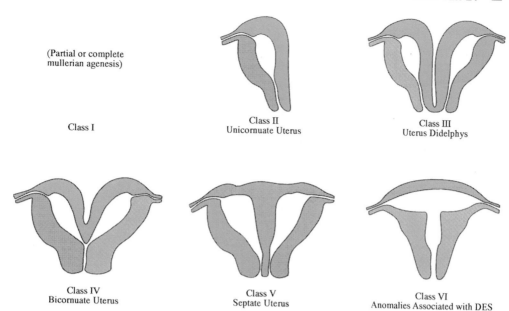

Class I

(Partial or complete mullerian agenesis)

Class II
Unicornuate Uterus

Class III
Uterus Didelphys

Class IV
Bicornuate Uterus

Class V
Septate Uterus

Class VI
Anomalies Associated with DES

Figure 24–3. Diagram of the six major classes of congenital uterine malformations. Many intermediate forms, which are not illustrated, exist. (Reprinted from *Seminars in Ultrasound, CT, and MRI* 1994; 15:4, with permission of the publisher.)

cervix, and the upper portion of the vagina. Disruption of this process leads to a variety of complex malformations of the uterus, one classification of which is illustrated in Figure 24–3. Classification of uterine anomalies is, however, subject to considerable controversy. It is important to remember that these anomalies exist not as discrete entities but rather as a continuum with incomplete or combined forms commonly encountered. Therefore, predicting prognosis and planning treatment is more dependent on a careful description of the malformation rather than an assignment to a precise category.

Most congenital uterine malformations occur without a known cause. A small number of cases are due to *in utero* exposure to diethylstilbestrol (DES), a synthetic hormone that was prescribed for a variety of pregnancy-related disorders from the late 1940s until 1970. Idiopathic uterine anomalies, unlike those associated with DES exposure, are often associated with renal anomalies, such as renal ectopia, ureteropelvic junction obstruction, and unilateral renal agenesis. This relationship reflects the close proximity of the müllerian ducts to the mesonephros and metanephros.

Many patients with congenital uterine anomalies are asymptomatic, and the malformation may remain unrecognized until discovered as an incidental finding. Anomalies are often revealed during evaluation for infertility, recurrent or spontaneous abortion, endometriosis, and hematometrocolpos (Fig. 24–4).

Agenesis/Hypoplasia

The diagnosis of müllerian agenesis of the uterus is based on primary amenorrhea and corresponding physical findings. Both ultrasonography and magnetic resonance imaging reveal the absence of the uterus, cervix, and upper vagina in a phenotypic female. Loops of small bowel fill in the space nor-

mally occupied by the uterus and cervix. Hypoplasia of müllerian duct structures occurs in degrees of severity. At the opposite end of the spectrum from agenesis, the uterus might appear nearly normal, whereas in other patients the uterus is premenarchal in size with a small endometrial stripe. The degree of hypoplasia determines the severity of the reproductive dysfunction. In most cases, surgical options are limited.

Unicornuate Uterus

A unicornuate uterus is characterized by a single uterine horn attached to a single tube. This anom-

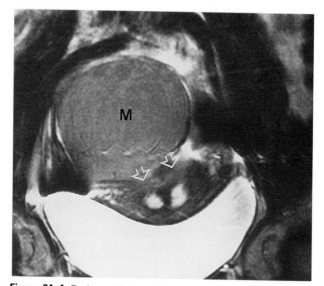

Figure 24–4. Endometriosis and septate uterus in a 41-year-old woman with chronic pelvic pain. T2-weighted magnetic resonance image, coronal plane. There is a septate uterus *(arrows)* and a homogeneous, relatively hypointense right ovarian mass (M). (Reprinted from *Seminars in Ultrasound, CT, and MRI* 1994; 15:4, with permission of the publisher).

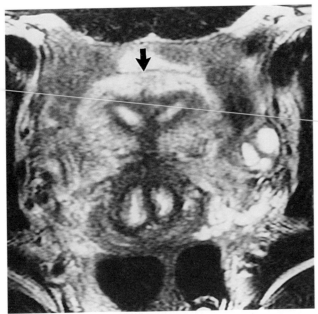

Figure 24–5. Septate uterus and septate cervix in a 33-year-old woman. T2-weighted magnetic resonance image, oblique axial projection. Two uterine cavities and a dividing septum within the cervix is noted. The external configuration of the uterine fundus is normal *(arrow)*.

aly is associated with a mild degree of reproductive dysfunction. Corrective surgical options are limited. Physical examination and ultrasonography generally fail to detect a unicornuate uterus. Diagnosis depends on hysterosalpingography, which depicts the absence of one uterine horn and the ipsilateral fallopian tube. This abnormal morphology is also demonstrable by magnetic resonance images.

Occasionally, a rudimentary horn is present. This component may or may not communicate with the main body of the uterus. This variation of unicornuate uterus may be asymptomatic. In some patients, however, a functioning endometrial layer that does not communicate with the main body of the uterus leads to endometriosis or hematometra and the need for surgical repair. Magnetic resonance imaging can provide a guide for surgical planning in these cases.

Uterus Didelphys

Uterus didelphys results from a failure of fusion of the two müllerian ducts. This anomaly is morphologically analogous to the juxtaposition of two unicornuate uteri. In a manner similar to that of unicornuate uterus, reproductive dysfunction is seen in only a minority of cases, and surgical options are limited. Ultrasonography usually demonstrates the separate uterine components. Hysterosalpingography requires cannulation of each cervix with separate injections of contrast material. Magnetic resonance imaging also defines the uterine morphology.

Bicornuate/Septate Uterus

Bicornuate and septate uteri are best discussed together because of similarities of internal structure and some overlap in imaging appearance. The components of a bicornuate uterus vary with the level of fusion of the two uterine horns. In the extreme, a bicornuate uterus is associated with two cervices if the separation extends far caudad. This is known as a *bicornuate bicollis* anomaly. Components that join together at a more cephalad level result in only a single cervix, termed *bicornuate unicollis*. Additionally, if the level of fusion extends higher still, the anomaly resembles a septate uterus. In practice, then, some cases of bicornuate bicollis anomaly cannot be distinguished from uterus didelphys and, at the other extreme, some cases of bicornuate unicollis cannot be distinguished from a septate uterus. True bicornuate uterus has a midline cleft of variable extent on the external surface of the uterine fundus.

A septate uterus results from complete fusion but incomplete resorption of a midline septum that varies in length and composition. The septum may be fibrous, myometrial, or both. The external morphology of the uterus is normal (Fig. 24–5).

The diagnosis of either a bicornuate or a septate uterus is suggested by the ultrasonographic demonstration of two separate endometrial cavities (Fig. 24–6). The same finding may be seen by hysterosalpingography. Compared with that of a septate uterus, the angle of separation between the two cavities in a bicornuate uterus is wide (greater than 90 degrees). However, this criterion is only about 85 per cent accurate because of overlap in the angle in both conditions. For the purpose of planning therapy, delineation of the external morphology of the uterus is more important than the configuration of the uterine cavities. Here, magnetic resonance

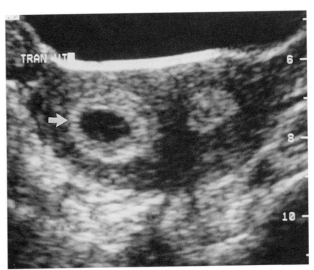

Figure 24–6. Bicornuate uterus with intrauterine pregnancy. Ultrasonogram, transverse plane. A gestational sac is present on the right *(arrow)*, and a decidual reaction is noted on the left. (Kindly provided by Carl Meyer, MD, Muncie, Indiana.)

TABLE 24–1. Summary of Differential Features Between Bicornuate and Septate Uterus

	BICORNUATE UTERUS	SEPTATE UTERUS
Internal morphology by hysterosalpingography	Horns are typically widely separated (> 90°)	Horns are less widely separated (< 90°)
External morphology by laparoscopy or magnetic resonance imaging	Abnormal	Normal
Rate of reproductive dysfunction	Intermediate	High

imaging is of particular value because of its ability to demonstrate both the internal and external configuration of the uterus. If two separate uterine horns are seen, the diagnosis of bicornuate uterus is established. If, on the other hand, the external morphology of the fundus is normal, the anomaly is that of a septate uterus.

Although delineation of the external uterine morphology is critical in order to determine treatment, the classification of the anomaly based on internal characteristics is somewhat arbitrary and of less importance clinically. The rate of pregnancy loss for a patient with a bicornuate uterus is intermediate between that of a uterus didelphys and that of a septate uterus. Determination of the external morphology of a uterus with a single cervix but two cavities is critical as it determines therapy. In the case of a septate uterus, the absence of a significant external cleft in the fundus allows for hysteroscopic resection of the septum. This is a less extensive procedure than the open laparotomy and metroplasty that is required for the treatment of a symptomatic bicornuate uterus. Table 24–1 summarizes these considerations.

THE MYOMETRIUM

Leiomyoma

Leiomyoma of the uterus is a benign smooth muscle neoplasm of the myometrium. The term *fibroid,* although commonly used to refer to this lesion, is less accurate. Leiomyoma occurs in up to 50 per cent of hysterectomy specimens and is particularly common in African-American women. Leiomyomas vary in size from microscopic foci to lesions 20 cm or more in diameter.

Symptoms may result from a leiomyoma of sufficient size in any location. Submucosal lesions, which are the least common, are most likely to cause abnormal uterine bleeding or infertility due to mass effect on the endometrial cavity. Typically, those tumors that produce pelvic pain, abnormal bleeding, or spontaneous abortion are multiple and range from 2 to 5 cm in diameter. Those that arise in the subserosal portion of the myometrium grow exophytically and have only a small stalk of attachment to the uterus. Degeneration of a leiomyoma, which occurs as a result of hemorrhage, necrosis, or hyalinization, is a cause of pelvic pain, especially in large lesions.

A leiomyoma may be detected on an abdominal radiograph as a result of a mass effect on bowel loops when the tumor is very large, calcified, or multiple. Calcification within a leiomyoma, often quite dense, is the result of hemorrhage or tumor necrosis (Fig. 24–7).

Hysterosalpingography typically demonstrates a smooth impression on the uterine cavity, a finding that does not always indicate a high risk for infertility but may be of significance in patients with recurrent spontaneous abortion (Fig. 24–8).

Computed tomography does not directly demonstrate noncalcified leiomyomas but does depict an enlarged, lobulated uterine configuration in cases of large or multiple lesions.

A leiomyoma is typically a solid hypoechoic, well-circumscribed, and slightly heterogeneous mass that attenuates sound slightly (Figs. 24–9 and 24–10A). Some lesions may be associated with enhanced through-transmission and, thus, may be mistaken for a cystic mass. Only occasionally is a leiomyoma slightly hyperechoic. When calcification is present in a leiomyoma, strong echoes with shadowing are seen. Deformity of the endometrial stripe may be present. A leiomyoma that extends from the serosal surface into the adnexa may be mistaken for an ovarian mass (Fig. 24–10). Sonohysterography, described later in this chapter, shows a smooth impression of a broad-based mass on the endometrial cavity.

Magnetic resonance imaging is particularly effec-

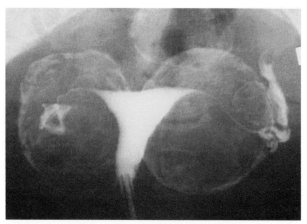

Figure 24–7. Bilateral large, calcified leiomyomas of the uterus. Hysterosalpingogram. There is no significant impression on the uterus from the calcified leiomyomas despite their large size.

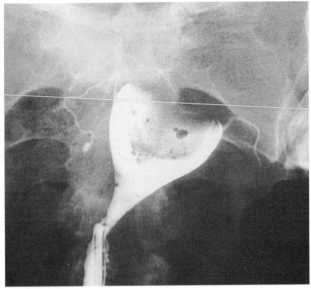

Figure 24–8. Leiomyoma, submucosal. Hysterosalpingogram. There is smooth impression on the uterine fundus. Note several air bubbles.

tive at detecting and characterizing a leiomyoma as well as other myometrial disorders. On T2-weighted images, a leiomyoma appears as a low-signal, well-circumscribed, spherical mass surrounded by myometrium (Fig. 24–11; see Fig. 24–13). The number and location of the lesions are generally better demonstrated by magnetic resonance imaging than by ultrasonography. This is particularly true in severely involved uteri but may be more critical in more mild cases in patients who are seeking to avoid hysterectomy. Magnetic resonance imaging can provide a guide to surgical planning for hysteroscopic myomectomy in patients with recurrent spontaneous abortion thought to be the result of a submucosal leiomyoma.

Magnetic resonance imaging is also effective at distinguishing between a solid adnexal mass that is ovarian in origin from a pedunculated one of uterine

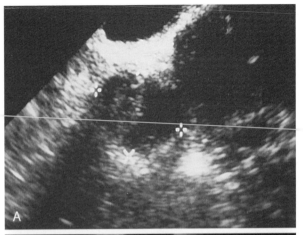

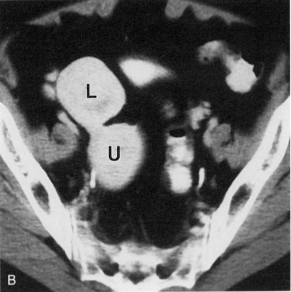

Figure 24–10. Pedunculated leiomyoma in a 59-year-old woman with a palpable right adnexal mass.

A, Transvaginal ultrasonogram, sagittal projection. A solid mass is present in the right adnexa *(cursors).* The right ovary could not be identified ultrasonographically.

B, Computed tomogram with contrast material enhancement. A subserosal leiomyoma (L) is attached by a short stalk to the uterus (U).

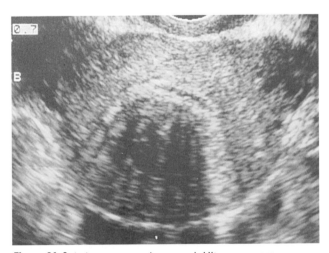

Figure 24–9. Leiomyoma, submucosal. Ultrasonogram, transverse projection. A central heterogeneous mass and areas of acoustic shadowing are noted.

origin. Magnetic resonance imaging can be valuable in cases in which a degenerating leiomyoma may be clinically and ultrasonographically indistinguishable from ovarian torsion or other adnexal disorders (Fig. 24–12). Finally, the ultrasonographic or magnetic resonance imaging features of a degenerated leiomyoma may be indistinguishable from those of a leiomyosarcoma, a far less common malignant smooth muscle tumor discussed below.

Adenomyosis

Adenomyosis represents heterotopic endometrial glandular and stromal tissue that infiltrates into the myometrium and incites a cellular reaction including smooth muscle proliferation. The condition is not uncommon, being found in more than 10 per

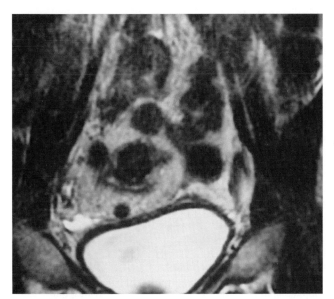

Figure 24–11. Multiple uterine leiomyomas. T2-weighted magnetic resonance image, coronal plane. There are multiple, round, homogeneous low-signal masses that are subserosal, mural, and submucosal.

cent of hysterectomy specimens. Adenomyosis tends to be more severe in late childbearing years.

Adenomyosis is occasionally referred to as *endometriosis interna* in order to distinguish it from *endometriosis externa,* described in Chapters 16 and 19, in which endometrial tissue is present outside the uterus itself. Endometriosis externa, which is usually referred to simply as endometriosis, occurs in 15 per cent of patients with adenomyosis. The pathophysiology of adenomyosis, however, differs fundamentally from that of endometriosis in that the heterotopic endometrium in the former arises from the basalis and is generally not responsive to hormonal treatment.

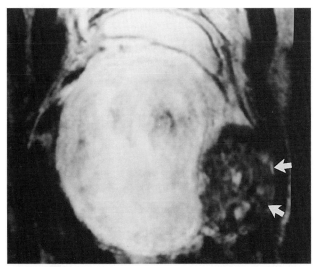

Figure 24–12. Leiomyoma of the uterus in a patient with a 24-week pregnancy. T2-weighted magnetic resonance image, coronal plane. An ovoid low signal mass of the myometrium *(arrows)* has a somewhat heterogeneous signal that suggests degeneration.

Patients with adenomyosis often experience dysmenorrhea or menorrhagia secondary to reactive changes in the surrounding myometrium. Thus, adenomyosis may mimic the clinical features of symptomatic leiomyomas. Determining the cause of symptoms is often difficult, as leiomyoma and adenomyosis frequently coexist. In most patients with adenomyosis, the uterus is enlarged but often not to a degree that is detectable on physical examination.

Hysterosalpingography is usually not performed for the investigation of adenomyosis, even though infertility may be present. When performed, however, small irregular outpouchings of contrast material may extend into the myometrium in some cases.

Ultrasonography documents uterine enlargement in adenomyosis. A generalized heterogeneity in the echo pattern of the myometrium may be noted, but this feature is nonspecific.

Magnetic resonance imaging using T2-weighted images demonstrates a diffuse increase in the thickness of the dark junctional zone. Severe cases of adenomyosis demonstrate extension of this low signal throughout the myometrium (Fig. 24–13). Although low-signal intensity is seen in both adenomyosis and leiomyoma, differentiation between the two can be based on the typically diffuse nature of the former and the circumscribed boundaries of the latter. Foci of high-signal intensity usually are a result of hemorrhage. In general, though, the imaging abnormalities encountered in adenomyosis are the result of smooth-muscle proliferation within the myometrium rather than hemorrhage.

The determination of an upper limit of normal for the thickness of the junctional zone in cases of suspected adenomyosis is controversial. Whereas a measurement of 6 mm yields a high sensitivity, specificity is optimized by an upper limit of 10 mm. The problem of defining imaging criteria is compounded by the nonuniformity of pathologic criteria. A small amount of extension of the endometrium into the myometrium is normal, and the pathologic condition is a matter of degree rather than detection of a specific finding. One must also remember that low signal of the junctional zone represents a high nuclear:cytoplasmic ratio, whereas the imaging findings of adenomyosis are related to smooth-muscle hypertrophy. Thus it may be somewhat misleading to think in terms of adenomyosis as causing a "thickening of the junctional zone."

Table 24–2 summarizes differential features of adenomyosis and leiomyoma.

Leiomyosarcoma

A leiomyosarcoma may arise from a pre-existing leiomyoma, but this is rare. Most leiomyosarcomas arise *de novo* from the smooth muscle of the myometrium. Most occur in older women, although they may be found in patients of any age. The clinical presentation varies with the size and location of the tumor. A diagnosis of leiomyosarcoma should be considered when an apparent leiomyoma enlarges

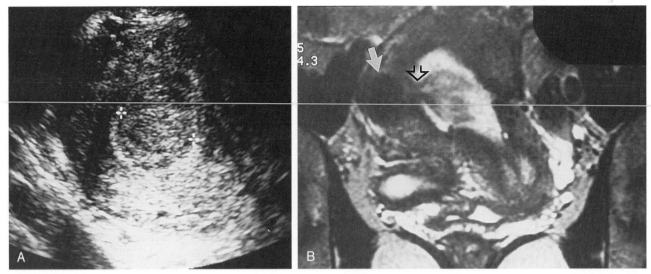

Figure 24–13. Adenomyosis, leiomyoma, and an endometrial polyp in a 39-year-old woman with abnormal bleeding.
    A, Transvaginal pelvic ultrasonogram. The polyp *(cursors)* is a moderately echogenic and heterogeneous mass within the endometrial cavity.
    B, T2-weighted magnetic resonance image, coronal plane. Adenomyosis appears as a widening of the junctional zone, especially in the fundus. An intramural leiomyoma *(white arrow)* is seen as a well-defined round hypointense mass within the myometrium. The polyp is a mass of low to intermediate intensity signal that projects within the high-signal–intensity endometrium. A narrow stalk *(open black arrow)* is apparent.

in a postmenopausal patient. Imaging of a leiomyosarcoma is apt to reveal a solid tumor of ill-defined margins. However, the internal architecture of a necrotic or hemorrhagic leiomyosarcoma is similar to that of the far more common degenerating leiomyoma.

THE ENDOMETRIUM

Abnormalities of the endometrium are effectively imaged by transvaginal ultrasonography, with emphasis on measurement of endometrial thickness in the sagittal plane. In North America, endometrial thickness is reported as the total of both sides of the endometrium and is, thus, actually a double-layer measurement. In Europe, only one-half of the ultrasonographic thickness is reported, which more accurately describes true thickness of the endometrium. Measurements given in this text are in terms of double layer and, thus, are twice the true thickness of the endometrium.

During the past several years, techniques that combine transvaginal pelvic ultrasonography with the instillation of saline into the uterine cavity have been advocated as a way to improve sensitivity and

specificity for endometrial disease. Various terms have been applied to this technique, including saline-infusion sonography, sonohysterography, and hysterosonography. Although specific methods vary, a catheter, usually 6 French in size, is inserted through the cervix into the lower uterine segment during a vaginal speculum examination. The speculum is removed, and saline is infused by gentle hand injection during transvaginal ultrasonography. The goal is to determine the true thickness of the endometrium and distinguish a focal process, such as an endometrial polyp, from diffuse disease, such as carcinoma.

As discussed previously in the section on normal anatomy, the endometrium in the premenopausal woman is thinnest immediately after menses and thickest in the late secretory phase of the cycle. Not infrequently, normal endometrial thickness approaches 20 mm. This wide range of normal in premenopausal women renders assessment of endometrial thickness both insensitive and nonspecific, unless the patient is symptomatic.

Synechiae

Synechiae are fibrous bands that occur within the endometrial canal, usually as a result of previous instrumentation, such as dilatation and curettage, or infection. These adhesions are associated with infertility and dysmenorrhea. Synechiae may be seen ultrasonographically if fluid is present within the uterus, either spontaneously or instilled during sonohysterography. Synechiae also are commonly imaged during hysterosalpingography for evaluation for infertility (Fig. 24–14).

TABLE 24–2. Differential Features of Adenomyosis and Leiomyoma

ADENOMYOSIS	LEIOMYOMA
Usually diffuse	Focal or multifocal
When focal, poorly defined	Well defined
When focal, tend to be oval	Round
Treated with hysterectomy	Hormonal, myomectomy, hysterectomy

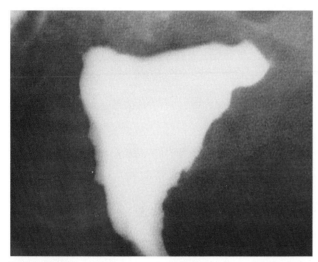

Figure 24–14. Synechiae and bilateral tubal obstruction. Hysterosalpingogram. There is a diffuse irregularity of the endometrial cavity with obstruction of the fallopian tubes at the level of the cornu.

Atrophy

Atrophy of the endometrium occurs normally as part of the postmenopausal decline in estrogen secretion. Some patients with atrophy, however, have bleeding as a result of the friability of the submucosal vessels. Atrophy accounts for up to three-fourths of all patients with postmenopausal bleeding. Ultrasonography detects an endometrium of less than 5 mm thickness.

Polyp

A polyp that arises from the mucosa of the endometrium is a common finding, occurring in up to 10 per cent of hysterectomy specimens. These lesions, which are almost always benign, are usually quite small and asymptomatic. Occasionally, though, a polyp is the cause of uterine bleeding. Endometrial polyps occur in adults of any age and may be seen after menopause.

The attachment of an endometrial polyp to the endometrium varies from a narrow, elongated stalk to a broad base (see Fig. 24–13B). The histologic composition of an endometrial polyp is variable. Most polyps are composed of unmodified endometrial tissue. In some polyps, however, the polypoid mass is composed of hyperplastic or carcinomatous endometrium. A focus of carcinoma in an otherwise benign polyp may occasionally be encountered. As discussed in a following section, carcinoma of the endometrium is usually a diffuse, rather than a focal, process. The internal architecture of a polyp may be solid or multicystic.

On hysterosalpingography, a polyp appears as a filling defect with a focal attachment to the mucosa. This must be differentiated from a submucosal leiomyoma, which has a relatively broad-based relationship to the mucosa. On conventional ultrasonography, the central endometrial stripe appears thickened in most cases. Most polyps appear as a multicystic mass, but a solid echogenic mass is also frequently seen (Fig. 24–15; see Fig. 24–13A). In either case, it may be difficult to see the polyp as a distinct entity against the surrounding endometrium, especially if the latter is hyperplastic. In this circumstance, saline infusion sonography may be of value in distinguishing a focal polyp from diffusely thickened endometrium (Fig. 24–16). Magnetic resonance images effectively reveal polyp and its stalk as structures of low-to-intermediate signal intensity (see Fig. 24–13B).

Adenocarcinoma

Endometrial carcinoma accounts for 90 per cent of uterine malignancies and is the most common gynecologic malignancy overall. Despite this high prevalence, endometrial carcinoma is less likely to be fatal than either carcinoma of the cervix or, especially, carcinoma of the ovary. This is because patients with endometrial carcinoma present earlier with bleeding and have organ-confined (Stage I) disease and are potentially cured by hysterectomy. Most patients with endometrial carcinoma are postmenopausal; the mean age at presentation is approximately 62 years. Risk factors include obesity, nulliparity, late menopause, estrogen-producing ovarian neoplasms, and unopposed exogenous estrogen administration. Tamoxifen, used to treat estrogen-receptor positive breast carcinoma, is a specific estrogen antagonist that increases the risk of endometrial carcinoma. This special circumstance is discussed at the end of this chapter.

The concept of defining a normal value for the thickness of the endometrium is based on the premise that the mean thickness for the most significant condition, carcinoma, is greater than 15 mm,

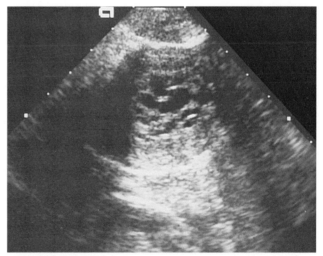

Figure 24–15. Endometrial polyp secondary to tamoxifen in a 56-year-old woman with uterine bleeding. Ultrasonogram. The polyp appears as a multicystic structure in the central portion of the uterus. Differential diagnosis includes hyperplasia, polyp, carcinoma, or a combination of these. Surgical excision confirmed a benign cystic polyp.

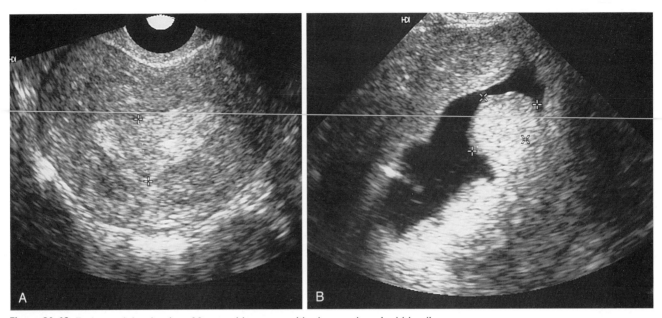

Figure 24–16. Endometrial polyp in a 36-year-old woman with abnormal vaginal bleeding.
A, Transvaginal ultrasonogram, sagittal projection. The endometrium is homogeneous but prominent *(cursors).*
B, Saline infusion sonography confirms a polyp *(cursors)* as the cause of the prominent endometrium seen in *(A).* A relatively broad base attaches the polyp to the posterior aspect of the endometrial cavity.

whereas normal thickness is approximately 6 mm. The normal state of limited endometrial activity in the postmenopausal woman and the relatively increased risk of endometrial carcinoma allow one to assess the patient in terms of the thickness of the endometrium. This is somewhat complicated in patients on supplemental exogenous hormones, usually estrogen, with or without progestin.

A patient with endometrial carcinoma usually develops abnormal bleeding. Prior to the widespread use of sonohysterography, an endometrial aspiration biopsy would be the initial diagnostic study. If the biopsy specimen were negative for carcinoma or hyperplasia, a presumed diagnosis of atrophy would be treated by hormonal modification. If, on the other hand, the biopsy specimen were positive for carcinoma, computed tomography of the abdomen for staging would be performed prior to hysterectomy. Sonohysterography is a contemporary approach, described later in this chapter, that characterizes a thickened endometrial stripe as either *focal* or *diffuse.* A focal abnormality suggests polyp as a cause, whereas a diffuse process is more likely the result of hyperplasia or carcinoma.

Magnetic resonance imaging rarely has a role in the prebiopsy evaluation of a patient with uterine bleeding because it cannot reliably differentiate benign from malignant endometrial disease. In a patient with a biopsy-proven carcinoma, magnetic resonance images typically show a thickened heterogeneous medium-to-high–signal intensity endometrium on T2-weighted images. If the tumor has extended into the myometrium, the normally well-defined low-signal junctional zone is disrupted (Fig. 24–17). However, depth of invasion is difficult to assess in many patients because of the similarity of

signal intensity found in both normal and neoplastic myometrium. The value of magnetic resonance images is further impaired by coexistent uterine atrophy and the fact that many postmenopausal women lack the characteristic zonal anatomic landmarks of the uterus.

Both computed tomography and magnetic resonance imaging are useful in the staging of endometrial carcinoma to detect pelvic extension and distant metastases. For patients thought to have local disease, however, assessment of the depth of myometrial invasion is best determined by histologic evaluation of the excised uterus. Depth of invasion greater than 50 per cent of the myometrial thickness (Stage IC) is associated with a high risk of

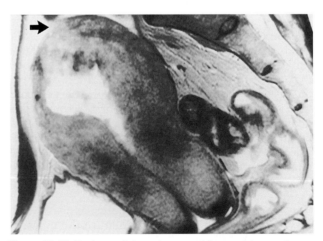

Figure 24–17. Endometrial carcinoma with extension to the serosa. T2-weighted magnetic resonance image, sagittal plane. Tumor diffusely infiltrates through the myometrium with trans-serosal disease noted at the fundus *(arrow).*

TABLE 24–3. International Federation of Gynecology and Obstetrics Staging of Endometrial Carcinoma

STAGE I	Confined to the uterine body
STAGE IA	Tumor limited to the endometrium
STAGE IB	Tumor invades less than half the myometrial thickness
STAGE IC	Tumor invades more than half the myometrial thickness
STAGE IIA, IIB	Uterine cervix involved
STAGE IIIA, IIIB, IIIC	Pelvic extension
STAGE IVA, IVB	Extrapelvic extension

TABLE 24–4. International Federation of Gynecology and Obstetrics Staging of Cervical Carcinoma

STAGE 0	*In situ*
STAGE IA, IB	Confined to cervix
STAGE IIA, IIB	Extends beyond cervix, upper two-thirds of vagina, or parametrial tissue
STAGE IIIA, IIIB	Extends to pelvic wall or lower one-third of vagina or causes ureteral obstruction
STAGE IVA, IVB	Extends beyond true pelvis or involves bladder or rectal mucosa

retroperitoneal lymph node involvement and a poor prognosis. These patients generally undergo a retroperitoneal lymph node dissection at the time of the initial surgery. The staging classification for endometrial carcinoma is shown in Table 24–3.

THE CERVIX

Carcinoma

The ease of direct visualization of the cervix limits the role of diagnostic imaging in the management of cervical disorders. This section discusses the potential role for imaging in the setting of cervical carcinoma.

Cervical carcinoma is almost always due to squamous cell carcinoma and has a peak incidence early in the 5th decade of life. Although there are multiple risk factors, the most important is a history of multiple sexual partners, probably related to transmission of human papillomavirus. The death rate from this disorder has declined dramatically over the past several decades, largely as a result of widespread use of cytologic sampling of the cervix, the Papanicolaou smear.

The patient with suspected cervical carcinoma is diagnosed by biopsy. Imaging, if it is used at all, is limited to staging. The key feature for cervical carcinoma in determining management is the presence or absence of parametrial disease (Stage IIB vs. IIA disease). Patients without parametrial extension (Stage IIA) are candidates for surgical treatment. Patients with stage IIB disease, on the other hand, are usually treated with radiation. The presence of parametrial involvement is determined by physical examination and surgical findings. Computed tomography has not been effective in differentiating Stage IIA from Stage IIB because of a high false-positive rate. Computed tomography may, however, be useful in detecting ureteral and periureteral involvement as well as enlargement of retroperitoneal lymph nodes. Table 24–4 summarizes the staging classification for carcinoma of the cervix.

Magnetic resonance imaging can be used to evaluate the parametrium for tumor extension (Fig. 24–18). However, this technique has not been shown to be more accurate than physical examination in this regard.

IMAGING OF THE PATIENT WITH POSTMENOPAUSAL BLEEDING

Atrophy is a dominant cause of postmenopausal bleeding. Neither biopsy nor dilatation and curettage are required in these patients. Polyps, hyperplasia, or carcinoma of the endometrium, on the other hand, must be considered as causes of postmenopausal bleeding in those patients who do not have atrophy.

Transvaginal ultrasonography is of value in the initial assessment of the patient with postmenopausal bleeding. An endometrial thickness of 4 mm or less supports the diagnosis of **atrophy** and indicates the need for hormonal treatment without biopsy. If the thickness of the endometrium exceeds 4 mm, differentiation between *focal* or *diffuse* thickening can be accomplished by sonohysterography. A focal area of thickening suggests the diagnosis of a **polyp,** which might be retrieved by hysteroscopic resection. On the other hand, diffuse thickening suggests a diagnosis of either endometrial **hyperplasia** or **carcinoma** and the need for an endometrial biopsy.

In a postmenopausal patient without bleeding, an endometrial width that exceeds 8 mm is usually

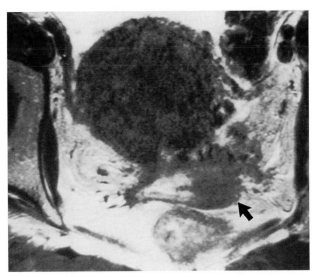

Figure 24–18. Cervical carcinoma, stage IIB. T2-weighted fast spin echo magnetic resonance image, transverse plane. Tumor *(arrow)* infiltrates the fat of the left parametrium.

investigated by sonohysterography or biopsy to investigate the possibility of endometrial carcinoma.

Patients receiving exogenous replacement hormones, with or without bleeding, pose a special problem both in terms of risk for endometrial carcinoma and the lack of an established range of normal for endometrial thickness. Unopposed estrogen therapy carries a clearly increased risk of endometrial carcinoma. In this setting, an endometrium that is slightly prominent should be considered potentially abnormal. Generally, however, unopposed estrogen is reserved for those women who have undergone hysterectomy. Hormone replacement regimens that include a progestational agent in addition to estrogen are safer in terms of the risk of endometrial carcinoma. In patients on sequential agents, the endometrium is best evaluated immediately after menses when it is at its thinnest width.

TAMOXIFEN EFFECT

Tamoxifen is an antiestrogenic drug that is used in patients with estrogen-receptor positive carcinoma of the breast in an effort to decrease the rate of tumor recurrence postoperatively. It has also been proposed for prophylactic use in patients at high risk for carcinoma of the breast. This agent has a paradoxical effect on the uterus, presumably representing an inherent agonist mechanism. Patients taking tamoxifen are prone to the development of both hyperplastic polyps, often with central cystic areas, and endometrial carcinoma (see Fig. 24–15). Any thickening of the endometrium in these patients should be considered as suspicious for carcinoma, especially in the setting of abnormal bleeding.

BIBLIOGRAPHY

Bourne, T. H., Lawton, F., Leather, A., Granberg, S., Campbell, S., and Collins, W. P.: Use of intracavity saline instillation and transvaginal ultrasonography to detect tamoxifen-associated endometrial polyps. Ultrasound Obstet Gynecol 4:73–75, 1994.

Buttram, V. S., and Gibbons, W. E.: Müllerian abnormalities: A proposed classification (an analysis of 144 cases). Fertil. Steril 32:40, 1979.

Cohen, J. R., Luxman, D., Sagi, J., Yovel, I., Wolman, I., and David, M. P.: Sonohysterography for distinguishing endometrial thickening from endometrial polyps in postmenopausal bleeding. Ultrasound Obstet Gynecol 4:2272, 1994.

Comerci, J. T., Jr., Fields, A. L., and Runowicz, D. D.: Continuous low-dose combined hormone replacement therapy and the risk of endometrial cancer. Gynecol. Oncol. 64:425, 1997.

Corley, D., Rowe, J., and Curtis, M. T.: Postmenopausal bleeding from unusual endometrial polyps in women on chronic tamoxifen therapy. Obstet. Gynecol. 79:111, 1992.

Doi, T., Yamashita, Y., Yasunaga, T., Fujiyoshi, K., Tsunawaki, A., Takahashi, M., Katabuchi, H., Tanaka, N., and Okamura, H.: Adenoma malignum: MR imaging and pathologic study. Radiology 204:39, 1997.

Emanuel, M. H., Ankum, W. M., Verdel, M. J. C., and Hart, A., A. M.: The reproducibility of the results of transvaginal sonography of the uterus in patients with abnormal uterine bleeding. Ultrasound Obstet. Gynecol. 8:346, 1996.

Ferenczy, A.: Anatomy and histology of the uterine corpus. In Kurman, R. J.: Blaustein's Pathology of the Female Genital Tract, 4th ed. New York, Springer-Verlag, 1994, pp. 327–366.

Goldstein, S. R.: Use of ultrasonohysterography for triage of perimenopausal patients with unexplained uterine bleeding. Am. J. Obstet. Genecol. 170:565, 1994.

Granberg, S. K., Wickland, M., and Karsson, B.: Endometrial thickness as measured by endovaginal ultrasonography for identifying endometrial abnormality. Am. J. Obstet. Gynecol. 164:47, 1991.

Hann L. E., Giess, C. S., and Bach, A. M.: Endometrial thickness in tamoxifen-treated patients: Correlation with clinical and pathologic findings. AJR 168:657, 1997.

Hawighorst, H., Knapstein, P. G., Weikel, W., Knopp, K. V., Schaeffer, U., Brix, G., Essig, M., Hoffmann, U., Zuna, I., Schönberg, S., and Kaick, G. V.: Cervical carcinoma: Comparison of standard and pharmacokinetic MR imaging. Radiology 201:531, 1996.

Hulka, C. A., Hall, D. A., McCarthy, K., and Simeone, J. F.: Endometrial polyps, hyperplasia, and carcinoma in postmenopausal women: Differentiation with endovaginal sonography. Radiology 191:755, 1994.

Kinkel, K., Ariche, M., Tardivon, A. A., Spatz, A., Castaigne, D., Lhommé, C., and Vanel, D.: Differentiation between recurrent tumor and benign conditions after treatment of gynecologic pelvic carcinoma: Value of dynamic contrast-enhanced subtraction MR imaging. Radiology 204:55, 1997.

Kobayashi, S., Takeda, K., Sakuma, H., Kinosada, Y., and Nakagawa, T.: Uterine neoplasms: Magnetization transfer analysis of MR images. Radiology 203:377, 1997.

Kurman, R. J., Zaino, R. J., and Norris, H. J.: Endometrial carcinoma. In Kurman, R. J.: Blaustein's Pathology of the Female Genital Tract, 4th ed. New York, Springer-Verlag, 1994, pp. 439–486.

Lev-Toaff, A. S., Toaff, M. E., Liu, J. B., and Merton, D. A.: Value of sonohysterography in the diagnosis and management of abnormal uterine bleeding. Radiology 201:179, 1996.

Levine, D., Gosink, B. B., and Johnson, L. A.: Change in endometrial thickness in postmenopausal women undergoing hormone replacement therapy. Radiology 197:603, 1995.

Morrow, C. P., Curtin, J. P., and Towsend, D. E.: Tumors of the cervix. In Morrow, C. P., Curtin, J. P., and Towsend, D. E.: Synopsis of Gynecologic Oncology, 4th ed. Churchill Livingstone, 1997, pp. 111–152.

Morrow, C. P., Curtin, J. P., and Towsend, D. E.: Tumors of endometrium. In Morrow, C. P., Curtin, J. P., and Towsend, D. E.: Synopsis of Gynecologic Oncology, 4th ed. Churchill Livingstone, 1997, pp. 153–188.

Outwater, E. K., Siegelman, E. S., and Deerlin, V. V.: Adenomyosis: Current concepts and imaging considerations. AJR 170:437, 1998.

Procope, B. J.: Aetiology of postmenopausal bleeding. Acta Obstet. Gynecol. Scand. 50:311, 1971.

Robby, S. J., Bernhardt, P. F., and Parmley, T.: Embryology of the female genital tract and disorders of abnormal sexual development. In Kurman, R. J.: Blaustein's Pathology of the Female Genital Tract, 4th ed. New York, Springer-Verlag, 1994, pp. 3–29.

Saidi, M. H., Sadler, R. K., Theis, V. D., Akright, B. D., Farhart, S. A., and Villanueva, G. R.: Comparison of sonography, sonohysterography, and hysteroscopy for evaluation of abnormal uterine bleeding. J. Ultrasound Med. 16:587, 1997.

Schwartz, L. B., Synder, J., Horan, C., Porges, R. F., Nachtigall, L. E., and Goldstein, S. R.: The use of transvaginal ultrasound and saline infusion sonohysterography for the evaluation of asymptomatic postmenopausal breast cancer patients on tamoxifen. Ultrasound Obstet. Gynecol. 11:48, 1998.

Scheidler, J., Heuck, A. F., Steinborn, M., Kimmig, R., and Reiser, M. F.: Parametrial invasion in cervical carcinoma: Evaluation of detection at MR imaging with fat suppression. Radiology 206:125, 1997.

Takahashi, S., Murakami, T., Narumi, Y., Kurachi, H., Tsuda, K., Kim, T., Enomoto, T., Tomoda, K., Miyake, A., Murata, Y., and Nakamura, H.: Preoperative staging of endometrial carcinoma: Diagnostic effect of T2-weighted fast spin echo MR imaging. Radiology 206:539, 1998.

Wagner, B. J., and Woodward, P. J.: Congenital uterine anomalies. Semin. Ultrasound CT MR 15:4, 1994.

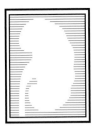
25

The Male Genital Tract: Prostate and Seminal Vesicle

The prostate, bladder, seminal vesicles, and vas deferens account for most of the pathology of the male pelvis. Among these organs, adenocarcinoma of the prostate and benign prostatic hyperplasia account for the highest prevalence of disease and the most significant socioeconomic impact. Infertility is yet another common clinical problem that may be caused by congenital or acquired diseases of the ejaculatory ducts and seminal vesicles. Finally, infection and inflammation may impact any of these structures.

ANATOMY

Prostate Gland

An understanding of prostate anatomy is fundamental to understanding the role of imaging in detecting prostate cancer. The concept of zonal, rather than lobar, anatomy of the prostate originated several decades ago when it was noted that regions of the prostate differed not only embryologically and histologically but also in their predisposition to cancer. The prostate is composed of several anatomic layers (Fig. 25–1). The outermost of these consists of the *periprostatic venous plexus* that surrounds the prostate on all but its posterior aspect where it is interrupted by the anterior and posterior layers of *Denonvillier's fascia*. The tough, fibrous *prostatic capsule* is encountered next. Deep to the capsule is the *peripheral zone*, which is composed primarily of acinar glandular tissue. The peripheral zone accounts for approximately 70 per cent of the gland's volume and is the site of origin for over 70 per cent of prostate cancers. Anteriorly, the peripheral zone is interrupted by relatively acellular tissue that comprises the *fibroelastic zone*, which is a base of support for the prostate's attachment to the bony

pelvis by the *puboprostatic ligament*. Deep to the peripheral zone is the *central zone*, which is composed principally of stromal cells. Only 10 per cent of prostate carcinomas arise in the central zone. Deep to the central zone and concentric with the prostatic urethra are the bilobed *transitional zones*, the most frequent sites for hyperplastic nodules as well as the zones in which approximately 20 per cent of prostate carcinomas arise. As men age, the transitional zone enlarges from approximately 5 per cent of the gland's volume in youth to up to 90 per

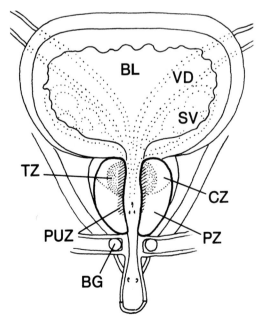

FIGURE 25–1. Zonal anatomy of the prostate. Coronal view: *BL* = bladder, *VD* = vasa deferens, *SV* = seminal vesicles, *CZ* = central zone, *PZ* = peripheral zone, *BG* = bulbourethral glands, *PUZ* = periurethral zone, *TZ* = transitional zone.

cent of volume in senescence. The *periurethral zone* represents the short ducts lining the prostatic urethra.

The prostate is ovoid and tapers inferiorly. The base of the prostate lies against the base of the bladder and is broader than the prostatic apex, which extends inferiorly to the urogenital diaphragm. This terminology can be confusing because it is exactly the inverse of bladder anatomy where the apex is superior to the base. The peripheral zone extends from the base to the apex, whereas the central gland, including both central and transitional zones, ends more superiorly. The prostatic apex is important because the capsule of the prostate is discontinuous due to the hiatus caused by the prostatic urethra. Thus, the apex is a common site of recurrent disease after radical prostatectomy.

The paired *neurovascular bundles* are found within the periprostatic tissue nestled in the lateral grooves between the rectum and the prostate at approximately 5 and 7 o'clock when the prostate is viewed transversely. They are nestled between the prostate and rectum. The bundle is composed of the prostatic arteries and veins as well as the cavernosal nerves, which supply erectile function to the penis. The neurovascular bundle is also a relatively common site of extracapsular extension because of multiple perforating vessels and the propensity of prostate cancer to spread along perineural pathways.

Lymphatic drainage from the prostate is to the obturator, external iliac, and internal iliac lymph node groups. Involvement of the para-aortic and even mediastinal nodes can occur if lymphatic spread of tumor is present.

Seminal Vesicles, Vas Deferens, and Ejaculatory Ducts

The paired seminal vesicles, which extend laterally from the superior aspect of the prostate base, are outpouchings of the paired vas deferens (see Fig. 20–2). The ejaculatory ducts form at the junction of the seminal vesicles and vas deferens and traverse the peripheral zone and then the central zone of the prostate gland before ending in the *verumontanum (colliculus seminalis)* in the prostatic urethra. On cross section, the seminal vesicles have a "bow tie" appearance near their junction with the base of the prostate. By ultrasonography, the normal seminal vesicle is homogeneously hypoechoic with fine internal echoes and, often, internal septations. The normal volume of the seminal vesicles is approximately 14 mL. The seminal vesicles are a common site of extracapsular spread of cancer either by direct extension from the prostate or through the ejaculatory ducts.

PROSTATE GLAND
Adenocarcinoma

Adenocarcinoma of the prostate is the most common non–skin cancer found in American men, with over 310,000 new diagnoses each year. Prostate cancer ranks between lung and colon cancer as the second leading cause of male cancer deaths in the United States, with over 45,000 deaths per year. Epidemiologic evidence indicates that better screening methods, an aging population, as well as known or suspected environmental factors account for the increasing frequency of prostate cancer.

Although prostate cancer is a very common microscopic finding at autopsy, it does not usually progress to a lethal form of the disease. American men have a lifetime risk of 2.9 per cent of dying of prostate cancer, although approximately 9.5 per cent of men are diagnosed with the disease during their lifetime. These data are to be compared with a lifetime risk of approximately 42 per cent of having histologic evidence of prostate cancer. The prevalence of prostate cancer varies with the country of origin, diet, exposure to sunlight, and, possibly, endogenous testosterone levels. For example, the rate of prostate cancer deaths is much higher in Scandinavian countries than it is in Japan, even though the frequency of microscopic cancers is comparable. This discrepancy may be related to diet, genetics, or sunlight exposure. Exposure to sunlight is inversely correlated with the frequency of cancer in the United States, so that southern states report lower rates of prostate cancer than northern states. High-fat diets have also been implicated in prostate cancer. Japanese immigrants to Hawaii who arrive with low rates of prostate cancer deaths experience rising prostate cancer death rates in each subsequent American-born generation, presumably the result of a change to a fatty, western diet. African-American males have a higher rate of prostate cancer and die more frequently of the disease than do American men of other racial origin. As is true in pancreatic, breast, and colon cancer, members of specific families also exhibit a tendency to develop prostate cancer.

The suspicion of prostate cancer is based on a combination of clinical symptoms, the serum level of prostate-specific antigen (PSA), digital rectal examination, and transrectal ultrasonography. Biopsy is required for diagnosis. Although the majority of prostate cancers are clinically silent, the most common symptom is a change in the pattern of voiding. Bone pain is an unusual presentation and may indicate the presence of metastatic disease. Increasingly, the diagnosis first comes to light as a result of a positive screening PSA test in an asymptomatic individual. This test measures the amount of antigen present in the blood and is influenced by both normal and neoplastic prostatic tissue. PSA is a glycoprotein protease produced in the cytoplasm of prostate epithelial cells that promotes liquefaction of sperm. PSA levels rise not only with carcinoma of the prostate but also with increasing age, enlargement of the transition zone in benign prostatic hyperplasia, and certain non-neoplastic conditions, including prostatitis and urinary tract infection.

Thus, a patient with severe prostatic hyperplasia will likely also have an elevated PSA blood level.

Prostatic biopsy is the only method of confirming prostate cancer. The prostate can be biopsied with a needle placed either transrectally or transperineally under palpation or by using ultrasonographic guidance. Automated spring-loaded needles are generally used to obtain multiple histologic cores. The pathologist determines the percentage or length of each core involved by cancer and also the grade of the tumor. The histologic diagnosis of prostate cancer is sometimes an incidental result of transurethral resection of the prostate for benign enlargement.

Prostate Ultrasound Evaluation. Although prostatic ultrasound was first used in the late 1960s it was not until the early 1980s that it was widely applied. Most modern transducers are composed of a single curved array that produce sagittal or oblique coronal projections through the prostate depending on how the probe is rotated. The transducer frequency is generally 5 to 7 MHz. A color Doppler study is also commonly integrated into the probe.

The probe is sheathed with a condom and rubber bands are applied at the neck of the transducer to entrap a water bath that ensures that the prostate is within the focal zone of the transducer. Degassed water is used to fill this water bath, and any bubbles introduced in the filling process are removed. A second sheath ensures sterility. Coupling gel is used between the two sheaths and on the external surface of the second sheath.

The peripheral zone is generally more echogenic than the central gland (Fig. 25–2). The ejaculatory ducts are usually seen as paired hypoechoic structures in the midline within the peripheral zone. Rotating the probe to demonstrate the long axis of the ejaculatory ducts serves to resolve any concern

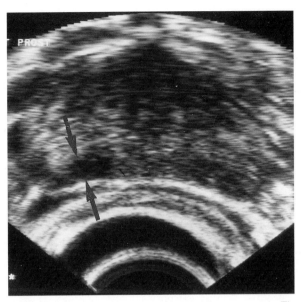

FIGURE 25–3. Adenocarcinoma, prostate. Ultrasonogram. The tumor is seen as a peripheral hypoechoic nodule *(arrows)*.

about their normalcy. The periprostatic venous plexus, also known as *Santorini's* or the *dorsal venous plexus,* can usually be seen as hypoechoic structures surrounding the prostate.

A tumor may appear as a hypoechoic mass within the peripheral zone (Fig. 25–3). However, not all hypoechoic masses represent cancers and not all cancers are hypoechoic. Hyperplasia, prostatitis, ischemia, and some nonspecific abnormalities also appear as hypoechoic foci within the prostate. Between 30 and 60 per cent of hypoechoic nodules prove to be cancers on biopsy, depending on the population examined. Moreover, isoechoic cancers are quite common. While isoechoic lesions may not be detected on gray scale imaging, they may be inferred by asymmetry of the gland. Color Doppler ultrasonography may reveal increased flow in some of these otherwise obscure lesions, but this technique lacks specificity in that increased flow may also be detected in prostatitis, in vascular abnormalities, and even in normal prostatic parenchyma. Similarly, hyperechoic nodules also are nonspecific. Foci of bright, echogenic reflections that are clustered near the junction of the peripheral and central zones usually represent *corpora amylacea,* which are proteinaceous deposits that have hardened within the acini. Hyperechoic prostatic cancers tend to be more advanced than smaller hypoechoic lesions.

Tumors within the central gland are usually difficult to see. Subtle changes in symmetry may be the only clue to the presence of a cancer. Because the central gland is generally hypoechoic to begin with and is subject to hyperplastic changes, the ability of ultrasonography to identify prostate cancer in this region is particularly limited.

A complete transrectal ultrasound examination should include measuring maximal prostate dimensions (D) in the anteroposterior, transverse, and

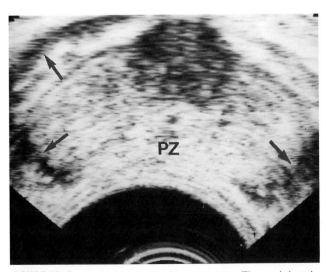

FIGURE 25–2. Normal prostate ultrasonogram. The peripheral zone *(PZ)* is more echogenic than the central gland. The periprostatic venous plexus *(arrows)* is seen at the periphery of the gland.

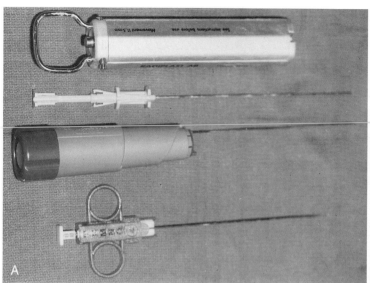

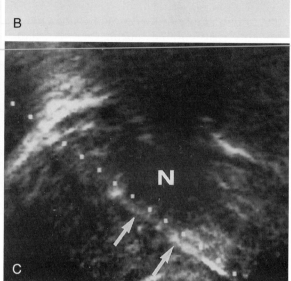

FIGURE 25–4. *A,* Prostate biopsy automated needles. Three different types of automated needles used for prostate biopsies. *From top to bottom:* Temno, Monopty, and Biopty devices.
   B, Close-up of the cutting needle with slot for tissue specimen. Pathologists can estimate the percent or length of each specimen occupied by tumor that provides a useful index regarding the size of the tumor.
   C, Needle in "fired" position within prostate. The echogenic needle is along the computer cursors *(arrows).* The needle is sampling the edge of a hypoechoic nodule *(N).*

craniocaudal planes. These are used to calculate the approximate prostatic volume using the formula D1 × D2 × D3 × 0.5. This value can be used for serial evaluation and for assessing PSA density. The prostate and seminal vesicles should be examined for asymmetry, and the peripheral zone should be inspected for hypoechoic nodules. Color Doppler evaluation, when available, can be used to note "vascular" areas. Finally, if cancer is suspected, any breaches in the prostatic capsule or into the neurovascular bundles should be recorded.

Transrectal ultrasonography is usually performed with the intent to biopsy (Fig. 25–4). The patient should have pre- and post-biopsy antibiotic coverage. Bowel cleansing is optional. The patient is put in the decubitus position or, if stirrups are available, in the lithotomy position. Automated core biopsy needles are preferred because they provide better histologic specimens. The needle is introduced through the rectal mucosa until it is just visualized on the image. The stylet is then "fired" to obtain the core. Three biopsy samples are obtained from the inferior, middle, and superior peripheral zone on each side using an automated needle with a needle guide for a total of six biopsy samples. The superior peripheral biopsy often includes a section of the transitional zone. Additionally, if seminal vesicle extension is suspected because a hypoechoic mass is located near the prostate base in the superior portion of the gland or because the seminal vesicles are asymmetric, the seminal vesicles should be biopsied. Any discrete hypoechoic mass should also be separately biopsied.

Each specimen is labeled by location to create a crude "map" of the prostate that includes the per cent or length of each core involved by tumor and the grade of tumor. For instance, when two adjoining biopsy sites yield cores containing significant amounts of Gleason sum 7 through 10 cancers, the implications are far more serious than when two discontinuous biopsy sites yield cores with small foci of Gleason 2 to 4 prostate cancer.

Transrectal biopsy is not entirely painless, and some consideration to pain control or amnesia is warranted. Moreover, the patient should be informed about the likelihood of finding blood in the stool and hematuria for up to 1 week or longer after prostate biopsy. Patients who have undergone seminal vesicle biopsy may experience hematospermia in the ejaculate. Infection and hematoma are additional risks to the procedure.

Endorectal Magnetic Resonance Imaging. To perform endorectal magnetic resonance imaging, an endorectal coil is inserted into the rectum. Approximately 100 mL of air is insufflated into the balloon that expands the surface coil itself. One milligram of intramuscular glucagon is administered to suppress rectal spasm. T2-weighted images are obtained with 3- to 4-mm slice thickness in the axial and coronal-oblique projection.

The normal peripheral zone is relatively high in signal intensity compared with the central gland (Figs. 25–5, 25–6). The periprostatic venous plexus and neurovascular bundle are generally very high in signal intensity, owing to the slow flow of blood within these structures. A tumor appears as a mass

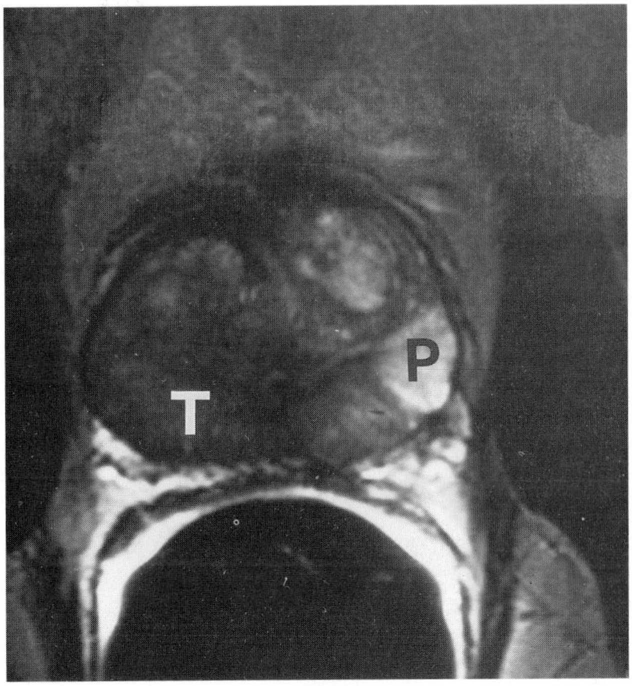

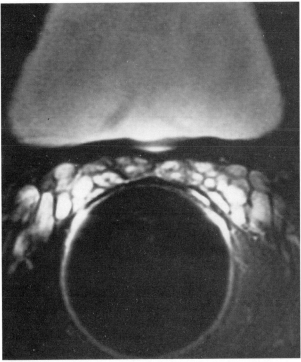

FIGURE 25–5. Adenocarcinoma, prostate. T2-weighted endorectal coil magnetic resonance image. The normal peripheral zone *(P)* demonstrates high signal intensity whereas the tumor *(T)* is low in single intensity. Note the margin of the tumor is smooth and there is no evidence of transcapsular invasion.

with relatively low signal intensity within the peripheral zone. Unfortunately, the presence of blood products up to 3 weeks after biopsy can produce spurious results. The time between biopsy and imaging, therefore, should be adjusted accordingly. After a tumor is identified, the periphery of the prostate should be carefully inspected for breaches through the capsule and the integrity of the neurovascular bundles evaluated. Small excrescences of tumor in the periprostatic fat are highly suggestive of extracapsular disease. Absence of normal high signal intensity in either the seminal vesicles or within the periprostatic venous plexus is also highly suggestive of extracapsular extension (Fig. 25–7). It is important to evaluate the apex of the prostate on

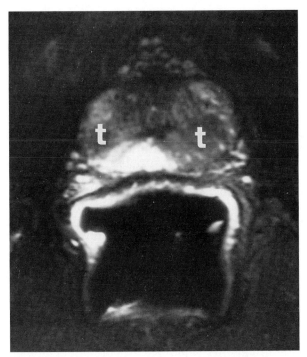

FIGURE 25–6. Adenocarcinoma, prostate. T2-weighted endorectal coil magnetic resonance image demonstrates two sites of tumor *(t)* within the peripheral zone. The margin of the left tumor, however, is partially obscured, making interpretation difficult.

FIGURE 25–7. Adenocarcinoma, prostate. T2-weighted magnetic resonance image of the normal seminal vesicles showing symmetric high signal intensity.

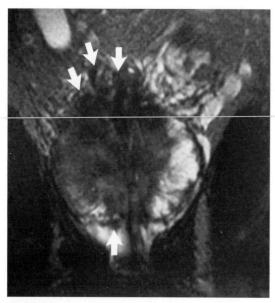

FIGURE 25–8. Adenocarcinoma, prostate. T2-weighted oblique coronal magnetic resonance image of the prostate demonstrates a large tumor that has spread through the base and apex *(arrows)* of the prostate.

coronal images for evidence of tumor. This site, which is difficult to evaluate by ultrasonography, is a common site for recurrence. The base of the prostate should also be evaluated for direct extension into the seminal vesicles (Fig. 25–8).

Several conflicting trends will impact the future of endorectal magnetic resonance imaging. Magnetic resonance technology is improving rapidly, and image quality should improve substantially. Moreover, other techniques, such as magnetic resonance spectroscopy, may achieve noninvasive "biopsies." On the other hand, the cost of endorectal magnetic resonance imaging, including the substantial cost of the endorectal coil itself, is a deterrent to its use in an increasingly cost-conscious medical environment.

Grading of Prostate Cancer. Two systems are generally employed for grading prostate cancer. In the United States, the Gleason grading system predominates. Using this approach, both the morphology of the prostatic tumor (e.g., well-circumscribed or diffuse), and the histologic character (e.g., cellularity, mitotic figures, pleomorphism, desmoplastic response) of the tumor are taken into account. Specific sections of the tumor are graded on a 1 to 5 scale, with 1 representing well-differentiated, well-circumscribed tumors and 5 representing pleomorphic, undifferentiated cells with a desmoplastic stroma. A Gleason score is the aggregate of the two predominant grades within a specimen, thus taking into account heterogeneity within a tumor. Gleason sum scores can range from 2 to 10. In Europe, a three-part grading system is employed. Grade 1 roughly corresponds to a Gleason score of 2 to 4; Grade 2 corresponds to a Gleason score to 5 to 7; and Grade 3 corresponds to a Gleason score of 8 to

10. In most studies, a Gleason score of 7+ or Grade 3 has a strikingly different clinical course than lower histologic grades. Men older than the age of 70 with prostate cancer with a Gleason score less than 7 have, on average, been shown to have a normal life span even if their prostate cancer is untreated. Other methods for predicting lethality include DNA ploidy, which is a measure of chromatin within cells, and tumor size.

Staging Transcapsular Extension. Once prostate cancer has been diagnosed and graded, staging is required. The Whitmore-Jewett system of staging is the most widely used in the United States. Increasingly, though, the American Joint Committee on Cancer (AJCC) system is used because it more closely reflects the current methods by which prostate cancer is diagnosed, is more universally accepted, and more accurately subclassifies the extent of disease. A comparison of the two staging schemes is shown in Table 25–1.

Transcapsular extension of prostate carcinoma is a contraindication for radical surgery. Digital rectal examination alone is only approximately 50 per cent accurate for local staging. Likewise, transrectal ultrasound evaluation is generally held to be inadequate to locally stage prostate cancer with positive predictive values ranging from 37 to 46 per cent in most studies. On the other hand, seminal vesicle asymmetry can suggest invasion and this can lead to a directed biopsy for confirmation. In this respect, a sensitivity of 92 per cent has been reported, although there is a substantial false-positive rate of 12 per cent (McSherry et al., 1991). Likewise, if the neurovascular bundle is absent on one side, a biopsy specifically guided to this region may lead to confirmation of extracapsular disease. On balance, however, transrectal ultrasound evaluation is not sufficient for local tumor staging in most cases.

Endorectal coil magnetic resonance imaging is more sensitive than ultrasonography in detecting extracapsular extension of prostatic carcinoma (see Fig. 25–5). However, early enthusiasm for a high level of accuracy with this technique has not been supported by multi-institutional clinical studies. Moreover, interobserver variability is an additional limitation of this technique (see Fig. 25–6). It is likely that magnetic resonance will never be adequate for detecting microscopic extension, and it is generally not considered sufficiently accurate to influence the treatment of patients with clinically localized prostate cancer. On the other hand, staging accuracy is improved when a number of different parameters, including PSA levels, Gleason score, and endorectal magnetic resonance imaging data, are considered in combination, rather than individually.

Endorectal magnetic resonance imaging is of value in patients who have already undergone cystoprostatectomy in whom the PSA level is rising. Local recurrence around the anastomosis can often be identified and biopsy directed to the appropriate site. A sensitivity of 100 per cent for the detection

TABLE 25–1. American Joint Committee on Cancer (AJCC) and Whitmore-Jewett Staging Systems for Staging Prostate Cancer

AJCC	DESCRIPTION	WHITMORE-JEWETT
T1	Clinically inapparent tumor not palpable or visible by imaging	A
T1a	Tumor incidental histologic finding in 5% or less of tissue resected	A1
T1b	Tumor incidental histologic finding in more than 5% of tissue resected	A2
T1c	Tumor identified by needle biopsy	No equivalent
T2	Tumor confined within the prostate	B
T2a	Tumor involves one half of a lobe or less	B1N
T2b	Tumor involves more than one half of a lobe but not both lobes	B1
T2c	Tumor involves both lobes	B2
T3	Tumor extends through the prostatic capsule	C
T3a	Unilateral extracapsular extension	C1
T3b	Bilateral extracapsular extension	C1
T3c	Tumor invades the seminal vesicles	C1
T4	Tumor is fixed or invades adjacent structures other than the seminal vesicles	C2
T4a	Tumor invades any of bladder neck, external sphincter, or rectum	C2
T4b	Tumor invades levator muscles and/or is fixed to the pelvic wall	C2
N1	Microscopic regional lymph node metastases	D1
N2	Gross regional lymph node metastases	D1
N3	Extraregional lymph node metastases	
M1	Elevated acid phosphatase on three consecutive exams	
M2	Visceral (V) or bone (B) metastases	D2

of anastomotic recurrence has been reported (Silverman et al., 1997). However, many of these recurrences were palpable. Experience in an unselected, general population is likely to decrease the sensitivity of this technique.

Staging Lymph Nodes Metastases. The first stage of a radical prostatectomy is to sample lymph nodes from the medial aspect of the external iliac artery to the obturator fossa. Suspicious nodes are studied by frozen section. If any are positive for tumor, no further surgery is performed. On the other hand, a negative frozen section interpretation is followed by prostatectomy. Because lymph node sampling is an integral part of the radical prostatectomy, the need for further imaging studies has been questioned.

Nevertheless, it is legitimate to question the ability of imaging techniques to accurately detect lymphadenopathy in prostate cancer. It has been well established that computed tomography is insensitive in detecting involved lymph nodes and is often falsely positive. Overall accuracy of nodal staging with computed tomography is approximately 67 per cent. False-negative results arise from the reliance on lymph node size as the criterion for positivity. Lymph nodes containing metastatic prostate cancer are often of normal size and, thus, escape detection (Fig. 25–9). If 6 mm is used as the criterion for the maximum size in any dimension of a normal lymph node, the false-positive rate increases and many percutaneous biopsies are required. False-positive diagnoses result from enlarged, but hyperplastic, lymph nodes that do not contain tumor. Any enlarged lymph node should be subject to biopsy percutaneously and the sample stained with PSA to pinpoint the prostate as the source of any tumor that might be present. The yield of abdominal and pelvic computed tomography

is diminishingly low when performed in patients whose PSA is less than 20 ng/mL (Huncharek and Muscat, 1996). Thus, computed tomography is best reserved for the surgical candidate with a negative bone scan but who might have extraprostatic disease because of a PSA level greater than 20 ng/mL.

Magnetic resonance imaging has been shown to be equal to computed tomography in detecting enlarged lymph nodes. However, magnetic resonance images have the added potential benefit of providing longitudinal as well as transverse dimensions of lymph nodes. The longitudinal direction may be

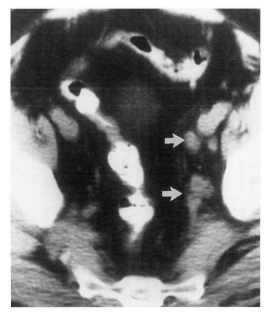

FIGURE 25–9. Adenocarcinoma, prostate with involvement of obturator lymph nodes. The obturator lymph nodes *(arrows)* measure only 5 to 8 mm in diameter but were involved by tumor. They grew progressively on subsequent studies.

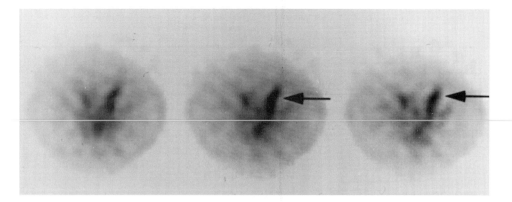

FIGURE 25-10.
Adenocarcinoma, prostate, with lymph node metastases. ProstaScint single photon emission computed tomographic images demonstrate uptake in left-sided lymph nodes *(arrows)* before surgery. The computed tomogram was negative in this area. Surgery confirmed the presence of tumor. Note the confounding effects of bone and blood pool activity.

more sensitive than the transverse dimension because it is in the same axis as the flow of lymph and, hence, metastatic disease. The possibility has been suggested that the enhancement properties of enlarged lymph nodes on dynamic magnetic resonance images may indicate a metastatic cause rather than hyperplasia (Jager et al., 1997).

A monoclonal antibody, CYT-356, labeled with indium and marketed as ProstaScint has been shown to have increased sensitivity over computed tomography for the detection of nodal prostatic metastases. Although this agent accumulates in nodal metastases, activity also normally accumulates in the bone marrow and in the blood pool. Single photon emission computed tomography is usually required, and the images can be difficult to interpret without experience (Fig. 25-10). Nonetheless, ProstaScint represents an entirely new class of imaging agents available for staging prostate cancer that surpasses anatomic imaging in specificity. One application of this agent is to direct laparascopic lymph node biopsy to areas that are abnormal on the ProstaScint scan or to detect sites of recurrent disease after therapy.

Staging Bone Metastases. Bone scans have been an established staging technique in prostate cancer for over 25 years. Because the bone metastases associated with prostate cancer are usually osteoblastic, there is avid uptake of a bone-seeking radionuclide agent in metastatic bony deposits. In diffuse disease there can be such uniform uptake in the skeleton that the bone scan may initially look normal. This is referred to as a "super scan" (Fig. 25-11). One clue to its presence is greatly elevated PSA levels and the absence of renal excretion of the bone imaging agent on the bone scan.

The routine use of bone scans has been challenged by studies showing that the risk of bone metastases is low in patients with PSA values less than 10 ng/mL. The yield from bone scans in this population is insufficient to warrant their routine use. However, this point of view is not accepted by all urologists, some of whom use symptomatology and other considerations as indicators for the use of bone scans in an individual patient. In selected patients with high-grade disease and a significant risk of recurrence, a scan for use as a baseline reference may prove advantageous prospectively.

The routine use of a radiographic bone survey for metastases is not justified. Film radiography should be restricted to areas of known metastases or new symptoms to assess for fracture or compression.

Evaluation of the skeletal system can also be performed with computed tomography and magnetic resonance imaging. Magnetic resonance imaging is more sensitive than plain films for early disease and can accurately depict abnormalities such as epidural extension of tumor from a vertebral body metastasis. Computed tomography is an excellent method for following the influence of therapy on the progression or regression of individual metastases (Fig. 25-12).

Benign Prostatic Hyperplasia

Benign prostatic hyperplasia is commonly identified incidentally on imaging studies including excretory urography, ultrasonography, computed tomography,

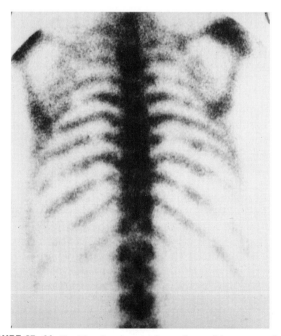

FIGURE 25-11. Positive bone scan in patient with metastatic prostate cancer. Note there is diffuse uptake of activity throughout the spine and ribs and absence of renal activity. These findings suggest a "super scan" indicative of diffuse metastatic disease.

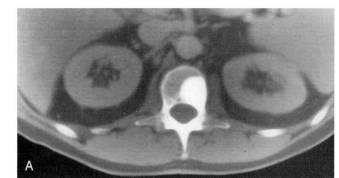
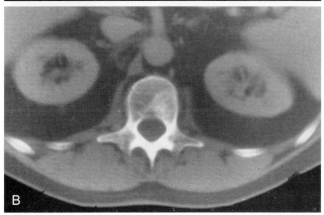

FIGURE 25–12. Adenocarcinoma, prostate, metastatic to bone. Serial computed tomograms demonstrate ability to measure effect of therapy.

A, Initial study demonstrates an osteoblastic metastasis in the L-2 vertebral body.

B, Three months after combined hormonal therapy, the metastasis is almost completely resolved.

and magnetic resonance imaging. However, direct imaging of the prostate gland plays a minor role in the diagnosis and management of this disease because actual measurements of prostate size are usually not necessary. However, as benign prostatic hyperplasia progresses, both bladder outlet and upper tract obstruction ensue. In regard to the latter, upper urinary tract imaging is of particular value in assessing the degree of obstruction. Obstructive uropathy is discussed in detail in Chapter 9.

Prostatitis

Prostatitis is a clinical entity characterized by pain, chills, malaise, irritative voiding symptoms, and,

occasionally, fever. Imaging is usually not required and, indeed, may be contraindicated because of the risk of bacteremia. An imaging study may become necessary, however, when a prostatic abscess is suspected because of fever or other symptoms that persist after an appropriate period of treatment. Transrectal ultrasonography is the preferred method to confirm such a complication (Fig. 25–13). Abscesses are generally peripheral in location, although infections after transurethral prostatectomy may be in the central portions of the gland. Increased blood flow within an infected prostate gland can be demonstrated by color Doppler ultrasonography. As part of an endorectal ultrasonographic procedure, an abscess can be aspirated and its contents

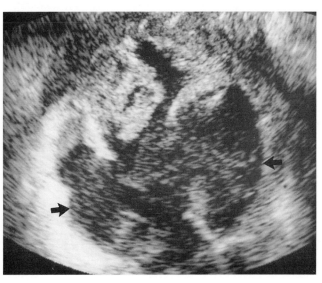

FIGURE 25–13. Prostatic abscess in a 40-year-old male with pelvic pain and fever. Transrectal ultrasonogram. There is a large irregular fluid collection with echogenic contents *(arrows)*. Transrectal needle aspiration yielded purulent material.

cultured. In very ill patients in whom a large prostatic abscess is suspected, computed tomography is preferred over ultrasonography to avoid the manipulation that accompanies transrectal ultrasound examination. With computed tomography, an abscess appears as a fluid density structure that enlarges the prostate and presses against the capsule.

~~Tuberculosis or other granulomatous infections of~~ the prostate gland, including malakoplakia, may cause widespread damage to the prostate. Here, computed tomography or magnetic resonance imaging may provide information on the extent of involvement.

Cyst

A large midline cyst within the prostate is often due to a prostatic utricle. This müllerian duct remnant forms as a diverticulum that arises posteriorly from the prostatic urethra. Complications include obstructive voiding symptoms, stone formation, and infection. Rarely, the utricle compresses and obstructs the ejaculatory ducts and, thereby, causes infertility. A prostatic utricle is often asymptomatic and does not warrant treatment. When symptomatic, they can be unroofed by transurethral instru-

mentation or drained under ultrasonographic guidance.

SEMINAL VESICLES, VAS DEFERENS, AND EJACULATORY DUCTS

Anomalies and Cysts

A variety of congenital abnormalities affect the seminal vesicles. A seminal vesicle may be unilaterally absent or become multicystic in association with agenesis of the ipsilateral kidney (Fig. 25–14; see Fig. 3–32). Multiloculated seminal vesicle cysts may form when the ejaculatory duct is atretic. Occasionally, a seminal vesicle enlarges and becomes cystic when the ureter inserts ectopically into the seminal vesicle rather than the bladder. In this situation, the ipsilateral kidney is obstructed and/or dysplastic. Often, when one seminal vesicle is the site of a congenital abnormality, the contralateral seminal vesicle is more likely to be mildly affected (see Fig. 25–14). The seminal vesicles may be atretic or cystic in association with congenital absence of the vas deferens, another cause of male infertility. However, even seminal vesicles that appear normal by imaging studies may not function normally and be a

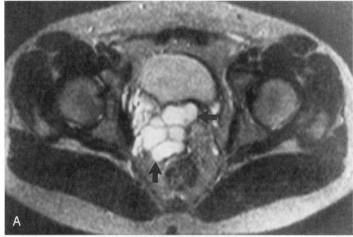
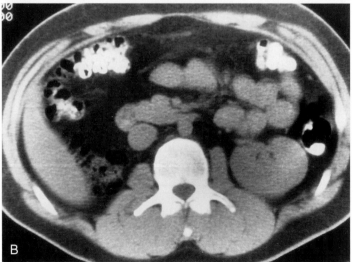

FIGURE 25–14. Seminal vesicle cyst associated with agenesis of the right kidney in a 34-year-old male undergoing evaluation for infertility.

A, T2-weighted magnetic resonance image demonstrates a multicystic seminal vesicle *(arrow).* The contralateral seminal vesicle is not seen.

B, Computed tomogram demonstrates absence of the right kidney.

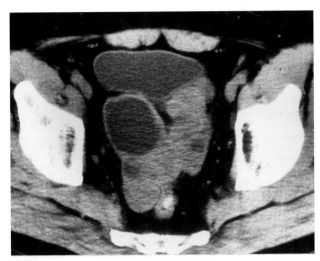

FIGURE 25–15. Echinococcal abscess, seminal vesicle, in a febrile male from the Middle East. Computed tomogram. Aspiration established the diagnosis.

cause of infertility. Calcification of the vas deferens is commonly seen in patients with diabetes mellitus. Occasionally, an infection within the seminal vesicles leads to an abscess or phlegmon (Fig. 25–15).

Ejaculatory duct cysts may cause obstruction of the ejaculatory duct and lead to infertility. Symptoms include perineal pain and hematospermia. The normal ejaculatory duct is not visualized by ultrasonography. An ejaculatory duct cyst is anechoic or hypoechoic and can be differentiated from an obstructed ejaculatory duct because the latter is tubular while the former is spherical.

Magnetic resonance imaging has been suggested as a superior method to identify blockages within the seminal vesicles because of its multiplanar capa-

bilities. However, magnetic resonance is limited by the absence of real-time imaging and the inability to perform drainage procedures. T2-weighted images are the preferred method of imaging an obstructed ejaculatory duct. Seminal vesicography also establishes the patency of the ejaculatory ducts but is more invasive and risks damaging the spermatic cord.

Neoplasm

Primary tumors, such as adenocarcinoma, sarcoma, or lymphoma, rarely occur in the seminal vesicles. Secondary tumors are most likely due to melanoma or drop metastases from a peritoneal tumor, as might occur in appendiceal adenocarcinoma (Fig. 25–16). The imaging appearance of an asymmetric mass in the region of the seminal vesicles is not specific. Biopsy can be performed percutaneously or through the transrectal approach using ultrasound for guidance.

BIBLIOGRAPHY

Prostate

Amis, E. S., Jr.: Role of CT and CT-guided nodal biopsy in staging of prostatic cancer. Radiology 190:309, 1994.

Barozzi, L., Pavlica, P., Menchi, I., de Matteis, M., and Canepari, M.: Prostatic abscess: Diagnosis and treatment. AJR 170:753, 1998.

Bartolozzi, C., Menchi, I., Lencioni, R., Serni, S., Lapini, A., Barbanti, G., Bozza, A., Amorosi, A., Manganelli, A., and Carini, M.: Local staging of prostate carcinoma with endorectal coil MRI: Correlation with whole-mount radical prostatectomy specimens. Eur. Radiol. 6:339, 1996.

Chelsky, M. J., Schnall, M. D., Siedmon, E. J., and Pollack, H. M.: Use of endorectal surface coil magnetic resonance imaging for local staging of prostate cancer. J. Urol. 150:391, 1993.

Cheng, D., and Tempany, C. M. C.: MR imaging of the prostate and bladder. Semin. Ultrasound, CT MR 19:67, 1998.

Choyke, P. L.: Imaging of prostate cancer. Abdom. Imaging 20:505, 1995.

Chybowski, F. M., Keller, J. J. L., Bergstrahl, E. J., and Oesterling, J. E.: Predicting radionuclide bone scan findings in patients with newly diagnosed, untreated prostate cancer: Prostate specific antigen is superior to all other clinical parameters. J. Urol. 145:313, 1991.

D'Amico, A. V.: The role of MR imaging in the selection of therapy for prostate cancer. Magn. Reson. Imaging Clin. North Am. 4:471, 1996.

D'Amico, A. V., Whittington, R., Malkowicz, S. B., Schultz, D., Schnall, M., Tomaszewski, J. E., and Wein, A.: Combined modality staging of prostate carcinoma and its utility in predicting pathologic stage and postoperative prostate specific antigen failure. Urology 49(3A Suppl):23, 1997.

Epstein, J.: Pathology of adenocarcinoma of the prostate. In Walsh, P. C., Retik, A. B., Vaughan, E. D., Jr., and Wein, A. J. (eds.): Campbell's Urology, 7th ed. Philadelphia, W. B. Saunders, 1998, pp. 2497–2505.

Flanigan, R. C., McKay, T. C., Olson, M., Shankey, T. V., Pyle, J., and Waters, W. B.: Limited efficacy of preoperative computed tomographic scanning for the evaluation of lymph node metastasis in patients before radical prostatectomy. Urology 48:428, 1996.

Hamper, U. M., Sheth, S., Walsh, P. C., Holtz, P. M., and Epstein, J. I.: Capsular transgression of prostatic carcinoma: Evaluation with transrectal US with pathologic correlation. Radiology 178:791, 1991.

Honig, S. C.: New diagnostic techniques in the evaluation of

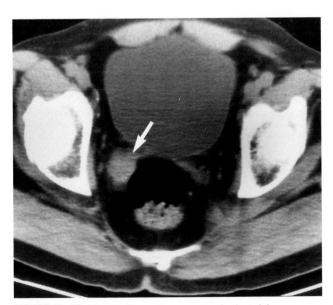

FIGURE 25–16. Metastatic melanoma, seminal vesicle. Computed tomogram. There is asymmetry of the seminal vesicle (arrow). Diagnosis was established by transrectal biopsy.

anatomic abnormalities of the infertile male. Urol. Clin. North Am. *21*:417, 1994.

Hricak, H., Dooms, G. C., Jeffrey, R. B., Avalone, A., Jacobs, D., Benton, W. K., Narayan, P., and Tanagho, E. A.: Prostatic carcinoma: Staging by clinical assessment, CT and MRI imaging. Radiology *162*:331, 1987.

Huncharek, M., and Muscat, J.: Serum prostate-specific antigen as a predictor of staging abdominal/pelvic computed tomography in newly diagnosed prostate cancer. Abdom. Imaging *21*:364, 1996.

Jager, G. J., Ruijter, E. T., van de Kaa, C. A., de la Rosette, J. J., Oosterhof, G. O., Thornbury, J. R., Ruijs, S. H., and Barentsz, J. O.: Dynamic TurboFLASH subtraction technique for contrast-enhanced MR imaging of the prostate: Correlation with histopathologic results. Radiology *203*:645, 1997.

Kahn, D., Williams, R. D., Seldin, D. W., Libertino, J. A., Hirschhorn, M., Dreicer, R., Weiner, G. J., Bushnell, D., and Gulfo, J.: Radioimmunoscintigraphy with [111]indium labeled CYT-356 for the detection of occult prostate cancer recurrence. J. Urol. *152*:1490, 1994.

Langlotz, C. P.: Benefits and costs of MR imaging of prostate cancer. Magn. Reson. Imaging Clin. North Am. *4*:533, 1996.

Le Marchand, L., Kolonel, L. N., Wilkens, L. R., Myers, B. C., and Hirohata, T.: Animal fat consumption and prostate cancer: A prospective study in Hawaii. Epidemiology *5*:276, 1994.

Levran, Z., Gonzalez, J. A., Diokno, A. C., Jafri, S. Z., and Steinert, B. W.: Are pelvic computed tomography, bone scan and pelvic lymphadenectomy necessary in the staging of prostatic cancer? Br. J. Urol. *75*:778, 1995.

McSherry, S. A., Levy, F., Schiebler, M. L., Keefe, B., Dent, G. A., and Mohler, J. L.: Preoperative prediction of pathological tumor volume and stage in clinically localized prostate cancer: Comparison of digital rectal examination, transrectal ultrasonography and magnetic resonance imaging. J. Urol. *146*:85, 1991.

Narayan, P., and Carroll, P. R.: Prostate cancer: Effect of postbiopsy hemorrhage on interpretation of MR images. Radiology *195*:385, 1995.

Oesterling, J. E., Martin, S. K., Berstrahl, E. J., and Lowe, F. C.: The use of prostate specific antigen in staging patients with newly diagnosed prostate cancer. JAMA *269*:67, 1993.

Oyen, R. H., Van Poppel, H. P., Ameye, F. E., Van de Voorde, W. A., Baert, A. L., and Baert, L. V.: Lymph node staging of localized prostatic carcinoma with CT and CT-guided fine needle aspiration biopsy: Prospective study of 285 patients. Radiology *190*:315, 1994.

Partin, A. W., Kattan, M. W., Subong, E. N., Walsh, P. C., Wojno, K. J., Oesterling, J. E., Scardino, P. T., and Pearson, J. D.: Combination of prostate-specific antigen, clinical stage, and Gleason score to predict pathological stage of localized prostate cancer: A multi-institutional update. JAMA *277*:1445, 1997.

Perrotti, M., Kaufman, R. P., Jr., Jennings, T. A., Thaler, H. T., Soloway, S. M., Rifkin, M. D., and Fisher, H. A.: Endo-rectal coil magnetic resonance imaging in clinically localized prostate cancer: Is it accurate? J. Urol. *156*:106, 1996.

Platt, J. F., Bree, R. L., and Schwab, R. E.: The accuracy of CT in the staging of carcinoma of the prostate. AJR *149*:315, 1987.

Presti, J. C., Jr., Hricak, H., Narayan, P. A., Shinohara, K., White, S., and Carroll, P. R.: Local staging of prostatic carcinoma: Comparison of transrectal sonography and endorectal MR imaging. AJR *166*:103, 1996.

Schiebler, M. L., Schnall, M. D., Pollack, H. M., Lenkinski, R. E., Tomaszewski, J. E., Wein, A. J., Whittington, R., Rauschning, W., and Hessel, H. Y.: Current role of MRI imaging in the staging of adenocarcinoma of the prostate. Radiology *189*:339, 1993.

Schiebler, M. L., Yankaskas, B. C., Tempany, C., Spritzer, C. E., Rifkin, M. D., Pollack, H. M., Holtz, P., and Zerhouni, E. A.: MRI imaging in adenocarcinoma of the prostate: Interobserver variation and efficacy for determining stage C disease. Invest. Radiol. *27*:575, 1992.

Seltzer, S. E., Getty, D. J., Tempany, C. M., Pickett, R. M., Schnall, M. D., McNeil, B. J., and Swets, J. A.: Staging prostate cancer with MR imaging: A combined radiologist-computer system. Radiology *202*:219, 1997.

Silverman, J. M., and Kreb, S. T. L.: Recurrence of prostatic cancer in men who have undergone radical prostatectomy. AJR *168*:379, 1997.

Sodee, D. B., Conant, R., Chalfant, M., Miron, S., Klein, E., Bahnson, R., Spirnak, J. P., Carlin, B., Bellon, E. M., and Rogers, D.: Preliminary imaging results using In-111 labeled CYT-356 (Prostascint) in the detection of recurrent prostate cancer. Clin. Nucl. Med. *21*:759, 1996.

Tempany, C. M., Zhou, X., Zerhouni, E. A., Rifkin, M. D., Quint, L. E., Piccoli, C. W., Ellis, J. H., and McNeil, B. J.: Staging of prostate cancer: Results of Radiology Diagnostic Oncology Group project comparison of three MR imaging techniques. Radiology *192*:47, 1994.

Terris, M. K., McNeal, J. E., and Stamey, T. A.: Invasion of the seminal vesicles by prostatic cancer: Detection with transrectal sonography. AJR *155*:811, 1990.

Van Arsdalen, K. N., Broderick, G. A., Malkowicz, S. B., and Wein, A. J.: Laparoscopic lymphadenectomy based on magnetic resonance imaging: Is a unilateral dissection adequate for staging prostate cancer? Tech. Urol. *2*:93, 1996.

Yu, K. K., Hricak, H., Alagappan, R., Chernoff, D. M., Bacchetti, P., and Zaloudek, C. J.: Detection of extracapsular extension of prostate carcinoma with endorectal and phased-array coil MR imaging: Multivariate feature analysis. Radiology *202*: 697, 1997.

Seminal Vesicles, Vas Deferens, and Ejaculatory Ducts

Alpern, M. B., Dorfman, R. E., Gross, B. H., Gottlieb, C. A., and Sandler, M. A.: Seminal vesicle cysts: Association with adult polycystic kidney disease. Radiology *180*:79, 1991.

Ramchandani, P., Banner, M. P., and Pollack, H. M.: Imaging of the seminal vesicles. Semin. Roentgenol. *1*:83, 1993.

Secaf, E., Nuruddin, R. N., Hricak, H., McClure, R. D., and Demas, B.: MR imaging of the seminal vesicles. AJR *156*:989, 1991.

van den Ouden, D., Blom, J. H. M., Bangma, C., and de Spiegeleer, A. H. V. C.: Diagnosis and management of seminal vesicle cysts associated with ipsilateral renal agenesis: A pooled analysis of 52 cases. Eur. Virol. *33*:433, 1998.

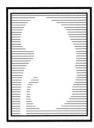

26

Scrotum

Most diseases of the scrotum yield more than one imaging pattern, with considerable overlap among the various conditions. Although this is true for various categories of disease, it is most evident with respect to detection of an intratesticular mass, which almost always results in orchiectomy for both diagnosis and treatment. This chapter, therefore, discusses imaging of the scrotum based on pathologic entities rather than on imaging patterns.

IMAGING TECHNIQUES

Ultrasonography

Ultrasonography is well suited to the evaluation of the scrotum. The area of interest is superficial and well within the range of high-frequency transducers, which permit high-resolution imaging and excellent sensitivity for the detection of intrascrotal disease. Linear transducers with a frequency greater than 5 mHz are generally considered essential for the production of quality ultrasonographic images of the scrotum. With excellent near-field resolution, a stand-off pad is required only rarely. Usually, the sonographer merely supports the scrotum with a gloved hand and scans from an anterior approach with the other hand. Alternatively, a towel can be placed between the legs to elevate the scrotum. Because of the mobility of the intrascrotal contents, such real-time evaluation is essential in producing images that allow precise localization

and characterization of both normal and abnormal structures. Flow-sensitive techniques, including spectral, color, and amplitude Doppler, may be useful in certain conditions, especially suspected torsion, focal infarction, and varicocele. These are discussed in detail in later sections of this chapter.

Radionuclide Imaging

Radionuclide imaging of the scrotum has been used for many years in the assessment of acute scrotal pain, based on the ability of technetium pertechnetate to demonstrate flow to the testes. Decreased perfusion to the symptomatic side on a combination of dynamic and static images has a specificity and sensitivity for testicular torsion approaching 95 per cent. However, radionuclide techniques are disadvantageous in that they do not characterize nonischemic disease, require the use of ionizing radiation, and are usually more time-consuming than ultrasonography. Additionally, scintigraphy often fails in the same situations in which ultrasonography is technically limited, such as intermittent or incomplete torsion and in imaging of young children. For these reasons, as well as advances in ultrasonography, especially the flow-sensitive techniques of color and amplitude Doppler, the use of radionuclide techniques has declined.

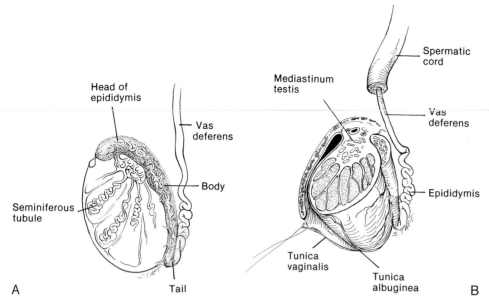

Figure 26–1. The testis and epididymis.

A, One to three seminiferous tubules fill each compartment and drain into rete testis in the mediastinum. Twelve to 20 efferent ductules become convoluted in the head of the epididymis and drain into a single coiled duct of the epididymis. The vas is convoluted in its first portion.

B, Cross section of the testis showing the mediastinum and septations continuous with the tunica albuginea. The parietal and visceral tunica vaginalis are confluent where the vessels and nerves enter the posterior aspect of the testis. (From Walsh, P. C., Retik, A. B., Vaughan, E. D., and Wein, A. J.: Campbell's Urology, 7th ed. Philadelphia, W. B. Saunders Co., 1998, p. 124.)

Magnetic Resonance Imaging

Although seldom needed, magnetic resonance imaging can be useful in selected situations of suspected scrotal disease. A flat surface coil generally results in high-quality images. Patients with equivocal ultrasonographic findings may benefit from the global visualization and high tissue contrast that is possible with standard multiplanar spin-echo sequences.

ANATOMY

Normal Anatomy

Figure 26–1 illustrates many of the anatomic features discussed in this section.

The scrotum is made up of the skin externally and the dartos muscle internally. Internal to the dartos are the layers of the spermatic fascia, which include the cremasteric muscle. The inner aspect of the spermatic fascia overlies the parietal portion of the tunica vaginalis, which is an extension of the peritoneum. The tunica vaginalis also covers much of the testis and epididymis. This covering is called the visceral layer. The potential space between the parietal and visceral layers of the tunica vaginalis may occasionally be the site of abnormal fluid accumulation, usually in response to inflammation (hydrocele or pyocele) or trauma (hematocele).

The visceral layer of the tunica vaginalis cannot be separated from the tunica albuginea, which itself is attached to the testicular parenchyma. Septa project into the testis from the tunica albuginea, grouping the seminiferous tubules into lobules. The mediastinum testis is a longitudinally oriented extension of the tunica albuginea that lies posteriorly within the testis. The tubules converge in the mediastinum before exiting to the epididymis. The septa are not identified ultrasonographically. The mediastinum, on the other hand, forms an eccentric echo-genic line of a few millimeters thickness that is located posteriorly and oriented along the long axis of the testis (Fig. 26–2). The background appearance of the testis itself is moderately echogenic and homogeneous owing to the numerous interfaces created by the seminiferous tubules.

Each testicular or spermatic artery arises from the aorta slightly below the renal artery. These paired vessels are extremely tortuous as they course within the spermatic cord. The epididymal arteries arise from the testicular arteries within the spermatic cord. As a result, torsion produces decreased flow to both the epididymis and the testis. The tunica albuginea receives much of its blood supply from a network of capillaries that is at least partially independent of the testicular artery. The internal arterial network of the testis consists of both centripetal and centrifugal vessels, which account for the detection of flow in both directions by means of

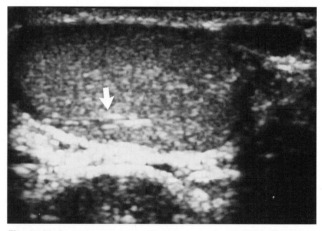

Figure 26–2. Normal testis. Ultrasonogram, longitudinal projection. A portion of the mediastinum *(arrow)* is noted within the homogeneous intermediate echogenicity of the parenchyma.

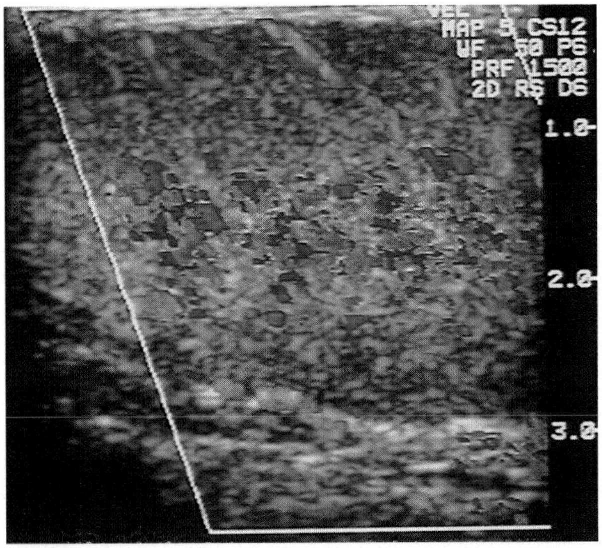

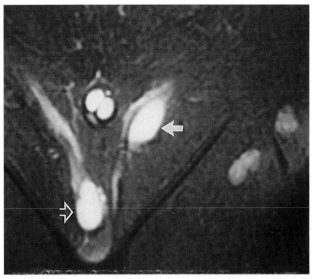

Figure 26–3. Normal testis. Color Doppler ultrasonogram, longitudinal projection. Normal bidirectional flow is demonstrated.

Figure 26–4. Undescended testis in an obese 12-year-old boy with nonpalpable left testis. T2-weighted magnetic resonance image with fat suppression, coronal plane. The right testis *(open arrow)* is normal. The left testis *(closed arrow)* is located in the lower inguinal canal.

both spectral and color Doppler techniques (Fig. 26–3).

A tortuous collection of anastamoses of testicular and epididymal veins, the pampiniform plexus, is juxtaposed to the testicular artery within the spermatic cord. In most individuals, the left testicular vein drains to the left renal vein, and the right testicular vein drains to the inferior vena cava at a level slightly below the renal veins. Dilatation of the pampiniform plexus, or scrotal varicocele, occurs in as many as 15 per cent of the general male population. Most men with varicocele are asymptomatic. Some, however, have oligospermia or other impairment of testicular function, as discussed later.

The epididymis is composed of the efferent duct-ules and the tortuous epididymal duct. It is slightly less homogeneous and slightly less echogenic than the testis. For descriptive purposes, the epididymis is divided into three parts: the superior bulbous head, called the globus major; a slender body; and a small prominence inferiorly, known as the tail or globus minor. The head is the easiest to recognize ultrasonographically and is approximately 1 cm in diameter. Although rarely recognized ultrasono-graphically, the vas deferens exits at the epididy-mal tail.

Cryptorchidism

The processus vaginalis, an extension of the perito-neum, allows for testicular descent from the abdo-men into the scrotum. Anomalous interruption of descent may occur at any level. Usually, this results in a testis within the inguinal canal. As many as 4 per cent of newborns have an undescended testis. However, this rate drops to less than 1 per cent by 6 months of age as a result of spontaneous descent after birth. Impaired function and an increased risk of malignant neoplasm are possible sequelae of

cryptorchidism. The risk of malignancy exists in the contralateral testis as well and persists to a lesser degree even after surgical treatment of the unde-scended testis.

The need for imaging of the patient with an unde-scended testis is not universally agreed upon. If imaging is undertaken, ultrasonography should be performed initially because most undescended tes-tes lie within the inguinal canal. Here, the testis appears as an ovoid, homogeneous, well-circum-scribed structure that is usually smaller than the normal, descended testis. When required to detect an intra-abdominal testis, magnetic resonance im-aging or computed tomography has a sensitivity and specificity in the range of 90 to 95 per cent (Figs. 26–4, 26–5).

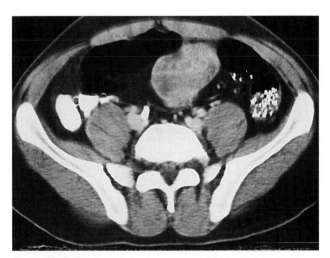

Figure 26–5. Seminoma in an undescended testis in a 25-year-old male. Computed tomogram with contrast material enhancement. The large, heterogeneous mass in the retroperitoneum caused hydronephrosis.

TUBULAR ECTASIA

Tubular ectasia is an acquired dilatation of the rete testis that may represent a postinflammatory obstruction or may be related to vasectomy in some patients. The condition may be chronic and/or subclinical and does not require treatment.

Tubular ectasia was unrecognized prior to the use of high-resolution scrotal ultrasonography. Thus, published descriptions are limited. The imaging features of tubular ectasia include dilated tubules that converge toward the junction of the epididymis and the testis (Fig. 26–6). These dilated tubules parallel the mediastinum testis and are often seen bilaterally, although asymmetrically.

Occasionally, individual tubules are difficult to resolve, and the ultrasonographic image is that of an intratesticular mass. Usually, however, the elongated shape as well as the location of the abnormality indicates the correct diagnosis. In those situations in which neoplasm cannot be excluded, magnetic resonance imaging can be of value. T2-weighted images demonstrate a hyperintense or isointense focus corresponding to the ultrasonographic abnormality (Fig. 26–7). The high-signal intensity is not characteristic of neoplasm, which tends to be hypointense relative to the background signal intensity of the testis on T2-weighted images, as discussed later.

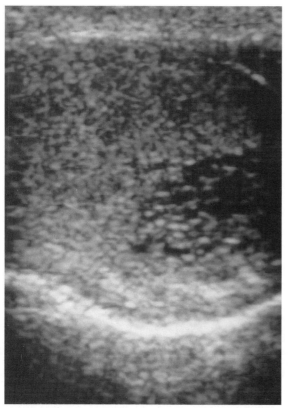

Figure 26–6. Tubular ectasia. Ultrasonogram. Serpentine anechoic channels converge toward the periphery of the testis near the junction with the epididymis.

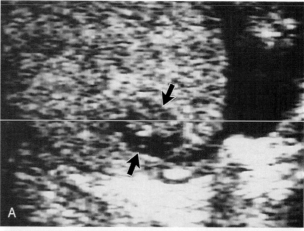

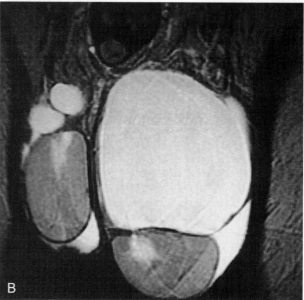

Figure 26–7. Epididymal cysts and tubular ectasia in a 63-year-old male with a palpable scrotal mass.

A, Transverse ultrasonogram of the left testis shows mass-like configuration of the dilated rete testis *(arrows).*

B, T2-weighted magnetic resonance image, coronal section. Bilateral epididymal cysts and bilateral areas of high intratesticular signal intensity are consistent with tubular ectasia.

INFLAMMATION

Epididymo-orchitis and Hydrocele

Epididymitis is the most common inflammatory condition of the scrotum. Causative organisms, which are often not isolated, include those of sexually transmitted disease, such as *Neisseria gonorrhoeae* and *Chlamydia trachomatis,* as well as standard urinary tract pathogens, such as *Escherichia coli.* Tuberculosis or other granulomatous infections, while less common, may be more likely to require surgery due to the relative chronicity of the process and a greater likelihood of unsuccessful antibiotic treatment. Symptoms of epididymitis include dysuria, pain, swelling and, occasionally, fever.

Mild cases of epididymitis are not associated with any imaging abnormality. In patients with moder-

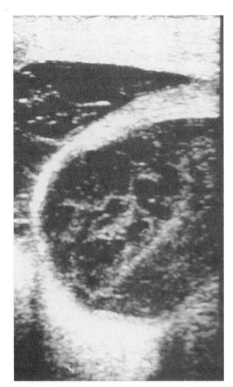

Figure 26–8. Epididymitis with abscess and pyocele in a 71-year-old male with pain and swelling. Ultrasonogram, longitudinal projection. Complex fluid is contained within a pyocele and epididymal abscess.

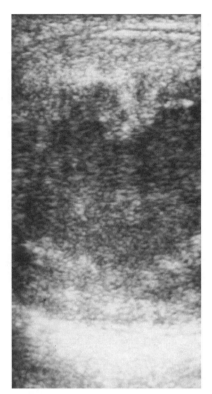

Figure 26–9. Epididymitis due to tuberculosis in a patient with chronic pain. Ultrasonogram. The epididymis is enlarged and exhibits a heterogeneous pattern.

ate to severe disease, ultrasonographic findings include skin thickening, swelling, hypoechogenicity, and the presence of a hydrocele represented by an anechoic crescentic-shaped collection of fluid surrounding the testis (Figs. 26–8, 26–9). The fluid accumulation is within the parietal and visceral layers of the tunica vaginalis. This finding, however, is not specific for epididymitis in that many other conditions, including trauma, vasculitis, and testicular tumor, are associated with the presence of a hydrocele. Indeed, a small amount of fluid in this location may be normal.

In epididymitis, color Doppler may show an increased blood flow to the epididymis (Fig. 26–10). If the testis is uninvolved, blood flow is normal. As discussed later, the occasional clinical similarities between epididymitis and torsion sometimes require assessment of testicular blood flow to differentiate these conditions.

Orchitis without epididymitis is rare and is usually associated with a viral infection, such as mumps. Approximately 20 per cent of patients with epididymitis also have orchitis. Generally, this association indicates a more severe form of epididymitis. Because it is quite difficult to exclude orchitis, severe forms of epididymitis in which testicular involvement is suspected or proven are referred to as epididymo-orchitis. Ultrasonographic findings, in addition to those of the epididymis described earlier, vary from normal in mild cases of testicular involvement to the demonstration of an enlarged testis

with heterogeneous hypoechogenicity and, as well, abscess formation. Color Doppler blood flow imaging demonstrates a patchy hyperemia, with focal areas of decreased perfusion and infarction in some cases (Fig. 26–11).

Sarcoidosis

Involvement of the scrotum by sarcoidosis is uncommon and is usually encountered in patients with

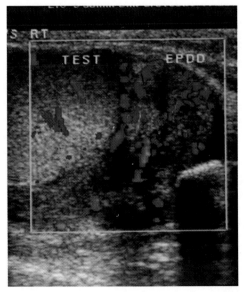

Figure 26–10. Epididymitis. Color Doppler ultrasonogram, longitudinal projection. Enlargement and hyperemia of the epididymal tail are noted.

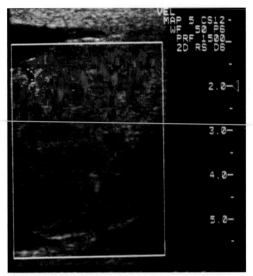

Figure 26–11. Epididymo-orchitis with regional infarction in a 56-year-old male with 4 hours of pain and swelling. Color Doppler ultrasonogram, longitudinal projection. There is anterior hyperperfusion and heterogeneity with decreased perfusion of the deeper portion of the testis. Swelling and hydrocele are also noted.

a previously known diagnosis. Rarely, sarcoidosis presents initially in the scrotum. The epididymis is more likely to be affected by sarcoidosis than is the testis. Isolated testicular involvement is unusual.

A generalized increase in epididymal size may be seen, with or without a defined mass. Within the testis, a focal site of disease may appear as a solitary mass and, thereby, mimic a germ cell tumor. If this finding is encountered in an African-American, the commonness of sarcoidosis and the rarity of testicular germ cell tumor in this racial group should be kept in mind in formulating a differential diagnosis. Sarcoidosis commonly occurs in multiple sites in the testis, a pattern that overlaps with findings seen in lymphoma and metastases, as discussed later (Fig. 26–12).

INTRATESTICULAR NEOPLASMS

In contrast to the masses of the female gonad, the great majority of testicular masses are neoplastic. The most common intratesticular neoplasms are classified into three groups: *germ cell tumors* (approximately 90 per cent), *gonadal stromal tumors* (approximately 5 per cent), and *secondary tumors* (approximately 5 per cent). The latter group includes lymphoma, leukemia, and metastases.

Percutaneous biopsy is virtually never undertaken for primary tumors of the testicle, as orchiectomy is a relatively minor procedure, the prior probability of malignancy is high, and sampling error would have to be considered to account for any biopsy that failed to demonstrate a malignant tumor. On the other hand, percutaneous biopsy may be of value in a patient with a known primary malignancy such as lymphoma or prostate or lung carcinoma.

Germ Cell Tumors

Differentiation from a totipotential germ cell initially proceeds along one of two lines, yielding either a *seminoma* or a *nonseminomatous tumor*. The delineation of these two tumor types has a practical importance as well: the seminoma is generally sensitive to therapeutic radiation whereas nonseminomatous tumors are not.

The prevalence of testicular germ cell tumors has increased over the past 25 years owing, perhaps, to the younger age at which males are engaging in regular sexual activity or to an unexplained increase in the prevalence of cryptorchidism. The most common presentation is that of a palpable, painless mass. Less often, the patient complains of chronic pain or a sense of heaviness. As many as 15 per cent of patients develop acute symptoms, including pain caused by a hematoma that develops after little or no trauma to the scrotum. A small percentage of patients, especially those with aggressive nonseminomatous germ cell tumors, presents with evidence of distant metastases, including pleural effusion, hydronephrosis, or pathologic bone fracture.

There are a variety of staging systems in use for testicular germ cell tumors. Most are based on three groupings: localized disease confined to the testis, abdominal/pelvic nodal disease, and distant metastases. Staging is based either on clinical findings, including radiologic data, or on pathologic findings based on biopsy-confirmed information.

Lymph node metastasis from primary testicular malignancy often first develops at the level of the renal hilum. This reflects the fact that lymphatic drainage parallels venous drainage and arterial supply. The most frequent site of detectable hematologic metastases is the lungs. Other metastatic sites occur in highly aggressive tumors, which are more

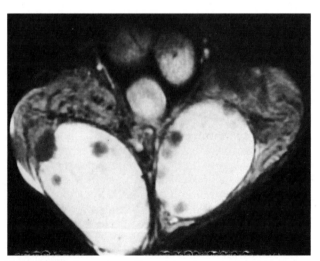

Figure 26–12. Sarcoidosis. T2-weighted magnetic resonance image, coronal plane. The epididymis is enlarged. The testes contain multiple masses of low signal intensity. Lymphoma and metastases would produce a similar pattern of abnormalities.

often associated with nonseminomatous germ cell tumors rather than with seminoma.

Seminoma. Seminoma, which accounts for approximately 40 per cent of all testicular neoplasms, tends to occur in a pure form in contrast to the often mixed components of nonseminomatous tumors. Peak prevalence is in men in the fourth decade of life, but the range extends to patients older than 70 years of age.

Although the tumor typically has a well-margined gross appearance, there is no capsule, and infiltration is usually seen on microscopic examination.

The ultrasonographic appearance of seminoma is generally that of a reasonably well-circumscribed hypoechoic mass that is of homogeneous echotexture (Figs. 26–13, 26–14). Multiple small calcifications, 1 to 2 mm in diameter, are detected in about one-third of cases. Larger aggregates of calcification are less common. As a tumor enlarges, areas of heterogeneity corresponding to hemorrhage or necrosis often appear.

In some patients with seminoma, the primary intratesticular tumor may not be identified as a discrete mass despite a large tumor burden elsewhere in the body, such as within retroperitoneal lymph nodes. In this circumstance, an ill-defined heterogeneity may be identified ultrasonographically representing an area that, on histologic examination, is fibrosis rather than tumor. This pattern has been called the "burnt out" seminoma and refers to a neoplasm that has become inactive at the

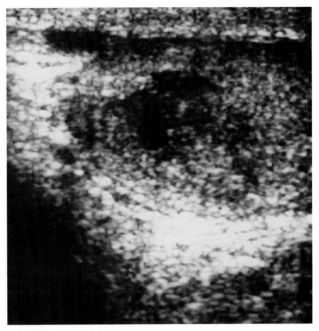

Figure 26–14. Seminoma. The testicular mass is of slightly heterogeneous echotexture.

site of the primary tumor but continues to exhibit malignant behavior elsewhere.

Most patients with clinical Stage I seminoma, in which the disease is thought to be macroscopically confined to the scrotum but in which microscopic tumor is possible in retroperitoneal lymph nodes of normal size, are treated with orchiectomy followed by radiation to the para-aortic retroperitoneum and the ipsilateral pelvic nodes. In this case, the role of therapeutic radiation is prophylactic. Patients with enlarged retroperitoneal nodes (Stage II) demonstrated by computed tomography are also treated with radiation, unless the nodes are very large, in which case chemotherapy may also be used.

Nonseminomatous Germ Cell Tumors. The other germ cell tumors of the testis include *embryonal carcinoma, choriocarcinoma, mature* and *immature teratoma,* and *yolk sac* or *endodermal sinus tumor.* Nonseminomatous germ cell tumors are much more likely to occur as a mixture of two or more of the individual components rather than as isolated pure tumors. Even when they occur as pure tumors, there are no specific ultrasonographic features.

The mean age at presentation for nonseminomatous germ cell tumor is 27 years. As a group, the stage at presentation is higher than that for seminoma. A nonseminomatous germ cell tumor is more likely than seminoma to be poorly defined and heterogeneous in its ultrasonographic appearance (Fig. 26–15). Calcifications, represented by small echogenic foci with acoustic shadowing, are seen ultrasonographically in more than one-half of tumors.

Most patients with germ cell neoplasm are cured. Advanced stage disease is associated with a fatality rate of higher than 25 per cent. Patients with non-

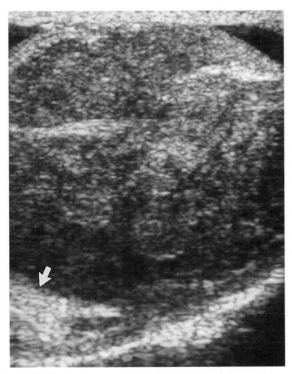

Figure 26–13. Seminoma. A slightly heterogeneous echotexture replaces almost the entire testis. A small amount of testicular parenchyma remains *(arrow).*

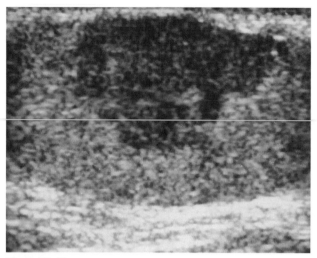

Figure 26–15. Mixed nonseminomatous germ cell tumor in a 24-year-old male with a palpable scrotal mass. Ultrasonogram. The tumor is heterogeneous and hypoechoic and has somewhat ill-defined margins.

seminomatous germ cell tumors are usually treated with chemotherapy if there is evidence for disease outside the scrotum, either at the time of initial presentation or on follow-up. This stage is documented either by imaging evidence of enlarged nodes or by lymphadenectomy in patients where the nodes are not grossly enlarged. Patients in whom no nodal disease is found are often managed with surveillance rather than with chemotherapy. Such surveillance usually includes serial serum tumor markers. Of these, the most commonly used are alpha-fetoprotein (AFP), which is elevated in 75 per cent of patients, and human chorionic gonadotropin (hCG), which is elevated in 60 per cent of patients.

Many histologic combinations are possible in mixed nonseminomatous germ cell tumors. The prognosis for an individual patient based on the histologic characteristics of the primary tumor is, however, difficult to predict. One exception is the *mature teratoma,* which rarely occurs in its pure form without other nonseminomatous components. In this situation the prognosis is more favorable than that of a mixed tumor. However, in contrast to mature teratoma of the ovary, the histologic designation of mature teratoma of the testicle is not necessarily associated with uniformly benign behavior, except in children.

Testicular Microlithiasis. Calcification occurs in the majority of testicular germ cell tumors. In most circumstances, the calcification is secondary to the tumor itself. However, in a small group of individuals, numerous small calcifications within the testicular parenchyma, termed *testicular microlithiasis,* predate the development of the neoplasm. This idiopathic condition is almost always bilateral, although sometimes asymmetric. As a result of improved ultrasonographic equipment, testicular microlithiasis has been increasingly recognized in recent years.

The significance of testicular microlithiasis is controversial. Backus et al. (1994) described a 40 per cent incidence of germ cell tumors among patients with testicular microlithiasis. These tumors were approximately evenly divided between seminoma and nonseminomatous germ cell tumors. The significance of this observation is undermined by the fact that the population studied was partially selected and composed mostly of patients with palpable tumors. It is now realized that most patients with isolated testicular microlithiasis are asymptomatic. Thus, the true risk of malignancy in the setting of testicular microlithiasis without a palpable mass is unknown. To emphasize this uncertainty, Rucker (1998) investigated a population defined by the presence of testicular microlithiasis and found a prevalence of germ cell tumor in only 5 per cent.

That there is a causal relationship between germ cell tumor and testicular microlithiasis is supported by a number of other observations (Fig. 26–16). *Intratubular germ cell neoplasia* is a form of preinvasive neoplasia similar in some respects to carcinoma *in situ* in other organs. Two of every three patients with intratubular germ cell neoplasia have testicular microlithiasis. Intratubular germ cell neoplasia is found both in the normal parenchyma of a testis that contains an adjoining germ cell tumor and in the normal testis of a patient with a contralateral germ cell tumor. It is also seen with increased frequency in cryptorchid testes and in patients with oligospermia, conditions that are associated with an increased risk of germ cell tumor. In view of these observations, serial ultrasonograms for patients with testicular microlithiasis who do not have a detectable mass on initial presentation is considered prudent.

Ultrasonographically, numerous echogenic foci

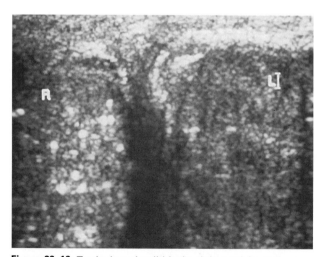

Figure 26–16. Testicular microlithiasis, right testicle, and embryonal carcinoma, left testicle. Ultrasonogram. Transverse projection. Echogenic foci in the right testicle are indicative of testicular microlithiasis. A few calcifications are present in the left testicle. The predominant finding, however, is that of heterogeneous replacement of the left testis with a malignant tumor.

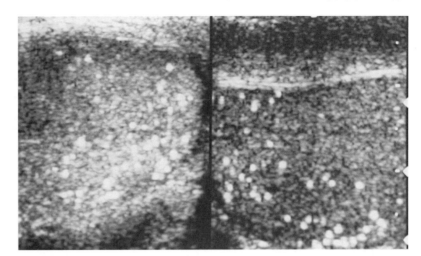

Figure 26–17. Testicular microlithiasis. Ultrasonograms of both testicles. Small echogenic foci are seen bilaterally.

are identified in testicular microlithiasis. Shadowing is usually not present, presumably because of the small size of the calcific deposits (Fig. 26–17). Most patients have too many calcifications to count. Some, on the other hand, have only a few foci in each testis. Unilateral testicular microlithiasis is very rare.

Sex Cord–Stromal Tumor

Sex cord–stromal tumors account for about 5 per cent of testicular neoplasms and are characterized as either *Leydig cell, Sertoli cell,* or *granulosa cell.* Combinations of these cell types and undifferentiated forms also occur.

Clinical behavior, rather than histologic appearance, defines the approximately 10 per cent of sex cord–stromal tumors that are malignant. Clinical symptoms may also suggest a particular diagnosis. For example, Leydig cell tumors are the most common of the sex cord–stromal tumors and are associated with gynecomastia in 30 per cent of men and with precocious puberty in boys. Despite manifestations of hormonal activity, most of these tumors are detected as palpable masses or incidental findings.

It is not possible by ultrasonography to differentiate among either the various types of sex cord–stromal tumors or between sex cord–stromal tumors and the far more common germ cell tumors. Ultrasonographically, these tumors appear as hypoechoic masses in most instances. Some Sertoli cell tumors, however, may be multiple and more densely calcified than is typical for a germ cell tumor.

Secondary Tumor

Solid organ metastases to the testis are rare and are almost always seen in patients with a known history of advanced carcinoma. Prostate and lung carcinoma combined account for more than one-half of primary lesions that produce clinically apparent testicular metastases.

Compared with a solid organ primary neoplasm, hematologic malignancy is more likely to affect the testis. Here, again, the patient usually has an established diagnosis prior to the development of a testicular mass. Leukemic involvement of the testis is noteworthy in that it may occur in the setting of clinical remission elsewhere in the body. Myeloma of the testis is rare.

Lymphoma is the most common hematologic malignancy to cause clinically apparent testicular masses. Owing to the relative decreased prevalence of germ cell tumor among older men, lymphoma is the most common testicular mass in men older than 60 years of age. Although lymphoma is itself unilateral in slightly more than half of cases, it accounts for the majority of cases of bilateral masses because of the relative infrequency of bilateral primary testicular neoplasms.

Testicular involvement by lymphoma commonly appears ultrasonographically as multiple ill-defined hypoechoic masses. Diffuse infiltration may also occur, however, in which cases the entire testis is replaced by a typically homogeneous process. Metastasis from a solid primary tumor, leukemia, or myeloma produce ultrasonographic features that are similar to those of lymphoma (Fig. 26–18).

Epidermoid Cyst

Epidermoid cyst, or epidermal inclusion cyst, is a cystic lesion filled with keratinized debris with a well-defined wall lined by squamous epithelium. Infiltration into the adjacent testis does not occur. Of uncertain origin, this lesion is neither a teratoma nor a testicular germ cell tumor, although there are some histologic similarities between these entities. Additionally, no association with intratubular germ cell neoplasia has been established. Most pathologists consider an epidermoid cyst to be benign. Surgical excision is curative.

Epidermoid cyst presents at any age but is unusual in children. Most patients have a painless palpable mass. Traditionally, epidermoid cyst was thought to represent only 1 per cent of testicular masses. However, a series of over 100 ultrasonographically detected testicular masses found that 5

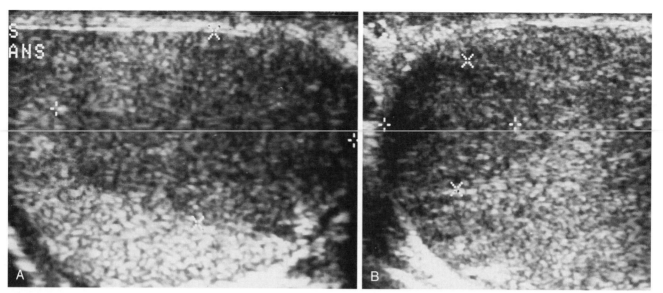

Figure 26–18. Testicular myeloma, bilateral, in a 48-year-old male with scrotal swelling. Ultrasonograms, transverse projections of right *(A)* and left *(B)* testes. Hypoechoic masses *(cursors)* are present in both testes.

per cent were epidermoid cysts (Eisenmenger et al., 1993). This increased prevalence presumably represents the fact that some epidermoid cysts were unrecognized prior to the frequent use of scrotal ultrasonography.

Ultrasonographically, more than 80 per cent of epidermoid cysts have a defined rim with either hypo- or hyperechoic contents. A multilayered appearance has been described but is not universally present (Fig. 26–19). The appearance is characteristic enough to suggest the diagnosis as support for a limited excision and frozen section tissue diagnosis rather than an orchiectomy.

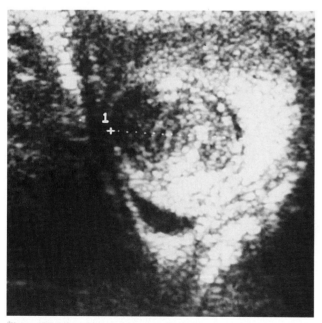

Figure 26–19. Epidermoid cyst presenting as a palpable mass. Ultrasonogram, transverse plane. There is a well-circumscribed mass *(cursors)* with a defined rim and a laminated appearance.

EXTRATESTICULAR NEOPLASMS

Most extratesticular masses are non-neoplastic and benign. These include cystic lesions, such as spermatocele and epididymal cyst, and inflammatory ones, such as chronic epididymitis. In an unselected adult population, approximately 3 per cent of extratesticular solid masses are malignant.

Adenomatoid Tumor

The most common extratesticular solid mass in an adult is an adenomatoid tumor. These benign and usually clinically unimportant lesions occur anywhere along the spermatic cord but often arise from the epididymis. The ultrasonographic appearance of an adenomatoid tumor is of a well-circumscribed, slightly heterogeneous mass (Fig. 26–20).

Embryonal Rhabdomyosarcoma

Although rare overall, embryonal rhabdomyosarcoma is the most common paratesticular mass in children. This aggressive neoplasm may arise anywhere in the pelvis, including the bladder base, prostate, and spermatic cord. The age of the patient and the typically large size of the fast-growing mass at the time of presentation suggest an accurate diagnosis.

NON-NEOPLASTIC MASSES

Testicular Cysts

Tunica Albuginea Cyst. A tunica albuginea cyst is a simple cyst of idiopathic origin. Because it presents as a palpable mass, ultrasonography is required to exclude a germ cell tumor or other neoplasm. Typically, several millimeters in diameter and often multiple, a tunica albuginea cyst meets

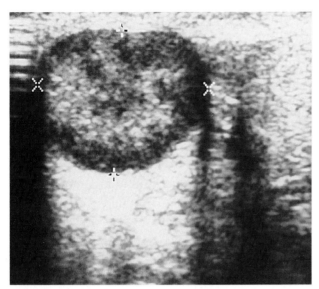

Figure 26–20. Adenomatoid tumor. Ultrasonogram, longitudinal plane. A heterogeneous mass *(cursors)* is situated superior to the head of the epididymis.

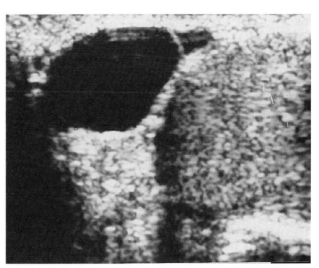

Figure 26–22. Epididymal cyst. Ultrasonogram, longitudinal projection. An uncomplicated cyst of the epididymal head is present. The adjacent testis is normal.

the ultrasonographic criteria of a simple cyst. If, however, such a lesion fails to completely satisfy the criteria for a simple cyst, surgical excision is required for diagnosis (Fig. 26–21).

As discussed in a previous section, tubular ectasia may occasionally appear as an eccentric intratesticular cyst. Usually, though, the characteristic features described earlier establish the correct diagnosis.

Extratesticular Cysts

Epididymal Cyst/Spermatocele. Cysts of the epididymis are encountered in as many as 30 per cent of men presenting for scrotal ultrasonography. Some epididymal cysts are undoubtedly the result of obstruction by acute or chronic epididymitis,

trauma, or previous vasectomy. However, most patients do not have a specific history indicating a precursor event. Often, an epididymal cyst is quite small and is an incidental finding. In a patient referred for a palpable testicular mass, the ultrasonographic identification of a typical extratesticular epididymal cyst obviates further intervention unless for large size, trauma, or infection (Fig. 26–22; see Fig. 26–7).

Spermatocele is a specific type of epididymal cyst that contains spermatozoa. Ultrasonographically, a spermatocele cannot be reliably differentiated from epidydimal cyst, and the distinction is rarely of clinical importance.

VASCULAR DISORDERS
Varicocele

A varicocele results from dilatation of the veins of the pampiniform plexus. This abnormality occurs in

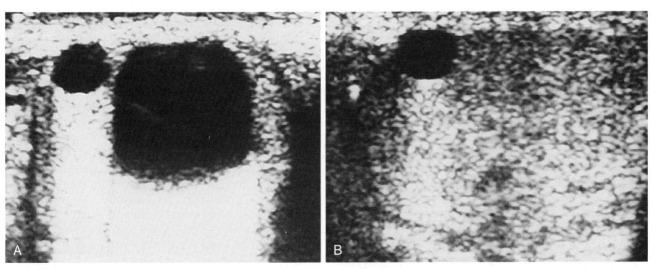

Figure 26–21. Tunica albuginea cysts in a 25-year-old male with a palpable scrotal mass. Ultrasonograms, transverse *(A)* and longitudinal *(B)* projections. The internal echogenicity of the larger mass raises the possibility of a germ cell tumor. However, the presence of a second cyst containing uncomplicated fluid favors a benign diagnosis for both.

15 per cent of men and is usually asymptomatic. The exact pathophysiology of a varicocele is not certain, although incompetence of the valves of the gonadal vein has been implicated. A striking left-sided predominance presumably represents the difference in venous drainage between testicles. The left testicular vein drains directly into the renal vein rather than into the inferior vena cava as is the case with the right testicular vein. However, as many as 10 per cent of patients have bilateral varicoceles, and in 5 per cent of patients the abnormality is right-sided.

Some patients may have mild chronic pain or a sense of testicular fullness caused by the varicocele. The most important clinical manifestation, however, is decreased fertility. A varicocele is found in 40 per cent of infertile men. The size of a varicocele does not correlate with the degree of infertility nor with the prognosis for improvement after treatment. Therefore, an aggressive search should be undertaken in patients with infertility to detect a subclinical varicocele in order that appropriate treatment might be accomplished. Treatment by either surgical ligation or percutaneous embolization of the gonadal vein leads to improved semen quality in most patients.

Most commonly, a varicocele is detected as an incidental finding by ultrasonography. Varicoceles appear as serpentine anechoic channels adjacent to the testis. Doppler techniques show flow signal in the vessels unless thrombosis has occurred (Fig. 26–23). Doppler techniques must be optimized for the detection of slow flow in order to avoid a false-positive diagnosis of thrombosis. From a practical point of view, the clinical significance of thrombosis is limited unless a patient is being monitored after treatment for a known varicocele. Respiratory phasicity is seen in a varicocele, reflecting systemic venous circulation. Because current instruments offer very high resolution, one must not render a diagnosis of varicocele merely on the basis of the

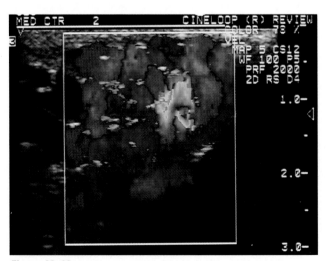

Figure 26–23. Varicocele. Color Doppler ultrasonogram, longitudinal projection. An intrascrotal serpentine grouping of dilated vessels inferior to the testis is noted.

identification of a paratesticular vein. At least two or three vessels, which are 2 to 3 mm in diameter, need to be identified to establish the diagnosis. Sensitivity for the detection of a varicocele is enhanced by examining the patient standing in order to distend the vessels to a greater degree than might be achieved with the patient supine. Valsalva's maneuver may also enhance detection.

Torsion, Ischemia, and Infarction

Testicular torsion results from the combination of a forceful cremasteric contraction and an anatomic variant in which the tunica vaginalis attaches abnormally high within the scrotum. The latter variant, sometimes called the "bell-clapper" anomaly, allows excessive mobility of the testis that is followed by twisting of the inferior spermatic cord and eventual compromise of venous and arterial blood flow. Depending on the degree and duration of torsion, infarction may result.

Any age may be affected, although late puberty is the most common. Although cremasteric contraction is usually the result of sexual activity, trauma, or vigorous physical activity, many patients report an acute onset of severe unilateral scrotal pain without a precipitating event. The urologist may make a confident clinical diagnosis in some patients based on the history and physical examination findings, and imaging is not required prior to surgery. In some patients, however, the clinical diagnosis is not certain, with differential considerations including epididymo-orchitis, trauma, or even tumor. Time is of the essence in the diagnosis of testicular torsion. After 6 hours of symptoms, the testis is not viable and must be removed in as many as 70 per cent of patients. The goal of early diagnosis, therefore, is to achieve prompt surgical detorsion and orchiopexy rather than orchiectomy.

For many years, scintigraphy with technetium pertechnetate was used with a sensitivity that approached 100 per cent for testicular ischemia. Specificity was lower, however, and varied with the population selected. Scintigraphy is also time-consuming and involves exposure to ionizing radiation.

With the development of high-resolution ultrasonographic equipment, efforts were directed toward characterizing the morphologic findings that would allow a reliable diagnosis of testicular ischemia. Unfortunately, however, ultrasonographic findings are not specific. Hydrocele, skin thickening, testicular enlargement, heterogeneity, and hypoechogenicity are seen in patients with orchitis or traumatic contusion as well as with torsion-induced ischemia. In addition, the ischemic, but not yet infarcted, testis often has a normal ultrasonographic appearance. If striking gray-scale ultrasonographic findings are present, the testis is often infarcted and beyond salvage (Fig. 26–24).

Color Doppler techniques have been shown to be accurate in the detection of testicular ischemia. The finding of absent or asymmetric blood flow in the

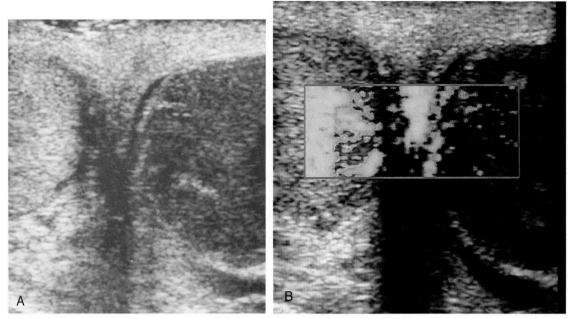

Figure 26–24. Testicular infarction in a 36-year-old male with several days of scrotal pain.
A, Gray-scale ultrasonogram. The echotexture of the left testis is markedly heterogeneous.
B, Power (amplitude) color Doppler ultrasonogram. There is markedly decreased flow to the left testis.

symptomatic testis allows sensitivity and specificity in the range of 95 per cent for the diagnosis of testicular torsion (see Fig. 26–24; Fig. 26–25). A false-negative result may occur in a case of intermittent or incomplete torsion in which flow may be visually normal at the time of the ultrasonographic examination, but torsion recurs or worsens in the hours or days that follow. A false-positive examination is likely to be related to a lack of quantification and the degree to which the examination depends on the assessment of the contralateral testis as a baseline. To minimize these pitfalls, extreme care must be practiced in keeping Doppler settings constant when comparing the two sides. Although the predisposing anomaly is bilateral in 50 per cent of patients and requires bilateral orchiopexy as part of the treatment for ischemic torsion, simultaneous bilateral acute torsion is extremely rare.

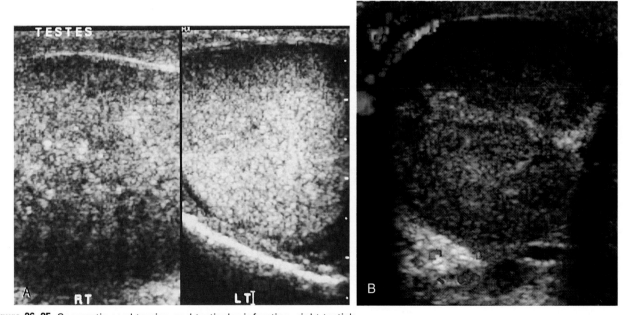

Figure 26–25. Spermatic cord torsion and testicular infarction, right testicle.
A, Ultrasonogram, transverse plane, of both testes. There is moderate heterogeneity and hypoechogenicity of the right testis compared to the left testis.
B, Color Doppler ultrasonogram, longitudinal plane, right testicle. Paratesticular flow is noted, but there is no appreciable flow within the testis itself.

In some patients, demonstration of flow within the normal, asymptomatic testis cannot be detected, precluding comparison with the symptomatic side. In this circumstance, the finding of absent flow to the symptomatic testis cannot be taken as evidence for ischemia, as it does not differ from baseline. This is especially problematic in children. Power or amplitude Doppler is exquisitely sensitive to flow and may offer a solution in some patients in which this problem is encountered, although approximately 40 per cent of prepubertal boys have no detectable flow with either technique.

Testicular infarction due to torsion has been referred to as "missed," "delayed," or "chronic" torsion. Missed torsion is to be avoided as a medical term, as it implies that the practitioner failed to make a timely diagnosis. In fact, many cases of infarction are due to delay by the patient in seeking medical attention, often in cases in which the torsion was partial or intermittent initially and then progressed to more severe ischemia and infarction. In cases of testicular infarction following long-standing torsion, there is increased perfusion of the dartos muscle. The radionuclide image that results is composed of a photopenic defect that corresponds to the infarcted testis surrounded by a zone of increased activity that represents increased soft-tissue perfusion. This appearance has been called the *rim sign of subacute torsion*. However, epididymo-orchitis, hematoma, and tumor may cause the same findings.

Focal infarction is not a common sequela of torsion but may follow epididymo-orchitis or vasculitis (see Fig. 26–11). Focal areas of flow are occasionally seen in patients with torsion who have a subacute infarction and have partially restored flow by way of collateral vessels.

BIBLIOGRAPHY

Albrecht, T., Lotzof, K., Hussain, H. K., Shedden, D., Cosgrove, D. O., and de Bruyn, R.: Power Doppler US of the normal prepubertal testis: Does it live up to its promises? Radiology 203:227, 1997.

Backus, M. L., Mack, L. A., Middleton, W. D., King, B. F., Winter, T. C., III, and True, L. D.: Testicular microlithiasis: Imaging appearance and pathologic correlation. Radiology 192:781, 1994.

Berg, N. B., Schenkman, N. S., Skoog, S. J., and Davis, C. J., Jr.: Testicular masses associated with congenital adrenal hyperplasia: MRI findings. Urology 47:252, 1996.

Borer, J. G., Nitti, V. W., and Glassberg, K. I.: Mixed gonadal dysgenesis and dysgenetic male pseudohermaphroditism. J. Urol. 153:1267, 1995.

Brown, D. L., Benson, C. B., Doherty, F. J., Doubilet, P. M., DiSalvo, D. N., Alstyne, G. A., Vickers, M. A., and Loughlin, K. R.: Cystic testicular mass caused by dilated rete testis: Sonographic findings in 31 cases. AJR 158:1257, 1992.

Cheng, H. C., Kahn, M. A., Bogdanov, A., Kwon, K., and Weissleder, R.: Relative blood volume measurements by magnetic resonance imaging facilitate detection of testicle torsion. Invest. Radiol. 32:763, 1997.

Coley, B. D., Frush, D. P., Babcock, D. S., O'Hara, S. M., Lewis, A. G., Gelfand, M. J., Bove, K. E., and Sheldon, C. A.: Acute testicular torsion: Comparison of unenhanced and contrast-enhanced power Doppler US, color Doppler US, and radionuclide imaging. Radiology 199:441, 1996.

Dieckman, K. P., and Loy, V.: Epidermoid cyst of the testis: A review of clinical and histogenetic considerations. Br. J. Urol. 73:436, 1994.

Eisenmenger, M., Donner, L. G., Kratzik, C. H., Marberger, M.: Epidermoid cysts of the testis: Organ-preserving surgery following diagnosis by ultrasonography. Br. J. Urol. 72:955, 1993.

Finkelde, D. T.: Epidermoid cyst of the testis. Aust. N. Z. J. Surg. 64:62, 1994.

Frush, D. P., Babcock, D. S., Lewis, A. G., Paltiel, H. J., Rupich, R., Bove, K. E., and Sheldon, A. C.: Comparison of color Doppler sonography and radionuclide imaging in different degrees of torsion in rabbit testes. Acad. Radiol. 2:945, 1995.

Frush, D. P., Kliewer, M. A., and Madden, J. F.: Testicular microlithiasis and subsequent development of metastatic germ cell tumor. AJR 167:889, 1996.

Hamm, B., Fobbe, F., and Loy, V.: Testicular cysts: Differentiation with US and clinical findings. Radiology 168:19, 1988.

Heidenreich, A., Engelmann, U. H., Vietsch, H. V., and Derschum, W.: Organ-preserving surgery in testicular epidermoid cysts. J Urol 153:1147, 1995.

Heiken, J. P., Forman, H. P., and Brown, J. J.: Neoplasms of the bladder, prostate, and testis. Radiol. Clin. North Am. 32:81, 1994.

Herbener, T. E.: Ultrasound in the assessment of the acute scrotum. J. Clin. Ultrasound 24:405, 1996.

Hilton, S., Herr, H. W., Teitcher, J. B., Begg, C. B., and Castellino, R. A.: CT detection of retroperitoneal lymph node metastases in patients with clinical stage I testicular nonseminomatous germ cell cancer: Assessment of size and distribution criteria. AJR 169:521, 1997.

Hinman, F., Jr.: Testis. In Hinman, F., Jr. (ed.): Atlas of Urosurgical Anatomy. Philadelphia, W. B. Saunders Co., 1993, pp. 471–525.

Holden, A., and List, A.: Extratesticular lesions: A radiological and pathological correlation. Australas. Radiol. 38:99, 1994.

Horowitz, M. B., and Abiri, M. M.: Case of the day. Radiographics 17:793, 1997.

Horstman, W. G.: Scrotal imaging. Urol. Clin. North Am. 24:653, 1997.

Horwich, A.: Testicular germ cell tumors: An introductory overview. In Horwich, A. (ed.): Testicular Cancer: Investigation and Management. London, Chapman & Hall, 1991, pp. 1–14.

Hrebinko, R. L., and Bellinger, M. F.: The limited role of imaging techniques in managing children with undescended testes. J. Urol. 150:458, 1993.

Kaveggia, F. F., Strassman, M. J., Apfelbach, L., Hatch, J. L., and Wirtanen, G. W.: Diffuse testicular microlithiasis associated with intratubular germ cell neoplasia and seminoma. Urology 48:794, 1996.

Keener, T. S., Winter, T. C., Nghiem, H. V., and Schmiedl, U. P.: Normal adult epididymis: Evaluation with color Doppler US. Radiology 202:712, 1997.

Kim, S. H., Pollack, H. M., Cho, K. S., Pollack, M. S., and Han, M. C.: Tuberculous epididymitis and epididymo-orchitis: Sonographic findings. J. Urol. 150:81, 1993.

Kirby, C. L., Rosenberg, H. K., Horrow, M. M., Stassi, J., and Gerber, W. L.: Doppler evaluation after closed testicular detorsion. J. Ultrasound Med. 16:S19, 1998.

Konez, O.: The ring sign. Radiology 207:439, 1998.

Kramolowsky, E. V., Beauchamp, R. A., and Milby, W. P., III.: Color Doppler ultrasound for the diagnosis of segmental testicular infarction. J. Urol. 150:972, 1993.

Maghnie, M., Vanzulli, A., Paesano, P., Bragheri, R., Palladini, G., Preti, P., Maschio, A. D., and Severi, F.: The accuracy of magnetic resonance imaging and ultrasonography compared with surgical findings in the localization of the undescended testis. Arch. Pediatr. Adolesc. Med. 148:699, 1994.

Malvica, R. P.: Epidermoid cyst of the testicle: An unusual sonographic finding. AJR 160:1047, 1993.

Mansfield, J. T., and Cartwright, P. C.: Bilateral testis tumors in an infant: Synchronous teratoma and epidermoid cyst. J. Urol. 153:1077, 1995.

Marsman, J. W. P.: The aberrantly fed varicocele: Frequency, venographic appearance, and results of transcatheter embolization. AJR 164:649, 1995.

Mazzu, D., Jeffrey, R. B., Jr., and Ralls, P. W.: Lymphoma and leukemia involving the testicles: Findings on gray-scale and color Doppler sonography. AJR *164:*645, 1995.

Miller, R. L., Wissman, R., White, S., and Ragosin, R.: Testicular microlithiasis: A benign condition with a malignant association. Clin. Ultrasound *24:*197, 1996.

Murphy, K. J., and Rubin, J. M.: Power Doppler: It's a good thing. Semin. Ultrasound CT MRI *18:*13, 1997.

Nistal, M., and Paniagua, R.: Non-neoplastic diseases of the testis. In Bostwick, D. C., and Eble, J. N. (eds.): Urologic Surgical Pathology, 1st ed. St. Louis, Mosby–Year Book, Inc., 1997, pp 457–566.

Older, R. A., and Watson, L. R.: Tubular ectasia of the rete testis: A benign condition with a sonographic appearance that may be misinterpreted as malignant. J. Urol. *152:*477, 1994.

Oliver, R. T. D.: A comparison of the biology and prognosis of seminoma and nonseminoma. In Horwich, A. (ed.): Testicular Cancer: Investigation and Management. London, Chapman and Hall, 1991, pp. 51–68.

Oliver, R. T. D., Ong, J., Blandy, J. P., and Altman, D. G.: Testis conservation studies in germ cell cancer justified by improved primary chemotherapy response and reduced delay, 1978–1994. Br. J. Urol. *78:*199, 1996.

Parra, B. L., Venable, D. D., Gonzalez, E., and Eastham, J. A.: Testicular microlithiasis as a predictor of intratubular germ cell neoplasia. Urology *48:*797, 1996.

Petros, J. A., Andriole, G. L., Middleton, W. D., and Picus, D. A.: Correlation of testicular color Doppler ultrasonography, physical examination and venography in the detection of left varicoceles in men with infertility. J. Urol. *145:*785, 1991.

Robinowitz, R., and Hulbert, W. C., Jr.: Acute scrotal swelling. Urol. Clin. North Am. *22:*101, 1995.

Ross, J. H., Kay, R., and Elder, J.: Testis sparing surgery for pediatric epidermoid cysts of the testis. J. Urol. *149:*353, 1993.

Rucker, P. T., and Wagner, B. J.: Frequency of testicular microlithiasis associated with germ cell tumors. J. Ultrasound Med. *16:*S19, 1998.

Sadler, B. T., Greenfield, S. P., Wan, J., and Glick, P. L.: Intra-scrotal epidermoid cyst with extension into the pelvis. J. Urol. *153:*1265, 1995.

Scheinfeld, J.: Nonseminomatous germ cell tumors of the testis: Current concepts and controversies. Urology *44:*2, 1994.

Schwerk, W. B., Schwerk, W. N., and Rodeck, G.: Testicular tumors: Prospective analysis of real-time US patterns and abdominal staging. Radiology *164:*369, 1987.

See, W. A., and Hoxie, L.: Chest staging in testis cancer patients: Imaging modality selection based upon risk assessment as determined by abdominal computerized tomography scan results. J. Urol. *150:*874, 1993.

Shapeero, L. G., and Vordermark, J. S.: Epidermoid cysts of testes and role of sonography. Urology *41:*75, 1993.

Siegel, M. J.: The acute scrotum. Radiol. Clin. North Am. *35:*959, 1997.

Simmons, P. D., Mead, G. M., Lee, A. H. S., Theaker, J. M., Dewbury, K., and Smart C. J.: Orchiectomy after chemotherapy in patients with metastatic testicular cancer. Cancer *75:*1018, 1995.

Slavis, S. A., Kollin, J., Miller, J. B.: Pyocele of scrotum: Consequence of spontaneous rupture of testicular abscess. Urology *33:*313, 1989.

Ulbright, T. M.: Neoplasms of the testis. In Bostwick, D. C., and Eble, J. N. (eds.): Urologic Surgical Pathology, 1st ed. St. Louis, Mosby–Year Book, Inc., 1997, pp. 567–645.

Weingarten, B. J., Kellman, G. M., Middleton, W. D., and Gross, M. L.: Tubular ectasia within the mediastinum testis. J. Ultrasound Med. *11:*349, 1992.

Weissman, B. N., Wong, M., and Smith, D. N.: The Radiological Society of North America 82nd Scientific Assembly and Annual Meeting: Image interpretation session: 1996. Radiographics *17:*243, 1997.

Wilbert, D. M., Schaerfe, C. W., Stern, W. D., Strohmaier, W. L., and Bichler, K. H.: Evaluation of the acute scrotum by color-coded Doppler ultrasonography. J. Urol. *149:*1475, 1993.

Wood, A., and Dewbury, K. C.: Case report: paratesticular rhabdomyosarcoma: Colour Doppler appearances. Clin. Radiol. *50:*130, 1995.

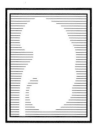

CHAPTER 27

Nephrographic Analysis

Enhancement of the renal parenchyma with contrast material provides information regarding arterial perfusion of the kidney as well as the functional and structural integrity of the nephrons. This chapter analyzes the mechanisms by which this information is derived.

DEFINITIONS

Angiographic/Cortical Nephrogram

Approximately 80 per cent of renal blood flows to the cortex; the remaining 20 per cent perfuses the medulla, pelvocalyceal system, and sinus fat. As a result, a bolus of contrast material flowing to the kidney renders the renal cortex radiodense relative to the medulla during that brief period (up to 30 seconds) in which distribution of contrast material is predominantly in the cortical microvasculature (Fig. 27–1). This phenomenon of selective cortical opacification is known as the *angiographic* or *cortical nephrogram.*

The density of the angiographic/cortical nephrogram depends on the amount of contrast material in the bolus and on the site of injection. Optimal visualization occurs with selective injection of contrast material (usual dose = 35 mg/kg of iodine) through a catheter in the renal artery and rapid sequence filming (Fig. 27–2).

The angiographic/cortical nephrogram can also be imaged during dynamic computed tomographic scanning for a period of approximately 30 seconds after intravenous injection of a bolus of approxi-

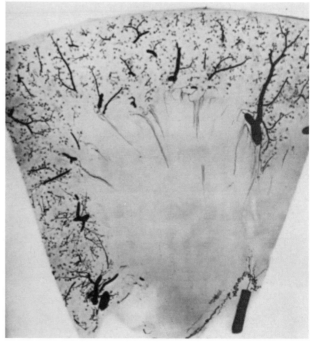

FIGURE 27–1. Microradiograph of a renal lobe from a human kidney that was injected post mortem with barium. The predominant vasculature is in the cortex. This distribution of blood vessels is the basis for the angiographic/cortical nephrogram.

mately 200 mg/kg of iodine (Fig. 27–3). The angiographic/cortical nephrogram may sometimes be visualized during standard excretory urography when a film of optimal technical quality is exposed within

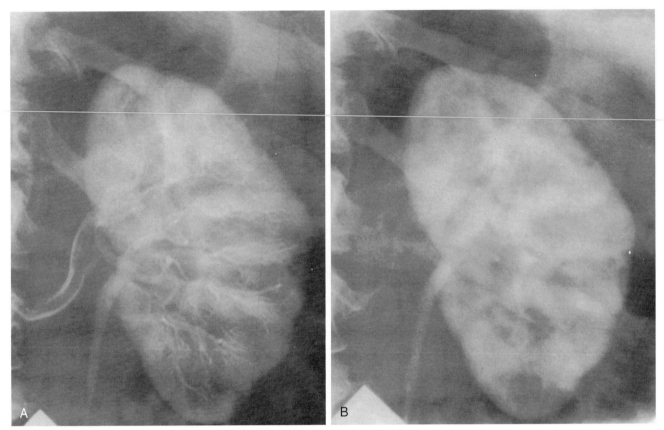

FIGURE 27–2. Angiographic/cortical nephrogram. The centrilobar and septal cortex are opacified, whereas the medulla of each lobe remains relatively radiolucent. This reflects predominant blood flow to the cortex in the first few seconds after injection of contrast material.
  A, Selective renal arteriogram, late arterial phase.
  B, Selective renal arteriogram, capillary phase.

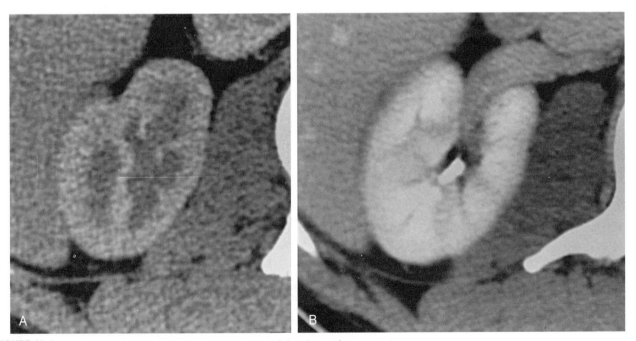

FIGURE 27–3. Helical computed tomogram, contrast material–enhanced.
  A, Upper pole image obtained at 15 seconds demonstrates parenchymal enhancement limited to the renal cortex, the *angiographic/cortical nephrogram.*
  B, Upper pole image obtained at approximately 120 seconds after contrast material injection demonstrates enhancement of both renal cortex and medulla, the *urographic/parenchymal nephrogram,* as well as opacification of the pelvocalyceal system, the *pyelographic phase.* (Same case illustrated in Fig. 1–8.)

30 seconds of the rapid injection of a bolus of contrast material into a peripheral vein (usual dose = approximately 300 mg/kg of iodine).

The magnetic resonance equivalent of the angiographic/cortical nephrogram can be seen within 30 seconds of an intravenous bolus injection of a gadolinium chelate. Rapidly acquired, breath-hold, T1-weighted sequences depict the cortex as hyperintense to the medulla owing to the T1-shortening effects of low-dose gadolinium chelate soon after the bolus arrives in the microvasculature of the cortex (Fig. 27–4).

Urographic/Parenchymal Nephrogram

The radiodensity of the medulla increases as the lumina of the proximal tubules fill with contrast material cleared from the plasma by glomerular filtration. There are two populations of nephrons with different proximal tubule and loop of Henle lengths (Fig. 27–5). One population is composed of short proximal tubules and loops of Henle whose extent is limited to the cortex and the juxtacortical medulla. The second population has long proximal tubules and loops of Henle that extend from the corticomedullary region to the apex of the renal lobe at the level of the papilla. This anatomic arrangement ensures that the full thickness of the renal parenchyma is opacified by contrast material filtering into both sets of proximal tubules. Within approximately 1 minute after injection of contrast material into a peripheral vein, the radiodensity of the medullae of the renal lobes, when imaged by radiographic or computed tomographic techniques, equals that of the cortices. It is this homogeneous density of the entire renal parenchyma that is known as the *urographic* or *parenchymal nephrogram* (Fig. 27–6).

The radiodensity of the urographic/parenchymal nephrogram in a normal, unobstructed kidney is a

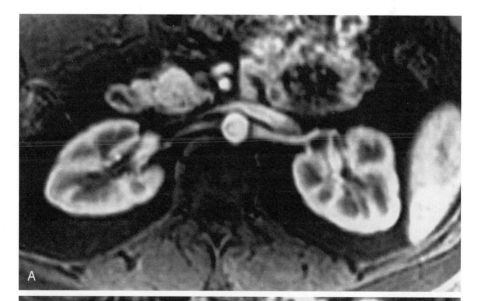
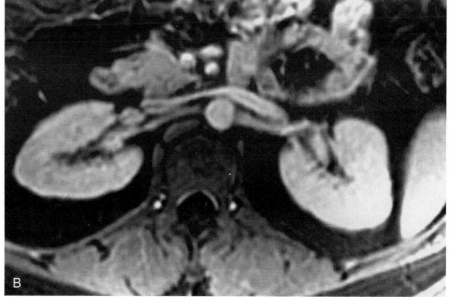

FIGURE 27–4. Angiographic/cortical and urographic/parenchymal nephrograms demonstrated by magnetic resonance imaging. Fat suppressed spoiled gradient echo breath-held sequences.

A, Early dynamic enhanced magnetic resonance image demonstrates cortical enhancement after a bolus injection of gadolinium chelate. The aorta, renal arteries, and left renal vein are also seen.

B, The urographic/parenchymal nephrogram develops as the cortical and medullary signal intensities equilibrate at approximately 1 minute after injection of contrast material.

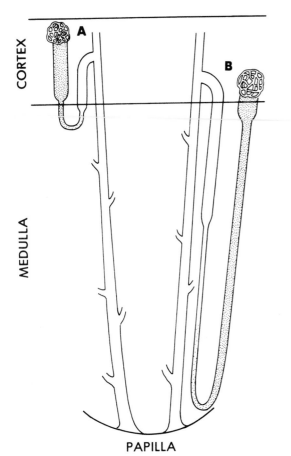

FIGURE 27–5. Distribution of nephrons and collecting ducts in the renal cortex and medulla. One population of nephrons *(A)* is limited to the cortex and adjacent parts of medulla. A second population *(B)* is composed of juxtamedullary glomeruli with tubules that extend deep into the medulla. Contrast material in the proximal tubules of both populations renders the full thickness of the renal parenchyma radiopaque and is the basis of the urographic/parenchymal nephrogram.

function of the *filtered fraction,* which is the product of the plasma concentration of contrast material and the glomerular filtration rate. The plasma concentration, in turn, varies with the amount of contrast material administered and the time elapsed after injection. The density of the urographic/parenchymal nephrogram is greatest approximately 1 minute after the bolus injection of contrast material (usual dose = 300 mg/kg of iodine) at which time the peak plasma level is reached. Beyond this point, the density of the nephrogram diminishes as the plasma level of the contrast material falls. Therefore, after each successive unit of time, fewer iodine-bearing molecules are cleared. Furthermore, the continued flow of contrast material from the nephrons and collecting ducts into the pelvocalyceal system contributes to the decrease in parenchymal density beyond 1 minute.

Technical considerations also influence perceived nephrographic density. Film with low-contrast characteristics, high-kilovoltage x-ray beams, and a large amount of overlying tissue reduce apparent radiodensity. Liver overlying a portion of the right kidney and intestinal gas overlying the left kidney may cause differences in the baseline radiodensity of the kidneys as well as in the radiodensity of the subsequent nephrograms. These variables undermine the value of comparing the nephrographic density of one kidney with that of another as an index of abnormality and also make the practice of using the intensity of the nephrogram as a measure of renal function unreliable.

The urographic/parenchymal nephrogram is best visualized during excretory urography with a film obtained approximately 1 minute after the bolus injection of contrast material. Linear tomography and a well-coned, low-kilovoltage x-ray beam enhance the quality of the image.

The urographic/parenchymal nephrogram is also seen during computed tomography once contrast material enters the tubules and obliterates the sharply defined corticomedullary junction that is a feature of the angiographic/cortical nephrogram (see Fig. 27–3B).

With magnetic resonance imaging, the urographic/parenchymal nephrogram becomes apparent as the medulla equilibrates with the cortex after the intravenous injection of a bolus of gadolinium chelate (see Fig. 27–4). As the gadolinium concentrates in collecting ducts, the medulla may become very hypointense owing to profound T2* (susceptibility weighted) shortening. If a highly T2-weighted gradient-echo sequence is employed, the cortex will be initially hypointense and become even darker as the intratubular concentration of gadolinium chelate increases.

Value of Nephrographic Analysis

The angiographic/cortical nephrogram, as a microvascular phenomenon, requires only an intact vascular system. Abnormality of the angiographic/cortical nephrogram, therefore, is a useful indicator of a disturbance in blood flow to the kidney.

The urographic/parenchymal nephrogram, in the simplest sense, permits accurate evaluation of the fundamentals of renal radiology: the kidney's size, position, and contour. A normal urographic/parenchymal nephrogram requires, in addition to normal blood flow, functional and structural integrity of the nephrons and an unobstructed flow of filtrate through the tubules. Therefore, information regarding these more complex aspects of the kidney can also be derived from nephrographic analysis.

The following sections of this chapter discuss the nephrogram in the context of renal perfusion, the dynamics of urine formation, and the structural integrity of the renal parenchyma. The appearance of the various nephrographic abnormalities and the principles that explain them apply regardless of whether the nephrogram is imaged by excretory urography, angiography, computed tomography, or magnetic resonance imaging.

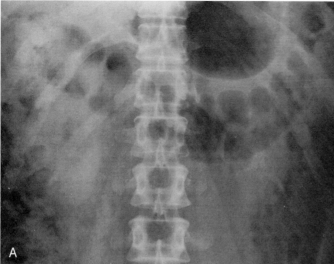

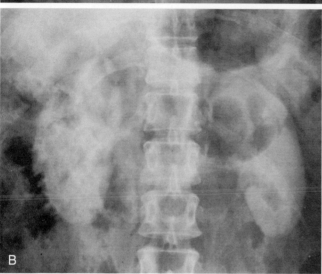
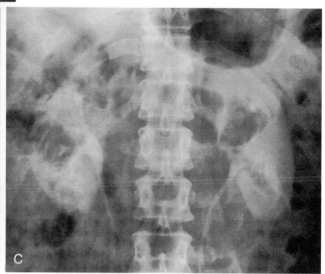

FIGURE 27-6. Urographic/parenchymal nephrogram.
A, Preliminary film. Bowel preparation is poor.
B, Excretory urogram, 1-minute film. There is intense radiodensity of the renal parenchyma, reflecting contrast material that is passing through the nephrons and the collecting ducts.
C, Excretory urogram, 5-minute film. The intensity of the nephrogram has diminished, owing to both the decrease in the plasma concentration of contrast material and the forward flow of opacified urine into the pelvocalyceal system.

ANALYSIS OF RENAL PERFUSION

Main Renal Artery Narrowing

In film radiography, there is frequently a difference in the baseline nephrographic density between the kidneys, caused by uneven distribution of overlying bowel gas and soft tissue. Because of this, a difference in radiodensity is not a reliable indicator of renal ischemia due to main renal artery stenosis unless the difference is of great magnitude (Fig. 27-7). With aortography, unequal nephrograms may result from incomplete mixing of the bolus of contrast material with the aortic blood before its flow to the kidneys. On the other hand, a reduced rate of nephrographic enhancement in one kidney compared with the other during computed tomography is presumptive evidence of decreased renal blood flow, assuming that unilateral renal parenchymal disease or obstructive uropathy is excluded.

Over time, the urographic/parenchymal nephrogram becomes increasingly dense in some patients with severe renal artery stenosis. This reflects an abnormality in the dynamics of urine formation, initiated by reduced renal perfusion pressure. This is discussed further later in this chapter in the section on Increasingly Dense Nephrogram. Other aspects of ischemia due to focal main renal artery disease are discussed in Chapter 6.

Main Renal Artery Occlusion

The nephrogram in acute total occlusion of the main renal artery, as seen with an embolism or trauma, is either absent or extremely faint (Fig. 27-8). In complete acute occlusion without collateral flow, no nephrogram is seen and renal infarction ensues. Any opacification that does occur is the result of collateral blood flow. If the collateral flow bypasses the occluding lesion itself, contrast material passes into the distal part of the main renal artery. Thus, the entire population of nephrons is perfused, although at a level greatly reduced from normal, and a faint nephrogram develops.

There are circumstances in which the only collaterals that form in response to main renal artery occlusion are those of the perirenal capsular circula-

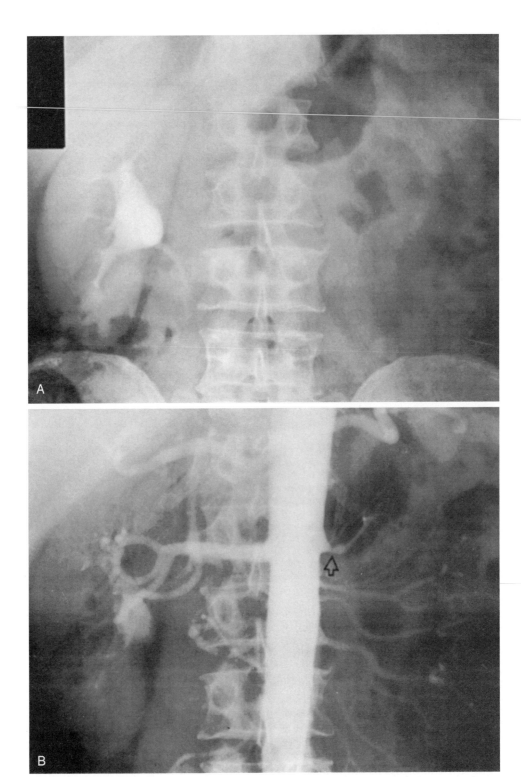

FIGURE 27–7. Diminished nephrographic density due to left main renal artery narrowing. The decreased radiodensity of the left urographic/parenchymal nephrogram relative to the right signals severe reduction in perfusion.

A, Excretory urogram, 4-minute film. In addition to the reduced radiodensity of the nephrogram, the left kidney is small and has delayed opacification of the pelvocalyceal system.

B, Aortogram. There is a high-grade stenosis of the left main renal artery *(arrow)* with post-stenotic dilatation.

(Courtesy of Department of Diagnostic Radiology, Hammersmith Hospital, Royal Postgraduate Medical School, London, England.)

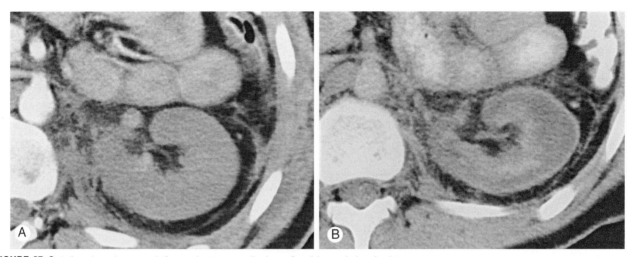

FIGURE 27-8. Infarction due to a left renal artery occlusion after blunt abdominal trauma.
   A, Computed tomogram, contrast material–enhanced examination performed immediately after trauma. The nephrogram is absent.
   B, Computed tomogram, contrast material–enhanced, obtained 2 weeks later. Some function in the subcapsular area, the *cortical rim nephrogram,* and the central juxtamedullary area has been restored by collateral arterial circulation. (Same patient illustrated in Fig. 29–10.)

tion. These collaterals are variably derived from the inferior adrenal, lumbar, gonadal, iliac, intercostal, or phrenic arteries. When this occurs, a 2- to 4-mm rim of outer cortex opacifies during contrast material–enhanced studies (Fig. 27–9). This opacification, known as the *cortical rim sign,* represents that portion of the subcapsular renal cortex that is perfused by capsular artery collateral circulation. The remainder of the kidney does not increase in density.

Segmental Renal Artery Occlusion

The considerations described for acute total occlusion of the main renal artery also apply to acute

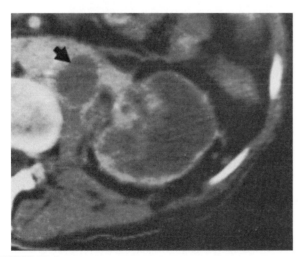

FIGURE 27-9. Occlusion of the left main renal artery by metastatic deposit from lung carcinoma. The low-density metastasis *(arrow)* has occluded the left renal artery, causing smooth enlargement of the kidney and an absent nephrogram except where collateral circulation continues to perfuse the cortex. A cortical rim nephrogram results. Computed tomogram, contrast material–enhanced. (Courtesy of Stuart London, M.D., Oakland, California.)

total occlusion of one or more of the major segmental branches of the renal artery (Figs. 27–10, 27–11). Here, the nephrogram will be absent or markedly reduced only in the affected region. One pole or a set of ventral or dorsal lobes may be involved. A cortical rim sign limited to the affected area may also be seen in acute segmental renal artery occlusion. Power Doppler ultrasonography demonstrates a similar pattern of absent blood flow that mimics the appearance of lobar or wedge-shaped hypoperfusion.

Interlobar or Arcuate Artery Occlusion

Occlusion of an interlobar or arcuate artery leads to infarction of a part or all of a renal lobe in a characteristic wedge-shaped pattern. During the period immediately after occlusion, the bulk of the infarcted tissue is preserved, although no blood flows to the area. This results in a triangle-shaped angiographic/cortical and urographic/parenchymal nephrogram defect without deformity of the renal contour (Fig. 27–12). Within 3 weeks, the affected area will be transformed into a deep, broad-based scar as the infarcted tissue is resorbed. As in segmental renal artery occlusion, power Doppler ultrasonography reveals a wedge-shaped pattern of absent flow. This process is discussed in detail in Chapter 5.

Acute Cortical Necrosis

Acute cortical necrosis is a unique perfusion abnormality in which the cortical microvasculature is obliterated. In some instances, the process is incomplete, leading to a patchy angiographic/cortical nephrogram and a homogeneous urographic/parenchymal nephrogram. In most circumstances, however, there is complete necrosis of the cortex and

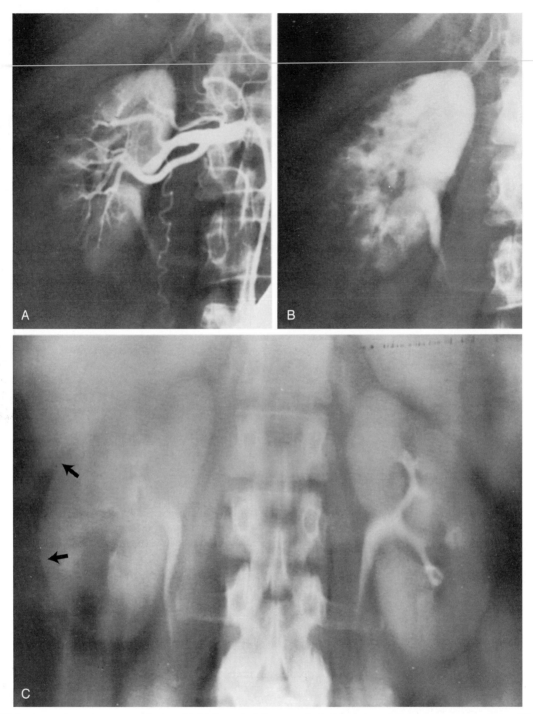

FIGURE 27–10. Segmental renal artery occlusion. Multiple emboli have occluded both interlobar and arcuate arteries. The nephrogram is absent in those portions of the kidney served by the occluded vessels. Collateral blood flow through capsular arteries causes a rim of nephrographic density in the cortex *(arrows)*.

   A, Selective right renal arteriogram, arterial phase. There are numerous points of occlusion.

   B, Selective right renal arteriogram, nephrographic phase. The distribution of the perfusion abnormality is well visualized.

   C, Excretory urogram. Tomogram. The nephrogram is absent in the lateral portion of the right kidney except for the cortical rim sign *(arrows)*. (Same patient illustrated in Fig. 9–16.)

   (Courtesy of Professor César Pedrosa and E. Ramirez, M.D., Hospital Clinico de San Carlos, Madrid, Spain.)

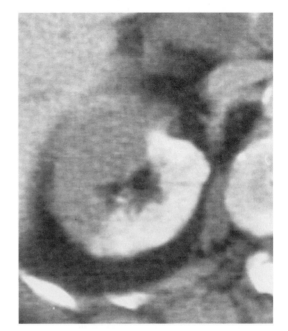

FIGURE 27–11. Acute occlusion of the segmental renal artery to the ventrolateral portion of the right kidney. The dorsomedial portion of the kidney continues to be perfused, whereas the affected part of the kidney has an absent nephrogram.

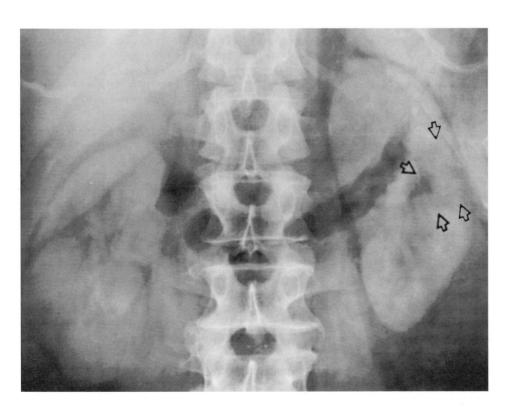

FIGURE 27–12. Acute lobar infarction in a 61-year-old man who experienced sudden left groin and flank pain with microscopic hematuria. Excretory urography was performed 3 days later. A triangular radiolucent nephrographic defect with its base on the renal margin is present in the interpolar region (arrows). Excretory urogram, early film. (Same patient illustrated in Figs. 5–18, 5–20, 5–21.) (Courtesy of Ira Kanter, M.D., Peralta Hospital, Oakland, California.)

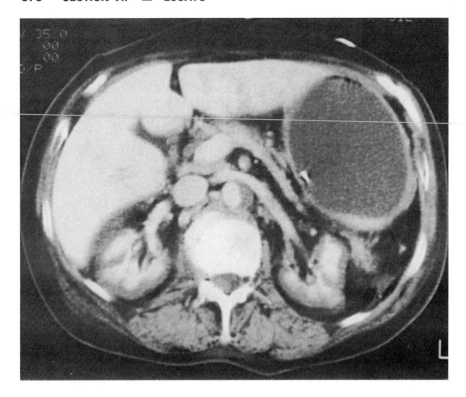

FIGURE 27–13. Acute cortical necrosis in a 74-year-old woman with recent surgery for thoracic and abdominal aortic dissection. Computed tomogram with contrast material enhancement demonstrates absence of enhancement of the cortex and selective enhancement of the medulla. (Same patient illustrated in Fig. 8–7.)

the nephrogram does not develop at all (Fig. 27–13). However, even in this circumstance medullary enhancement may occur, presumably as a result of the continued function of viable juxtamedullary nephron units.

In other cases of acute cortical necrosis, the outer margin of the cortex receives blood from the perirenal capsular arterial system, which acts like a collateral pathway in acute main or segmental renal artery occlusion. When this happens, arterial blood perfuses the outer rim and the juxtamedullary portion of the cortex; however, the central zone between them infarcts. The result is a distinctive nephrogram characterized by a middle zone of nonenhanced cortex located between the opacified outer rim and the inner cortex and medulla. Chapter 8 includes an additional discussion of acute cortical necrosis.

ANALYSIS OF THE DYNAMICS OF URINE FORMATION

Normal Time-Density Curve

The density of the urographic/parenchymal nephrogram is greatest approximately 1 minute after a bolus of contrast material is injected into a peripheral vein. Thereafter, the nephrogram becomes progressively less dense. Fading of the nephrogram is due to the continuous flow of contrast material out of the nephrons and collecting ducts and into the pelvocalyceal system, while at the same time decreasing amounts of contrast material enter the tubules as plasma concentration falls. Thus, over time the decrease in nephrographic density or gadolinium-induced change in signal intensity parallels the plasma decay curve of contrast material concentration. There is a 50 per cent reduction in the plasma level concentration of iodinated contrast material approximately every 50 minutes. This is discussed in Chapter 1.

Abnormalities that affect the dynamics of urine formation may disturb the normal time-density pattern of nephrogram decay. Three abnormal time-density patterns are recognized: (1) immediate, faint, and persistent; (2) increasingly dense; and (3) immediate, dense, and persistent.

Immediate, Faint, Persistent Nephrogram

With this nephrographic pattern, peak density is seen on the first film exposed at the completion of contrast material injection but is not commensurate with the amount of contrast material injected. The nephrogram, although faint, persists for several hours.

The immediate, faint, persistent nephrogram occurs when glomerular filtration is severely impaired by a reduction in the number of functioning nephrons. The faintness of the nephrogram reflects a low plasma clearance rate of contrast material. In fact, a high dose of contrast material is required if the nephrogram is to be seen at all during excretory urography.

The renal diseases associated with an immediate, faint, persistent nephrogram are often associated with a high urea load and impaired sodium reabsorption in the proximal tubules. These cause a diuresis that also contributes to the faintness of the nephrogram. Persistence of the nephrogram reflects a very slow rate of decay of plasma contrast material owing to impaired glomerular filtration.

An immediate, faint, persistent nephrogram is seen in patients with *chronic glomerular disease* and in those who have had a sudden loss of glomerular function as a result of widespread obliteration of the renal microvasculature, such as in *atheroembolic renal disease* (Fig. 27–14).

Increasingly Dense Nephrogram

In this nephrographic pattern, the nephrogram is absent or faint to begin with, but becomes increasingly dense over a period of hours to days. The mechanism for each of the many causes of an increasingly dense nephrogram is an increase in tubule transit time of filtrate combined with diminished clearance of contrast material from plasma. Leakage of contrast material into the renal interstitial space is an additional possible factor that may contribute to an increasingly dense nephrogram in certain etiologies.

Acute extrarenal obstruction, as occurs with ureteral calculus, is the most common cause of an increasingly dense nephrogram (Fig. 27–15). Pathophysiologically, a downstream ureteral obstruction leads to an increase in hydrostatic pressure that extends back to the nephron. The subsequent reduced glomerular filtration rate lowers the amount of contrast material entering the tubules during any given period, producing the reduced density of the nephrogram during the first few minutes of the excretory urogram or computed tomogram. However, continued reabsorption of water by the tubules compensates for the elevated hydrostatic pressure within the tubules, and thus glomerular filtration does not cease completely. There are other factors, less important and inconstant, that help to compensate for the increased hydrostatic pressure that follows acute extrarenal obstruction. These include distention of the collecting structures proximal to the obstructing lesion and leakage of urine into the renal sinus, interstices, lymphatics, or veins through rents in the fornices of the calyces. The net result is the continued formation of an iodine-bearing glomerular filtrate that moves sluggishly forward. Because of this, the nephrogram gradually increases over many hours, and calyceal opacification is delayed.

Diminished perfusion pressure of the kidney, as seen in systemic arterial hypotension or severe main renal artery stenosis, is another cause of an increasingly dense nephrogram. Here, a decrease in arterial perfusion pressure at the level of the glomerular capillary bed reduces the rate of contrast material clearance from the plasma into the proximal tubule lumina. Renal underperfusion also promotes increased reabsorption of salt and water by the tubules, causing the volume of tubule filtrate to diminish. The net effect of these alterations is a slow accumulation of contrast material molecules with an increasingly dense nephrogram.

In the case of systemic hypotension, the nephrograms of both kidneys become increasingly dense (Fig. 27–16). Only on restoration of normal blood pressure is there rapid pelvocalyceal opacification and the return of normal nephrographic density. This nephrographic pattern is most often seen in the clinical setting of an adverse reaction to contrast material. (See discussion in Chapter 7.) An increasingly dense nephrogram due to diminished perfusion pressure secondary to severe main renal artery stenosis, on the other hand, is usually unilateral and is accompanied by other radiologic signs of ischemia (Fig. 27–17), as discussed in Chapter 6.

Other, less common, causes of an increasingly dense nephrogram include *acute tubular necrosis,* which is often associated with contrast material–

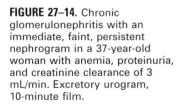

FIGURE 27–14. Chronic glomerulonephritis with an immediate, faint, persistent nephrogram in a 37-year-old woman with anemia, proteinuria, and creatinine clearance of 3 mL/min. Excretory urogram, 10-minute film.

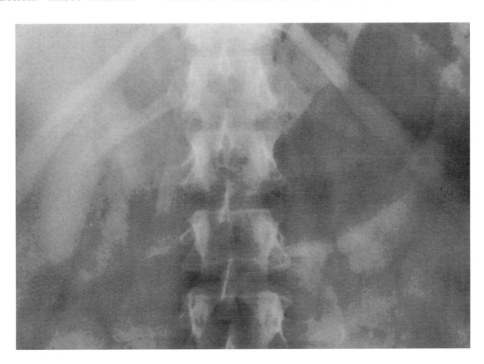

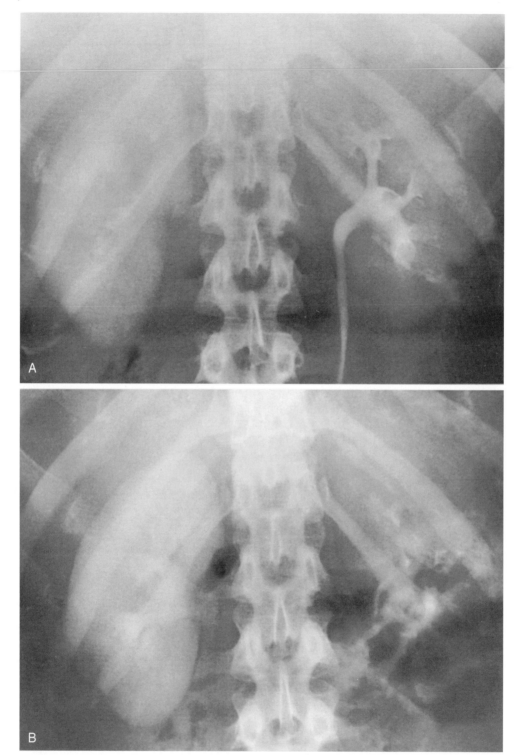

FIGURE 27–15. Acute extrarenal obstruction with an increasingly dense nephrogram. The patient was a young woman with a right distal ureteral stone.
   A, Excretory urogram, 10-minute film. The right nephrogram is already more dense than the left.
   B, Excretory urogram, 4-hour film. The density of the nephrogram has increased. (Same patient illustrated in Fig. 9–17.)

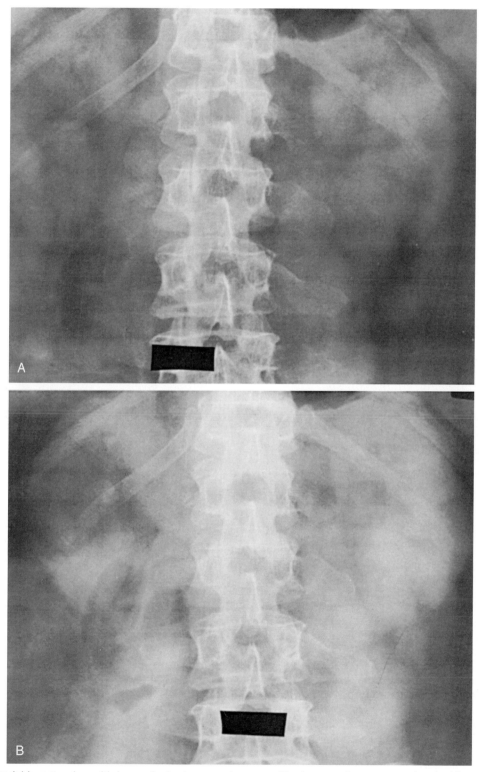

FIGURE 27–16. Arterial hypotension with increasingly dense nephrogram. The hypotension was associated with an adverse response to contrast material.

 A, Excretory urogram, 5-minute film. There is impaired nephrographic density and absent pelvocalyceal opacification.

 B, Excretory urogram, 10-minute film. The nephrographic density has increased, but the pelvocalyceal system remains unopacified. (Same patient illustrated in Fig. 7–22.)

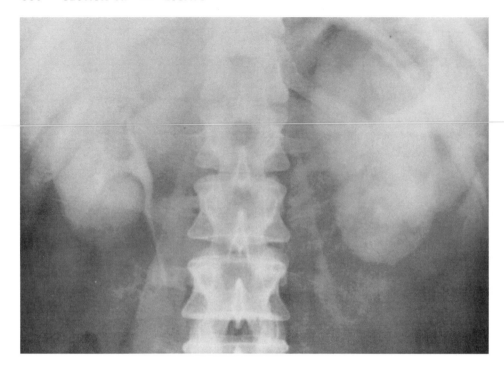

FIGURE 27–17. Renovascular ischemia of the left kidney associated with an increasingly dense urographic nephrogram. The nephrogram of the left kidney is more dense than that of the right, and the calyces are faintly opacified. Excretory urogram, delayed film.

induced nephrotoxicity; *intratubular obstruction,* as might be seen in acute urate or myeloma nephropathy or Tamm-Horsfall proteinuria; *acute glomerular disease;* and *acute renal vein thrombosis.*

Immediate, Dense, Persistent Nephrogram

In this pattern, the nephrogram is at least as dense as would be normally expected at 1 minute. Rather than fading, however, the level of density persists, and often slightly increases over a period of hours to days. When this pattern is associated with nonoliguric acute renal failure, the collecting system may opacify.

The mechanism for the production of an immediate, dense, persistent nephrogram has not been clarified. The early appearance of a dense nephrogram suggests unimpaired glomerular filtration. Because nephrographic density remains rather constant despite anuria or oliguria, there must be return of filtered contrast material to the circulation. This is believed to occur through diffusion of tubule fluid into the interstitial space and then into the systemic circulation through veins and/or lymphatics. Another mechanism that may contribute to an immediate, dense, persistent nephrogram is blockage of tubule lumina by casts and cellular debris shed from damaged tubule epithelium. This might add an obstructive component that could account for the slight increase in nephrographic density over time that is seen in some of these patients.

Acute tubular necrosis is most commonly associated with an immediate, dense, persistent nephrogram (Fig. 27–18). The evolution of this pattern following an initially normal excretory urogram suggests the development of contrast material–induced nephrotoxicity.

Severe acute pyelonephritis is another condition in which an immediate, dense, persistent nephrogram with little or no collecting system opacification is sometimes observed. Here, the abnormality is almost always unilateral. Bilateral involvement is a rare, chance event. A striated urographic/parenchymal nephrogram is frequently encountered in patients with severe acute pyelonephritis, especially with computed tomography, as discussed in the following section of this chapter and in Chapter 9.

The reader is cautioned against using any of the various abnormal time-density nephrographic patterns described here as specific presentations of any given renal abnormality or as hard and fast rules in formulating a diagnosis. As always, careful integration of all radiologic, laboratory, and clinical data remains basic to accurate diagnosis.

Striated Urographic/Parenchymal Nephrogram

Inhomogeneity of the urographic/parenchymal nephrogram, characterized by fine linear bands of alternating lucency and density uniformly oriented in a direction similar to that of tubules and collecting ducts, is encountered occasionally as a transitory phenomenon in a number of different circumstances.

Stasis of urine in tubules underlies the development of nephrographic striations in *acute extrarenal obstruction.* During the course of a contrast material–enhanced imaging study, the striated pattern emerges from a background of faint but homogeneous density, becomes progressively more apparent, reaches a plateau, and then fades (Fig. 27–19). The exact nature of the striae is unclear. The abnormality is either dense striae representing hyper-

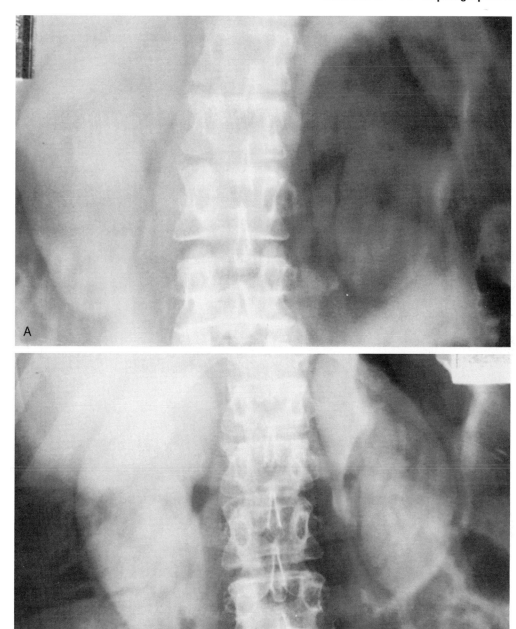

FIGURE 27–18. Acute tubular necrosis with an immediate, dense, persistent nephrogram.

A, Excretory urogram, 2-minute film. The nephrogram is denser than normally seen at 2 minutes.

B, Excretory urogram, 16-hour film. The nephrogram persists and becomes slightly denser over time. (Same patient illustrated in Fig. 8–5.)

(Courtesy of Professor Thomas Sherwood, M.B., University of Cambridge, Cambridge, England.)

concentration of contrast material in dilated medullary rays or linear lucencies caused by unopacified calyceal urine that has been forced retrograde into some of the collecting ducts dilated by obstruction.

The striated nephrogram in *severe acute pyelonephritis* represents an acute tubulointerstitial nephritis in medullary or cortical rays served by incompetent papillary orifices, as described in Chapter 9. Here, the acute inflammatory cell infil-trate increases interstitial pressure, which diminishes the perfusion and contrast enhancement of the affected portions of the kidney. This is seen as striated areas of relative radiolucency in the early stages of a contrast material–enhanced study. On delayed images, these linear radiolucent striations gradually become radiodense as iodine-containing urine slowly accumulates in collecting ducts that are partially obstructed by inflammatory exudate.

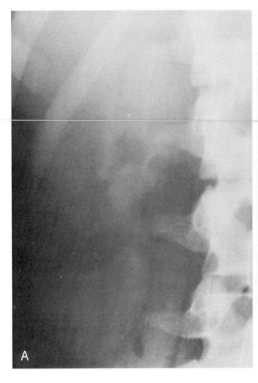
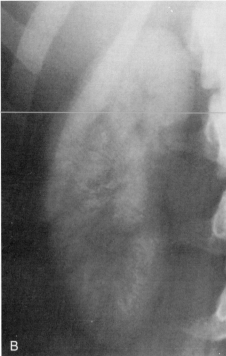

FIGURE 27–19. Striated nephrogram in acute obstructive uropathy.

A, Excretory urogram, 5-minute film. Delayed opacification.

B, Excretory urogram, 45-minute film. Striae are well illustrated. (Same patient illustrated in Fig. 9–22.)

Ectasia of collecting ducts is the fundamental structural kidney abnormality in *autosomal recessive (infantile) polycystic kidney disease,* as discussed in Chapter 8. As contrast material initially passes through the nephrons, adjacent dilated collecting ducts in the cortical and medullary rays appear as striated nephrographic radiolucencies because they are filled with nonopacifed urine (see Figs. 8–13, 8–15). Eventually, the collecting ducts opacify. However, the striated pattern may persist as the bundles of nephrons that are interposed with the cortical and medullary rays lose their radiopacity and become radiolucent relative to the collecting ducts.

The basis for a striated urographic nephrogram described in isolated case reports in *hypotension,*

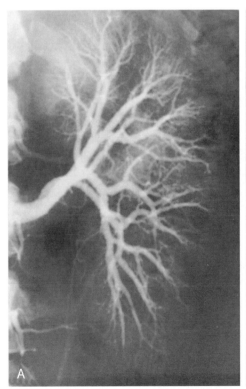
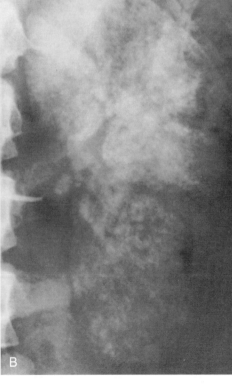

FIGURE 27–20. Patchy urographic/parenchymal nephrogram in acute lupus nephritis.

A, Selective renal arteriogram. Arterial phase. The kidney is enlarged, and the intrarenal arteries are stretched.

B, Selective renal arteriogram. Nephrogram phase. There is a patchy nephrogram indicative of diffuse, obliterative changes in the microvasculature.

intratubular block, renal contusion, and *renal vein thrombosis* is entirely speculative. Suggestions for its existence have included prolonged tubule transit time and hyperconcentration due to decreased glomerular filtration (hypotension), increased interstitial pressure (renal vein thrombosis, renal contusion), intratubular block (Tamm-Horsfall proteinuria), and vasospasm (renal contusion).

Patchy Urographic/Parenchymal Nephrogram

Inhomogeneous urographic/parenchymal nephrograms have been described in obliterative diseases of the renal microvasculature, such as *polyarteritis nodosa, scleroderma,* and *necrotizing angiitis,* and in *catheter-induced vasospasm* (Fig. 27–20). In these diseases, the nephrogram consists of patchy densities and does not have an orderly pattern of striations. This reflects random occlusive events in the microvasculature of the kidney.

ANALYSIS OF THE INTEGRITY OF RENAL STRUCTURE

The radiologist's ability to detect structural abnormalities of the kidney depends on identifying disruption of the homogeneity of the urographic nephrogram. This is best accomplished using computed tomography.

The urographic/parenchymal nephrogram is deformed by processes that cause loss of renal tissue (*reflux nephropathy, lobar infarction*), displacement of normal parenchyma (*chronic obstructive uropathy, autosomal dominant [adult] and autosomal recessive [infantile] polycystic kidney disease, medullary cystic disease, simple cyst, focal hydronephrosis*), or replacement of parenchyma (*benign or malignant neoplasm and inflammatory mass*). Each of these diseases is discussed in detail in other chapters.

BIBLIOGRAPHY

Bowley, N. B.: Renal opacification during intravenous urography in acute cortical necrosis (the nephrogram in cortical necrosis). Br. J. Radiol. *54*:24, 1981.

Cohan, R. H., Sherman, L. S., Korobkin, M., Bass, J. C., and Francis, I. R.: Renal masses: Assessment of corticomedullary-phase and nephrographic-phase CT scans. Radiology *196*:445, 1995.

Frank, J. A., Choyke, P. L., Austin, H. A., and Girton, M. E.: Functional MR of the kidney. Magn. Reson. Med. *22*:319, 1991.

Frank, P. H., Nuttall, J., Brander, W. L., and Prosser, D.: The cortical rim sign of renal infarction. Br. J. Radiol. *47*:875, 1974.

Fry, I. K., and Cattell, W. R.: The nephrographic pattern during excretion urography. Br. Med. Bull. *28*:227, 1972.

Glazer, G. M., and London, S. S.: CT appearance of global renal infarction. J. Comput. Assist. Tomogr. *5*:847, 1981.

Goergen, T. G., Lindstrom, R. R., Tan, H., and Lilley, J. J.: CT appearance of acute renal cortical necrosis. AJR *137*:176, 1981.

Hann, L., and Pfister, R. C.: Renal subcapsular rim sign: New etiologies and pathogenesis. AJR *138*:51, 1982.

Hattery, R. R., Williamson, B., Jr., Hartman, G. W., LeRoy, A. J., and Witten, D. M.: Intravenous urographic technique. Radiology *167*:593, 1988.

Ishikawa, I., Onouchi, Z., Saito, Y. K., Kitada, H., Shinoda, A., Ushitani, K., Tabuchi, M., and Suzuki, M.: Renal cortex visualization and analysis of dynamic CT curves of the kidney. J. Comput. Assist. Tomogr. *5*:695, 1981.

Lee, J. K. T., McClennan, B. L., Melson, G. L., and Stanley, R. J.: Acute focal bacterial nephritis: Emphasis on gray scale sonography and computed tomography. AJR *135*:87, 1980.

Martin, D. C., and Jaffe, N.: Prolonged nephrogram due to hyperuricaemia. Br. J. Radiol. *44*:806, 1971.

Newhouse, J. H., and Murphy, R. X., Jr.: Tissue distribution of soluble contrast: Effect of dose variation and changes with time. AJR *136*:463, 1981.

Newhouse, J. H., and Pfister, R. C.: The nephrogram. Radiol. Clin. North Am. *17*:213, 1979.

Paul, G. J., and Stephenson, T. F.: The cortical rim sign in renal infarction. Radiology *122*:338, 1977.

Rubin, B. E., and Schliftman, R.: The striated nephrogram in renal contusion. Urol. Radiol. *1*:119, 1979.

Saunders, H. S., Dyer, R. B., Shifrin, R. Y., Scharling, E. S., Bechtold, R. E., and Zagoria, R. J.: The CT nephrogram: Implications for evaluation of urinary tract disease. RadioGraphics *15*:1069, 1995.

Sherwood, T., Doyle, F. H., Boulton-Jones, M., Joekes, A. M., Peters, D. K., and Sissons, P.: The intravenous urogram in acute renal failure. Br. J. Radiol. *47*:368, 1974.

Tomiak, M. M., Foley, W. D., and Jacobson, D. R.: Variable-mode helical CT: Imaging protocols. AJR *164*:1525, 1995.

Wicks, J. D., Bigongiari, L. R., Foley, W. D., and Walter, J.: Parenchymal striations in renal vein thrombosis: Arteriographic demonstration. AJR *129*:95, 1977.

Young, S. W., Noon, M. A., and Marincek, B.: Dynamic computed time-density study of normal human tissue after intravenous contrast administration. AJR *129*:36, 1981.

Young, S. W., Noon, M. A., Nassi, M., and Castellino, R. A.: Dynamic computed tomography body scanning. J. Comput. Assist. Tomogr. *4*:168, 1980.

Radiologic Assessment of a Renal Mass: Implications for Patient Management

PATHOLOGIC AND THERAPEUTIC BACKGROUND
SIMPLE CYST
HEMORRHAGIC CYST, INFECTED CYST, ABSCESS
MALIGNANCY

BENIGN NEOPLASM, NON-NEOPLASTIC TUMOR, AND INFLAMMATORY MASS
MISCELLANEOUS CONSIDERATIONS
SUMMARY

Renal masses are discussed in Chapter 12 in the context of the diagnostic set, "Large, Unifocal, Unilateral" with an emphasis on the pathologic characteristics and the radiologic analogues of individual entities that present as a mass in the kidney. This chapter approaches the same subject in the context of differential diagnosis, levels of diagnostic confidence, and implications for patient care.

Technological developments in imaging have led to an unprecedented accuracy in the detection and characterization of a mass arising in the kidney. The value of these advances can hardly be disputed. It is also clear, however, that the various imaging modalities applied to a given patient often result in uncertain interpretion or wasted resources. Radiologic characteristics of different pathologic entities may overlap. Some features are highly diagnostic for a certain pathologic diagnosis, whereas others are equivocal. The use of multiple imaging modalities frequently produce data that are either redundant or contradictory. Further, radiologic interpretation is sometimes confounded by small lesion size. In any of these circumstances, the diagnostic radiologic effort may fail to provide data that usefully inform subsequent therapeutic choices and/or patient outcome.

Contemporary imaging has also opened Pandora's box, revealing conditions that previously had gone undetected. These include the discovery of a small solid mass or a hyperdense fluid-filled mass in the kidney of an asymptomatic patient. Many of these small solid masses prove to be cancer at an early stage and, indeed, their early detection may account for the improvement in survival rates for renal cancer that have been reported (Kessler et al., 1994; Guinan et al., 1995). The true significance of these apparent salutary effects of computed tomography

and ultrasonography, however, are yet to be determined, as emphasized by questions regarding lead-time bias of early detection and the biologic activity of incidentally discovered small lesions (Black and Ling, 1990).

The discussion of the role of the radiologic evaluation of a renal mass in clinical decision in this chapter is based on the following assumptions: (1) that radiologic data are *indirect* analogues of pathologic features; (2) that a final tissue diagnosis is considered the province of the pathologist, not the radiologist; and (3) that a proper radiologic diagnosis is a prediction of a final tissue diagnosis with an implied level of probability based on what is known about the inherent pathologic characteristics of the proposed diagnosis, on the sensitivity of the modality or modalities used, and, to a lesser extent, on the prevalence and demographic features of the diagnoses under consideration.

PATHOLOGIC AND THERAPEUTIC BACKGROUND

There is an inherent linkage between the pathology of a mass, its radiologic analogue, and its therapeutic implication. For example, a radiologic diagnosis of a simple nephrogenic cyst can be made with near 100 per cent confidence and carries an implication of no subsequent therapy, considering the benign nature of this entity. Similarly, a highly confident radiologic diagnosis of a renal malignancy militates for surgical excision, usually with radical techniques.

Using this formulation, the various pathologic entities that constitute renal masses and their likely therapeutic implications fall into four categories, as outlined in Table 28-1.

The obligation of the radiologist is to not only know the radiologic analogues for each of these pathologic entities but also to have a firm sense

The material presented in this chapter has been previously published in Radiology, 202:297, 1997, and is reproduced by permission of the Radiologic Society of North America.

TABLE 28–1. Pathologic Entities That Constitute Renal Masses and Their Therapeutic Implications

Pathology	Therapeutic Implication
Renal cyst	No intervention
Hemorrhage or infection in a renal cyst, abscess	Variable: no intervention; needle aspiration, culture, antibiotic, and follow-up
Malignancy (e.g., carcinoma, Wilms' tumor, metastasis, lymphoma)	Surgical excision (except known metastasis or lymphoma)
Benign neoplasm, non-neoplastic or inflammatory mass	Variable: no intervention; nephron sparing surgery; follow-up; antibiotic

of the level of certainty inherent in the observed radiologic features. It is the interaction of these two elements of the radiologic diagnosis that contributes to an appropriate therapeutic decision.

The criteria in the sections that follow assume a lesion size large enough for radiologic characterization. Lesions that are too small to characterize radiologically are discussed in a subsequent section.

SIMPLE CYST

Pathologic Features. The pathologic characteristics of a simple nephrogenic cyst include one or more chambers lined by low cuboidal or flattened epithelium, a 1- to 2-mm-thick fibrous wall and a serous fluid content that is clear, is slightly yellow, and may contain a small amount of protein. Uncommonly, thin septa divide the cyst into multiple chambers, which may or may not communicate with each other. Calcium may deposit in the wall or septa of a simple, nephrogenic cyst in the absence of any complication such as hemorrhage or infection.

Radiologic Analogues. The ultrasonographic analogues of a simple cyst include an anechoic mass with a well-defined far wall and enhanced sound through transmission.

By computed tomography or magnetic resonance imaging the content of the mass is characteristic for water. Cysts do not enhance. Any change in the attenuation value of a cyst after injection of contrast material is minimal, usually measuring less than 15 Hounsfield Units. However, technical factors may influence this number. For example, slice thickness, milliamperage, and the shape and size of the measured region of interest must be held constant when comparing unenhanced with enhanced images. Further, attenuation values vary with the location of a region of interest within a cyst as well as with the spatial relationship of a cyst to nearby renal and extrarenal structures.

By all modalities, including excretory urography, the wall of the cyst is so thin that it borders on imperceptible and the interface with surrounding renal parenchyma is sharply marginated. Cysts that protrude from the surface of the kidney can be encircled on their periphery by an effaced wedge of renal parenchyma. This is the so-called *beak* or *claw* sign. A true beak sign must be distinguished from the thick wall of a cystic neoplasm by ascertaining on contiguous slices that the tissue of the beak is continuous with the remainder of the renal parenchyma. It must be remembered that a beak sign is not specific for a simple cyst. Rather, it represents both the renal origin and slow growth of an expansive mass of any pathologic type.

Septa, when present, are few in number, filamentous, and often have an undulating appearance (Fig. 28–1A). Calcification is sometimes deposited on the periphery of the cyst or in the septa as a fine curvilinear density best evaluated by computed tomography (Fig. 28–2).

Confidence Levels. Rigid adherence to all of these imaging criteria using ultrasonography, computed tomography, or magnetic resonance imaging permits the diagnosis of a simple nephrogenic cyst with a degree of accuracy approaching 100 per cent. This high level of confidence applies even to those lesions that have septations and/or calcification, as described earlier, but only if all other criteria for the radiologic diagnosis of a simple cyst are fulfilled. Excretory urography, alone, is insufficient for a high confidence radiologic diagnosis of simple nephrogenic cyst. Any deviation from the imaging criteria for simple cyst may indicate that the lesion is a cyst complicated by hemorrhage or infection or is an abscess or cystic neoplasm. These are discussed in the sections that follow.

Clinical Implications. Simple nephrogenic cyst requires no therapeutic intervention except in the rarest of circumstances when these lesions produce pain or obstruction. Thus, a simple cyst can be diagnosed with a very high level of confidence and requires no further evaluation or therapeutic intervention.

HEMORRHAGIC CYST, INFECTED CYST, ABSCESS

Pathologic Features. A simple nephrogenic renal cyst may become hemorrhagic as a result of trauma, varices in the cyst wall, bleeding diatheses, or unknown reasons. The contents of these liquefied and encapsulated masses contain rust-colored, puttylike material confined by a thick fibrous wall that is frequently calcified. A fibrin ball, which is sometimes moveable, may form within the cavity. The mass may be unilocular or be divided into multiple locules separated by thick septa. There are also

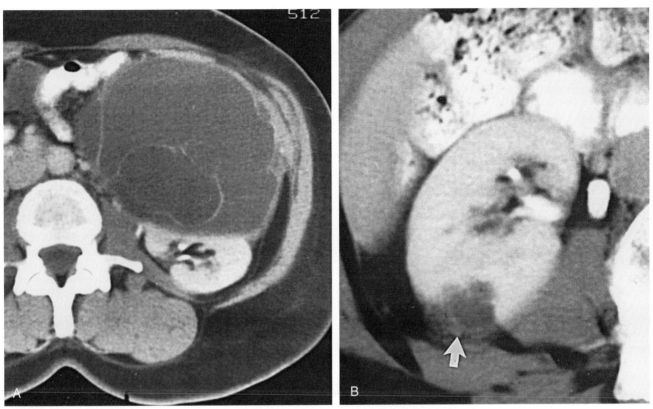

FIGURE 28–1. The filamentous, undulating septa within a simple cyst *(A)* are distinct from the thicker septa with a focal nodule *(arrow)* within a renal carcinoma *(B)*. Computed tomograms, contrast material–enhanced.

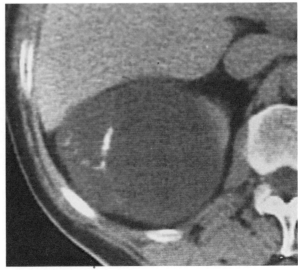

FIGURE 28–2. Thin, linear deposition of calcium in the septa of a simple cyst. Computed tomogram, contrast material–enhanced.

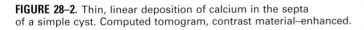

simple nephrogenic cysts with normal gross morphology whose contents, although clear, have a protein content that imparts computed tomographic, magnetic resonance, or ultrasonographic features that may simulate hemorrhagic cyst.

A renal cyst may also become infected by hematogenous dissemination of bacteria, by ascending urinary tract infection with or without vesicoureteral reflux, or as a result of surgical manipulation. In this circumstance, the wall thickens and occasionally calcifies. The infected cyst contains pus and debris. Similar pathologic characteristics are encountered in an abscess that has evolved from pyelonephritis into a mature stage of liquefaction and encapsulation.

Radiologic Analogues. The radiologic analogue for a complicated cyst or an abscess may include features that suggest a substantial fluid component. However, these are lesions that deviate from the strict criteria for a simple nephrogenic cyst. Deviations take the form of impaired sound transmission and internal echoes by ultrasonography and increased attenuation values by computed tomography. Magnetic resonance signal intensity is higher than expected for a simple cyst on T1-weighted images and variable on T2-weighted images. Other atypical features that may be seen include a thickened wall, thick or irregular mural calcification, a fluid-debris level, and thick septations (Figs. 28–3A and 28–4A, B).

Acute hemorrhage may give rise to characteristic computed tomographic or magnetic resonance findings. The attenuation values of cyst contents are in the range of 50 to 90 Hounsfield units depending on dilution and may be homogeneous. With time, this value diminishes and becomes equal to or slightly less than adjacent renal parenchyma. On magnetic resonance images, acute hemorrhage within a cyst may initially appear as low signal intensity on T1-weighted images and increase in signal intensity with time. On T2-weighted images, the appearance is usually high in signal intensity, but less so than would be seen in a simple cyst. A fluid-debris level may develop over time, with the dependent component generally lower in signal intensity than the nondependent component.

The radiologic appearance of the simple cyst with high protein content meets all computed tomographic criteria discussed previously for the simple uncomplicated nephrogenic cyst except for an attenuation value sufficiently increased so as to be readily seen as more dense than unenhanced renal parenchyma (Fig. 28–5). These lesions may have ultrasonographic findings that are those of either a simple or complicated cyst.

Confidence Levels. All of the pathologic entities discussed in this section create radiologic images that deviate from the strict criteria required for the diagnosis of a simple, uncomplicated nephrogenic cyst. In other words, a diagnosis of simple cyst is precluded when these radiologic features are present. Management should be influenced most by abnormal findings, even subtle ones, rather than normal findings. Further, as will be discussed in subsequent sections, the radiologic characteristics associated with cyst hemorrhage and infection, and abscess, as well as uncomplicated cyst with high density fluid content, overlap with radiologic findings that may be associated with malignant tumors. Therefore, an accurate prospective diagnosis of these lesions based on imaging data alone cannot be made.

Clinical Implications. The confident diagnosis of hemorrhagic or infected simple cyst and abscess requires pathologic examination of surgically excised tissue. Whether this is actually accomplished in a given patient varies with individual circumstances, such as the patient's age, clinical presentation, and other medical and/or social considerations. In some, serial follow-up may suffice, whereas in

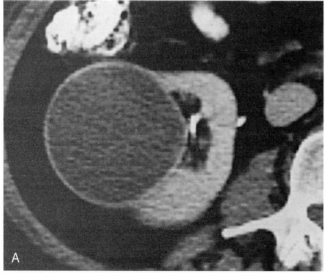 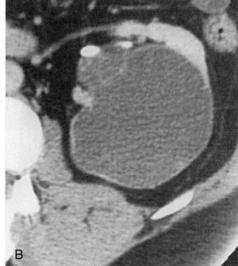

FIGURE 28–3. Similar patterns of thick, slightly irregular, enhancing wall in a complicated cyst *(A)* and in a renal carcinoma *(B)*. Computed tomograms, contrast material–enhanced.

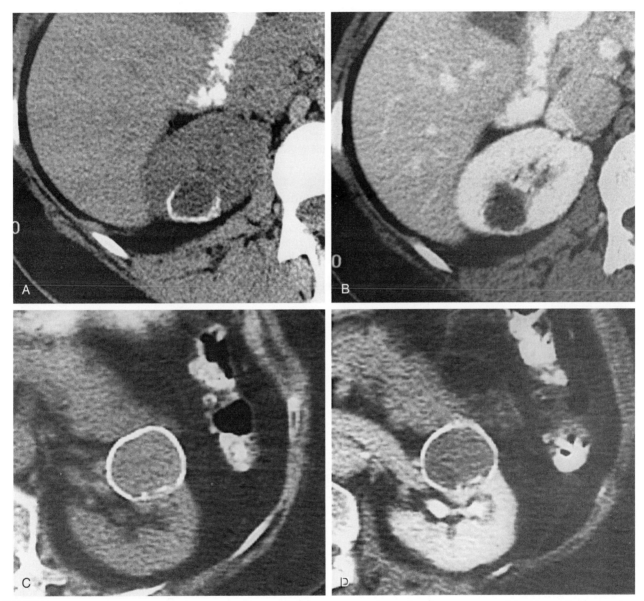

FIGURE 28–4. Similar patterns of thick peripheral rim of calcification in unenhanced and contrast material–enhanced computed tomographic scans of a complicated cyst *(A, B)* and a renal carcinoma *(C, D)*.

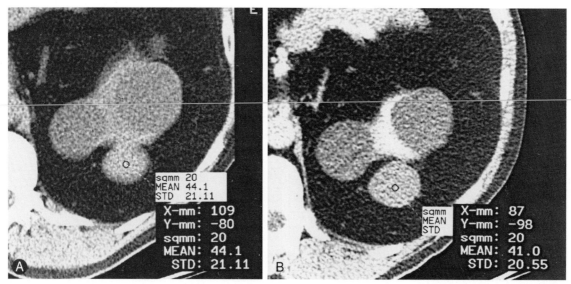

FIGURE 28–5. Similar patterns of hyperdensity and nonenhancement in a simple cyst before (A) and after (B) contrast material enhancement. The attenuation values were 44.1 and 41.0 Hounsfield units, respectively. The hyperdense cyst is also visually of greater density than that of two other cysts in the same region. (Same illustration as Fig. 12–54.)

others nephron-sparing surgical excision of the lesion may be the choice. A mass with the imaging characteristics described in this section detected in the clinical setting of infection may be further investigated by percutaneous needle aspiration. A positive culture would justify appropriate antibiotic therapy based on the confident diagnosis of abscess or infected cyst.

The clinical implications of a high density mass that meets all other criteria of a simple cyst are discussed subsequently in the section on Miscellaneous Considerations.

MALIGNANCY

Pathologic Features. The gross pathologic features of a malignant neoplasm in the kidney include regional enlargement that is of a spherical or ball-shaped geometry in those entities that characteristically grow by expansion (e.g., carcinoma, Wilms' tumor) or of a bean-shaped geometry in those lesions that typically grow by infiltration of the renal interstitium (e.g., transitional cell carcinoma of the collecting system invading the kidney). In any form of malignancy, evidence of spread into adjacent soft tissues, regional lymph nodes, or distant organs may be present. Intratumoral fat at a macroscopic level is extremely rare in renal malignancy.

Expansive tumors may be uniformly solid or contain areas of hemorrhage and necrosis. In some instances, a previously solid tumor will evolve into a mass composed almost exclusively of necrotic tissue surrounded by a thick irregular rim of viable tissue, whereas in other cases, foci of hemorrhage and necrosis become filled with loculated blood or debris-containing fluid. Multiple locules of varying size may compose the bulk of the tumor.

Carcinoma may also develop *de novo* as a unicameral or multilocular cystic mass with malignant cells lining the single cyst or multiple locules. In Wilms' tumor that presents as a multilocular mass the malignant cells are within the septa. The content of these cystic malignancies is either bloody fluid, sometimes with debris, or clear, colorless fluid devoid of solid elements. The wall of these cystic tumors, however, is invariably thicker than a simple cyst and may be irregular with one or more mural nodules as well.

Malignant tumors that grow by infiltration enlarge the kidney while preserving the reniform shape. These usually remain solid throughout their natural history.

Radiologic Analogues. Radiologic analogues for malignant tumors of the kidney include focal enlargement (either ball or bean shaped) and either uniform or patchy enhancement of the tumor to a lesser degree than adjacent normal renal parenchyma. In analyzing enhancement patterns, caution should be exercised when early-phase contrast material–enhanced helical computed tomography is used. With this technique, small, hypervascular renal tumors may be missed because they are as dense as the surrounding renal cortex. Therefore, a complete evaluation of the renal parenchyma for small tumors using dynamic techniques requires repeat scanning at a time when contrast material has moved from the microvasculature of the cortex into the nephrons, thereby opacifying the medulla as well as the cortex. This entails obtaining images at 90 or more seconds after a bolus of contrast material is injected. Fresh bleeding into the tumor may cause hyperdensity relative to normal renal tissue on unenhanced computed tomographic scans. Foci of old hemorrhage or necrosis may be of lower attenuation values than adjacent areas of viable tumor and remain unenhanced after contrast material is given. Evidence of spread as seen by venous or adjacent soft tissue invasion, adenopathy, or distant metastases may be present. Ultrasonographic features characteristic of a malignant renal tumor include internal echoes and impaired sound transmission, as evidenced by poor definition of the far wall of the tumor or the absence of increased sound through transmission beyond the tumor.

Tumors that grow as unicameral cysts *de novo* and those that have undergone extensive necrosis with only a rim of viable tissue may simulate some of the imaging features of a simple cysts. Therefore, careful analysis and strict application of the criteria for simple cyst, described previously, are always required to detect the features that indicate either a malignant tumor or those conditions described earlier as complicated cysts or cyst look-alikes (see Figs. 28–3B, 28–4C, D). Lesions demonstrated as anechoic by ultrasonography must also exhibit enhanced sound through transmission and the ab-

sence of any internal or mural structures to support a diagnosis of simple cyst (Fig. 28–6). Computed tomographic features indicative of cystic malignancy include tumor content with an attenuation value greater than that of water, enhancement after contrast material administration to a degree greater than the technical variation expected for a simple cyst, mural nodule(s) with or without enhancement, thick and/or irregular wall with or without calcification, and nonperipheral calcification (Fig. 28–7; see Fig. 28–3B).

Malignant tumors that develop *de novo* as multilocular cystic masses have imaging characteristics of multiple water-filled locules with thick septa that are either smooth or nodular (Fig. 28–8; see Fig. 28–1B). The septa often enhance after contrast material administration, as demonstrated on computed tomography or magnetic resonance imaging. Septal

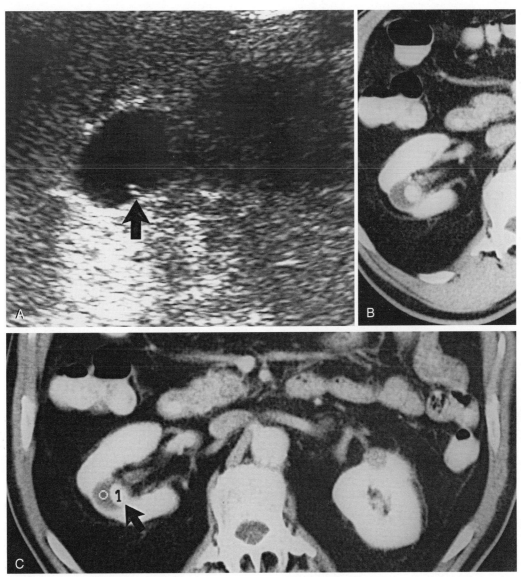

FIGURE 28–6. *A,* Simple cyst with a mural nodule *(arrow).* Ultrasonogram, left kidney, sagittal projection. This finding alone militates for surgical removal despite other findings indicative of simple cyst.

B and *C,* Cystic adencarcinoma with mural nodule *(arrow).* Computed tomograms, contrast material–enhanced. The cystic component measured 17.1 Hounsfield units. (Figure 28–6B also illustrated in Fig. 12–23.)

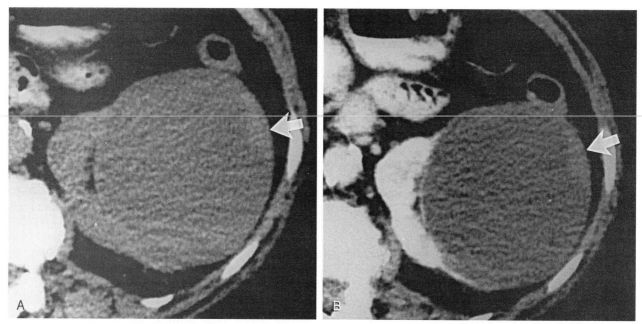

FIGURE 28–7. Mural nodule in renal carcinoma.
  A, Unenhanced computed tomogram scan demonstrates a mural nodule *(arrow)* of slightly higher density than the tumor.
  B, Computed tomogram with contrast material enhancement demonstrates enhancement of the nodule but not of the tumor.

calcification may occur. These findings are identical with those of benign multilocular cystic nephroma, as discussed subsequently.

Confidence Levels. Characterization of a renal mass with the imaging features described in the preceding paragraph implies a level of probability for malignancy that approaches 100 per cent, espe-

cially if evidence of aggressive growth such as necrosis or spread beyond the kidney is present. The greatest likelihood for error lies in the assessment of those malignant tumors whose imaging characteristics simulate some features of simple cyst, with an implication that these may represent benign disease. An incorrect interpretation can be avoided

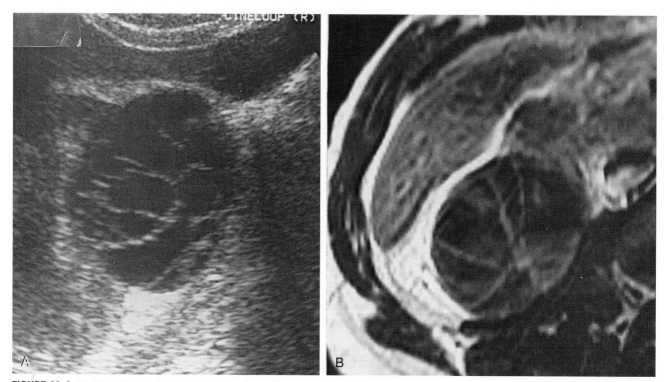

FIGURE 28–8. Multilocular cystic renal carcinoma with imaging characteristics by both ultrasonography *(A)* and magnetic resonance imaging with contrast material enhancement *(B)* of multiple, water-filled locules with thick, smooth, enhancing septa. These findings are identical to those of benign multilocular cystic nephroma.

only by strict adherence to the criteria just discussed if management errors are to be avoided.

Clinical Implications. The radiologic findings described in this section for malignancy overlap those for hemorrhagic and infected renal cyst as well as those for abscess. There is also considerable overlap with the radiologic features for benign neoplasms and non-neoplastic masses, which are described subsequently. Therefore, these radiologic findings should lead to surgical excision to establish the final diagnosis unless there are unusual clinical circumstances that militate for biopsy, as discussed subsequently, or the clinical setting suggests infection as a basis for the mass. In the latter circumstance, needle aspiration of pus or infected tissue may obviate surgical excision.

BENIGN NEOPLASM, NON-NEOPLASTIC TUMOR, AND INFLAMMATORY MASS

Pathologic Features. Oncocytoma and multilocular cystic nephroma are two benign tumors of the kidney with gross pathologic features that are purported to be characteristic. For oncocytoma, these include a solid tumor whose color is that of normal kidney, a frequently present central stellate-shaped scar, and the absence of hemorrhage or necrosis. For multilocular cystic nephroma, characteristic features include multiple locules filled with clear fluid; septa that are thick, smooth, and vascularized; and occasional herniation of some locules of the tumor into the renal pelvis. Although such features, indeed, are characteristic of these two benign neoplasms, they are not unique. Except for herniation into the renal pelvis of a loculated portion of a multilocular cystic nephroma, similar gross pathologic features may occur in some malignant renal tumors, particularly renal carcinoma and Wilms' tumor, as previously described. Other rare, benign tumors of the kidney (e.g., juxtaglomerular cell tumor or leiomyoma), also share gross pathologic features with malignant renal tumor.

Angiomyolipoma and congenital arteriovenous malformation (hemangioma), on the other hand, are two renal masses that do have unique pathologic characteristics that form the basis for distinctive radiologic analogues. For angiomyolipoma, macroscopic aggregates of fat are estimated to be present in 95 per cent of cases. In arteriovenous malformation, virtually the entire mass is composed of flowing blood passing through a single, enlarged feeding artery into either a cluster of blood vessels (*cirsoid arteriovenous malformation*) or a large vascular chamber (*cavernous arteriovenous malformation*) and then exiting through an enlarged vein or veins, usually without increased circulation time.

Inflammatory renal masses are composed of either an interstitial infiltrate of acute inflammatory cells (acute pyelonephritis) or their breakdown products (abscess) or the formation of granulomas (focal xanthogranulomatous pyelonephritis, malakoplakia, or tuberculosis). Gross pathologic features of these lesions may simulate neoplasm to the extent that there is regional enlargement of the kidney (either ball or bean shaped) by tissue that is either solid or of mixed solid and fluid composition. Among the inflammatory masses, focal xanthogranulomatous pyelonephritis is distinctive pathologically based on the usual obstructing calculus in the renal pelvis and associated calicectasis surrounded by xanthomatous granulomas.

Radiologic Analogues. Radiologic features that have been described for oncocytoma include a solid tumor that enhances evenly after contrast material administration, a central, stellate-shaped area of diminished enhancement, and arteries arranged in a rim and spoke-wheel pattern on angiography. All of these findings also may be observed in renal carcinoma. Conversely, a pattern of uneven or patchy enhancement, usually associated with hemorrhage or necrosis in a renal carcinoma, may be found in an oncocytoma as a result of scar forming in an eccentric location within the tumor.

The radiologic findings in multilocular cystic nephroma include a multiloculated mass with thick, smooth, enhancing septa and, occasionally, herniation of some locules into the renal pelvis. The fluid within the locules usually has the same attenuation values or signal characteristics as does water, but variation may occur in some locules. Whereas herniation of locules into the renal pelvis is probably unique, the other radiologic findings of multilocular cystic nephroma may be encountered in renal carcinoma or Wilms' tumor.

Radiologic detection of intratumoral fat by either computed tomography or magnetic resonance imaging, on the other hand, is virtually diagnostic of angiomyolipoma. Contrariwise, ultrasonography does not lend itself to the confident diagnosis of angiomyolipoma because the pattern of increased echogenicity associated with fat may be duplicated by tumors that contain no fat, most notably renal carcinoma. The conventional computed tomographic features of an arteriovenous malformation are indistinguishable from those of a solid, enhancing tumor. Likewise, gray-scale ultrasonographic images of a cirsoid arteriovenous malformation are consistent with those of a solid tumor. The ultrasonographic image of a cavernous arteriovenous malformation, on the other hand, indicates that the mass is composed of uncomplicated fluid and is, thus, discordant with a solid tumor. The true nature of an arteriovenous malformation of either type is established by modalities that detect blood flow, such as angiography, color Doppler ultrasonography, arterial phase dynamic helical computed tomography, or magnetic resonance imaging. Major hematuria in a child or young adult often provides the clinical impulse to use these modalities in the search for the diagnosis of arteriovenous malformation.

Inflammatory renal masses may have the same radiologic features as malignancies (Fig. 28–9). Discrimination between the two, therefore, is often not possible on the basis of radiologic appearance alone.

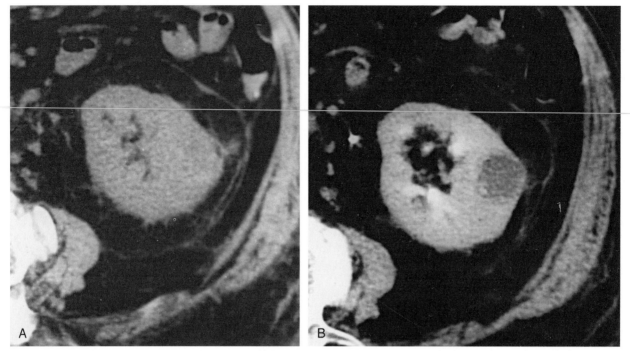

FIGURE 28–9. Inflammatory mass that has the same characteristics as a renal carcinoma on unenhanced *(A)* and contrast material–enhanced *(B)* computed tomographic scans. Because the clinical setting in this patient was that of urinary tract infection, needle aspiration was performed and yielded a positive culture for bacteria.

One exception to this generalization is focal xanthogranulomatous pyelonephritis, which usually demonstrates an obstructing calculus in the collecting system, associated calicectasis, and occasional enhancement of a rim of inflammatory tissue immediately surrounding the dilated calyx.

Confidence Levels/Clinical Implications. Because of the overlap in features associated with malignancy, the radiologic diagnosis of oncocytoma or multilocular cystic nephroma does not have a level of confidence high enough to obviate excisional biopsy at a minimum to establish the true diagnosis. An exception to this might be that circumstance in which herniation of fluid density locules into the renal pelvis from a multiloculated tumor is encountered in the appropriate demographic setting associated with multilocular cystic nephroma (e.g., a young man or a middle-aged woman).

On the other hand, the detection of fat within a renal tumor is the basis for a highly confident radiologic diagnosis of angiomyolipoma, given the extreme rarity of intratumoral fat in renal carcinoma. In this situation, the radiologist must assess the relationship of the fat to the remainder of the tumor to be certain that the fat is truly intratumoral and not perirenal fat entrapped by a renal tumor invading the perirenal space or renal sinus. With the radiologic diagnosis of angiomyolipoma, a determination of maximum diameter of the lesion will guide therapeutic options in view of the increased likelihood of hemorrhage in an angiomyolipoma greater than 4 cm in diameter.

The demonstration of blood flow within a mass that is essentially composed entirely of blood vessels establishes the diagnosis of arteriovenous malformation with sufficient confidence to permit consideration of nonsurgical therapeutic interventions, such as embolization.

Contrariwise, a confident diagnosis of inflammation as a cause for a renal mass cannot usually be made solely on the basis of radiologic findings, which simulate various forms of neoplasm. Diagnostic strategies (e.g., aspiration) can be adjusted accordingly only when these radiologic findings are encountered in the clinical context of infection.

MISCELLANEOUS CONSIDERATIONS

Small, Asymptomatic Renal Mass. The discovery of small (<3 cm diameter), solid tumors in the kidneys of asymptomatic individuals has been one consequence of contemporary imaging. Published series of excised incidentally discovered masses suggest their potential seriousness in that approximately 85 per cent of these are renal carcinomas and that approximately 8 per cent have metastasized at the time of diagnosis (Hajdu et al., 1980; Talamo and Shonnard, 1980, Hellsten et al., 1981). On the other hand, histologic and cytologic studies of these tumors have confirmed the previously established correlation between small tumor size, low grade of malignancy, and lack of aggressive behavior (Montie, 1991; Tsukamoto et al., 1991; Frank et al., 1993; Kessler et al., 1994; Guinan et al., 1995). In the absence of a clear understanding of the natural history of small renal carcinomas and their lethal potential, there are no established guidelines for their management. Individual circumstances, such as a patient's age, life expectancy, coexisting medical problems, and tolerance for the unknown, as well as general economic concerns, enter into the decision as to whether an incidentally discovered small lesion should be excised or followed with serial images seeking evidence of growth.

Small, Hyperdense Mass. Another conundrum created by modern imaging of the kidney is the discovery of the small (<3 cm diameter) mass that projects from the surface of the kidney and fulfills the established computed tomographic criteria of a simple cyst except for being hyperdense relative to unenhanced renal parenchyma. It has been stated that an incidentally discovered mass of this description is a simple cyst containing fluid that has been altered either by previous hemorrhage or by an inherently high protein content (Bosniak, 1986). This pathogenesis has also been used to explain the ultrasonographic findings of echogenicity and impaired sound transmission that are sometimes present in these hyperdense masses. With this assumed high level of confidence in the diagnosis of simple cyst, it has been suggested that these lesions do not require excision for diagnosis and that in some circumstances follow-up studies might be pursued (Bosniak, 1991). Radiologists should be aware, however, that the actual number of published cases in which hyperdense masses of these characteristics have been excised and studied pathologically number only 18, of which 17 have been benign cysts and 1 a renal carcinoma (Curry et al., 1982; Fishman et al., 1983; Pearlstein, 1983; Coleman et al., 1984; Dunnick et al., 1984; Sussman et al., 1984; Zirinsky et al., 1984; Foster et al., 1988; Hartman et al., 1992). Based on this limited experience, it can be argued that the relative prevalence of cyst and carcinoma represented by hyperdense masses is not clearly established even though chance alone greatly favors the diagnosis of simple cyst when the relative prevalence of cysts over tumors in the general population is taken into account. Given this uncertainty, management decisions, including excision, serial follow-up, or dismissal should be individualized.

Needle Biopsy. Most solid malignancies of the kidney are composed of a heterogeneous cell population in which the histologic and cytologic features in some parts of the tumor are unequivocally high grade malignancy, whereas in other areas the cells are classified as either of a low or indeterminate grade. Pathologic diagnosis based on needle biopsy of most tumors, therefore, is subject to sampling error. A biopsy specimen that is positive clearly militates for surgical removal of the tumor. However, in view of the potential for sampling error a negative biopsy specimen should *not* obviate surgical removal. With this perspective, needle biopsy detracts from, rather than enhances, the efficiency of a diagnostic evaluation and should be employed only in exceptional circumstances. These would include patients who are poor operative risks, patients who have one kidney, or who have multiple

tumors in one or both kidneys and to confirm renal metastases in patients with a known primary malignancy, including lymphoma. When needle biopsy is performed, multiple samples should be obtained to reduce sampling error.

Masses Too Small to Characterize. A common occurrence in clinical radiology is the detection of small (<1 cm) lesions within the kidney. These are often too small to avert partial-volume artifacts that become likely at this size even if 5-mm-thick slice collimation is employed. It is simply impractical to label these "indeterminate" with the implication that they may be malignant. Because the vast majority of incidental lesions will be cysts and at least some of the remaining solid lesions will be very slow growing or benign, it seems reasonable to suggest that lesions that are too small to characterize likely represent cysts and need not be followed. Risk factors such as previous renal tumor, known primary malignancy, age of patient, positive family history, unusual occupational exposure, or other medical or psychologic factors may justify follow-up studies in some patients.

SUMMARY

The relationships between the gross pathology of neoplastic and non-neoplastic renal masses and their radiologic analogues described in this chapter establish specific guidelines for the impact of radiologic studies on clinical management.

A tumor that contains fat, as determined by computed tomography or magnetic resonance imaging, can be confidently diagnosed as an angiomyolipoma without further diagnostic intervention. The size of the lesion should be used to influence clinical decisions related to the fact that angiomyolipomas larger than 4.0 cm in diameter are more likely to hemorrhage than those below that size. High confidence can also be assigned to those renal masses that exhibit the radiologic analogues for arteriovenous malformation using imaging modalities that document their vascular nature. These findings should be sufficient for therapeutic decisions directed toward embolization or surgical excision when clinically warranted.

If a mass can be characterized as a simple cyst by satisfying all of the required computed tomographic or ultrasonographic criteria, no further diagnostic interventions are required. This includes the radiologic findings of thin rim of peripheral calcification and thin septa with or without calcification.

An equally high level of confidence is associated with the broad range of computed tomographic, ultrasonographic, or magnetic resonance imaging findings that indicate malignant tumor. These militate for radical surgery. However, the same findings are also encountered in hemorrhagic and infected renal cyst, abscess, benign neoplasms, and inflammatory mass. Therefore, surgical excision, the extent of which will vary according to individual circumstances, is usually required to establish these diagnoses. Exceptions to the need for a tissue diagnosis might be considered in the patient in whom a renal mass is detected in the clinical setting of infection and in the patient with either a small asymptomatic renal mass or a small hyperdense mass that meets the other criteria of a simple cyst. Here again, individual circumstances may lead to such alternatives as aspiration of the mass for culture, interval follow-up seeking evidence of growth, or dismissal.

A four-part classification for cystic renal masses with diagnostic and therapeutic implications was proposed and later modified by Bosniak (Bosniak, 1986 and 1991). There is general agreement that a lesion classified as Category I manifests radiologic characteristics described in this chapter that imply a high probability of a diagnosis of simple cyst with an implication of no further required intervention. According to Bosniak, Category II lesions are considered "minimally complex" and include cysts that contain a "small amount" of peripheral or septal calcification; hyperdense cysts that are homogeneous and do not enhance with use of contrast material; septated cysts with all septa less than 2 mm thick and no thickening or nodularity; and clinically infected cysts that can be confirmed by needle puncture. Most Category II lesions are benign and, therefore, nonsurgical. Typically, they do not require further imaging or follow-up. Cystic masses are classified as Category III on the basis of thick, irregular calcification, especially if centrally located; hyperdensity with heterogeneity, enhancement after use of contrast material, or internal echogenicity by ultrasonography; thick, irregular, or nodular septa; multiple locules; and mural nodularity, thickening, or enhancement. In Category III lesions, differentiation of a benign from a malignant cystic mass cannot be reliably made by radiologic criteria. Surgery is required for diagnosis, although a renal sparing procedure may be justified. Characteristics of Category IV lesions are similar to those of Category III but are more unequivocally associated with malignancy. Category IV lesions are therefore typically treated by nephrectomy. Although the general principles of this classification system are useful, several difficulties must be kept in mind (Wilson et al., 1996). There has been at least one example of a Category II hyperdense mass that was a carcinoma of the kidney (Hartman et al., 1992). Some parameters that distinguish Category II from Category III are qualitative, as, for example, "small amount" of calcification. Thus, observers may be inconsistent in assigning a lesion to Category II or III (Siegel et al., 1997). As emphasized in this chapter, considerations such as pretest probability and clinical circumstances unique to a given patient may support serial imaging follow-up for some Category II lesions if surgery is not to be performed.

BIBLIOGRAPHY

Agrons, G. A., Wagner, B. J., Davidson, A. J., and Suarez, E. S.: Multilocular cystic renal tumor in children: Radiologic-pathologic correlation. Radiographics 15:653, 1995.

Amendola, M. A., Bree, R. L., Pollack, H. M., Francis, I. R., Glazer, G. M., Jafri, S. Z. H., Tomaszewski, J. E.: Small renal cell carcinomas: Resolving a diagnostic dilemma. Radiology 166:637, 1988.

Aronson, S., Frazier, H. A., Baluch, J. D., Hartman, D. S., and Christenson, P. J.: Cystic renal masses: Usefulness of the Bosniak classification. Urol. Radiol. 13:83, 1991.

Bennington, J. L., and Beckwith, J. B.: Tumors of the upper urinary tract. In Tumors of the Kidney, Renal Pelvis, and Ureter. Washington, D.C., Armed Forces Institute of Pathology, 1975, pp. 25–192.

Bennington, J. L., and Beckwith, J. B.: Mesenchymal tumors of the kidney. In Tumors of the Kidney, Renal Pelvis, and Ureter. Wasington, D.C., Armed Forces Institute of Pathology, 1975, pp. 201–242.

Black, W. C., and Ling, A.: Is earlier diagnosis really better? The misleading effects of lead time and length biases. AJR 155:625, 1990.

Bosniak, M. A.: The current radiological approach to renal cysts. Radiology 158:1, 1986.

Bosniak, M. A.: Difficulties in classifying cystic lesions of the kidney. Urol. Radiol. 13:91, 1991.

Bosniak, M. A.: The small (<3.0 cm) renal parenchymal tumor: Detection, diagnosis, and controversies. Radiology 179:307, 1991.

Bosniak, M. A., Birnbaum, B. A., Krinsky, G. A., and Waisman, J.: Small renal parenchymal neoplasms: Further observations on growth. Radiology 197:589, 1995.

Bosniak, M. A., Megibow, A. J., Hulnick, D. H., Horii, S., and Raghavendra, B. N.: CT diagnosis of renal angiomyolipoma: The importance of detecting small amounts of fat. AJR 151:497, 1988.

Bosniak, M. A., and Rofsky, N. M.: Problems in the detection and characterization of small renal masses. Radiology 198:638, 1996.

Chovnick, S. D., and Silvert, D. S.: Infected solitary cyst of the kidney. J. Urol. 83:7, 1960.

Choyke, P. L.: MR imaging in renal cell carcinoma. Radiology 169:572, 1998.

Choyke, P. L., Glenn, G. M., Walther, M. M., Zbar, B., Weiss, G. H., Alexander, R. B., Hayes, W. S., Long, J. P., Thakore, K. N., and Linehan, W. M.: The natural history of renal lesions in von Hippel-Lindau disease: A serial CT study in 28 patients. AJR 159:1229, 1992.

Chung, C. J., Lorenzo, R., Rayder, S., Schemankewitz, E., Guy, C. D., Cutting, J., and Munden, M.: Rhabdoid tumors of the kidney in children: CT findings. AJR 164:697, 1995.

Cohan, R. H., Dunnick, N. R., Degesys, G. E., and Korobkin, M.: Computed tomography of renal oncocytoma. J. Comput. Assist. Tomogr. 8:284, 1984.

Cohan, R. H., Sherman, L. S., Korobkin, M., Bass, J. C., and Francis, I. R.: Renal masses: Assessment of corticomedullary phases and nephrographic phase CT scan. Radiology 197:445, 1995.

Coleman, B. G., Arger, P. H., Mintz, M. C., Pollack, H. M., and Banner, M. P.: Hyperdense renal masses: A computed tomographic dilemma. AJR 143:291, 1984.

Crotty, K. L., Orihuela, E., and Warren, M. M.: Recent advances in the diagnosis and treatment of renal arteriovenous malformations and fistulas. J. Urol. 150:1355, 1993.

Curry, N. S.: Small renal masses (lesions smaller than 3 cm): Imaging evaluation and management. AJR 164:355, 1995.

Curry, N. S., Brock, G., Metcalf, J. S., and Sens, M. A.: Hyperdense renal mass: Unusual CT appearance of a benign renal cyst. Urol. Radiol. 4:33, 1982.

Curry, N. S., Reining, J., Schabel, S. I., Ross, P., Vujic, I., and Gobien, R. P.: An evaluation of the effectiveness of CT vs other imaging modalities in the diagnosis of atypical renal masses. Invest. Radiol. 19:447, 1984.

Curry, N. S., Schabel, S. I., and Betsill, W. L.: Small renal neoplasms: Diagnostic imaging, pathologic features, and clinical course. Radiology 158:113, 1986.

Curry, N. S.: Atypical cystic renal masses. Abdom. Imaging 23:230, 1998.

Davidson, A. J., Choyke, P. L., Hartman, D. S., and Davis, C. J.:

Renal medullary carcinoma associated with sickle cell trait: Radiologic findings. Radiology 195:83, 1995.

Davidson, A. J., and Davis, C. J.: Fat in renal adenocarcinoma: Never say never. Radiology 188:316, 1993.

Davidson, A. J., Hayes, W. S., Hartman, D. S., McCarthy, W. F., and Davis, C. J.: Renal oncocytoma and carcinoma: Failure of differentiation with CT. Radiology 186:693, 1993.

Dinney, C. P. N., Awad, S. A., Gajewski, J. B., Belitsky, P., Lannon, S. G., Mack, F. G., and Millard, O. H.: Analysis of imaging modalities, staging systems, and prognostic indicators for renal cell carcinoma. Urology 39:122, 1992.

Dunnick, N. R.: Renal lesions: Great strides in imaging. Radiology 182:305, 1992.

Dunnick, N. R., Korobkin, M., and Clark, W. M.: CT demonstration of hyperdense renal carcinoma. J. Comput. Assist. Tomogr. 8:1023, 1984.

Dunnick, N. R., Korobkin, M., Silverman, P. M., and Foster, W. L.: Computed tomography of high density renal cysts. J. Comput. Assist. Tomogr. 8:458, 1984.

Einstein, D. M., Herts, B. R., Weaver, R., Obuchowski, N., Zep, R., and Singer, A.: Evaluation of renal masses detected by excretory urography: Cost-effectiveness of sonography versus CT. AJR 164:371, 1995.

Fishman, M. C., Pollack, H. M., Arger, P. H., and Banner, M. P.: High protein content: Another cause of CT hyperdense benign renal cyst. J. Comput. Assist. Tomogr. 7:1103, 1983.

Forman, H. P., Middleton, W. D., Melson, G. L., and McClennan, B. L.: Hyperechoic renal cell carcinomas: Increase in detection at US. Radiology 188:431, 1993.

Foster, W. L., Roberts, L., Halvorsen, R. A., and Dunnick, N. R.: Sonography of small renal masses with indeterminate density characteristics on computed tomography. Urol. Radiol. 10:59, 1988.

Fowler, J. E., and Perkins, T.: Presentation, diagnosis and treatment of renal abscess: 1972–1988. J. Urol. 151:847, 1994.

Frank, W., Guinan, P., Stuhldreher, D., Saffrin, R., Ray, P., and Rubenstein, M.: Renal cell carcinoma: The size variable. J. Surg. Oncol. 54:163, 1993.

Frishman, E., Orron, D. E., Heiman, Z., Kessler, A., Kaver, I., and Graif, M.: Infected renal cysts: Sonographic diagnosis and management. J. Ultrasound Med. 13:7, 1994.

Glass, R. B. J., Davidson, A. J., Fernbach, S. K.: Clear cell sarcoma of the kidney: CT sonographic and pathologic correlation. Radiology 180:715, 1991.

Goldman, S. M., and Hartman, D. S.: The simple cyst. In Hartman, D. S. (ed.): Renal Cystic Disease. Philadelphia, W. B. Saunders, 1989, pp. 6–37.

Guinan, P. D., Vogelzang, N. J., Fremgen, A. M., Chmiel, J. S., Sylvester, J. L., Sener, S. F., and Imperato, J. F.: Renal cell carcinoma: Tumor size, stage and survival. Members of the Cancer Incidence and End Results Committee. J. Urol. 153:901, 1995.

Hajdu, S. I., Thomas, A. G., Talamo, T. S., and Shonnard, J. W.: Small renal adenocarcinoma with metastases. J. Urol. 124:132, 1980.

Hartman, D. S.: Pediatric renal tumors. In Taveras, J., Ferucci, J. (eds.): Radiology Diagnosis, Imaging, Intervention. Philadelphia, J. B. Lippincott, 1986, pp. 1–9.

Hartman, D. S., Aronson, S., and Frazer, H.: Current status of imaging indeterminate renal mass. Radiol. Clin. North Am. 29:475, 1991.

Hartman, D. S., Lesar, M. S. C., Madewell, J. E., and Davis, C. J.: Mesoblastic nephroma: Radiologic-pathologic correlation of 20 cases. AJR 136:69, 1981.

Hartman, D. S., Weatherby, E., Laskin, W. B., Brody, J. M., Corse, W., and Baluch, J. D.: Cystic renal cell carcinoma: CT findings simulating a benign hyperdense cyst: Case report. AJR 159:1235, 1992.

Hélénon, O., Chretien, Y., Paraf, F., Melki, P., Denys, A., and Moreau, J. F.: Renal cell carcinoma containing fat: Demonstration with CT. Radiology 188:429, 1993.

Hellsten, S., Berge, T., and Wehlin, L.: Unrecognized renal cell carcinoma. Scand. J. Urol. Nephrol. 15:269, 1981.

Hill, G. S.: Renal Infection. In Hill, G. S. (ed.): Uropathology. New York, Churchill Livingstone, 1989, pp. 333–430.

Honda, H., Onitsuka, H., Naitov, S., Hasoo, K., Kamoi, I., Hanada, K, Kumazawa, J., and Masuda, K.: Renal arteriovenous malformations: CT features. J. Comput. Assist. Tomogr. 15:261, 1991.

Hopper, K. D., Holabinko, J. N., Ten Have, T. R., and Hartman, D. S.: Variability of Hounsfield Unit measurements based on CT of a renal cyst (abstract). Radiology 197(P):147, 1995.

Jamis-Dow, C. A., Choyke, P. L., Jennings, S. B., Linehan, W. M., Thakore, K. N., and Walther, M. M.: Small (<3 cm) renal masses: Detection with CT versus US and pathologic correlation. Radiology 198:785, 1996.

Kenneley, M. J., Grossman, H. B. and Cho, K. J.: Outcome analysis of 42 cases of renal angiomyolipoma. J. Urol. 152:1988, 1994.

Kessler, O., Mukamel, E., Hadar, H., Gillon, G., Konechezky, M., and Servadio, C.: Effect of improved diagnosis of renal cell carcinoma on the course of the disease. J. Surg. Oncol. 57:201, 1994.

Kier, R., Taylor, K. J. W., Feyock, A. L., and Ramos, I. M.: Renal masses: Characterization with Doppler US. Radiology 176:703, 1990.

Kinder, P. W., and Rous, S. N.: Infected renal cysts from hematogenous seeding: A case report and review of the literature. J. Urol. 120:239, 1978.

Kurosaki, Y., Tanaka, Y., Kuramoto, K., and Itai, Y.: Improved CT fat detection in small kidney angiomyolipomas using thin sections and single voxel measurements. J. Comput. Assist. Tomogr. 17:745, 1993.

Lemaitre, L., Robert, Y., Dubrulle, F., Claudon, M., Duhamel, A., Danjou, P., and Mazeman, E.: Renal angiomyolipoma: Growth followed up with CT and/or US. Radiology 197:598, 1995.

Levine, E., Huntrakoon, M., and Wetzel, L. H.: Small renal neoplasms: Clinical, pathologic, and imaging features. AJR 153:69, 1989.

Limjoco, U. R., and Strauch, A. E.: Infected solitary cyst of the kidney: Report of a case and review of the literature. J. Urol. 96:625, 1966.

Marotti, M., Hricak, H., Fritzsche, P., Crooks, L. E., Hedgcock, M. W., and Tanagho, E. A.: Complex and simple renal cysts: Comparative evaluation with MR imaging. Radiology 162:679, 1987.

McGowan, A. J., and Ippolito, J. J.: Infected solitary renal cyst. J. Urol. 93:359, 1965.

Millan, J. C.: Tumors of the kidney. In Hill, G. S. (ed.): Uropathology. New York, Churchill Livingstone, 1989, pp. 623–702.

Montie, J. E.: The incidental renal mass: Management alternatives. Urol. Clin. North Am. 18:427, 1991.

Morra, M. N., and Das, S.: Renal oncocytoma: A review of histogenesis, histopathology, diagnosis and treatment. J. Urol. 150:295, 1993.

Pearlstein, A. E.: Hyperdense renal cysts. J. Comput. Assist. Tomogr. 7:1029, 1983.

Quinn, M. J., Hartman, D. S., Friedman, A. C., Sherman, J. L., Lawtin, E. N., Pyatt, R. S., Ho, C. K., Csere, R., and Fromowitz, F. B.: Renal oncocytoma: New observations. Radiology 153:49, 1984.

Quint, L. E., Glazer, G. M., and Chenevert, T. L.: In vivo and in vitro MR imaging of renal tumors: Histopathologic correlation and pulse sequence optimization. Radiology 169:359, 1988.

Ritchie, A. W., and deKernion, J. B.: Incidental renal neoplasms: Incidence in Los Angeles County, treatment and prognosis. Prog. Clin. Biol. Res. 269:347, 1988.

Rosenberg, E. R., Korobkin, M., Foster, W., Silverman, P. M., Bowie, J. D., and Dunnick, N. R.: The significance of septations in a renal cyst. AJR 144:593, 1985.

Segal, A. J., and Spitzer, R. M.: Pseudo thick-walled renal cyst by CT. AJR 132:827, 1979.

Siegel, C. L., McFarland, E. G., Brink, J. A., Fisher, A. J., Humphrey, P., and Heiken, J. P.: CT of cystic renal masses: Analysis of diagnostic performance and interobserver variation. AJR 169:813, 1997.

Smelka, R. C., Shoenut, J. P., Kroeker, M. A., MacMahon, R., and Greenberg, H. M.: Renal lesions: Controlled comparison between CT and 1.5-T MR imaging with nonenhanced and gadolinium-enhanced fat suppressed spin-echo and breath-hold FLASH techniques. Radiology 182:425, 1992.

Smith, S. J., Bosniak, M. A., Megibow, A. J., Hulnick, D. H., Horii, S., and Raghavendra, B. N.: Renal cell carcinoma: Earlier discovery and increased detection. Radiology *170*:699, 1989.

Steiner, M. S., Goldman, S. M., Fishman, E. K., and Marshall, F. F.: The natural history of renal angiomyolipoma. J. Urol. *150*:1782, 1993.

Strotzer, M., Lehner, K. B., and Becker, K.: Detection of fat in a renal cell carcinoma mimicking angiomyolipoma. Radiology *188*:427, 1993.

Subramanyam, B. R., Lefleur, R. S., and Bosniak, M. A.: Renal arteriovenous fistulas and aneurysm: Sonographic findings. *149*:261, 1983.

Sussman, S., Cochran, S. T., Pagani, J. J., McArdle, C., Wong, W., Austin, R., Curry, N., and Kelly, K. M.: Hyperdense renal masses: A CT manifestation of hemorrhagic renal cysts. Radiology *150*:207, 1984.

Takebayashi, S., Aida, N., and Matsui, K.: Arteriovenous malformations of the kidneys: Diagnosis and followup with color Doppler sonography in six patients. AJR *157*:991, 1991.

Talamo, T. S., and Shonnard, J. W.: Small renal adenocarcinoma with metastases. J. Urol. *124*:132, 1980.

Talner, L. B., Davidson, A. J., Lebowitz, R. L., Dalla Palma, L., and Goldman, S. M.: Acute pyelonephritis: Can we agree on terminology? Radiology *192*:297, 1994.

Tosaka, A., Ohya, K., Yamada, K., Ohashi, H., Kitahara, S., Sekine, H., Takehara, Y., and Oka, K.: Incidence and properties of renal masses and asymptomatic renal cell carcinoma detected by abdominal ultrasonography. J. Urol. *144*:1097, 1990.

Tsukamoto, T., Kumamoto, Y., Yamazaki, K, Miyao, N., Takahashi, A., and Masumori, N.: Clinical analysis of incidentally found renal cell carcinomas. Eur. Urol. *19*:109, 1991.

Warshauer, D. M., McCarthy, S. M., and Street, L.: Detection of renal masses: Sensitivities and specificities of excretory urography/linear tomography, US, and CT. Radiology *169*: 363, 1988.

Wills, J. S.: Management of small renal neoplasms and angiomyolipoma: A growing problem. Radiology *197*:583, 1995.

Wilson, T. E., Duelle, E. A., Cohan, R. H., Wojno, K., and Korobkin, M.: Cystic renal masses: A reevaluation of the usefulness of the Bosniak classification system. Acad. Radiol. *3*:564, 1996.

Yamashita, Y., Takahashi, M., Watanabe, O., Yoshimatsu, S., Ueno, S., Ishimaru, S., Kan, M., Takano, S., and Minumiya, N.: Small renal cell carcinoma: Pathologic and radiologic correlation. Radiology *184*:493, 1992.

Zagoria, R. J., Wolfman, N. T., Karstaedt, N., Hinn, G. C., Dyer, R. B., and Chen, Y. M.: CT features of renal cell carcinoma with emphasis on relation to tumor size. Invest. Radiol. *14*:261, 1990.

Zagoria, R. J., and Dyer, R. B.: The small renal mass: Detection, characterization, and management. Abdom. Imaging *23*:256, 1998.

Zirinsky, K., Auh, Y. H., Rubenstein, W. A., Williams, J. J., Pasmantier, M. W., and Kazam, E.: CT of hyperdense renal cysts: Sonographic correlation. AJR *143*:151, 1984.

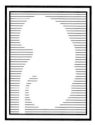

29

Radiologic Evaluation of Urinary Tract Trauma

KIDNEY
URETER

BLADDER
URETHRA

KIDNEY

The kidney is frequently injured in blunt abdominal trauma, although most damage is minor and does not require specific treatment. When renal injury is serious, abnormalities in other organs are often present. This is particularly so in patients with penetrating trauma in whom 80 per cent have multiple organ involvement. In contradistinction, only 20 to 30 per cent of patients with blunt trauma have an injury of other organs.

Abnormal kidneys are more susceptible to injury than normal kidneys, presumably because of their often enlarged size and diminished mobility. Kidneys with tumor, hydronephrosis due to any cause, fusion abnormalities (viz., horseshoe kidney), ectopia, and polycystic disease may be severely injured in association with mild trauma.

None of the several grading systems for renal trauma have been widely accepted. Typically, renal injury is graded as minor, moderate, or major with several subsets to fill out specific elements. In the absence of one dominant classification, it is especially important to precisely describe each injury.

Minor injury (75 to 85 per cent) includes superficial laceration that does not involve the collecting system, focal contusion, small intrarenal hematoma, segmental infarction, and a small subcapsular or perinephric hematoma. Minor injuries are usually treated conservatively.

Moderate injury (10 per cent) applies to a laceration that extends to and communicates with the collecting system, a moderate to large perirenal hematoma, and renal fracture. Surgical intervention in these patients is usually determined by the patient's hemodynamic status as well as by the size and stability of extrarenal blood and urine collections.

Major injury (5 per cent) includes a shattered kidney, vascular pedicle injury (including arterial thrombosis or laceration and venous avulsion), avulsion of the ureteropelvic junction, and laceration of the renal pelvis. Major renal trauma is typically treated surgically in an attempt to maintain parenchymal viability or to control life-threatening hemorrhage. Angiographic embolization may be a suitable alternative to surgery for control of hemorrhage.

Clinical Setting

The clinical findings of renal trauma are variable and include microscopic or gross hematuria, flank pain, tenderness, hypotension, and shock. Radiologic evaluation is indicated in patients with gross hematuria, in patients with microscopic hematuria and hypotension, and in all patients with suspected renal injury associated with penetrating trauma.

Radiologic Techniques

Computed Tomography. Computed tomography is the imaging modality of choice for the evaluation of suspected renal trauma. Images should be obtained after a bolus of 100 to 150 mL of contrast material. Unenhanced studies are rarely required. Power injection maximizes parenchymal density and enhances detection of active bleeding. Spiral technique permits the rapid acquisition of 8- to 10-mm scans throughout the abdomen and pelvis. Bowel opacification is essential for the detection of nonrenal trauma.

Angiography. The availability of computed tomography coupled with the realization that most renal injuries are best managed conservatively has greatly diminished the need for angiography in renal trauma. In selected patients, however, angiography may provide both diagnostic and therapeutic advantage.

Arteriovenous aneurysm (fistula) is an arterial to venous shunt, often hemodynamically significant, that complicates some cases of blunt or penetrating renal trauma. Hematuria or hypertension may result. Angiography not only accurately identifies this abnormality but also provides access for transcatheter embolization of the aneurysm. Arteriovenous aneurysm is to be distinguished from congenital arteriovenous malformation, which is discussed in detail in Chapter 12.

An initial midstream aortogram should be performed to evaluate the number and status of the renal arteries. Although an aortogram alone may provide adequate assessment of the kidneys, optimal evaluation often requires selective renal artery injections. Digital subtraction imaging is the method of choice. Filming sequence must be timed to include arterial, capillary and venous phases.

Radiologic Findings

Parenchymal Abnormalities

Contusion is caused by a blunt force that disrupts the renal microvasculature and leads to bleeding in the interstitial space. The contusion may involve the entire kidney or be limited to one area. Renal enlargement develops in the contused region, but the reniform shape is preserved, as is characteristic of all interstitial processes. Likewise, nephrographic density is diminished in affected portions (Fig. 29–1). These changes are similar to those seen in renal infarction, which are discussed further in Chapter 9.

Hematoma refers to a discrete collection of blood within the renal parenchyma. A hematoma is manifested by computed tomography as a round or oval mass with a poorly marginated border. An acute hematoma is hyperdense relative to unenhanced normal parenchyma and has an attenuation value of 50 to 60 Hounsfield units. With time, the attenuation value decreases to that of water.

Laceration refers to tearing of the kidney by a shearing or crushing force. This is distinguished from a *renal incision* caused by penetrating trauma. Laceration is diagnosed when a blood-filled cleft extends through the renal capsule (Fig. 29–2). Extravasation of contrast material and/or urine indicates that a laceration extends into the collecting system.

Fracture indicates separation of renal parenchyma into fragments. Typically, the capsule is disrupted and a perinephric hematoma forms (see Fig. 29–1). If the fracture is between major vascular branches, there may be only a small amount of hemorrhage. Renal function is preserved in each of the separated fracture fragments unless devascularization has occurred (Fig. 29–3; see Fig. 29–1).

Juxtarenal Abnormalities

Subcapsular hematoma is typically a biconvex-shaped collection of blood between the renal parenchyma and the capsule. High pressure within the subcapsular space flattens the renal parenchyma and may interfere with renal perfusion and urine formation. As a result, an ipsilateral prolonged nephrogram and a delayed pyelogram may be noted (Fig. 29–4). Most subcapsular hematomas resolve with conservative management. However, some persist, organize, calcify, and cause renovascular hypertension, a phenomenon known as *Page kidney*. This is also discussed in Chapter 21. Biconvex, lentiform peripheral calcification is characteristic of

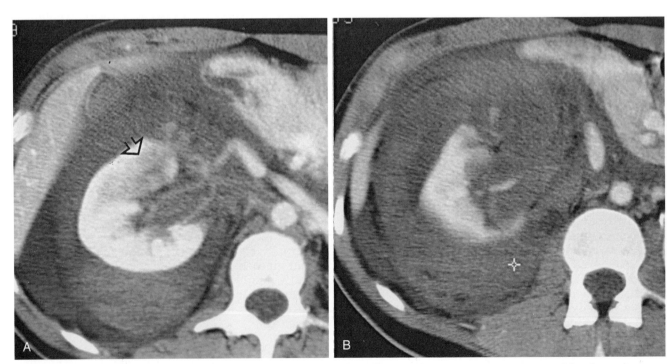

FIGURE 29–1. Contusion, fracture, and perirenal hematoma, right kidney. Computed tomograms, contrast material–enhanced.

A, There is an ill-defined focal decrease in parenchymal enhancement in the ventral aspect of the upper pole *(arrow).* Blood in the perinephric space surrounds the kidney.

B, The lower pole is separated from the upper pole and is distorted by the perinephric hemorrhage.

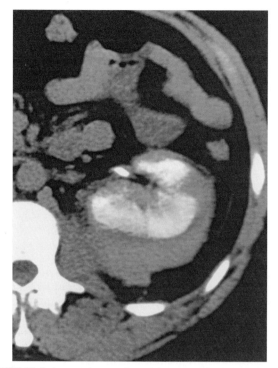

FIGURE 29–2. Laceration, perirenal hematoma, and persistent nephrogram, left kidney. Computed tomogram, contrast material–enhanced. A hematoma-filled cleft extends through the renal capsule into the perinephric space. The perinephric hemorrhage causes delayed excretion of contrast material, resulting in a persistent, dense nephrogram.

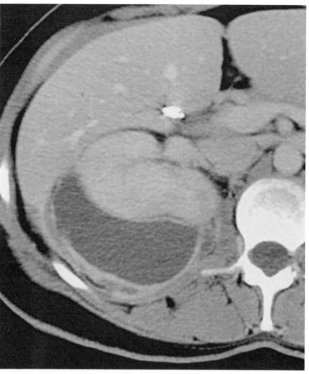

FIGURE 29–4. Subcapsular hematoma with delayed nephrogram and pyelogram, right kidney. Computed tomogram, contrast material–enhanced. Compression of the kidney by the hematoma causes delayed contrast material excretion.

FIGURE 29–3. Fracture, right kidney, with infarction and a small perinephric hematoma. Computed tomogram, contrast material–enhanced. There is a fracture through the ventral aspect of the upper pole of the right kidney extending through the capsule. The fractured segment is devascularized and therefore does not enhance. A small perinephric hemorrhage surrounds the kidney.

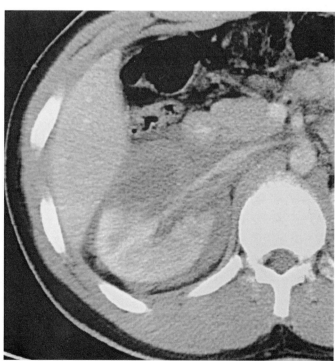

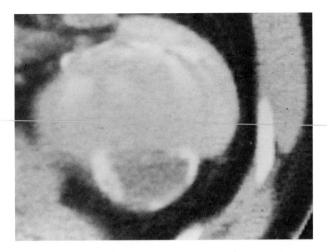

FIGURE 29–5. Calcified subcapsular hematoma. Computed tomogram, contrast material–enhanced. There is a peripheral biconvex calcification compressing the renal parenchyma.

chronic subcapsular hematoma (Fig. 29–5; see also Fig. 21–22).

Perirenal hematoma refers to blood that has accumulated between the renal capsule, which is usually disrupted, and the renal fascia (see Figs. 29–1 through 29–3). The renal fascia provides a tamponade effect that usually slows or stops bleeding. Unlike subcapsular hematoma, perinephric hematoma often completely surrounds the kidney and rarely extends into the contralateral perinephric space by way of fascial communications located anterior to the lower aorta and inferior vena cava. A perirenal hematoma can become quite large and fill the cone of renal fascia extending into the true pelvis. The kidney typically is not compressed nor is function compromised. Small amounts of blood in the perirenal fat produce streaks of soft tissue density within the perirenal fat.

As discussed in Chapter 21, there are bridging septa or renorenal fascia in the perinephric space. These may contain the spread of a perinephric hematoma, thereby creating a localized collection of blood that is indistinguishable from a subcapsular hematoma. Differentiation between these two, however, does not impact management.

Collecting System Abnormalities

Hematoma in the pelvis is characterized as a filling defect with a density on computed tomography between that of unenhanced and enhanced renal parenchyma (Fig. 29–6). A large pelvic blood clot is likely to cause an acute obstruction. A pelvic hematoma often forms a cast of the collecting system with a resultant "hand-in-glove" appearance on an excretory urogram or retrograde pyelogram (Fig. 29–7). Another characteristic of collecting system

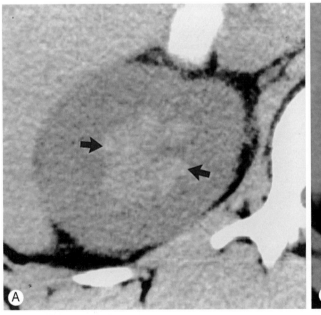
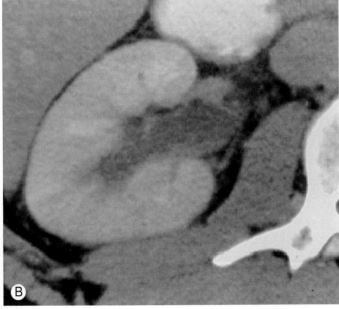

FIGURE 29–6. Pelvic hematoma, right kidney.
A, Computed tomogram, unenhanced. The hematoma *(arrows)* fills the pelvis and is of greater density than the surrounding unenhanced renal parenchyma.
B, Computed tomogram, contrast material–enhanced. The hematoma is less dense than enhanced parenchyma.

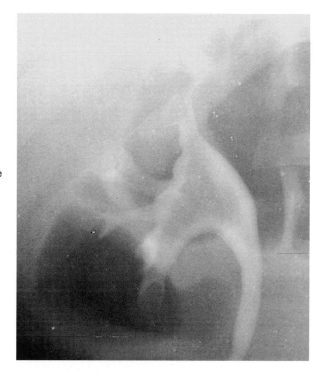

FIGURE 29–7. Pelvic hematoma, right kidney. Excretory urogram. The blood clot, relatively radiolucent within the opacified pelvis, conforms to the shape of the renal pelvis and calyces, resulting in a "hand-in-glove" appearance.

blood clot is that it changes in appearance on serial examinations owing to thrombolysis caused by urinary urokinase. The differential diagnosis of pelvic filling defects is discussed in Chapters 14 through 16.

Extravasation of contrast material from a ruptured pelvocalyceal system is usually seen only when there has been major parenchymal laceration (Fig. 29–8). Extravasation with normal renal parenchyma may be seen as a complication of concomitant ureteral obstruction or ureteropelvic junction avulsion (Fig. 29–9).

Avulsion of the ureteropelvic junction is uncommon and indicates severe trauma. Computed tomography demonstrates contrast material extravasation into an inferomedially located urinoma on delayed images. Identification of an unopacified ureter within the urinoma confirms the ureteropelvic junction transection.

Vascular Abnormalities

Arterial occlusion involves either the main renal artery or one of its branches and is usually due to stretching of the vessel with or without an intimal tear. In either situation there is a decrease in blood flow followed by thrombosis and infarction.

An acute main renal artery occlusion is seen as an absent nephrogram on contrast material–enhanced computed tomography (Fig. 29–10A). A thin rim of peripheral cortical enhancement may occur (see Fig. 29–10B). This *cortical rim nephrogram* represents perfusion of juxtacapsular nephrons through collateral arterial pathways. This subject is also discussed in Chapter 9.

Occlusion of branches of the renal artery usually results in segmental or lobar infarction recognized

as a wedge-shaped nephrographic defect. The base of the triangle abuts the capsule with the apex centrally (Fig. 29–11). Other abnormal nephrographic patterns are determined by the specific vessel that is involved. An occlusion of the major ventral or dorsal branch of the main renal artery leads to an absent nephrogram in the corresponding ventral or dorsal renal set of lobes (Fig. 29–12). If, on the other hand, an accessory renal artery is occluded, the nephrographic abnormality is usually confined to either the upper or lower poles. See Chapters 5 and 6 for further discussion of renal infarction.

Avulsion of the renal pedicle is associated with an absent nephrogram and an associated hematoma. Abrupt termination of the artery is demonstrated either by angiography or computed tomography. This uncommon injury may be fatal.

Aneurysm or *pseudoaneurysm* from trauma is rare and almost always is the result of penetrating injury. Whereas large aneurysms can be identified utilizing computed tomography or ultrasonography, including color Doppler imaging, definitive diagnosis usually requires angiography (Figs. 29–13, 29–14).

Arteriovenous aneurysm (fistula) sometimes complicates penetrating renal trauma, especially biopsy. Clincal findings, when present, include hematuria, flank or abdominal bruit, renovascular hypertension, and high-output cardiac failure. A small arteriovenous aneurysm usually requires angiography for visualization (see Fig. 29–14). Large lesions are readily detected by computed tomography, ultrasonography including color Doppler imaging, magnetic resonance imaging, or radionuclide studies (Fig. 29–15).

Text continued on page 709

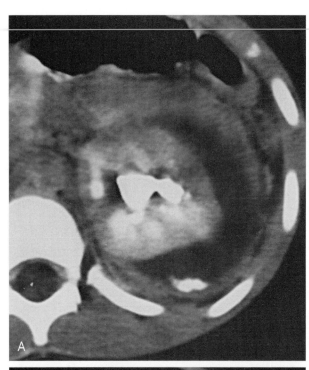

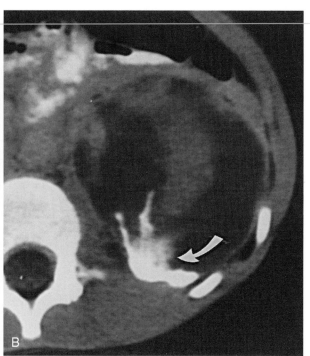

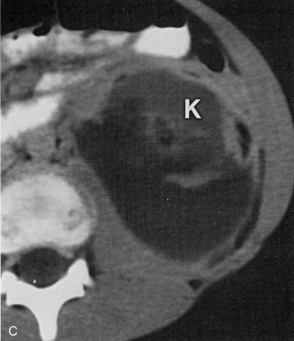

FIGURE 29–8. Fracture, left kidney, in a 7-year-old child after a bicycle accident. Computed tomogram, contrast material–enhanced.

A, Upper renal pole is intact and excretes urine.

B, Urine in the perirenal space *(arrow)* indicates a tear of the collecting system.

C, The lower pole of the kidney (K) is nonperfused owing to arterial occlusion or avulsion and is displaced by perirenal urine and blood.

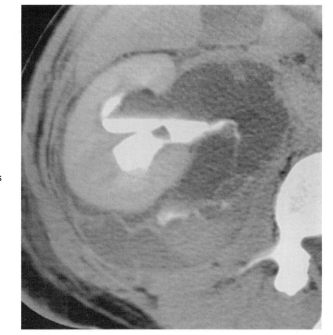

FIGURE 29–9. Extravasation of contrast material after instrumentation of right kidney. Computed tomogram, contrast material–enhanced. Contrast material extravasates from the pelvis into a urinoma, which is predominantly medial to the kidney.

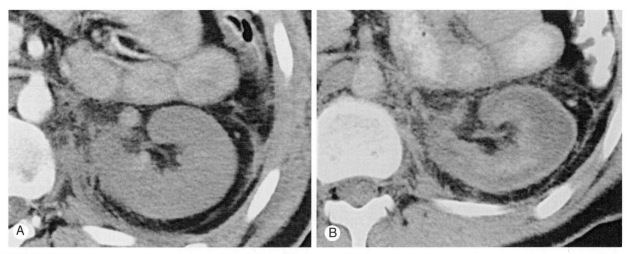

FIGURE 29–10. Infarction due to left renal artery occlusion after blunt abdominal trauma.

 A, Computed tomogram, contrast material–enhanced examination performed immediately after trauma. The nephrogram is absent.

 B, Computed tomogram, contrast material–enhanced, obtained 2 weeks later. Some function in the subcapsular area (cortical rim nephrogram) and the central juxtamedullary area has been restored by collateral arterial circulation. (Same patient illustrated in Fig. 27–8.)

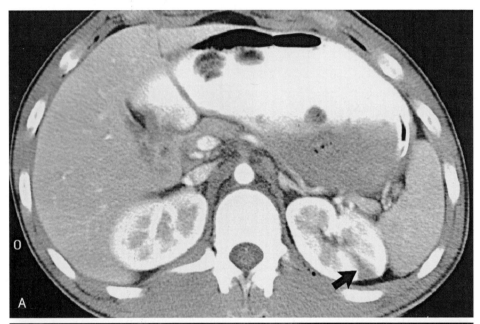

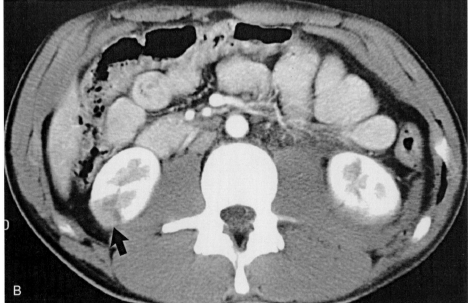

FIGURE 29–11. Lobar infarctions from emboli complicating thoracic aortic dissection in a patient with blunt thoracic trauma.

A and *B,* Computed tomograms, contrast material–enhanced. There are bilateral wedge-shaped zones of absent perfusion *(arrows).* The base of the triangle abuts the capsule, and the apex is central.

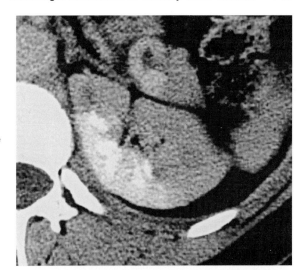

FIGURE 29–12. Infarction, ventral portion of the left kidney. Computed tomogram, contrast material–enhanced. Interruption of the artery to the ventral portion of the kidney results in nonperfusion. Renal contour remains normal.

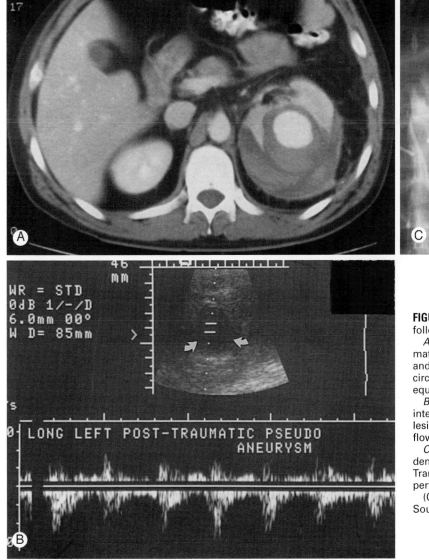

FIGURE 29–13. Pseudoaneurysm, left kidney, following stab wound.

A, Computed tomogram with contrast material enhancement demonstrates intrarenal and perirenal hemorrhage and a well-circumscribed central lesion that enhances equally with the aorta.

B, Ultrasonogram with Doppler interrogation. There is a "cystic" intrarenal lesion *(arrows)* with pulsatile disorganized flow.

C, Selective renal arteriogram directly demonstrates the pseudoaneurysm *(arrows).* Transcatheter embolization for control can be performed at this time.

(Courtesy of Philip Ralls, M.D., University of Southern California, Los Angeles, California.)

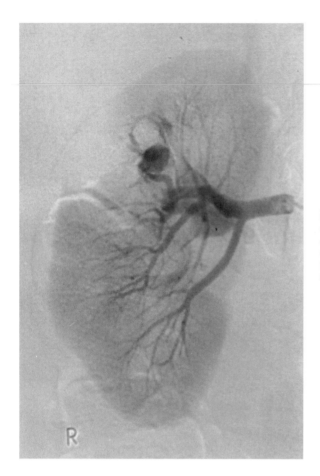

FIGURE 29–14. Pseudoaneurysm, lobar infarction and small arteriovenous aneurysm (fistula), right kidney. Selective renal arteriogram performed 8 days after a stab wound. There is a 1-cm pseudoaneurysm and an adjacent peripheral triangular zone of absent perfusion. Early visualization of the inferior vena cava indicates arteriovenous shunting at the site of the aneurysm.

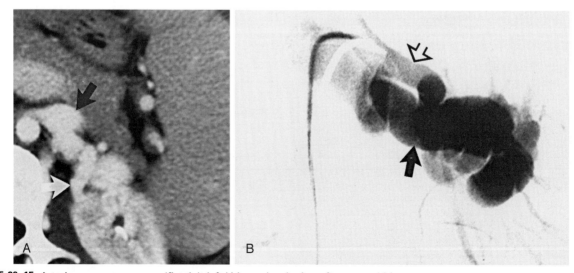

FIGURE 29–15. Arteriovenous aneurysm (fistula), left kidney, developing after a renal biopsy.
A, Computed tomogram, contrast material–enhanced. During the arterial phase of a dynamic scan, both the renal artery *(white arrow)* and renal vein *(black arrow)* are simultaneously opacified.
B, Selective left renal arteriogram, arterial phase. Renal artery *(open arrow)*; renal vein *(closed arrow)*.

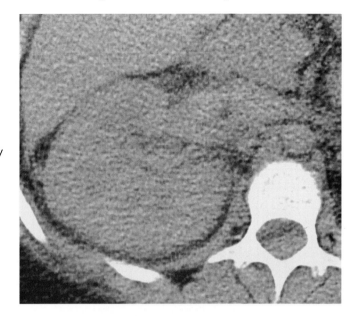

FIGURE 29–16. Renal vein thrombosis, right kidney. Computed tomogram, contrast material–enhanced. The kidney is globally enlarged. Both the nephrogram and pyelogram are absent. Venous thrombosis was confirmed by selective renal venography.

Renal vein thrombosis secondary to trauma is uncommon. Cases of isolated venous thrombosis demonstrate renal enlargement, delayed function, and attenuation of the intrarenal collecting system (Fig. 29–16). Thrombosis may be detected with computed tomography, magnetic resonance imaging, ultrasonography including color Doppler imaging, or selective renal venography.

URETER

Ureteral injuries are almost always the result of penetrating or iatrogenic trauma, either surgical or endourologic. Penetrating injuries of the ureter are usually associated with injuries to other organs, including the psoas muscle, bowel, liver, spleen, or major blood vessel. The ureters, on the other hand, are well protected from the effects of blunt abdominal trauma.

Surgical injury to the ureter includes ligation, contusion, laceration, devascularization, and periureteral hematoma. Those surgical procedures most often associated with ureteral injury include hysterectomy and other gynecologic procedures, aortic aneurysm resection, abdominal perineal resection, excision of pelvic tumors, lysis of adhesions, orthopedic procedures, and lumbar disk surgery.

Endourologic procedures that may result in ureteral injury include ureteroscopy, ureteral stone extraction, retrograde pyelography, ureterolithotomy, and ureteral stent placement.

Clinical Setting

The signs and symptoms of ureteral trauma relate to severity of the injury and whether both ureters are involved. Anuria usually follows bilateral ureteral injury. Unilateral injuries may not be recognized immediately unless there is a high degree of clinical suspicion. Acute symptoms, such as flank pain and fever, usually correlate with obstruction and/or extravasation. Hematuria is frequently absent. Sequelae of ureteral injury include stricture, hydronephrosis with variable postobstructive atrophy, and urinoma.

Ureteral stenting is successful in many cases of small ureteral lacerations. When associated with severe obstruction or large retroperitoneal fluid collections, nephrostomy and percutaneous drainage also may be required. Long-standing severe ureteral injuries may require excision of the traumatized ureter and reimplantation.

Radiologic Techniques

Traditionally, excretory urography has been the principal technique for the evaluation of suspected ureteral trauma (Fig. 29–17). The sensitivity for detecting ureteral injury and extravasation is dependent, however, on several factors, including the magnitude of extravasation and renal function.

Computed tomography with contrast material enhancement is now the preferred technique for evaluating ureteral trauma. This technique is extremely sensitive for detecting renal obstruction, diminished function, and extraluminal contrast material and is ideally suited for identifying perirenal and periureteral fluid collections (Figs. 29–18 through 29–20). At the same time, computed tomography depicts the other abdominal organs that are at risk for injury.

Once an abnormality is identified by computed tomography, retrograde or antegrade pyelography may provide more precise definition of the site and nature of the injury and, at the same time, facilitate stent placement (see Fig. 29–20*B*).

Radiologic Findings

The radiologic appearance of ureteral trauma is dependent on the mechanism of injury, the extent

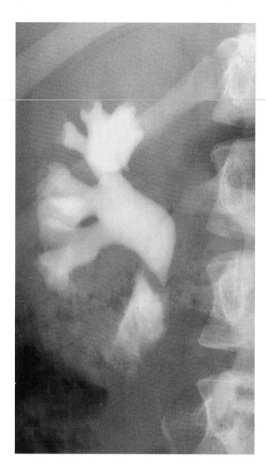

FIGURE 29–17. Rupture, right ureter, secondary to instrumentation. Excretory urogram. Contrast material extravasates from the proximal ureter into the retroperitoneum.

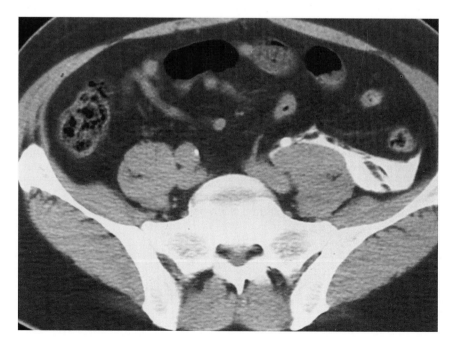

FIGURE 29–18. Periureteral extravasation of contrast material. Computed tomogram, contrast material–enhanced. Contrast material adjacent to the left ureter and psoas muscle is present within the retroperitoneum.

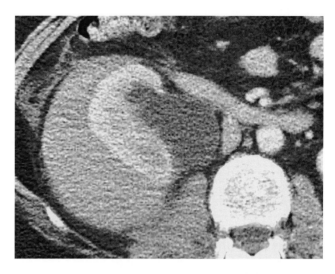

FIGURE 29–19. Perirenal hemorrhage and hydronephrosis after pelvic surgery. Computed tomogram, contrast material–enhanced, nephrogram phase. A 38-year-old woman had right flank pain for 10 days after hysterectomy. The high attenuation blood compresses and displaces the kidney. The renal pelvis is dilated.

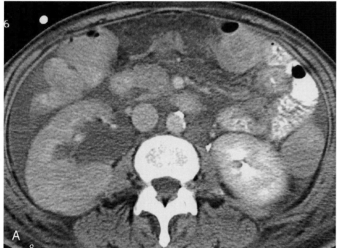

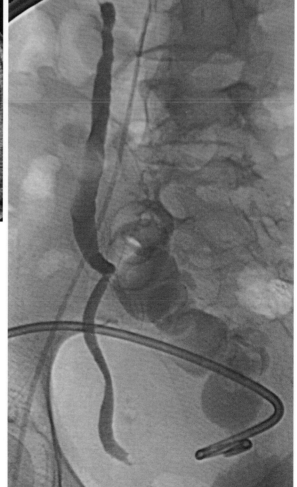

FIGURE 29–20. Ligation of right ureter after hysterectomy.
   A, Computed tomogram, contrast material–enhanced. The kidney is enlarged, and there is delayed excretion of contrast material and a dilated pelvis. Ascites is also present.
   B, Antegrade nephrostogram. There is abrupt termination of the right distal ureter near the expected ureterovesicle junction. Contrast material within the colon, a suprapubic drainage catheter, and a catheter within the inferior vena cava are also present.

of damage, and the time elapsed from the injury to the imaging study. Cases of ureteral laceration imaged immediately after trauma frequently show periureteric extravasation (see Figs. 29–17, 29–18). Other manifestations include varying degrees of obstruction, urinoma formation, blood in the perinephric space, and renal atrophy (see Figs. 29–19, 29–20).

BLADDER

Bladder injury, most commonly rupture, results from penetrating, blunt, or iatrogenic trauma. Approximately 10 per cent of patients with pelvic fracture have an associated bladder injury. Although several detailed classifications for bladder rupture exist, the two most clinically significant categories are *intraperitoneal* and *extraperitoneal.*

Intraperitoneal bladder rupture occurs at the dome of the bladder. This follows a sudden rise in intravesical pressure, as occurs with blunt abdominal trauma, especially in the presence of a distended bladder. Individuals involved in an automobile accident while wearing a lap-type seat belt are at particular risk for intraperitoneal bladder rupture. Children, whose distended bladder typically protrudes into the lower abdomen, are also more likely to experience this type of bladder injury. Approximately 25 per cent of patients with intraperitoneal bladder rupture have no associated pelvic fracture.

Extraperitoneal rupture of the bladder due to blunt trauma is almost always associated with a spicule of bone from a fracture of the anterior pelvic arch lacerating the bladder base. In some cases the bladder tear occurs at a site that is remote from the pelvic fracture, suggesting a compression and bursting mechanism rather than a direct laceration.

Penetrating trauma (e.g., from a bullet or knife) may result in intraperitoneal rupture, extraperitoneal rupture, or combined bladder injury. Injury to other viscera often occurs.

Clinical Setting

Bladder injury may be accompanied by lower abdominal or suprapubic pain. Hematuria is almost always present, often with clots. Despite an urge to void, the patient may be unable to urinate.

Intraperitoneal bladder rupture is usually repaired surgically as an emergency. Most extraperitoneal bladder ruptures close spontaneously and are, therefore, usually managed conservatively with an indwelling bladder catheter. Patients with external penetrating trauma are often subjected to surgical exploration to evaluate associated injury to bowel, blood vessels, and other viscera.

Radiologic Techniques

Retrograde cystography is the preferred technique for evaluating suspected bladder injury. It is essential to first exclude an associated urethral injury by performing a retrograde urethrogram, as described in the following section. Once urethral patency is established and a preliminary radiograph obtained, dilute (25 to 30 per cent) contrast material is instilled slowly into the bladder using a gravity drip. The study should be performed under fluoroscopic control, if possible. Otherwise, an initial radiograph is obtained after instillation of approximately 100 mL of contrast material and serial radiographs thereafter are required to monitor the course of the examination. The earliest images, obtained either by fluoroscopy or radiography, must be carefully evaluated for leakage of contrast material outside the bladder lumen. If this is not detected, additional contrast material up to a volume of between 300 and 400 mL is given. Oblique projections assist in the detection of a small amount of extravesical contrast material, but these may be difficult to obtain in the setting of acute trauma. A radiograph after draining the bladder is essential at the completion of the study to detect those cases in which there is delayed leakage of contrast material outside the bladder.

Computed tomographic cystography may be used in place of conventional cystography in those patients undergoing abdominal and pelvic computed tomography. The bladder should be filled with 300 mL of very dilute contrast material before 10-mm contiguous sections through the bladder are obtained. Post-void images should be obtained. Computed tomographic evaluation of the bladder using only contrast material excreted after an intravenous injection is insensitive in detecting bladder injury unless delayed scans are obtained during optimal bladder distention.

Radiologic Findings

Diagnosis of intraperitoneal bladder injury depends on the demonstration of contrast material entering the peritoneal cavity from the bladder. The contrast material surrounds loops of bowel and intraperitoneal viscera and fills the paracolic gutters (Fig. 29–21).

Contrast material leakage in an *uncomplicated* extraperitoneal rupture is limited to the pelvic extraperitoneal space (Fig. 29–22). A *complex* extraperitoneal injury is characterized by spread of contrast material beyond this space and into the scrotum, perineum, retroperitoneum, thigh, penis, or anterior abdominal wall (Fig. 29–23). Severe, complex extraperitoneal injury may be confused with an intraperitoneal bladder rupture.

URETHRA

The urethra is subject to injury by blunt, penetrating, or iatrogenic causes. Injury of the male urethra is classified either as a *posterior urethral injury,* which is typically associated with pelvic fracture, or as an *anterior urethral injury,* which is usually not

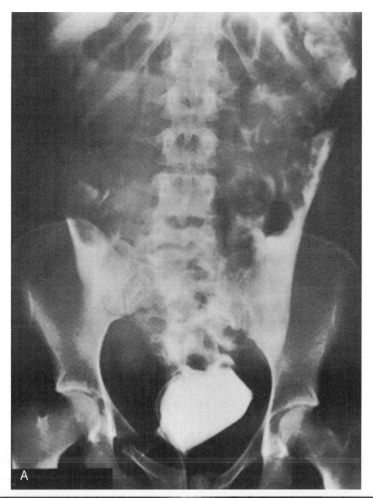

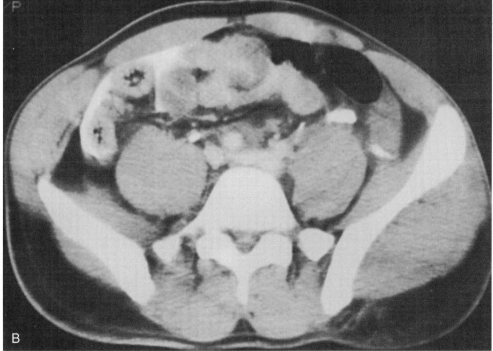

FIGURE 29–21. Bladder rupture, intraperitoneal, in two patients.
   A, A cystogram demonstrates contrast material outlining loops of small and large bowel.
   B, Computed tomogram, contrast material–enhanced. Contrast material surrounds loops of bowel.

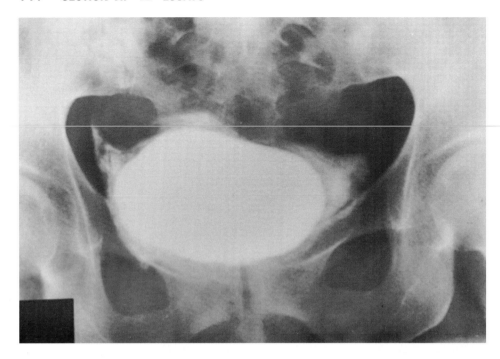

FIGURE 29–22. Bladder rupture, *simple* extraperitoneal. Cystogram. The leakage of contrast material from the bladder is limited to the perivesical extraperitoneal space of the pelvis.

associated with pelvic fracture. Posterior urethral and bladder injuries sometimes coexist.

Posterior urethral injury occurs in as many as 10 per cent of males with pelvic fracture. The urethra is subject to a shearing force when a pelvic fracture disrupts the urogenital diaphragm and the puboprostatic ligaments, resulting in displacement of the prostate gland.

The radiologic classification of urethral injury is based on the following definitions, which are illustrated in Figure 29–24:

Type 1. The posterior urethra is intact but stretched, narrowed, and elongated. The prostate is displaced proximally owing to the disruption of the puboprostatic ligaments. Resultant hematoma elevates the bladder high in the pelvis. No contrast material is present in the periurethral tissue.

Type II. Disruption of the urethra occurs above the urogenital diaphragm at the junction of the posterior and membranous urethra, which is intact.

Type III. The membranous urethra is disrupted with extension of the injury to the proximal bulbous urethra and/or disruption of the urogenital diaphragm. This is the most frequent posterior urethral injury.

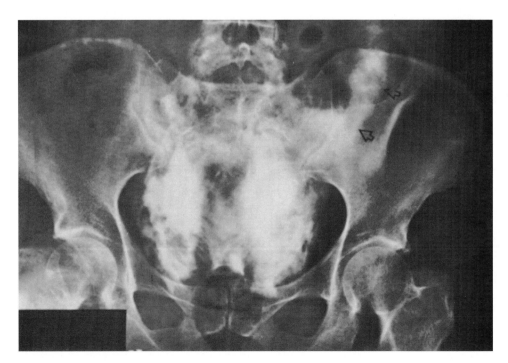

FIGURE 29–23. Bladder rupture, *complex* extraperitoneal. Cystogram. Contrast material has dissected from the perivesical extraperitoneal space superiorly into the pararenal compartment of the retroperitoneum *(arrows)*.

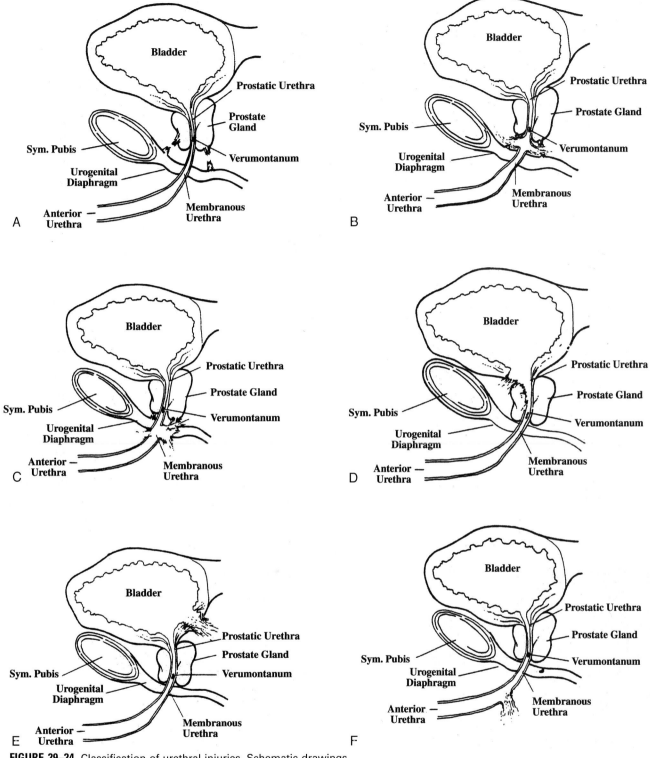

FIGURE 29–24. Classification of urethral injuries. Schematic drawings.
   A, Type I.
   B, Type II.
   C, Type III.
   D, Type IV.
   E, Type IVA.
   F, Type V.
(From Goldman, S. M., Sandler, C. M., Corriere, N. J., Jr., and McGuire, E. J.: Blunt urethral trauma: A unified, anatomical mechanical classification. J. Urol. *157*:85–89, 1997. Reproduced with kind permission of the authors and *Journal of Urology.*)

Type IV. The bladder neck is injured with extension into the urethra. These injuries are uncommon but may involve the internal urethral sphincter. This is especially important in women who are dependent on the internal urethral sphincter for urinary continence. Occasionally, there is an injury of the bladder base with periurethral extravasation simulating a Type IV injury. This is classified as a **Type IVA** injury.

Type V. This is an anterior urethral injury.

Types II, III, and IV urethral tears may be *partial* or *complete*. During urethrography, filling of the bladder indicates a partial tear. Strictures resulting from partial tears tend to be shorter than those associated with complete disruption.

Trauma to the anterior urethra is less common than is trauma to the posterior urethra. Injury of the anterior urethra results from a direct blow to the perineum or a straddle injury involving the bulbous urethra. Straddle injuries most often occur as a result of falling astride a parallel bar, the frame of a bicycle, or the top of a fence rail or steel beam. Typically, there is no associated pelvic fracture.

The force of a straddle injury compresses the bulbous urethra against the inferior pubis, resulting in contusion or partial or complete urethral tear. The corpus spongiosum may also be affected. If Buck's fascia is disrupted, the hematoma may spread into the scrotum, perineum, or anterior abdominal wall. Spread beyond, however, is limited by Colles' fascia.

Urethral injury from surgical instrumentation, long-term transurethral bladder catheterization, or radiation may cause a stricture to form over time. Stricture related to a long-term transurethral bladder catheter follows pressure necrosis and is most likely to occur at the penoscrotal junction or the bulbomembranous segment.

Combined Urethral and Bladder Injury. Bladder injury is present in as many as 20 per cent of males with posterior urethral injury. Bladder involvement may be demonstrated at the time of retrograde urethrography if the urethral injury is incomplete and some bladder opacification occurs. An attempt should not be made to completely distend the bladder with contrast material during retrograde urethrography once a posterior urethral injury is detected. Rather, the examination of the bladder should be performed after a suprapubic catheter is in place.

Penetrating Urethral Injury. Penetrating wounds of the perineum or buttocks may involve either the anterior or the posterior urethra. The anterior urethra is more commonly involved. Examination of the patient with suspected penetrating injury of the urethra should follow the previously described guidelines for retrograde urethrography. Most require surgical exploration and antibiotic therapy.

Female Urethral Injury. Urethral injury in the female is relatively rare because of short length and lack of ligamentous fixation to adjacent structures. A urethrovaginal fistula is a complication of penetrating urethral trauma.

Clinical Findings

The classic clinical findings in posterior urethral injury include blood at the urethral meatus, inability to void spontaneously, and a superior displacement of the prostate gland on rectal examination. The absence of these findings, however, does not preclude a urethral injury. Complications from these injuries include incontinence, impotence, and recurrent strictures.

With minor injury of the anterior urethra blood is not necessarily present at the urethral meatus. A severe straddle injury can rupture Buck's fascia with spread of the hematoma into the perineum and scrotum. This may result in a butterfly hematoma dorsal to the scrotum within the perineum.

Type I injuries require no surgical intervention. With Types II and III injuries, repair may be immediate (primary) or delayed (approximately 3 months after the trauma). Delayed repair requires suprapubic bladder drainage and a one- or two-stage urethroplasty. Delayed repair is probably associated with fewer complications, such as incontinence or impotence, than is primary repair.

A mild anterior urethral injury may be treated with an indwelling catheter, whereas a severe injury usually requires a suprapubic cystostomy. Complicating strictures are often repaired using anterior urethroplasty.

Radiologic Techniques

Radiologic examination of the urethra in the setting of acute trauma must be performed with carefully monitored retrograde instillation of contrast material. Any attempt to catheterize the urethra beyond the fossa navicularis carries the risk of creating a false passage, conversion of a partial to a complete tear, contamination of a hematoma, or hemorrhage in the prostate. A small Foley catheter is placed in the distal urethra. The balloon is inflated within the fossa navicularis using 2 mL of saline solution. Radiographs should be obtained in an oblique projection with the patient facing the radiologist. The catheter is stretched over the leg using mild traction. Ten to 20 mL of 30 per cent contrast material is injected, preferably under fluoroscopic control.

In a patient with suspected urethral injury who has been catheterized before the performance of a retrograde urethrogram, the urethra should be evaluated by pericatheter urethrography (Fig. 29–25). This technique requires a pediatric feeding tube to be introduced into the penile urethra alongside the catheter. Contrast material is then injected into the feeding tube utilizing fluoroscopic control. Oblique films similar to the retrograde urethrogram should be obtained. In this procedure, the catheter is recognized as a prominent urethral filling defect

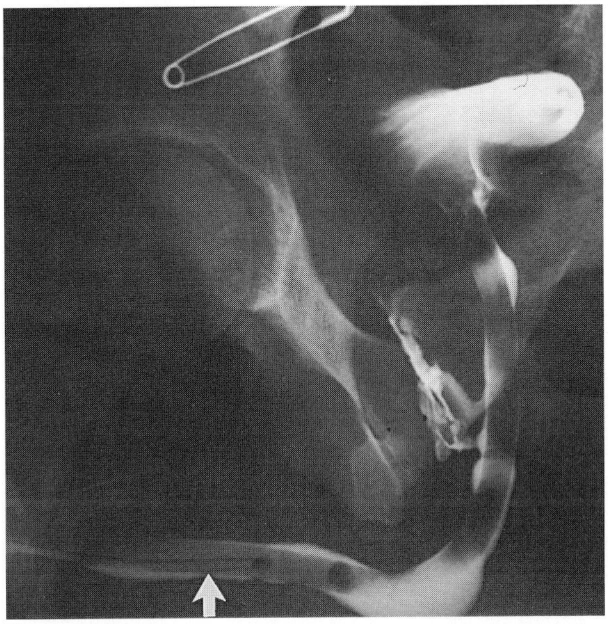

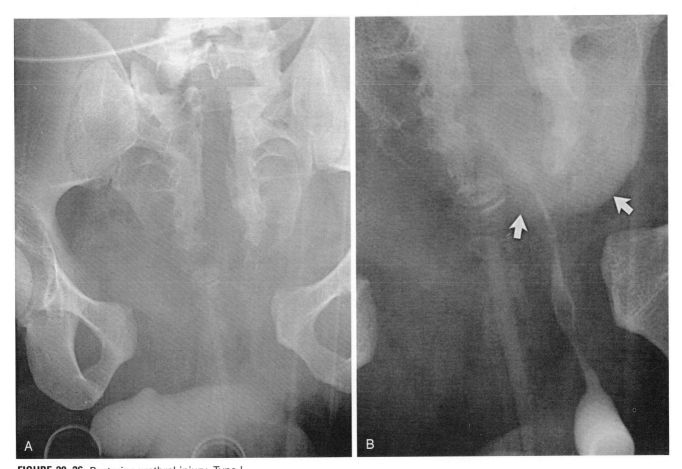

FIGURE 29–25. Extravasation from the bulbous urethra after surgical repair of a traumatic urethral injury. Pericatheter urethrogram. Patients with suspected urethral trauma who have already been catheterized can be evaluated by injecting contrast material through a pediatric feeding tube *(arrow)* that has been placed in the distal penile urethra adjacent to the catheter. There is extravasation from the bulbous urethra indicating a surgical leak. The offset of the two pubic rami was from the initial trauma.

FIGURE 29–26. Posterior urethral injury, Type I.
 A, Plain film. Diastasis of the pubic symphysis and a vertical fracture of the sacrum are present.
 B, Retrograde urethrogram. The posterior urethra is stretched and the faintly opacified bladder *(arrows)* is elevated from adjacent pelvic hemorrhage. There is no extravasation.

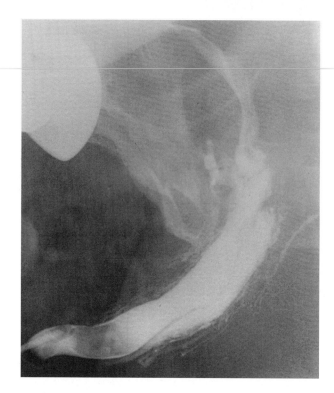

FIGURE 29–27. Posterior urethral injury. Type III, partial. Retrograde urethrogram. There is contrast material extravasation above and below the urogenital diaphragm. Contrast material within the bladder indicates that the rupture is partial.

FIGURE 29–28. Type IVA bladder injury. Cystogram. Contrast material extravasates from the bladder base to surround the proximal urethra. Note also diastasis of the symphysis pubis and sacroiliac joint. This injury represents an extraperitoneal bladder rupture, but extension of the injury into the proximal urethra cannot be excluded.

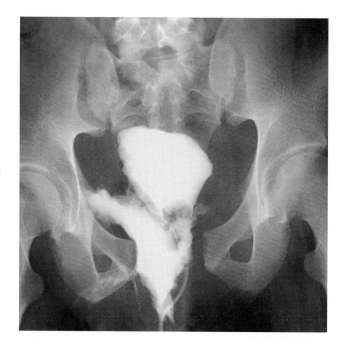

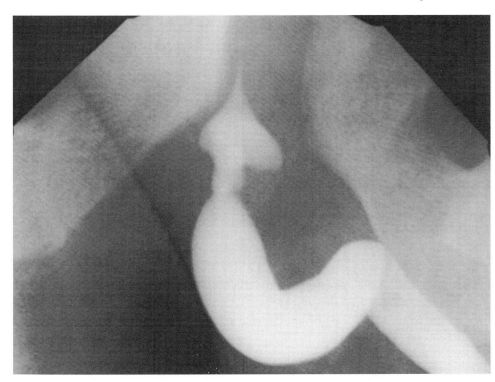

FIGURE 29–29. Urethral stricture, post-traumatic. Retrograde urethrogram demonstrates a proximal bulbar urethral stricture.

(see Fig. 29–25). Areas of urethral extravasation typically are obvious.

Radiologic Findings

Posterior Urethra

Abnormal radiologic findings in the urethra correspond to the preceding descriptions for the classification of urethral injury, as illustrated in Figure 29–24.

With Type I injury the urethra is elongated and there is no leakage of contrast material (Fig. 29–26). A Type II injury manifests contrast material extending from the urethral lumen into the extraperitoneal space of the pelvis above the urogenital diaphragm. In a Type III rupture, contrast material is detected either below or above and below the urogenital diaphragm (Fig. 29–27). Contrast material also may be seen overlying the perineum and scrotum. With incomplete Type II or III injuries, contrast material also fills the bladder. Associated abnormalities relating to the bladder or pelvis as well as findings of other abdominal trauma may be present. A Type IV injury exhibits contrast material extravasation at the bladder base and adjacent to the proximal urethra (Fig. 29–28). Distinction between a Type IV and a Type IVA injury may be very difficult to make radiologically.

The radiologic evaluation for the late complications of urethral trauma includes an assessment of the integrity of the urethral lumen, the presence of false passages, bladder incontinence, and stricture formation. Stricture may form after either partial or complete urethral tear (Fig. 29–29).

Anterior Urethra

The urethrogram is normal in contusion of the anterior urethra. Severe straddle injury leads to partial or complete urethral rupture. With partial rupture, contrast material is present outside the bulbous urethra but the continuity of the urethra is maintained. If Buck's fascia is torn, contrast material may extend into the scrotum, perineum, or anterior abdominal wall. With complete rupture no contrast material is present in the proximal bulbous urethra. A stricture may form as a long-term complication of straddle injury. These occur generally in the proximal bulbous urethra and are usually short, measuring 0.5 cm or less (see Fig. 29–29).

BIBLIOGRAPHY

Renal

Baumann, L., Greenfield, S. P., Aker, J., Brody, A., Karp, M., Allen, J., and Cooney, D.: Nonoperative management of major blunt renal trauma in children: In-hospital morbidity and long-term follow-up. J. Urol. *148*:691, 1992.

Blankenship, B., Earls, J. P., and Talner, L. B.: Renal vein thrombosis after vascular pedicle injury. AJR *168*:1574, 1997.

Brennan, F. J., and Goff, W. B.: Seatbelt injury to a pelvic kidney as demonstrated on CT. J. Comput. Assist. Tomogr. *17*:664, 1993.

Eastham, J. A., Wilson, T. G., and Ahlering, T. E.: Radiographic assessment of blunt renal trauma. J. Trauma *31*:1527, 1991.

Eastham, J. A., Wilson, T. G., Larsen, D. W., and Ahlering, T. E.: Angiographic embolization of renal stab wounds. J. Urol. *148*:268, 1992.

Fanney, D. R., Casillas, J., and Murphy, B. J.: CT in the diagnosis of renal trauma. RadioGraphics *10*:29, 1990.

Fisher, R. G., Ben-Menachem, Y., and Whigham, C. Stab wounds of the renal artery branches: Angiographic diagnosis and treatment by embolization. AJR *152*:1231, 1989.

Goldman, S. M., and Wagner, L. K.: Radiographic management of abdominal trauma in pregnancy. AJR *166*:763, 1996.

Herschorn, S., Radomski, S. B., Shoskes, D. A., Mahoney, J., Hirshberg, E., and Klotz, L.: Evaluation and treatment of blunt renal trauma. J. Urol. *146*:274, 1991.

Heyns, C. F., and Vollenhoven, P. V.: Increasing role of angiography and segmental artery embolization in the management of renal stab wounds. J. Urol. *147*:1231, 1992.

Kawashima, A., Sandler, C. M., Corriere, J. N., Jr., Rodgers, B. M., and Goldman, S. M.: Ureteropelvic injuries secondary to blunt abdominal trauma. Radiology *205*:487, 1997.

Knudson, M. M., McAninch, J. W., Gomez, R., Lee, P., and Stubbs, H. A.: Hematuria as a predictor of abdominal injury after blunt trauma. Am. J. Surg. *164*:482, 1992.

Leppäniemi, A., Lamminen, A., Tervahartiala, P., Salo, J., Haapainen, R., and Lehtonen, T.: MRI and CT in blunt renal trauma: An update. Semin. Ultrasound CT MRI *18*:129, 1997.

Lupetin, A. R., Mainwaring, B. L., and Daffner, R. H.: CT diagnosis of renal artery injury caused by blunt abdominal trauma. AJR *153*:1065, 1989.

Miller, K. S., and McAninch, J. W.: Radiolographic assessment of renal trauma: Our 15-year experience. J. Urol. *154*:352, 1995.

Mirvis, S. E.: Trauma. Radiol. Clin. North Am. *34*:1225, 1996.

Morey, A. F., Bruce, J. E., and McAninch, J. W.: Efficacy of radiographic imaging in pediatric blunt renal trauma. J. Urol. *156*:2014, 1996.

Nunez, D., Jr., Becerra, J. L., Fuentes, D., and Pagson, S.: Traumatic occlusion of the renal artery: Helical CT diagnosis. AJR *167*:777, 1996.

Pollack, H. M., and Wein, A. J.: Imaging of renal trauma. Radiology *172*:294, 1989.

Shuman, W. P.: CT of blunt abdominal trauma in adults. Radiology *205*:297, 1997.

Sivit, C. J., Taylor, G. A., Bulas, D. I., Kushner, D. C., Potter, B. M., and Eichelburger, M. R.: Post-traumatic shock in children: CT findings associated with hemodynamic instability. Radiology *182*:723, 1992.

Teigen, C. L., Venbrux, A. C., Quinlan, D. M., and Jeffs, R. D.: Late massive hematuria as a complication of conservative management of blunt renal trauma in children. J. Urol. *147*:1333, 1992.

Wolfman, N. T., Bechtold, R. E., Scharling, E. S., and Meredith, J. W.: Blunt upper abdominal trauma: Evaluation by CT. AJR *158*:493, 1992.

Ureter

Hall, S. J., and Carpinito, G. A.: Traumatic rupture of renal pelvis obstructed at the ureteropelvic junction: Case report. J. Trauma *37*:850, 1994.

Horrow, M. M., Tuncali, K., and Kirby, C. L.: Imaging of ureteroscopic complications. AJR *168*:633, 1997.

Mulligan, J. M., Cagiannos, I., Collins, J. P., and Millward, S. F.: Ureteropelvic junction disruption secondary to blunt trauma: Excretory phase imaging (delayed films) should help prevent a missed diagnosis. J. Urol. *159*:67, 1998.

Selzman, A. A., and Spirnak, J. P.: Iatrogenic ureteral injuries: A 20-year experience in treating 165 injuries. J. Urol *155*:878, 1996.

Bladder

Lis, L. E., and Cohen, A. J.: CT cystography in the evaluation of bladder trauma. J. Comput. Assist. Tomogr. *14*:386, 1990.

Mee, S. L., McAninch, J., and Federle, M. P.: Computerized tomography in bladder rupture: Diagnostic limitations. J. Urol *137*:207, 1987.

Sandler, C. M., Hall, J. T., Rodriguez, M. B., and Corriere, J. N., Jr.: Bladder injury in blunt pelvic trauma. Radiology *158*:633, 1986.

Sivit, C. J., Cutting, J. P., and Eichelberger, M. R.: CT diagnosis and localization of rupture of the bladder in children with blunt abdominal trauma: Significance of contrast material extravasation in the pelvis. AJR *164*:1243, 1995.

Urethra

Follis, H. W., Koch, M. O., and McDougal, W. S.: Immediate management of prostatomembranous urethral disruptions. J. Urol. *147*:1259, 1992.

Goldman, S. M., Sandler, C. M., Corriere, N. J., Jr., and McGuire, E. J.: Blunt urethral trauma: A unified, anatomical-mechanical classification. J. Urol. *157*:85, 1997.

Herschorn, S., Thijssen, A., and Radomski, S. B.: The value of immediate or early catheterization of the traumatized posterior urethra. J. Urol. *148*:1428, 1992.

Netto, N. R., Ikari, O., and Zuppo, V. P.: Traumatic rupture of the female urethra. Urology *22*:601, 1983.

Perry, M. O., and Husmann, D. A.: Urethral injuries in female subjects following pelvic fractures. J. Urol. *147*:139, 1992.

APPENDIX

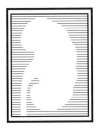

Urographic Contrast Material: Historical Development and Chemical Characteristics

In 1897, Tuffier placed a rigid metal stylet through a ureteral catheter and thereby outlined the course of the ureter on a radiograph of the abdomen. In so doing, he began the history of the development of urographic contrast material. Reports of modifications of this method rapidly followed, first describing the use of flexible wires to outline the margins of the renal pelvis and later, replacement of metallic rods and wires with a diverse group of materials for retrograde instillation into the ureter. These materials included colloidal silver, bismuth, iodine-silver emulsions, thorium, potassium iodide, sodium iodide, sodium bromide, and strontium chloride. Even air, oxygen, and carbon dioxide were used as contrast agents. All of these techniques were abandoned after short periods of use, principally because of complications, usually of a common nature, such as infection and tissue trauma, but also because of exotic problems such as air embolism,

silver deposits in the kidneys, and generalized argyry (silver poisoning).

The concept of radiographically visualizing the urinary tract by renal excretion rather than retrograde introduction of a radiopaque substance was discussed in a report of bladder opacification after oral or intravenous administration of 10% sodium iodide (Osborne et al., 1923). Osborne and Rowntree (Figs. A–1, A–2), dermatologists at the Mayo Clinic, had been studying the therapeutic potential of iodine-containing compounds for the treatment of syphilis and other infections. It occurred to them that the known radiopacity and renal excretion of iodine might make this substance useful in rendering the urinary tract opaque to x-radiation. Charles G. Sutherland (Fig. A–3) was the only co-author of this landmark article who was a radiologist. The value of the Mayo Clinic approach, which used sodium iodide, was soon confirmed by others. Other

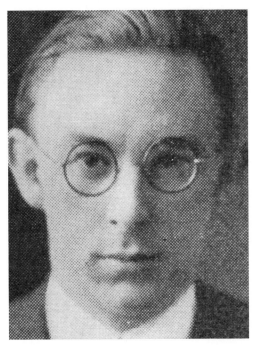

FIGURE A–1. Earl D. Osborne, M.D. (Courtesy of the late Glen W. Hartman, M.D., Mayo Clinic, Rochester, Minnesota.)

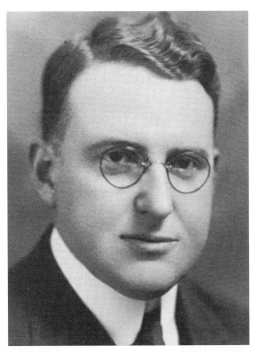

FIGURE A–2. Leonard G. Rowntree, M.D. (Courtesy of the late Glen W. Hartman, M.D., Mayo Clinic, Rochester, Minnesota.)

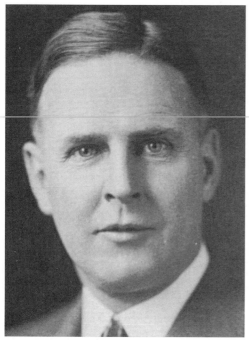

FIGURE A–3. Charles G. Sutherland, M.D. (Courtesy of the late Glen W. Hartman, M.D., Mayo Clinic, Rochester, Minnesota.)

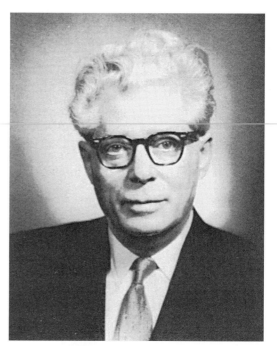

FIGURE A–5. Moses Swick, M.D.

forms of iodine, bromide, and sodium iodide–urea complexes were investigated during the 1920s. However, none of these agents consistently opacified the kidneys and ureters, large amounts of material were required for minimal density, and systemic reactions were common. Clearly, improvements were needed.

During this period of testing inorganic iodide radiopaque materials, two German chemists, Arthur Binz and C. Räth, were synthesizing pyridine compounds as potential therapeutic agents in the treatment of infections. One of these compounds, Selectan-neutral (Fig. A–4), was excreted by both the biliary system and the kidneys and therefore was used as treatment for infections of the gallbladder and urinary tract. Clinical trials were conducted in a hospital in Hamburg-Altona at which a young American urologist, Moses Swick (Fig. A–5), was working under the direction of Prof. Dr. Lichwitz. Swick, noting that Selectan-neutral was composed of 54 per cent iodine, realized the potential for urinary tract opacification and conducted simultane-

ous excretion, toxicity, and radiologic studies. Nausea, vomiting, headache, and diplopia limited the usefulness of Selectan-neutral. Paying particular attention to the diplopia, Swick reasoned that the toxicity might be diminished by modification of the *N*-methyl group at position 1. This change, along with other suggestions designed to increase solubility of the drug, was proposed to Binz, who synthesized sodium 5-iodo-2-pyridone-*N*-acetate, or Uroselectan, containing 42 per cent iodine (Fig. A–6). This new material was tested by Swick, who by then had transferred to the service of Prof. von Lichtenberg at St. Hedwig's Krankenhaus in Berlin. It was found to offer improved water solubility over Selectan-neutral, was well tolerated, and provided a degree of opacification of the urinary tract that was never before achieved. Swick and von Lichtenberg reported their results to the German Urologic Congress, which met in Munich in 1929. This report set the stage for the era of modern excretory urography. Uroselectan, marketed in the United States

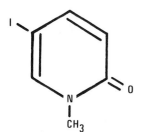

Mol. Wt.: 238
Iodine Content: 54%
Trade Name: Selectan-neutral

N-methyl-5-iodo-2-pyridone

FIGURE A–4. Chemical characteristics of Selectan-neutral.

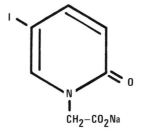

Mol. Wt.: 301
Iodine Content: 42%
Trade Names: Uroselectan
Iopax

Sodium 5-iodo-2-pyridone-N-acetate

FIGURE A–6. Chemical characteristics of Uroselectan (Iopax).

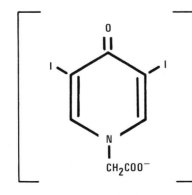

FIGURE A–7. Chemical characteristics of Uroselectan B (Neo-Iopax).

Mol. Wt.: 493
Iodine Content: 51.5%
Generic Name: sodium iodomethamate, U.S.P.
Iodoxyl, B.P.
Trade Names: Neo-Iopax
Uroselectan B

Disodium 1-methyl-3,5-diiodo-
4-pyridone-2,6-dicarboxylate

as Iopax, was modified by Binz into disodium 1-methyl-3,5-diiodo-4-pyridone-2,6-dicarboxylate (Fig. A–7), which offered increased iodine content. The modified version was sold as Uroselectan B in Europe and as Neo-Iopax in the United States.

In 1930, Bronner, Hecht, and Schüller introduced sodium iodomethanesulfonate (Abrodil in Europe, Skiodan in the United States). At about the same time, Iopax was modified into 3,5-diiodo-4-pyridone-N-acetic acid diethanolamine salt, or Diodrast (Fig. A–8). Neo-Iopax and Diodrast were accepted rapidly as the contrast agents of choice for excretory urography; their predominance continued until the introduction of the benzoic acid derivative, acetrizoate, some 20 years later.

Whereas it was not until 1950 that acetrizoate was introduced into clinical radiology, the conceptual basis for the radiologic use of this compound was laid by Moses Swick in the early 1930s. Swick originated the idea of using an organic nucleus that was a normal product of metabolism (not a synthetic substance) as a carrier for a radiopaque element. He proposed the detoxification product of benzoic acid, sodium orthoiodohippurate, or Hippuran, as an iodine carrier that would be excreted by the kidneys. The Billings Gold Medal of the American Medical Association was awarded to Swick in 1933 for the introduction of this concept. Hippuran could be administered orally and did opacify the urinary tract. Unfortunately, its usefulness was impaired by adverse systemic effects related to the addition of iodine to the hippuric acid molecule. Additional factors that limited its use were obscuration of the urinary tract by the orally administered opaque material in the gut and the limitation of radiopacity imposed by one iodine atom on each molecule of Hippuran. Despite these drawbacks, the value of binding iodine to the 6-carbon benzoic acid ring rather than the 5-carbon pyridone-derived ring was established.

During the period of 1948–1950, V. H. Wallingford and his colleagues at the Research Laboratories of Mallinckrodt Chemical Works, St. Louis, studied a group of normal detoxication products obtained by acetylation of aminobenzoic acid. These workers reported on the synthesis and clinical usefulness of sodium 3-acetamido-2,4,6-triiodobenzoate, or acetrizoate (Fig. A–9). This was one of a group of iodinated acylaminobenzoic acids tested by Wallingford and associates that was selected as potentially useful for excretory urography because of its high iodine content (sodium salt, 65.8%), high water solubility, and urinary excretion. Initial biochemical, toxicologic, and clinical trials showed acetrizoate to be of low toxicity and efficacious for urinary tract opacification. Other studies indicated that this compound was excreted principally by glomerular filtration and that visualization of the urinary tract was more satisfactory than that possible with agents generally in use at that time. This achievement was due to acetrizoate's high iodine content

FIGURE A–8. Chemical characteristics of Diodrast.

$H_2N^+(CH_2CH_2OH)_2$

Mol. Wt.: 510
Iodine Content: 49.8%
Generic Names: iodopyracet, U.S.P.
diodone, B.P.
Trade Names: Diodrast
Umbradil

3,5-diiodo-4-pyridone-N-acetic
acid, diethanolamine salt

$CO_2^-Na^+$

I

I

NHCOCH$_3$

I

Sodium 3-acetamido-2,4,6-triiodobenzoate

Mol. Wt.: 479
Iodine Content: 65.8%
Generic Name: sodium acetrizoate, U.S.P.
Trade Name: Urokon

FIGURE A–9. Chemical characteristics of Urokon.

and low toxicity relative to Diodrast. Acetrizoate was marketed as Urokon and began to replace Diodrast in clinical urography.

In the formulation of acetrizoate, the 5 position on the benzoic ring was unsubstituted (see Figs. A–9 and A–13). In 1955, J. O. Hoppe and his colleagues at the Sterling-Winthrop Research Institute reported their evaluation of a large number of di- and tri-iodinated benzoic acid derivatives in which the 5 position was substituted with a variety of radicals. Of the compounds studied, one stood out as fulfilling requirements for a urographic compound in humans, namely, high radiopacity, high water solubility, low toxicity, and a minimum of pharmacodynamic activity. This substance, 3,5-diacetamido-2,4,6-triiodobenzoic acid, or diatrizoate, was registered by Winthrop Laboratories. The sodium salt was marketed as Hypaque (Fig. A–10). Development of sodium diatrizoate was reported independently by the Schering group in West Germany. As clinical experience and laboratory investigations into contrast material pharmacology accumulated, the relative safety of sodium diatrizoate compared with sodium acetrizoate and other previously used contrast agents (e.g., Diodrast and Neo-Iopax) became apparent. Every water-soluble urographic contrast agent in clinical use today is a modification or derivative of tri-iodinated, fully saturated benzoic acid.

The ionic urographic contrast agents most commonly in use are monomers that ionize into a cation (sodium or *N*-methylglucamine) and a benzoate anion that bears three atoms of iodine. The formulas, chemical characteristics, and generic and trade names of these agents are illustrated in Figures A–10 through A–12. Table A–1 lists the sodium and iodine content of these preparations. All of these substances are fully substituted benzoic acid derivatives. The several agents are distinguished one from the other by the radical at position 3 or 5 and/or by the sodium or *N*-methylglucamine (meglumine) cation at position 1 (Fig. A–13).

A major factor in the toxicity of ionic monomers is their high osmolality (greater than 2000 mOsm/kg water in some products) relative to that of physiologic solutions (approximately 290 mOsm/kg water). Hyperosmolality of this magnitude is responsible for the injection site pain, heat, flushing, and nausea that are associated with contrast material injection. Serious adverse systemic reactions also are related in some way to the osmolality of contrast agents. Other alterations that are considered due to hyperosmolality of ionic monomeric forms of contrast material include crenation of erythrocytes, increase in pulmonary artery pressure, injury to venous and capillary endothelium, disruption of the blood-brain barrier, and increase in circulating blood volume with associated alterations in heart rate. Depression of the kidney's ability to extract para-aminohippuric acid, changes in renal blood flow, decrease in glomerular filtration rate, abnormal urine enzyme output, and changes in urinary electrolyte excretion are a

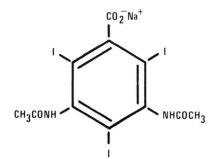

$CO_2^-Na^+$

I

I

CH$_3$CONH

NHCOCH$_3$

I

Sodium 3,5-diacetamido-2,4,6-triiodobenzoate

Mol. Wt.: 636
Iodine Content: 59.8%
Generic Name: sodium diatrizoate, U.S.P.
Trade Name: Hypaque

FIGURE A–10. Chemical characteristics of Hypaque.

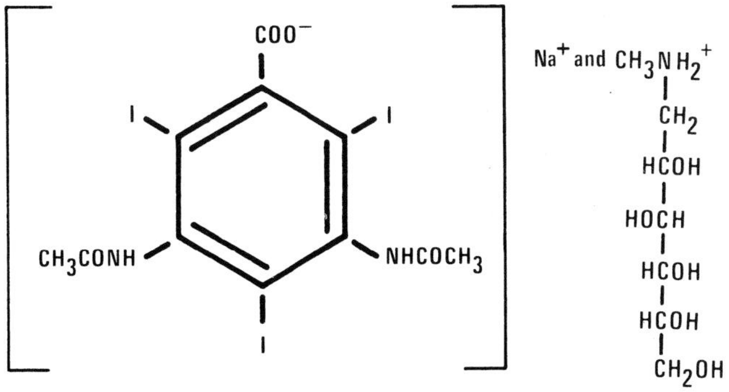

FIGURE A-11. Chemical characteristics of Renografin 60 (Urografin).

Sodium and N-methylglucamine 3,5-diacetamido-2,4,6-triiodobenzoate

Mol. Wt.: 810
Iodine Content: 47.6%
Generic Name: meglumine and sodium diatrizoate, U.S.P.
Trade Names: Renografin 60 Urografin

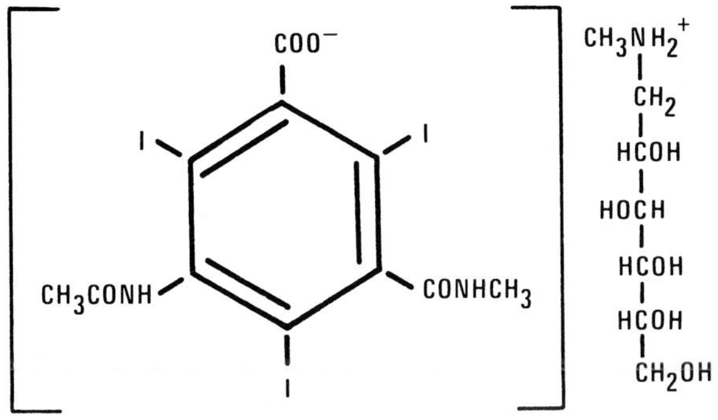

N-methylglucamine-5-acetamido-2,4,6-triiodo-N-methylisophthalamate

Mol. Wt.: 810
Iodine Content: 62%
Generic Name: meglumine iothalamate, U.S.P.
Trade Name: Conray

FIGURE A-12. Chemical characteristics of Conray.

TABLE A-1. Commonly Used Contrast Material for Excretory Urography and Computed Tomography

GENERIC NAME	TRADE NAME	SODIUM CONTENT (mEq/mL)	IODINE CONTENT (mg/mL)	OSMOLALITY (mOsm/kg H_2O)
Ionic Monomers (Ratio 1.5)				
Sodium diatrizoate	Hypaque 50	0.8	300	1515
Meglumine and sodium diatrizoate	Renografin 60	0.16	292	1420
Sodium iothalamate	Conray 400	1.05	400	2300
Meglumine iothalamate	Conray		282	1400
Nonionic Monomers (Ratio 3)				
Iopamidol	Isovue 300		300	616
Iohexol	Omnipaque		300	709
Ioversol	Optiray		320	702
Iopromide	Ultravist		300	620
Ionic Dimers (Ratio 3)				
Meglumine and sodium ioxaglate	Hexabrix	0.15	320	600
Nonionic Dimers (Ratio 6)				
Iodixanol	Visipaque	0.48	320	290

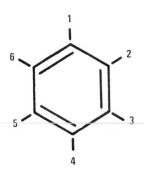

Position 1 – carboxyl group (–CO₂H) as sodium or
N-methylglucamine salt
Positions 2, 4, 6 – iodine
Position 3 – acetamido
Position 5 – acetamido (diatrizoate)
N-methyl carbamyl (iothalamate)
N-methyl acetamido (metrizoate)

FIGURE A–13. Basic benzene ring common to all modern contrast agents. Variations at positions 3 and 5 distinguish the generic designation of various compounds. Variation at position 1 determines the form of the salt.

result of contrast material administration in both humans and laboratory animals. Hyperosmolality accounts for some, if not all, of these effects.

Although these toxic reactions to contrast material have not been of sufficient magnitude to prevent the widespread vascular use of monomeric ionic forms of contrast material in large doses, the need for agents of lower osmolality has been apparent for a long time. In 1969, the Swedish radiologist Torsten Almén (Fig. A–14) opened a new era in the history of water-soluble radiopaque compounds by theorizing that osmolality would be lower and radiopacity would be maintained with iodine-bearing compounds that were *nonionizing*. Metrizamide (Amipaque) was the first of the water-soluble nonionic monomeric compounds based on this concept to gain clinical use, principally for opacification of the subarachnoid space.

The development of low-osmolality water-soluble contrast agents for intravascular use that have followed Almén's concepts has been along three lines. The first was focused on a single benzene ring that is fully saturated with both iodine atoms (positions 2, 4, and 6) and hydrophilic radicals (positions 1, 3, and 5). The latter render the molecules water soluble without ionization. The architecture of nonionic monomers is illustrated in Figure A–15. These retain the same radiopacity as ionic monomers with three atoms of iodine on each molecule. The reduction of the number of particles in solution from two to one, however, substantially reduces the osmolality of these compounds. Characteristics of various nonionic monomers are listed in Table A–1 and illustrated in Figures A–16 through A–19.

A second line of development of low-osmolality contrast agents has been dimers of tri-iodinated benzene rings, as illustrated in Figure A–20. The first product developed as a dimer, sodium-meglumine ioxaglate (Hexabrix), has one ionizing carboxyl group and is classified as an ionic, or monoacid, dimer (Fig. A–21). The ionic dimeric contrast agent is characterized further in Table A–1.

The development of low-osmolality contrast agents has progressed along a third line with dimers that achieve water solubility by full substitution with hydrophilic radicals at all sites except for the six sites at which atoms of iodine are attached. This yields a product that is compounded with an osmolality essentially equivalent to that of plasma. The generic structure of this compound and its chemical characteristics are illustrated in Figures A–22 and A–23.

The new classes of low-osmolality contrast agents are conveniently characterized by the ratio of the number of atoms of iodine to the number of particles in solution for each molecule. This expression re-

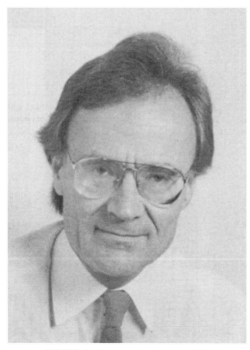

FIGURE A–14. Torsten Almén, M.D.

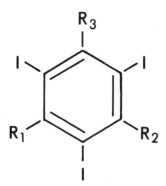

FIGURE A–15. Generic structure of radiopaque nonionic monomers. R_1, R_2, and R_3 are hydrophilic, nonionizing radicals.

FIGURE A–16. Chemical characteristics of Isovue.

Mol. Wt.: 777
Iodine Content: 49%
Generic Name: iopamidol, U.S.P.
Trade Name: Isovue

(S)-N,N'-bis[2-hydroxy-1-(hydroxymethyl)ethyl]-2,4,6-triiodo-5-lactamidoisophthalamide

Mol. Wt.: 821
Iodine Content: 46%
Generic Name: iohexol, U.S.P.
Trade Name: Omnipaque

FIGURE A–17. Chemical characteristics of Omnipaque.

N,N'-bis(2,3-dihydroxypropyl)-5-[N-(2,3-dihydroxypropyl)-acetamidol]-2,4,6-triiodoisophthalamide

Mol. Wt.: 807
Iodine Content: 47%
Generic Name: ioversol, U.S.P.
Trade Name: Optiray

FIGURE A–18. Chemical characteristics of Optiray.

N,N'-bis(2,3-dihydroxypropyl)-5-[N-(2-hydroxyethyl)-glycolamidol]-2,4,6-triiodoisophthalamide

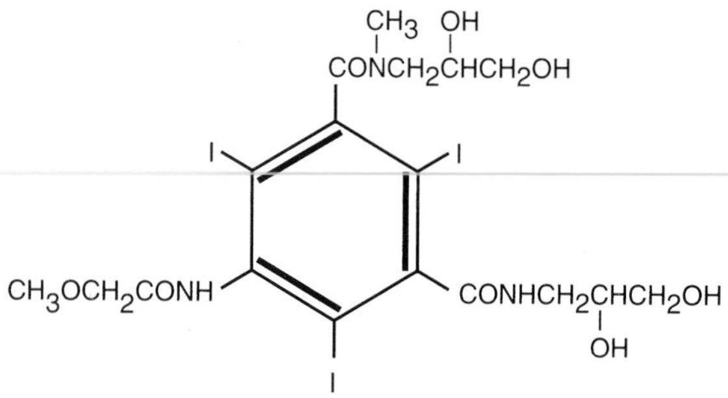

CH₃ OH
CONCH₂CHCH₂OH

CH₃OCH₂CONH

CONHCH₂CHCH₂OH
OH

5-Methoxyacetylamino-2,4,6-triiodoisophthalic acid
[(2,3-dihydroxy-N-methylpropyl)-(2,3-dihydroxypropyl)]diamide

Mol. Wt.: 791
Iodine Content: 48%
Generic Name: iopromide, U.S.P.
Trade Name: Ultravist

FIGURE A–19. Chemical characteristics of Ultravist.

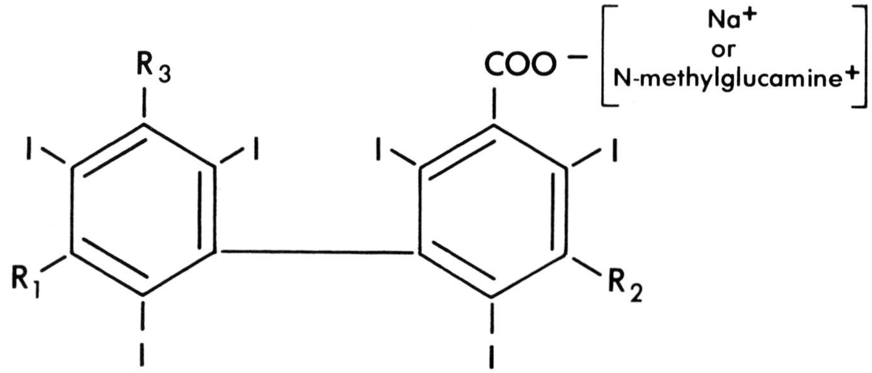

R₃

R₁

R₂

COO⁻ [Na⁺ or N-methylglucamine⁺]

FIGURE A–20. Generic structure of a mono-acid dimer contrast agent. R₁, R₂, and R₃ are hydrophilic, nonionizing radicals.

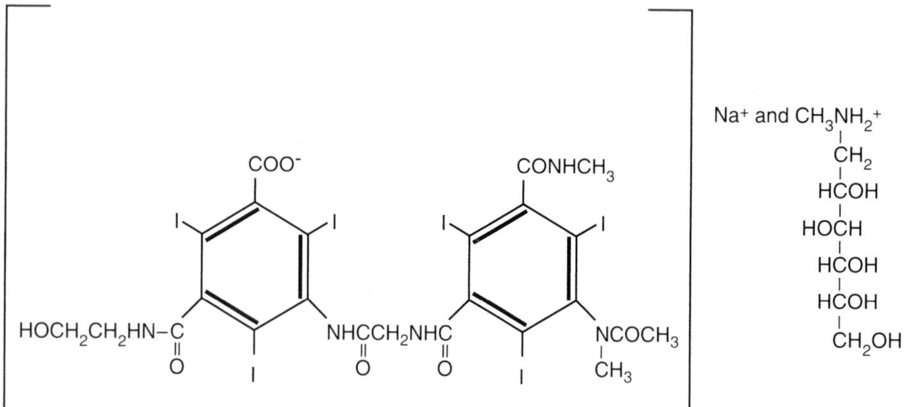

COO⁻

CONHCH₃

HOCH₂CH₂HN–C
O

NHCCH₂NHC
O   O

NCOCH₃
CH₃

Na⁺ and CH₃NH₂⁺
CH₂
HCOH
HOCH
HCOH
HCOH
CH₂OH

Iodine Content: 32%
Generic Name: ioxaglate meglumine and sodium
Trade Name: Hexabrix

N-(2-hydroxyethyl)-2,4,6-triiodo-5-[2-[2,4,6-triiodo-3-(N-methylacetamido)-isophthalamic acid, compounded with 1-deoxy-1-(methylamino)-D-glucitol (1:1) and sodium N-(2-hydroxyethyl)-2,4,6-triiodo-5-[2-(2,4,6-triiodo-3-(N-methylacetamido)-5-(methylcarbamoyl)benzamido]acetamido]-isophthalamate.

FIGURE A–21. Chemical characteristics of Hexabrix.

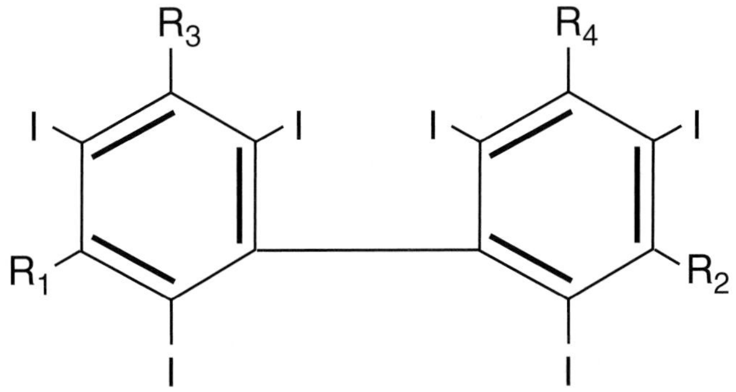

FIGURE A–22. Generic structure of a nonionic dimer contrast agent. R_1, R_2, R_3, and R_4 are hydrophilic, nonionizing radicals.

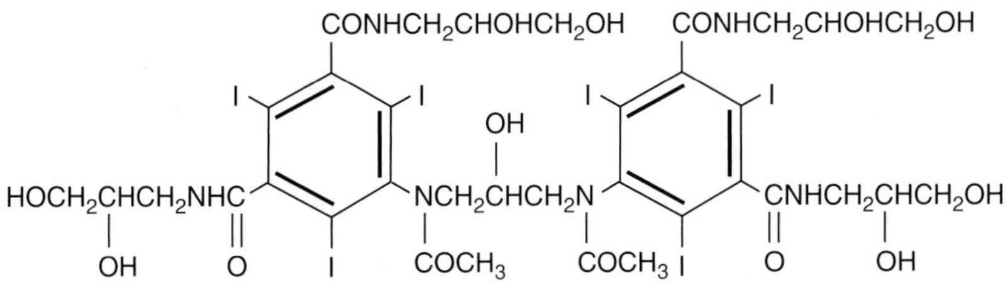

Mol. Wt.: 1550.20
Iodine Content: 49.1%
Generic Name: iodixanol
Trade Name: Visipaque

5,5'-[(2-hydroxy-1,3-propanediyl)bis(acetylimino)]bis[N,N'-bis(2,3-dihydroxypropyl)-2,4,6-triiodo-1,3-benzenecarboxamide]

FIGURE A–23. Chemical characteristics of Visipaque.

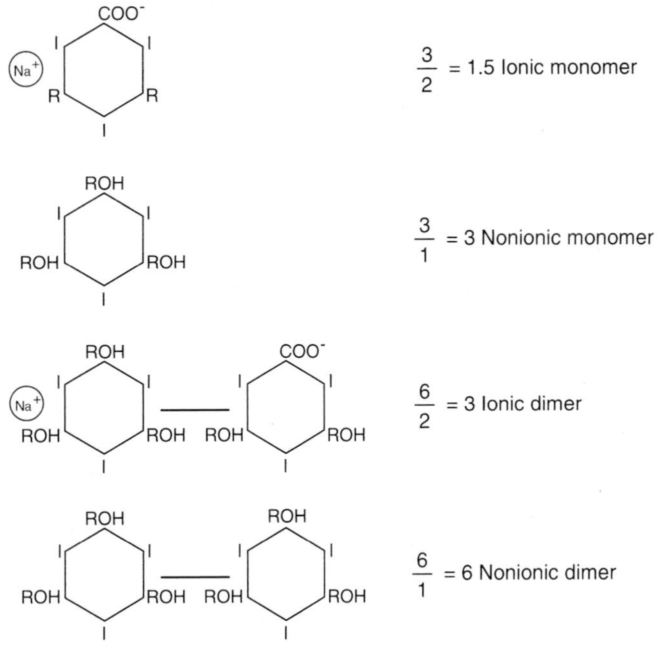

$\dfrac{3}{2}$ = 1.5 Ionic monomer

$\dfrac{3}{1}$ = 3 Nonionic monomer

FIGURE A–24. Contrast material classification by ratio number.

$\dfrac{6}{2}$ = 3 Ionic dimer

$\dfrac{6}{1}$ = 6 Nonionic dimer

lates, respectively, radiodensity to osmolality. Ionic monomers are *ratio 1.5* compounds by virtue of their three atoms of iodine for every two particles in solution. Nonionic monomers (three atoms of iodine to one particle in solution) and ionic dimers (six atoms of iodine to two particles in solution) are *ratio 3* compounds. Nonionic dimers (six atoms of iodine to one particle in solution) are *ratio 6* compounds. This nomenclature is summarized in Figure A–24.

BIBLIOGRAPHY

Almén, T.: Contrast agent design. J. Theor. Biol. *24*:216, 1969.

Almén, T.: Experience from 10 years of development of water-soluble nonionic contrast media. Invest. Radiol. *15*:S283, 1980.

Almén, T.: Development of nonionic contrast media. Invest. Radiol. 20(Suppl.):S2, 1985.

Almén, T.: Visipaque—a step forward: A historical review. Acta Radiol. *36*(Suppl. 399):2, 1995.

Bettmann, M.: Clinical summary with conclusions: Ionic versus nonionic contrast agents and their effects on blood components. Invest. Radiol. *23*(Suppl. 2):S378, 1988.

Bettmann, M. A.: Guidelines for use of low-osmolality contrast agents. Radiology *172*:901, 1989.

Bettmann, M. A.: Ionic versus nonionic contrast agents for intravenous use: Are all the answers in? Radiology *175*:616, 1990.

Brennan, R. E., Rapoport, S., Weinberg, I., Pollack, H. M., and Curtis, J. A.: CT determined canine kidney and urine, iodine concentrations following intravenous administration of sodium diatrizoate, metrizamide, iopamidol and sodium ioxaglate. Invest. Radiol. *17*:95, 1982.

Bruwer, A. J. (ed.): Classic Descriptions in Roentgenology. Springfield, IL, Charles C Thomas, 1964, pp. 1606–1614.

Cochran, S. T., Ballard, J. W., Katzberg, R. W., Barbaric, A. L., Spataro, R., Iwamoto, K., and Lee, J. J.: Evaluation of iopamidol and diatrizoate in excretory urography: A double-blind study. AJR *151*:523, 1988.

Cohan, R. H., and Dunnick, N. R.: Intravascular contrast media: Adverse reactions. AJR *149*:665, 1987.

Danford, R. O., Talner, L. B., and Davidson, A. J.: Effect of graded osmolalities of saline solution and contrast media on renal extraction of PAH in the dog. Invest. Radiol. *4*:301, 1969.

Davidson, A. J.: Lysozymuric response to contrast agents. Invest. Radiol. *3*:65, 1968.

Davidson, A. J., Abrams, H. L., and Stamey, T. A.: Renal extraction of PAH in man following aortography. Radiology *85*:1043, 1965.

Dawson, P.: Chemotoxicity of contrast media and clinical adverse effects: A review. Invest. Radiol. 20(Suppl.):S84, 1985.

Dawson, P., Grainger, R. G., and Pitfield, J.: The new low-osmolar contrast media: A simple guide. Clin. Radiol. *34*:321, 1983.

Dawson, P., Heron, C., and Marshall, J.: Intravenous urography with low-osmolarity contrast agents: Theoretical considerations and clinical findings. Clin. Radiol. *35*:173, 1984.

Evill, C. A., and Benness, G. T.: Solute excretion during intravenous urography: A comparison of sodium and methylglucamine iothalamates. Invest. Radiol. *10*:148, 1975.

Fountaine, H., Harnish, P., Andrew, E., and Grynne, B.: Safety, tolerance, and pharmacokinetics of iodixanol injection, a nonionic, isosmolar, hexa-iodinated contrast agent. Acad. Radiol. *3*:S475, 1996.

Gale, M. E., Robbins, A. H., Hamburger, R. J., and Widrich, W. C.: Renal toxicity of contrast agents: Iopamidol, iothalamate and diatrizoate. AJR *142*:333, 1984.

Gavant, M. L., and Siegle, R. L.: Iodixanol in excretory urography: Initial clinical experience with a nonionic, dimeric (ratio 6:1) contrast medium. Radiology *183*:515, 1992.

Grainger, R. G.: The clinical and financial implications of the low-osmolar radiological contrast media. Correspondence. Clin. Radiol. *35*:422, 1984.

Hoppe, J. O., Larsen, A. A., and Coulston, F.: Observations on the toxicity of a new urographic contrast medium, sodium 3,5-diacetamido-2,4,6-triiodobenzoate (Hypaque sodium) and related compounds. J. Pharmacol. Exp. Ther. *116*:394, 1956.

Hryntschak, T.: Studien Zur röentgenologischen Darstellung von Nierenparenchym und Nierenbecken auf intravenösem Wege. Z. Urol. Nephrol. *23*:893, 1929.

Katayama, H., Yamaguchi, K., Kozuka, T., Takashima, T., Seez, P., and Matsuura, K.: Adverse reactions to ionic and nonionic contrast media: A report from the Japanese committee on the safety of contrast media. Radiology *175*:621, 1990.

Kaye, B., Howard, J., Foord, K. D., and Cumberland, D. C.: Comparison of the image quality of intravenous urograms using low-osmolar contrast media. Br. J. Radiol. *61*:589, 1988.

Kennison, M. C., Powe, N. R., and Steinberg, E. P.: Results of randomized controlled trials of low- versus high-osmolality contrast media. Radiology *170*:381, 1989.

Khoury, G. A., Hopper, J. C., Varghese, Z., Farrington, K., Dick, R., Irving, J. D., Sweny, P., Fernando, O. N., and Moorhead, J. F.: Nephrotoxicity of ionic and non-ionic contrast material in digital vascular imaging and selective renal arteriography. Br. J. Radiol. *56*:631, 1983.

Kolbenstvedt, A., Andrew, E., Christophersen, B., Golman, K., Kvarstein, B., and Lien, H. H.: Metrizamide in high dose urography. Acta Radiol. (Diagn.) *10*:39, 1979.

Lalli, A. F., Williams, B., and Maynard, E.: Iohexol in urography. Urol. Radiol. *5*:95, 1983.

Langecker, H., Harward, A., and Junkman, K.: 3,5-Diacetylamino-2,4,6-trijodensoesäure als Röntgenkontrastmittel. Arch. Exp. Path. Pharmakol. *222*:584, 1954.

Larsen, A. A., Moore, C., Sprague, J., Cloke, B., Moss, J., and Hoppe, J. O.: Iodinated 3,5-diaminobenzoic acid derivatives. J. Am. Chem. Soc. *78*:3210, 1956.

Lasser, E. C.: Pretreatment with corticosteroids to prevent reactions to IV contrast material: Overview and implications. AJR *150*:257, 1988.

Lasser, E. C., Walters, A., Reuter, S. R., and Lang, J.: Histamine release by contrast media. Radiology *100*:683, 1971.

Lasser, E. C., and Berry, C. C.: Nonionic versus ionic contrast media: What do the data tell us? AJR *152*:945, 1989.

Lenarduzzi, G., and Pecco, R.: Iniezioni endovenose di ioduro di sodio (richerche radiologische sperimentali). Arch. Radiol. *3*:1055, 1927.

Lichtenberg, A., and Swick, M.: Klinische Prüfung des Uroselectans. Klin. Wochenschr. *8*:2089, 1929.

Longhran, C. F.: Clinical intravenous urography: Comparative trial of ioxaglate and iopamidol. Radiology *161*:455, 1986.

Magill, H. L., Clarke, E. A., Fitch, S. J., Boulden, J. F., Ramirez, R., Siegle, R. L., and Somes, G. W.: Excretory urography with iohexal: Evaluation in children. Radiology *161*:625, 1986.

McChesney, E. W., and Hoppe, J. O.: Studies of the tissue distribution and excretion of sodium diatrizoate in laboratory animals. AJR *78*:137, 1957.

McClennan, B.: Ionic versus nonionic contrast media: Safety, tolerance and rationale for use. Urol. Radiol. *11*:200, 1989.

McClennan, B. L.: Low-osmolality contrast media: Premises and promises. Radiology *162*:1, 1987.

Miller, D. L., Chang, R., Wells, W. T., Dowjat, B. A., Malinovsky, R. M., and Doppman, J. L.: Intravascular contrast media: Effect of dose on renal function. Radiology *167*:607, 1988.

Mindell, H. J., and Gibson, T. C.: ECG abnormalities during excretory urography: The effect of stress. AJR *150*:1327, 1988.

Moore, T. D., and Mayer, R. F.: Hypaque: An improved medium for excretory urography: A preliminary report of 210 cases. South. Med. J. *48*:135, 1955.

Moreau, J.-F., Droz, D., Sabto, J., Jungers, P., Kleinknecht, D., Hinglais, N., and Michel, J.-R.: Osmotic nephrosis induced by water-soluble triiodinated contrast media in man. Radiology *115*:329, 1975.

Mudge, G. H.: Some questions on nephrotoxicity. Invest. Radiol. *5*:407, 1970.

Narath, P. A.: Renal Pelvis and Ureter. New York, Grune & Stratton, 1951.

Neuhaus, D. R., Christman, A. A., and Lewis, H. B.: Biochemical studies on Urokon (sodium 2,4,6-triiodo-3-acetylaminobenzoate), a new pyelographic medium. J. Lab. Clin. Med. *35*:43, 1950.

O'Reilly, P. H., Jones, D. A., and Farah, N. B.: Measurement of the plasma clearance of urographic contrast media for the determination of glomerular filtration rate. J. Urol. *139*:9, 1988.

Osborne, E. D., Sutherland, C. G., Scholl, A. J., and Rowntree, L. G.: Roentgenography of urinary tract during excretion of sodium iodide. JAMA *80*:368, 1923.

Palmer, F. J.: The RACR survey of intravenous contrast media reactions final report. Aust. Radiol. *32*:426, 1988.

Porporis, A. A., Elliott, G. V., Fischer, G. L., and Mueller, C. B.: The mechanism of Urokon excretion. AJR *72*:995, 1954.

Rapoport, S., Bookstein, J. J., Higgins, C. B., Carey, P. H., Sovak, M., and Lasser, E. C.: Experience with metrizamide in patients with severe anaphylactoid reactions to ionic contrast agents. Radiology *143*:321, 1982.

Rockoff, S. D., Brasch, R., Kuhn, C., and Chraplyvy, M.: Contrast media as histamine liberators: I. Mast-cell histamine release *in vitro* by sodium salts of contrast media. Invest. Radiol. *5*:503, 1970.

Rockoff, S. D., Kuhn, C., and Chraplyvy, M.: Contrast media as histamine liberators: IV. *In vitro* mast-cell histamine release by methylglucamine salts. Invest. Radiol. *6*:186, 1971.

Rockoff, S. D., Kuhn, C., and Chraplyvy, M.: Contrast media as histamine liberators: V. Comparison of *in vitro* mast-cell histamine release by sodium and methylglucamine salts. Invest. Radiol. *7*:177, 1972.

Rollins, M., Bonte, F. J., Rose, F. A., and Keating, D. R.: Clinical evaluation of a new compound for intravenous urography. AJR *73*:771, 1955.

Root, J. C., and Strittmatter, W. C.: Hypaque, a new urographic contrast medium. AJR *73*:768, 1955.

Roseno, A.: Die intravenöse Pyelographic: II. Mitteilung. Klin. Ergebnisse. Klin. Wochenschr. *8*:1165, 1929.

Schrott, K. M., Behrends, B., Clauss, W., Kaufman, J., and Lehnert, J.: Iohexal in der Auscheidungsurographic: Ergelbnisse des drug-monitoring. Forshr. Med. *104*:153, 1986.

Sherwood, T., and Lavender, J. P.: Does renal blood flow rise or fall in response to diatrizoate? Invest. Radiol. *4*:327, 1969.

Siegle, R. L., and Gavant, M. L.: Comparison of iodixanol with iohexol in excretory urography. Acad. Radiol. *3*:S524, 1996.

Spataro, R. F., Fischer, H. W., and Baylan, L.: Urography with low osmolality contrast media: Comparative urinary excretion of iopamidol, Hexabrix and diatrizoate. Invest. Radiol. *17*:494, 1982.

Spataro, R. F., Katzberg, R. W., Fischer, H. W., and McMannis, M. J.: High-dose clinical urography with low-osmolality contrast agent Hexabrix: Comparison with conventional agent. Radiology *162*:9, 1987.

Swick, M.: Darstellung der Niere und Harmwege im Röntgenbild durch intravenöse Einbringung eines neuen Kontrastoffes, des Uroselectans. Klin. Wochenschr. *8*:2087, 1929.

Swick, M.: Intravenous urography by means of the sodium salt of 5-iodo-2-pyridon-n-acetic acid. JAMA *95*:1403, 1930.

Swick, M.: Excretion urography by means of the intravenous and oral administration of sodium orthoiodohippurate: With some physiological considerations: Preliminary report. Surg. Gynecol. Obstet. *56*:62, 1933.

Swick, M.: Excretion urography: With particular reference to a newly developed compound: Sodium orthoiodohippurate. JAMA *101*:1853, 1933.

Swick, M.: Intravenous urography in children. Radiology *26*:539, 1936.

Swick, M.: The discovery of intravenous urography: Historical and developmental aspects of the urographic media and their role in other diagnostic and therapeutic areas. Bull. N.Y. Acad. Med. *42*:128, 1966.

Swick, M.: Radiographic media in urology. Surg. Clin. North Am. *58*:977, 1978.

Talner, L. B., and Davidson, A. J.: Renal hemodynamic effects of contrast media. Invest. Radiol. *3*:310, 1968.

Talner, L. B., and Davidson, A. J.: Effect of contrast media on renal extraction of PAH. Invest. Radiol. *3*:229, 1968.

Talner, L. B., Rushmer, H. N., and Coel, M. N.: The effect of renal artery injection of contrast material on urinary enzyme excretion. Invest. Radiol. *7*:311, 1972.

Thompson, W. M., Foster, W. L., Jr., Halvorsen, R. A., Dunnick, N. R., Rommel, A. J., and Bates, M.: Iopamidol: New, nonionic contrast agent for excretory urography. AJR *142*:329, 1984.

Törnquist, C., and Holtäs, S.: Renal angiography with iohexol and metrizoate. Radiology *150*:331, 1984.

Volkmann, J.: Zur röntgenographischen Darstellung der Harnwege durch intravenöse Verabreiehung schattengebender Mittel. Dtsch. Med. Wochenschr. *50*:1413, 1924.

Wallingford, V. H.: The development of organic iodine compounds as x-ray contrast media. J. Am. Pharm. Assoc. *42*:721, 1953.

Wallingford, V. H., Decker, H. G., and Kruty, M.: X-ray contrast media: I. Iodinated acylaminobenzoic acids. J. Am. Chem. Soc. *74*:4365, 1952.

Webb, J. A. W.: The role of the distal nephron mechanisms in the distribution of contrast medium in the urine. Br. J. Radiol. *57*:381, 1983.

Webb, J. A. W.: The effect of intravenous contrast medium on glomerular filtration rate. Br. J. Radiol. *57*:387, 1983.

Wilcox, J., Evill, C. A., Sage, M. R., and Beness, G. T.: Urographic excretion studies with nonionic contrast agents: Iopamidol vs. iothalamate. Invest. Radiol. *18*:297, 1983.

Winfield, A. C., Dray, R. J., Kirchner, F. K., Jr., Muhletater, C. A., and Price, R. R.: Iohexol for excretory urography: A comparative study. AJR *141*:571, 1983.

Williams, T. C.: Detoxication Mechanisms. New York, John Wiley & Sons, 1947.

Wolf, G. L., Arenson, R. L., and Cross, A. P.: A prospective trial of ionic vs nonionic contrast agents in routine clinical practice. Comparison of adverse effects. AJR *152*:939, 1989.

Index

Note: Page numbers in *italics* refer to illustrations; page numbers followed by the letter t refer to tables.

Angiitis *(Continued)*
  necrotizing, 683
Angioendothelioma, 270
Angiography, *20,* 20–21, *21*
  computed tomographic, 17, *18*
  magnetic resonance, 20, *20*
Angiokeratoma corporis diffusum universale, 180
Angiomyolipoma, 292–297
  angiography in, *295,* 295–297, *296*
  clinical implications of, 694
  clinical setting in, 293
  computed tomography in, 293–294, *294–297*
  confidence levels in diagnosis of, 694
  definition of, 292–293
  excretory urography in, 293, *293*
  fat in, 292–294, *293–297*
  hemorrhage in, 295, *296*
  in tuberous sclerosis complex, 245–247, *246*
  magnetic resonance imaging in, 294–295, *297*
  radiologic analogues of, 693
  radiologic findings in, 293–297, *293–297*
  renal, pathologic features of, 693
  ultrasonography in, 294, *297*
  uroradiologic elements in, 294
Angiotensin II, in renovascular hypertension, 33
Angiotensin-converting enzyme inhibitor (ACEI), in
    renovascular hypertension, 33
Angiotensin-converting enzyme inhibitor (ACEI) renography,
    33–34
  interpretation of, 33, *34*
  pitfalls of, 33
Anterior pararenal space, abnormalities of, 549, *550*
  anatomy of, 539
Anterior perivesical space, 485
Anterior urethral valve, 521, *523*
Antigen, prostate-specific, 638
Antihistamines, for contrast material reaction, 9
Anuria, in acute cortical necrosis, 166, *166*
  in acute tubular necrosis, 162, *163*
Aortography, *20,* 20–21
Apatite calculus, characteristics of, 364t
Appendicitis, bladder in, 503
Arcuate arteries, *45,* 46
  arteriosclerosis of, 138–140, *140*
  development of, 48, *49*
  occlusion of, *200*
    nephrographic analysis of, 673
  radiologic findings in, in aging, 140, *141*
  thrombosis of, in lobar infarction, 95
Arcuate veins, 48
Arrhythmia, contrast material–induced, 11
Arterial dysplasia, aneurysmal, 438
  definition of, 109–110
Arterial hypotension. See *Hypotension, arterial.*
Arterial infarction. See *Renal artery(ies), infarction of.*
Arterial stenosis, and ischemia, 109–117
  clinical setting in, 110–111
  definition of, 109–110
  radiologic findings in, *111–116,* 111–117
  uroradiologic elements in, 116
  causes of, 110
Arteriography, *20,* 20–21, *21*
  renal, selective, 21, *21*
    contrast material in, 21
Arterioles, afferent, *46,* 47
Arteriosclerosis, clinical setting in, 136–137
  definition of, 136
  generalized, 136–141
    differential diagnosis of, 153
  in acquired cystic kidney disease, 145
  radiologic findings in, 137–141, *137–141*
  uroradiologic elements in, 136
Arteriovenous aneurysm (fistula), 438
  acquired, congenital arteriovenous malformation vs, 319
  angiography of, 440, *442*
  signs/symptoms of, 438–439

Arteriovenous aneurysm (fistula) *(Continued)*
  spontaneous, 438
  traumatic, 703, *708*
    angiography of, 699–700
Arteriovenous malformation, 319–321
  angiography of, *318,* 319–321, *320, 321*
  cavernous, 319, *320,* 693
  cirsoid, *318,* 319, *321,* 693
  clinical implications of, 694
  clinical setting in, 319
  computed tomography of, 319, *320, 321*
  confidence levels in diagnosis of, 694
  definition of, 319
  excretory urography of, *318,* 319, *320*
  pathologic features of, 693
  radiologic analogues of, 693
  radiologic findings in, *318,* 319–321, *320, 321*
  ultrasonography of, *318,* 319, *320*
  uroradiologic elements in, 319
Arteritis, drug abuse and, 136, 138, *140*
Ask-Upmark kidney, 88, 124
Aspiration, of simple cyst, 308
Atheroembolic renal disease, 142–143
  clinical setting in, 142–143
  definition of, 142
  differential diagnosis of, 153
  nephrogram in, 677
  radiologic findings in, 143
  uroradiologic elements in, 143
Atherosclerosis, aneurysm in, 438
  definition of, 109
  in renal ischemia, aortography of, *115*
Atrophy, in chronic renal infarction, 117, *122*
  postinflammatory. See *Postinflammatory atrophy.*
  postobstructive. See *Postobstructive atrophy.*
  radiation-induced, 123, *123*
  reflux. See *Reflux atrophy.*
Autonephrectomy, tuberculous, 350, *353*
    multicystic dysplastic kidney disease vs., 265
    uroepithelial, *409*
Azotemia, medullary cystic disease in, *150*

Bacteriuria, in acute pyelonephritis, 214
Bartter's syndrome, 180–181
  nephrocalcinosis in, 329
Basalis tissue, 625
Beak sign, 305, *307,* 686
Beckwith-Wiedemann syndrome, *180,* 181
  differential diagnosis of, 181
"Bell-clapper" anomaly, 660
Benign prostatic hyperplasia, 644–645
Benzene ring, *728*
Bergman's sign, 390, *396*
Beta-iodomethyl-19-norcholesterol (NP-59), in adrenal imaging,
    35, *36,* 573
Bicornuate bicollis, 628
Bicornuate unicollis, 628
Bicornuate uterus, *627, 628,* 628–629
  septate uterus vs., 629t
Bilharzial polyps, 407
Bilharziasis. See *Schistosomiasis.*
Biopsy, renal, arteriovenous aneurysm after, *708*
  of mass, 695
    perinephric/paranephric hemorrhage after, *551*
  transrectal, 640, *640*
Bladder, 485–514
  adenocarcinoma of, 497
  anatomy of, 485–486
  anomalies of, 486–491
  apex of, 485
  base of, 485
  blood clot in, 493, *493*
  calculus of, 491–493, *492*

Lymphocele, bladder compression in, 511
Lymphoma, 249–253
    adrenal, 591
        metastases of, *592*
    bladder, 502, 510, *510*
    clinical setting in, 249
    computed tomography of, *250,* 251, *251*
    definition of, 249
    differential diagnosis of, 253
    excretory urography of, *250*
    magnetic resonance imaging of, *252,* 253
    non-Hodgkin's, *250–252*
        bladder in, *510*
        with periureteral spread, *397*
    radiologic findings in, 249–253, *250–252*
    renal sinus, 451, *451*
    retroperitoneal, and obstructive uropathy, *209*
        necrotic lymph nodes with, 562, *564*
    testicular, 657
    ultrasonography of, *250,* 251–253, *252*
    uroradiologic elements in, 253

Macrophages, Hansemann's, in malakoplakia, 257
Magnesium ammonium phosphate calculus, formation of, 363
Magnetic resonance angiography, 20, *20*
Magnetic resonance imaging, 17–20, *19, 20*
    contrast material in, 19
    endorectal, 640–642, *641, 642*
    endoscopic, in prostate cancer staging, 642
    motion compensation/suppression in, 17–19
Malakoplakia, 257–258
    angiography of, 258
    bladder, mural thickening in, 507, *508*
    clinical setting in, 257
    computed tomography of, 258, *258*
    definition of, 257
    differential diagnosis of, 265
    pelvocalyceal, 411–413
        clinical setting in, 412
        definition of, 411–412
        differential diagnosis of, 427
        radiologic findings in, *412,* 412–413
    radiologic findings in, 257–258, *258*
    ultrasonography of, 257
    uroradiologic elements in, 258
Malignant hypertension, in nephrosclerosis, 141
Mass(es), abdominal, in multicystic dysplastic kidney disease, 260–263, *262*
    adnexal, radiologic evaluation of, 619–622, *620, 621*
    adrenal, conditions simulating, 571–572
        diagnostic sets for, 600t, 601t
    cystic, Type II pyelocalyceal diverticulum as, *418,* 419
    flank, in chronic obstructive uropathy, *462,* 463
    in mural hemorrhage, 414, *414*
    non-neoplastic, 304–321
        renal enlargement in, patterns of, 268t
    parapelvic, adenocarcinoma as, *450*
    perirenal space, pelvocalyceal/ureteral effacement in, 480
    renal. See *Renal mass.*
    renal sinus, pelvocalyceal/ureteral effacement in, 480
    scrotal, non-neoplastic, 658–659, *659*
Matrix, in calculogenesis, 363
Matrix calculus, radiologic findings in, 371
    ultrasonographic diagnosis of, 372
Meatal stenosis, congenital, 521
Medial fibroplasia, 110, *115,* 440, *445*
Medial umbilical ligament, 488
Median umbilical ligament, 485
Medulla, adrenal, anatomy of, 571
    renal, architecture of, *45,* 45–46, *46*
        development of, 44
        fetal, echogenicity of, 54, *55*
Medullary carcinoma, 270
    clinical findings in, 271

Medullary cystic disease, 148–149
    clinical setting in, 148–149
    definition of, 148
    differential diagnosis of, 153
    radiologic findings in, 149, *150, 151*
    uroradiologic elements in, 149
Medullary hyperplasia, 584–585
Medullary sponge kidney, 329–335
    autosomal recessive (infantile) polycystic kidney disease vs., 183
    differential diagnosis of, 356
    excretory urography of, 333, *333–337*
    focal, 335, *337*
    in children, 335, *336*
    in transitional cell carcinoma, 335, *337*
    nephrocalcinosis in, 329, *338*
    papillary blush in, 333–335
    ultrasonography of, *336*
Megacalyces, congenital, 470–472
        diagnosis of, 471–472
        pathogenesis of, 471
        pelvocalyceal/ureteral dilatation in, 472, *472*
        primary megaureter with, 476
        radiologic findings in, 472, *472*
        renal function in, 472
Megacystis-megaureter syndrome, 467
Megalocytic interstitial nephritis, 257
Megalourethra, 521
Megaureter, primary, 473–475, *474, 475*
        congenital megacalyces with, 476
        differential diagnosis of, 476
        vesicoureteral reflux with, 476
Meglumine, 5t
    diuretic effect of, 4
Meglumine iothalamate, 5t
Melanoma, metastatic, of seminal vesicle, 647, *647*
    of uroepithelium, *397*
    primary, of adrenal glands, 599
Membranoproliferative glomerulonephritis, 158
MEN (multiple endocrine neoplasia) syndrome, pheochromocytoma in, 584–585
Menstrual cycle, proliferative phase of, 625
    secretory phase of, 625
Mesenchymal/juxtaglomerular cell tumor, 303–304
    angiography of, 304
    benign, clinical setting in, 388
    clinical setting in, 303–304
    computed tomography of, 304
    definition of, 303
    differential diagnosis of, 321–322
    excretory urography of, 304
    radiologic findings in, 304
    retroperitoneal, 552–554, *553–555*
        features of, 552t
    ultrasonography of, 304
    uroradiologic elements in, 304
Mesoblastic nephroma, 299–303
    clinical findings in, 302
    computed tomography of, *302,* 302–303
    definition of, 299–302
    differential diagnosis of, 321
    excretory urography of, 302
    polyhydramnios in, 302, *303*
    radiologic findings in, *302,* 302–303, *303*
    ultrasonography of, 303, *303*
    uroradiologic elements in, 303
Mesoderm, intermediate, 41
Mesodermal tumors, benign, 388
Mesonephric duct, 41–42, *42*
    remnants of, 42, 42t
Mesonephric tubules, remnants of, 42, 42t
Mesonephros, 41–42, *42*
Metaiodobenzylguanidine (MIBG), in adrenal imaging, 35, *36, 37, 37,* 573
    in pheochromocytoma imaging, *586,* 586–587
Metanephric blastema, 42, *42*

ISBN 0-7216-7144-6

90038